Nursing
Care Plans

Transitional Patient & Family Centered Care

Nursing Care Plans

Transitional Patient & Family Centered Care

6TH EDITION

LYNDA JUALL CARPENITO, RN, MSN, CRNP

Family Nurse Practitioner
ChesPenn Health Services
Chester, Pennsylvania

Nursing Consultant
Mullica Hill, New Jersey

 Wolters Kluwer | Lippincott Williams & Wilkins
Health
Philadelphia · Baltimore · New York · London
Buenos Aires · Hong Kong · Sydney · Tokyo

Acquisitions Editor: Patrick Barbera
Supervising Product Manager: Annette Ferran
Production Project Manager: Marian Bellus
Project Manager: Karen Ettinger
Design Coordinator: Paul Fry
Manufacturing Coordinator: Karin Duffield
Prepress Vendor: S4Carlisle

6th Edition

9 8 7 6 5 4 3 2 1

Printed in USA

Library of Congress Cataloging-in-Publication Data

Carpenito, Lynda Juall, author.
  Nursing care plans / Lynda Juall Carpenito. — Sixth edition.
     p. ; cm.
  Preceded by: Nursing care plans & documentation / Lynda Juall Carpenito-Moyet. Ed. 5. c2009.
  Includes bibliographical references and index.
  ISBN 978-1-4511-8787-8 (alk. paper)
  I. Title.
  [DNLM: 1. Patient Care Planning.   2. Nursing Process.   3. Nursing Records.   WY 100.1]
  RT49
  610.73—dc23
                                                                      2013020995

DISCLAIMER

Care has been taken to confirm the accuracy of the information presented and to describe generally accepted practices. However, the author(s), editors, and publisher are not responsible for errors or omissions or for any consequences from application of the information in this book and make no warranty, expressed or implied, with respect to the currency, completeness, or accuracy of the contents of the publication. Application of this information in a particular situation remains the professional responsibility of the practitioner; the clinical treatments described and recommended may not be considered absolute and universal recommendations.

The author(s), editors, and publisher have exerted every effort to ensure that drug selection and dosage set forth in this text are in accordance with the current recommendations and practice at the time of publication. However, in view of ongoing research, changes in government regulations, and the constant flow of information relating to drug therapy and drug reactions, the reader is urged to check the package insert for each drug for any change in indications and dosage and for added warnings and precautions. This is particularly important when the recommended agent is a new or infrequently employed drug.

Some drugs and medical devices presented in this publication have Food and Drug Administration (FDA) clearance for limited use in restricted research settings. It is the responsibility of the health care provider to ascertain the FDA status of each drug or device planned for use in his or her clinical practice.

LWW.com

To My Mother: Elizabeth Julia Juall

Every year brings me a new appreciation and admiration for this woman

In her 90s there is not much she does not do

She has role-modeled unconditional love, respect for all, forgiveness, and independence

She is determined she can, and she does! Gardening, water aerobics, casino blackjack

She is one generation of my family's Hungarian Woman Warriors, and I proudly walk in their footprints, carry their swords to battle injustice, and cherish deeply our loved ones.

> *Love your daughter*
> *Lynda*

Contributors

Carie Bilicki, RE, MSN, ACNS-BC, OCN
Clinical Nurse Specialist
Froedtert Health
Milwaukee, Wisconsin

(Initial Cancer Diagnosis, Breast Surgery, Chemotherapy, Radiation)

Choosing nursing as my career, and solidifying my commitment to the profession, I earned my Bachelor of Science in Nursing in 1995 from Alverno College in Milwaukee, Wisconsin. I pursued my Masters in Nursing, board certified as a Clinical Nurse Specialist. Sixteen years into the profession, nursing remains my passion and my constant drive of excellence for my patients. Nursing was beyond a choice for my career, it is a privilege to help patients and families in sometimes the most vulnerable times of their lives. I am passionate in my commitment to nursing, ensuring high quality patient care. In my current role, I manage and coordinate breast cancer women's needs across the care continuum.

Education does not stop with a degree; education in nursing is continuous, and it is the personal ownership of the nurse to continue to pursue. I have a deep personal commitment to nursing and the specialty of oncology. I remain professionally active on a local and national level. I have taken my nursing work beyond hospital walls as host of Nursestalk (nursestalk.com) a health-related talk show that can be seen on YouTube.

Deborah H. Brooks, MSN, ANP-BC, CNN-NP
Nurse Practitioner
Division of Nephrology
Medical Center University of South Carolina,
South Carolina

(RC of Acute Urinary Retention, RC of Renal Insufficiency, RC of Renal Calculi, Hemodialysis, Peritoneal Dialysis Acute Kidney Failure [Injury], Chronic Kidney Disease, Nephrectomy)

I have worked in nephrology nursing since 1980, including acute and chronic inpatient and outpatient hemodialysis. I was the supervisor for the home dialysis program at UNC for 10 years. Our patient population included both hemodialysis and peritoneal dialysis, and the age range was pediatrics to geriatrics. At MUSC, I was the inpatient case manager for nephrology and the research coordinator for AASK, a long-term nephrology multicenter NIH study. Currently, I am the nurse practitioner for nephrology at MUSC and work in clinical, educational, and research areas.

Professionally, I have been involved in the American Nephrology Nurses Association, ANNA, at the national and local chapter level as a speaker, author, consultant, and local chapter officer. I'm currently on the editorial board of the Nephrology Nursing Journal. I serve on the Nephrology Nursing Certification Commission, (NNCC), as a board member for the nurse practitioner certification exam and am certified as both a nephrology nurse and nephrology nurse practitioner.

Jeanne M. Fenn, MS, MEd, RN, CPNP, CDE
Pediatric Nurse Practitioner
University of Arizona Medical Center Diamond
Children's
Tucson, Arizona

(Infant, Children, Adolescent Generic Care Plans)

I have been a nurse for over 35 years. After working in adult health early in my career, I found my niche in pediatrics. For the past 32 years, I have been able to work in a variety of pediatric nursing roles, including staff nurse, educator, clinical nurse specialist, and now as a pediatric nurse practitioner. I received my BSN and MEd at the University of Arizona. In 2009, I received my MSN as a Pediatric Nurse Practitioner at Arizona State University. I have been rewarded in so many ways throughout the years as I have worked with children, families, and health care staff. I have been selected as a 1997 "Fabulous Fifty Nurse" Tucson, Arizona, finalist for the Diabetes Educator of the Year in 2005, Washington, D.C., and the March of Dimes, Arizona Nurse of the Year for Community Service in 2007. Currently, I work with children and families with asthma and diabetes. I serve as an adjunct faculty member at the University of Arizona, College of Nursing. I have been a contributing editor for Lynda Juall Carpenito since 2009.

Kimberly Dupree Harrelson, BSN, RN, CRRN
Student in Doctorate of Nursing Practice (DNP)
program
Senior Study Research Coordinator (RN) for the
Blood Pressure in Dialysis Study (BID Study)
The Medical University of South Carolina (MUSC)
Charleston, South Carolina

(Laminectomy)

Being a nurse has provided me not only the sense of self-enlightenment, but has also given me the grand opportunity to show others how actions such as being compassionate, showing empathy, and most importantly, having the ability to show patients and / or families the vulnerable side of nursing by being the "friend" who sits quietly while holding an inconsolable patient's hand, and which I believe truly encompasses the meaning of what it is to be a nurse.

I have had the wonderful opportunity to practice as a Registered Nurse on various units for a little over 10 years. Three years later, I transferred to a newly built Neurosurgical Unit and have practiced there 7 years now and am hopeful to have many more gratifying years in such a valued profession. My nursing passion and career began at quite a young age, as at the age of 22, little did I know about life's many wonderful and sometimes unexpected experiences, or how sneaky and devious life's little lessons can pop up when least expected. Even so, I continue this journey and persevere as my inherited tenacity and quite often stubborn side has given me the strength and willfulness needed to push myself toward the ultimate goal and sacrifice of which my hard work will assist in leading to a life filled with much happiness, contentment, and overall achievement.

I have spent 7 years with my "Neuro-Family" and gained such a respect for the intricate complexities of the central nervous system. The amount of knowledge gained thus far has guided me to my present position as a Senior Study Research Coordinator at The Medical University of South Carolina, to my obtaining a position in a new nursing specialty. MUSC has also provided me with a wonderful opportunity by furnishing the necessary framework needed to complete my educational ambition of becoming a Family Nurse Practitioner. I have high hopes of completing my Doctorate in Nursing Practice by August 2015.

Gabrielle A. Jurecky, RN, MSN/Ed.
Clinical Leader Diamond 5
University of Arizona Medical Center Diamond Children's
Tucson, Arizona

(Infant, Children Adolescent Care Plan)

I have been a pediatric nurse for over 24 years. I obtained my bachelor's from the University of Arizona, College of Nursing in May 1989. I then received my Master of Science in Nursing specialization in Health Care Education in July 2009 from the University of Phoenix. I am a PALS and CPR instructor for my facility, and I have my ANCC certification in pediatrics. I have been awarded and recognized by my colleagues in various disciplines. These award include 2003 Fabulous Fifty Nurses Award, Tucson, Arizona; 2006 Candle Lighters Nurse of the Year Award; 2008 Top 5 Nurses for Life Award recipient; and 2011 Awarded Best Evidence Based Project in State of Arizona.

Pediatrics and the care of the child and family has been my nursing focus for most of my career, and since 2006 I have been an adjunct faculty member of the University of Arizona, College of Nursing. I have been a contributing editor for Lynda Juall Carpenito in Nursing Diagnosis: Application to Clinical Practice since 2006. For the last three years, I have been a clinical leader and nurse educator for Diamond Children's Medical Center, pediatric general floor.

Elizabeth Knoll, RN, MSN, CMSRN
Nursing Faculty
Muskegon Community College
Department of Nursing
Muskegon, Michigan

(Myasthenia Gravis, Guillain Barre Syndrome)

I believe as nurses we are privileged to be present through the life transitions of our clients and communities, and that caring and a commitment to excellence are essential components of nursing practice. Since obtaining my BSN from Wayne State University in 1986, I have had a diverse background in nursing. I have practiced in various settings from a major medical center in Detroit, Michigan, to rural home care, outpatient oncology, and medical-surgical nursing. I also have served as an educator for the implementation of acute care electronic medical records, and obtained various specialty certifications for my areas of clinical focus. After obtaining my MSN from Michigan State University, I began my current role as full-time medical-surgical faculty in the ADN program at Muskegon Community College. I continue to practice as a medical-surgical staff nurse.

Shana McClone, MSN, ACNS-BC
Clinical Nurse Specialist
Aurora St. Luke's South Shore
Cudahy, Wisconsin

(Asthma, Chronic Obstructive Pulmonary Disease, Pneumonia, Thoracic Pulmonary Surgery [co-contributor with author])

I started my practice as a medical surgical staff nurse in 1999. I became a float pool nurse and gained many experiences. I became certified as a med-surg nurse in 2004 and continue to be very active in assisting nurses to achieve certification. I believe in the power of the medical surgical staff nurse. Additionally, I completed Adult-Health CNS certification within three months of graduation. I believe that patients provide the professional nurse opportunities to learn and grow. This has molded my experience in fall prevention and pain education. It has granted permission to set aside judgments and assumptions in order to obtain the entire story and treat the patient holistically. This approach builds trust, rapport, and credibility with patients, peers, families, and friends.

Suzanne Pach, RN, MSN, FNP-C
Stroke Nurse Practitioner
University of South Carolina
Charleston, South Carolina

(Parkinson's Disease, Cerebrovascular Accident)

I have been employed with the Medical University of South Carolina (MUSC) for 12 years. Prior to nursing, I earned my degree as a Medical Technologist and worked in laboratory medicine for over 12 years.

I first began working in the Microbiology and Immunology Laboratory at MUSC 12 years ago and decided to go back to school to obtain my Family Nurse Practitioner's degree. While working on my Master's, I worked as an Orthopedic/Trauma nurse for 5 years. I have been working as a nurse practitioner for 4 years. I first started out working for Endocrinology mainly working with patients with diabetes. In 2011, I joined the Stroke Neurology team. There are two units that I am responsible for: a neurology step down unit and a neurology floor. We take care of patients from all over South Carolina that need specialized stroke care via our REACH telemedicine network. Our stroke team is currently working on obtaining Comprehensive Stroke Certification from the Joint Commission.

Amy Salgado, RN, MSN
Clinical Coordinator–Carondelet-PCOA Transitional Care Navigation Program
Carondelet Health Network
Tucson, Arizona

(RC of Bleeding, RC of Decreased Cardiac Output, RC of Dysrhythmias, RC of Hypovolemia, RC of Pulmonary Edema, Heart Failure, Hypertension, Acute Coronary Syndrome, Peripheral Arterial Disease [Atherosclerosis])

Nursing has been a personal interest to me, and I have always looked upon it with respect. I believe that the role of a nurse can be very challenging and hectic at times, as well as rewarding and fulfilling. The definition of a great nurse, in my opinion, needs to have good interpersonal skills, a great listener, empathetic, eager to learn, and strives to improve themselves. It is also extremely important to understand patient's needs with compassion. With the evolving needs of the patients and the constantly changing healthcare industry, nurses still are the first line of defense in caring, educating, and providing priceless hands-on advocacy.

Patients are faced with increased healthcare concerns, multipharmacy prescriptions and complexity when it comes to their care. Times are changing, patients, now more than ever, need to be empowered to recognize and understand the importance of self-advocacy. Transitional care programs are becoming more accepted in the healthcare industry. It is exciting to be part of this innovating health care phenomenon.

Lisa Wallen, RN, ANP-BC, Certified Wound Specialist
Senior Wound Specialist
Strong Hyperbaric and Wound Center
University of Rochester
Rochester, New York

(Pressure Ulcers)

Healing of wounds is an old art of both medical and nursing sciences. However, until recent times care for nonhealing, chronic wounds was limited to pain relief and simple dressings with limited focus on resolution and healing. Patients were left with debilitating and disfiguring ulcers and little hope of healing. When I started my nursing career over 30 years ago, these patients were treated with home remedies such as Maalox and sugar or dry heat to desiccate these tissues. Much progress and promising new treatments have been developed to promote healing and improve the lives of these patients. This new road toward advanced sciences and improved outcomes has been very exciting and interesting to me as an advanced nurse practitioner and wound specialist. I can now use human skin grown in a lab or add growth factors and other advanced modalities to promote healing and hope for recovery. I greatly enjoy the ability to heal and vastly improve the lives of my patients. The satisfaction of seeing a painful nonhealing wound transform into precious new living tissues is very gratifying. Wound healing is indeed a healing art and a rewarding career.

Teresa Wilson, MS, APRNC-OB, CNS, BC
Perinatal Clinical Nurse Specialist
Women's Care Services
Carondelet St. Joseph's Hospital
Tucson, Arizona

(Perinatal Nursing Care Plan. Postpartum Nursing Care Plan)

Nursing was more than a choice for me, it was a calling. It has been my path for over 30 years, and the care of women and infants has been my passion. I earned a Bachelor of Science in Nursing from the University of Iowa in 1983, and obtained my Master of Science in Maternal-Newborn Nursing from the University of Arizona in 1990. From both programs, I encountered nursing leaders and scholars who inspired and mentored me. I have worked in Mother / Baby units, with antepartum patients, special care nursery, and Labor and Delivery. I taught childbirth education for a number of years as well. Working within all of the areas of women and infant care was my goal from the start of my career, so I could better understand all the facets of the childbearing experience.

Through my years of clinical practice and education, I arrived at my definition of a great nurse. He or she is someone who is always focused on giving excellent and safe hands-on care to patients and families, approaching each patient / family with empathy and seeing them as individuals with their own unique strengths and needs. Always demanding and always evolving, nursing is rightfully one of the most respected professions in the world. As healthcare has changed so has nursing to collectively be the patient's advocate, teacher, care giver, and protector in a high tech and complex system.

Currently, as a Perinatal Clinical Nurse Specialist, I combine a management role with the coordination of professional development, writing of policies, managing perinatal data, mentoring other nurses, and promoting excellence and patient safety. Being able to function as a leader in so many dimensions of nursing is what makes being a CNS so satisfying. Although I no longer give direct patient care at the bedside, I can influence the mastery of the nurses who do and promote ever better care. I serve as adjunct faculty for an ADN and a BSN nursing program and have been the local chapter chair of AWHONN (Association for Women's Health, Obstetric & Neonatal Nursing).

Preface

Nursing is primarily assisting individuals, sick or well, in activities that contribute to health or its recovery, or to a peaceful death, and that they perform unaided when they have the necessary strength, will, or knowledge. Nursing also helps individuals carry out prescribed therapy and to be independent of assistance as soon as possible (Henderson & Nite, 1960).

Historically, nurses have represented the core of the health care delivery system (including acute, long-term, and community agencies), but their image continues to be one of individuals whose actions are dependent on physician supervision. Unfortunately, what Donna Diers wrote over 15 years ago is still relevant today: "Nursing is exceedingly complicated work since it involves technical skill, a great deal of formal knowledge, communication ability, use of self, timing, emotional investment, and any number of other qualities. What it also involves—and what is hidden from the public—is the complex process of thinking that leads from the knowledge to the skill, from the perception to the action, from the decision to the touch, from the observation to the diagnosis. *Yet it is this process of nursing care, which is at the center of nursing's work, that is so little described . . .*" (Diers, 1981, p. 1, emphasis supplied).

Physicians regularly and openly explain their management plans to the public, especially to clients and their families. Nurses, however, often fail to explain the nursing care plan to clients and family. This book provides both a framework for nurses to provide responsible nursing care and guidelines for them to document and communicate that care. These care plans should not be handwritten. They must be reference documents for practicing nurses. Write or free text the different care the client needs in addition to the standard.

The focus of this 6th edition of *Nursing Care Plans* is transitional nursing care for individuals and their families in an acute care facility. In order for transitions to home or a community care facility to be timely, appropriate, and safe, many factors must be considered. In every care plan, the following elements have been highlighted to enhance the transition process:

- **Transitional Risk Assessment Plan** to begin at admission to assess individual's vulnerability for infection, pressure ulcers, falls, and delayed transition. Evidence-based risk assessment tools for each potential hospital-acquired condition are illustrated on the inside back cover.
- **Clinical Alerts** are placed in the plans to advise the clinical or student nurse of a serious event that requires immediate action.
- **Clinical Alert Reports** are a list of clinical observations or findings that are communicated to the novice or student nurses and / or medical assistants before they begin care that needs to be monitored for. Changes in status need to be reported in a timely and sometimes urgent fashion.
- **Carp's Cues** notes from the author to emphasize a certain principle of care.
- **STAR** is an acronym for Stop, Think, Act, Review. This is a process to be utilized "when something just is not right."
- **SBAR** is an acronym (Situation, Background, Assessment, Recommendation) for the method of concisely organizing a communication to another professional regarding a concern about a client / family status or situation.
- **Transition to Home / Community Care** is an element in each care plan placed before the last diagnosis, *Risk for Ineffective Self-Health Management*, that focuses the nurse on evaluating for the presence of risk factors that can delay transition.

Also new this edition is Unit II, which contains frequently occurring nursing diagnoses* and collaborative problems that supplement the care plans in Unit III. For example, if an individual is admitted for Acute Coronary Syndrome and has also recently lost his sister to cancer, the nurse can refer to Unit II to the *Grieving* nursing diagnosis. In another situation, an individual had a total knee replacement and also has type II diabetes mellitus. In Unit II, the collaborative problem *Risk for Complications of Hypo / Hyperglycemia* would be added to the problem list. The entire care plan for Diabetes Mellitus would not be indicated because the priorities of care would be in the Total Knee Replacement Care Plan. *Risk for Complications of Hyper / Hypoglycemia*, would be added to monitor blood glucose levels.

This book also incorporates the findings of a validation study, a description of which (method, subjects, instrument findings) is presented in the section titled *Validation Project*, following the Preface. These findings should be very useful for practicing nurses, students of nursing, and departments of nursing.

The Bifocal Clinical Practice Model underpins this book and serves to organize the nursing care plans in Unit III. Chapter 1 describes and discusses the Bifocal Clinical Practice Model, which differentiates nursing diagnoses from other problems that nurses treat. In this chapter, nursing diagnoses and collaborative problems are explained and differentiated. The relationship of the type of diagnosis to outcome criteria and nursing interventions is also emphasized.

Communication is emphasized as the critical key to preventing adverse events in Chapter 2. The imperative of timely, clinically pertinent communication is emphasized with SBAR and reducing the barriers to "speaking up." Chapter 3 focuses on early identification of high-risk individuals and / or family. The eight hospital-acquired conditions that are deemed preventable by the Centers for Medicare and Medicaid Services are presented. Nurses' unique role in their prevention is discussed.

The preparation of individual / family for care at home or transition to a community care facility is the focus of Chapter 4. The assessment of risk factors in the individual and his or her support system and home environment is presented for early identification of potential barriers to a timely, safe transition. Chapter 5 gives an overview of the 11 steps in care planning and takes the student nurse through each phase of this process. The purpose is to reduce writing of care plans but instead for the student to use the care plan as a reference and then to add or delete based on other comorbidities and / or their clinical assessments. The process of identification of priority diagnoses is described.

What is the most important thing to do for this patient right now? is the focus of Chapter 6. Case studies are used to emphasize that what might seem to be most important from a nurse's perspective may not be what the individual or the families are most distressed about. Moral distress in nurses is described with preventive strategies. Professional nursing practice must represent the art and the science of the profession. The care plans in this book represent the science of nursing. A nurse who is a scientist but has not incorporated the art of this profession into his / her practice is providing care but is not caring. This chapter will emphasize caring as a critical component of our profession.

Unit III presents care plans that represent a compilation of the complex work of nursing in caring for individuals (and their families) experiencing medical disorders or surgical interventions or undergoing diagnostic or therapeutic procedures. It uses the nursing process to present the type of nursing care that is expected to be necessary for clients experiencing similar situations. The plans provide the nurse with a framework for providing initial, or essential, care. The intent of this book is to assist the nurse to identify the responsible care that nurses are accountable to provide. The incorporation of recent research findings further enhances the applicability of the care plans. By using the Bifocal Clinical Practice Model, the book clearly defines the scope of independent practice.

Section 4 is new to this edition and outlines five specialty care plans for newborns, children, adolescents, the family in the postpartum period, and individuals with mental health disorders. Diagnostic clusters of nursing diagnoses and collaborative problems are presented for each specialty plan. The reader can access the complete plans on thePoint, the website for additions and supplements to this book, at http:// thePoint.lww.com/Carpenito6e.

---

* Nursing diagnoses contain definitions designated as NANDA-I and characteristics and factors identified with a blue asterisk from Nursing Diagnoses: Definitions and Classification 2012–2014. Copyright © 2012, 2009, 2007, 2003, 2001, 1998, 1996, 1994 by NANDA International. Used by arrangement with Blackwell Publishing Limited, a company of John Wiley & Sons, Inc.

Additional Resources

Additional resources to accompany this edition such as printable client information guides like "Getting Started to Quitting Smoking" can be accessed at thePoint at http://thePoint.lww.com/Carpenito6e

The author invites comments and suggestions from readers. Correspondence can be directed to the publisher or to the author's email at juall46@msn.com.

References

Diers, D. (1981). Why write? Why publish? *Image*, 13, 991–997.

Henderson, V., & Nite, G. (1960). *Principles and practice of nursing* (5th ed.). New York: Macmillan, p. 14.

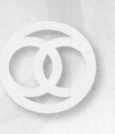

Validation Project

Background

In 1984, this author published diagnostic clusters under medical and surgical conditions (Carpenito, 1984). These diagnostic clusters represented nursing diagnoses and collaborative problems described in the literature for a medical or surgical population. After the initial diagnostic clusters were created, they were reviewed by clinicians who practiced with specific corresponding populations.

Since 1984, numerous other authors (Doenges, 1991; Holloway, 1988; Sparks, 1993; Ulrich, 1994) have generated similar groupings. Prior to 1993, none of the clusters have been studied to determine their frequency of occurrence. In other words, are some diagnoses in the diagnostic cluster treated more frequently than others? To this date in 2013, this validation study by this author remains to be the only research with this clinical focus.

Reasons for Study

In the last 10 years, the health care delivery system has experienced numerous changes. Specifically, clients are in the acute care setting for shorter periods. These client populations all share a high acuity. This acuity is represented with multiple nursing diagnoses and collaborative problems. However, do all these diagnoses have the same priority? Which diagnoses necessitate nursing interventions during the length of stay?

Care planning books report a varied number of diagnoses to treat under a specific condition. For example, in reviewing a care plan for a client with a myocardial infarction, this author found the following number of diagnoses reported: Ulrich, 16; Carpenito, 11; Doenges, 7; Holloway, 4. When students review these references, how helpful are lists ranging from 4 to 16 diagnoses? How many diagnoses can nurses be accountable for during a client's length of stay?

The identification of nursing diagnoses and collaborative problems that nurses treat more frequently than others in certain populations can be very useful data to:

- Assist nurses with decision making
- Determine the cost of nursing services for population sets
- Plan for resources needed
- Describe the specific responsibilities of nursing

Novice nurses and students can use these data to anticipate the initial care needed. They can benefit from data reported by nurses experienced in caring for clients in specific populations.

These data should not eliminate an assessment of an individual client to evaluate if additional nursing diagnoses or collaborative problems are present and establish priority for treatment during the hospital stay. This individual assessment will also provide information to delete or supplement the care plans found in this book. The researched data will provide a beginning focus for care.

By identifying frequently treated nursing diagnoses and collaborative problems in client populations, institutions can determine nursing costs based on nursing care provided. Nurse administrators and managers can plan for effective use of staff and resources. Knowledge of types of nursing diagnoses needing nursing interventions will also assist with matching the level of preparation of nurses with appropriate diagnoses.

To date, the nursing care of clients with medical conditions or postsurgical procedures has centered on the physician-prescribed orders. The data from this study would assist departments of nursing to emphasize the primary reason why clients stay in the acute care setting—*for treatment of nursing diagnoses and collaborative problems.* The purpose of this study is to identify which nursing diagnoses and collaborative problems are most frequently treated when a person is hospitalized with a specific condition.

Method

Settings and Subjects

The findings presented are based on data collected from August 1993 to March 1994. The research population consisted of registered nurses with over two years' experience in health care agencies in the United States and Canada. A convenience sample of 18 institutions represented five U.S. geographical regions (Northeast, Southeast, North-Midwest, Northwest, Southwest) and Ontario province in Canada. The display lists the participating institutions. The target number of R responses was 10 per condition from each institution. The accompanying table illustrates the demographics of the subjects.

Instrument

A graphic rating scale was developed and pilot-tested to measure self-reported frequencies of interventions provided to clients with a specific condition. Each collaborative problem listed under the condition was accompanied by the question *When you care for clients with this condition, how often do you monitor for this problem?*

Each nursing diagnosis listed under the condition was accompanied by the question: *When you care for clients with this condition, how often do you provide interventions for this nursing diagnosis?*

The respondent was asked to make an X on a frequency scale of 0% to 100%. Scoring was tabulated by summing the scores for each question and calculating the median.

PARTICIPATING INSTITUTIONS

Allen Memorial Hospital
1825 Logan Avenue
Waterloo, Iowa 50703

Carondelet St. Joseph's Hospital
350 N. Wilmont Road
Tucson, Arizona 85711-2678

The Evanston Hospital
Burch Building
2650 Ridge Avenue
Evanston, Illinois 60201

Huron Valley Hospital
1601 East Commerce Road
Milford, Michigan 48382-9900

Lehigh Valley Hospital
Cedar Crest & I-78
Allentown, Pennsylvania 18105-1556

Memorial Medical Center of Jacksonville
3625 University Blvd., South
Jacksonville, Florida 32216

Presbyterian Hospital
200 Hawthorne Lane
Charlotte, North Carolina 28233-3549

St. Francis Medical Center
211 St. Francis Drive
Cape Girardeau, Missouri 63701

St. Joseph Hospital
601 N. 30th Street
Omaha, Nebraska 68131

St. Peter Community Hospital
2475 Broadway
Helena, Montana 39601

San Bernardino County Medical Center
780 E. Gilbert Street
San Bernardino, California 92415-0935

Sioux Valley Hospital
1100 South Euclid Avenue
Sioux Falls, South Dakota 57117-5039

University of Minnesota Hospital
420 Delaware Street, S.E.
Minneapolis, Minnesota 55455

University of New Mexico Hospital
2211 Lomas Blvd., N.E.
Albuquerque, New Mexico 87131

Victoria Hospital
800 Commissioners Road, East
London, Canada N6A 4G5

Wills Eye Hospital
900 Walnut Street
Philadelphia, Pennsylvania 19107

Wilmer Ophthalmological Institute
Johns Hopkins Hospital
Baltimore, Maryland 21287-9054

Winthrop-University Hospital
259 First Street
Mineola, New York 11501

Data Collection

Prior to data collection, the researcher addressed the requirements for research in the institution. These requirements varied from a review by the nursing department's research committee to a review by the institutional review board (IRB).

After the approval process was completed, each department of nursing was sent a list of the 72 conditions to be studied and asked to select only those conditions that were regularly treated in their institution. Only those questionnaires were sent to the respective institutions. Study institutions received a packet for those selected conditions containing 10 questionnaires for each condition. Completed questionnaires were returned by the nurse respondent to the envelope, and the envelope sealed by the designated distributor. Nurse respondents were given the option of putting their questionnaire in a sealed envelope prior to placing it in the larger envelope.

Since two of the study institutions did not treat ophthalmic conditions, questionnaires related to these conditions were sent to two institutions specializing in these conditions.

Findings

Of the 19 institutions that agreed to participate, 18 (including the two ophthalmic institutions) returned the questionnaires. The target return was 160 questionnaires for each condition. The range of return was 29% to 70%, with the average rate of return 52.5%.

Each condition has a set of nursing diagnoses and collaborative problems with its own frequency score. The diagnoses were grouped into three ranges of frequency: 75% to 100%—frequent; 50% to 74%—often; <50%—infrequent. Each of the 72 conditions included in the study and this book has the nursing diagnoses and collaborative problems grouped according to the study findings.

Future Work

This study represents the initial step in the validation of the nursing care predicted to be needed when a client is hospitalized for a medical or surgical condition. It is important to validate which nursing diagnoses and collaborative problems necessitate nursing interventions. Future work will include the identification of nursing interventions that have priority in treating a diagnosis, clarification of outcomes realistic for the length of stay, and evaluation and review by national groups of nurses.

DEMOGRAPHICS OF RESPONDENTS

Questionnaires	
Sent	9,920
Returned	5,299
% returned	53.4%
Average Age	39
Average Years in Nursing	15

Level of Nursing Preparation	
Diploma	22.7%
AD	25.7%
BSN	36.5%
MSN	12.4%
PhD	1.5%
No indication	1.2%

References

Carpenito, L. J. (1984). *Handbook of nursing diagnosis.* Philadelphia, PA: J. B. Lippincott.
Carpenito, L. J. (1991). *Nursing care plans and documentation.* Philadelphia, PA: J. B. Lippincott.
Doenges, M., & Moorhouse, M. (1991). *Nurse's pocket guide: Nursing diagnoses with interventions.* Philadelphia, PA: F. A. Davis.
Holloway, N. M. (1988). *Medical surgical care plans.* Springhouse, PA: Springhouse.
Sparks, S. M., & Taylor, C. M. (1993). *Nursing diagnoses reference manual.* Springhouse, PA: Springhouse.
Ulrich, S., Canale, S., & Wendell, S. (1994). *Medical-surgical nursing: Care planning guide.* Philadelphia, PA: W. B. Saunders.

Acknowledgments

The Validation Project could not have been completed without the support of the following nurses who coordinated the data collection in their institutions:

Tammy Spier, RN, MSN
Department of Nursing Services
Department of Staff Development
Allen Memorial Hospital
Waterloo, Iowa

Donna Dickinson, RN, MS
Carol Mangold, RN, MSN
Carondelet St. Joseph's Hospital
Tucson, Arizona

Kathy Killman, RN, MSN
Liz Nelson, RN, MSN
The Evanston Hospital
Evanston, Illinois

Margaret Price, RN, MSN
Lynn Bobel Turbin, RN, MSN
Nancy DiJanni, RN, MSN
Huron Valley Hospital
Milford, Michigan

Pat Vaccaro, RN, BSN, CCRN
Deborah Stroh, RN
Mary Jean Potylycki, RN
Carolyn Peters, RN
Sue DeSanto, RN
Christine Niznik, RN
Carol Saxman, RN
Kelly Brown, RN
Judy Bailey, RN
Nancy Root, RN
Cheryl Bitting, RN
Carol Sorrentino, RN
Lehigh Valley Hospital
Allentown, Pennsylvania

Loretta Baldwin, RN, BSN
Karin Prussak, RN, MSN, CCRN
Bess Cullen, RN
Debra Goetz, RN, MSN
Susan Goucher, RN

Sandra Brackett, RN, BSN
Barbara Johnston, RN, CCRN
Lisa Lauderdale, RN
Randy Shoemaker, RN, CCRN
Memorial Medical Center of Jacksonville
Jacksonville, Florida

Karen Stiefel, RN, PhD
Jerre Jones, RN, MSN, CS
Lise Heidenreich, RN, MSN, FNP, CS
Christiana Redwood-Sawyer,
  RN, MSN
Presbyterian Hospital
Charlotte, North Carolina

Pauline Elliott, RN, BSN
St. Francis Medical Center
Cape Girardeau, Missouri

Dena Belfiore, RN, PhD
Dianne Hayko, MSRN, CNS
St. Joseph Hospital
Omaha, Nebraska

Jennie Nemec, RN, MSN
St. Peter Community Hospital
Helena, Montana

Eleanor Borkowski, RN
Tina Buchanan, RN
Jill Posadas, RN
Deanna Stover, RN
Margie Bracken, RN
Barbara Upton, RN
Kathleen Powers, RN
Jeanie Goodwin, RN
San Bernardino County Medical Center
San Bernardino, California

Kathy Karpiuk, RN, MNE
Monica Mauer, RN
Susan Fey, RN

Joan Reisdorfer, RN
Cheryl Wilson, Health Unit
  Coordinator
Gail Sundet, RN
Pat Halverson, RN
Ellie Baker, RN
Jackie Kisecker, RN
Cheri Dore-Paulson, RN
Kay Gartner, RN
Vicki Tigner, RN
Jan Burnette, RN
Maggie Scherff, RN
Sioux Valley Hospital
Sioux Falls, South Dakota

Keith Hampton, RN, MSN
University of Minnesota Hospital
Minneapolis, Minnesota

Eva Adler, RN, MSN
Jean Giddens, RN, MSN, CS
Dawn Roseberry, RN, BSN
University of New Mexico Hospital
Albuquerque, New Mexico

Carol Wong, RN, MScN
Cheryl Simpson, RN
Victoria Hospital
London, Canada

Heather Boyd-Monk, RN, MSN
Wills Eye Hospital
Philadelphia, Pennsylvania

Fran Tolley, RN, BSN
Vicky Navarro, RN, MAS
Wilmer Ophthalmological Institute
Johns Hopkins Hospital
Baltimore, Maryland

Joan Crosley, RN, PhD
Winthrop-University Hospital
Mineola, New York

My gratitude also extends to each of the nurses who gave their time to complete the questionnaires. A sincere thank you to Dr. Ginny Arcangelo, at the time of the research was the Director of the Family Nurse Practitioner Program at Thomas Jefferson University in Philadelphia, for her work as the methodology consultant to the project.

A study of this magnitude required over 9,000 questionnaires to be produced, duplicated, and distributed. Over 100,000 data entries were made, yielding the findings found throughout this edition.

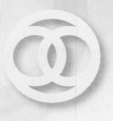

Acknowledgments

This 6th edition was made possible with the creative input of my editor, Patrick Barbera and the timely assistance of Annette Ferran from Lippincott Williams & Wilkins. Due to the unprecedented changes in health care in the last four years, this edition encompassed more than a usual revision due to the addition of four new chapters and a new Unit II.

The process of this labor-intensive revision and the frustrations when one ventures into new territory were made easier by one person, Karen Ettinger, the project manager. She tolerated my late-night emails, my unknown number of revised table of contents, missing deadlines, etc. She knows more about me than she probably wants to, but thank you, Karen, for being a genuine, caring person and one of the most competent project managers I have experienced in over 20 years.

Gracias to my patient friends, who understood the chaos of the last year that held me absent from doing other things: Maureen, Ginny, Judy, Karen, Donna, and Zalphia.

On a personal level, my son Olen Juall Carpenito and his wife, Heather, have given me two special gifts—my grandsons Olen, Jr. and Aiden. They light up my world every day. Love, Ona.

Contents

Section 2   Individual Collaborative Problems   211

Unit III Client and Family Centered Care Plans   297

Section 3 Diagnostic and Therapeutic Procedures 803

Section 4 Specialty Diagnostic Clusters 873

Unit I

Introduction to Client and Family Centered Care

"Continuum of Care is a concept involving an integrated system of care that guides and tracks client care over time through a comprehensive array of health services spanning all levels of intensity and all phases of illness from diagnosis to the end of life" (Zazworsky, personal communications).

All health care facilities are in this rapidly changing environment from the acute care hospital to the primary care medical home. Community care also provides skilled care facilities and home health agencies.

Principles of Client and Family Centered Care

- Competent, trustworthy staff
- Care is respectful
- Dignity is protected
- All care processes are explained clearly and understood
- Family / support persons are involved
- Physical and emotional comfort are priorities
- Decisions are made collaboratively and differences respected
- Transition process begins on admission
- Preparation for safe and comfortable transition to home

The focus of this book is to:

- Provide evidence-based, caring care that is a priority for the condition and length of stay.
- Guide the student nurse or clinician to identify high-risk individuals for adverse events.
- Emphasize elements to address for timely and safe transition from the acute care setting.

In order for the individual and family to be prepared to assume care that is safe and correct at home, five components must be addressed in an ongoing process beginning on admission to transition to home care and follow-up in a medical home. All of these components are integrated in all the care plans in this edition.

Components of Effective, Safe Transition

1. On admission, identification of individuals / support persons who have barriers to a timely, effective transition
2. On admission, identification of individuals who are high risk for an adverse outcome / event during hospitalization
3. Early identification of support persons or absence of (or unavailable) and their ability to continue care in the home setting
4. Deliberate, ongoing preparation to provide care in the home settings and teaching of when to seek advice
5. Identification of follow-up care: When? Where? etc.

The motives for preventing adverse events (falls, infections, readmissions) may for some in health care be primarily financial. The Centers of Medicare and Medicaid have clearly set forward financial penalties for adverse event occurrences which are deemed preventable.

These reforms are long overdue. Clerical nurses would benefit from viewing these critical changes not as burdens but instead as opportunities to integrate them into the core of every interaction with a client and family. As you give the individual a consultation, briefly explain why this piece is needed and, if indicated, what will need to be done after discharge. For example, as you change a dressing, have the individual and family member view the incision. Point out how it is healing and advise what needs to be reported after discharge. Make each moment a teachable moment.

Chapter 1

The Bifocal Clinical Practice Model

The classification activities of the North American Nursing Diagnosis Association International (NANDA-I) have been instrumental in defining nursing's unique body of knowledge. This unified system of terminology:

* Provides consistent language for oral, written, and electronic communication
* Stimulates nurses to examine new knowledge
* Establishes a system for automation and reimbursement
* Provides an educational framework
* Allows efficient information retrieval for research and quality assurance
* Provides a consistent structure for literature presentation of nursing knowledge
* Clarifies nursing as an art and a science for its members and society
* Establishes standards to which nurses are held accountable

Appendix A of this text provides a list of nursing diagnoses grouped under Functional Health Patterns.

Clearly, nursing diagnosis has influenced the nursing profession positively. Integration of nursing diagnosis into nursing practice, however, has proved problematic. Although references to nursing diagnosis in the literature have increased exponentially since the first meeting in 1973 of the National Group for the Classification of Nursing Diagnoses (which later became NANDA-I), nurses have not seen efficient and representative applications. For example, nurses have been directed to use nursing diagnoses exclusively to describe their clinical focus. Nevertheless, nurses who strongly support nursing diagnosis often become frustrated when they try to attach a nursing diagnosis label to every facet of nursing practice. Some of the dilemmas that result from the attempt to label as nursing diagnoses all situations in which nurses intervene are as follows:

1. *Using nursing diagnoses without validation.* When the nursing diagnoses are the only labels or diagnostic statements the nurse can use, the nurse is encouraged to "change the data to fit the label." For example, using the Imbalanced Nutrition category for all clients who are given nothing-by-mouth status. Risk for Injury also frequently serves as a "wastebasket" diagnosis because all potentially injurious situations (e.g., bleeding) can be captured within a Risk for Injury diagnosis.
2. *Renaming medical diagnoses.* Clinical nurses know that an important component of their practice is monitoring for the onset and status of physiologic complications and initiating both nurse-prescribed and physician-prescribed interventions. Morbidity and mortality are reduced and prevented because of nursing's expert management.

If nursing diagnoses are to describe all situations in which nurses intervene, then clearly a vast number must be developed to describe the situations identified in the International Code of Diseases (ICD-10). Table 1.1 represents examples of misuse of nursing diagnoses and the renaming of medical diagnoses. Examination of the substitution of nursing diagnosis terminology for medical diagnoses or pathophysiology in Table 1.1 gives rise to several questions:

* Should nursing diagnoses describe all situations in which nurses intervene?
* If a situation is not called a nursing diagnosis, is it then less important or scientific?
* How will it serve the profession to rename medical diagnoses as nursing diagnoses?
* Will using the examples in Table 1.1 improve communication and clarify nursing?

Table 1.1 Diagnostic Errors: Renaming Medical Diagnoses with Nursing Diagnosis Terminology

Medical Diagnosis	Nursing Diagnosis
Myocardial Infarction	Decreased Cardiac Output
Shock	Decreased Cardiac Output
Adult Respiratory Distress	Impaired Gas Exchange
Chronic Obstructive Lung Disease	Impaired Gas Exchange
Asthma	Impaired Gas Exchange
Alzheimer's Disease	Impaired Cerebral Tissue Perfusion
Increased Intracranial Pressure	Impaired Cerebral Tissue Perfusion
Retinal Detachment	Disturbed Sensory Perception: Visual
Thermal Burns	Impaired Tissue Integrity
Incisions, Lacerations	Impaired Skin Integrity
Hemorrhage	Deficient Fluid Volume
Congestive Heart Failure	Excess Fluid Volume

3. *Omitting problem situations in documentation.* If a documentation system requires the use of nursing diagnosis exclusively, and if the nurse does not choose to "change the data to fit a category" or "to rename medical diagnoses," then the nurse has no terminology to describe a critical component of nursing practice. Failure to describe these situations can seriously jeopardize nursing's effort to justify and affirm the need for professional nurses in all health care settings (Carpenito, 1987).

Bifocal Clinical Practice Model

Nursing's theoretical knowledge derives from the natural, physical, and behavioral sciences, as well as the humanities and nursing research. Nurses can use various theories in practice, including family systems, loss, growth and development, crisis intervention, and general systems theories.

The difference between nursing and the other health care disciplines is nursing's depth and breadth of focus. Certainly, the nutritionist has more expertise in the field of nutrition and the pharmacist in the field of therapeutic pharmacology than any nurse. Every nurse, however, brings a knowledge of nutrition and pharmacology to client interactions. The depth of this knowledge is sufficient for many client situations; when it is insufficient, consultation is required. No other discipline has this varied knowledge, explaining why attempts to substitute other disciplines for nursing have proved costly and ultimately unsuccessful. Figure 1.1 illustrates this varied expertise.

The Bifocal Clinical Practice Model (Carpenito, 1987) represents situations that influence persons, groups, and communities as well as the classification of these responses from a nursing perspective. The situations are organized into five broad categories: pathophysiologic, treatment-related, personal, environmental, and maturational (Figure 1.2). Without an understanding of such situations, the nurse will be unable to diagnose responses and intervene appropriately.

Clinically, these situations are important to nurses. Thus, as nursing diagnoses evolved, nurses sought to substitute nursing terminology for these situations; for example, Impaired Tissue Integrity for burns and High Risk for Injury for dialysis. Nurses do not prescribe for and treat these situations (e.g., burns and dialysis). Rather, they prescribe for and treat the *responses* to these situations.

The practice focus for clinical nursing is at the response level, not at the situation level. For example, a client who has sustained burns may exhibit a wide variety of responses to the burns and the treatments. Some responses may be predicted, such as High Risk for Infection; others, such as fear of losing a job, may not be predictable. In the past, nurses focused on the nursing interventions associated with treating burns rather than on those associated with the client's responses. *This resulted in nurses being described as "doers" rather than "knowers"; as technicians rather than scientists.*

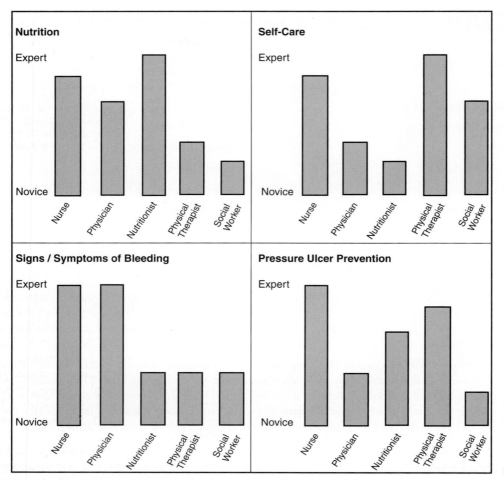

FIGURE 1.1 Knowledge of multidisciplines of selected topics.

Nursing Diagnoses and Collaborative Problems

The Bifocal Clinical Practice Model describes the two foci of clinical nursing: nursing diagnoses and collaborative problems.

A nursing diagnosis is a clinical judgment about individual, family, or community responses to actual or potential health problems / life processes. Nursing diagnosis provides the basis for selection of nursing interventions to achieve outcomes for which the nurse has accountability (NANDA, 2008). Collaborative problems are certain physiologic complications that nurses monitor to detect onset or changes of status. Nurses manage collaborative problems using physician-prescribed and nursing-prescribed interventions to minimize the complications of the events (Carpenito, 1997). Figure 1.3 illustrates the Bifocal Clinical Practice Model.

Pathophysiologic
Myocardial infarction
Borderline personality disorder
Burns

Treatment-related
Anticoagulants
Dialysis
Arteriogram

Personal
Dying
Divorce
Relocation

Environmental
Overcrowded school
No handrails on stairs
Rodents

Maturational
Peer pressure
Parenthood
Aging

FIGURE 1.2 Examples of pathophysiologic, treatment-related, personal, environmental, and maturational situations.

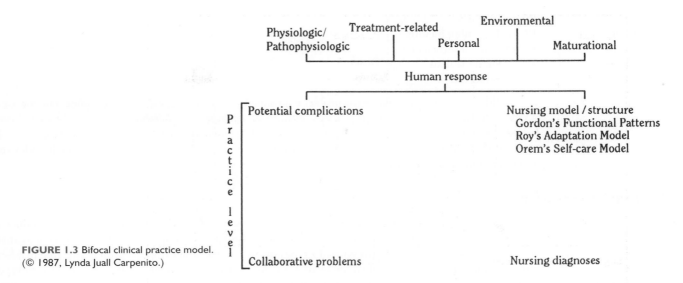

FIGURE 1.3 Bifocal clinical practice model. (© 1987, Lynda Juall Carpenito.)

The nurse makes independent decisions for both collaborative problems and nursing diagnoses. The difference is that in nursing diagnoses, nursing prescribes the definitive treatment to achieve the desired outcome, while in collaborative problems, prescription for definitive treatment comes from both nursing and physicians / nurse practitioners. Some physiologic complications (such as Risk for Infection and Impaired Skin Integrity) are nursing diagnoses because nurses can order the definitive treatment. In a collaborative problem, the nurse uses surveillance to monitor for the onset and change in status of physiologic complications, and manages these changes to prevent morbidity and mortality. These physiologic complications are usually related to disease, trauma, treatments, medications, or diagnostic studies. Thus, collaborative problems can be labeled Risk for Complications of (specify),** for example, Risk for Complications of Hemorrhage or Risk for Complications of Renal Failure.

Monitoring, however, is not the sole nursing responsibility for collaborative problems. For example, in addition to monitoring a client with increased intracranial pressure, the nurse also restricts certain activities, maintains head elevation, implements the medical regimen, and continually addresses the client's psychosocial and educational needs.

The following are some collaborative problems that commonly apply to certain situations:

Situation	Collaborative Problem
Myocardial Infarction	Risk for Complications (RC) of Dysrhythmias
Craniotomy	RC of Increased Intracranial Pressure
Hemodialysis	RC of Fluid / Electrolyte Imbalance
Surgery	RC of Hemorrhage
Cardiac Catheterization	RC of Allergic Reaction

If the situation calls for the nurse to monitor for a cluster or group of physiologic complications, the collaborative problems may be documented as

RC of Cardiac

or

RC of Postop: Urinary retention
RC of Hemorrhage
RC of Hypovolemia

**Previously labeled Potential Complications: (specify)

RC of Hypoxia
RC of Thrombophlebitis
RC of Renal insufficiency
RC of Paralytic ileus
RC of Evisceration

A list of common collaborative problems grouped under conditions that necessitate nursing care appears in Appendix A. *Not all physiologic complications, however, are collaborative problems.* Nurses themselves can prevent some physiologic complications such as infections from external sources (e.g., wounds and catheters), contractures, incontinence, and pressure ulcers. Thus, such complications fall under the category of nursing diagnosis.

Nursing Interventions

Nursing interventions are treatments or actions that benefit a client by presenting a problem, reducing or eliminating a problem, or promoting a healthier response. Nursing interventions can be classified as either of two types: nurse-prescribed or physician / nurse practitioner**-prescribed. Independent interventions are nurse-prescribed; delegated interventions are physician / NP-prescribed. Both types of interventions, however, require independent nursing judgment. By law, the nurse must determine if it is appropriate to initiate an intervention regardless of whether it is independent or delegated (Carpenito, 1997).

Carpenito (1987) stated that the relationship of diagnosis to interventions is a critical element in defining nursing diagnoses. Many definitions of nursing diagnoses focus on the relationship of selected interventions to the diagnoses. A certain type of intervention appears to distinguish a nursing diagnosis from a medical diagnosis or other problems that nurses treat. The type of intervention distinguishes a nursing diagnosis from a collaborative problem and also differentiates between actual risk / high risk and possible nursing diagnoses. Table 1.2 outlines definitions of each type and the corresponding intervention focus. For example, for a nursing diagnosis of Impaired Tissue Integrity related to immobility as manifested by a 2-cm epidermal lesion on the client's left heel, the nurse would order interventions to monitor the lesion and to heal it. In another client with a surgical wound, the nurse would focus on prevention of infection and promotion of healing.

Risk for Infection would better describe the situation than Impaired Tissue Integrity. *Nursing diagnoses are not more important than collaborative problems, and collaborative problems are not more important than nursing diagnoses.*

Table 1.2 • Differentiation Among Types of Diagnoses

Diagnostic Statement	Corresponding Client Outcome or Nursing Goals	Focus of Intervention
Actual Diagnosis Three-part statement, including nursing diagnostic label, etiology, and signs / symptoms	Change in client behavior moving toward resolution of the diagnosis or improved status	Reduce or eliminate problem
Risk / High-Risk Diagnosis Two-part statement, including nursing diagnostic label and risk factors	Maintenance of present conditions	Reduce risk factors to prevent an actual problem
Possible Diagnosis Two-part statement, including nursing diagnostic label and unconfirmed etiology or unconfirmed defining characteristics	Undetermined until problem is validated	Collect additional data to confirm or rule out signs / symptoms or risk factors
Collaborative Problems Potential or actual physiologic complication	Nursing goals	Determine onset or status of the problem Manage change in status

---

**Nurse practitioners have the legal authority to prescribe medical interventions, thus can diagnose and treat collaborative problems.

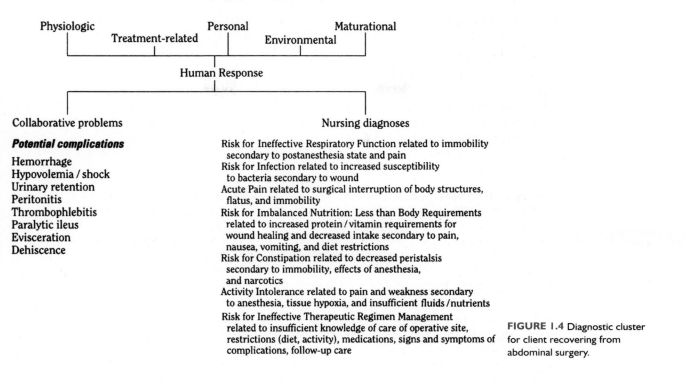

FIGURE 1.4 Diagnostic cluster for client recovering from abdominal surgery.

Priorities are determined by the client's situation, not by whether it is a nursing diagnosis or a collaborative problem.

A *diagnostic cluster* represents those nursing diagnoses and collaborative problems that have a high likelihood of occurring in a client population. The nurse validates their presence in the individual client. Figure 1.4 represents the diagnostic cluster for a client after abdominal surgery. Unit II contains diagnostic clusters for medical and surgical conditions or goals.

Goals / Outcome Criteria

In a nursing care plan, goals (outcome criteria) are "statements describing a measurable behavior of client / family that denote a favorable status (changed or maintained) after nursing care has been delivered" (Alfaro, 1989). Outcome criteria help to determine the success or appropriateness of the nursing care plan. If the nursing care plan does not achieve a favorable status even though the diagnosis is correct, the nurse must change the goal or change the plan. If neither option is indicated, the nurse confers with the physician / nurse practitioner for delegated orders. Nursing diagnoses should *not* represent situations that require physician / NP orders for treatment. Otherwise how can nurses assume accountability for diagnosis and treatment? For example, consider a client with a nursing diagnosis:

Risk for Impaired Cerebral Tissue Perfusion related to effects of recent head injury and these goals:

The client will demonstrate continued optimal cerebral pressure as evidenced by

* Pupils equally reactive to light and accommodation
* No change in orientation or consciousness

If this client were to exhibit evidence of increased intracranial pressure, would it be appropriate for the nurse to change the goals? What changes in the nursing care plan would the nurse make to stop the cranial pressure from increasing? Actually, neither action is warranted. Rather, the nurse should confer with the physician / NP for delegated orders to treat increased intracranial pressure. When the nurse formulates client goals or outcomes that require delegated medical orders for goal achievement, the situation is not a nursing diagnosis but a collaborative problem. In this case, the client's problem would be described better as a collaborative problem:

Risk for Complications of Increased Intracranial Pressure

Collaborative Outcomes

The individual will be monitored for early signs and symptoms of increased intracranial pressure and will receive interventions to achieve physiologic stability.

Indicators of physiologic stability:

- Alert, oriented, calm
- Pupils, equal, reactive to light and accommodation
- Pulse 60–100 bpm
- Respirations 16–20 bpm
- BP >90/60, <140/90 mm Hg
- No nausea / vomiting
- Mild to no headache

These collaborative goals represent the nursing accountability for monitoring for physiologic instability and providing interventions (nursing and medical) to maintain or restore stability.

SUMMARY   The Bifocal Clinical Practice Model provides nurses with a framework to diagnose the unique responses of a client and significant others to various situations. Clear definition of the two dimensions of nursing enhances the use and minimizes the misuse of nursing diagnoses. The Bifocal Clinical Practice Model describes the unique knowledge and focus of professional nursing.

Chapter 2

Communication: The Critical Key to Preventing Adverse Events

The literature identifies that clinical mistakes and adverse events are caused by human error, at-risk behavior, or reckless behavior. In this chapter, root causes for errors creating adverse events in a safe culture will be discussed.

Sentinel Events

Sentinel events are described as "any unexpected event in a health care setting that causes death or serious injury to a patient and is not related to the natural cause of the patient's illness" (Sherwood & Barnsteiner, 2012, p. 395). Since 2008, the Joint Commission has compiled a report of sentinel events and root causes. Reporting is voluntary and represents only a small portion of actual events (2012). The principle of root cause is that clinical adverse events are not caused by a single human error "but by a combination of factors relating to organizational practices, structured by which errors are missed and adverse incidents are not prevented" (Nicolini et al., 2012). The Joint Commission identified the most frequent root causes of sentinel events. Inadequate communication appears as the third most frequent cause of these events since 2009 (Joint Commission, 2012).

Examples of Failure to Communicate

Incident 1

When a student performs a catheterization, contaminates the catheter, and inserts it anyway.
    Cause: Failure to communicate the need for assistance or the need to stop and start the procedure again.

Incident 2

An individual's condition is declining and the physician / NP does not respond to the nurse's assessment and need for evaluation. The client's further decline is the result of the nurse not notifying the next in the chain of command (manager, chief of staff).

Incident 3

A nurse observes a protocol violation that will increase the risk of infection (e.g., contamination of venous access during dressing change). Does the nurse stop the person or ignore it? Would it matter if it was the surgeon or a nurse breaking practice?

Incident 4

An individual falls while trying to access the bathroom. Was the person's risk factors for fall clearly communicated during the "hand-off" report?

Incident 5

During "hand-off," personal discussions and accessing instead of "hands-on" information, does someone acknowledge that this time must be reserved for pertinent clinical information?

Incident 6

The emergency room nurse calls to advise the nurse a new admission is on his way to the unit. Does the nurse alert the ER nurse that she or he needs to hold the person there for a half hour more or does she or he rush through some treatments instead?

Barriers to "Speaking Up"

What prevents a nurse from calling a physician / NP when needed, reporting on negligent staff members, asking for help, discussing poor prognoses with a family, or end-of-life care?

- Fear
- Inexperience
- Not taken seriously
- Retaliation
- Intimidation
- Disruptive response

In 2008, the Joint Commission issued a sentinel event alert regarding behaviors that undermine a culture of safety (The Joint Commission, 2008a).

Intimidating and disruptive behaviors can foster medical errors, contribute to poor client satisfaction and to preventable adverse outcomes, increase the cost of care, and cause qualified clinicians, administrators, and managers to seek new positions in more professional environments. Safety and quality of client care is dependent on teamwork, communication, and a collaborative work environment. To assure quality and to promote a culture of safety, health care organizations must address the problem of behaviors that threaten the performance of the health care team.

Intimidating and disruptive behaviors include overt actions such as verbal outbursts and physical threats, as well as passive activities such as refusing to perform assigned tasks or quietly exhibiting uncooperative attitudes during routine activities. Intimidating and disruptive behaviors are often manifested by health care professionals in positions of power. Such behaviors include reluctance or refusal to answer questions, return phone calls or pages; condescending language or voice intonation; and impatience with questions. Overt and passive behaviors undermine team effectiveness and can compromise the safety of clients. All intimidating and disruptive behaviors are unprofessional and should not be tolerated.

Carp's Cues

In 2005, one study reported that 40% of clinicians related that they kept quiet or remained passive rather than question a known aggressive intimidator (Institute of Safe Medication Practices). Most nurses can relate numerous incidents, when during morning report (hands-off), the nurse reports a change in an individual's condition during the night that was not reported to the physician because of "fear of the response."

Disruptive Behavior

Hospitals are mandated to have a policy that (The Joint Commission, 2008b):

- Defines disruptive and inappropriate behavior
- Outlines a process for managing disruptive and inappropriate behaviors.

Everyone is entitled to having a "bad day" on occasion within limits. Disruptive behavior is a pattern of inappropriate, abusive conduct that harms and intimidates others. In health care settings, this behavior compromises the quality care and / or client safety.

Any member of the health care team can be disruptive (a nurse, manager, administrator, medical assistant, physician, nurse practitioner, etc.). It is unacceptable at any level and there needs to be a culture of zero tolerance. Even in an atmosphere where disruptive behavior is expected and tolerated, individual nurses can choose to speak up.

Everyone can develop the skills to communicate effectively and also preserve his or her dignity.

 ## Carp's Cues

"So for most nurses, the first step in addressing disruptive behavior is internal. It starts with an absolute belief that nobody deserves to be yelled at for making or witnessing a mistake, much less while doing their job correctly and competently" (Lyndon et al., 2012).

Effective Communication

"Communication failures are the leading cause of inadvertent patient harm" (Leonard, Graham, Bonacum, 2004, p. i86). "Analysis of 2455 sentinel events reported to the Joint Commission for Hospital Accreditation revealed that the primary root cause in over 70% was communication failure" (JCAH, 2004, quoted in Leonard et al., 2004, p. i86).

> "Effective communication and teamwork is essential for the delivery of high quality, safe patient care. Communication failures are an extremely common cause of inadvertent patient harm. The complexity of medical care, coupled with the inherent limitations of human performance, make it critically important that clinicians have standardized communication tools, create an environment in which individuals can speak up and express concerns, and share common 'critical language'" (Leonard et al., 2004, p. i85).

As described earlier in this chapter, it is "equally important. . .creating an environment that feels 'safe' to team members so they will speak up when they have safety concerns" (Leonard et al., 2004, p. i86).

SBAR

> "Human factors science tells us that the inherent limitations of human memory, effects of stress and fatigue, the risks associated with distractions and interruptions, and limited ability to multitask ensure that even skilled, experienced providers will make mistakes" (Leonard et al., 2004, p. i86).

Developed at Kaiser Permanente in Denver (Leonard et al., 2004), SBAR uses a brief and concise structure to communicate critically important information. SBAR stands for situation, background, assessment, recommendation.

> "Briefly and concisely, critically important pieces of information can be transmitted in a predictable structure. Not only is there familiarity in how people communicated, but the SBAR structure helps develop desired critical thinking skills. The person initiating the communication knows that before they pick up the telephone that they need to provide an assessment of the problem and what they think an appropriate solution is" (Leonard et al., 2004, p. i86).

> "Thus, a nurse at the bedside may not be able to put a concise label or description on what is clinically unfolding, but very probably knows 'something is wrong, and I need your help.' Lowering the threshold to obtain help, and treating the request respectfully and legitimately creates a much safer system" (Leonard et al., 2004, p. i86).

Table 2.1 outlines the format of SBAR with examples.

Table 2.1   SBAR Guidelines
When calling the physician / nurse practitioner, follow the SBAR process:

(S) Situation: What is the situation you are calling about? What is going on with the client?

- Identity, self, unit, client, room number
- Briefly state the problem, what is it, when it happened or started, and how severe.

(B) Background: Pertinent background information related to the situation could include the following:

- The admitting diagnosis and date of admission
- List of current medications, allergies, IV fluids, and labs
- Most recent vital signs
- Lab results: provide the date and time test was done and results of previous tests for comparison
- Other clinical information
- Code status

(A) Assessment: What is your assessment of the situation? What do you think the problem is?

(R) Recommendation: What is your recommendation or what do you want?

Examples:

- "I need you to come now and see the individual."
- Order change
- Notification that their client has been admitted
- Need to transfer to ICU
- Any tests needed?
- Need to talk to individual family about code status

STAR

When confronted with a change in a client's condition, utilize the STAR approach:

STAR	**Stop**	
	Think	What is wrong with this situation? How does this individual's condition change for the worse?
	Act	If unsure, consult with an experienced nurse.
		Recommend: State what your next action is (e.g., reassess or implement SBAR).

Prior to notifying or discussing an individual with a physician / NP, discuss the situation with the manager or coordinator if indicated.

Carp's Cues

Avoid having experienced colleagues call instead of yourself, which will only continue your fears and inexperience. Students can be assisted with a clinical nurse or faculty listening, while the student talks. The faculty person can add data if needed. This is an invaluable lesson that must be practiced as a student.

- Consider the following prior to making the call:
  - Selecting the appropriate physician / NP
  - Assess the person yourself before calling
  - Open the electronic health record of the person
  - Relate allergies, pertinent medications, p.o. status fluids, lab results
  - Report vital signs, focus on changes
  - Clarify code status or if it is unknown

Unit II and the care plans contain numerous examples of SBAR.

"Medical care is extremely complex, and this complexity coupled with inherent human performance limitations, even in skilled, experienced, highly motivated individuals, ensures there will be mistakes" (Leonard et al., 2004, p. i86).

"Effective teamwork and communication can help prevent these inevitable mistakes from becoming consequential, and harming patients and providers" (Leonard et al., 2004, p. i86).

The Hand-Off Process

The hand-off is a term used to describe the transfer of information (along with authority and responsibility) during transitions in care across the continuum (Friesen et al., 2008). This hand-off, also known as shift report, transfer report, sign over, is utilized at:

- Change of shift on a unit
- Transfer to another care of facility
- Discharge to a community agency

Effective hand-offs support the transition of critical information and specifically identifies high risk and clinical unstable individuals. Unfortunately, the literature describes adverse events and safety risks occurring when the hand-off process is compromised, incomplete and / or missing.

All health care facilities have a format / process for hand-offs; however, the quality and accuracy of the hand-off is primarily dependent on the involved clinicians. Nurses engaged in hand-offs can increase the accuracy and clarity of the dialogue. Refer to Table 2.2 for strategies to increase the effectiveness of the hand-off. The usual data, name, room, age, medical diagnoses, meds, treatment will also be presented.

Table 2.2 Tips to Increase the Effectiveness of Hand-offs

1. Establish that the dialogue will be limited to that which will improve the care to individuals.
   • Avoid negative discussions of family, visitors, individuals
   • Avoid socialization
   • Avoid criticizing staff, personnel, etc.
2. Relate to the priorities of care for the individual.
   • Frequency of vital signs
   • Changes in condition
   • Physician / NP involvement
   • Last prn medication dose, time
   • Risk status for falls, pressure ulcers
3. Report what teaching has been done to prepare for transition.
   • Individual / family involvement
   • Individual / families understanding of condition, progress, code status

Carp's Cues

Nursing care is 24 hours/7 days a week. Care of an individual is not completed when a shift is over. The care continues and thus, it is a "hand-off."

Sometimes, a treatment may have to be handed over to the next nurse. Work as a 24-hour team and less frustration will occur. Nursing is a difficult profession with huge responsibilities. Lend a hand to your nursing colleague because it is the right thing to do.

Note: Nurses, who habitually hand-off incomplete care without cause is a management problem.

SUMMARY

Despite the explosion of technology as electronic medical records, invasive lines with alarms, bed alarms, cardiac alarms, PCA pumps, the safety and comfort of individuals and their families depend primarily on the expertise of the bedside nurse.

The nurse's personal sense of authority applies the same standard of care to the president of the local bank as to the man addicted to prescription pain medications who is complaining of pain postabdominal surgery. The expert nurse knows when "something is not right" or when "wrong is wrong" and speaks up.

Chapter 3

Early Identification of High-Risk Individuals and / or Family

On admission, all individuals will have a nursing assessment of vital signs, functional health patterns, and body systems (e.g., skin, respiratory, cardiac) using the Nursing Admission Data Base. Refer to Appendix B for an example.

After the initial assessment, determine the likelihood that the individual will have an uncomplicated complex transition. For the majority of clients, the transition will be uncomplicated as described as:

- Will usually return to their own home or someone else's for a short stay
- Having care needs that can managed by the individual or support system and do not require complex planning, teaching, or referrals

 Carp's Cues

Individuals / families that were providing good care at home for long-term chronic conditions may be able to resume this care with little help. Keep in mind that a change in the individual's status or support system situation can change a transition process to uncomplicated from complex.

To differentiate between a predicted uncomplicated or complex transition, the following assessments are indicated:

- Medication reconciliation and barriers to adherence
- Factors that are barriers to effective transition to home care
- Factors that increase the individual's risk for injury, falls, pressure ulcers, and / or infection during hospitalization

Medication Reconciliation and Barriers to Adherence

Medication errors occur 46% of the time during transitions, admission, transfer, or discharge from a clinical unit / hospital. Almost 60% of individuals have at least 1 discrepancy in their medication history completed on admission (Cornish et al., 2005). "The most common error (46.4%) was omission of a regularly used medication. Most (61.4%) of the discrepancies were judged to have no potential to cause serious harm (p. 424). However, 38.6% of the discrepancies had the potential to cause moderate to severe discomfort or clinical deterioration" (p. 424).

Medication reconciliation on admission to the health care facilities often entails:

- Name of medication (prescribed, over the counter)
- Prescribed dose
- Frequency (daily, bid, tid, as needed)

> **CLINICAL ALERT**
>
> A list of medications that have been prescribed by a provider does not represent a process of medication reconciliation. A family member recently took an older relative to the ER with chest pain. A typed list of her medications was given to the ER nurse. No discussion occurred about her medication.
>
> Unfortunately, one of two hypertension medications she regularly took was not entered in the electronic health record. Since her blood pressure was elevated on admission and persisted, another antihypertensive medication was ordered. After two deep, another medication was added with good results.
>
> The first medication that was added was the medication she was already taking prior to admission. So essentially, no new medication was added as a result of the error. She spent three unnecessary days in the hospital with increased costs to Medicare and would have definitely rather been home eating her own food and having a good night's sleep in her own bed.

According to the Joint Commission (p. 1),

> Medication reconciliation is the process of comparing a client's medication orders to all of the medications that the patient has been taking. This reconciliation is done to avoid medication errors such as omissions, duplications, dosing errors, or drug interactions. It should be done at every transition of care in which new medications are ordered or existing orders are rewritten. Transitions in care include changes in setting, service, practitioner, or level of care. The process comprises five steps: (1) develop a list of current medications; (2) develop a list of medications to be prescribed; (3) compare the medications on the two lists; (4) make clinical decisions based on the comparison; and (5) communicate the new list to appropriate caregivers to the patient.

Table 3.1 outlines a comprehensive list of medications to review during medication reconciliations.

Critical to acquiring a list of medications authorized in Table 3.1 are the additional assessment questions, which are the defining elements for medication reconciliation: *versus a list of medications reported to be taking.*

The individual / family member is asked the following:

For each medication reported ask:

- What is the reason you are taking each medication?
- Are you taking the medication as prescribed? Specify once a day, twice a day, etc.
- Are you skipping any doses? Do you sometimes run out of medications?
- How often are you taking the medication prescribed "if needed as a pain medication"?
- Have you stopped taking any of these medications?
- How much does it cost you to take your medications?
- Are you taking anybody else's medication?

Table 3.1 Sources of Medication History

The medication history can be obtained from a variety of sources:
- The client
- A list the patient may have
- The medications themselves, if brought in from home
- A friend or family member
- A medical record
- The individual's pharmacy

Factors that increase are barriers to effectively transition to home

Individuals, on admission to an acute care setting, necessitate an assessment to determine the presence of barriers to a timely transition to home care (or a community health setting).

Barriers that effectively transition from acute care setting are:

- Personal
- Support system
- Home environment

Personal Barriers

Determine if any of these barriers to self-care are responsible for this admission. Access the appropriate resource in the institution as early as possible to initiate resolving or reducing barriers (e.g., social service, home care).

Individuals are assessed for disabilities and compromised functioning at admission. Assess if the individual:

- Is homeless
- Has no medical insurance
- Unable to live alone
- Physically impaired
- Mentally compromised
- Can read, level of comprehension
- Understand English
- Is abusing drugs, alcohol

Support System Barriers

Preparing family members / support persons for home care is addressed in each care plan in Unit III. If a support system is not present, nonexistent, or incapable to providing home care, refer to the appropriate resource in the institution as early as possible (e.g., social service, home care agency).

Determine the present status of a support system. Assess:

- What kind of assistance is needed for homecare 24/7 (e.g., daily visits, phone calls, etc.)?
- Is there a support system? Who?
- Are they willing / available to provide assistance?
- Will they arrange for assistance from others?
- Are they capable of providing needed care at home (e.g., elderly spouse)?

Home Environment

If there are barriers to home care due to the environment, refer to the appropriate resource in the institution as early as possible (e.g., social service, home health agency).

Determine the status of the home environment. Assess:

- Where does the person live? Home alone? Shelter? Homeless? With others?
- Can equipment for home care be accessed? Insurance coverage? Home barriers?
- Is the person capable accessing home / apartment? Stairs?
- Is there access to a bathroom without using stairs?
- If there is a temporary alternative (e.g., family member's home)?

Factors that increase the individual's risk of injury, falls, pressure ulcers and / or infection during hospitalization and preventable hospital-acquired conditions

The Centers for Medicare and Medicaid Services (CMS) in 2008 published "Roadmap for Implementing Value Driven Healthcare in the Traditional Medicare Fee-for-Service-Program."

The Centers for Medicare and Medicaid Services (CMS) objective is "to improve the accuracy of Medicare's payment under the acute care hospital inpatient prospective payment system . . . while providing additional incentives for hospitals to engage in quality improvement efforts (CMS, 2008).

Of equal importance is that additional payments will be denied for the treatment of the following fourteen hospital acquired conditions (CMS, 2008)

- Stage II and IV pressure ulcers
- Falls and trauma such as fractures, dislocations, intracranial injuries, crushing injuries, burns, and other injuries
- Manifestations of poor glycemic control (e.g., ketoacidosis, hyperosmolar coma, hypoglycemic coma, secondary diabetes with ketoacidosis, or hyperosmolarity)
- Catheter-associated UTIs
- Vascular catheter-associated infections
- Surgical-site infection, mediastinitis, following coronary artery bypass graft (CABG)
- Surgical-site infection following bariatric surgery for obesity (laparoscopic gastric bypass, gastroenterostomy, laparoscopic gastric restrictive surgery)
- Surgical-site infection following certain orthopedic procedures (spine, neck, shoulder, elbow)
- Surgical-site infection following cardiac implantable electronic device (CIED)
- Foreign objects retained after surgery
- Deep vein thrombosis (DVT) pulmonary embolism (PE) following certain orthopedic procedures (total knee replacement, hip replacement)
- Iatrogenic puemothorax with venous catherization
- Air embolism
- Blood incompatibility

Buerhaus and Kurtzman wrote (2008, p. 30):

> Most hospital nurses are salaried; hospitals consider those salaries a cost of doing business. In most hospitals, nurses represent about 40% of the direct-care budget. By contrast, physicians are revenue generators because hospitals charge the CMS and other payers for the costs of the resources used to produce medical care provided by or ordered by physicians. Until now, there hasn't been a mechanism under Medicare payment policies for measuring nurses' specific economic contribution to hospitals. CMS-1533-FC offers a mechanism for doing so; to the degree that nursing care prevents costly complications, hospitals will not lose money. In this way, the new Medicare payment rule has the potential to more clearly demonstrate nurses' economic value to hospitals.

A white paper* on Preventing Never Events / Evidence-Based Practice reported the following (Leonardi, Faller, & Siroky, 2011, p. 8):

- 1 in 25 clients suffer injury at a cost of $17–29 billion per year (AHRQ, 2010)
- 1.5 million injuries occurred in 2008 from medical errors at an average cost $13,000/injury or a total of $19.5 billion (Shreve et al., 2010)
- 7% of admissions had some type of medical injury according to inpatient billing records (Shreve et al., 2010)
- 42,243 clients (0.2% of inpatients) developed a hospital-acquired infection
- Approximately 1.7 million hospital-acquired infections, the most common complications of hospital care (McGlynn, 2008) occur each year in hospitals, leading to about 100,000 deaths (AHRQ, 2010)

Studies have demonstrated a correlation of lowered rates of complication, nurse to client ratios and high quality nursing care (Leonardi et al., 2011; Aiken et al., 2010; Moore et al., 2010; Kane, Shamliyan, Mueller, Duval, & Wilt, 2007; Unruh & Fottler, 2006). The white paper concluded that the number of nurses on a unit strengthens patient safety (Leonardi et al., 2011). In addition to adequate nursing staffing, the following were noted to enhance quality (Leonardi et al., 2011, p. 15; Savitz, Jones, & Bernard, 2005):

- Unfinished or incomplete care
- Use of standardized technique, such as hand washing, skin preparation, wound dressings
- Prudent monitoring of invasive medical devices, such as catheters, chest tubes, IVs

---

*A white paper in nursing is an authoritative report of research or expert opinion to understand an issue, solve a problem, or make a decision.

- Systematic skin inspection, cleaning, and positioning
- Adherence to care pathways / protocols
- Other measure that reflect communications, collaboration, documentation, and teamwork

High-Risk Nursing Diagnoses for Preventable Hospital-Acquired Conditions

This edition has identified the importance of prevention of eight conditions identified by CMS. Using evidence-based guidelines the following can be accessed:

- Nursing diagnoses that represent prevention of infection, falls, pressure ulcers, and delayed discharge
- Collaborative problems that identify individuals at high risk for air emboli, deep vein thrombosis, sepsis
- Medical condition, postsurgical care, and treatment plan specifically identify adverse events that are associated with clinical diagnoses or situations
- Standardized risk assessment tools for falls, infection, and pressure ulcers that are incorporated in every care plan

Table 3.2 illustrates examples of prevention of hospital-acquired conditions or detection of complications.

Table 3.2 Examples of Prevention of Hospital-Acquired Conditions or Detection of Complications

Unit II

Section 1: Nursing Diagnoses
- Risk for surgical site infection
- Risk for catheter site infection
- Risk for pressure ulcers

Section 2: Collaborative Problems
- Risk for complication of deep vein thrombosis
- Risk for complications of fat embolism
- Risk for complications of sepsis

Unit III: Medical / Surgical / Treatment Plans
- Seizure disorders
- Risk for aspiration
- Total hip replacement
- Risk for complication of dislocation
- Long-term access devices
- Risk for complication of an embolism

SUMMARY

Nurses have been the primary health care professionals in all health care facilities for decades. Unfortunately, the impact of scientific, caring nursing has eluded measurement and thus has been invisible. Individuals are admitted to hospitals for medical or surgical care that requires professional nursing. If professional nursing was not indicated, their medical condition would be managed by the primary care provider or specialist in an ambulatory setting. If professional nursing care is not indicated past a surgical procedure, it completed as a same-day surgery. *The reason an individual is admitted to an intensive care unit is for specialized nursing care. The reason individuals are transitioned to their home is that they no longer need professional nursing care in the hospital. The reason an individual transfers to a skilled care facility is that he or she needs a type of professional and skilled nursing care. The assumption that individuals are admitted to hospitals primarily for medical care is erroneous. They need professional nursing expertise in order for medical management to be successful.*

As a profession, nurses have rights and responsibilities. This author has addressed the responsibilities of nursing associated with medical and surgical conditions and treatments. In addition, the rights of clinicians are addressed with multiple strategies so that other members of the health care team stop and listen when the nurse "speaks up."

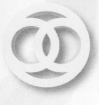

Chapter 4

Preparation of Individual / Family for Care at Home

Nurses may view this new emphasis on a safe, timely transition as a means "to save finances" for the health care institution or the third-party payer. When health care funds dwindle, the recipients, unfortunately, suffer the most.

Carp's Cues

Ask one of your relatives or neighbors who has been on medicine for over five years, how the benefits have declined on the need to have supplemental insurance.

Each day an individual stays in the hospital, the following effects occur:

- Sleep deprivation
- Deconditioning
- Increase in infections
- Family disruption
- Sensory overload
- Nutritional deficits

Types of Literacy

Functional Illiteracy

Functional illiteracy is when someone who has minimal reading and writing skills does not have the capacity for health literacy to manage ordinary everyday needs and requirements of most employments.

Individuals who are illiterate (who cannot read or write) are easier to identify than someone who is functionally illiterate.

Health Literacy

Health literacy is the capacity to obtain, process, and understand basic health information and services needed to make appropriate health decisions (Ratzan & Parker, 2000) and to follow instructions for treatment (White, 2003). In 2003, the National Assessment of Adult Literacy (NAAL) reported that 9 out of 10 English-speaking adults in the U.S. do not have health literacy (Kutner, Greenberg, Jiny, & Paulson, 2006). A large study on the scope of health literacy at two public hospitals found (Williams et al., 1995):

- Half of English-speaking patients could not read and understand basic health education material
- 60% could not understand a routine consent form
- 26% could not understand the appointment card
- 42% failed to understand directions for taking their medications

Table 4.1 Red Flags for Low Literacy
• Frequently missed appointments
• Incomplete registration forms
• Noncompliance with medication
• Unable to name medications, explain purpose, or dosing
• Identifies pills by looking at them, not reading label
• Unable to give coherent, sequential history
• Asks fewer questions
• Lack of follow-through on tests or referrals

Source: DeWalt et al., 2010

The AMA's committee of Health Literacy found inadequate health literacy was most prevalent in the elderly and individuals who report poor overall health (1999). The report concluded that individuals who reported "the worst health status have less understanding about their medical conditions and treatment" (1999, p. 57).

Carp's Cues

"Social and educational levels have little relationship to health literacy" (Speros, 2004, p. 638). Individuals will hide the literacy problems if allowed. Many individuals are at risk of understanding, but it is hard to identify them (DeWalt et al., 2010).

Table 4.1 illustrates the red flag of low literacy.

The Complexity of the Health Care System

The Health Care System increasing the expectations of clients to self-manage their conditions continues to increase in areas of (DeWalt et al., 2010):

• Self-assessment of health status (e.g., peak flow meters, glucose testing)
• Self-treatment (act on information) (e.g., insulin adjustments, wound care)
• Prevention (e.g., nutrition, exercise, dental care, cancer screenings)
• Access Health Care System (e.g., decisions to go to ER, when to call primary care, referral process, follow-up instructions, navigation of insurance / Medicare coverage)

Figure 4.1 illustrates the complex process clients and families encounter in the health care system (DeWalt et al., 2010).

Strategies to Improve Comprehension

CLINICAL ALERT
Research shows that individuals remember and understand less than half of what clinicians explain to them (Williams et al., 1995; Roter, Rune, & Comings, 1998).
Testing general reading levels does not ensure client understanding in the clinical setting (AMA, 2007).

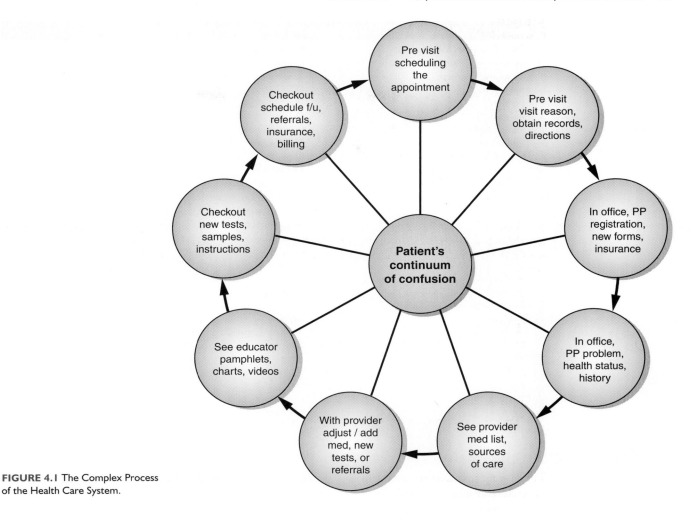

FIGURE 4.1 The Complex Process of the Health Care System.

Principles of Health Care Teaching

For comprehension to occur, the nurse must accept that there is limited time and that the use of this time is enhanced by:

- Using every contact time to teach something
- Creating a relaxed encounter
- Using eye contact
- Slowing down—break it down into short statements
- Limited content—focus on 2 or 3 concepts
- Using plain language (refer to Box 4.1)
- Engaging individual / family in discussion
- Using graphics
- Explaining what you are doing to the individual / family and why
- Asking them to tell you about what you taught. Tell them to use their own words.

Use the Teach-Back Method. Refer to Figure 4.2.

- Explain / Demonstrate
  - Explain one concept (e.g., medication, condition, when to call PCP)
  - Demonstrate one procedure (e.g., dressing charge, use of inhaler)

Box 4.1   REPLACING MEDICAL JARGON / WORDS WITH PLAIN WORDS

Medical Jargon / Words	Plain Words
Hepatic	Livers
Pulmonary Function	Lungs
Medications	Pills
Nutrition	Food
Beverages	Drinks
Dermatologist	Skin doctor
Opthalmology	Eye doctor
Dermatitis	Rash
Conjunctivitis	Eye infection
Gastrointestinal Specialist	Stomach doctor
Antihypertensive Medicine	Blood pressure medications
Anticoagulant	Blood thinner
Enlarge	bigger infection
Lesion	sore
Lipids	fats
Menses	period
Osteoporosis	decrease in the inside of the bone
Depression	feeling sad
Normal range	good
Toxic	high levels
Anti-inflammatory	helps swelling and irritation go away
Dose	how much medicine you should take
Contraception	helps you not get pregnant
Generic	general name for a type of medication
Oral	by mouth
Monitor	keeps track of
Referral	see another doctor / nurse practitioner

- Assess
  - I want to make sure, I explained _____ clearly, can you tell me _____
  - Tell me what I told you
  - Show me how to _____
  - Avoid asking, Do you understand?
- Clarify
  - Add more explanation if you are not satisfied the person understands or can perform the activity
  - If the person cannot report the information, don't repeat the same explanation; rephrase it

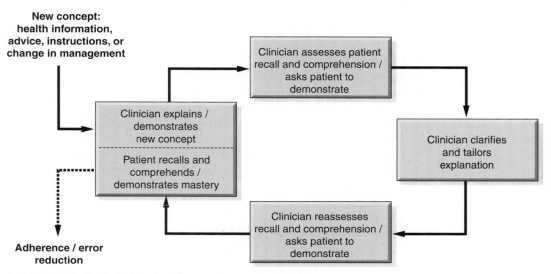

FIGURE 4.2 The Teach-Back Process (Source: Berkman et al., 2004).

Carp's Cues

Be careful the person / family does not think you are testing him or her. Assure them it is important that you help them to understand that the teaching method can help you teach and also diagnose educational needs.

- Teach-Back Questions (Examples)
  - When should you call your PCP?
  - How do you know your incision is healing?
  - What foods should you avoid?
  - How often should you test your blood sugar?
  - What should you do for low blood sugar?
  - What weight gain should you report to your PCP?
  - Which inhaler is your rescue inhaler?
  - Is there something you have been told to do that you do not understand?
  - What should you bring to your PCP office?
  - Is there something you have a question about?

Carp's Cues

Use every opportunity to explain a treatment, a medication, the condition and / or restrictions. For example, as you change a dressing:

- Explain and ask the individual / family member to redress the wound.
- Point out how the wound is healing and what would indicate signs of infection.

Teach-Back Method: A Strategy to Improve Understanding

- Reminder Card
  - Who—*me*
  - What—*anything important I want them to understand*
  - When—*every time*
  - Why—*I need to know they understand*
  - How—Focus on "need to know" and "need to do"
- Demonstrate / draw pictures
- Provide simple written education materials
- Break content into short sentences
- Go slow
- Use Teach-Back every day with all assigned clients who are capable of recall
- Practice with and improve one's Teach-Back skills
- Understanding
  - Based on the person's response or demonstration, there is confidence that the person / family can apply the teaching to safe self-care at home.

Carp's Cues

When individual / family do not understand what was said or demonstrated, the teach-back needs to be revised in a manner that will improve understanding. Teach-Back has the potential to improve health outcomes because if done correctly, it forces the nurse to limit the information to need to know. The likelihood of success is increased when the individual is not overwhelmed.

Elements to Teach for Optional Self-Care or Care at Home

The Condition

- Medical Conditions
  - What do you know about your condition?
  - How do you think this condition will affect you after you leave the hospital?
  - What do you want to know about your condition?

- Surgical Procedure
  - What do you know about the surgery you had?
  - Do you have any questions about your surgery?
  - How will surgery affect you after you leave the hospital?

Medications

- Renew all the medications that the client will continue to take at home
- Explain what OTC not to take
- Finish all the meds like antibiotics
- Do not to take any medications that are at home unless approved by PCP
- Ask client to bring all his or her medications to next visit to PCP (e.g., prescribed, OTC, vitamins, herbal medicines)
- Depending on the literacy level of the individual / family, provide
  - A list of each medication, what used for, times to take, with food or without food
  - Create a pill card with columns
    - Pictures of pill
    - Simple terms for used for
    - Time using symbols with pictures of pills in spaces

Figure 4.3 illustrates a pill card. For a printable pill card to use with clients, refer to thePoint at http://thePoint.lww.com/Carpenito6e.

> **CLINICAL ALERT**
> - Warn a client that if a pill looks different, check with pharmacy.
> - Emphasize not to take any other medications except those on list unless approved by PCP.
> - In the author's primary care practice, hospitalized clients may be given a different medication in the same class due to formulary restrictions. When the client has a follow-up used in the office, during medication reconciliation, it is discovered he or she is taking two beta-blockers, one prescribed in the hospital and the one previously taken.

Name: Sarah Smith **Date Created: 12/15/07**
Pharmacy phone number: 123-456-7890

Name	Used For	Instructions	Morning	Afternoon	Evening	Night
Simvastatin 20mg	Cholesterol	Take 1 pill at night				●
Furosemide 20mg	Fluid	Take 2 pills in the morning and 2 pills in the evening	⊖ ⊖		⊖ ⊖	
Insulin 70/30	Diabetes (Sugar)	Inject 24 units before breakfast and 12 units before dinner	24 units		12 units	

FIGURE 4.3 Example of a Pill Card (Source: DeWalt et al., 2010).

Financial Implications of Prescribed Medication

- Does the person have insured medication coverage? If yes, does it cover the medication ordered? If yes, what is the copay? Can the person afford this?
- If there is no insurance or no medication coverage, how will the person access these medications?
- Is there an inexpensive generic available?
- Which medications are critical?

> **CLINICAL ALERT**
> - Most pharmaceutical companies provide free branded medications (not generic) through patient assisted programs.
> - Applications can be accessed via the pharmaceutical website. Social service departments can also assist with this process.
> - Some medications can be acquired free (e.g., oral diabetic medications, antibiotics), or low cost (e.g., Target).
> - Advise individual / family to call PCP office if they do not want to continue a medication before they stop taking it, to discuss why (e.g., side effects).

Diet

- Ask individual / family to report if there are any dietary limitations
- Ensure there are written directions
- Explain why some foods / beverages are to be avoided (e.g., avoid olives, pickles on a low-salt diet)

Activities

- Provide instructions on activities permitted and restrictions
- When they can drive
- Return to work; what kind of job do they have?

Treatments

- Explain each treatment to be continued at home
- Equipment needed, frequency of treatment.
- Write down what signs and symptoms should be reported (e.g., decrease in output for catheter)

Evaluation

- Can this treatment be provided safely by the individual or caregiver?
- If not, consult with the transition specialist in the health care agency.

> **CLINICAL ALERT**
> If a home health agency is referred to, validate that their arrival will be timely in order to begin the treatment on time.

SUMMARY   The positive outcomes achieved in the acute care setting will quickly evaporate if the individual / family is not prepared to continue care at home. Teach-Back is an effective strategy to focus on "need to know" rather than overwhelming everyone, leading them to be confused and stressed. Fear and uncertainty are a very common reason individuals return to the emergency room and are often readmitted.

Chapter 5

11 Steps to Care Planning

Care plans have one primary purpose: to provide directions for the nursing staff for a particular client. Abbreviated care plans are usually in the electronic health record. For students and nurses inexperienced in caring for a client with a particular condition or after a certain surgical procedure, these directions (care plan) need to be detailed.

For example, a client who has diabetes mellitus is having abdominal surgery. An inexperienced nurse or student will need to refer to the generic care plan for a surgical client and to the single collaborative problem *Risk for Complications of Hypo / Hyperglycemia* (low or high blood glucose). An experienced nurse will not need to read a care plan for abdominal surgery but will need to know that the client also has diabetes and will need blood glucose monitoring.

 Carp's Cues

Some hospitals have problem lists for each client. This would list problems associated with general surgery and an additional problem of hyper / hypoglycemia.

Step 1: Assessment

If you interview your assigned client before you write your care plan, complete your assessment using the form recommended by your faculty. If you need to write a care plan before you can interview the client, go to Step 2. After you complete your assessment, circle all information that points to client strengths. Write all the strengths on an index card.

Strengths are factors that will help the client recover, cope with stressors, and progress to his or her original health prior to hospitalization, illness, or surgery. Examples of strengths include:

- Positive spiritual framework
- Positive support system
- Ability to perform self-care
- No eating difficulties
- Effective sleep habits
- Alert, good memory
- Financial stability
- Relaxed most of the time

Write all the strengths on the back of the index card.

Risk factors are situations, personal characteristics, disabilities, or medical conditions that can hinder the client's ability to heal, cope with stressors, and progress to his or her original health prior to hospitalization, illness, or surgery. Examples of risk factors include

- Obesity
- Fatigue
- Limited ability to speak or understand English
- Limited literacy

- Memory problems
- Hearing problems
- Self-care problems before hospitalization
- Difficulty walking
- Financial problems
- Tobacco use
- Alcohol problem
- Moderate to high anxiety most of the time
- Frail, elderly
- Presence of chronic diseases
  - Arthritis
  - Diabetes mellitus
  - HIV
  - Multiple sclerosis
  - Depression
  - Cardiac disorder
  - Pulmonary disease

Step 2: Same Day Assessment

If you have not completed a screening assessment of your assigned client, determine the following as soon as possible by asking the client, family, or nurse assigned to your client:

- Before hospitalization:
  - Could the client perform self-care?
  - Did the client need assistance?
  - Could the client walk unassisted?
  - Did the client have memory problems?
  - Did the client have hearing problems?
  - Did the client smoke cigarettes?
- What conditions or diseases does the client have that make him or her more vulnerable to:
  - Falling
  - Infection
  - Nutrition / fluid imbalances
  - Pressure ulcers
  - Severe or panic anxiety
  - Physiologic instability (e.g., electrolytes, blood glucose, blood pressure, respiratory function, healing problems)
- When you meet the assigned client, determine if any of the following risk factors are present:
  - Obesity
  - Impaired ability to speak / understand English
  - Communication difficulties, limited literacy
  - Moderate to high anxiety

Write significant data on the index card. Go to Step 3.

In some nursing programs, students do not have the opportunity to see or assess their assigned client prior to the clinical day. Therefore they must assess the client on their first clinical day.

Step 3: Create Your Initial Care Plan

Why is your client in the hospital? Go to the index in this book and look up the medical condition or surgical procedure. If you find the condition or surgical procedure, go to Step 4.

If the condition your client is hospitalized for is not in the index, refer to the generic medical care plan at the beginning of Section 1. If your client had surgery, refer to the generic surgical or ambulatory care plan at the beginning of Section 2.

Step 4: Additional Problems

If the medical condition or risk factor puts your client at high risk for a physiologic complication such as electrolyte imbalances or increased intracranial pressure or for nursing diagnoses such as Impaired Skin

Integrity, Risk for Infection Transmission, or Self-Care Deficit, go to the individual indexes for collaborative problems and / or nursing diagnoses. You will find the problem or nursing diagnoses there. Go to Step 5.

Author's Note
These individual indexes provide numerous options when your assigned client has risk factors and medical conditions in addition to the primary reason he or she is hospitalized.

Step 5: Review Standard Plan

- Initiate The Transitional Risk Assessment Plan on your assigned client. Using your assessment of the individual's risk factors, determine if the individual is :
  - High Risk for Injury
  - High Risk for Infection
  - High Risk for Falls
  - High Risk for Ineffective Self-Health Management (delayed transition)
- Review each section of the care plan. Review your client's risk factors on your index card.
- Review the collaborative problems listed. These are the physiologic complications that you need to monitor. Do not delete any because they all relate to the condition or procedure that your client has had. You will need to add how often you should take vital signs, record intake and output, change dressings, etc. Ask the nurse you are assigned with for prescribed frequencies for monitoring and treatment or where this information is noted.
- Review each intervention for collaborative problems. Are any interventions unsafe or contraindicated for your client? For example, if your client has edema and renal problems, the fluid requirements may be too high for him or her.

Author's Note
Review the collaborative problems on the standard plan. *Also* review all additional collaborative problems that you found in the separate index that relate to your assigned client.

Step 6: Review the Nursing Diagnoses on the Standard Plan

Review each nursing diagnosis on the plan:

- Does it apply to your assigned client?
- Does your client have any risk factors (see your index card) that could make this diagnosis worse or increase the risk?

Interventions

Review the intervention for each nursing diagnosis:

- Are they relevant for your client?
- Will you have time to provide them?
- Are any interventions not appropriate or contraindicated for your assigned client?
- Can you add any specific interventions?
- Do you need to modify any interventions because of risk factors (see index card)?

Author's Note
Remember that you cannot individualize a care plan for a client until you spend time with him or her, but you can add and delete any inappropriate interventions based on your preclinical knowledge of this client (e.g., medical diagnosis, coexisting medical conditions).

Goals / Outcome Criteria

Review the goals listed for the nursing diagnosis:

- Are they pertinent to your client?
- Can the client demonstrate achievement of the goal on the day you provide care?
- Do you need more time?

Delete goals that are inappropriate for your client. If the client will need more time to meet the goal, add "by discharge." If the client can accomplish the goal by a certain day, write "by (insert date)" after the goal.

Hint: Faculty and references may have different words to describe goals. Ask your faculty which terminology they use.

Using the same diagnosis, *Risk for Injury related to unfamiliar environment and physical or mental limitations secondary to the condition, therapies, and diagnostic tests,* consider this goal:

The client will not sustain an injury.

Indicators

- Identify factors that increase risk of injury.
- Describe appropriate safety measures.

If it is realistic for your client to achieve all the goals on the day of your care, you should add the date to all of them. If your client is confused, you can add the date to the main goal, but you would delete all the indicators because the client is confused. Or you could modify the goal by writing:

Family member will identify factors that increase the client's risk of injury.

Author's Note
Consult with clinical faculty to assure this is acceptable.

Step 7: Prepare the Care Plan (Written or Printed)

If agreed upon by the instructor, you can prepare the care plan by doing the following:

- Select the care plan from this book.
- Create a problem list for your assigned client using the nursing diagnoses and collaborative problems from the care plan you selected.
- Add additional nursing diagnoses and / or collaborative problems as indicated.
- Be prepared to provide rationales for why some interventions are not relevant or contraindicated.

Step 8: Initial Care Plan Completed

Now that you have a care plan of the collaborative problems and nursing diagnoses, which are associated with the primary condition for which your client was admitted? If your assigned client is a healthy adult undergoing surgery or was admitted for an acute medical problem and you have not assessed any significant risk factors in Step 1, you have completed the initial care plan. Go to Step 10.

Step 9: Additional Nursing Diagnoses and Collaborative Problems

The following questions can help to determine if the client or family has additional diagnoses that need nursing interventions:

- Are additional collaborative problems associated with coexisting medical conditions that require monitoring (e.g., hypoglycemia)?
- Are there additional nursing diagnoses that, if not managed or prevented now, will deter recovery or affect the client's functional status (e.g., High Risk for Constipation)?
- What problem does the client perceive as priority?
- What nursing diagnoses are important but treatment for them can be delayed without compromising functional status?

You can address nursing diagnoses not on the priority list by referring the client for assistance after discharge (e.g., counseling, weight loss program).

Author's Note

Priority identification is a very important but difficult concept. Because of shortened hospital stays and because many clients have several chronic diseases at once, nurses cannot address all nursing diagnoses for every client. Nurses must focus on those for which the client would be harmed or not make progress if they were not addressed. Ask your clinical faculty to review your list. Be prepared to provide rationales for your selections. Refer to the index for additional information on priorities.

Step 10: Evaluate the Status of Your Client (After You Provide Care)

Collaborative Problems

Review the nursing goals for the collaborative problems:

- Assess the client's status.
- Compare the data to established norms (indicators).
- Judge if the data fall within acceptable ranges.
- Conclude if the client is stable, improved, unimproved, or worse.

Is your client stable or improved?

- If yes, continue to monitor the client and to provide interventions indicated.
- If not, has there been a dramatic change (e.g., elevated blood pressure, decreased urinary output)? Have you notified the physician or advanced practice nurse? Have you increased your monitoring of the client?

Review the Clinical Alert Report and communicate this data to your clinical faculty and to the nurse assigned to your client.

Nursing Diagnosis

Review the goals or outcome criteria for each nursing diagnosis. Did the client demonstrate or state the activity defined in the goal? If yes, then communicate (document) the achievement on your plan. If not and the client needs more time, change the target date. If time is not the issue, evaluate why the client did not achieve the goal. Was the goal:

- Not realistic because of other priorities
- Not acceptable to the client

Author's Note

Ask your clinical faculty where to document evaluation of goal achievement.

Step 11: Document the Care as Instructed (e.g., Electronic Record)

Chapter 6

What Is the Most Important Thing To Do for This Client Right Now?

Carp's Cues

Often nurses attempt to define priorities by exclusively using a physiologic model such as accuracy, circulation, etc. Of course, physiologic instability when critical or increasing is a priority. However, other physiologic dysfunctions such as constipation, infections, unstable gait, or confusion can also be priorities. In addition, an emotional crisis or disruptive behavior can be priorities. Thus, it is more useful clinically to view priorities as having three components.

Priorities can be described as having three components. Table 6.1 differentiates the three types of clinical priorities.

Urgent Priority

Of the three types of priorities, urgent priorities acquire immediate attention. Integrated into Unit II, nursing diagnoses and collaborative. In Unit III care plans are Clinical Alerts to advise the clinician or student nurse that a clinical situation necessitates immediate action.

Priority of Set Diagnoses

Carp's Cues

"Priority identification is a very important but difficult concept. Because of shortened hospital stays and because clients have several chronic diseases, nurses cannot address most of the nursing diagnoses and collaborative problems for each client. Nurses must focus on those for which the client would be harmed," more stressed or not progress to a timely, successful transition.

Priority Diagnoses

Initially it is important to differentiate between priority diagnoses and nonpriority diagnoses. A priority set of nursing diagnoses is described in Table 6.1.
    Fundamentally, the set contains:

- All of the nursing diagnoses and collaborative problems identified in the diagnostic cluster for the client's medical condition that necessitated admission or surgical procedure
- Additional collaborative problems associated with coexisting medical conditions that require monitoring
- Additional nursing diagnoses that, if not managed or prevented now, will deter recovery, negatively affect the person's / family's functional states, and/or delay a timely, successful transition

Table 6.1 Differentiate the Types of Clinical Priorities

- Urgent priorities
  - New changes or worsening of an individual's condition or a potential for violent situations that requires immediate action (e.g., contact physician / NP for immediate action, access Rapid Response team or Code team, security alert)
- Priority Set of Diagnoses
  - A group of nursing diagnoses or collaborative problems that, if not managed, will deter progress to achieve positive outcomes and to a timely, successful transition
  - Are associated with their primary medical or surgical condition
  - May contain additional necessary diagnoses or collaborative problems if indicated by medical or personal problems
- Stressful or Disruptive Response Priorities
  - Stressful responses
    - Moderate anxiety or fear
    - Family crisis
  - Disruptive responses
    - Protocol / rule violations (e.g., smoking, equipment tampering)
    - Anger (perceived as nonthreatening)
    - Repetitive, unreasonable demands

Refer to Table 6.2 for an example of one client's priority set of diagnoses.

Even though the individual has diabetes mellitus, the care plan for diabetes mellitus in Unit III should not be activated. Some critical deficits in knowledge about diabetes mellitus such as differentiation of high vs. low glucose levels and what to do must be addressed during hospitalization. Other teaching that is needed for management of diabetes mellitus can be done posttransition in the primary care setting or in individual or group classes. A home health nursing consult maybe indicated.

Carp's Cues

Because students will have one or two client assignments, more teaching can be addressed. Caution, however: Is the individual physically and cognitively able to comprehend the content? Support systems can also be instituted if indicated.

Stressors / Barriers

All hospitalized individuals / families have stressors. The key is, are they interfering with the person's ability to recover and progress to transition to home care? In addition, some stressors need acknowledgement and dialogue because "it just is right." When someone is admitted with injuries from a car accident, the nurse should allow the person an opportunity to share. Opening an opportunity to share never means "we have the solution," but only that we are willing to listen to the pain of others.

Table 6.2 Example of a Client's Set of Diagnoses

A client's priority set includes Primary Condition Necessitating Admission, Coexisting Medical Conditions with Related Collaborative Problems, and Personal Risks Factors as a Nursing Diagnosis	
Admitting Diagnosis: Pneumonia	Insert diagnostic cluster
Coexisting Medical Condition: Diabetes Mellitus	Risk for Complications of Hypo / Hyperglycemia
Personal Stressors / Barriers (e.g., cannot read)	Risk for Self-Health Management related to low literacy

Stressful or Disruptive Behavior Response Priorities

 Carp's Cues

This is a new addition to the author's defining of priorities of care. This is a result of numerous accounts of nurses' experiences with disrespectful, repetitive, unrealistic demanding and / or threatening behavior of clients and / or families. It also represents some personal experiences as a nurse practitioner in primary care.

Zero Tolerance Clinical Situations

All individuals and their support systems are in a high stress situation. Inappropriate or rude incidents need to be treated as an incident unless they are on a zero tolerance list. Refer to Table 6.3.

The Joint Commission and other organizations have identified disruptive behaviors of a nurse, manager, physician, or nurse practitioner that can or have caused adverse events to occur. When nurses are recipients of threatening, demanding or unrealistic, rude demands by individuals / families, care is compromised. Abusive individuals and families will receive the standard of care but it will create barriers that may delay a response to a request and avoidance of the client's room.

Health systems have evolved from an environment that tolerated disruptive and disrespectful behavior from some physicians and administrators to one with policies to support an environment of respect and true colleagueship. Unfortunately, this has not occurred when the nurse is a recipient and disruptive, abusive behavior by individuals and families. Frequently, the reports of the behavior are ignored and nurse's attempts to reduce the behavior are criticized. The "customer" is not always right. Nurses must be assured that administration will protect them and preserve their dignity.

Carp's Cues

In an environment where administrative support is lacking, let the most competent, experienced nurse have the assignment. This may increase the likelihood of successful outcomes.

"Stress-full" Behavior

Illness by its nature is disruptive to one's life. Hospitalization compounds these disruptions. Stressors experienced by all individuals and their families are

- Fear of the unknown
- Isolation
- Loss of privacy
- Exposure of body parts
- Sleep disruption
- Invasive procedures by "strangers"

  Additional stressors for some may be:

- Financial burden of situation
- Preexisting coping problems
- Language barriers

Table 6.3 Zero Tolerance Clinical Situations*

- "Personal" insults (e.g., racial, gender)
- Deliberate violation of infection prevention
- Tampering of equipment (e.g., patient controlled anesthesia pump)
- Repetitive, deliberate vulgar language / actions (e.g., inappropriate exposing of genitals)
- Throwing any object at personnel
- Deliberate contamination of bodily fluids (e.g., urinating or spitting on floor or in garbage can)

*Some mentally impaired / confused individuals may be unaware of their behaviors.

Unit I References

Agency for Healthcare Research and Quality. (2008). *Reducing errors in health care: Translating research into practice*. Retrieved from http://ahrq.hhs.gov/qual/errors.htm

Agency for Healthcare Research and Quality. (2010). *2009 National healthcare quality report* (AHRQ Publication No. 10-0003). Rockville, MD: Author. Retrieved from http://www.ahrq.gov/qual/nhqr09/nhqr09.pdf

Aiken, L. H., Sloane, D. M., Cimiotti, J. P., Clarke, S. P., Flynn, L., Seago, J. A., …Smith, H. L. (2010). *Implications of the California nurse staffing mandate for other states*. Retrieved from http://www.nationalnursesunited.org/assets/pdf/hsr_ratios_study_042010.pdf

Alfaro-LeFevre, R. (1989). *Apply the Nursing Process: A step by step guide* (2nd ed.). Philadelphia, PA: Lippincott Williams & Wilkins.

American Medical Association. (1999). Health Literacy: Report of the Council on Scientific Affairs. *JAMA, 28*(6), 552–557.

American Medical Association. (2007). *Health literacy and patient safety: Help patients understand: Manual for clinicians* (2nd ed.). Chicago, IL: Author.

Berkman, N. D., DeWalt, D. A., Pignone, M. P., Sheridan, S. L., Lohr, K. N., Lux, L., Sutton, S. F., Swinson, T., Bonito, A. J. (2004). Literacy and health outcomes. (Evidence report/technology assessment #87.) (AHRQ Publication No. 04-E007-2). Rockville, MD: Agency for Healthcare Research and Quality.

Buerhaus, P. I., & Kurtzman, A. (2008). New medicare payment rules: Danger or opportunity for nursing? *American Journal of Nursing, 10*(6), 30–35.

Carpenito, L. J. (1983). *Nursing diagnosis: Application to clinical practice*. Philadelphia, PA: J.B. Lippincot.

Carpenito, L. J. (1987). *Nursing diagnosis: Application to clinical practice* (3rd ed.). Philadelphia, PA: J.B. Lippincott.

Carpenito, L. J. (1997). *Nursing diagnosis: Application to clinical practice* (7th ed.). Philadelphia, PA: J.B. Lippincott.

Carpenito, L. J. (1999). *Nursing diagnosis: Application to clinical practice* (8th ed.). Philadelphia, PA: Lippincott Williams & Wilkins.

Centers for Medicare and Medicaid Services. (2008). *Proposed changes to the hospital inpatient prospective payment systems and fiscal year 2009*. Retrieved from http://www.cms.hhs.gov/AcuteInpatientPPS/downloads/CMS-1390-P.pdf

Centers for Medicare and Medicaid Services. (2008). *Roadmap for implementing value driven healthcare in the traditional Medicare fee for service program*. Retrieved from https://www.cms.gov/QualityInitiativesGenInfo/downloads/VBPRoadmap_QEA_1_16_508.pdf

Cornish, P., Knowles, S., Tam, V., Shadowitz, S., Juurlink, D., & Etchells, E. (2005). Unintended medication discrepancies at the time of hospital admission. *Archives of Internal Medicine, 165*(4), 424–429.

DeWalt, D. A., Callahan, L. F., Hawk, V. H., Broucksou, K. A., Hink, A., Rudd, R., & Brach, C. (2010, April). *Health Literacy Universal Precautions Toolkit* (Prepared by North Carolina Network Consortium, The Cecil G. Sheps Center for Health Services Research, The University of North Carolina at Chapel Hill, under Contract No. HHSA290200710014.) (AHRQ Publication No. 10-0046-EF). Rockville, MD: Agency for Healthcare Research and Quality.

Friesen, M. A., White, S. V., Byers, J. F. (2008). Handoffs: Implications for Nurses. Chap. 34 in *Patient Safety and Quality: An Evidence-Based Handbook for Nurses*. Hughes, R. G., ed. Rockville, MD: Agency for Healthcare Research and Quality.

Joint Commission on Accreditation of Healthcare Organizations. (2004). *Sentinel event statistics*. Retrieved from www.jacho.org/accredited+organizations/ambulatory+care/sentinel+events/sentinel+events+statistics

The Joint Commission. (2008a). *Improving America's hospitals*. (The Joint Commission's Annual Report on Quality and Safety). Retrieved July 15, 2013, from http://www.jointcommission.org/assets/1/6/2008_Annual_Report.pdf

The Joint Commission. (2008b). *Patient safety goals*. Retrieved July 23, 2013, from, www.jcrinc.com/common/PDFs/fpdfs/pubs/pdfs/JCReqs/JCP-07-07-S1.pdf

The Joint Commission. (2012). *Improving Ameirica's hospitals*. (The Joint Commission's Annual Report on Quality and Safety.) Retrieved July 20, 2013, from http://www.jointcommission.org/2012_patient_quality and safety

Kane, R. L., Shamliyan, T., Mueller, C., Duval, S., & Wilt, T. (2007). *Nurse staffing and quality of patient care.* (Evidence report/technology assessment #151.) (Prepared by the Minnesota Evidence-based Practice Center under Contract No. 290-02-0009.) (AHRQ Publication No. 07-E005). Rockville, MD: Agency for Healthcare Research and Quality. Retrieved from www.ahrq.gov/downloads/pub/evidence/pdf/nursestaff/nursestaff.pdf

Kutner, M., Greenberg, E., Jin, Y., & Paulsen, C. (2006). *The health literacy of America's adults: Results from 2003 National Assessment of Adult's Literacy.* Washington, D. C: U.S. Department of Education, National Center for Education Statistics.

Leonard, S., Graham, S., & Bonacum, D. (2004). The human factor: The critical importance of effective teamwork and communication in providing safe care. *Quality and Safety in Health Care, 13,* i85–i90.

Leonardi, B. C., Faller, M., & Siroky, K. (2011). *Preventing never events/evidence-based practice* (White paper). San Diego, CA: AMN Healthcare. Retrieved from http://amnhealthcare.com/uploadedFiles/MainSite/Content/Healthcare_Industry_Insights/Healthcare_News/Never_Events_white_paper_06.16.11.pdf

Lyndon, A., Sexton, J. B., Simpson, K. R., Rosenstein, A., Lee, K. A., & Wachter, R. M. (2012). Predictors of likelihood of speaking up about safety concerns in labour and delivery. *BMJ Quality and Safety, 21*(9), 791–799.

McGlynn, E. A. (2008, April). *Health care efficiency measures: Identification, categorization, and evaluation* (AHRQ Publication No. 08-0030). Rockville, MD: Agency for Healthcare Research and Quality. Retrieved from http://www.ahrq.gov/qual/efficiency/

Moore, L. J., Moore, F. A., Todd, S. R., Jones, S. L., Turner, K. L., & Bass, B. L. (2010). Sepsis in general surgery. The 2005–2007 National Surgical Quality Improvement Program perspective. *Archives of Surgery, 145*(7), 695–700.

National Association of Adult Literacy. (2005). *The Health Literacy of America's Adults: Results from the 2003 National Assessment of Adult Literacy.* Retrieved July 28, 2013, from http://nces.ed.gov/naal/fr_definition.asp

NANDA Nursing Diagnoses: Definitions and Classification. (2007–2008). Philadelphia, PA: North American Nursing Diagnosis Association.

Nicolini, D., Mengis, J., & Swan, J. (2012). Understanding the role of objects in cross-disciplinary collaboration. *Organization Science, 23*(3), 612–629.

Nicolini, D., Waring, J., & Mengis, J. (2011). Policy and practice in the use of root cause analysis to investigate clinical adverse events: Mind the gap. *Social Science & Medicine, 73*(2), 217–225.

North American Nursing Diagnosis Association. (2009). *Nursing Diagnoses: Definitions and Classifications* (2009-2010). Philadelphia: Author.

Ratzan, S. C., & Parker, R. M. (2000). Introduction. In C. R. Selden, M. Zorn, S. C. Ratzan, & R. M. Parker (Eds.), *National Library of Medicine, Current Bibliographies in Medicine: Health Literacy* (NLM Publication No. CBM 2000-1). Bethesda, MD: National Institutes of Health, U.S. Department of Health and Human Services.

Rost, K., & Roter, D. (1987). Predictors of recall of medication regimens and recommendations for lifestyle changes in elderly patients. *Gerontologist, 27*(4), 510–515.

Roter, D. L., Rude, R. E., & Comings, J. (1998). Patient Literacy: A Barrier to Quality of Care. *Journal of General Internal Medicine, 13*(12), 850–851.

Savitz, L. A., Jones, C. B., & Bernard, S. (2005). Quality indicators sensitive to nurse staffing in acute care settings. In: Henriksen, K., Battles, J. B., Marks, E. S., & Lewin, D. I., (Eds.), *Advances in Patient Safety: From Research to Implementation* (Volume 4: Programs, Tools, and Products). Rockville, MD: Agency for Healthcare Research and Quality.

Sherwood, G., & Barnsteiner, J. (Eds.). (2012). *Quality and safety in nursing: A competency approach to improving outcomes.* Ames, IA: Wiley-Blackwell.

Shreve, J., Van Den Bos, J., Gray, T., Halford, M., Rustagi, K., & Ziemkiewicz, E. (2010). *The economic measurement of medical errors.* (Published by Society of Actuaries' Health Section and sponsored by Milliman, Inc). Retrieved from http://www.soa.org/files/pdf/research-econ-measurement.pdf

Speros, C. (2004). Health literacy: Concept and analysis. *Journal of Advanced Nursing, 50*(6), 633–640.

Unruh, L. Y., & Fottler, M. D. (2006). Patient turnover and nursing staff adequacy. *Health Services Research, 41*(2), 599–612.

White, S. (2003). *Assessing the nation's health literacy: Key concepts and findings of the National Assessment of Adult Literacy (NAAL)* NAAL. Retrieved July 26, 2013, from http://www.ama-assn.org/resources/doc/ama-foundation/hl_report_2008.pdf

Williams, M. V., Parker, R. M., Baker, D. W., Parikh, N. S., Pitkin, K., Coates, W. C., Nurss, J. R. (1995). Inadequate functional health literacy among patients at two public hospitals. *Journal of the American Medical Association, 274*(21), 1677–1682.

Unit II

Manual of Nursing Diagnoses

Section I

Individual Nursing Diagnoses

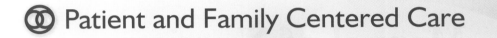 **Patient and Family Centered Care**

ACTIVITY INTOLERANCE

NANDA-I Definition

Insufficient physiologic or psychological energy to endure or complete required or desired daily activities

Defining Characteristics

Major (Must Be Present)

An altered physiologic response to activity

Respiratory
Exertional dyspnea*
Excessively increased rate
Shortness of breath
Decreased rate

Pulse
Weak
Excessively increased
Rhythm change
Decreased
Failure to return to preactivity level after 3 minutes
EKG changes reflecting arrhythmias or ischemia*

Blood Pressure
Abnormal blood pressure response to activity
Failure to increase with activity
Increased diastolic pressure greater than 15 mm Hg

Minor (May Be Present)

Verbal report of weakness*
Pallor or cyanosis

---

*Definitions designated as NANDA-I and characteristics and factors identified with a blue asterisk are from *Nursing Diagnoses: Definitions and Classification 2012–2014*. Copyright © 2012, 2009, 2007, 2003, 2001, 1998, 1996, 1994 by NANDA International. Used by arrangement with Blackwell Publishing Limited, a company of John Wiley & Sons, Inc.

Verbal reports of vertigo
Verbal report of fatigue*
Confusion

Related Factors

Any factors that compromise oxygen transport, physical conditioning, or create excessive energy demands that outstrip the client's physical and psychological abilities can cause activity intolerance. Some common factors follow.

Pathophysiologic

Related to imbalance between oxygen supply/demand* secondary to (examples below)
Related to compromised oxygen transport system secondary to (examples below)

Cardiac
Cardiomyopathies
Dysrhythmias
Acute coronary syndrome
Congenital heart disease
Congestive heart failure
Angina
Valvular disease

Respiratory
Chronic obstructive pulmonary disease (COPD)
Bronchopulmonary dysplasia
Atelectasis

Circulatory
Anemia
Hypovolemia
Peripheral arterial disease
Related to increased metabolic demands secondary to (examples below)

Acute or Chronic Infections
Viral infection
Endocrine or metabolic disorders
Mononucleosis
Hepatitis

Chronic Diseases
Renal
Inflammatory
Neurologic
Hepatic
Musculoskeletal
Related to inadequate energy sources secondary to inadequate diet (examples below)

Treatment Related

Related to increased metabolic demands secondary to (e.g., cancer surgery)
Related to compromised oxygen transport secondary to (e.g., hypovolemia, immobility*)

Situational (Personal, Environmental)

Related to inactivity secondary to (e.g., depression, inadequate social support, sedentary lifestyle*)
Related to increased metabolic demands secondary to assistive equipment (walkers, crutches, braces)
Related to inadequate motivation secondary to (e.g., fear of falling, depression, obesity, pain, dyspnea, generalized weakness*)

Goal

NOC
Activity Intolerance

The client will progress in activity to (specify level of activity desired), evidenced by these indicators:

- Identify factors that aggravate activity intolerance.
- Identify methods to reduce activity intolerance.
- Maintain blood pressure within normal limits 3 minutes after activity.

Interventions

NIC
Activity Tolerance, Energy Management Therapy, Exercise Promotion, Sleep Enhancement, Mutual Goal Setting

Elicit From Client Their Personal Goals to Improve Their Health

R: Mutual goal-setting results in improved well-being and goal attainment.

Monitor the Client's Response to Activity and Record Response

- Take resting pulse, blood pressure, and respirations.
- Consider rate, rhythm, and quality (if signs are abnormal—e.g., pulse above 100—consult with physician about advisability of increasing activity).
- If signs are normal or if physician approves, have client perform the activity.
- Take vital signs immediately after activity.
- Have client rest for 3 minutes; take vital signs again.

  R: Response to activity can be evaluated by comparing preactivity blood pressure, pulse, and respiration with postactivity results. These, in turn, are compared with recovery time.

  R: Strenuous activity may increase the pulse by 50 beats. This rate is still satisfactory as long as it returns to resting pulse within 3 minutes.

- Discontinue the activity if the client responds with:
  - Complaints of chest pain, vertigo, or confusion
  - Decreased pulse rate
  - Failure of systolic blood pressure to increase
  - Decreased systolic blood pressure
  - Increased diastolic blood pressure by 15 mm Hg
  - Decreased respiratory response

> **CLINICAL ALERT**
> - Immediately report if any of the above occur

R: Abnormal clinical responses can be indicators of compromised cardiac or respiratory ability.

If No Abnormal Responses Occur, Increase the Activity Gradually

- Increase tolerance for activity by having the client perform the activity more slowly, for a shorter time with more rest pauses, or with more assistance.
- Minimize the deconditioning effects of prolonged bed rest and imposed immobility:
  - Begin active range of motion (ROM) at least twice a day. For the client who is unable, the nurse should perform passive ROM.
  - Gradually increase tolerance by starting with 15 minutes the first time out of bed.
  - Promote ambulation with or without assistive devices.
  - If the client cannot stand without buckling the knees, he or she is not ready for ambulation; help the client to practice standing in place with assistance.
  - Choose a safe gait. (If the gait appears awkward but stable, continue; stay close by and give clear coaching messages, e.g., "Look straight ahead, not down.")
  - Allow the client to gauge the rate of ambulation.
  - Provide sufficient support to ensure safety and prevent falling.

  R: Activity tolerance develops cyclically through adjusting frequency, duration, and intensity of activity until the desired level is achieved. Increasing activity frequency precedes increasing duration and intensity (work demand). Increased intensity is offset by reduced duration and frequency. As tolerance for more intensive activity of short duration develops, frequency is once again increased.

R: Rest relieves the symptoms of activity intolerance. The daily schedule is planned to allow for alternating periods of activity and rest and coordinated to reduce excess energy expenditure.

Promote a Sincere "Can-Do" Attitude

- Allow the client to set the activity schedule and functional activity goals. If the goal is too low, negotiate (e.g., "Walking 25 ft seems low. Let's increase it to 50 ft. I'll walk with you.").
- Plan a purpose for the activity, such as sitting up in a chair to eat lunch.
- Help client to identify progress.

   R: Do not underestimate the value of praise and encouragement as effective motivational techniques.

Related to Insufficient Knowledge of Adaptive Techniques Needed Secondary to COPD

- Teach pulmonary hygiene routine.
- Teach the proper method of controlled coughing:
  - Breathe deeply and slowly while sitting up as upright as possible.
  - Use diaphragmatic breathing.
  - Hold the breath for 3 to 5 seconds; then slowly exhale as much of this breath as possible through the mouth. (Lower rib cage and abdomen should sink down with exhaling.)
  - Take a second deep breath, hold, and cough forcefully from deep in the chest (not from the back of the mouth or throat); use two short, forceful coughs.
- Rest after coughing sessions.
- Instruct the client to practice controlled coughing four times a day: 30 minutes before meals and at bedtime. Allow 15 to 30 minutes of rest after coughing session and before meals.

   R: Clearing and defense of the airways are of utmost importance in meeting tissue demands for increased oxygen during periods of rest and periods of increased activity.

- Consult with respiratory therapy if indicated.

   R: People with COPD can benefit from specific breathing exercises, which involve retraining of breathing patterns, and from general exercise programs that support normal daily activities.

   R: Symptom-limited endurance training has been shown effective for improving performance and reducing perceived breathlessness (Punzal, Ries, Kaplan, & Prewitt, 1991). The minimal duration and frequency of exercise required to improve performance appears to be 20 to 30 minutes three to five times per week. Not all people, however, are candidates for exercise reconditioning.

- Refer to Getting Started to Quit Smoking on the Point at http://thePoint.lww.com/Carpenito6e.

   R: Being hospitalized has been found to increase readiness to quit and to lead to long-term quitting. Smoking cessation should be considered of highest priority in any program of comprehensive care of clients who smoke (Chouinard & Robichaud-Ekstrand, 2005).

- Teach the client to modify approaches to activities to regulate energy expenditure and reduce cardiac workload.
- Take rest periods during activities, at intervals during the day, and for 1 hour after meals; sit rather than stand when performing activities; when performing a task, rest every 3 minutes for 5 minutes to allow the heart to recover; stop an activity if exertional fatigue or signs of cardiac hypoxia, such as markedly increased pulse rate, dyspnea, or chest pain, occur.

   R: People with impaired cardiac function can achieve some immediate gains in activity tolerance by modifying their approach (e.g., pacing activities, avoiding isometric work, limiting the duration of dynamic work by taking frequent rests).

- Instruct the client to avoid certain types of exertion: isometric exercises (e.g., using arms to lift self, carry objects) and Valsalva maneuver (e.g., bending at the waist in a sit-up fashion to rise from bed, straining during a bowel movement).

   R: When a person forcefully expires against a closed glottis, changes occur in intrathoracic pressure that dramatically affect venous return, cardiac output, arterial pressure, and heart rate.

TRANSITION PLAN

Initiate health teaching and referrals as indicated.

- For those with COPD, teach to observe sputum; note changes in color, amount, and odor; and advise to call primary provider if sputum changes to yellow or green.
- Discuss the need for annual influenza immunizations. Ensure they have had pneumococcal vaccination.

  R: Clients with COPD are susceptible to infection and must detect symptoms early and consult with primary provider for treatment (frequently, early antibiotic therapy is necessary). Strategies to increase resistance to infection include immunizations, avoiding environmental irritants and crowds, and maintaining optimal nutrition and hydration.

- Instruct to consult with primary care provider for a long-term exercise program.
- Refer to *Risk for Falls* for more specific muscle strengthening strategies.

  R: Regular exercise programs can prevent deconditioning and falls and increase exercise tolerance and muscle strength.

Clinical Alert Report

- Advise ancillary staff / student to report the client's progress with attention to complaints of chest pain, vertigo, change in orientation, response to activity (pulse rate, blood pressure, respiratory response).

IMPAIRED COMMUNICATION**

Definition

The state in which a person experiences, or is at risk to experience, difficulty exchanging thoughts, ideas, wants, or needs with others

Defining Characteristics

Major (Must Be Present)

Inappropriate or absent speech or response
Impaired ability to speak or hear

Minor (May Be Present)

Incongruence between verbal and nonverbal messages
Stuttering
Slurring
Word-finding problems
Weak or absent voice
Statements of being misunderstood or not understanding
Dysarthria
Aphasia
Language barrier

**This diagnosis is not presently on the NANDA-I list but has been added for clarity and usefulness.

Related Factors

Pathophysiologic

Related to impaired motor function of muscles of speech secondary to:

Cerebrovascular accident
Oral or facial trauma
Tumor (of the head, neck, or spinal cord)
Nervous system diseases (e.g., myasthenia gravis, multiple sclerosis, muscular dystrophy)
Vocal cord paralysis/quadriplegia

Related to impaired ability to produce speech secondary to:

Respiratory impairment (e.g., shortness of breath)
Laryngeal edema/infection
Oral deformities

Related to auditory impairment

Treatment Related

Related to impaired ability to produce speech secondary to:

Endotracheal intubation
Surgery of the head, face, neck, or mouth
Tracheostomy/tracheotomy/laryngectomy
Pain (especially of the mouth or throat)

Situational (Personal, Environmental)

Related to no access to or malfunction of hearing aid
Related to unavailable interpreter
Related to hearing impairment

Goal

NOC
Communication

The client will report improved satisfaction with ability to communicate as evidenced by the following indicators:

- Demonstrates increased ability to understand.
- Demonstrates improved ability to express self.
- Relates feelings of reduced frustration and isolation.
- Uses alternative methods of communication, as indicated.

Interventions

NIC
Communication Enhancement: Speech, Hearing, Active Listening; Socialization Enhancement: Active Listening, Culture Brokerage

Determine How the Client Usually Communicates

- Assess ability to comprehend, speak, read, and write.
- Provide alternative methods of communication.
  - Use a computer, pad and pencil, hand signals, eye blinks, head nods, and bell signals.
  - Make flash cards with pictures or words depicting frequently used phrases (e.g., "Wet my lips," "Move my foot," "I need a glass of water" or "I need a bedpan").
  - Encourage the person to point, use gestures, and pantomime.

  R: Effective communication may require using alternative forms of communication and can help decrease anxiety, isolation, and alienation; promote a sense of control; and enhance safety.

> **CLINICAL ALERT**
> - Some form of effective communication must be established.

Identify Factors That Promote Communication

- Provide a nonrushed environment.
- Use techniques to increase understanding.
  - Face the client and establish eye contact if possible.
  - Look at the client when speaking, enunciate words and speak slowly.
  - Use uncomplicated one-step commands and directives.
  - Have only one person talk (following a conversation among multiple parties can be difficult).
  - Encourage the use of gestures and pantomime.
  - Match words with actions; use pictures.
  - Validate that the client understands the message.
  - Give information in writing to reinforce.

  R: The nurse should make every attempt to understand the client. Each success, regardless of how minor, decreases frustration and increases motivation. Communication is the core of all human relations. Impaired ability to communicate spontaneously is frustrating and embarrassing (Underwood, 2004).

Reduce Factors That Contribute Impaired Communication

Effects of Hearing Loss

Ask the Person What Mode of Communication He or She Desires

- Record on care plan the method to use (may be combination of the following):
  - Writing
  - Speech-reading (or lip-reading)
  - Speaking
  - Gesturing
  - Sign language

  R: Successful interaction with deaf or hearing-impaired clients requires knowing background issues, including age of onset, choice of language, cultural background, education level, and type of hearing loss.

Assess Ability to Receive Verbal Messages

- If client can hear with a hearing aid, make sure that it is on and functioning.
- If client can hear with only one ear, speak slowly and clearly directly into the good ear. It is more important to speak distinctly than loudly.

  R: Many older adults with hearing impairments do not wear hearing aids. Those who wear them must be encouraged to use them consistently, clean and maintain them, and replace batteries.

- If the person can lip-read:
  - Look directly at the person and talk slowly and clearly.
  - Avoid standing in front of light—have the light on your face so the person can see your lips.
  - Use facial gestures.
  - Minimize conversations if the person is fatigued or use written communication.

  R: Not all deaf people have the skill and language level to read lips. Only 30% to 40% of the English language is visible. Lip- or speech-reading is difficult and fatiguing in the hospital.

- If client can read and write, provide pad and pencil at all times. If client can understand only sign language, have an interpreter with him or her as much as possible.

  R: When using an interpreter, some things may be omitted or misunderstood. Whenever possible, give information in writing as well as through the interpreter.

- Use factors that promote hearing and understanding.
  - Talk distinctly and clearly, facing the person.
  - Minimize unnecessary sounds in the room.
  - Have only one person talk.
  - Be aware of background noises (e.g., close the door, turn off the television or radio).

- Repeat, then rephrase a thought, if the person does not seem to understand the whole meaning.
- Use gestures to enhance communication.
- Encourage the person to maintain contact with other deaf people to minimize feelings of social isolation.
- Write as well as speak all important messages.
- Validate the person's understanding by asking questions that require more than "yes" or "no" answers. Avoid asking, "Do you understand?"

  R: Hearing aids magnify all sounds. Therefore, extraneous sounds (e.g., rustling of papers, minor squeaks) can inhibit understanding of voiced messages.

- Access DEAFNET, a computer system that allows clients to type messages to a computer at the phone company, which a voice synthesizer translates verbally.

Related to Effects of Aphasia on Expression or Interpretation

Use Techniques That Enhance Verbal Expression

- Do not talk too fast or say too much. Keep phrases simple, and speak slowly.
- Acknowledge when you understand, and do not be concerned with imperfect pronunciation at first.
- Do not pretend you understand if you do not.
- Observe nonverbal cues for validation (e.g., answers "yes" and shakes head "no").
- Allow person time to respond; do not interrupt; supply words only occasionally.

  R: Deliberate actions can improve speech. As speech improves, confidence increases and the client will make more attempts to speak.

- Teach techniques to improve speech.

  - Ask to slow speech down and say each word clearly, while providing the example.
  - Encourage client to speak in short phrases.
  - Suggest a slower rate of talking, or taking a breath before beginning to speak.
  - Ask client to write down message, or to draw a picture, if verbal communication is difficult.
  - Focus on the present; avoid controversial, emotional, abstract, or lengthy topics.

  R: Poor communication can cause frustration, anger, hostility, depression, fear, confusion, and isolation.

- Consult with speech therapist for specific exercises.
- Acknowledge client's frustration and improvements.

  R: Good communicators are also good listeners, who listen for both facts and feelings. Just being present and available, even if one says or does little, can effectively communicate caring to another.

Identify Factors That Promote Comprehension

- Modify your speech.

  - Speak slowly; enunciate distinctly.
  - Use common adult words.
  - Do not use slang or sayings: say what you mean.
  - Do not change subjects or ask multiple questions in succession.
  - Repeat or rephrase requests.
  - Try to use the same words with the same task (e.g., bathroom vs. toilet, pill vs. medication).

  R: Improving the client's comprehension can help decrease frustration and increase trust. Clients with aphasia can correctly interpret tone of voice. Using alternative forms of communication can help to decrease anxiety, isolation, and alienation (Iezzoni et al., 2004).

Teach Communication Techniques and Consistent Approaches to Significant Others/Family

- Encourage family to share feelings concerning communication problems.
- Explain the need to include the person in family decision making.
- Seek consultation with a speech pathologist early in treatment regimen.

R: Speech represents the fundamental way for humans to express needs, desires, and feelings. If only one person expresses information without any feedback from a listener, effective communication cannot be said to have happened.

Related to Foreign Language Barrier

Assess Ability to Communicate in English** (Ability to Read, Write, Speak, and Comprehend)

R: Knowledge of a foreign language depends on four elements: how to speak, understand, read, and write the language.

Access a Translator

- Use a *fluent* translator when discussing important matters (e.g., taking a health history, signing an operation permit). Reinforce communications through the translator with written information. Allow the translator to spend as much time as the person wishes.
- If a translator is unavailable, plan a daily visit from someone who has some knowledge of the person's language. (Many hospitals and social welfare offices keep a "language bank" with names and phone numbers of persons who are willing to translate.)
- Avoid using family members to translate if possible.

  R: Family members may not translate all communications. The client may not want the family member to have access to certain information.

- Use a telephone translating system when necessary.

  R: Effective communication is critical and must be ensured with persons who do not speak or understand English.

Identify Factors That Promote Communication Without a Translator

- Face the person and give a pleasant greeting, in a normal tone of voice.
- Talk clearly and somewhat slower than normal (do not overdo it).

  R: An attempt on the nurse's part to communicate over a language barrier encourages the client to do the same.

- Do not evaluate understanding based on "yes" or "no" responses.

  R: An answer of "yes" may be an effort to please rather than a sign of understanding.

- If the person does not understand or speak (respond), try an alternative communication method.
  - Use gestures or actions.
  - Use pictures or drawings.

Be Cognizant of Possible Cultural Barriers

- Be careful when touching the person; some cultures may consider touch inappropriate.
- Be aware of different ways the culture expects men and women to be treated (cultural attitudes may influence whether a man speaks to a woman about certain matters, or vice versa).

  R: Communicating through touch or holding varies among cultures. Some cultures view touch as an extremely familiar gesture, some shy away from touching a given part of the body (e.g., a pat on the head may be offensive), and some consider it appropriate for men to kiss one another and for women to hold hands.

> **TRANSITION PLAN**
> Initiate health teaching and referrals as indicated.
> - Teach communication techniques and repetitive approaches to significant others to use at home.

**English is used as an example of the dominant language.

IMPAIRED VERBAL COMMUNICATION

NANDA-I Definition

Decreased, delayed, or absent ability to receive, process, transmit, and/or use a system of symbols

Defining Characteristics

Difficulty or inability to speak words but can understand others
Articulation or motor planning deficits

Related Factors

See *Impaired Communication*.

Goal

NOC
Communication:
Expressive Ability

See *Impaired Communication*.

Interventions

NIC
Active Listening,
Communication
Enhancement: Speech
Deficit

- Identify a method for communicating basic needs.
  - See *Impaired Communication* for general interventions.

  R: Communication is the core of all human relations. Impaired ability to communicate effectively is frustrating and embarrassing.

- Identify factors that promote communication.

> **CLINICAL ALERT**
> - Some form of effective communication must be established.

- Seek consultation with a speech pathologist early in the treatment regimen.

  R: Expert consultation will be needed during hospitalization and to prepare for transition.

- For clients with dysarthria:
  - Reduce environmental noise (e.g., radio, TV) to increase the caregiver's ability to listen to words.
  - Do not alter your speech or messages.

  R: The client's comprehension is not affected; speak on an adult level.

  - Encourage the client to make a conscious effort to slow down speech and to speak louder (e.g., "Take a deep breath between sentences").
  - Ask the client to repeat unclear words; observe for nonverbal cues to gain an understanding.
  - If the client is tired, ask questions that require only short answers.

  R: Interventions focus on decreasing the tension and conveying an understanding of how difficult the situation is for the client and significant others. Simple questions that can be answered with "yes" or "no" enhance communication and reduce energy expenditure.

  - If speech is unintelligible, teach use of gestures, written messages, and communication cards.

  R: Dysarthria is a disturbance in the voluntary muscular control of speech. People with dysarthria usually do not have problems with comprehension.

- For those who cannot speak (e.g., endotracheal intubation, tracheostomy):
  - Reassure that speech will return, if it will. If not, explain available alternatives (e.g., esophageal speech, sign language).
  - Do not alter your speech, tone, or type of message; speak on an adult level.
  - Read lips for cues.

  R: The person's ability to understand is not affected.

- Attempt to assign same caregivers to reduce frustration.
- For the client with limited speaking ability (e.g., can make simple requests but not lengthy statements), encourage letter writing or keeping a diary to express feelings and share concerns.

  R: Perhaps the most basic human need, after survival, is to communicate with others. Communication provides security by reinforcing that clients are not alone and that others will listen. Poor communication can cause frustration, anger, hostility, depression, and fear.

- Record the method of communication that is used.
  - Record directions for specific measures (e.g., "allow him to keep a urinal in bed," "uses word cards," "points for bedpan," alphabet board, picture board writing materials).

    R: Written directions will help to reduce communication problems and frustration.

TRANSITION PLAN

Initiate health teaching and referrals as indicated.

- Teach communication techniques and repetitive approaches to significant others to use at home.
- Ensure that speech therapy will continue after discharge to home.

ACUTE CONFUSION

NANDA-I Definition

Abrupt onset of reversible disturbances of consciousness, attention, cognition, and perception that develop over a short period of time

Defining Characteristics

Major (Must Be Present)

Abrupt onset of:

Fluctuation in cognition*
Fluctuation in level of consciousness*
Fluctuation in psychomotor activity*
Increased agitation*
Reduced ability to focus
Disorientation
Increased restlessness*
Hypervigilance
Incoherence
Fear
Anxiety
Excitement

Symptoms are worse at night or when fatigued or in new situations.

Minor (May Be Present)

Illusions
Hallucinations*
Delusions
Misperceptions*

Related Factors

Pathophysiologic

Related to abrupt onset of cerebral hypoxia or disturbance in cerebral metabolism secondary to (Miller, 2009) :

Fluid and Electrolyte Disturbances

Dehydration	Hypokalemia
Acidosis/alkalosis	Hyponatremia/hypernatremia
Hypercalcemia/hypocalcemia	Hypoglycemia/hyperglycemia

Nutritional Deficiencies

Folate or vitamin B_{12} deficiency	Niacin deficiency
Anemia	Magnesium deficiency

Cardiovascular Disturbances

Acute coronary syndrome	Heart block
Congestive heart failure	Temporal arteritis
Dysrhythmias	Subdural hematoma

Respiratory Disorders

Chronic obstructive pulmonary disease: Tuberculosis and pneumonia
Pulmonary embolism

Infections

Sepsis   Urinary tract infection (especially elderly)   Meningitis, encephalitis

Metabolic and Endocrine Disorders

Thyroid disorders	Postural hypotension
Adrenal disorders	Hypothermia/Hyperthermia
Pituitary disorders	Hepatic or renal failure
Parathyroid disorders	

Central Nervous System (CNS) Disorders

Cerebral vascular accident	
Multiple infarctions	Head trauma
Tumors	Seizures and postconvulsive states
Normal-pressure hydrocephalus	

Treatment Related

Related to a disturbance in cerebral metabolism secondary to:

Surgery
Side effects of certain medication:

Diuretics	Barbiturates, Opioids	Sulfa drugs
Digitalis	Methyldopa	Ciprofloxacin
Propranolol	Disulfiram	Metronidazole
Atropine	Lithium	Acyclovir
Oral hypoglycemic	Phenytoin	H2 receptor antagonists
Anti-inflammatories	Benzodiazepines	Anticholinergic
Antianxiety agents	Phenothiazines	

Over-the-counter cold, cough, and sleeping preparations

Situational (Personal, Environmental)

Related to disturbance in cerebral metabolism secondary to:

Withdrawal from alcohol, opioids, sedatives, hypnotics
Heavy metal or carbon monoxide intoxication

Related to:

Pain　　　　　　Immobility　　　　　Unfamiliar situations
Depression

Goal

NOC
Cognition, Cognitive Orientation, Distorted Thought Self-Control

The person will have diminished episodes of delirium as evidenced by the following indicators:

- Be less agitated
- Participate in ADLs
- Be less combative

Interventions

NIC
Delirium Management, Calming Technique, Reality Orientation, Environmental Management: Safety

- Assess for causative and contributing factors, by referring to related factors above.

  R: "Delirium may be present when admitted to hospital, any care setting, or may develop during a stay. It usually develops over 1–2 days." (Cook & Lloyd, 2010)

- Identify if the client's behavior is (Cook & Lloyd, 2010):
  - Hyperactive (fast/loud speech, impatient, anger, restlessness, uncooperative, nightmares, wandering, persistent thoughts, easily startled)
  - Hypoactive (unawareness, lethargy, decreased alertness, slow/sparse speech, apathy, staring, decreased motor activity)
  - Mixed responses

  R: Delirium can present with hyperactive, hypoactive, or mixed signs and symptoms. Hypoactive behavior is often unrecognized as manifestations of acute confusion. (Cook & Lloyd, 2010)

> **CLINICAL ALERT**
> - Implement falls prevention protocol with *Risk for Falls*.

- If client is not confused, assess for the presence of prehospitalization risk factors (Cook& Lloyd, 2010).
  - Severe illness
  - Visual / hearing impairments
  - Physically frail
  - Medication side effects
  - Fracture of neck of femur
  - Dehydration/ sepsis
  - Excess alcohol use
  - Some cognitive impairment

- If confusion is present, use *Risk for Acute Confusion.*

  R: Old age is not a risk factor for acute confusion. Avoid accepting old age as a cause for acute confusion.

- Educate family, significant others, and caregivers about the situation and coping methods (Cook & Lloyd, 2010; Young, 2001).
  - Explain the cause of acute confusion.
  - Explain that the client does not realize the situation.
  - Explain the need to remain patient, flexible, and calm.
  - Stress the need to respond to the client as an adult.
  - Explain that the behavior is part of a disorder and is not voluntary.

  R: Differentiating between acute (reversible) and chronic (irreversible) confusion is important for family and caregivers (Miller, 2009).

- Maintain standards of empathic, respectful care.
  - Be an advocate. Function as a role model with coworkers.
  - Expect empathic, respectful care and monitor its administration.
  - Attempt to obtain information for conversation (likes, dislikes; interests, hobbies; work history). Interview early in the day.
  - Encourage significant others and caregivers to speak slowly with a low voice pitch and at an average volume (unless hearing deficits are present), with eye contact, and as if expecting the client to understand.

  R: Communication can be enhanced with useful and meaningful topics as one adult to another.

CLINICAL ALERT
- Confused individuals are very vulnerable to abuse.
- Monitor for and address unacceptable staff behavior toward client.
- The following SBAR indicates its use to communicate in such a situation.

SBAR

Situation: I overheard Ms. Wood, a CNA, yelling at Mr. Smith. Mr. Smith is a 70-year-old client, who became acutely confused after abdominal surgery. He was oriented and communicated appropriately prior to surgery

Background: This is the first incident of this type that I witnessed with Ms. Wood and I am unaware of previous similar occurrences.

Assessment: The behavior of Ms. Wood is unacceptable and abusive.

Recommendation: "I overheard you in a loud voice telling Mr. Smith to stop calling out for help. Mr. Smith was not confused before his surgery and now is. He must be very frightened. He probably would be comforted with quiet, kind words."

The response/reaction of Ms. Wood will determine if this incident needs additional management interventions.

- Assess for nonverbal signs of pain (e.g., grimacing, moaning when re-positioned).

    R: Communication difficulties prevent usual assessment foci.

- Provide respect and promote sharing.
    - Pick out meaningful comments and continue talking.
    - Call the client by name and introduce yourself each time you make contact; use touch if welcomed.
    - Use the name the client prefers; avoid "Pops" or "Mom," which is unacceptable and can increase confusion.
    - Convey to the client that you are concerned and friendly (through smiles, an unhurried pace, humor, and praise; do not argue; use light touch if comforting).

    R: This demonstrates unconditional positive regard and communicates acceptance and affection to a person who has difficulty interpreting the environment (Hall, 1994).

- Provide sufficient and meaningful sensory input.
    - Reduce noise and multiple conversations in room.
    - Keep the client oriented to time and place.
    - Refer to time of day and place each morning.
    - Provide the client with a clock and calendar large enough to see.
    - Ensure that corrective lenses are available and used.
    - Use nightlights or dim lights at night.
    - Provide the client with the opportunity to see daylight and dark through a window, or take the client outdoors.

    R: Sensory input is carefully planned to promote orientation and reduce misinterpretations.

- Reduce or eliminate:
    - Fatigue
    - Change in routine, environment, or caregiver
    - Frustration from trying to function beyond capabilities or from being restrained
    - Pain, discomfort, illness, or side effects from medications
    - Competing or misleading stimuli (e.g., mirrors, television, costumes)

    R: Studies have shown that these factors contribute to delirium (Feldt & Griffin, 1999; Sanberg et al., 2001; Segatore & Adams, 2001).

- Do not endorse confusion.
    - Do not argue with the client.
    - Determine the best response to confused statements.
    - Sometimes the confused client may be comforted by a response that reduces his or her fear; for example, "I want to see my mother," when his or her mother has been dead for 20 years. The nurse may respond with, "I know that your mother loved you."

- Direct the client back to reality; do not allow him or her to ramble.
- Remember to acknowledge your entrance with a greeting and your exit with a closure (e.g., "I will be back in 10 minutes").

R: Unconditional positive regard communicates acceptance and affection to a person who has difficulty interpreting the environment.

- Consult with physician / nurse practitioner regarding:
  - Discontinue or reduce dosage of medications that increase disturbances of cognition (e.g., sedatives, analgesics).
  - Avoid cauterizations / intravenous lines if possible.

    R: Tethering lines are restrictive, confusing, and pose an increased risk of infection and trauma.

  - Implement medication plan to prevent constipation (e.g., stool softeners).

    R: Constipation is uncomfortable and will increase confused behavior.

- Use adaptive devices (e.g., lighting, glasses, and hearing aids).

  R: Adaptive devices can diminish confusing sensory input.

- Promote mobility as much as possible. Provide appropriate walking aids and ensure that they are accessible at all times.

  R: Frequent ambulation simulates normal ADLs and reduces the hazards of immobility on physical and cognitive function.

- Ensure optimal sleep patterns. Refer to *Disturbed Sleep Pattern.*

  R: Attention to optimal mobility and restorative sleep can improve daytime functioning.

- Encourage the family to bring in familiar objects from home (e.g., photographs, afghan).
  - Ask the client to tell you about the picture.
  - Focus on familiar topics.
- Discuss current events, seasonal events (e.g., snow, water activities); share your interests (e.g., travel, crafts).

  R: Strategies that emphasize normalcy can contribute to positive self-esteem and reduce confusion.

- In teaching a task or activity—such as eating—break it into small, brief steps by giving only one instruction at a time.

  R: Memory loss and diminished intellectual functioning create a need for simple instructions and consistency.

- Prevent injury to the individual by referring to *Risk for Injury* for strategies for assessing and manipulating the environment for hazards.

TRANSITION PLAN

Initiate health teaching and referrals as indicated.

- Refer caregivers to appropriate community resources.

  R: *A variety of community services may be needed for management at home.*

Clinical Alert Report

- Advise ancillary staff / student to report an increase in anxiety and/or confusion.

  R: *An increase in confusion and/or anxiety can represent deterioration in physiological stability.*

CHRONIC CONFUSION

NANDA-I Definition

Irreversible, long-standing, and/or progressive deterioration of intellect and personality characterized by decreased ability to interpret environmental stimuli; decreased capacity for intellectual thought processes; and manifested by disturbances of memory, orientation, and behavior

Defining Characteristics

Major (Must Be Present)

Progressive or long-standing:

Cognitive or intellectual losses
Altered perceptions
Poor judgment
Loss of language abilities
Affective or personality losses
Progressively lowered stress threshold
Purposeless behavior
Violent, agitated, or anxious behavior
Compulsive repetitive behavior
Withdrawal or avoidance behavior

Related Factors

Pathophysiologic (Hall, 1991)

Related to progressive degeneration of the cerebral cortex secondary to:

Alzheimer's disease*   Multi-infarct dementia (MID)*
Combination

Related to disturbance in cerebral metabolism, structure, or integrity secondary to:

Pick's disease   Creutzfeldt-Jakob disease
Toxic substance injection   Degenerative neurologic disease
Brain tumors   Huntington's chorea
Multiple sclerosis   Psychiatric disorders
End-stage diseases (AIDS, cirrhosis, cancer, renal failure, cardiac failure, and chronic obstructive pulmonary disease)

Goal

NOC
Cognitive Ability, Cognitive Orientation, Distorted Thought Self-Control, Surveillance: Safety, Emotional Support, Environmental Management, Fall Prevention, Calming Technique

The person will participate to the maximum level of independence in a therapeutic milieu as evidenced by the following indicators:

* Decreased frustration
* Diminished episodes of combativeness, sexual disinhibition
* Increased hours of sleep at night
* Stabilized or increased weight

Interventions

NIC
Dementia Management:
Multisensory Therapy,
Cognitive Stimulation,
Calming Technique,
Reality Orientation,
Environmental
Management: Safety

- Refer to Interventions under *Acute Confusion*.
- Promote the client's safety. Refer to *Risk for Falls*.

    R: Confused persons are at high risk for injury.

> **CLINICAL ALERT**
> • Implement falls prevention protocol with *Risk for Falls*.

- Assess who the person was before the onset of confusion.
    - Educational level, career
    - Hobbies, lifestyle
    - Coping styles

    R: Assessing the client's personal history can provide insight into current behavior patterns and communicates the nurse's interest. Specific personal data can improve individualization of care (Hall, 1991).

- Observe the client to determine baseline behaviors.
    - Best time of day
    - Response time to a simple question
    - Amount of distraction tolerated
    - Judgment
    - Insight into disability
    - Signs/symptoms of depression
    - Routine

    R: Baseline behavior can be used to develop a plan for activities and daily care routines.

- When planning for care for this client, distinguish between behavioral excesses (such as disruptive vocalization or aggression) and behavioral deficits (such as lack of social interaction or lack of self-care) (Allen-Burge et al., 1999).

    R: Strategies differ for addressing behavioral excesses vs. deficits (Allen-Burge et al., 1999).

- Address disruptive behaviors by focusing of the underlying unmet need (Cohen-Mansfield, 2000).
    - For aggression triggered by pain or discomfort, address for sources of pain (e.g., constipation, UTI).
    - For pacing triggered by boredom, plan opportunities to engage client in an activity.
    - For repetitive questioning or statements triggered by a need to communicate, increase meaningful dialogue with client during all caregiving encounters.

    R: The focus on the client's needs rather than on behavior helps to target more appropriate interventions (Cohen-Mansfield, 2000).

- Consult with physician/nurse practitioner to evaluate the use of neuroleptic or other sedatives as first-line therapy regarding side effects of sedation, risk for falls, and extrapyramidal signs. If prescribed, discuss a lower dose.

    R: Studies have shown that the neuroleptic treatment for chronic confusion leads to reduced well-being and quality of life and may even accelerate cognitive decline (Douglas et al., 2004).

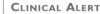

> **CLINICAL ALERT**
> • Caution: It is easier to sedate a client with disrupting behaviors than to utilize a nonpharmaceutical approach.
> • Sedation does not address the underlying origins of disrupting behavior; it only silences the individual.

- Promote the client's sense of integrity (Miller, 2009).
    - Adapt communication to client's level.
        - Avoid "baby talk" and a condescending tone of voice.

- Use simple sentences and present one idea at a time.
  - If the client does not understand, repeat the sentence using the same words.
- Use positive statements; avoid "don'ts."
- Unless a safety issue is involved, do not argue.
- Avoid general questions such as, "What would you like to do?" Instead, ask, "Do you want to go for a walk or work on your rug?"
- Be sensitive to the feelings the client is trying to express.
- Avoid questions you know the client cannot answer.
- If possible, demonstrate to reinforce verbal communication.
- Use touch to gain attention or show concern unless a negative response is elicited.
- Maintain good eye contact and pleasant facial expressions.
- Determine which sense dominates the client's perception of the world (for e.g., auditory, kinesthetic, olfactory, or gustatory). Communicate through the preferred sense.

   R: Alzheimer's disease–related dementia affects communication abilities (i.e., receptive and expressive).

> **CLINICAL ALERT**
> - Confused individuals are very vulnerable to abuse.
> - Monitor for and address unacceptable staff behavior toward client.

- Consult with physician / nurse practitioner regarding whether certain treatments are needed.
  - Discontinue or reduce dosage of medications that increase disturbances of cognition (e.g., sedatives, analgesics).
  - Avoid cauterizations / intravenous lines if possible.
  - Consider an intermittent access device instead of continuous IV therapy.

   R: Tethering lines are restrictive, confusing. and pose an increased risk of infection and trauma.

  - If catheter is necessary, place urinary collection bag at the end of the bed with catheter between rather than draped over legs. Velcro bands can hold the catheter against the leg.
  - Implement medication plan to prevent constipation (e.g., stool softeners).

   R: Constipation is uncomfortable and will increase confused behavior.

- Assess for nonverbal signs of pain (e.g., grimacing, moaning when re-positioned).

   R: Communication difficulties prevent usual assessment foci.

- Use adaptive devices (e.g., optimal lighting, glasses, and hearing aids).

   R: Adaptive devices can diminish confusing sensory input.

- Promote mobility as much as possible. Provide appropriate walking aids and ensure that they are accessible at all times.

   R: Frequent ambulation simulates normal ADLs and reduces the hazards of immobility on physical and cognitive function and improves mood and confidence (Douglas et al., 2004).

- Ensure optimal sleep patterns. Refer to *Disturbed Sleep Pattern.*

   R: Attention to optimal mobility and restorative sleep can improve daytime functioning.

- Select modalities involving the five senses (hearing, sight, smell, taste, and touch) that provide favorable stimuli for the client. Elicit from family some of client's favorites (e.g., music, object, TV show, fragrances).

   R: Research has validated that nonpharmaceutical interventions for chronic confusion should be the first-line approach no pharmaceutical treatments (Douglas et al., 2004).

  - Ask the family to bring in a non-candle source of lavender scent (e.g., oil, lotion).

   R: Lavender proves effective in promoting mental relaxation.

  - Allow an opportunity to draw using colored pencils.

   R: Drawing allows self-expression and opportunities to make choices (e.g., what to draw, what colors).

  - Ask the family to bring in recordings of the client's favorite music.

   R: Studies have shown that playing favorite music improves social interactions, memories, and a reduction in abnormal vocalizations.

- If combative, determine the source of fear and frustration.
  - Fatigue
  - Misleading or inappropriate stimuli
  - Change in routine, environment, caregiver
  - Pressure to exceed functional capacity
  - Physical stress, pain, infection, acute illness, discomfort

    R: Fatigue is the most frequent cause of dysfunctional episodes. Physical stressors can precipitate a dysfunctional episode (e.g., urinary tract infections, caffeine, constipation).

- If an aggressive episode occurs:
  - Address the client by surname. Assume a dependent position relative to the client.
  - Distract the client with cues that require automatic social behavior (e.g., "Mrs. Smith, would you like some juice now?").
  - Document antecedents, behavior observed, and consequences.

    R: With careful recording of the episode, these strategies can reduce aggression and may prevent future episodes.

- Implement techniques to lower the stress threshold (Hall & Buckwalter, 1987; Miller, 2009).
  - Reduce competing or excessive stimuli.
    - Keep the environment simple and uncluttered.
    - Use simple written cues to clarify directions for use of radio and television.
    - Eliminate or minimize unnecessary noise.

    R: Overstimulation, understimulation, or misleading stimuli can cause dysfunctional episodes because of impaired sensory interpretation (Hall, 1994).

- Plan and maintain a consistent routine. Attempt to assign the same caregivers.
  - Elicit from family members the specific methods that help or hinder care.
  - Determine a daily routine with the client and family.

    R: Consistency can reduce confusion and increase comfort.

- Focus on the client's ability level.
  - Do not request performance of function beyond ability.
  - Use simple sentences; demonstrate activity.
  - Do not ask questions that the client cannot answer.
  - Avoid open-ended questions (e.g., "What do you want to eat?" "When do you want to take a bath?").
  - Offer simple choices (e.g., "Do you want a cookie or crackers?").
  - Use finger foods (e.g., sandwiches) to encourage self-feeding.

    R: Attempting to perform functions that exceed cognitive capacity will result in fear, anger, and frustration (Hall, 1994).

- Minimize fatigue (Hall, 1994).
  - Allow the person to cease an activity at any time.
  - Be alert to expressions of fatigue and increased anxiety; immediately reduce stimuli.

    R: Fatigue can increase confusion.

TRANSITION PLAN
Initiate health teaching and referrals as needed.
- Support groups
- Community-based programs (e.g., day care, respite care)
- Alzheimer's association (www.alz.org)
- Long-term care facilities

Clinical Alert Report
- Advise ancillary staff / student to report an increase in anxiety and/or confusion.
  R: An increase in confusion and/or anxiety needs a focused assessment to determine causes.

CONSTIPATION

NANDA-I Definition

Decrease in normal frequency of defecation accompanied by difficult or incomplete passage of stool and/or passage of excessively hard, dry stool

Defining Characterisitcs

Major (Must Be Present)

Hard, formed stool*
Defecation fewer than two times a week
Prolonged and difficult evacuation

Minor (May Be Present)

Distended abdomen*
Generalized fatigue*
Decreased bowel sounds
Straining on defecation
Palpable rectal mass*
Feeling of inadequate emptying*

Related Factors

Pathophysiologic

Related to defective nerve stimulation, weak pelvic floor muscles, and immobility secondary to:

Spinal cord lesions
Spinal cord injury
Spina bifida

Cerebrovascular accident (CVA, stroke)
Neurologic diseases (multiple sclerosis, Parkinson's)
Dementia

Related to decreased metabolic rate secondary to (e.g., obesity, uremia, diabetic neuropathy, hypothyroidism)
Related to decreased response and an urge to defecate secondary to (e.g., cognitive/affective disorders)
Related to painful defecation
Related to decreased peristalsis secondary to hypoxia (cardiac, pulmonary)
Related to motility disturbances secondary to irritable bowel syndrome

Treatment Related

Related to side effects of (specify) (e.g., iron, diuretics, narcotics [codeine, morphine], anticholinergics, phenothiazines, antidepressants)
Related to effects of anesthesia and surgical manipulation on peristalsis
Related to habitual laxative use
Related to mucositis secondary to radiation

Situational (Personal, Environmental)

Related to decreased peristalsis secondary to (e.g., immobility, stress, pregnancy, insufficient exercise)
Related to irregular evacuation patterns
Related to inadequate diet (lack of roughage, fiber, thiamine) or fluid intake

Goal

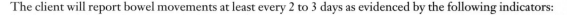

NOC
Bowel Elimination,
Hydration, Knowledge:
Diet

The client will report bowel movements at least every 2 to 3 days as evidenced by the following indicators:

- Describe components for effective bowel movements.
- Explain rationale for lifestyle change(s).

Interventions

NIC
Bowel Management,
Fluid Management,
Constipation/Impaction
Management, Nutrition
Therapy

Assess Contributing Factors

- Refer to *Related Factors*.

> **CLINICAL ALERT**
> - Constipation is often viewed as expected and benign.
> - Constipation can be responsible for undiagnosed pain and exacerbating confusion in individuals who cannot communicate.
> - Mostly all episodes of constipation can be prevented.

- If fecal impaction is present:
  - If fecal impaction is suspected, perform a digital rectal examination (DRE).

    R: Caution regarding producing the Valsalva maneuver, which can cause hypotension.

  - Remove fecal impaction. Refer to procedure manual as needed.
  - Make the client comfortable and allow to take rest.
  - The client may require temporary use of a stool softener or mild cathartic.
- If severe constipation is present:
  - Consult with physician / nurse practitioner for treatment.

Promote Corrective Measures

- Regular time for elimination
  - Review daily routine.
  - Provide a stimulus to defecation (e.g., coffee, prune juice).
  - Advise the client to attempt to defecate about 1 hour or so after meals and that remaining in the bathroom for a suitable length of time may be necessary.

  R: The gastrocolic and duodenocolic reflexes stimulate mass peristalsis two or three times a day, most often after meals.
- Adequate exercise
  - Review the current exercise pattern.
  - Provide frequent ambulation of hospitalized client when tolerable.
  - Perform range-of-motion exercises for the client who is bedridden.

  R: Regular physical activity promotes muscle tonicity needed for fecal expulsion. It also increases circulation to the digestive system, which promotes peristalsis and easier feces evacuation.
- Balanced diet
  - Avoid food low in fiber (e.g., starches, white bread, pasta, white rice, dairy products, processed foods).

    R: Low-fiber foods pass slowly in the large intestines and thus become dry, hard, and difficult to defecate.

  - Review list of foods high in fiber:
    - Fresh fruits, fruit juices, and vegetables with skins
    - Beans (navy, kidney, lima), nuts, and seeds
    - Whole-grain breads, cereal, and bran
  - Include approximately 800 g of fruits and vegetables (about four pieces of fresh fruit and large salad) for normal daily bowel movement. Avoid cooked fruits.

- Suggest moderate use of bran at first (may irritate GI tract, produce flatulence, cause diarrhea or blockage). Explain the need for fluid intake with bran.

  R: Diets high in unrefined fibrous food produce large, soft stools that decrease the colon's susceptibility to disease. Diets low in fiber and high in concentrated refined foods produce small, hard stools that increase the colon's susceptibility to disease. An increase in fiber without optimal hydration will worsen constipation.

- Adequate fluid intake
  - Encourage fluid intake of at least 2 L (8 to 10 glasses) unless contraindicated.
  - Discuss fluid preferences.
  - Set up regular schedule for fluid intake.
  - Recommend drinking a glass of hot water 30 minutes before breakfast, which may stimulate bowel evacuation.
  - Advise avoiding grapefruit juice, apple juice, coffee, tea, cola, and chocolate drinks as daily fluid intake.

    R: Sufficient fluid intake, at least 2 L daily, is necessary to maintain bowel patterns and to promote proper stool consistency.

- Optimal position
  - Provide privacy (close door, draw curtains around the bed, play the television or radio to mask sounds, have a room deodorizer available).
  - Use the bathroom instead of a bedpan if possible. Allow suitable position (sitting and leaning forward, if not contraindicated).
  - Assist the client onto the bedpan if necessary; elevate the head of the bed to high Fowler's position or elevation permitted.

    R: Flexing the hip pulls the anal canal open, which decreases resistance of feces movement. An upright position uses gravity to promote feces movement. Elevating the legs can increase intra-abdominal pressure.

TRANSITION PLAN

Initiate health teaching and referrals as indicated.

- Explain the relationship of lifestyle changes to constipation. Emphasize that constipation can be prevented.

  R: Sedentary lifestyle, inadequate fluid intake, inadequate dietary fiber, and stress can contribute to constipation.

- Go to thePoint at http://thePoint.lww.com/Carpenito6e and print Getting Started to Prevent Constipation.

Clinical Alert Report

- Advise ancillary staff / student to report early signs of constipation (e.g., difficulty in passing stools) and if client reports more than 2 days have passed without a bowel movement.

DIARRHEA

NANDA-I Definition

Passage of loose, unformed stools

Defining Characteristics*

At least three loose, liquid stools per day
Urgency
Cramping/abdominal pain
Hyperactive bowel sounds

Related Factors

Pathophysiologic

Related to malabsorption* or inflammation* secondary to (specify):

Colon cancer	Crohn's disease	Gastritis
Diverticulitis	Peptic ulcer	Spastic colon
Irritable bowel	Celiac disease (sprue)	Ulcerative colitis

Related to lactose deficiency, dumping syndrome
Related to increased peristalsis secondary to increased metabolic rate (hyperthyroidism)
Related to infectious process* secondary to:

Trichinosis	Shigellosis	Dysentery
Typhoid fever	Cholera	Infectious hepatitis
Malaria	Microsporidia	Cryptosporidium

Related to excessive secretion of fats in stool secondary to liver dysfunction
Related to inflammation and ulceration of gastrointestinal mucosa secondary to high levels of nitrogenous wastes (renal failure)

Treatment Related

Related to malabsorption or inflammation secondary to surgical intervention of the bowel
Related to side effects* of (specify) (e.g., diuretics, antibiotics)
Related to tube feedings

Situational (Personal, Environmental)

Related to stress or anxiety

Goal

NOC
Bowel Elimination, Electrolyte & Acid–Base Balance, Fluid Balance, Hydration, Symptom Control

The client/parent will report less diarrhea as evidenced by the following indicators:

- Describe contributing factors when known.
- Explain rationale for interventions.

Interventions

NIC
Bowel Management, Diarrhea Management, Fluid/Electrolyte Management, Nutrition Management, Enteral Tube Feeding

- Monitor for dehydration
  - Hourly output less than 5 mL/kg/hour
  - Dark-colored urine
  - Low serum potassium, low serum sodium
  - Dizziness, headache

  R: *Undetected hypovolemia can cause electrolyte imbalances and decreased blood flow to heart, brain, and kidneys.*
- Closely monitor the elderly for dehydration.

  R: *The body compensates for fluid losses by concentrating urine and increasing the thirst response. As one ages, these mechanisms are less effective, thus dehydration can occur more rapidly with severe complications of dysrhythmias and decreased cardiac output. (Porth, 2010)*
  - Monitor perianal tissue for redness/excoriation. Use a barrier cream.

    R: *Gastric enzymes can irritate and excoriate perianal tissue.*

CLINICAL ALERT
• Early signs of dehydration in the elderly require interventions.

• Reduce diarrhea.
  • Avoid milk (lactose) products, fat, whole grains, fried and spicy foods, and fresh fruits and vegetables.
  • Gradually add semisolids and solids (crackers, yogurt, rice, bananas, and applesauce).

  R: Foods with complex carbohydrates (e.g., rice, toast, and cereal) facilitate fluid absorption into the intestinal mucosa.

• Encourage liquids (e.g., tea, water, apple juice, flat ginger ale).
• Caution against the use of very hot or cold liquids.
• See *Deficient Fluid Volume* for additional interventions.

  R: Soft drinks (nondietetic or dietetic) and sport drinks are unsatisfactory for fluid replacement for moderate or severe fluid loss because of their high sugar and salt content (Bennett, 2000).

• Reduce GI side effects of tube feeding.
  • Control the infusion rate (depending on delivery set).
  • Administer smaller, more frequent feedings.
  • Change to continuous-drip tube feedings.
  • Administer more slowly if signs of gastrointestinal intolerance occur.
  • If formula has been refrigerated, warm it in hot water to room temperature.
  • Dilute the strength of feeding temporarily.
  • Follow the standard procedure for administration of tube feeding.
  • Follow tube feeding with the specified amount of water to ensure hydration.
  • Be careful of contamination/spoilage (unused but opened formula should not be used after 24 hours; keep unused portion refrigerated).

  R: High-solute tube feedings may cause diarrhea if not followed by sufficient water.

TRANSITION PLAN
Conduct health teaching as indicated.
• Avoid dietetic foods.

  R: Foods containing large amounts of the hexitol, sorbitol, and mannitol that are used as sugar substitutes in dietetic foods, candy, and chewing gum can cause diarrhea.
• Explain safe food handling (e.g., required temperature storage, washing of food preparation objects after use with raw food, and frequent hand washing).
• Instruct the client to call primary care provider if diarrhea lasts more than 24 hours.
• Instruct the client to seek IMMEDIATE medical care if blood and mucous are in stool and if fever is present.

  R: Acute bloody diarrhea (dysentery) has certain causative pathogens (e.g., campylobacter jejuni, shigella, and salmonella) that require antibiotic therapy (Spies, 2009).

Clinical Alert Report
• Advise ancillary staff / student to report an increase in diarrhea and/or decrease in urinary output.
  R: Dehydration can occur in vulnerable clients (e.g., elderly, weakened).

RISK FOR DISUSE SYNDROME

NANDA-I Definition

At risk for deterioration of body systems as the result of prescribed or unavoidable musculoskeletal inactivity

Defining Characteristics

Presence of a cluster of actual or risk nursing diagnoses related to inactivity:

Risk for Impaired Skin Integrity
Risk for Constipation
Risk for Altered Respiratory Function
Risk for Ineffective Peripheral Tissue Perfusion
Risk for Infection
Risk for Activity Intolerance
Risk for Impaired Physical Mobility
Risk for Injury
Powerlessness
Disturbed Body Image

Related Factors

Pathophysiologic

Related to decreased sensorium/unconsciousness
Related to neuromuscular impairment secondary to (specify)

Treatment Related

Related to:

Surgery (amputation, skeletal)   Mechanical ventilation
Traction/casts/splints   Invasive vascular lines
Prescribed immobility

Situational (Personal, Environmental)

Related to:

Depression   Debilitated state
Fatigue   Pain

Goal

NOC
Endurance, Immobility
Consequences:
Physiological, Immobility
Consequences: Psycho-
Cognitive, Mobility, Joint
Movement

The client will not experience complications of immobility as evidenced by the following indicators:

- Intact skin/tissue integrity
- Maximum pulmonary function
- Maximum peripheral blood flow
- Full range of motion
- Bowel, bladder, and renal functioning within normal limits
- Uses of social contacts and activities when possible
- Make decisions regarding care when possible
- Share feelings regarding immobile state

Interventions

NIC
Bed Rest Care,
Bowel Management,
Activity Therapy,
Energy Management,
Mutual Goal Settings,
Exercise Therapy, Fall
Prevention, Pressure
Ulcer Prevention, Body
Mechanics Correction,
Self-Care Assistance,
Skin Surveillance,
Positioning, Coping
Enhancement, Decision
Making, Support
Therapeutic Play

Identify Causative and Contributing Factors

- Pain; refer also to *Impaired Comfort*.
- Fatigue; refer also to *Fatigue*.
- Decreased motivation; refer also to *Activity Intolerance*.
- Depression; refer also to *Ineffective Coping*.

Promote Optimal Respiratory Function

- Vary the position of the bed, thus gradually changing the horizontal and vertical position of the thorax, unless contraindicated.
- Assist client to reposition, turning frequently from side to side (hourly if possible).
- Encourage deep breathing and controlled coughing exercises five times every hour.

R: Bed rest decreases chest expansion and cilia activity and increases mucus retention, increasing risks of pneumonia.

Maintain Usual Pattern of Bowel Elimination

- Refer to *Constipation* for specific interventions.

Prevent Pressure Ulcers

- Refer to *Risk for Impaired Skin Integrity*.

  R: Principles of pressure ulcer prevention include reducing or rotating pressure on soft tissue. If pressure exceeds intracapillary pressure (approximately 32 mm Hg), capillary occlusion causes tissue damage. (Porth, 2010)

Promote Factors That Improve Venous Blood Flow

- Elevate extremity above the level of the heart (may be contraindicated in cases of severe cardiac or respiratory disease).
- Ensure that the client avoids standing or sitting with legs dependent for long periods.
- Consider the use of below-knee elastic stockings to prevent venous stasis.
- Avoid pillows behind the knees or suggest a bed that is elevated at the knees.
- Tell the client to avoid crossing the legs.
- Remind the client to change positions, move extremities, or wiggle fingers and toes every hour.
- Ensure that the client avoids garters and tight elastic stockings above the knees.
- Monitor legs for edema, tissue warmth, and redness daily.

  R: Increased serum calcium resulting from bone destruction caused by lack of motion and weight-bearing increases blood coagulability. This, in addition to circulatory stasis, makes the client vulnerable to thrombosis formation. (Porth, 2010)

> **CLINICAL ALERT**
> - Any change in peripheral circulation, onset of edema, tissue warm, or c/o of leg aches/pains need immediate attention to rule out thrombosis.

Maintain Limb Mobility and Prevent Contractures

- Increase limb mobility.
  - Perform range-of-motion exercises (frequency to be determined by client's condition).
- Position the client in alignment to prevent complications.
  - Point toes and knees toward ceiling when the client is supine. Keep them flat when in a chair.
  - Use footboard.
  - Instruct the client to wiggle toes, point them up and downward, rotate ankles inward and outward every hour.

    R: These strategies prevent footdrop, a serious complication of immobility.

  - Avoid prolonged periods of hip flexion (i.e., sitting position).
  - Keep arms abducted from the body with pillows.

- Keep elbows in slight flexion.
- Keep wrist neutral, with fingers slightly flexed and thumb abducted and slightly flexed.
- Change position of shoulder joints during the day (e.g., abduction, adduction, range of circular motion).

R: Compression of nerves by casts, restraints, or improper positions can cause ischemia and nerve degeneration. Compression of the radial nerve results in wrist drop and possible permanent nerve damage after 6 to 8 hours. (Hockenberry & Wilson, 2009)

- Consult with physical therapy.

R: Joints without range of motion develop contractures in 3 to 7 days, because flexor muscles are stronger than extensor muscles.

- Prevent urinary stasis and calculi formation.
  - Provide a daily fluid intake of 2,000 mL or more (unless contraindicated).

R: The peristaltic contractions of the ureters are insufficient when in a reclining position; thus, there is stasis of urine in the renal pelvis. Interventions to maintain hydration prevent hypercoagulability and clot formation and urine concentration of stone-forming elements. (Porth, 2010)

Reduce and Monitor Bone Demineralization

- Promote weight-bearing when possible (tilt-table).
- Maintain vigorous hydration.

R: The upright position improves bone strength, increases circulation, and prevents postural hypotension (Porth, 2010).

Promote Sharing and a Sense of Well-Being

- Encourage the client to share feelings and fears regarding restricted movement.
- Encourage the client to wear own clothes, rather than pajamas, and unique adornments (e.g., baseball caps, colorful socks) to express individuality.
- Be creative; vary the physical environment and daily routine when possible.
  - Update bulletin boards, change pictures on the walls, and move furniture within the room.
  - Maintain a pleasant, cheerful environment (e.g., plenty of light, flowers).
  - Place the client near a window, if possible.
  - Provide reading material (print or audio), radio, and television.
  - Plan an activity daily to give the client something to look forward to; always keep promises.
  - Discourage the use of television as the primary source of recreation unless it is highly desired.
  - Consider using a volunteer to spend time reading to the client or helping with an activity.
  - Encourage suggestions and new ideas (e.g., "Can you think of things you might like to do?").

R: Decreased activity reduces social contacts, reduces problem-solving ability, and decreases coping ability and orientation to time. Strategies are focused on increasing visual and auditory stimuli, engaging in decision making and activities to reduce monotony.

TRANSITION PLAN

Initiate health teaching and referrals as needed.

- Refer to community health nurse for a home evaluation.

Clinical Alert Report

- Advise ancillary staff / student to report changes in mobility, respirations, bowel movements, and skin condition and any complaints of leg pain.

  R: Early detection of complications of immobility can initiate strategies to reverse these complications or prevent further deterioration.

RISK FOR DRY EYE**

NANDA-I Definition

At risk for eye discomfort or damage to the cornea and conjunctiva due to reduced quantity or quality of tears to moisten the eye

Risk Factors

Pathophysiologic

Related to:

Autoimmune diseases (rheumatoid arthritis, diabetes mellitus, thyroid disease, gout, osteoporosis, etc.)*
Collagen vascular disease
Structural eyelid problems
Neurological lesions with sensory or motor reflex loss (lagophthalmos, lack of spontaneous blink reflex due to decreased consciousness and other medical conditions)*
Ocular surface damage*
Deficient tear-producing glands
Tear gland damage from inflammation
Difficulty in blinking due to eyelid problems (e.g., ectropion [turning out]; entropion [turning in])

Treatment Related

Related to:

Pharmaceutical agents such as angiotensin-converting enzyme inhibitors, antihistamines, diuretics, steroids, antidepressants, tranquilizers, analgesics, sedatives, neuromuscular blockage agents,* surgical operations,* oral contraceptives
Anti-inflammatory agents (e.g., ibuprofen, naproxen, decongestants)
Post–laser eye surgery
Tear gland damage from radiation
Post–cosmetic eyelid surgery
Mechanical ventilation therapy*

Goals

NOC
Knowledge: Illness Care, Infection Control, Symptom Control, Hydration

The client will exhibit minimal or no sign / symptoms of complications of dry eye as evidenced by the following indicators:

- Pink conjunctiva
- No increase in drainage or purulent drainage
- Clear cornea

Interventions

NIC
Eye Care Infection Protection; Medication Administration: Eye, Comfort Level, Hydration, Anxiety Reduction (family)

- Identify high-risk clients
  - Unconscious
  - Sedated for >48 hours
  - Paralyzed
  - Ventilatory support

  R: The above conditions prevent eye closure, lack of random eye movements, and diminished or loss of blink reflex. The exposure and drying of the eye can result in superficial keratopathy. This can compromise the integrity of

---

**Note: The focus in this book for this diagnosis is prevention of corneal abrasion in a health care setting.

the surface of the cornea resulting in ulceration, perforation, and scarring. The effects of mechanical ventilation increase intraocular pressure resulting in edema. (Joyce, 2002)

- Monitor for keratitis.
  - Red and watery eyes
  - Pain in the eye (if can report)
  - White to gray area on cornea (late sign)

R: Keratitis is an inflammation of the cornea caused by corneal exposure and a compromise in the normal tear film and / or bacterial or viral infections (Joyce, 2002).

> **CLINICAL ALERT**
> • Report any changes in the eye appearance or report of eye pain or blurring (if able) immediately.

- Provide eye care as prescribed.
  - Eye drops, lubricants, antibiotics
  - Patches, gauze, eye shields, polyethylene covers

R: Studies have reported the effectiveness of these preventive practices. The use of polyethylene covers has been found to be most effective. (Joyce, 2002)

> **CLINICAL ALERT**
> • If no eye care protocol has been prescribed, consult with physician / nurse practitioner (NP) immediately.
>   *R: Cornea drying can occur quickly in high-risk clients after 48 hours.*

- Prevent infection.
  - Wear gloves with all eye care.
  - Instruct family not to touch or wipe the eye area of an individual.
  - Gently pull lower lid and instill drops or a line of ointment in pocket of the lid.
  - Avoid any contamination of eye care products. Never touch dropper or tube tip to eyelid. If this occurs, discard the medicine.
  - Offer to demonstrate to a new nurse or student nurse.

R: Every attempt is made to prevent contamination of the eye. Eye drops can become contaminated when the container is e-xposed to bacteria.

- Evaluate hydration status frequently.

R: Mild dehydration can make dry eyes worse (Yanoff & Duker, 2009).

- Prior to seeing client, explain to client and / or significant others the reason for the eye care treatments (e.g., use of shields, polyethylene covers [plastic wrap]).

R: The client's appearance with eye patches or polyethylene covers can be very disturbing to significant others.

SBAR

Situation: Certain clients are at high risk for corneal injury and infection. Protocols provide interventions to be followed.

Background: Not applicable to this situation.

Assessment: "I observed when you were instilling eye drops into Mr. Blue; the tip of the container touched his eyelid."

Recommendation: "This medication container has been contaminated and must be discarded and a new one needs to be ordered from the pharmacy."

TRANSITION PLAN

Initiate health teaching as indicated.

- Advise to see primary care provider or an eye specialist if there are signs and symptoms of dry eyes, infection, and eye pain.

  R: Prolonged dry eyes can cause eye infections, scarring of the cornea surface, and vision problems. Eye complaints must be addressed immediately.

Clinical Alert Report

- Advise ancillary staff / student to report any c/o of eye pain.
  R: Eye pain can indicate an infection or corneal abrasion.

RISK FOR FALLS

NANDA-I Definition

At risk for increased susceptibility to falling that may cause physical harm

Risk Factors

Pathophysiologic

Related to altered cerebral function secondary to hypoxia
Related to syncope, vertigo, or dizziness
Related to impaired mobility secondary to (e.g., cerebrovascular accident, arthritis, Parkinsonism)
Related to loss of limb
Related to impaired vision
Related to hearing impairment
Related to fatigue
Related to orthostatic hypotension

Treatment Related

Related to lack of awareness of environmental hazards secondary to (e.g., confusion)
Related to improper use of aids (e.g., crutches, canes, walkers, wheelchairs)
Related to tethering devices (e.g., IV, Foley, compression therapy, telemetry)
Related to prolonged bed rest
Related to side effects of medication(s)

Situational (Personal, Environmental)

Related to history of falls

CLINICAL ALERT
- History of falls is a high-risk factor for future falls.

Related to improper footwear
Related to unstable gait

Older Adult

Related to faulty judgments, secondary cognitive deficits
Related to sedentary lifestyle and loss of muscle strength

Goal

NOC

Risk Control, Fall
Occurrence, Fall
Prevention Behavior,
Personal Safety
Behavior, Safe Home
Environment

The client will not injure himself or herself during hospital stay as evidenced by the following indicators:

* Identify factors that increase risk of injury.
* Describe appropriate safety measures.
* Will agree to ask for help when needed.

Interventions

NIC

Fall Prevention;
Environmental
Management: Safety,
Health Education;
Surveillance: Safety,
Risk Identification;
Technology
Management;
Medication
Management; Family
Involvement Promotion;
Environmental
Management: Home
Preparation

Involve All Hospital Personnel on Every Shift in the Fall Prevention Program

R: Approximately 14% of all falls in hospitals are accidental, another 8% are unanticipated physiologic falls, and 78% are anticipated physiologic falls.

* Always glance into the room of a high-risk person when passing his or her room.
* Alert other departments of high-risk individuals when off unit for tests, procedures.
* Address fall prevention and risks with every hand-off and transfer.
* Seek to identify reversible risk factors in all individuals. Be aware of changing client conditions and a change in risk status.
* Identify in a private conference room the number of falls on the unit monthly (e.g., poster).

   R: Intradisciplinary approach to fall prevention is effective when falls are viewed not as inevitable accidents but as preventable events.

Identify the Client's Risk for Falls

* Assess the person's ability to Timed Up and Go (TUG) (Podsiadlo & Richardson, 1991).
   * Have the person wear his or her usual footwear and use any assistive device he or she normally uses.
   * Have the person sit in the chair with his or her back to the chair and his or her arms resting on the arm rests.
   * Ask the person to stand up from a standard chair and walk a distance of 10 feet (3 meters).
   * Have the person turn around, walk back to the chair, and sit down again.
   * Timing begins when the person starts to rise from the chair and ends when he or she returns to the chair and sits down.
   * The person should be given one practice trial and then three actual trials if needed. The times from the three actual trials are averaged.
   * Predictive Results
      <10 sec Freely mobile
      <20 sec Mostly independent
      20–29 sec Variable mobility
      >30 sec Impaired mobility

      R: Numerous researchers have reported that the TUG test is reliable (87% sensitivity and specificity) for community-dwelling older adults (Beling & Roller, 2009). Loss of strength in legs and ankles is a common cause of falls in older persons; however, it is not an outcome of aging but one of a sedentary lifestyle. It is not inevitable; it is preventable.

* Identify high-risk individuals and initiate the institution's standard and protocol to prevent falls.

   R: Standard interventions to prevent any individual from falling are instituted on admission. In addition, high-risk individuals are identified using the institution's protocol (e.g., red slippers, colored bracelet). Refer to the last page of this book.

* Ensure that tables and chairs with side arms are stable.

   R: Persons with lower extremity weakness will benefit from sturdy chairs.

Reduce or Eliminate Contributing Factors for Falls

Related to Unfamiliar Environment

* Orient the client to his or her environment (e.g., location of bathroom, bed controls, call bell). Leave a light on in the bathroom at night. Ensure that path to bathroom is clear.

   R: Orientation helps provide familiarity; a light at night helps the client find the way safely.

- Teach him or her to keep the bed in the low position with side rails up at night.

  R: The low position makes it easier for the client to get in and out of bed.

- Make sure that the telephone, eyeglasses, urinal, and frequently used personal belongings are within easy reach.

  R: Keeping objects at hand helps prevent falls due to overreaching and overextending.

- Instruct the client to request assistance whenever needed.

  R: Getting needed help with ambulation and other activities reduces a client's risk of injury.

- For individuals with difficulty accessing toilet:
  - If urgency exists, evaluate for a urinary tract infection.

    R: New onset urinary urgency can be a sign of an infection.

  - Provide an opportunity to use bathroom / urinal / bedpan every 2 hours while awake, at bedtime, and upon awakening.

    R: Thirty percent of falls are related to attempting to access the bathroom and can be prevented by timed toileting schedule (Alcee, 2000).

- Frequently scan floor for wet areas, objects on floor.

Related to Gait Instability / Balance Problems

- Explain that gait and balance problems are due to underuse and deconditioning, NOT AGING.
  - Alert clients that they may not be able to prevent a fall if they trip.

    R: Weak leg muscles and decreased range of motion (ROM) in ankles prevent a safe recovery from a trip.

  - Explain that deficiencies in vitamin D interferes with one's postural balance, propulsion, and navigation.

    R: Vitamin D supplements improve gait performance and prevent falls by more than 22% in older adults (Annweiler, Montero-Odasso et al., 2010).

  - Seek to include a vitamin D level in next laboratory tests. Explain that the normal range is 30–100 nmol/L.

    R: Researchers have reported that the level should be at least 60 nmol/L is needed to affect a reduction of falls (Annweiler, Montero-Odasso et al., 2010).

  - Refer to Getting Started for strategies and exercises to improve gait and balance on thePoint at http://thePoint.lww.com/Carpenito6e.
- Instruct the client to wear slippers with nonskid soles and to avoid shoes with thick, soft soles.

  R: These precautions can help prevent falls from slipping. Thick soles require adequate lifting of feet as one walks or the soles will catch and trip the person.

- Ensure that mobility aids are available and reachable. Wheelchairs should always be locked. Remind that IV poles are on wheels and are not sturdy.

  R: Falls occur when an individual is reaching for a mobility aid or for a wheelchair not in the locked position.

- Ensure that call bell, TV controls, and telephone are within reach.

  R: Stretching and reaching can contribute to rolling out of bed.

Related to Tethering Devices (IVs, Foley, telemetry, compression devices)

- Evaluate if tethering devices can be discontinued at night.
- Can the IV be converted to a saline port?
- If the client is competent, teach him or her how to safely ambulate with devices to bathroom or advise to call for assistance.

  R: Individuals can become entangled in lines and tubes and fall.

Related to Orthostatic Hypotension

- Explain orthostatic hypotension as what happens when one stands and blood flow momentarily shifts to the lower body. When the body cannot compensate rapidly to this shift of fluids, dizziness and even fainting are experienced because of inadequate blood flow to brain (Porth, 2011).

  R: By emphasizing that more time is needed to prevent dizziness, the client's understanding of how to prevent dizziness and falls may increase.

- Explain the following reasons why dizziness occurs when a person changes positions (Porth, 2010):
  - Reduced blood volume as blood loss, dehydration

    R: Low blood volume causes cardiac output to decrease when a person stands, decreasing blood to brain.
  - Medication-induced hypotension, diuretics, some antihypertensives, psychotropics
  - Aging, usually over 70

    R: As one ages, the physiologic response needed to control blood flow when one stands is slowed; thus dizziness results when position changes are too rapid.
  - Prolonged bed rest

    R: Causes loss of vascular and skeletal muscular tone, which are needed to return the blood in the lower body to the heart and brain.
  - Neurologic disorders as Parkinson's, autonomic failure of unknown etiology

    R: Conditions that affect autonomic nervous system function, such as increased heart rate and constricted peripheral veins / arterioles, prevent the body's compensatory mechanisms from responding quickly when one stands.
- Teach to:
  - Change positions slowly.

    R: Gradual position change allows the body to compensate for venous pooling, which is needed to return blood to the heart.
  - Move from lying to an upright position in stages.
    - Sit up in bed. Dangle first one leg, then the other, over the side of the bed.
    - Allow a minute before going on to another position.
    - Place a chair, walker, cane, or other assistive device nearby to use to steady oneself when getting out of bed.
  - Sleep with the head of the bed elevated.
  - Avoid stooping to pick something up from the floor; use an assistive device available from an orthotics department or a self-help store.

    R: Prolonged bed rest promotes a reduction in plasma volume (after 3–4 days), decreased venous tone, peripheral vasoconstriction, and muscle weakness (after 2 weeks).
- Teach to avoid dehydration and vasodilatation.
  - Replace fluids during periods of excess fluid loss (e.g., hot weather).
  - Minimize diuretic fluids (e.g., caffeinated drinks like coffee, tea, cola).
  - Minimize alcohol consumption.
  - Avoid sources of intense heat (e.g., direct sun, hot showers, baths, electric blankets).

  R: Adequate hydration is necessary to prevent decreased circulating volume. Certain fluids are diuretics and reduce body fluids. Heat and alcohol can cause vasodilation.
- Teach to reduce postprandial hypotension.
  - Avoid high carbohydrate meals.
  - Take antihypertensive medications after meals rather than before.
  - Eat small, frequent meals.
  - Remain seated or lie down after meals.

  R: Studies have shown that in healthy older adults, blood pressure is reduced by 20 mm Hg within 1 hour of eating the morning or afternoon meal. This is thought to result from an impaired baroreflex compensatory response to splanchnic blood pooling during digestion.

Related to Medication Side Effects
- Review the person's medication reconciliation completed on admission.
  - Question regarding alcohol use.

    R: Alcohol can potentiate side effects of sombulence / dizziness.
  - Question if the person has side effects when taking certain meds.
  - Question if, in the person's opinion, he or she is taking a medication for pain that is not working.

    R: Some medications might need to be discontinued because of side effects or ineffective therapeutic response.

- Review with pharmacist / physicians / NP the present medications and evaluate those that can contribute to dizziness and if they should be discontinued, have dose reduced, or replaced with an alternative (Riefkohl et al., 2003).
  - Antidepressants (e.g., SSRIs)
  - Antipsychotics
  - Benzodiazepines
  - Antihistamines (e.g., Benadryl, hydroxyzine)
  - Anticonvulsants
  - Nonsteroidal anti-inflammatory drugs
  - Muscle relaxants
  - Narcotic analgesics
  - Antiarrhythmics (type 1A)
  - Digoxin

R: The use of medications is one of the many different factors that can contribute to balance problems and the risk of falls. Published research suggests an association between the use of these drugs or drug class and an increased risk of falling (Riefkohl et al., 2003).

Related to Confused / Uncooperative / Impaired Cognition

- Consider use of electronic devices in bed, chair, video surveillance.
- Follow institutional policy for side rails.
- Consider use of sitter.
- Move person to a more observable room.
- Plan to complete shift documentation in room of high-risk person.

R: In some cases, extra measures are necessary to ensure a client's safety and prevent injury to him or her and others. The cost of extra surveillance will be less than the cost of injury related to a fall.

If Person Falls or Reports a Fall

> **CLINICAL ALERT**
> - Call out for help immediately and continue to attend to the client.

- Implement the following:
  - Do not move initially.
  - IF PERSON HIT HEAD OR IF UNKNOWN, IMMOBILIZE CERVICAL SPINE.
  - Assess if loss of consciousness was experienced, c/o of pain, is confused.
  - Take baseline vital signs, blood glucose.
  - Determine baseline Glasgow Coma Scale.
  - Assess risk for intracranial bleed (anticoagulants, thrombocytopenia, coagulopathy).
  - Assess for lacerations, fractures, contusions, decreased ROM.
  - Clean and dress any wounds.
  - Implement neuro checks q 2 hours × 24 hours.
  - Contact the appropriate physician / NP to discuss findings and implications.

  R: Immediate assessment with notification of medical staff is indicated in order to determine the extent of injuries and the need for diagnostic tests and or treatments.

SBAR

Situation: Ask client and witnesses what happened, at what time? location? who witnessed?

Background: Prior fall risk score? hx of falls?

Assessment: Evaluate the following:

Side rails up / down	Fall risk alerts present (placards, wrist band)	
Position of bed	Call light reachable	Sitter present
Nonskid footwear	Use of assistive devices	Visitors present
Presence of clutter	Bed alarm on	Presence of IV, Foley
Staffing ratios		

Recommendation: Communicate identified factors that caused or contributed to the fall.

- Engage in a post-fall huddle within 1 hour of fall. Involve all staff. Avoid all discussions of blaming. Refer to the Appendix for a sample of Post-Fall Huddle Guidelines.

  R: Post-fall huddles can identify falls amenable to prevention interventions as client education, staff heightened awareness, and reduction of risk factors (Gray-Miceli, Johnson, & Strumpf, 2005).

CLINICAL ALERT
- If the institution does not engage in a formal post-fall huddle, any nurse, student, or client care team member can review this form and provide the team with valuable data concerning the circumstances of the fall and strategies to be implemented to prevent future falls.

TRANSITION PLAN
Teach strategies to decrease risk of falling at home.
- Go to thePoint at http://thePoint.lww.com/Carpenito6e and access Getting Started for take-home guidelines to prevent falls at home and exercises to improve muscle strength and balance.

Clinical Alert Report
- Advise ancillary staff / student to report any incident of an almost fall or accident, attempts of a vulnerable client to get out of bed without assistance, other risk situations (e.g., attempts of incapable visitors to assist a client).

  R: Ancillary staff are in an optimal position to witness high-risk situations, which can be addressed to prevent injury.

Documentation
- Progress notes
- Multidisciplinary client education record
- Client teaching and response are stable
- Post-fall documentation
  - Document circumstances, assessment, and interventions in health record
  - Complete incident report

FATIGUE

NANDA-I Definition

An overwhelming sustained sense of exhaustion and decreased capacity for physical and mental work at the usual level

Defining Characteristics*

Reports an unremitting and overwhelming lack of energy
Perceived need for additional energy to accomplish routine tasks
Reports inability to maintain usual routines
Reports feeling tired
Compromised concentration
Compromised libido

Increased physical complaints
Decreased performance
Disinterest in surroundings
Lethargy; drowsiness
Reports inability to maintain usual level of physical activity
Increase in rest requirements
Reports guilt for not keeping up with responsibilities
Reports inability to restore energy even after sleep
Introspection
Listlessness

Related Factors

Many factors can cause fatigue; combining related factors may be useful (e.g., *Related to muscle weakness, accumulated waste products, inflammation, and infections secondary to hepatitis*).

Pathophysiologic

Related to hypermetabolic state secondary to (e.g., viruses such as Epstein-Barr, fever, pregnancy*)
Related to inadequate tissue oxygenation secondary to (e.g., chronic obstructive lung disease, congestive heart failure (CHF), anemia,* peripheral vascular disease)
Related to biochemical changes secondary to:

Endocrine / metabolic disorders (e.g., diabetes mellitus, pituitary disorders, acquired immunodeficiency syndrome [AIDS], hypothyroidism, Addison's disease)
Chronic diseases (e.g., renal failure, cirrhosis, Lyme disease)

Related to muscular weakness / wasting secondary to (e.g., myasthenia gravis, Parkinson's disease, multiple sclerosis, AIDS, amyotrophic lateral sclerosis)
Related to hypermetabolic state, competition between body and tumor for nutrients, anemia, and stressors associated with cancer
Related to malnutrition*
Related to nutritional deficits* or changes in nutrient metabolism secondary to (e.g., nausea, side effects of medications, vomiting, gastric surgery, diarrhea, diabetes mellitus)
Related to chronic inflammatory process secondary to (e.g., AIDS, cirrhosis, arthritis, inflammatory bowel disease, lupus erythematosus, renal failure, hepatitis, Lyme disease)

Treatment Related

Biochemical changes secondary to (e.g., chemotherapy, radiation therapy, side effects of [specify])
Related to surgical damage to tissue and anesthesia
Related to increased energy expenditure secondary to (e.g., amputation, gait disorder, use of walker, crutches)

Situational (Personal, Environmental)

Related to prolonged decreased activity and deconditioning secondary to (specify)
Related to excessive role demands
Related to overwhelming emotional demands
Related to extreme stress*
Related to sleep disturbance

Goals

NOC
Activity Tolerance, Endurance, Energy Conservation

The person will participate in activities that stimulate and balance physical, cognitive, affective, and social domains as evidenced by the following indicators:

- Discuss the causes of fatigue.
- Share feelings regarding the effects of fatigue on life.
- Establish priorities for daily and weekly activities.

Interventions

NIC
Energy Management,
Environmental
Management, Mutual
Goal Setting, Socialization
Enhancement, Coping
Enhancement

Nursing interventions for this diagnosis are for people with fatigue regardless of etiology that cannot be eliminated. The focus is to assist the client and family to adapt to the fatigue state.

Assess Causative or Contributing Factors

- If fatigue has related factors that can be treated, refer to the specific Nursing Diagnosis as:
  - Lack of sleep; refer to *Disturbed Sleep Pattern*.
  - Poor nutrition; refer to *Imbalanced Nutrition*.
  - Sedentary lifestyle; refer to *Sedentary Lifestyle*.
  - Inadequate stress management; refer to *Stress Overload*.
  - Chronic excessive role or social demands; refer to *Ineffective Coping*.

Explain the Causes of Fatigue

R: In many chronic diseases, fatigue is the most common, disruptive, and distressing symptom because it interferes with self-care activities.

Allow Expression of Feelings Regarding the Effects of Fatigue on Life

Assist the Client to Identify Strengths, Abilities, and Interests

- Identify areas of success and usefulness; emphasize past accomplishments.
- Assist the client in developing realistic short- and long-term goals (progress from simple to more complex; use a "goals poster" to indicate type and time for achieving specific goals).

  R: Focusing the client on strengths and abilities may provide insight into positive events and lessen the tendency to overgeneralize the severity of disease, which can lead to depression.

- Help the client identify how he or she can help others (e.g., listening to clients' problems, using the computer to access information, making phone calls).

  R: Reciprocity or returning support to one's support system is vital for balanced and healthy relationships (Tilden & Weinert, 1987).

  R: Clients with fatigue have difficulty with reciprocity.

Assist the Client to Identify Energy Patterns

- Analyze together the 24-hour fatigue levels using a scale of 0–10 (10 = severe fatigue).
  - Times of peak energy
  - Times of exhaustion
  - Activities associated with increasing fatigue

Explain the Purpose of Pacing and Prioritization

- Explore what activities the client views as important to maintain self-esteem.
- Attempt to divide vital activities or tasks into components (e.g., preparing menu, shopping, storing, cooking, serving, cleaning up); the client can delegate some parts and retain others.
- Plan important tasks during periods of high energy (e.g., prepare all meals in the morning).

R: Quality or type of activity reportedly is more important than quantity. Informal activities promoted well-being the most, followed by formal structured activities, and last by solitary activities, which were found to have little or no effect on life satisfaction (Longino & Kart, 1982).

Teach Energy Conservation Techniques

- Modify the environment.
  - Replace steps with ramps.
  - Install grab rails.
  - Elevate chairs 3 to 4 inches.
  - Organize kitchen or work areas.
  - Reduce trips up and down stairs (e.g., put a commode on the first floor).

- Use a taxi instead of driving self.
- Delegate housework (e.g., employ a high-school student for a few hours after school).

R: Strategies can be utilized to decrease energy used in activities of daily living.

- Discuss with individual some type of appropriate exercise component that could be integrated into his or her life.

R: Research has shown that exercise lowers levels of fatigue and improved quality of life for persons with cancer (Conn et al., 2006).

Provide Significant Others Opportunities to Discuss Feelings in Private Regarding:

- Changes in person with fatigue
- Caretaking responsibilities
- Financial issues
- Changes in lifestyle, role responsibilities, and relationships
- See *Caregiver Role Strain* for additional strategies for caregivers if indicated.

TRANSITION PLAN
Initiate health teaching and referrals as indicated.
- Counseling
- Community services (Meals On Wheels, housekeeper)
- Financial assistance

Clinical Alert Report

- Advise ancillary staff / student to report c/o of increased fatigue or reluctance to ambulate.
  R: Increase fatigue needs further assessment by the nurse to r/o infection, overexertion, dehydration, nutritional deficits.

DEFICIENT FLUID VOLUME

NANDA-I Definition

Decreased intravascular, interstitial, and / or intracellular fluid. This refers to dehydration, water loss alone without change in sodium

Carp's Cues

Deficient Fluid Volume frequently is used to describe people who are NPO, in hypovolemic shock, or experiencing bleeding. This author recommends its use only when a client can drink but has an insufficient intake for metabolic needs. If the client cannot drink or needs intravenous therapy, refer to the collaborative problems in Section 2: *Risk for Complications of Hypovolemia* and *Risk for Complications of Electrolyte Imbalances*.

Defining Characteristics

Major (Must Be Present, One or More)

Insufficient oral fluid intake   Dry skin* / mucous membranes*
Negative balance of intake and output   Weight loss

Minor (May Be Present)

Increased serum sodium

Concentrated urine or urinary frequency

Thirst* / nausea / anorexia

Decreased urine output* or excessive urine output

Related Factors

Pathophysiologic

Related to excessive urinary output (e.g., uncontrolled diabetes, diabetes insipidus)

Related to increased capillary permeability and evaporative loss from burn wound (nonacute)

Related to losses secondary to (e.g., abnormal drainage, diarrhea, excessive menses, fever or increased metabolic rate)

Situational (Personal, Environmental)

Related to nausea / vomiting

Related to decreased motivation to drink liquids secondary to (e.g., depression, fatigue)

Related to high-solute tube feedings

Related to difficulty swallowing or feeding self secondary to (e.g., oral or throat pain, fatigue)

Related to excessive loss through (specify)

Related to excessive use of (e.g., laxatives or enemas, diuretics, alcohol, or caffeine)

Older Adult

Related to increased vulnerability secondary to decreased fluid reserve and decreased sensation of thirst

Goal

NOC
Electrolyte and Acid–Base Balance, Fluid Balance, Hydration

The client will maintain urine-specific gravity within normal range as evidenced by the following indicators:

- Increase fluid intake to a specified amount according to age and metabolic needs.
- Identify risk factors for fluid deficit and relate need for increased fluid intake as indicated.
- Demonstrate no signs and symptoms of dehydration.

Interventions

NIC
Fluid/Electrolyte Management, Fluid Monitoring

Assess Causative Factors

Prevent Dehydration in High-Risk Clients

- Monitor client intake; ensure at least 2,000 mL of oral fluids every 24 hours unless contraindicated. Offer fluids that are desired hourly.
- Teach the client to avoid coffee, tea, grapefruit juice, sugared drinks, and alcohol.

  R: Output may exceed intake, which already may be inadequate to compensate for insensible losses.

  R: Large amounts of sugar, alcohol, and caffeine act as diuretics that increase urine production and may cause dehydration.

- Monitor output; ensure at least 0.5 mL/kg per hour.

  R: Monitoring of output will help to evaluate hydration status early.

- Weigh the client daily at the same time. A 2% to 4% weight loss indicates mild dehydration; 5% to 9% weight loss indicates moderate dehydration.

  R: To monitor weight effectively, weight should be measured at the same time on the same scale with the same clothes.

- Monitor urine and serum electrolytes, blood urea nitrogen, osmolality, creatinine, hematocrit, and hemoglobin.

  R: These laboratory studies will reflect hydration status.

- Advise older people scheduled to fast before diagnostic studies to increase fluid intake 8 hours before fasting.

  R: This will reduce the risks of dehydration.

- Review the client's medications. Do the medications contribute to dehydration (e.g., diuretics)? Do they require increased fluid intake (e.g., lithium)?

  R: Certain medications can contribute to dehydration.

TRANSITION PLAN

Initiate health teaching as indicated.

- Give verbal and written directions for types of fluids and amounts needed at home.
- Include the client / family in keeping a written record of fluid intake, output, and daily weights, if indicated.
- Explain the need to increase fluids during exercise, fever, infection, and hot weather.
- Teach the client / family how to observe for dehydration (especially in infants, elderly) and to intervene by increasing fluid intake.

  R: Careful monitoring after discharge will be needed for at-risk clients.

Clinical Alert Report

- Advise ancillary staff / student to report a decrease in usual urine output and oral intake.

  R: Early signs of changes in fluid intake can be addressed before dehydration occurs.

Documentation

- Intake, output flow records

EXCESS FLUID VOLUME

NANDA-I Definition

Increased isotonic fluid retention

Carp's Cues

Excess Fluid Volume is frequently used to describe pulmonary edema, ascites, or renal failure. These are all collaborative problems that should not be renamed as *Excess Fluid Volume*. Refer to Section 2 for collaborative problems such as *Risk for complications of renal / urinary dysfunction* or *pulmonary edema* or *hepatic dysfunction*. The interventions below focus on preventing or reducing peripheral edema. Nursing interventions center on teaching the client or family how to minimize edema and protect tissue.

Defining Characteristics

Major (Must Be Present, One or More)

Edema (peripheral, sacral)
Taut, shiny skin

Minor (May Be Present)

Intake greater than output
Weight gain

Related Factors

Pathophysiologic

Related to portal hypertension, lower plasma colloidal osmotic pressure, and sodium retention secondary to:

Liver disease   Cirrhosis   Ascites

Cancer

Related to venous and arterial abnormalities secondary to:

Varicose veins	Phlebitis	Infection
Peripheral vascular disease	Immobility	Trauma
Thrombus	Lymphedema	Neoplasms

Treatment Related

Related to sodium and water retention secondary to corticosteroid therapy
Related to inadequate lymphatic drainage secondary to mastectomy

Situational (Personal, Environmental)

Related to excessive sodium intake / fluid intake
Related to a malnutrition
Related to dependent venous pooling / venostasis secondary to (e.g., standing or sitting for long periods, immobility, tight cast or bandage)
Related to venous compression from pregnant uterus
Related to impaired venous return secondary to increased peripheral resistance and decreased efficiency of valves secondary to (e.g., aging, obesity)

Goals

NOC
Electrolyte Balance,
Fluid Balance, Hydration

The client will exhibit decreased edema (specify site), as evidenced by the following indicators:

- Relate causative factors.
- Relate methods of preventing edema.

Interventions

NIC
Electrolyte
Management, Fluid
Management, Fluid
Monitoring, Skin
Surveillance, Nutritional
Counseling, Weight
Reduction Assistance

Identify Contributing and Causative Factors

- Refer to Related Factors.

Reduce or Eliminate Causative and Contributing Factors

High Salt Diet
- Request a consult of nutritionist.
- Explain why salt intake contributes to leg edema.

  R: Excess dietary salt causes fluid retention, which increases capillary filtration pressure, which results in peripheral edema.

- Assess dietary intake and habits that may contribute to fluid retention.
- Explain high-sodium foods, including salted snacks, bacon, cheese, olives, pickles, soy sauce, processed lunchmeats, monosodium glutamate (MSG), canned vegetables, ketchup, and mustard.
- Teach how to read labels for sodium content. Go to thePoint at http://thePoint.lww.com/Carpenito6e for a printout of Getting Started to Decrease Salt in Foods.
- Avoid canned vegetables; choose fresh or frozen.
- Cook without salt; use spices (e.g., lemon, basil, tarragon, mint) to add flavor.

- Use vinegar in place of salt to flavor soups, stews, etc. (e.g., 2 to 3 teaspoons of vinegar to 4 to 6 quarts, according to taste).
- Ascertain whether the client may use salt substitute (caution that he or she must use the exact substitute prescribed).

R: High-sodium intake leads to increased water retention. Drugs, such as antacids, are also high in sodium.

Dependent Venous Pooling

- Assess for evidence of dependent venous pooling or venous stasis.
- Encourage alternating periods of horizontal rest (legs elevated) with vertical activity (standing); this may be contraindicated in CHF.
  - Keep the edematous extremity elevated above the level of the heart whenever possible (unless contraindicated by heart failure).
  - Keep the edematous arms elevated on two pillows or with IV pole sling.
  - Elevate the legs whenever possible, using pillows under them (avoid pressure points, especially behind the knees).
  - Discourage leg and ankle crossing.

  R: These strategies reduce venous stasis by promoting lymphatic flow movement back into circulatory system.

- Reduce constriction of vessels.
  - Assess clothing for proper fit and constrictive areas.
  - Instruct the client to avoid panty girdles / garters, knee-highs, and leg crossing and to practice elevating the legs when possible.
- Consider using antiembolism stockings or Ace bandages; measure the legs carefully for stockings / support hose.*
- Apply stockings while lying down (e.g., in the morning before arising).
- Check extremities frequently for adequate circulation and evidence of constrictive areas.
- Explain the effects of excess weight on edema.

  R: Edema inhibits blood flow to the tissue, resulting in poor cellular nutrition and increased susceptibility to injury. Compression stockings increase venous return. Obesity interferes with venous return.

Venous Pressure Points

- Assess for venous pressure points associated with casts, bandages, and tight stockings.
  - Observe circulation at edges of casts, bandages, and stockings.
  - For casts, insert soft material to cushion pressure points at the edges.
- Check circulation frequently.
- Shift body weight in the cast to redistribute weight within (unless contraindicated).
  - Encourage client to do this every 15 to 30 minutes while awake to prevent venostasis.
  - Encourage wiggling of fingers or toes and isometric exercise of unaffected muscles within the cast.
  - If the client cannot do this alone, assist him or her at least hourly to shift body weight.

  R: These strategies increase circulation and venous return.

Inadequate Lymphatic Drainage

Refer to Breast Surgery Care Plan for specific interventions to prevent injury to extremity(ies).

- Explain the reason for the lymphatic drainage (e.g., trauma, surgery). Emphasize the need to prevent injury and infection.
- Keep the extremity elevated on pillows.
  - If the edema is marked, the arm should be elevated, *but not in adduction* (this position may constrict the axilla).
  - The elbow should be higher than the shoulder.
  - The hand should be higher than the elbow.
- Measure blood pressure in the unaffected arm.
- Do not give injections or start IV fluids in the affected arm.
- Protect affected limb from injury.
- Teach the client to avoid using strong detergents, carrying heavy bags, holding cigarettes, injuring cuticles or hangnails, reaching into hot ovens, wearing jewelry or a wristwatch, or using Ace bandages.

- Advise the client to apply lanolin or a similar cream, often daily, to prevent dry, flaky skin.
- Encourage the client to wear a Medic-Alert tag engraved with *Caution: lymphedema arm—no tests / no needle injections*.
- Caution the client to visit a physician if the arm becomes red, swollen, or unusually hard.
- After a mastectomy, encourage ROM exercises and use of the affected arm to facilitate development of a collateral lymphatic drainage system (explain that lymphedema often decreases within 1 month, but that the client should continue massaging, exercising, and elevating the arm for 3 to 4 months after surgery).

R: Compromised lymph drainage compromises the body defenses against infection. Trauma to tissue can increase lymphedema.

> **CLINICAL ALERT**
> - Promptly report any change in skin integrity. Immediate attention is needed to prevent serious complication (e.g., cellulitis, abscesses, thrombosis).

Immobility

- Plan passive or active ROM exercises for all extremities every 4 hours, including dorsiflexion of the foot to massage veins.
- Change the client's position at least every 2 hours, using the four positions (left side, right side, back, abdomen), if not contraindicated (see *Impaired Skin Integrity*).
- If the client must remain in high Fowler's position, assess for edema of buttocks and sacral area; help the client shift body weight every 2 hours to prevent pressure on edematous tissue.

R: Contracting skeletal muscles increases lymph flow. Exercise increases muscle efficiency.

Protect Edematous Skin From Injury

- Inspect skin for redness and blanching.
- Reduce pressure on skin areas; pad chairs; use knee-high stockings and footstools.
- Prevent dry skin.
- Use soap sparingly.
- Rinse off soap completely.
- Use a lotion to moisten skin.

R: Edema inhibits blood flow to the tissues, resulting in poor cellular nutrition and increased susceptibility to injury.

> **TRANSITION PLAN**
> Initiate health teaching and referrals as indicated.
> - Consider home care or visiting nurses referral to follow at home.
> - Give clear verbal and written instructions for all medications: what, when, how often, why, side effects; pay special attention to drugs that directly influence fluid balance (e.g., diuretics, steroids).
> - Write down instructions for diet, activity, and use of Ace bandages, stockings, etc.
> - Have the client demonstrate the instructions.
> - Instruct to weigh self daily and record the weight.
> - Instruct to call a primary care provider for a weight gain greater than 2 pounds per day or increased shortness of breath at night or on exertion. Explain that these signs may indicate early heart problems and will require medication to prevent them from worsening.
>
> *R: Home management of edema will require specific instructions and monitoring. Readmission for CHF is often due to failure to take medications or ignoring early signs of an exacerbation.*

> ### *Clinical Alert Report*
> * Advise ancillary staff / student to report any signs / symptoms of edema, redness, tissue irritation / breakdown.
>   *R: Ancillary staff can assess for changes in skin / tissue when providing care (e.g., bathing.)*

RISK FOR IMBALANCED FLUID VOLUME

NANDA-I Definition

At risk for a decrease, increase, or rapid shift from one to the other of intravascular, interstitial, and / or intracellular fluid that may compromise health. This refers to body fluid loss, gain, or both.

Risk Factors*

Abdominal surgery   Pancreatitis
Receiving apheresis   Intestinal obstruction
Sepsis   Ascites
Burns   Traumatic injury (e.g., fractured hip)

Carp's Cues

This diagnosis can represent several clinical conditions, such as edema, hemorrhage, dehydration, and compartmental syndrome. If the nurse is monitoring a client for imbalanced fluid volume, labeling the specific imbalance as a collaborative problem, such as hypovolemia, compartment syndrome, increased intracranial pressure, gastrointestinal bleeding, or postpartum hemorrhage, would be more useful clinically. For example, most intraoperative clients would be monitored for hypovolemia. If the procedure were neurosurgery, then cranial pressure would also be monitored. If the procedure were orthopedic, compartment syndrome would be addressed.

GRIEVING

NANDA-I Definition

A normal complex process that includes emotional, physical, spiritual, social, and intellectual responses and behaviors by which individuals, families, and communities, incorporate an actual, anticipated, or perceived loss into their daily lives.

Defining Characteristics

Major (Must Be Present)

The client reports an actual or perceived loss (person, pet, object, function, status, or relationship) with varied responses such as the following:

Denial   Disorganization
Suicidal thoughts   Feelings of worthlessness
Guilt   Numbness
Crying   Disbelief
Anger   Anxiety
Sorrow   Helplessness
Despair

Related Factors

Many situations can contribute to feelings of loss. Some common situations follow.

Pathophysiologic

Related to loss of function or independence secondary to:

Loss of body part (planned, sudden)
Congenital anomaly
Sudden loss of function (e.g., amputation, ostomy)
Illness
Trauma
Visible scars

Treatment Related

Related to losses associated with:

Long-term dialysis
Surgery (e.g., mastectomy)

Situational (Personal, Environmental)

Related to losses associated with the death of (e.g., someone, pet)
Related to the losses associated with (e.g., chronic pain, terminal illness)
Related to losses in lifestyle associated with (e.g., empty nest, divorce, separation)

Maturational

Related to losses / changes attributed to aging as:

Friends
Function
Relocation (e.g., assisted living, living with adult children)
Occupation, retirement

 Carp's Cues

Grieving, Anticipatory, and *Complicated Grieving* represent three types of responses of individuals or families experiencing a loss. *Grieving* describes normal grieving after a loss and participation in grief work. *Anticipatory Grieving* describes engaging in grief work before an expected loss. Refer to Palliative Care Plan for Interventions for Anticipated Grieving *Complicated Grieving* represents a maladaptive process in which grief work is suppressed or absent or a client exhibits prolonged exaggerated responses. The nurse should consult with physician / NP for a mental health consultation.

In many clinical situations, the nurse expects a grief response (e.g., loss of body part, death of significant other). Other situations that evoke strong grief responses are sometimes ignored or minimized (e.g., abortion, newborn death, death of one twin or triplet, death of secret lover, suicide, loss of children to foster homes, or adoption).

Goals

NOC
Coping, Family Coping, Grief Resolution, Psychosocial Adjustment, Life Change

• The client will express his or her grief.

Indicators

• Describe the meaning of the death or loss to him or her.
• Share his or her grief with significant others.

Interventions

Promote a Trust Relationship

Carp's Cues

Too often nurses believe that they must have the answers for individuals who are suffering. This belief creates a barrier and the nurse is afraid she or he will say the wrong thing, so nothing is said. A nurse can gently touch a grieving person and say, "I am sorry for your loss," "I am so sorry you have cancer." This communication can create a flood of emotion and tears. This nurse should be proud that she or he is willing to enter this darkness because the true professional nurse is one who can sit in the cave of darkness and not talk about the light.

- Create a therapeutic milieu (convey that you care). "I am sorry." Provide a presence of simply "being" with the bereaved.
- Communicate clearly, simply, and to the point.
- Never try to lessen the loss (e.g., "She didn't suffer long"; or "You can have another baby").
- Offer support and reassurance.
- Establish a safe, secure, and private environment.
- Provide privacy but be careful not to isolate the client or family inadvertently.

R: Grief work cannot begin until the client acknowledges the loss. Nurses can encourage this acknowledgment by engaging in open, honest dialogue, providing the family an opportunity to view the dead person, and recognizing and validating the grief (Vanezis & McGee, 1999).

> **CLINICAL ALERT**
>
> The following tasks of *Grieving* have been identified by Worden (2002) and can assist the nurse in identifying the client's current progression in the grief process:
>
> Task 1: To accept the reality of loss
> Task 2: To feel the pain of grief
> Task 3: To adjust to an environment in which the deceased is missing
> Task 4: To emotionally relocate the deceased and move on with life

Assess the Present Grief Response

- Ambivalence, Anger, Denial, Depression, Fear, Guilt

Explain the Normalcy of the Emotional and Physical Responses to a Significant Loss

- Emotional Responses: Numbness, shock, anger, frustration, irritation, misdirected hostility, denial, sadness, fear, loneliness, relief, guilt, yearning, helplessness, out of control, "Nothing seems real."
- Physical responses: Shakiness, edginess, insomnia, lack of energy, weakness
- Dry mouth, increased perspiration, stomach hollowness, "butterflies"
- Headache, chest or throat pain or tightness, breathlessness

R: Research findings have refuted the notion that grief is neat, orderly, linear, and completed at an arbitrary point (Wright & Hogan, 2008). Acknowledging that grief responses are expected and normal can support an anxious, grieving client (Hooyman & Kramer, 2006).

R: Grief in older adults is often related to losses within the self, such as changes in roles or body image or decreased body function. These losses sometimes are less easily accepted than is the loss of a significant other (Miller, 2009).

Demonstrate Respect for the Client's Culture, Religion, and Values

R: Bereavement is a universal stressor, but the magnitude of stress and its meaning vary cross-culturally. The dominant US culture assumes that the death of a child is more stressful than that of an older relative. This belief can encourage nurses to ignore the profound grief when one loses an older mother or father.

Promote Family Cohesiveness

R: Understanding and strengthening families at the end of life and during bereavement are essential for health maintenance or restoration (O'Mallon, 2009).

- Support the family at its level of functioning.

    R: Each family member has his or her own perception of making sense of a loved one's death (O'Mallon, 2009).

- Encourage self-exploration of feelings with family members.

- Explain the need to discuss behaviors that interfere with relationships.

- Recognize and reinforce the strengths of each family member.

    R: Social supports, strong religious beliefs, and good prior mental health are resources that decrease psychosocial and physical dysfunction (Hooyman & Kramer, 2006; Miller, 2009).

CLINICAL ALERT

Complicated / unresolved grief may be difficult to determine because the grief experience has no clearly defined end point, nor is there a "right way" to grieve (Varcarolis, 2011). Some people do experience factors that interfere with the natural progress of grief work and, therefore, its resolution. Rando (1984) outlines eight variations of unresolved grief:

1. *Absent grief*: as if the death had never occurred
2. *Inhibited grief*: can mourn only certain aspects of the loss
3. *Delayed grief*: cannot experience grief at the time of loss (e.g., "I must be strong for my children now.")
4. *Conflicted grief*: often associated with a previous dependent or ambivalent relationship
5. *Chronic grief*: ongoing intense grief reaction, sometimes serves to keep the deceased "alive" through grief
6. *Unanticipated grief*: cannot grasp the full implications of loss; extreme bewilderment, anxiety, self-reproach, and depression
7. *Abbreviated grief*: often confused with unresolved grief, this shortened but normal form of grief might occur when significant grief work has been done before the loss
8. *Disenfranchised grief*: usually associated with a socially unacceptable or negated loss (e.g., suicide, AIDS)

Identify Clients at High Risk for Complicated Grieving Reactions

Identify Predisposing Factors Attributed to *Complicated Grieving* as Follows (Bateman, 1999; Worden, 2002)

- A socially unspeakable or negated loss (e.g., suicide, AIDS-related death, illegal substance abuse)

    R: Rando (1984) describes the social factors that can contribute to unresolved grief such as social negation of the loss (e.g., abortion, newborn, death of twin, death of frail elderly parent) and socially defined as inappropriate to discuss (e.g., death of lover, suicide).

- New feelings of dependency and neediness associated with the loss
- History of depressive illness or previous complicated grief reactions
- Sudden, uncertain, or overcomplicated circumstances surrounding the loss
- A highly ambivalent, narcissistic, or dependent relationship with the deceased

    R: The more dependent the client was on the deceased person, the more difficult the resolution (Varcarolis, 2011).

- Family conflicts

    R: Unresolved conflicts disrupt successful grief work (Varcarolis, 2011).

- Isolation: geographical, social, emotional

CLINICAL ALERT
Gay men who have experienced multiple AIDS-related losses (e.g., loss of friends and community, disintegrating family structures, and social networks) may receive little understanding from heterosexuals (Cotton et al., 2006; Mallinson, 1999). Disenfranchised grief occurs when social stigma is associated with a death or illness (e.g., illegal behavior, suicide, AIDS); the client may be alone, emotionally isolated, or fearful of public expressions of grief (Bateman, 1999).

Refer High-Risk Individuals / Families for Counseling

R: Research validates that professional interventions and professionally supported voluntary and self-help services are capable of reducing the risk of psychiatric and psychoanalytic disorders resulting from bereavement (Bonanno & Lilienfeld, 2008; Boyd, 2005). Promote Physical Well-Being: Nutrition, Sleep / Rest, Exercise for Survivors of Suicide.

Provide Health Teaching and Referrals, as Indicated

Advise to Make an Appointment with Primary Care Provider

Teach the Client and Family Signs of Resolution

- Grieving client no longer lives in the past but is future oriented and establishes new goals.
- Grieving client redefines relationship with the lost object / person.
- Grieving client begins to resocialize.

Identify Agencies that May be Helpful (e.g., Community Agencies, Religious Groups)

RISK FOR COMPROMISED HUMAN DIGNITY

NANDA-I Definition

At risk for perceived loss of respect and honor

Risk Factors

Treatment Related

Related to multiple factors associated with hospitalization, institutionalization, supervised group living environments, or any health care environment.

Examples of factors are:

- Unfamiliar procedures
- Intrusions for clinical procedures
- Multiple, unfamiliar personnel
- Assistance needed for personal hygiene
- Painful procedures
- Unfamiliar terminology

Situational (Personal, Environmental)

Related to the nature of restrictions and environment of incarceration

Carp's Cues

Risk for compromised human dignity was accepted by NANDA-I in 2006.

This nursing diagnosis presents a new application for nursing practice. All clients are at risk for this diagnosis. Providing respect and honor to all clients, families, and communities is a critical core element of professional nursing. Prevention of compromised human dignity must be a focus of all nursing interventions. It is the central concept of a caring profession.

This author recommends that this diagnosis be developed and integrated into a Standard Care of the Nursing Department for all clients and families. The outcomes and interventions apply to all individuals, families, and groups. This Department of Nursing Standards of Practice could also include *Risk for Infection*, *Risk for Infection Transmission*, *Risk for Falls*, and *Risk for Compromised Family Coping*.

Goal

Refer to Generic Medical Care Plan.

Interventions

Refer to Generic Medical Care Plan.

BOWEL INCONTINENCE

NANDA-I Definition

Change in normal bowel habits characterized by involuntary passage of stool

Defining Characteristics*

Constant dribbling of soft stool
Fecal odor
Fecal staining of bedding
Fecal staining of clothing
Inability to delay defecation
Inability to recognize urge to defecate
Inattention to urge to defecate
Recognizes rectal fullness but reports inability to expel formed stool
Red perianal skin
Self-report of inability to recognize rectal fullness
Urgency

Related Factors

Pathophysiologic

Related to rectal sphincter abnormality secondary to:

Anal or rectal surgery   Obstetric injuries
Peripheral neuropathy   Anal or rectal injury

Related to overdistention of rectum secondary to chronic constipation
Related to loss of rectal sphincter control* secondary to:

Cerebral vascular accident   Spinal cord compression
Spinal cord injury   Multiple sclerosis
Progressive neuromuscular disorder

Related to impaired reservoir capacity* secondary to chronic rectal ischemia, inflammatory bowel disease

Treatment Related

Related to impaired reservoir capacity secondary to colectomy, radiation proctitis*

Situational (Personal, Environmental)

Related to inability to recognize, interpret, or respond to rectal cues secondary to impaired cognition, depression*

Goal

NOC
Bowel Continence,
Tissue Integrity

The client will evacuate a soft, formed stool every other day or every third day:

- Relate bowel elimination techniques.
- Describe fluid and dietary requirements.

Interventions

NIC
Bowel Incontinence
Care, Bowel Training,
Bowel Management,
Skin Surveillance

Assess Contributing Factors

- Refer to Related Factors.

Assess the Client's Ability to Participate in Bowel Continence

- Ability to reach toilet
- Control of rectal sphincter
- Intact anorectal sensation
- Orientation, motivation

R: To maintain bowel continence, a client must have access to a toileting facility, be able to contract puborectals and external anal sphincter muscles, have intact anorectal sensation, be able to store feces consciously, and must be motivated and able to recognize bowel cues.

Plan a Consistent, Appropriate Time for Elimination

- Institute a daily bowel program for 5 days or until a pattern develops, then move to an alternate-day program (morning or evening).
- Provide privacy and a nonstressful environment.
- Offer reassurance and protect from embarrassment while establishing the bowel program.

    R: Long-standing constipation or fecal impaction causes overdistention of the rectum by feces. This causes continuous reflex stimulation, which reduces sphincter tone. Incontinence will be either diarrhea leaking around the impaction or leaking of feces from a full rectum.

- Implement prompted voiding program.

    R: Research has shown prompted voiding results in an increase in bowel continence.

- Assess perirectal tissue.

    R: GI enzymes can erode tissue, cause discomfort, and increase the risk of infections.

Consult With Physical Therapy for a Bowel Elimination Program

Explain Fluid and Dietary Requirements for Good Bowel Movements

- Ensure that client drinks 8 to 10 glasses of water daily.
- Design a diet high in bulk and fiber. Refer to *Constipation* for specific dietary instructions.

    R: Stool consistency and volume are important for continence. Large volumes of loose stool overwhelm the continence mechanism. Small, hard stools that do not distend or stimulate the rectum do not alert the client of the need to defecate. (Bliss et al., 2001)

- Teach the client about caffeine and explain why it should be avoided.

    R: Research demonstrates that caffeine increases urgency and bowel incontinence (Hansen et al., 2006).

Explain Effects of Activity on Peristalsis

* Assist in determining the appropriate exercises for the client's functional ability.

    R: Exercise increases gastrointestinal motility and improves bowel function.

TRANSITION PLAN

Initiate health teaching as indicated.

* Explain the hazards of using stool softeners, laxatives, suppositories, and enemas.
* Explain the signs and symptoms of fecal impaction and constipation.
* Ensure comprehension of a bowel program before discharge. If the client is functionally able, encourage independence with the bowel program; if not, incorporate assistive devices or attendant care, as needed.
* Explain the effects of stool on the skin and ways to protect the skin (refer to *Diarrhea* for interventions).

    R: Laxatives cause unscheduled bowel movements, loss of colon tone, and inconsistent stool consistency. Enemas can overstretch the bowel and decrease tone. Stool softeners are not needed with adequate food or fluid intake.

Clinical Alert Report

* Advise ancillary staff / student to report the number of bowel movements, character, and skin condition.

    R: Ancillary staff are present for toileting activities and can be directed to assess for changes.

RISK FOR INFECTION

NANDA-I Definition

At risk for being invaded by pathogenic organisms

Risk Factors

See Related Factors.

Related Factors

Various health problems and situations can create favorable conditions that would encourage the development of infections.* Some common factors follow.

Pathophysiologic

Related to compromised host defenses secondary to:

Cancer	Altered or insufficient leukocytes	Arthritis
Respiratory disorders	Periodontal disease	Renal failure
Hematologic disorders	Hepatic disorders	Diabetes mellitus*

AIDS
Alcoholism
Immunosuppression*
Immunodeficiency secondary to (specify)

Related to compromised circulation secondary to:

Lymphedema   Obesity*   Peripheral vascular disease

Treatment Related

Related to a site for organism invasion secondary to:

Surgery	Invasive lines	Dialysis
Intubation	Total parenteral nutrition	Enteral feedings

Related to compromised host defenses secondary to:

Radiation therapy
Organ transplant
Medication therapy (specify) (e.g., chemotherapy, immunosuppressants)

Situational (Personal, Environmental)

Related to compromised host defenses secondary to:

History of infections	Malnutrition*	Prolonged immobility
Stress	Increased hospital stay	Smoking

Related to a site for organism invasion secondary to:

Trauma (accidental, intentional)	Postpartum period
Bites (animal, insect, human)	Thermal injuries
Warm, moist, dark environment (skin folds, casts)	

Related to contact with contagious agents (nosocomial or community acquired)

Goal

NOC
Infection
Severity, Wound
Healing: Primary
Intention, Immune
Status, Knowledge
Infection Control

The person will report risk factors associated with infection and precautions needed as evidenced by the following indicators:

- Demonstrate meticulous hand-washing technique by the time of discharge.
- Describe methods of transmission of infection.
- Describe the influence of nutrition on prevention of infection.

Interventions

NIC
Infection Control,
Infection Protection,
Wound Care,
Incision Site Care,
Health Education,
Environmental
Management: Worker
Safety, Environmental
Management

Identify Clients at High Risk for Health Care Acquired Infections (HAI)

Use Appropriate Universal Precautions for Every Client

R: Assume everyone is potentially infected or colonized with an organism that could be transmitted in the health care setting (Siegel, 2007).

- Hand hygiene
  - Wash hands before and after all contact with client, objects in room, and specimens.
    R: Hand washing is one of the most important means to prevent the spread of infection.
  - Use with soap and water. If hands were not in contact with anyone or thing in the client's room, use an alcohol-based hand rub (Siegel, 2007).
- Personal protective equipment (PPE)
  - Wear PPE when the client interaction indicates that contact with blood / body fluids may occur.
    R: This will prevent contamination of clothing and skin during the process of care.
  - Before leaving room, remove and discard all PPE in the room or cubicle.

- Gloves
  - Wears gloves when providing direct client care.

    R: Gloves provide a barrier from contact with infectious secretions and excretions.

    - Wear gloves for potential contact with nonintact skin, mucous membranes blood, and body fluids. Handle the blood of all clients as potentially infectious.
    - Remove gloves properly to prevent hand contamination. Deposit gloves in the proper container in the client's room.
    - After removing gloves, wash hands with soap and water.
    - Do not substitute alcohol-based hand rubs when the physical action of washing and rinsing hands with antimicrobial or nonantimicrobial soap and water is needed. Alcohol, chlorhexidine, and other antiseptic agents have poor activity against some organisms (e.g., spores *C. difficile*) (Siegel, 2007, p. 78).
- Masks
  - Use PPE (masks, goggles, face shields) to protect the mucous membranes of your eyes, mouth, nose during procedures and client-care activities that may generate splashes or sprays of blood, body fluids, secretions, and excretions.
- Gowns
  - Wear a gown for direct contact with uncontained secretions or excretions.

    R: Gowns are needed to prevent soiling or contamination of clothing during procedures and client-care activities.

    - Remove gown and perform hand hygiene before leaving the client's room / cubicle.
    - Do not reuse gowns even with the same client.

R: These precautions prevent the transmission of pathogens to the caregiver and then to others (e.g., other clients, visitors, other staff).

Educate All Staff, Visitors, Clients on the Importance Preventing Droplet and Formit Transmission From Themselves to Others

- Offer a surgical mask to persons who are coughing.

  R: Surgical masks decrease contamination of the surrounding environment.

- Cover the mouth and nose during coughing and sneezing.
- Use tissues to contain respiratory secretions with prompt disposal into a no-touch receptacle. Wash hands with soap and water.
- Turn the head away from others and maintain spatial buffer, ideally >3 feet, when coughing.

R: These measures are targeted to all clients with symptoms of respiratory infection and their accompanying family members or friends beginning at the point of initial encounter with a health care setting (e.g., reception / triage in emergency departments, ambulatory clinics, health care provider offices) (www.cdc.gov/flu/professionals/infection-control/resphygiene.htm).

> **CLINICAL ALERT**
> - If a client or visitors refuse to comply with infection prevention requirements, report situation to manager or infection control officer.

Determine the Client Placement Based on (Siegel, 2007, p. 81):

- Route of transmission of known or suspected infectious agent
- Risk factors for transmission in the infected client
- Risk factors for adverse outcomes resulting from an HAI in other clients in the area or room
- Availability of single-client rooms
- Client options for room-sharing (e.g., placing clients with the same infection in the same room)

> **CLINICAL ALERT**
> - Immediately report any situation that increases the risk of infection transmission to clients, visitors, or staff.

Assess Client Care Equipment, Instruments, Devices, Environment for Contamination From Blood or Body Fluids. Follow Policies and Procedures for Containing, Transporting, Handling, Cleaning

Prior to Confirmation of Infectious Agent, Initiate Specific Precautions for the Suspected Agent:

- Meningitis: droplet, airborne precautions
- Maculopapular rash with cough, fever
- Rubella: airborne precautions
- Abscess
- MRSA: contact, droplet precautions
- Cough / fever / pulmonary infiltrate in HIV infected or someone high risk of HIV infection
- Tuberculosis: airborne / contact (respirators)

R: Prevention strategies are indicated when high-risk infections are suspected but not yet confirmed.

Reduce Entry of Organisms Into Clients

Surgical Site Infection (SSI)

- Identify individuals at high risk for delayed wound healing:
  - Malnourishment
  - Tobacco use
  - Obesity
  - Anemia
  - Diabetes
  - Cancer
  - Corticosteroid therapy
  - Renal insufficiency
  - Hypovolemia
  - Hypoxia
  - Surgery >3 hours
  - Night or emergency surgery
  - Zinc, copper, magnesium deficiency
  - Immune system compromise

  R: Intervention can be implemented to control or influence the degree of risk associated with predictors and confounding factors.

- Maintain normothermia
  - Monitor temperature every 4 hours; notify physician / NP if temperature is greater than 100.8° F.

  R: Hypothermia also increases the risk of surgical wound infection. Hypothermia directly impairs immune function, including T-cell-mediated antibody production.

  R: Thermoregulatory vasoconstriction decreases subcutaneous oxygen tension and increases the risk of wound infection (Sessler, 2006).

- Monitor for inadequate tissue oxygen in high-risk clients (e.g., pulse oximetry).

  R: Deceased tissue oxygen impairs tissue repair (Sessler, 2006).

- Advise smokers that the risk of wound infection is tripled in smokers (Sessler, 2006).
- Monitor for hyperglycemia in diabetic and nondiabetic clients.

  R: Surgical site infections have been found to double in both diabetic and nondiabetic postcardiac surgical clients when blood glucose exceeds 200 mg/dL in the first 48 hours (Sessler, 2006).

- Consult with physician / NP for interventions to achieve rigorous postoperative glucose control.

  R: Aggressive insulin infusion protocol has been shown to reduce wound infections, multiple organ failure, sepsis, and mortality in critical care clients (Sessler, 2006).

Reduce or Eliminate Noxious Stimuli

Pain
- Plan care to avoid unpleasant or painful procedures before meals.
- Medicate clients for pain 30 minutes before meals according to physician / NP's orders.
- Provide a pleasant, relaxed atmosphere for eating (no bedpans in sight; do not rush); try a "surprise" (e.g., flowers with meal).
- Arrange the plan of care to decrease or eliminate nauseating odors or procedures near mealtimes.

Fatigue
- Teach or assist client to rest before meals.
- Teach client to spend minimal energy preparing food (cook large quantities and freeze several meals at a time; request assistance from others).

Odor of Food
- Teach client to avoid cooking odors—frying food, brewing coffee—if possible (take a walk; select foods that can be eaten cold).
- Suggest using foods that require little cooking during periods of nausea.
- Suggest trying sour foods.

R: Unpleasant sights or odors can stimulate the vomiting center.

Decrease Stimulation of the Vomiting Center

- Reduce unpleasant sights and odors.
- Teach client to practice deep breathing and voluntary swallowing to suppress the vomiting reflex. Restrict activity.
- Offer small amounts of clear fluids and foods and beverages with ginger.

  R: Ginger has been found to be effective for treatment of nausea.

- Restrict liquids with meals to avoid overdistending the stomach; also, avoid fluids 1 hour before and after meals.
- Encourage client to sit in fresh air or use a fan to circulate air.

  R: The above strategies reduce gastric pressure and decrease stimuli that induce nausea and vomiting.

- Instruct the person to sit down after eating. Loosen clothing. Advise client to avoid lying flat for at least 2 hours after eating.

  R: A person who must rest should sit or recline so the head is at least 4 inches higher than the feet to reduce gastro reflex.

- Advise client to listen to music.

  R: Music can serve as a diversional adjunct to antiemetic therapy (Ezzone et al., 1998).

- Offer muscle relaxation and distraction techniques to adult cancer patients.
- Both muscle relaxation and distraction techniques have been found to decrease nausea and vomiting in adults receiving chemotherapy (Miller & Kearney, 2004; Vasterling et al., 1993).

> **TRANSITION PLAN**
> - Reinforce strategies utilized in hospital to prevent / reduce nausea.
> - Advise client to call primary care provider if nausea or vomiting continue or recur.

> *Clinical Alert Report*
> - Advise ancillary staff / student to report increases in nausea, decrease oral intake, and / or vomiting (description, amount, presence of blood).
>   *R: Barriers to effective nutritional intake need to be addressed. Emesis needs to be assessed for evidence of bleeding.*
> **Document**
> - Intake
> - Vomiting episodes, character of emesis

UNILATERAL NEGLECT

NANDA-I Definition

Impairment in sensory and motor response, mental representation, and special attention of the body, and the corresponding environment characterized by inattention to one side and over-attention to the opposite side. Left-side neglect is more severe and persistent than right-side neglect.

Defining Characteristics

Major (Must Be Present, One or More)

Neglect of involved body parts and / or extrapersonal space (hemispatial neglect), and / or denial of the existence of the affected limb or side of body (anosognosia)

Minor (May Be Present)

Difficulty with spatial-perceptual tasks
Hemiplegia (usually of the left side)

Related Factors

Pathophysiologic

Related to the impaired perceptual abilities secondary to:

Cerebrovascular accident (CVA)*
Brain injury / trauma
Cerebral aneurysms
Cerebral tumors

Refer to CVA for goals and interventions for *Unilateral Neglect*

IMBALANCED NUTRITION: LESS THAN BODY REQUIREMENTS

NANDA-I Definition

Intake of nutrients insufficient to meet metabolic needs

Carp's Cues

Nurses are usually the primary diagnosticians and are usually the primary professional for improving nutritional status. *Imbalanced Nutrition* is not a difficult diagnosis to validate. However, before interventions can be determined, it is necessary to identify the contributing factors, which are usually multiple and complex.

Nurses should not use this diagnosis to describe people who are NPO or cannot ingest food. For example, *Imbalanced Nutrition: Less Than Body Requirements related to parenteral therapy and NPO status.*

This diagnosis represents a situation with which nurses are intricately involved (parenteral therapy). From a nutritional perspective, however, what interventions do nurses prescribe to improve the nutritional status of an NPO client? Parenteral nutrition in a client who is NPO influences several actual or potential responses that nurses treat, representing both nursing diagnoses, such as *Risk for Infection* and *Impaired Comfort,* and the collaborative problems *RC of Hypovolemia* and *RC of Negative Nitrogen Balance.*

Many factors influence food habits and nutritional status: personal, family, cultural, financial, functional ability, nutritional knowledge, disease and injury, and treatment regimens. *Imbalanced Nutrition: Less Than Body Requirements* describes people who can ingest food but eat an inadequate or imbalanced quality or quantity. For instance, the diet may have insufficient protein or excessive fat. Quantity may be insufficient because of increased metabolic requirements (e.g., cancer, pregnancy, trauma or interference with nutrient use [e.g., impaired storage of vitamins in cirrhosis]).

Defining Characteristics

Major (Must Be Present, One or More)

The client who is not NPO reports or is found to have food intake less than the recommended daily allowance (RDA) with or without weight loss

and / or

Actual or potential metabolic needs in excess of intake with weight loss

Minor (May Be Present)

Weight 10% to 20% or more below ideal for height and frame

Triceps skinfold, mid-arm circumference, and mid-arm muscle circumference less than 60% standard measurement

Muscle weakness and tenderness

Mental irritability or confusion

Decreased serum prealbumin

Related Factors

Pathophysiologic

Related to increased caloric requirements and difficulty in ingesting sufficient calories secondary to (e.g.):

Burns (postacute phase)	Cancer	Infection
Trauma	Chemical dependence	
GI complications / deformities	AIDS	

Related to dysphasia secondary to:

CVA	Muscular dystrophy	Amyotrophic lateral sclerosis
Parkinson's disease	Cerebral palsy	Neuromuscular disorders
Möbius syndrome	Cleft lip / palate	

Related to decreased absorption of nutrients secondary to:

Crohn's disease

Lactose intolerance

Necrotizing enterocolitis

Cystic fibrosis

Related to decreased desire to eat secondary to altered level of consciousness

Related to self-induced vomiting, physical exercise in excess of caloric intake, or refusal to eat secondary to anorexia nervosa

Related to reluctance to eat for fear of poisoning secondary to paranoid behavior

Related to anorexia, excessive physical agitation secondary to bipolar disorder

Related to anorexia and diarrhea secondary to protozoal infection

Related to vomiting, anorexia, and impaired digestion secondary to pancreatitis

Related to anorexia, impaired protein and fat metabolism, and impaired storage of vitamins secondary to cirrhosis

Related to anorexia, vomiting, and impaired digestion secondary to GI malformation or necrotizing enterocolitis

Related to anorexia secondary to gastroesophageal reflux

Related to anorexia secondary to indigestion, bloating, pain

Related secondary to gastric ulcer

Treatment Related

Related to protein and vitamin requirements for wound healing and decreased intake secondary to surgery, surgical reconstruction of mouth, radiation therapy, medications (chemotherapy), wired jaw

Related to inadequate absorption as a medication side effect of (specify) (e.g., colchicine, neomycin, pyrimethamine, para-aminosalicylic acid, antacid)

Related to decreased oral intake, mouth discomfort, nausea, and vomiting secondary to (e.g., radiation therapy, tonsillectomy, chemotherapy, oral trauma)

Situational (Personal, Environmental)

Related to decreased desire to eat secondary to (specify):

Social isolation
Depression
Nausea and vomiting
Stress
Allergies
Excessive chronic alcohol intake

Related to increased metabolic rate with decreased intake secondary to the effects of substance abuse (e.g., cocaine, amphetamines)

Related to inability to procure food (physical limitation or financial or transportation problems)

Related to inability to chew (e.g., damaged or missing teeth, ill-fitting dentures)

Related to diarrhea* secondary to (specify)

Key Concepts

Nutritional Disturbances in individuals with cancer are (Cunningham & Huhmann, 2011):

- Cancer-induced alterations in nutrient intake
  - Changes in appetite
  - Changes in taste and smell
  - Early satiety
  - Cancer cachexia
  - Changes in electrolyte balance
- Cancer-induced changes in energy balance
  - Changes in energy expenditure
  - Changes in nutrient metabolism
  - Changes in GI tract
  - Changes in body storage
- Treatment-induced alterations in nutrient intake
  - Changes in appetite
- Treatment-induced changes in energy balance
  - Changes in energy expenditure
  - Changes in the GI tract

Pediatric Considerations

- Changes in nutritional needs characterize each growth period (see Table II.1).
- Nonadolescent children should not be put on diets. The goal for growing children is to maintain, not lose, weight. Healthy food choices of fruit, vegetables, and low-fat snacks (e.g., pretzels) can replace

Table II.1	Age-Related Daily Nutritional Requirements
Age	**Daily Nutritional Requirements**
Infants	*100–120 kcal/kg/day for growth*
Newborn	12–18 oz formula or breast milk
2–3 months	20–30 oz formula or breast milk
4–5 months	25–35 oz formula or breast milk; strained vegetables and fruits; egg yolks
6–7 months	28–40 oz formula or breast milk; above solids, plus meat, finger foods
8–11 months	24 oz formula or breast milk; three regular meals, chopped table food
1–2 years	24 oz formula or breast milk; 100 cal/kg same as 8–11 months
Children	
Preschool (3–5 years)	90 cal/kg; 1.2 g/kg protein Basic food groups Calcium 800 mg

School (6–12 years)	80 cal/kg; 1.2 g/kg protein
	Basic food groups (as preschool)
	    1.5–2 g calcium
	    400 units vitamin D
	    1.5–3 L water

Adolescent (13–17 years)	2,200–2,400 cal for girls
	3,000 cal for boys
	Basic food groups (as preschool)
	    50–60 g protein
	    1,200–1,500 mg calcium (to age 25)
	    400 units vitamin D

Adults	1,600 to 3,000 calorie range (based on physical activity, emotional state, body size, age, and individual metabolism) Basic food groups Men need increased protein, ascorbic acid, riboflavin, and vitamins E and B_6 Women need the above as well as increased iron, calcium, and vitamins A and B_{12}

Pregnant women (second and third trimesters)	Daily calorie requirement
	    11–15 years: 2,500
	    16–22 years: 2,400
	    23–50 years: 2,300
	Increase protein 10 g or 1 serving meat
	1.2–3.5 g calcium
	Increase vitamins A, B, and C

Lactating women	30–60 mg iron
	2,500–3,000 cal (500 more than regular diet)
	Basic food groups
	    4 servings protein
	    5 servings dairy
	    4+ servings grain
	    5+ servings vegetables
	        2+ servings vitamin C-rich
	        1+ green leafy
	        2+ others
	Fluids 2–3 qt (1 qt milk)
	Increase in vitamins A and C, niacin

Older than 65 years	Basic food groups (same as adult) Caloric requirements decrease with age (1,600–1,800 for women, 2,000–2,400 for men), but dependent on activity, climate, and metabolic needs Ensure intake of essential amino acids, fatty acids, vitamins, elements, fiber, and water 60 mg ascorbic acid 40–60 mg protein 1,200 mg calcium (1,500 mg for women not taking estrogen) 10 mg iron

foods high in salt, fats, and sugar. Refer to *Ineffective Health Maintenance* for specific interventions for weight loss.

- As BMI increases, so does the prevalence of iron deficiency in overweight children and adolescents (Nead, Halterman, Kaczorowski, Auinger, & Weitzman, 2004)

Goal

NOC
Nutritional Status,
Teaching: Nutrition,
Symptom Control

The client will ingest daily nutritional requirements in accordance with activity level and metabolic needs as evidenced by the following indicators:

- Relate importance of good nutrition. For healing and preventing complications.
- Identify deficiencies in daily intake.
- Relate methods to increase appetite.

Interventions

NIC
Nutrition Management,
Weight Gain Assistance,
Nutritional Counseling

Ensure a Nutritional Assessment Is Done on Admission According to Protocols

R: Nutritional Assessments are required within 24 hours of admission to a hospital and within 14 days of admission to a long-term facility (Joint Commission, 2010).

Evaluate the Appropriateness of Attempting to Increase Food / Fluid Intake in Individuals at the End-of-Life

R: Researchers report that "increased caloric intake may neither reverse weight loss nor improve survival" in individuals with end-stage disease (e.g., cancer, CHF, COPD, renal failure). Refer to Palliative Care Plan.

> **CLINICAL ALERT**
> - Specialized nutritional interventions "are not recommended for individuals who are adequately nourished, who are not anticipated to be unable to eat for 10 to 14 days or who have uncontrolled disease" (Macfie, 2004, as cited in Cunningham & Huhmann, 2011).
> - Consideration of these criteria may assist with ethical concerns regarding providing or withholding nutritional supplements (Cunningham & Huhmann, 2011).
> - Refer to Palliative Care Plan.

STAR   **Stop**

Think   The family is upset because Mr. Platte does not want to eat or drink. Attempts are made constantly for him to eat or drink. Mr. Platte has end-stage liver failure.

Act   Explain to family his failing condition. Gently explain that food or fluids are not going to improve his condition. Share that you have observed these attempts and that Mr. Platte becomes more agitated when attempts are made to feed him food or liquids. Explain that his body systems are now unaware of the sensation of appetite or thirst. Share that measures such as mouth care and lip lubrication can provide increased comfort.

Review   If family is insistent in continuing attempts to feed him, consult with palliative care specialist.

Carp's Cues

If you are inexperienced with this situation, do not attempt to intervene. Consult with an experienced colleague, your instructor, physician / NP.

SBAR   ***Situation:*** I am concerned about Mr. Platte, a 78-year-old man in end-stage hepatic failure. His family is trying to force him to eat and drink. He is listless and becomes agitated during these attempts. Now they are asking about a "feeding tube." All my attempts to explain his condition and his failing status have not changed their attempts.

Background: He is listless and becomes agitated during these attempts.

Assessment: The problem seems to be that the family is in denial or do not understand that food / fluids will not improve him.

Recommendation: I am requesting that you (physician / NP) speak to the family about Mr. Platte's condition and progressive deterioration. I would like to consult the palliative care specialist regarding his care.

Explain the Need for Adequate Consumption of Carbohydrates, Fats, Protein, Vitamins, Minerals, and Fluids

R: Nutrients provide energy sources, build tissue, and regulate metabolic processes.

- When indicated, consult with a nutritionist to establish appropriate daily caloric and food type requirements for the client. (Dudek, 2009; Hockenberry & Wilson, 2009).

  R: The body requires a minimum level of nutrients for health and growth. During the lifespan, nutritional needs vary.
- Assess if there are cultural preferences in regard to food.
- Address the factors that are causing or contributing to decrease intake.
  - Related to decreased oral intake, mouth discomfort, nausea, and vomiting. Secondary to (e.g., alcohol abuse, drug use, depression, side effects of treatments).
  - Related to inability to chew.
  - Access a dental consult.
  - Related to decreased oral intake, mouth discomfort, nausea, and vomiting. Secondary to (e.g., radiation therapy, tonsillectomy, chemotherapy).
  - Refer to specific care plans for radiation or chemotherapy. Refer to *Impaired Oral Mucous Membranes* in Section 1.
  - Related to factors associated with aging.

Assess for Factors That Contribute to Nutritional Deficiencies in Older Clients (Lutz & Przytulski, 2011)

- Explain that their sense of smell and taste will diminish with aging, which may result in decreased intake due to bland taste and oversalting of foods.

  R: Seventy-five percent of individuals over 85 years old have decreased sense of smell. Smell is required for the sense of taste to function (Lutz & Przytulski, 2011).
- Explain the need to drink sufficient fluids even when not thirsty. Hydration can be evaluated by color of urine (e.g., goal is light yellow).

  R: The thirst sensation is diminished and can result in uncompensated dehydration.
- Explain delayed gastric emptying can create bloating and decreased intake.

  R: Intestinal motility decreases with aging.
- Advise to reduce fluids with meals and to increase foods higher in protein (e.g., eggs, milk, cheese).
- Related to barriers of food procurement / preparation

  R: Barriers affect functional ability, financial, transportation, and kitchen facilities.
- Refer to nutritionist / social services for an assessment and interventions.

Evaluate If Lactose Intolerance Is Present

R: The prevalence of primary lactose intolerance varies according to race. As many as 25% of the white population (prevalence in those from southern European roots) is estimated to have lactose intolerance, whereas among black, Native American, and Asian American populations, the prevalence of lactose intolerance is estimated at 75% to 90%. (Roy, 2011)

Identify Factors Such as Pain, Fatigue, Analgesic Use, and Immobility That Can Contribute to Anorexia

R: Identifying a possible cause enables interventions to eliminate or minimize it.

- Provide the following generic interventions for clients with decreased appetite regardless of etiology:
  - When possible, attempt to have some socialization during mealtime (e.g., suggest to family that they eat with client if appropriate).

    R: In nursing home settings, resident's nutritional status is significantly better in those who eat in the general dining room rather than isolated in their own rooms (Simmons & Levy-Storms, 2005).
  - Encourage the client to rest before meals.

    R: Fatigue further reduces an anorectic client's desire and ability to eat.
  - Offer frequent, small meals instead of a few large ones; offer foods served cold.

    R: Even distribution of total daily caloric intake helps prevent gastric distention, possibly increasing appetite.
  - With decreased appetite, restrict liquids with meals and avoid fluids 1 hour before and after meals.

    R: Restricting fluids with meals helps prevent gastric distention.
  - Encourage and help the client to maintain good oral hygiene.

    R: Poor oral hygiene leads to bad odor and taste, which can diminish appetite.
  - Arrange to have high-calorie and high-protein foods served at the times that the client usually feels most like eating.

    R: Presenting high-calorie and high-protein food when the client is most likely to eat increases the likelihood that he or she will consume adequate calories and protein.
  - Decrease amounts of food on tray, if it is anticipated that the person will eat only some.

    R: Unrealistic amounts of food can discourage the client before he or she starts.

Provide for Supplemental Dietary Needs Amplified by Acute Illness

R: Metabolic demands are increased by the catabolic processes that occur through stages of acute illness, usually increasing nutritional demand (Gary & Fleury, 2002).

Take Steps to Promote Appetite

- Determine the client's food preferences and arrange to have them provided, as appropriate.
- Eliminate any offensive odors and sights from the eating area.
- Control any pain and nausea before meals.
- Encourage the client's support people to bring permitted foods from home, if possible.

  R: Diet planning focuses on avoiding nutritional excesses. Reducing fats, salt, and sugar can reduce the risk of heart disease, diabetes, certain cancers, and hypertension.
- Give the client printed materials outlining a nutritious diet. Refer to Getting Started to Eating Better on thePoint at http://thePoint.lww.com/Carpenito6e. Print it and give to client / family.

  R: Self-help materials can be used at home for reinforcement.
- Promote foods that stimulate eating and increase protein consumption.
- Maintain good oral hygiene (brush teeth, rinse mouth) before and after eating.

  R: Maintaining good oral hygiene before and after meals decreases microorganisms that can cause foul taste and odor, inhibiting appetite.
- Offer frequent small feedings (six per day plus snacks). Restrict fluids with meals.

  R: Small feedings and fluid restrictions with meals can help to prevent gastric distention, which can decrease appetite.
- Practice relaxation techniques prior to meals.
- To stimulate appetite (Cunningham & Huhmann, 2011):
  - Try a different food choice.
  - Avoid sight and smell of food prior to eating.
  - Eat sour foods.
  - Eat cold foods.
  - Use a straw.

- Increase seasoning.
- Use plastic utensils.
- To increase intake, teach the client to:
  - Arrange to serve the highest protein / calorie nutrients when the client feels most like eating (e.g., if chemotherapy is in the early morning, serve food in the late afternoon).
  - Eat dry foods (e.g., toast, crackers) on arising.
  - Try salty foods, if permissible.
  - Avoid overly sweet, rich, greasy, or fried foods.
  - Try clear, cool beverages. Sip slowly through a straw.
  - Try whatever the client feels can be tolerated.
  - Eat small portions low in fat. Eat more frequently.
  - Review high-calorie versus low-calorie foods. Avoid empty-calorie foods (e.g., soda).
  - Encourage significant others to bring in favorite home foods.
  - Try commercial supplements available in many forms (e.g., liquids, powder, pudding); keep switching brands until some are found that are acceptable to the client in taste and consistency.

R: Varied techniques should be attempted to increase intake of nutritious foods and beverages. Attempts to vary the taste and texture can improve appetite and prevent food aversion.

TRANSITION PLAN
Initiate health teaching and referrals, as indicated.

- Dietitian for meal planning
- Psychiatric therapy when indicated
- Community meal centers

  R: *Resources in the community can assist the client and family.*

Clinical Alert Report

Prior to providing care, advise ancillary staff / student to report the following to the professional nurse assigned to the client:

- Significant decline in food and / or fluid intake
- Urine darker than pale yellow

IMBALANCED NUTRITION: MORE THAN BODY REQUIREMENTS

NANDA-I Definition

Intake of nutrients that exceeds metabolic needs

Defining Characteristics

Major (Must Be Present, One or More)

Overweight (weight 10% over ideal for height and frame), or
Obese (weight 20% or more over ideal for height and frame)*
Triceps skinfold greater than 15 mm in men and 25 mm in women*

Minor (May Be Present)

Reported undesirable eating patterns
Intake in excess of metabolic requirements
Sedentary activity patterns

Related Factors

Pathophysiologic

Related to excessive intake in relation to metabolic needs *

Related to altered satiety patterns secondary to (specify)

Related to decreased sense of taste and smell

Treatment Related

Related to altered satiety secondary to:

Medications (corticosteroids, antihistamines, estrogens)

Radiation (decreased sense of taste and smell)

Situational (Personal, Environmental)

Related to risk of gaining more than 25 to 30 pounds when pregnant

Related to lack of basic nutrition knowledge

Maturational

Adult / Older Adult

Related to decreased activity patterns, decreased metabolic needs

 ### Carp's Cues

Using this single diagnosis to describe people who are overweight or obese places the focus of interventions on nutrition. Obesity is a complex condition with sociocultural, psychological, and metabolic implications. When the focus is primarily on limiting food intake, as with many weight-loss programs, bariatric surgery, the chance of permanent weight loss is slim. To be successful, a weight-loss program must focus on behavior modification and lifestyle changes.

Therefore, the approach to lifestyle changes to reduce weight and maintain it must focus on nutrition, exercise, and behavioral modification. *Imbalanced Nutrition: More Than Body Requirements* can be utilized to address healthier eating patterns. *Risk-Prone Health Behavior related to intake in excess of metabolic requirements* can focus on the need to increase metabolic requirements through exercise, decreased intake, and the emotional component of overeating. For some people with dysfunctional eating, *Ineffective Coping related to increase eating in response to stressors* would be valid and require a referral after discharge.

Imbalanced Nutrition: More Than Body Requirements does have clinical usefulness for people at risk for or who have experienced weight gain because of pregnancy, taste or smell changes, or medications (e.g., corticosteroids).

Goal

NOC
Nutritional Status,
Weight Control

The person will describe why he or she is at risk for weight gain as evidenced by the following indicators:

* Describe reasons for increased intake with taste or olfactory deficits.
* Discuss the nutritional needs during pregnancy.
* Discuss the effects of exercise on weight control.

Interventions

NIC
Nutritional
Management, Weight
Management, Teaching:
Individual, Behavioral
Modification, Exercise
Promotion

Initiate Discussion: "How Can You Be Healthier?"

* Focus on client's response (e.g., stop smoking, exercise more, eat healthier, and cut down on drinking).
* Refer to index for interventions for the targeted lifestyle change.

  R: The nurse should be cautioned against applying a nursing diagnosis for an overweight or obese person who does not want to participate in a weight-loss program. Motivation for weight loss must come from within.

- If appropriate, gently and expertly teach the hazards of obesity but must respect a person's right to choose, the right of self-determination.

  R: Individuals who are very ill are probably not ready for discussions about lifestyle changes.

- Prior to discharge, provide the client with the appropriate "Getting Started" take-home information. Access these on thePoint at http://thePoint.lww.com/Carpenito6e.
- Identify clients who are at risk for diminished taste and smell (e.g., elderly, radiation therapy, and certain cancers) (Lutz & Przytulski, 2011).
- For affected clients, explain the effects of decreased sense of taste and smell on perception of satiety after eating (e.g., medications, radiation).
- Encourage client to (Lutz & Przytulski, 2011):
  - Complete oral hygiene before eating.
  - Evaluate intake by calorie counting, not feelings of satiety.
  - If not contraindicated, season foods heavily to satisfy decreased sense of taste. Experiment with seasonings (e.g., dill, basil).
  - Try lemon-flavored beverages.

    R: This will improve taste sensations.

- If client c/o of metallic taste, cook in microwave and in glass bowls.

  R: This will reduce metallic tastes.

- Eat food at room temperature or cold.

  R: This will lessen a bitter taste.

- When taste is diminished, concentrate on food smells.

  R: People with altered smell or taste may consume more food in an attempt to satisfy their taste (Dudek, 2009).

Explain the Rationale for Increased Appetite Owing to Use of Certain Medications (e.g., Steroids, Androgens)

R: The ability to lose weight while undergoing corticosteroid therapy likely depends on limiting sodium intake and maintaining reasonable caloric intake.

Discuss Nutritional Intake and Weight Gain during Pregnancy

- Discuss the total weight gain appropriate for the client (Institute of Medicine, 2009A).
  - 25 to 35 pounds if you were a healthy weight before pregnancy, with a BMI of 18.5 to 24.9.
  - 28 to 40 pounds if you were underweight before pregnancy with a BMI of less than 18.5.
  - 15 to 25 pounds if you were overweight before pregnancy with a BMI of 25 to 29.9.
  - 11 to 20 pounds if you were obese before pregnancy with a BMI of over 30.

  R: The extra weight gained during pregnancy is needed to nourish the developing fetus. It also stores nutrients for breastfeeding. The amount of weight you should gain depends on your weight and BMI (body mass index) before pregnancy.

- Explain healthy weight gain for each trimester (Institute of Medicine, 2009A).
  - 1 to 4.5 pounds during the first trimester
  - Approximately 1 to 2 pounds per week in the second trimester
  - Approximately 1 to 2 pounds per week in the third trimester

  R: Gaining weight at a steady rate within recommended boundaries can also lower your chances of having hemorrhoids, varicose veins, stretch marks, backache, fatigue, indigestion, and shortness of breath during pregnancy.

- Explain the problems that can occur with too much weight gain during pregnancy. (Institute of Medicine, 2009A).

  - Gestational diabetes
  - Leg pain
  - Varicose veins
  - High blood pressure
  - Backaches
  - Increased fatigue
  - Increased risk of cesarean delivery

- Stress the importance of not dieting, skipping meals but instead consume recommended portions and avoid high-fat / CHO foods.

    R: Dieting during pregnancy may result in insufficient maternal intake to provide the fetus with the necessary energy for growth. The fetus depends on the mother's dietary intake for growth and development, taking only iron and folate from maternal stores (Pillitteri, 2010).

TRANSITION PLAN

Initiate health teaching as indicated.

- Provide client with Getting Started to Healthy Eating on thePoint at http://thePoint.lww.com/Carpenito6e.
- Refer to a community weight loss program (e.g., Weight Watchers, Curves).
- Advise to consult primary care provider for continued assistance in weight loss.

    R: Strategies are needed after discharge to assist a person initiate / sustain a change in eating patterns and exercise patterns that will focus on why, where, and what is eaten and methods to reduce intake and increase activity.

Clinical Alert Report

- Advise ancillary staff / student to report types / amounts of foods ingested.

    R: Individuals can be malnourished even though they are eating (e.g., high fat, high carbohydrate).

Documentation

- Intake: types / amounts of food

IMPAIRED ORAL MUCOUS MEMBRANE

NANDA-I Definition

Disruption of the lips and / or soft tissue of the oral cavity

Defining Characteristics

Major (Must Be Present)

Disrupted oral mucous membranes

Minor (May Be Present)

Color changes—erythema, pallor, white patches, lesions, and ulcers
Moisture changes—increased or decreased saliva
Cleanliness changes—debris, malodor, discoloration of the teeth
Mucosal integrity changes—difficulty swallowing, decreased taste, difficulty weaning
Perception changes—difficulty swallowing, decreased taste, difficulty wearing dentures, burning, pain, and change in voice quality

Related Factors

Pathophysiologic

Related to inflammation secondary to (e.g., periodontal disease, oral cancer, infection)

Treatment Related

Related to drying effects of:

NPO more than 24 hours

Radiation to head or neck

Prolonged use of steroids or other immunosuppressives and other medications including opioids, anti-depressants, phenothiazines, antihypertensives, antihistamines, diuretics, and sedatives

Use of antineoplastic drugs

Oxygen therapy

Mouth breathing

Blood and marrow stem cell transplant

Related to mechanical irritation secondary to (e.g., endotracheal tube, nasogastric tube)

Situational (Personal, Environmental)

Related to chemical irritants* secondary to:

Acidic foods	Drugs
Noxious agents	Alcohol
Tobacco	High sugar intake

Related to mechanical trauma secondary to (e.g., broken or jagged teeth, ill-fitting dentures, braces)
Related to malnutrition*
Related to inadequate oral hygiene

Goal

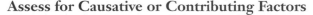

NOC
Oral Tissue Integrity, Oral Health Restoration, Chemotherapeutic Management, Oral Health Maintenance, Oral Health Promotion

The person will be free of oral mucosa irritation or exhibit signs of healing with decreased inflammation, as evidenced by the following indicators:

• Describe factors that cause oral injury.
• Demonstrate knowledge of optimal oral hygiene.
• Be free of oral discomfort during food and fluid intake.

Interventions

NIC
Oral Health Restoration, Chemotherapeutic Management, Oral Health Maintenance, Oral Health Promotion

Assess for Causative or Contributing Factors

Refer to Related Factors.

Evaluate Person's Ability to Perform Oral Hygiene. Allow Person to Perform as Much Oral Care as Possible. For high-risk clients, inspect the oral cavity for lesions (e.g., white patches broken teeth, signs of infection).

> **CLINICAL ALERT**
> • Too often, oral care and assessments are omitted in client care.

R: Researchers have reported that for clients with mechanical ventilation, only 32% had suctioning to manage oral secretions, 33% had their teeth brushed, 65% had swab cleansing, and 63% had a moisturizer applied to the oral mucosal tissues. In addition, nurses reported performing more oral care than actually completing (Cutler & Davis, 2005; Fields, 2008; Goss, Coty, & Myers, 2011).

Teach Preventive Oral Hygiene to Clients at Risk for Development of Mucositis (e.g., Radiation)

R: Mucosal damage usually occurs 7 to 14 days after the start of radiation and 3 to 9 days after the start of chemotherapy.

- Instruct client to:
  - Perform the regimen, including brushing, flossing, rinsing, and moisturizing, after meals and before sleep. If client resists, have him or her rinse mouth with water after meals.
  - Avoid mouthwashes with alcohol content, lemon / glycerin swabs, or prolonged use of hydrogen peroxide.

    R: These solutions can cause mucosal abnormalities, dryness, and discomfort (Meurman et al., 1996).

Promote Healing and Reduce Progression of Mucositis

- Inspect oral cavity three times daily with tongue blade and light; if mucositis is severe, inspect mouth every 4 hours.
- Use normal saline solution as a mouthwash.
- Floss teeth only once in 24 hours.
- Omit flossing if bleeding is excessive.
- Ensure that oral hygiene regimen is done every 1 to 2 hours while awake and every 4 hours during the night.

R: Systematically applied protocols may significantly decrease the incidence, severity, and duration of oral problems (ONS, 2007).

R: Salt and soda rinses are effective and the least costly selection for the prevention of treatment of mucositis. Foam brushes are not equal to toothbrushes for removing plaque and bacteria for cavity prevention. The effectiveness of mouthwash preparations over normal saline has not been supported in the literature (Dodd et al., 2000; ONS, 2007).

R: Proper hydration must be maintained to liquefy secretions and prevent drying of oral mucosa.

Reduce Oral Pain and Maintain Adequate Food and Fluid Intake

- Assess person's ability to chew and swallow.
- Administer mild analgesic every 3 to 4 hours as ordered by physician.
- Instruct client to:
  - Avoid commercial mouthwashes, citrus fruit juices, spicy foods, extremes in food temperature (hot, cold), crusty or rough foods, alcohol, and mouthwashes with alcohol.
  - Eat bland, cool foods (sherbets).
  - Drink cool liquids every 2 hours and PRN.
- Consult with dietitian for specific interventions.
- Refer to *Impaired Nutrition: Less Than Body Requirements* related to anorexia for additional interventions.
- Consult with physician / nurse practitioner for an oral pain-relief solution.
  - Xylocaine viscous 2% oral, swish and expectorate every 2 hours and before meals.

    R: If throat is sore, the solution can be swallowed; Xylocaine produces local anesthesia and, if swallowed, may affect the gag reflex. The dose of the viscous Xylocaine is not to exceed 25 mL per day (NCCN, 2008).

  - Gelclair is a concentrated gel that provides a protective barrier. Requires frequent applications because of limited duration. Prophylaxis is not recommended.
  - Topical morphine provides a reduction in pain severity and duration of pain. If the morphine is in an alcohol-based formula it may cause burning.

    R: Dry oral mucosa causes discomfort and increases the risk of breakdown and infection.

Discuss the Importance of Daily Oral Hygiene and Periodic Dental Examinations

- Explain the relationship of plaque to dental and gum disease and the need for daily brushing and flossing.
- Brush teeth (after meals and before sleep); use a soft-bristled toothbrush.
- Explain how to floss if needed.

R: Plaque, microbial flora found in the mouth, is the primary cause of dental cavities and periodontal disease. Daily removal of plaque through brushing and flossing can help prevent dental decay and disease.

Perform Oral Hygiene on Person Who Is Unconscious or at Risk for Aspiration as Often as Needed

R: Mechanically ventilated patients are at an increased risk of ventilatory-associated pneumonia (VAP) due to factors such as decreased level of consciousness; dry, open mouth; and microaspiration of secretions (Fields, 2008).

* Position client head of bed (HOB) >30 degrees unless medically contraindicated.
* Perform oral care with brushing every 8 hours.
* For people with dentures, remove dentures and clean as above. Leave dentures out and store in water (in denture cup) for people who are semicomatose.
* Do not use toothettes.

   R: The bristles of a toothbrush are much more effective at removing plaque than foam sticks (Pearson & Hutton, 2002).

* Apply lip lubricant and mouth moisturizer.

R: Oral health is influenced by microorganisms that grow in the plaque. With ventilators the microorganisms can transfer to the lungs and cause ventilator-associated pneumonia (Berry, Davidson, & Masters, 2007; Fields, 2008)

TRANSITION PLAN

Initiate health teaching and referrals as indicated.

* Teach person and family the factors that contribute to stomatitis and its progression.
* Teach diet modifications to reduce oral pain and to maintain optimal nutrition.
* Have client describe or demonstrate home care regimen.

   R: The frequency of oral health maintenance varies according to a person's health status and self-care ability, but minimum is in a.m. and at bedtime. High-risk clients (e.g., NG tubes, cancer, poorly nourished) should have oral assessments daily.

* Explain factors that contribute to oral disease are excessive use of alcohol and tobacco, microorganisms, inadequate nutrition (quantity, quality), inadequate hygiene, and trauma (ill-fitting dentures, sharp-edged teeth, sharp-edged prostheses, improper use of cleaning devices).
* Teach person and family the factors that contribute to stomatitis and its progression.
* Teach diet modifications to reduce oral pain and to maintain optimal nutrition.
* Have client describe or demonstrate home care regimen.
* Refer clients with tooth and gum disorders to a dentist.

If Pregnant:

* Stress the importance of good oral hygiene and continued dental examinations. Advise woman to increase intake of vitamin C.
* Remind client to advise dentist of her pregnancy.
* Explain that gum hypertrophy and tenderness are normal during pregnancy.

   R: Gum hypertrophy, tenderness, and bleeding during normal pregnancy may be the result of vascular swelling called epulis of pregnancy (Pillitteri, 2009).

Explain Risk Factors in Older Adults for Oral and Dental Disorders (Miller, 2009)

* Degenerative bone disease
* Dry mouth
* Diminished oral blood supply
* Vitamin deficiencies

R: Age-related changes and nutritional deficiencies increase vulnerability to oral ulcerations and infection (Miller, 2009; NCCN, 2007).

Explain That Some Medications Cause Dry Mouth

- Laxatives
- Antidepressants
- Analgesics
- Cardiovascular medications

- Antibiotics
- Anticholinergics
- Iron sulfate

R: Dry mouth contributes to tissue injury.

> **Clinical Alert Report**
>
> Advise ancillary staff / student to report any c/o mouth lesions, white patches, broken, sharp teeth.
>   *R: A focused assessment will be indicated.*

RISK FOR IMPAIRED ORAL MUCOUS MEMBRANE

Definition**

At risk for disruption of the lips and soft tissue of the oral cavity

Risk Factors

Pathophysiologic

Related to inflammation secondary to:

| Diabetes mellitus | Periodontal disease | Oral cancer | Infection |

Treatment Related

Related to drying effects of:

NPO more than 24 hours
Radiation to head or neck
Prolonged use of steroids or other immunosuppressives and other medications, including opioids, anti-depressants, phenothiazines, antihypertensives, antihistamines, diuretics, and sedatives
Use of antineoplastic drugs
Oxygen therapy
Mouth breathing
Blood and marrow stem cell transplant

Related to mechanical irritation secondary to:

| Endotracheal tube | NG tube |

Situational (Personal, Environmental)

Related to chemical irritants secondary to:

| Acidic foods | Drugs | Noxious agents |
| Alcohol | Tobacco | High sugar intake |

Related to mechanical trauma secondary to:

| Broken or jagged teeth | Ill-fitting dentures | Braces |

**This diagnosis is not presently on the NANDA-I list but has been added for clarity and usefulness.

Related to malnutrition
Related to inadequate oral hygiene
Related to lack of knowledge of oral hygiene

Goals / Interventions

Refer to Generic Medical Care Plan.

ACUTE PAIN

NANDA-I Definition

Unpleasant sensory and emotional experience arising from actual or potential tissue damage or described in terms of such damage (International Association for the Study of Pain); sudden or slow onset of any intensity from mild to severe with anticipated or predictable end and a duration of <6 months

Defining Characteristics

Self-Report of Pain Quality and Intensity

(Attempt to use with all patients.)

For Patients Unable to Provide Self-Report (in Order of Preference)

Presence of pathological condition or procedure known to cause pain. Physical responses such as diaphoresis, changes in blood pressure or pulse, pupil dilation, change in respiratory rate, guarding, grimacing, moaning, crying, or restlessness
Surrogate reporting (family members, caregivers)
Response to an analgesic trial

Related Factors

Biopathophysiologic

Related to uterine contractions during labor
Related to trauma to perineum during labor and delivery
Related to tissue trauma and reflex muscle spasms secondary to (specify)
Related to inflammation of, or injury (specify)
Related to effects of cancer on (specify)
Related to abdominal cramps, diarrhea, and vomiting secondary to (specify)
Related to inflammation and smooth muscle spasms secondary to renal calculi

Treatment Related

Related to tissue trauma and reflex muscle spasms secondary to:

Surgery   Diagnostic tests (venipuncture, invasive scanning, biopsy)

Carp's Cues

There is an ethical duty to relieve pain. Deandrea et al. reported that 40% of individuals with cancer pain are undertreated (2008). Nurses should be as aggressive in advocating for effective pain relief for their clients as they would be if the client were their child, mother, partner, or best friend. Those most in need for effective pain relief may be the poor, uneducated, substance abuser and others who are voiceless in the health care system.

Goal

NOC
Comfort Level, Pain
Control

The person will report or exhibit a satisfactory relief measure as evidenced by (specify):

- Increased participation in activities of recovery
- Reduction in pain behaviors (specify)
- Improvement in mood, coping

Interventions

NIC
Pain Management,
Medication
Management, Emotional
Support, Teaching:
Individual, Hot / Cold
Application, Simple
Massage

Reduce or Eliminate Factors That Increase Pain

Disbelief From Others

- Establish a supportive accepting relationship.
  - Acknowledge the pain.
  - Listen attentively to client's discussion of pain.
  - Convey that you are assessing pain because you want to understand it better (not to determine if it really exists).
- Assess the family for any misconceptions about pain or its treatment.

R: Trying to convince health care providers that he or she is experiencing pain will cause the client anxiety, which compounds the pain. Both are energy depleting.

Lack of Knowledge / Uncertainty

- Explain the cause of the pain, if known.
- Relate the severity of the pain and how long it will last, if known.
- Explain painful diagnostic tests and procedures in detail by relating the discomforts and sensations that the client will feel; approximate the duration.
- Support individual in addressing specific questions regarding diagnosis, risks, benefits of treatment, and prognosis. Consult with the specialist or primary care provider.

R: People who are prepared for painful procedures by explanations of the actual sensations experience less stress than those who receive vague explanations.

Fear

- Provide accurate information to reduce fear of addiction.
  - Explore reasons for the fear.
  - Explain the difference between drug tolerance and drug addiction.

R: Addiction is a psychological syndrome characterized by compulsive drug-seeking behavior generally associated with a desire for drug administration to produce euphoria or other effects, not pain relief. Addiction is believed to be rare, and there is no evidence that adequate administration of opioids for pain produces addiction (Pasero & McCaffery, 2011).

- Assist in reducing fear of losing control.
  - Include client in setting a realistic pain goal and in adopting strategies for pain control that are congruent with his or her beliefs and experiences.
  - Provide privacy for the client's pain experience.
  - Discuss the effect of relaxation techniques on medication effects.

R: Studies have shown that the human brain secretes endorphins, which have opiate-like properties that relieve pain. The release of endorphins may be responsible for the positive effects of placebos and noninvasive pain-relief measures.

Fatigue

- Determine the cause of fatigue (sedatives, analgesics, sleep deprivation).
- Explain that pain contributes to stress, which increases fatigue.
- Assess present sleep pattern and the influence of pain on sleep.
- Provide opportunities to rest during the day and with periods of uninterrupted sleep at night.

- Consult with prescriber for an increased dose of pain medication at bedtime.
- Explain the options of nonpharmaceutical interventions and the rationale.

R: Relaxation and guided imagery effectively manage pain by increasing sense of control, reducing feelings of helplessness and hopelessness, providing a calming diversion, and disrupting the pain–anxiety–tension cycle.

Explain the Various Noninvasive Pain-Relief Methods to the Client and Family and Why They Are Effective

R: The use of noninvasive pain-relief measures (e.g., relaxation, massage, distraction) can enhance the therapeutic effects of pain-relief medications (Fellowes et al., 2004).

- Discuss the use of heat applications, their therapeutic effects, indications, and related precautions.
  - Hot water bottle
  - Warm tub
  - Hot summer sun
  - Electric heating pad
  - Moist heat pack
  - Thin plastic wrap over painful area to retain body heat (e.g., knee, elbow)
- Discuss the use of cold applications,* their therapeutic effects, indications, and related precautions.
  - Cold towels (wrung out)
  - Ice bag
  - Ice massage
  - Cold water immersion for small body parts
  - Cold gel pack

R: Nonpharmacologic interventions provide clients with an increased sense of control, promote active involvement, reduce stress and anxiety, elevate mood, and raise the pain threshold (McGuire, Sheidler, & Polomano, 2000).

Provide Optimal Pain Relief With Prescribed Analgesics

- Use oral route when feasible, intravenous or rectal routes if needed.

  R: Oral administration is preferred when possible. Liquid medications can be given to those who have difficulty swallowing. Avoid intramuscular routes.

  R: If frequent injections are necessary, the IV route is preferred because it is not painful and absorption is guaranteed. IM routes have erratic absorption and cause unnecessary pain. Side effects (decreased respirations and blood pressure), however, may be more profound (Pasero & McCaffery, 2011).

- When possible use client controlled analgesics (PCA).

  R: Intramuscular injections are less effective at offering pain control than PCA administration (Chang et al., 2004). PCA increases one's sense of control and reduces feelings of helplessness and hopelessness.

- Use a preventive approach.
  - Medicate before an activity (e.g., ambulation) to increase participation, but evaluate the hazard of sedation.
  - Instruct client to request PRN pain medication before the pain is severe.
  - Collaborate with physician / nurse practitioner to order medications on a 24-hour schedule basis rather than PRN unless the person is sedated.

  R: The preventive approach may reduce the total 24-hour dose compared with the PRN approach; it provides a constant blood level of the drug, it reduces craving for the drug, and it reduces the anxiety of having to ask and wait for PRN relief.

- Determine the type of pain from the individual's description. Consult with physician or advance practice nurse to determine appropriate analgesia. The types of pain are (McMenamin, 2011):
  - Somatic pain is described as aching, gnawing, or throbbing pain.
  - Visceral or soft tissue pain is typically described as dull, aching, cramping, and generally not localized. It is caused by compression, infiltration, or distention of viscera.
  - Visceral and somatic pain are responsive to opioids and nonsteroidal anti-inflammatory drugs (NSAIDs).

R: Nociceptive pain can be somatic and visceral. Somatic pain results from the activation of peripheral nociceptors, as in muscle, joints, bone, or connective tissue. Visceral pain results from activation of nociceptors in the abdomen or thoracic cavity (McMenamin, 2011).

- Neuropathic pain is described as burning, stabbing, stinging, electric, pins and needles, shooting, or numbness.
- Opioids alone usually do not manage this type of pain. It is responsive to anticonvulsants (gabapentin), selective serotonin reuptake inhibitors (SSRIs), tricyclic antidepressants (TCAs), clonidine, Lidoderm patches®, and N-methyl-D-aspartate receptor antagonists (NMDAs) such as ketamine or methadone.

R: Neuropathic pain results when there is abnormal processing of input by the peripheral or central nervous system (McMenamin, 2011).

- Muscle spasm is described as cramping, spasm, or tightening and responds to muscle relaxants (e.g., Soma, Flexeril).

R: Multimodal analgesia, which utilizes two or three classes of analgesics, can be more effective than one class only. Lower doses of each class is more effective than higher doses of one class with fewer side effects (Pasero & McCaffery, 2011).

Assess Client's Response to the Pain-Relief Medication

- After administration, return in 30 minutes to assess effectiveness.
- Ask client to rate severity of pain before the medication and amount of relief received.
- Ask person to indicate when the pain began to increase. How long since the last pain medication? After a certain activity (e.g., ambulation, dressing change)?
- Advise person to request pain medication earlier. Plan pain-relief measures prior the activities.
- Consult with prescriber if a dosage or interval change is needed; the dose may be increased by 50% until effective.

R: Undertreatment of pain associated with cancer is reported to be 40% (Deandrea, Montanari, Moja, & Apolone, 2008). Pain management should be aggressive and individualized to eliminate any unnecessary pain with drugs administered on a regular schedule rather than PRN.

- If pain management is ineffective, collaborate with the prescriber to consider multimodal analgesia.

R: Multimodal analgesia is the use of combination of acetaminophen and NSAIDS in combination with other analgesics (Pasero & McCaffery, 2011).

- If individual has a history of substance / alcohol abuse, refer also to care plan for substance abuse.

Reduce or Eliminate Common Side Effects of Opioids

- Sedation
  - Assess whether the cause is the opioids, fatigue, sleep deprivation, or other medications (sedatives, antiemetics).
  - Assess for signs of respiratory depression (decreased level of consciousness, respiratory rate below 8, decreased oxygen saturation)
- Identify individuals at risk for adverse effects of opioids (e.g., renal insufficiency, hepatic insufficiency)

R: Clearance and excretion of opioids is delayed and high concentrations of the drug can accumulate (Pasero & McCaffery, 2011).

- Respiratory disorders, obstructive sleep apnea syndrome

R: Opioids decrease cough reflex and dry secretions increase the risk of aspiration (Pasero & McCaffery, 2011).

CLINICAL ALERT
- Carefully monitor high-risk individuals.
- Report signs of excessive sedation, early signs respiratory depression immediately.

- Constipation (Refer to Constipation.)
- Nausea and Vomiting (Refer to Nausea.)

- Dry Mouth
  - Explain that opioids decrease saliva production.
  - Instruct person to rinse mouth often, suck on sugarless sour candies, eat pineapple chunks or watermelon (if permissible), and drink liquids often.
  - Explain the necessity of good oral hygiene and dental care.

    R: Management of side effects can increase comfort level and use of medications.

Assist Family to Respond Optimally to Client's Pain Experience

- Give accurate information to correct misconceptions (e.g., addiction, doubt about pain).
- Provide each family member with opportunities to discuss fears, anger, and frustrations privately; acknowledge the difficulty of the situation.

  R: Helping the family to understand the pain experience can enhance positive coping (Pasero & McCaffery, 2011).

Minimize Procedural and Diagnostic Pain

- Anticipate pain and premedicate the client prior to painful procedures (e.g., sedation).
- Encourage the use of relaxation or guided imagery during procedures.

  R: Management of pain prior to a painful procedure can decrease the amount of analgesia needed and the effects of anxiety and fear, which will escalate the pain experience.

TRANSITION PLAN

Initiate health teaching and referrals as indicated.

- Review pain management strategies at home.
- Alert significant others on early signs of adverse effects and to call primary care provider.
- Instruct not to suddenly stop taking the pain medication.

  R: Tapering of opioids dose will prevent withdrawal symptoms. The longer the opioids have been taken, the longer it takes to wean off the medication (Pasero & McCaffery, 2011).

- Advise client to request specific instructions from prescriber.
- Discuss the need to prevent constipation.
  - Optimal hydration (8 to 10 cups unless contraindicated)
  - Stool softener, laxatives
  - Avoid bulk forming laxatives (e.g., psyllium)
- Discuss with client and family noninvasive pain-relief measures (relaxation, distraction, massage, music, topical analgesics).
- Teach the techniques of choice to the person and family.
- Explain the expected course of the pain (resolution) if known (e.g., fractured arm, surgical incision).

  R: Optimal pain management at home requires specific instructions to client and significant others.

Clinical Alert Report

- Advise ancillary staff / student to report any changes in respiratory status and cognition and complaints of pain to the charge nurse.
  R: Sedation and respiratory depression can occur with opioids use. Complaints of pain require a nursing assessment.

CHRONIC PAIN

NANDA-I Definition

Unpleasant sensory and emotional experience arising from actual or potential tissue damage or described in terms of such damage (International Association for the Study of Pain); sudden or slow onset of any intensity from mild to severe with anticipated or predictable end and a duration of >6 months

Defining Characteristics

Major (Must Be Present)

The client reports that pain has existed for more than 6 months (may be the only assessment data present).

Minor (May Be Present)

Discomfort
Guarded movement
Anger, frustration, depression because of situation
Muscle spasms
Redness, swelling, heat
Facial mask of pain
Color changes in affected area
Anorexia, weight loss
Reflex abnormalities
Insomnia

Related Factors

Related to tissue trauma and reflex muscle spasms secondary to:

Contractures
Arthritis
Fibromyalgia
Spinal cord disorders
Vasospasm
Occlusion
Vasodilatation (headache)

Related to inflammation of or injury of

Nerve	Muscle
Joint	Bursa
Tendon	Pancreas, liver, GI tract, brain

Related to effects of cancer on (specify)
Related to tissue trauma and reflex muscle spasms secondary to (specify)

 Carp's Cues

Chronic or persistent pain is common in 80% of older adults. One survey of 10,291 clients revealed prevalence of 10.1% for back pain, 7.1% for leg and foot pain, 4.1% for hand and arm pain and 3.5% for headache (Hardt et al., 2008). Chronic pain is responsible for 1/2 million working days lost in the United States each year. Forty percent of the elderly report persistent pain with arthritis as the most frequent cause. (Castillo-Bueno et al., 2010).

It is well known that chronic pain affects coping, sleep, sexual activity, socialization, family processes, nutrition, spirituality, and activity tolerance. Approximately 50% of clients with persistent pain also suffer from depression or anxiety disorder (Weisburg & Boatwright, 2007).

Currie and Wong found that the combination of chronic back pain and depression was associated with greater disability than either depression or chronic back pain alone (2004).

Goals

NOC
Comfort Level, Pain:
Disruptive Effects, Pain
Control, Depression
Control

The client will relate:

- Increased understanding of his or her disease / disorder and resources / skills needed to cope.
- Will commit to practice at least one noninvasive pain-relief measures such as:
  - Music therapy
  - Stretching exercises, yoga, and / or walking
  - Massage
  - Guided imagery
  - Relaxation therapy
  - Heat / cold therapy

Interventions

NIC
Pain Management,
Medication
Management, Exercise
Promotion, Mood
Management, Coping
Enhancement

- Establish a supportive accepting relationship.
  - Acknowledge the pain. Listen attentively to client's discussion of pain.
  - Convey that you are assessing pain because you want to understand it better (not determine if it really exists).
- Assess the family for any misconceptions about pain or its treatment.

  R: Trying to convince health care providers that he or she is experiencing pain will cause the client anxiety, which compounds the pain. Both are energy depleting.

- Determine the client's level of understanding of his or her condition, and causes of pain and pain-relieving techniques that he or she uses. Supplement the client's information and correct misconceptions.

  R: The chronic self-management program (CPSMP) focuses on increasing a client's understanding of his or her condition. This theory has validated that better knowledge of one's condition increases confidence and skill in managing a chronic condition. (Ledford, 1998)

- Determine with individual factors that decrease pain tolerance and / or factors that increase pain.
- Determine with client and family the effects of chronic pain on the client's life (Ferrell, 1995; Pasero & McCaffery, 2011).
  - Physical well-being (fatigue, strength, appetite, sleep, function, constipation, nausea)
  - Psychological well-being (anxiety, depression, coping, control, concentration, sense of usefulness, fear, enjoyment)
  - Spiritual well-being (religiosity, uncertainty, positive changes, sense of purpose, hopefulness, suffering, meaning of pain, transcendence)
  - Social well-being (family support, family distress, sexuality, affection, employment, isolation, financial burden, appearance, roles, relationships)

  R: Chronic pain is an intense experience for the client and family members. Interventions focus on helping families understand pain's effects on roles and relationships.

- Evaluate for the presence of depression.
  - Explain the relationship between chronic pain and mood disorders (e.g., anger, anxiety, depression).
  - Refer to primary care provider or specialist for management of depression.

  R: The client with chronic pain may respond with withdrawal, depression, anxiety, anger, frustration, and dependency, all of which can affect the family in the same way (Chronic Pain, 2011). Fifty percent of clients with chronic pain have depression or anxiety disorders. Major depression is thought to be four times greater in people with chronic back pain than in the general population (Sullivan, Reesor, Mikail, & Fisher, 1992). Currie and Wong found that the greater the rate of major depression, the greater pain severity (2004).

- Evaluate the client's sleep quality. Refer to *Disturbed Sleep Patterns* for interventions.

  R: Depression and insomnia are the most common comorbid disorders experienced by chronic pain patients (Wilson et al., 2002). Research suggests that interventions for insomnia and depression may yield improvements across a number of chronic pain-related variables, including pain intensity, affective / sensory pain ratings and anxiety (Tang et al., 2007).

- Provide pain relief with prescribed analgesics.
  - Determine preferred route of administration: oral, IM, IV, rectal.
  - Assess client's response to the medication. For those admitted to acute care settings:
    - After administration, return in 30 minutes to assess effectiveness.
    - Ask client to rate severity of pain before the medication and amount of relief received.
    - Consult with the physician / advanced practice nurse if a dosage or interval change is needed.
- Encourage the use of oral medications as soon as possible.
  - Consult with physician / NP for a schedule to change from IM to IV or oral.
  - Explain to client and family that oral medications can be as effective as IM.
- Explain how the transition will occur.
  - Begin oral medication at a larger dose than necessary (loading dose).
  - Continue PRN IV medication but use as a backup for pain unrelieved by oral medication.
  - Gradually reduce IM IV medication dose.
- Use the client's account of pain to regulate oral doses.
- Consult with physician / NP about possibly adding aspirin or acetaminophen to medication regimen.

  R: The oral route is preferred because it is convenient and cost effective. Intramuscular routes are painful and have unreliable absorption rates (McCaffery, 2003; Pasero & McCaffery, 2011).

- Discuss fears (individual, family) of addiction and under treatment of pain.
  - Explain tolerance versus addiction.

  R: Control of pain effectively requires clarifying misconception about addiction and overdose. Opioid tolerance and physical dependence are expected with long-term opioid treatment. Addiction is different and not usual in clients who use opioids for pain management (APS, 2005; Pasero & McCaffery, 2011).

- Reduce or **eliminate common side effects of opioids**. See *Acute Pain.*
- Assist **family to respond optimally to the client's pain experience**. See *Acute Pain.*
- Explain the various nonpharmaceutical pain-relief measures. Encourage client to try one method in the hospital

  R: The goal is for teaching the use of nonpharmaceutical chronic pain management techniques and to help client feel less dependent on pain killers and feel more empowered to be able to control their pain (Block, 2007).

- Discuss the value of exercise (e.g., walking, yoga, or stretching, water exercise).
  - Plan daily activities when pain is at its lowest level.

    R: Exercise walking is one way to benefit from regular exercise while not aggravating the structures in the lower back. Exercise improves muscle strength, which provides stability for joints (e.g., arthritis) (Hurkmans et. al, 2009).

  - If exercise aggravates pain, consider water exercises.

    R: Water exercising improves pain, stress, and depression symptoms in persons with widespread pain (e.g., fibromyalgia).

- Teach and demonstrate the effectiveness of distraction techniques.

  R: Distraction techniques focus one's attention away from negative or painful images to positive mental thoughts. Explain that the pain will return after the distraction is over.

  - Watching a favorite movie
  - Reading a book or listening to a book on tape
  - Listening to only music (20 minutes to 1 hour daily)

    R: Music therapy has been confirmed to reduce chronic pain (McCaffery, 2003), depression, disability, and feelings of helplessness over their pain (Siedliecki & Good, 2006).

  - Talking to a friend
- Discuss the use of heat applications (e.g., hot water bottle, warm tub, hot summer sun, electric heating pad, moist heat pack, topical analgesic gels / lotions, single-use air-activated heating pads, thin plastic wrap over painful area to retain body heat [e.g., knee, elbow]), their therapeutic effects, indications, and related precautions. Refer to rationale to explain benefits to the client.

  R: Heat causes blood flow to increase to an area, it brings along oxygen and nutrients that can help to speed healing. Heat relaxes muscles, which can decrease some types of pain sensations, and can increase flexibility and overall feeling of comfort. The sensation of heat on the skin stimulates the sensory receptors in the skin, and therefore reduces the perception of pain by decreasing transmissions of pain signals to the brain. Heat therapy application facilitates stretching the soft tissues around the spine, including muscles, connective tissue, and adhesions, which increases flexibility.

- Discuss the use of cold applications, their therapeutic effects, indications, and related precautions (e.g., cold towels [wrung out], ice bag, cold gel pack). Refer to rationale to explain benefits to the client.

  R: Cold therapy provides pain relief (analgesia) by decreasing muscle spasms and by inhibiting pain sensations by reducing the speed of impulses conducted by nerve fibers (Pasero & McCaffery, 2011).

- Teach relaxation breathing.
  - Find a quiet, comfortable place to sit or lie down in a dark room.
  - First, take a normal breath. Then try a deep breath: Breathe in slowly through your nose, allowing your chest and lower belly to rise as you fill your lungs. Let your abdomen expand fully. Now breathe out slowly through your mouth (or your nose, if that feels more natural).
  - Try to practice once or twice a day, always at the same time, in order to enhance the sense of ritual and establish a habit.
  - Try to practice at least 10 to 20 minutes each day.

  Accessed from http://www.health.harvard.edu/fhg/updates/update1006a.shtml

  R: When the body's stress response is activated, breathing becomes shallow. Breathing slowly and deeply activates the relaxation response.

TRANSITIONAL PLAN

Initiate health teaching and referrals as indicated.

- Discuss with client and family the various treatment modalities available:
  - Family therapy
  - Group therapy
  - Behavior modification
  - Biofeedback
  - Hypnosis
  - Acupuncture
  - Exercise program
- Access a multitude of stress relieving techniques at http://www.stress-relief-tools.com.

IMPAIRED PHYSICAL MOBILITY

NANDA-I Definition

Limitation in independent, purposeful physical movement of the body or of one or more extremities

Defining Characteristics**

Major (Must Be Present; 80% to 100%)

Compromised ability to move purposefully within the environment (e.g., bed mobility, transfers, ambulation)
Range-of-motion (ROM) limitations

Minor (May Be Present; 50% to 80%)

Imposed restriction of movement
Reluctance to move

**Levin, Krainovitch, Bahrenburg, & Mitchell, 1989

Related Factors

Pathophysiologic

Related to decreased muscle strength* and endurance* secondary to:

Neuromuscular impairment
Autoimmune alterations (e.g., multiple sclerosis, arthritis)
Muscular dystrophy
Partial paralysis (spinal cord injury, stroke)
Nervous system diseases (e.g., Parkinson's disease, myasthenia gravis, tumors)
Trauma
Cancer
Musculoskeletal impairment
Fractures
Connective tissue disease (systemic lupus erythematosus)

Related to joint stiffness* or contraction* secondary to:

Inflammatory joint disease
Post joint replacement or spinal surgery
Degenerative joint disease
Degenerative disc disease

Related to peripheral edema

Treatment Related

Related to external devices (casts or splints, braces, intravenous [IV] tubing)
Related to insufficient strength and endurance for ambulation with (specify) (e.g., prosthesis, crutches, walker)

Situational (Personal, Environmental)

Related to:

Fatigue	Deconditioning*
Depressive mood state*	Obesity
Decreased motivation	Dyspnea
Sedentary lifestyle*	Cognitive impairment*
Pain*	

 ## Carp's Cues

Impaired Physical Mobility describes a client with limited use of arm(s) or leg(s) or limited muscle strength. If more immobility is present, refer to *Risk for Disuse Syndrome*. Limitation of physical movement also can be the etiology of other nursing diagnoses, such as *Self-Care Deficit* and *Risk for Injury*. If the client has no limitations in movement but is deconditioned and has reduced endurance, as in CHF, COPD, refer to *Activity Intolerance*.

Goal

NOC
Ambulation, Joint Movement, Mobility, Fall Prevention Behavior Modification

The client will report increased strength and endurance of limbs as evidenced by the following indicators:

- Demonstrate the use of adaptive devices to increase mobility.
- Use safety measures to minimize potential for injury.
- Describe rationale for interventions.
- Demonstrate measures to increase mobility.
- Evaluate pain and effectiveness of management.

Interventions

Assess Causative Factors

Refer to Related Factors.

Consult With Physical Therapy for Evaluation

Promote Optimal Mobility and Movement

Promote Motivation and Adherence (Addams & Clough, 1998)

- Explain the problem and the objective of each exercise.
- Establish short-term goals. Ensure that initial exercises are easy and require minimal strength and coordination.
- Point out progress.

R: Mobility is one of the most significant aspects of physiologic functioning because it greatly influences maintenance of independence (Miller, 2009). Motivation can be increased if short-term goals are accomplished.

Ensure Effective Pain Management

R: Effective management of pain and depression is sometimes necessary. Inadequate pain relief may be a primary factor leading to depression in some people, but depression should not be discounted as a secondary feature of pain. Depression may require aggressive management, including drugs and other therapies.

Increase Limb Mobility and Determine Type of ROM Appropriate for the Client (Passive, Active Assistive, Active, Active Resistive)

- Perform passive or active assistive ROM exercises (frequency determined by client's condition).
  - Teach the client to perform active ROM exercises on unaffected limbs at least four times a day, if possible.
  - Perform passive ROM on affected limbs. Do the exercises slowly to allow the muscles time to relax, and support the extremity above and below the joint to prevent strain on joints and tissues.
- Support extremity with pillows to prevent or reduce swelling.
- Medicate for pain as needed, especially before activity or physical therapy.
- Encourage the client to perform exercise regimens for specific joints as prescribed by physician, nurse practitioner, or physical therapist (e.g., isometric, resistive).

R: Active ROM increases muscle mass, tone, and strength and improves cardiac and respiratory functioning. Passive ROM improves joint mobility and circulation and decreases the likelihood of contractures.

Position in Alignment to Prevent Complications

- If the client is in the lateral position, place pillow(s) to support the leg from groin to foot, and use a pillow to flex the shoulder and elbow slightly. If needed, support the lower foot in dorsal flexion with a towel roll or special boot.

  R: These measures prevent internal rotation and adduction of the femur and shoulder and prevent foot drop.

Maintain Good Body Alignment When Mechanical Devices Are Used

Traction Devices
- Assess for correct position of traction and alignment of bones.
- Allow weights to hang freely, with no blankets or sheets on ropes.
- Assess for changes in circulation; check pulse quality, skin temperature, color of extremities, and capillary refill (should be less than 3 seconds), feelings of numbness, tingling, and / or pain.
- Assess for signs of skin irritation (redness, ulceration, blanching).
- Assess skeletal traction pin sites for loosening, inflammation, ulceration, and drainage; clean pin insertion sites (procedure may vary with type of pin and protocols).

Casts

- Refer to Cast Care Plan.

Prosthetic Devices

- Refer to Amputation Care Plan.

Provide Progressive Mobilization

- Refer to *Activity Intolerance* for specific interventions.

R: Researchers have shown that early mobilization has better outcomes than bed rest after an injury, surgery, or as treatment of a medical condition.

Encourage Use of Affected Arm When Possible

- Consult with physical therapy for a plan.
- Encourage the client to use affected arm for self-care activities (e.g., feeding self, dressing, brushing hair).

R: A physical therapy evaluation is need for a plan, which can be reinforced and implemented on the unit to increase use of affected arm and motivation.

Ensure That the Client Can Ambulate Correctly With Adaptive Equipment (e.g., Crutches, Walkers, and Canes). Consult with PT.

R: Ambulatory aids must be used correctly and safely to ensure effectiveness and prevent injury.

TRANSITIONAL PLAN

Initiate health teaching and referrals as indicated.

- Ensure a referral for physical therapy and to a home health nursing service if needed.

  R: This will ensure an assessment in the home to determine if barriers to ambulation are present and to continue physical therapy.

Clinical Alert Report

- Advise ancillary staff / student to report c/o of increased fatigue or reluctance to ambulate.

  R: Increased fatigue needs further assessment by the nurse to r/o infection, overexertion, dehydration, nutritional deficits.

Documentation

- Response to ambulation.

IMPAIRED RELIGIOSITY

NANDA-I Definition

Impaired ability to exercise reliance on beliefs and / or participate in rituals of a particular faith tradition

Defining Characteristics

Individuals experience distress because of difficulty with adhering to prescribed religious rituals such as the following:

Religious ceremonies
Worship / religious services

RISK FOR IMPAIRED RELIGIOSITY

NANDA-I Definition

At risk for an impaired ability to exercise reliance on religious beliefs and / or participate in rituals of a particular faith tradition

Related Factors

Refer to *Impaired Religiosity*.

Goal

NOC
Spiritual Well-Being

The client will express continued satisfaction with religious activities, as evidenced by the following indicators:

- Continue to practice religious rituals.
- Describe increased comfort after assessment.

Interventions

NIC
Spiritual Support

Refer to *Impaired Religiosity* for interventions.

RISK FOR INEFFECTIVE RESPIRATORY FUNCTION

NANDA-I Definition

At risk for experiencing a threat to the passage of air through the respiratory tract and / or to the exchange of gases (O_2–CO_2) between the lungs and the vascular system

Risk Factors

Presence of risk factors that can change respiratory function (see Related Factors).

Related Factors

Pathophysiologic

Related to excessive or thick secretions secondary to:

Infection	Cardiac or pulmonary disease
Inflammation	Smoking
Allergy	Exposure to noxious chemical

Related to immobility, stasis of secretions, and ineffective cough secondary to:

Diseases of the nervous system (e.g., Guillain-Barré syndrome, multiple sclerosis, myasthenia gravis)
Central nervous system (CNS) depression / head trauma
Cerebrovascular accident (stroke)
Quadriplegia

Treatment Related

Related to immobility secondary to:

Sedating or paralytic effects of medications, drugs or chemicals (specify)
Anesthesia, general or spinal

Related to suppressed cough reflex secondary to (specify)
Related to effects of tracheostomy (altered secretions)

Situational (Personal, Environmental)

Related to immobility secondary to:

Surgery or trauma
Fatigue
Pain
Perception / cognitive impairment
Fear
Anxiety

Related to extremely high or low humidity

For infants, related to placement on stomach for sleep
Exposure to cold, laughing, crying, allergens, and smoke

 ## Carp's Cues

The author has added *Risk for Ineffective Respiratory Function* to describe a state that may affect the entire respiratory system, not just isolated areas, such as airway clearance or gas exchange. Allergy and immobility are examples of factors that affect the entire system; thus, it is incorrect to say *Impaired Gas Exchange related to immobility*, because immobility also affects airway clearance and breathing patterns. The nurse can use the diagnoses *Ineffective Airway Clearance* and *Ineffective Breathing Patterns* when nurses can definitely alleviate the contributing factors influencing respiratory function (e.g., ineffective cough, stress).

The nurse is cautioned not to use this diagnosis to describe acute respiratory disorders, which are the primary responsibility of medicine and nursing together (i.e., collaborative problems). Such problems can be labeled *RC of Acute hypoxia* or *RC of Pulmonary edema*. When a client's immobility is prolonged and threatens multiple systems—for example, integumentary, musculoskeletal, vascular, as well as respiratory—the nurse should use *Disuse Syndrome* to describe the entire situation.

Goal

NOC
Aspiration Control,
Respiratory Status

The client will have a respiratory rate within normal limits compared with baseline as evidenced by the following indicators:

- Express willingness to be actively involved in managing respiratory symptoms and maximizing respiratory function.
- Relate appropriate interventions to maximize respiratory status (varies depending on health status).
- Have satisfactory pulmonary function, as measured by pulmonary function tests.

Interventions

NIC
Airway Management,
Cough Enhancement,
Respiratory Monitoring,
Positioning

Eliminate or Reduce Causative Factors, If Possible

- Encourage ambulation as soon as consistent with the medical plan of care.
- If the client cannot walk, establish a regimen for being out of bed in a chair several times a day (e.g., 1 hour after meals and 1 hour before bedtime).

  R: Lying flat causes the abdominal organs to shift toward the chest, thereby crowding the lungs and making it more difficult to breathe.

- Increase activity gradually. Explain that respiratory function will improve and dyspnea will decrease with practice.

  R: Exercises and movement promote lung expansion and mobilization of secretions.

- For neuromuscular impairment:
  - Vary the position of the bed, thereby gradually changing the horizontal and vertical position of the thorax, unless contraindicated.
  - Assist the client to reposition, turning frequently from side to side (hourly if possible).

- In the hospital, especially if the client is on a ventilator, utilize beds with continuous lateral rotation (when available) (Swadener-Culpepper, 2010).
- Encourage deep-breathing and controlled-coughing exercises five times every hour.
- Teach the client to use a blow bottle or incentive spirometer every hour while awake.

  R: Incentive spirometry promotes deep breathing by providing a visual indicator of the effectiveness of the breathing effort.

- Ensure optimal hydration status and nutritional intake.

  R: Adequate hydration and humidity liquefy secretions, enabling easier expectoration and preventing stasis of secretions, which provide a medium for microorganism growth (Halm & Krisko-Hagel, 2008).

- For the client with a decreased level of consciousness:
  - Position the client from side to side with a set schedule (e.g., left side on even hours, right side on odd hours); do not leave the client lying flat on the back.

    R: Lying flat causes the abdominal organs to shift toward the chest, thereby crowding the lungs and making it more difficult to breathe.

  - Position the client on the right side after feedings (nasogastric [NG] tube feeding, gastrostomy) to prevent regurgitation and aspiration.
- Keep the head of the bed elevated 30 degrees unless contraindicated.
- See also *Risk for Aspiration.*

Prevent the Complications of Immobility

See *Disuse Syndrome.*

Clinical Alert Report
- Advise ancillary staff / student to report any change such as:
  - B/P more than 10 mm Hg, diastolic, and / or systolic
  - Observed difficulty breathing while eating, talking, and walking
  - Change in pulse irregular rhythm, rate <60 or >100
  - Decrease in urine output less than 5 mL/kg per hour
  - Onset of sweating, cool, pale skin changes
  - Pulse oximetry <90 or a significant decrease (e.g., 100 to 92)
  - Onset of restlessness, confusion, and mood changes
  R: These changes need further assessment to determine if physiologic instability is present.

TRANSITION PLAN
Initiate health teaching and referrals as indicated.
- Documentation
- Flow records
- Vital signs
- Pulse oximetry
- Sputum characteristics
- Effectiveness of cough

SELF-CARE DEFICIT SYNDROME

Definition**

State in which a client experiences an impaired motor function or cognitive function, causing a decreased ability in performing each of the five self-care activities

Defining Characteristics

Major (One Deficit Must Be Present in Each Activity)

Bathing Self-Care Deficit (Includes Washing Entire Body, Combing Hair, Brushing Teeth, Attending to Skin and Nail Care, and Applying Makeup)
Inability (or unwilling) to:**

Access bathroom	Dry body
Get bath supplies	Unable to obtain a water source
Wash body	Unable to regulate bath water

Dressing Self-Care Deficits (Includes Donning Regular or Special Clothing, Not Nightclothes)
Inability or unwilling to:**

Choose clothing put clothing on lower body
Put clothing on upper body
Put on necessary items of clothing
Maintain appearance at a satisfactory level
Pick up clothing
Put on shoes / remove shoes
Put on / remove socks
Use assistive devices
Use zippers
Fasten, unfasten clothing
Obtain clothing

Feeding Self-Care Deficit
Inability (or unwilling to):**

Bring food from a receptacle to the mouth
Complete a meal
Set food onto utensils
Handle utensils
Ingest food in a socially acceptable manner
Open containers
Pick up cup or glass
Prepare food for ingestion
Use assistive device

Instrumental Self-Care Deficits**
Difficulty using telephone
Difficulty accessing transportation
Difficulty laundering, ironing
Difficulty managing money
Difficulty preparing meals
Difficulty with medication administration
Difficulty shopping

**These diagnoses are not currently on the NANDA-I list but have been included for clarity and usefulness.

Toileting Self-Care Deficits

Unable or unwillingness to:**

Get to toilet or commode
Carry out proper hygiene
Manipulate clothing for toileting
Rise from toilet or commode
Sit on toilet or commode
Unable to flush toilet or empty commode

Instrumental ADLs

Difficulty to write checks and pay bills
Difficulty to handle cash transactions (simple, complex)
Difficulty with medication administration
Difficulty using telephone
Difficulty accessing transportation
Difficulty laundering, ironing
Difficulty managing money
Difficulty preparing meals
Difficulty shopping
Inadequate social supports:

Support people
Availability of help with transportation, shopping, money management, laundry, housekeeping, and
food preparation
Community resources

Related Factors

Pathophysiologic

Related to lack of coordination secondary to (specify)
Related to spasticity or flaccidity secondary to (specify)
Related to muscular weakness secondary to (specify)
Related to partial or total paralysis secondary to (specify)
Related to atrophy secondary to (specify)
Related to muscle contractures secondary to (specify)
Related to visual disorders secondary to (specify)
Related to nonfunctioning or missing limb(s)

Treatment Related

Related to external devices (specify) (e.g., casts, splints, braces, intravenous [IV] equipment)
Related to postoperative fatigue and pain

Situational (Personal, Environmental)

Related to cognitive deficits
Related to fatigue
Related to pain
Related to decreased motivation
Related to confusion
Related to disabling anxiety

**These diagnoses are not currently on the NANDA-I list but have been included for clarity and usefulness.

Maturational

Older Adult
Related to decreased visual and motor ability, muscle weakness

Assess for Related Factors

Ability to remember
Judgment
Ability to follow directions
Ability to identify / express needs

Carp's Cues

Self-care encompasses the activities needed to meet daily needs, commonly known as activities of daily living (ADLs), which are learned over time and become lifelong habits. Self-care activities involve not only what is to be done (hygiene, bathing, dressing, toileting, feeding), but also how much, when, where, with whom, and how (Miller, 2009).

In every client, the threat or reality of a self-care deficit evokes panic. Many people report that they fear loss of independence more than death. A self-care deficit affects the core of self-concept and self-determination. For this reason, the nursing focus for self-care deficit should be not on providing the care measure, but on identifying adaptive techniques to allow the client the maximum degree of participation and independence possible.

Currently not on the NANDA-I list, the diagnosis *Self-Care Deficit Syndrome* has been added here to describe a client with compromised ability in all five self-care activities. For this client, the nurse assesses functioning in each area and identifies the level of participation of which the client is capable. The goal is to maintain current functioning, to increase participation and independence, or both. The syndrome distinction clusters all five self-care deficits together to enable grouping of interventions when indicated, while also permitting specialized interventions for a specific deficit.

The danger of applying a Self-Care Deficit diagnosis lies in the possibility of prematurely labeling a client as unable to participate at any level, eliminating a rehabilitation focus.

It is important to classify the client's baseline functional level to evaluate changes in the client's ability to participate in self-care. Use the following scale to rate the client's ability to perform:

0 = Is completely independent
1 = Requires use of assistive device
2 = Needs minimal help
3 = Needs assistance and / or some supervision
4 = Needs total supervision
5 = Needs total assistance or unable to assist

BATHING SELF-CARE DEFICIT

NANDA-I Definition

Impaired ability to perform or complete bathing activities for self

Defining Characteristics*

Inability (or unwilling) to:**

Access bathroom	Dry body
Get bath supplies	Unable to obtain a water source
Wash body	Unable to regulate bath water

Goals, Interventions, and Rationales

Refer to Generic Medical Care Plan.

**These characteristics are not currently on the NANDA-I list but have been included for clarity and usefulness.

DRESSING SELF-CARE DEFICITS

NANDA-I Definition

Impaired ability to perform or complete dressing activities for self

Defining Characteristics

Inability or unwilling to:**

Choose clothing
Put clothing on lower body
Put clothing on upper body
Put on necessary items of clothing
Maintain appearance at a satisfactory level
Pick up clothing
Put on shoes / remove shoes
Put on / remove socks
Use assistive devices
Use zippers
Fasten, unfasten clothing
Obtain clothing

Goals, Interventions, and Rationales

Refer to Generic Medical Care Plan.

FEEDING SELF-CARE DEFICIT

NANDA-I Definition

Impaired ability to perform or complete self-feeding activities

Defining Characteristics*

Inability (or unwilling to):**

Bring food from a receptacle to the mouth
Complete a meal
Set food onto utensils
Handle utensils
Ingest food in a socially acceptable manner
Open containers
Pick up cup or glass
Prepare food for ingestion
Use assistive device

Goals, Interventions, and Rationales

Refer to Generic Medical Care Plan.

**These characteristics are not currently on the NANDA-I list but have been included for clarity and usefulness.

INSTRUMENTAL SELF-CARE DEFICITS

Definition

Impaired ability to perform certain activities or access certain services essential for managing a household

Defining Characteristics

Difficulty using telephone
Difficulty accessing transportation
Difficulty laundering, ironing
Difficulty managing money
Difficulty preparing meals
Difficulty with medication administration
Difficulty shopping

Goals, Interventions, and Rationales

Refer to Generic Medical Care Plan.

TOILETING SELF-CARE DEFICIT

NANDA-I Definition

Impaired ability to perform or complete toileting activities for self

Defining Characteristics*

Unable (or unwilling) to:**

Get to toilet or commode
Carry out proper hygiene
Manipulate clothing for toileting
Rise from toilet or commode
Sit on toilet or commode
Flush toilet or empty commode

Goals, Interventions, and Rationales

Refer to Generic Medical Care Plan.

IMPAIRED SKIN INTEGRITY (PRESSURE ULCER STAGE)

NANDA-I Definition

Altered epidermis and / or dermis

**These characteristics are not currently on the NANDA-I list but have been included for clarity and usefulness.

Defining Characteristics*

Destruction of skin layers
Disruption of skin surface
Invasion of body structures

Carp's Cues

Because tissue is composed of epithelium, connective tissue, muscle, and nervous tissue, *Impaired Tissue Integrity correctly* describes some pressure ulcers that are deeper than the dermis. Impaired Skin Integrity should be used to describe disruptions of epidermal and dermal tissue only. This author anticipates that Pressure Ulcer Stage__ and Risk for Pressure Ulcers will be submitted and approved by NANDA-I. These diagnoses would add diagnostic clarity for clinicians.

If a stage III or IV pressure ulcer requires surgical interventions, the nurse can continue to use the Pressure Ulcer diagnosis, which will continue to need specific nursing interventions.

This would represent a situation that a nurse manages with physician- and nurse-prescribed interventions. When a stage II or III pressure ulcer needs a dressing that requires a physician's order in an acute-care setting, the nurse should continue to label the situation a nursing diagnosis because it would be appropriate and legal for a nurse to treat the ulcer independently in other settings (e.g., in the community).

If a client is immobile and multiple systems are threatened (respiratory, circulatory, musculoskeletal as well as integumentary), refer to Care Plan for Immobility.

Related Factors

Pathophysiologic

Related to decreased blood and nutrients to tissues secondary to:

Peripheral vascular alterations	Arteriosclerosis
Obesity	Dehydration
Anemia	Malnutrition
Venous stasis	Edema*
Cardiopulmonary disorders	Emaciation

Treatment Related

Related to decreased blood and nutrients to tissues secondary to:

Therapeutic extremes in body temperature
Surgery
Obesity
NPO status

Related to imposed immobility secondary to sedation
Related to mechanical trauma

Therapeutic fixation devices

Wired jaw
Casts
Traction

Orthopedic devices / braces

Related to effects of radiation on epithelial and basal cells*
Related to effects of mechanical irritants or pressure secondary to:*

Inflatable or foam donuts	Dressings, tape, solutions
Tourniquets	External urinary catheters
Footboards	NG tubes
Restraints	Shear

Friction   Oral prostheses / braces
Endotracheal tubes   Contact lenses

Situational (Personal, Environmental)

*Related to chemical irritants * secondary to:*

Excretions
Secretions
Noxious agents / substances

Related to environmental irritants secondary to:

Radiation / sunburn
Humidity
Bites (insect, animal)
Poisonous plants
Temperature extremes*
Parasites
Inhalants

*Related to the effects of pressure of impaired physical mobility * secondary to:*

Pain
Fatigue
Motivation
Cognitive, sensory, or motor deficits

Related to dry, thin skin and decreased dermal vascularity secondary to aging

Carp's Cues

Pressure ulcers represent a major burden of sickness and reduced quality of life for patients and their caregivers. Increased morbidity and mortality associated with pressure ulcer development in hospitalized patients is documented in multiple studies. Hospital lengths of stay, readmission rates, and hospital charges are greater in patients who develop pressure ulcers than in those remaining ulcer-free. The development of a single pressure ulcer in U.S. hospitals can increase a patient's length of stay five-fold and increase hospital charges by $2,000 to $11,000. Recent European cost models to highlight the cost of illness associated with pressure ulcers have indicated that the total costs may consume between 1% in the Netherlands and 4% in the United Kingdom of health care expenditure (National Pressure Ulcer Advisory Panel, 2009).

Goal

NOC
Tissue Integrity

The client will demonstrate progressive healing of dermal ulcer as evidenced by the following indicators:

- Identify causative factors for pressure ulcers.
- Identify rationale for prevention and treatment.
- Participate in the prescribed treatment plan to promote wound healing.

Interventions

NIC
Teaching: Individual,
Surveillance

Identify the Stage of Pressure Ulcer Development (National Pressure Ulcer Advisory Panel, 2009)

Category / stage I: Nonblanchable erythema
Intact skin with nonblanchable redness of a localized area usually over a bony prominence. Darkly pigmented skin may not have visible blanching; its color may differ from the surrounding area. The area may be painful, firm, soft, warmer or cooler as compared with adjacent tissue. Category I may be difficult to detect in individuals with dark skin tones. May indicate "at risk" persons.

Category / stage II: Partial thickness

Partial-thickness loss of dermis presenting as a shallow open ulcer with a red pink wound bed, without slough. May also present as an intact or open / ruptured serum-filled or sero-sanginous filled blister. Presents as a shiny or dry shallow ulcer without slough or bruising*. This category should not be used to describe skin tears, tape burns, incontinence associated dermatitis, maceration or excoriation.

*Bruising indicates deep tissue injury.

Category / stage III: Full thickness skin loss

Full-thickness tissue loss. Subcutaneous fat may be visible but bone, tendon, or muscle are *not* exposed. Slough may be present but does not obscure the depth of tissue loss. *May* include undermining and tunneling. The depth of a Category / stage III pressure ulcer varies by anatomical location. The bridge of the nose, ear, occiput and malleolus do not have (adipose) subcutaneous tissue and Category / stage III ulcers can be shallow. In contrast, areas of significant adiposity can develop extremely deep Category / stage III pressure ulcers. Bone / tendon is not visible or directly palpable.

Category / stage IV: Full thickness tissue loss

Full-thickness tissue loss with exposed bone, tendon or muscle. Slough or eschar may be present. Often includes undermining and tunneling. The depth of a Category / stage IV pressure ulcer varies by anatomical location. The bridge of the nose, ear, occiput, and malleolus do not have (adipose) subcutaneous tissue and these ulcers can be shallow. Category / stage IV ulcers can extend into muscle and / or supporting structures (e.g., fascia, tendon or joint capsule) making osteomyelitis or osteitis likely to occur. Exposed bone / muscle is visible or directly palpable.

Additional Categories / Stages for the USA

Unstageable / Unclassified: Full thickness skin or tissue loss–depth unknown

Full thickness tissue loss in which actual depth of the ulcer is completely obscured by slough (yellow, tan, gray, green or brown) and / or eschar (tan, brown or black) in the wound bed. Until enough slough and / or eschar are removed to expose the base of the wound, the true depth cannot be determined; but it will be either a Category / stage III or IV. Stable (dry, adherent, intact without erythema or fluctuance) eschar on the heels serves as "the body's natural (biological) cover" and should not be removed.

Suspected Deep Tissue Injury–depth unknown

Purple or maroon localized area of discolored intact skin or blood-filled blister due to damage of underlying soft tissue from pressure and / or *shear*. The area may be preceded by tissue that is painful, firm, mushy, boggy, warmer or cooler as compared with adjacent tissue. Deep tissue injury may be difficult to detect in individuals with dark skin tones. Evolution may include a thin blister over a dark wound bed. The wound may further evolve and become covered by thin eschar. Evolution may be rapid exposing additional layers of tissue even with optimal treatment.

Devise a Plan for Pressure Ulcer Management Using Principles of Moist Wound Healing

- Cleanse skin only when soiled. (Daily cleansing of aged, dry or at-risk skin may remove naturally protective oils) (Bryant, 2000; Maklebust & Sieggreen, 2001).
- Wash reddened area gently with mild soap, rinse area thoroughly to remove soap, and pat dry.
- Maintain the moisture balance by:
  - Reducing environmental factors contributing to dry skin
  - Preventing incontinence
  - Managing wound exudates
  - Using a topical moisturizer.
- Protect the healthy skin surface with one or a combination of the following:
  - Apply a thin coat of liquid copolymer skin sealant.
  - Cover the area with moisture-permeable film dressing.
  - Cover the area with a hydrocolloid wafer barrier and secure with strips of 1-inch tape; leave in place for 2 to 3 days.
- Wound healing occurs most efficiently with the following extrinsic factors (Maklebust & Sieggreen, 2001):
  - Humidity affects the rate of epithelialization and the amount of scar formation. A moist environment provides optimal conditions for rapid healing.

- When wounds are left uncovered, epidermal cells must migrate under the scab and over the fibrous tissue below. When wounds are semi-occluded and the surface of the wound remains moist, epidermal cells migrate more rapidly over the surface.
- Appropriate use of dressings may promote a moist wound. Use of semi-occlusive film dressings or hydrocolloid barrier wafers mechanically protect and properly humidify wounds that are epidermal or dermal. These dressings bathe the wound in serous exudates and do not adhere to the wound surface when they are removed.

  R: The cardinal rule of healing is to keep the wound tissue moist and the surrounding skin dry. Use a dressing that will keep the wound occluded. Humidity affects the rate of epithelialization and the amount of scar formation. A moist environment provides optimal conditions for rapid healing.

- Assess the status of pressure ulcer (ASSESSMENT) (National Pressure Ulcer Advisory Panel, 2009)
  - **A Anatomic location:** Describe location using precise anatomic terms, as much as possible. Consider using a body diagram to clearly communicate location of the pressure ulcer.
  - **S Size, shape:** Use disposable measuring guide. Measure length, width, depth in centimeters at the longest or widest portion of the pressure ulcer. Depth is measured into deepest portion of wound. May use gloved finger or a carefully placed cotton-tipped applicator to measure depth and compare to measuring guide. Describe measurements utilizing face of clock 12-6 direction for length, 3-9 direction for width.
  - **S Stage:** Use National Pressure Ulcer Advisory Panel definitions and descriptions A pressure ulcer that is covered with eschar or necrotic tissue cannot be staged until the majority of the base is clearly identified. Pressure ulcers are never "backstaged" as the ulcer heals; the ulcer is described as a healing pressure ulcer with a notation of the highest stage.
  - **E Exudate:** Describe amount using terms such as none, light / scant, moderate, or large. Describe characteristics using terms such as serous, serosanguineous, sanguinous / bloody, or purulent.
  - **S Surrounding skin:** Assess and describe color, texture, temperature, presence of induration, maceration, or integrity of periwound skin.
  - **S Sinus tract, tunneling:** Measure length / depth using gloved finger or carefully placed cotton-tipped applicator. Describe location utilizing the face of a clock, as above.
  - **M Margins:** Note presence of undermining. Note presence of erythema or maceration. Undermining—tissue destruction around the perimeter of the wound under the intact surface / skin.
  - **E Edges:** Describe wound edges using terms such as indistinct, distinct attached, not attached, defined, undefined. or rolled under.
  - **N Nose (odor):** Some dressings or topical solutions can affect the odor.
  - **T Tissue:** Note characteristics of tissue in wound base, such as epithelial, granulation, slough, or necrotic tissue. Necrotic tissue can be further described as white / gray, yellow.

> **CLINICAL ALERT**
> - Notify physician / NP if changes in ulcer represent deterioration.

- For wound care, consult with a nurse wound care specialist needed.
  - Remove necrotic tissue.

    R: This delays wound healing by prolonging the inflammatory phase.

  - Cleanse wound bed to decrease bacterial count.

    R: Bacterial counts above 10_5 may produce infection by overwhelming the host.

  - Obliterate dead space in the wound.

    R: This prevents premature closure and abscess formation.

  - Absorb excess exudates.

    R: This can cause damage to surrounding skin, and increases the risk of infection in the wound bed.

  - Cover pressure ulcer with a sterile dressing (e.g., film dressing, hydrocolloid wafer dressing, moist gauze dressing). Do not occlude ulcers on immunocompromised patients.
  - Protect the healing wound from trauma and bacterial invasion.

    R: Appropriate use of dressings may promote moist wound. Use of semiocclusive film dressings or hydrocolloid barrier wafers mechanically protect and properly humidify wounds that are epidermal or dermal.

Consult With Nurse Specialist or Physician for Treatment of Necrotic, Infected, or Deep Pressure Ulcers

R: Surgical debridement may be needed.

For pain management, refer to *Acute Pain*.

For nutrition management, refer to *Impaired Nutrition*.

Clinical Alert Report

- Advise ancillary staff / student of the repositioning schedule for client and report any new signs of compromised skin as blanching, reddened skin, any areas that are painful, firm, soft, warmer or cooler as compared with adjacent tissue that does disappear with a position change. Advise that dark skin may appear darker, not reddened.

TRANSITION PLAN

Initiate health teaching and referrals as indicated.

- Instruct the client and family of :
  - Causes of pressure ulcers
  - Ways to prevent them
  - Dietary needs
  - Positioning
- Teach the client importance of good skin hygiene.
- Refer the client to a community nursing agency for assistance at home.

RISK FOR IMPAIRED SKIN INTEGRITY

Risk for Pressure Ulcer**

NANDA-I Definition

At risk for alteration in epidermis and / or dermis

Risk Factors

Pathophysiologic

Related to decreased blood and nutrients to tissues secondary to:

Diabetes mellitus:
    Peripheral vascular alterations
    Venous stasis
Cardiopulmonary disorders
Obesity
Emaciation
Dehydration*
Malnutrition
Edema*

Related to neuropathy

**If the person is at risk for pressure ulcers, use the new Nanda-I diagnosis *Risk for Pressure Ulcers* instead of *Risk for Impaired Skin Integrity*.

Treatment Related

Related to decreased blood and nutrients to tissues secondary to:

Therapeutic extremes in body temperature
NPO status
Surgery

Related to imposed immobility secondary to sedation
Related to mechanical trauma

Therapeutic fixation devices
    Wired jaw
    Casts
    Traction
Orthopedic devices / braces

Related to effects of radiation* on epithelial and basal cells
Related to effects of mechanical factors* or pressure secondary to:

Tourniquets	NG tubes
Footboards	Shear
Restraints	Friction
Dressings, tape, solutions	Endotracheal tubes
External urinary catheters	Oral prostheses / braces

Situational (Personal, Environmental)

Related to chemical irritants* secondary to:

Excretions	Secretions	Noxious agents / substances

Related to the effects of pressure of impaired physical mobility* secondary to:

Pain	Fatigue	Motivation
Cognitive, sensory, or motor deficits		

Related to vascular and neurological deficits secondary to tobacco use, excess alcohol intake
Related to dry, thin skin and decreased dermal vascularity secondary to aging

Goal

NOC
Tissue Integrity: Skin and Mucous Membrane

The client will demonstrate skin integrity free of pressure ulcers (if able) as evidenced by the following indicators:

- Participate in risk assessment.
- Express willingness to participate in prevention of pressure ulcers.
- Describe etiology and prevention measures.

Interventions (National Pressure Ulcer Advisory Panel, 2009)

NIC
Pressure Management, Pressure Ulcer Care, Skin Surveillance, Positioning

- Perform regular skin assessments as frequently as indicated.
- Skin inspection should include assessment for localized heat, edema, or induration (hardness), especially in individuals with darkly pigmented skin.
- Inspect areas at risk of developing ulcers with each position change.
  - Ears
  - Elbows
  - Occiput
  - Trochanter**
  - Heels

**Areas with little soft tissue over a bony prominence are at greatest risk.

- Ischia
- Sacrum
- Scapula
- Scrotum

- Ask individuals to identify any areas of discomfort or pain that could be attributed to pressure damage.
- Observe the skin for pressure damage caused by medical devices.
- Observe for blanching, nonblanching erythema, indurated or boggy skin.

  R: Blanching erythema is an early indicator of the need to redistribute pressure; nonblanching erythema is suggestive that tissue damage has already occurred or is imminent; indurated or boggy skin is a sign that deep tissue damage has likely occurred.

- Document all skin assessments, noting details of any pain possibly related to pressure damage.

  R: The frequency of inspection may need to be increased in response to any deterioration in overall condition.

Attempt to Modify Contributing Factors to Lessen the Possibility of a Pressure Ulcer Developing

Incontinence of Urine or Feces

- Determine the etiology of the incontinence.
- Maintain sufficient fluid intake for adequate hydration (approximately 2,500 mL daily, unless contraindicated); check oral mucous membranes for moisture and check urine specific gravity.
- Establish a schedule for emptying the bladder (begin with every 2 hours).
- If the client is confused, determine what his or her incontinence pattern is and intervene before incontinence occurs.
- Explain problem to the client; secure his or her cooperation for the plan.
- When incontinent, wash the perineum with a liquid soap.
- Apply a protective barrier to the perineal region (incontinence film barrier spray or wipes).
- Check the client frequently for incontinence when indicated.
- For additional interventions, refer to *Impaired Urinary Elimination*.

R: Maceration is a mechanism by which the tissue is softened by prolonged wetting or soaking. If the skin becomes waterlogged, the cells are weakened and the epidermis is easily eroded. Bowel incontinence is more damaging than urinary incontinence, due to the additional digestive enzymes found in stool. Care must be taken to prevent excoriation (Wilkinson & Van Leuven, 2007).

Skin Care

- Whenever possible, do not turn the individual onto a body surface that is still reddened from a previous episode of pressure loading.
- Do not use massage for pressure ulcer prevention or do not vigorously rub skin that is at risk for pressure ulceration.

  R: Massage is contraindicated in the presence of acute inflammation and where there is the possibility of damaged blood vessels or fragile skin.

- Use skin emollients to hydrate dry skin in order to reduce risk of skin damage. Protect the skin from exposure to excessive moisture with a barrier product.

  R: Excessive moisture will contribute to maceration when tissues are softened by prolonged wetting, which breaks down the protective layer of epidermis / dermis.

- Avoid use of synthetic sheepskin pads; cutout, ring, or donut-type devices; and water-filled gloves.

  R: These products are irritating and create pressure, which compromises circulation.

Nutrition for Pressure Ulcer Prevention

- Screen and assess the nutritional status of every individual at risk of pressure ulcers in each health care setting.
- Refer each individual with nutritional risk and pressure ulcer risk to a registered dietitian.
- Offer high-protein mixed oral nutritional supplements and / or tube feeding, in addition to the usual diet, to individuals with nutritional risk and pressure ulcer risk because of acute or chronic diseases, or following a surgical intervention.

- Administer oral nutritional supplements (ONS) and / or tube feeding (TF) in between the regular meals to avoid reduction of normal food and fluid intake during regular mealtimes.

  R: An individual with nutritional risk and pressure ulcer risk needs a minimum of 30–35 kcal per kg body weight per day, with 1.25–1.5; g/kg/day protein and 1 mL of fluid intake per kcal per day.

- Monitor serum prealbumin levels.
  - Less than 5 mg/dL predicts a poor prognosis.
  - Less than 11 mg/dL predicts high risk and requires aggressive nutritional supplementation.
  - Less than 15 mg/dL predicts an increase risk of malnutrition (Evans, 2005).

    R: Laboratory values, such as albumin, prealbumin, and transferin may not reflect the current nutritional state, especially in the critically ill client. Other assessment factors such as weight loss, illness severity, comorbid conditions, and gastrointestional function should be considered for a nutrition plan of care. (Doley, 2010)

Repositioning

- Assess the individual's skin condition and general comfort. If the individual is not responding as expected to the repositioning regime, reconsider the frequency and method of repositioning.

  R: Repositioning frequency will be determined by the individual's tissue tolerance, his or her level of activity and mobility, his or her general medical condition, the overall treatment objectives, and assessments of the individual's skin condition.

- Repositioning should be undertaken using the 30-degree tilted side-lying position (alternately, right side, back, left side) or the prone position if the individual can tolerate this and her or his medical condition allows. Avoid postures that increase pressure, such as the 90-degree side-lying position, or the semi-recumbent position.

- Ensure that the heels are free of the surface of the bed. Position knee in slight flexion. Uses a pillow under the calves so that heels are elevated (i.e., "floating").

  R: Heel protection devices should elevate the heel completely (offload them) in such a way as to distribute the weight of the leg along the calf without putting pressure on the Achilles tendon.

- Use transfer aids to reduce friction and shear. Lift—don't drag—the individual while repositioning.

  R: Shear is a parallel force in which one layer of tissue moves in one direction and another layer moves in the opposite direction. If the skin sticks to the bed linen and the weight of the body makes the skeleton slide down inside the skin (as with semi-Fowler's positioning), the subepidermal capillaries may become angulated and pinched, resulting in decreased perfusion of the tissue. (Porth, 2011)

  R: Friction is the physiologic wearing away of tissue. If the skin is rubbed against the bed linens, the epidermis can be denuded by abrasion.

- Avoid positioning the individual directly onto medical devices, such as tubes or drainage systems.
- Avoid positioning the individual on bony prominences with existing nonblanchable erythema.
- If sitting in bed is necessary, avoid head-of-bed elevation or a slouched position that places pressure and shear on the sacrum and coccyx.

  R: Reposition the individual in such a way that pressure is relieved or redistributed.

Repositioning the Seated Individual

- Position the individual so as to maintain his or her full range of activities.
- Select a posture that is acceptable for the individual, and minimizes the pressures and shear exerted on the skin and soft tissues. Place the feet of the individual on a footstool or footrest when the feet do not reach the floor.
- Limit the time an individual spends seated in a chair without pressure relief.

R: Prevention in individuals at risk should be provided on a continuous basis during the time that they are at risk.

Use of Support Surfaces to Prevent Pressure Ulcers

- Use a pressure-redistributing seat cushion for individuals sitting in a chair whose mobility is reduced.
- Limit the time an individual spends seated in a chair without pressure relief.
- Use alternating-pressure active support overlays or mattress as indicated.

R: A pressure-reducing surface must not be able to be fully compressed by the body. To be effective, a support surface must be capable of first being deformed and then redistributing the weight of the body across the surface. Comfort is not a valid criterion for determining adequate pressure reduction. A hand check should be performed to determine if the product is effectively reducing pressure. The palm is placed under the pressure-reducing mattress; if the client can feel the hand or the caregiver can feel the client, the pressure is not adequate.

R: Pressure-reducing devices must be used in conjunction with repositioning protocols, not in place of them (Defloor et al., 2005).

> **TRANSITION PLAN**
> Initiate health teaching as indicated.
> * Instruct the client and family in specific techniques to use at home to prevent pressure ulcers.
> * Consider the use of long-term pressure-relieving devices for permanent disabilities.
>   *R: Pressure reduction is the one consistent intervention that must be included in all pressure ulcer treatment plans.*

DISTURBED SLEEP PATTERN

NANDA-I Definition

Time-limited interruptions of sleep amount and quality due to external factors

Defining Characteristics

Major (Must Be Present)

Adults
Difficulty falling or remaining asleep

Minor (May Be Present)

Adults

Fatigue on awakening or during the day	Agitation
Dozing during the day	Mood alterations

Related Factors

Many factors can contribute to disturbed sleep patterns. Some common factors follow.

Pathophysiologic

Related to frequent awakenings secondary to:

Impaired oxygen transport
  Angina
  Respiratory disorders
  Peripheral arteriosclerosis
  Circulatory disorders
Impaired elimination; bowel or bladder
  Diarrhea
  Retention
  Constipation

Dysuria
Incontinence
Frequency
Impaired metabolism
Hyperthyroidism
Hepatic disorders
Gastric ulcers

Treatment Related

Related to interruptions (e.g., for therapeutic monitoring, lab tests)*
Related to physical restraints*
Related to difficulty assuming usual position secondary to (specify)
Related to excessive daytime sleeping or hyperactivity secondary to (specify medication)

Tranquilizers
Sedatives
Amphetamines
Monoamine oxidase inhibitors
Hypnotics

Barbiturates
Antidepressants
Corticosteroids
Antihypertensives

Situational (Personal, Environmental)

Related to lack of sleep privacy / control*
Related to lighting, noise, noxious odors*
Related to sleep partner (e.g., snoring)*
Related to unfamiliar sleep furnishing*
Related to ambient temperature, humidity*
Related to caregiving responsibilities*
Related to change in daylight–darkness exposure*
Related to excessive hyperactivity secondary to:

Bipolar disorder
Attention-deficit disorder

Panic anxiety
Illicit drug use

Related to excessive daytime sleeping
Related to depression
Related to inadequate daytime activities
Related to pain
Related to anxiety response
Related to environmental changes (specify)

Hospitalization (noise, disturbing roommate, fear)

Goal

NOC
Rest, Sleep, Well-Being

The client will report a satisfactory balance of rest and activity as evidenced by the following indicators:

- Complete at least four sleep cycles (100 minutes) undisturbed.
- State factors that increase or decrease the quality of sleep.

Interventions

NIC
Energy Management,
Sleep Enhancement,
Environmental
Management

- Discuss the reasons for differing individual sleep requirements, including age, lifestyle, activity level, and other possible factors.

    R: Although many believe that a person needs 8 hours of sleep each night, no scientific evidence supports this. Individual sleep requirements vary greatly. Generally, a person who can relax and rest easily requires less sleep to feel refreshed. With aging, less time is spent in the sleep cycle stages 3 & 4, which are the most restorative stages of sleep. The results are difficulty falling asleep and staying asleep. (Cole & Richards, 2007)

- Explain the effects of sleep deprivation (e.g., cognition, stress management).

  R: Sleep deprivation results in impaired cognitive functioning (e.g., memory, concentration, and judgment) and perception, reduced emotional control, increased suspicion, irritability, and disorientation. It also lowers the pain threshold and decreases production of catecholamines, corticosteroids, and hormones (Colten & Altevogt, 2006). Sleep disturbance is the leading cause of hospital complications, such as falls, delirium. (IOM, 2009)

- Explain the need for sleep cycle.

  R: Sleep cycle. A client typically goes through four or five complete sleep cycles each night. Awakening during a cycle may cause him or her to feel poorly rested in the morning.

- Assess with client and family their usual bedtime routine—time, hygiene practices, rituals such as reading—and adhere to it as closely as possible.

  R: Sleep is difficult without relaxation, which the unfamiliar hospital environment can hinder.

- Encourage or provide evening care:
  - Bathroom or bedpan
  - Personal hygiene (mouth care, bath, shower, partial bath)
  - Clean linen and bedclothes (freshly made bed, sufficient blankets)

  R: A familiar bedtime ritual may promote relaxation and sleep.

- Reduce or eliminate environmental distractions and sleep interruptions.
  - Noise
    - Close the door to the room.
    - Pull the curtains.
    - Unplug the telephone.
    - Use "white noise" (e.g., fan; quiet music; recording of rain, waves).
    - Eliminate 24-hour lighting.
    - Provide night lights.
    - Decrease the amount and kind of incoming stimuli (e.g., staff conversations).
    - Cover blinking lights with tape.
    - Reduce the volume of alarms and televisions.
    - Place the client with a compatible roommate, if possible.
  - Interruptions

    R: Researchers have reported that the chief deterrents to sleep in critical care clients were activity, noise, pain, physical condition, nursing procedures, lights, vapor tents, and hypothermia.

- Explain the need to avoid sedative and hypnotic drugs.

  R: Sleep medications can increase awakenings and fewer total sleep hours (LaReau et al., 2008). These medications begin to lose their effectiveness after a week of use, requiring increased dosages and leading to the risk of dependence.

- Cluster procedures to minimize the times you need to wake the client at night. If possible, plan for at least 4 periods of 90 minutes uninterrupted sleep.

  R: In order to feel rested, a person usually must complete an entire sleep cycle (70 to 90 minutes) four or five times a night.

SBAR *Situation:* Mr. Nelo has only slept _ hours the last 24 hours.

Background: He is not sleeping because . . . .

Assessment: He is c/o of more pain, wants a sleeping pill.

Recommendation: It would be useful to . . . e.g., stop vital signs 10 p.m. – 6 a.m. unless needed, change the times for medication administration.

Provide treatments before 10 p.m. and after 6 a.m. when possible.

- Discuss with physician / NP / PA the use of a "Sleep Protocol." This will allow the nursing staff the authority not to wake a person for blood draws or vital signs if appropriate and (Bartick, 2009):
  - Designate "quiet time" between 10 p.m. and 6 a.m.

- Lullabies were played over public address system.
- Overhead hallway lights went off on a timer at 10 p.m.
- Mute phones close to client rooms, avoid intercom use except in emergencies.
- Vital signs were taken at 10 p.m., and started again at 6 a.m. unless otherwise indicated.
- Medications are ordered bid, tid, qid, not "q" certain hours when possible.
- No administering a diuretic after 4 p.m.
- Avoiding blood transfusions during "quiet time" due to frequent monitoring.

  R: A small study reported that "Sleep Protocol" can reduce the number of clients reporting disturbed sleep 38% and a 49% reduction in clients needing sedatives (Bartick, 2009).

TRANSITION PLAN
Initiate health teaching as indicated.

- If poor sleep is contributing to daytime fatigue and pain, try the following tips to improve sleep and get the rest you need (Arthritis Foundation, 2012):
  - Maintain a regular daily schedule of activities, including a regular sleep schedule.
  - Exercise, but not late in the evening.
  - Set aside an hour before bedtime for relaxation.
  - Eat a light snack before bedtime. You should not go to bed hungry, nor should you feel too full.
  - Make your bedroom as quiet and as comfortable as possible. Maintain a comfortable room temperature. Invest in a comfortable mattress and / or try a body-length pillow to provide more support.
  - Use your bedroom only for sleeping and for being physically close to your partner.
  - Arise at the same time every day, even on weekends and holidays.
  - Avoid caffeine and alcohol before bedtime.
  - Avoid long naps. If a nap is needed to get you through the day, keep it short, and schedule it well in advance of your bedtime. Try exercising in the afternoon rather than napping.
  - Avoid sleeping pills.
  - Don't smoke. If you must smoke, don't smoke before bedtime.
  - Use a clock radio with an automatic shutoff to play soft music at bedtime. If you are not a heavy sleeper, wake up to music rather than a clanging alarm.
  - Take a warm bath before going to bed.
  - Listen to soothing music or a relaxation tape.
  - Read before bedtime if you like, but avoid suspenseful, action-filled novels or work-related material that can preoccupy your thoughts and cause a poor night's sleep.
  - Use earplugs or white noise to block distracting noises.
  - Before going to bed, write down your worries and make a "things to do" list. Then put it away for tomorrow so you can stop thinking about them.
  - If you don't go to sleep within 30 minutes after going to bed, or if you wake up in the middle of the night and can't get back to sleep, get up and go to a different room. Try a relaxation technique, read, or listen to soothing music.

Clinical Alert Report
Advise ancillary staff / student to report the amount of time spent sleeping include naps, nighttime.
  R: The quality and amount of sleep time with at least 4 periods of 90 minutes of uninterrupted sleep is the goal.

RISK FOR DISTURBED SLEEP PATTERN**

Definition

Risk for time-limited interruptions of sleep amount and quality due to external factors

Risk Factors

Many factors can contribute to disturbed sleep patterns. Some common factors follow.

Pathophysiologic

Related to frequent awakenings secondary to:

Impaired oxygen transport
   Angina
   Respiratory disorders
   Peripheral arteriosclerosis
   Circulatory disorders
Impaired elimination; bowel or bladder
   Diarrhea
   Retention
   Constipation
   Dysuria
   Incontinence
   Frequency
Impaired metabolism
Hyperthyroidism
Hepatic disorders
Gastric ulcers

Treatment Related

Related to interruptions (e.g., for therapeutic monitoring, lab tests)
Related to physical restraints
Related to difficulty assuming usual position secondary to (specify)
Related to excessive daytime sleeping or hyperactivity secondary to (specify medication)

Tranquilizers
Sedatives
Amphetamines
Monoamine oxidase inhibitors
Hypnotics
Barbiturates
Antidepressants
Corticosteroids
Antihypertensives

Situational (Personal, Environmental)

Related to lack of sleep privacy / control
Related to lighting, noise, and noxious odors
Related to sleep partner (e.g., snoring)
Related to unfamiliar sleep furnishing

**This diagnosis is not currently on the NANDA-I list but has been included for clarity and usefulness.

Related to ambient temperature, humidity
Related to caregiving responsibilities
Related to change in daylight-darkness exposure
Related to excessive hyperactivity secondary to:

Bipolar disorder
Attention-deficit disorder
Panic anxiety
Illicit drug use

Related to excessive daytime sleeping
Related to depression
Related to inadequate daytime activities
Related to pain
Related to anxiety response
Related to environmental changes (specify)

Hospitalization (noise, disturbing roommate, fear)

Goals and Interventions

Refer to Generic Medical Care Plan.

TRANSITION PLAN
Refer to Disturbed Sleep Pattern

Clinical Alert Report
Refer to Disturbed Sleep Pattern

SPIRITUAL DISTRESS

NANDA-I Definition

Impaired ability to experience and integrate meaning and purpose in life through connectedness with self, others, art, music, literature, nature, and / or a power greater than oneself

Defining Characteristics

Questions meaning of life, death, and suffering
Conveys meaning of life, death, and suffering
Reports no sense of meaning and purpose in life
Lacks enthusiasm for life, feelings of joy, inner peace, or love
Demonstrates discouragement or despair
Experiences alienation from spiritual or religious community
Expresses need to reconcile with self, others, God, or creator
Presents with sudden interest in spiritual matters (reading spiritual or religious books, watching spiritual or religious programs on television)
Displays sudden changes in spiritual practices (rejection, neglect, doubt, fanatical devotion)
Verbalizes that family, loved ones, peers, or health care providers opposed spiritual beliefs or practices
Questions credibility of religion or spiritual belief system
Requests assistance for a disturbance in spiritual beliefs or religious practice

Related Factors

Pathophysiologic

Related to challenge in spiritual health or separation from spiritual ties secondary to (e.g., hospitalization, pain, loss of body part or function, trauma, terminal illness, debilitating disease, miscarriage, stillbirth)

Treatment Related

Related to conflict between (specify prescribed regimen) and beliefs (e.g., isolation, surgery, termination, medical procedures, blood transfusion, dialysis, dietary restrictions, medications)

Situational (Personal, Environmental)

Related to death* or illness of significant other
Related to embarrassment of expressions of spirituality or religion, such as prayers, meditation, or other rituals
Related to barriers to practicing spiritual rituals

Restrictions of intensive care
Lack of privacy
Unavailability of special foods / diet or ritual objects
Confinement to bed or room

Related to spiritual or religious beliefs opposed by family, peers, health care providers
Related to divorce, separation from loved one, or other perceived loss

Carp's Cues

To promote positive spirituality with clients and families, the nurse must possess spiritual self-knowledge. For the nurse, self-evaluation must precede assessment of spiritual concerns, and assessment of spiritual health should be confined to the context of nursing. The nurse can assist people with spiritual concerns or distress by providing resources for spiritual help, by listening nonjudgmentally, and by providing opportunities for meeting spiritual needs (O'Brien, 2010; Wright, 2004).

Spirituality and religiousness are two different concepts. Burkhart and Solari-Twadell define spirituality as the "ability to experience and integrate meaning and self; others, art, music, literature, nature, or a power greater than oneself" (2001, p. 51). Religiousness is "the ability to exercise participation in the beliefs of a particular denomination of faith community and related rituals" (Burkhart & Solari-Twadell, 2001, p. 51). Although the spiritual dimension of human wholeness is always present, it may or may not exist within the context of religious traditions or practices.

Goal

NOC
Hope, Spiritual Well-Being

The client will find meaning and purpose in life, including and during illness as evidenced by the following indicators:

* The client expresses his or her feelings related to beliefs and spirituality.
* The client describes his or her spiritual belief system as it relates to illness.
* The client finds meaning and comfort in religious or spiritual practice.

Interventions

NIC
Spiritual Growth Facilitation, Hope Instillation, Active Listening, Presence, Emotional Support, Spiritual Support

Create an Environment of Trust (Puchalski & Ferrell, 2010)

* Be open to listening to the patient's story, not just the medical facts.
* Listen for the content, emotion and manner, and spiritual meanings.
* Give "permission" to discuss spiritual matters with the nurse by bringing up the subject of spiritual welfare, if necessary.
* Be fully present.

R: The nurse should practice with a confidence to initiate spiritual dialogues and as an advocate in recognizing and respecting the client's spiritual needs (Mauk & Schmidt, 2004).

Eliminate or Reduce Causative and Contributing Factors, If Possible

Feeling Threatened and Vulnerable Because of Symptoms or Possible Death
- Inform clients and families about the importance of finding meaning in illness.
- Suggest using prayer, imagery, and meditation to reduce anxiety and provide hope and a sense of control.

Failure of Spiritual Beliefs to Provide Explanation or Comfort During Crisis of Illness / Suffering / Impending Death
- Use questions about past beliefs and spiritual experiences to assist the client in putting this life event into wider perspective.
- Offer to contact the usual or a new spiritual leader.
- Offer to pray / meditate / read with the client if you are comfortable with this, or arrange for another member of the health care team if more appropriate.
- Provide uninterrupted quiet time for prayer / reading / meditation on spiritual concerns.

R: The nurse should practice with a confidence to initiate spiritual dialogues and as an advocate in recognizing and respecting the client's spiritual needs (Mauk & Schmidt, 2004).

Doubting Quality of Own Faith to Deal with Current Illness / Suffering / Death

- Be available and willing to listen when client expresses self-doubt, guilt, or other negative feelings.
- Silence, touch, or both may be useful in communicating the nurse's presence and support during times of doubt or despair.
- Offer to contact usual or new spiritual leader.

R: Research shows that people with higher levels of spiritual well-being tend to experience lower levels of anxiety. For many people, spiritual activities provide a direct coping action and may improve adaptation to illness (Puchalski & Ferrell, 2010).

Anger Toward God or Spiritual Beliefs for Allowing or Causing Illness / Suffering / Death
- Express to the client that anger toward God is a common reaction to illness / suffering / death.
- Help the client recognize and discuss feelings of anger.

R: The client may view anger at God and a religious leader as "forbidden" and may be reluctant to initiate discussions of spiritual conflicts (Kemp, 2006).

- Allow client to problem-solve to find ways to express and relieve anger.
- Offer to contact the usual spiritual leader or offer to contact another spiritual support person (e.g., pastoral care, hospital chaplain) if the client cannot share feelings with the usual spiritual leader.

Related to Conflict Between Religious or Spiritual Beliefs and Prescribed Health Regimen

Assess for Causative and Contributing Factors

- Lack of information about or understanding of spiritual restrictions
- Lack of information about or understanding of health regimen
- Informed, true conflict
- Parental conflict concerning treatment of their child
- Lack of time for deliberation before emergency treatment or surgery
- Practice as an advocate for the client and family.

R: The nurse should be the link between the family and other members of the health care team.

Eliminate or Reduce Causative and Contributing Factors, If Possible

Lack of Information About Spiritual Restrictions
- Have the spiritual leader discuss restrictions and exemptions as they apply to those who are seriously ill or hospitalized.
- Provide reading materials on religious and spiritual restrictions and exemptions.
- Encourage the client to seek information from and discuss restrictions with spiritual leader and / or others in the spiritual group.
- Chart the results of these discussions.

R: Interventions focus on providing information about all alternatives and the consequences of each option.

Lack of Information About Health Regimen

- Provide accurate information about health regimen, treatments, and medications.
- Explain the nature and purpose of therapy.
- Discuss possible outcomes without therapy; be factual and honest, but do not attempt to frighten or force the client to accept treatment.

  R: The nurse's role is as an advocate for the family.

Informed, True Conflict

- Encourage the client and physician / nurse practitioner to consider alternative methods of therapy. Support the client making an informed decision—even if the decision conflicts with nurse's own values.

  R: Interventions focus on providing information about all alternatives and the consequences of each option.

Parental Conflict Over Treatment of the Child

- If parents refuse treatment of the child, follow the interventions under informed conflict above.
- If parents still refuse treatment, the physician or hospital administrator may obtain a court order appointing a temporary guardian to consent to treatment.

  R: Court orders to save a child's life remove the parent's right to refuse (Hockenberry & Wilson, 2009).

- Call the spiritual leader to support the parents (and possibly the child).
- Encourage expression of negative feelings.

  R: The nurse should be the link between the family and other members of the health care team.

RISK FOR SPIRITUAL DISTRESS

NANDA-I Definition

At risk for an impaired ability to experience and integrate meaning and purpose in life through connectedness with self, others, art, music, literature, nature, and / or a power greater than oneself

Risk Factors

Refer to *Spiritual Distress*.

Goals

NOC
Refer to *Spiritual Distress*.

The person will express continued spiritual harmony as evidenced by the following indicators:

- Continue to practice usual spiritual rituals.
- Describe increased comfort after assistance.

Interventions

NIC
Refer to *Spiritual Distress*.

Refer to *Spiritual Distress*.

INEFFECTIVE TISSUE PERFUSION**
Definition

Decrease in oxygen resulting in failure to nourish tissues at capillary level

Carp's Cues

The use of any *Ineffective Tissue Perfusion* diagnosis other than *Peripheral* merely provides new labels for medical diagnoses, for example, renal failure, congestive heart failure, increased intracranial pressure labels that do not describe the nursing focus or accountability.

**This diagnosis is not currently on the NANDA-I list but has been included for clarity and usefulness.

These situations required both medical and nursing intervention to maintain or restore physiologic stability. Instead of using *Ineffective Tissue Perfusion*, the nurse should focus on the nursing diagnoses and collaborative problems applicable because of altered renal, cardiac, cerebral, pulmonary, or gastrointestinal (GI) tissue perfusion, such as *Risk for Complications of GI Bleeding* or *Activity Intolerance related to insufficient oxygenation secondary to COPD*.

For each of the specific body Tissue Perfusion diagnoses listed above, refer to the discussion under its Carp's Cues.

INEFFECTIVE PERIPHERAL TISSUE PERFUSION

NANDA-I Definition

Decrease in blood circulation to the periphery that may compromise health

Defining Characteristics

Major (Must Be Present, One or More)

Presence of one of the following types (see Key Concepts for definitions):

Claudication (arterial)*
Aching pain (arterial or venous)
Rest pain (arterial)
Diminished or absent arterial pulses* (arterial)
Skin color changes*
Pallor (arterial)
Reactive hyperemia (arterial)
Cyanosis (venous)
Skin temperature changes
Cooler (arterial)
Warmer (venous)
Decreased blood pressure (arterial)
Capillary refill longer than 3 seconds (arterial)*

Minor (May Be Present)

Edema* (venous)
Change in sensory function (arterial)
Change in motor function (arterial)
Trophic tissue changes (arterial)

Hard, thick nails
Loss of hair
Nonhealing wound

Related Factors

Pathophysiologic

Related to compromised blood flow secondary to:

Vascular disorders
   Arteriosclerosis
   Leriche's syndrome
   Venous hypertension
   Raynaud's disease / syndrome
   Aneurysm
   Varicosities
   Alcoholism
   Buerger's disease
   Deep vein thrombosis
   Sickle cell crisis

> Collagen vascular disease
> Cirrhosis
> Rheumatoid arthritis

Diabetes mellitus

Hypotension

Blood dyscrasias

Renal failure

Cancer / tumor

Treatment Related

Related to immobilization

Related to presence of invasive lines

Related to pressure sites / constriction (elastic compression bandages, stockings, restraints)

Related to blood vessel trauma or compression

Situational (Personal, Environmental)

Related to pressure of enlarging uterus on pelvic vessels

Related to pressure of enlarged abdomen on pelvic / peripheral vessels

Related to vasoconstricting effects of tobacco

Related to decreased circulating volume secondary to dehydration

Goal

NOC

Sensory Functions: Cutaneous, Tissue Integrity, Tissue Perfusion: Peripheral

The individual will report a decrease in pain as evidenced by the following indicators:

- Define peripheral vascular problem in own words.
- Identify factors that improve peripheral circulation.
- Identify necessary lifestyle changes.
- Identify medical regimen, diet, medications, activities that promote vasodilation.
- Identify factors that inhibit peripheral circulation.
- State when to contact physician or health care professional.

Interventions

NIC

Peripheral Sensation Management, Circulatory Care: Venous Insufficiency, Circulatory Care: Arterial Insufficiency, Positioning, Exercise Promotion, Smoking Cessation Assistance

- Assess causative and contributing factors
  - Tobacco use
  - Type 2 diabetes
  - Hypertension
  - Dyslipidemia
  - Obesity
  - Sedentary lifestyle
  - Metabolic syndrome
  - COPD
  - Mobility problems (e.g., arthritis)

  R: Peripheral arterial disease is typically due to aggressive atherosclerosis resulting from untreated cardiovascular disease (CVD) risk factors (Oka, 2006).

  - Discuss specifically with client his or her symptoms associated with mobility and are relieved by rest as pain, numbness and /or weakness in hips, buttocks, thigh, or calf (Oka, 2006).

  R: Only 30% to 50% of older adults report typical claudication symptoms (e.g., calf pain when walking relieved with rest). Older, male, diabetic clients may be asymptomatic. (McDermott et al.,1999)

  - Explain the effects of impaired peripheral circulation on causing substantial walking impairment, diminished quality of life, limb ischemia / amputation and increased CVD morbidity and mortality (Oka, 2006).

R: An explanation of the probable course of impaired peripheral circulation can increase motivation to modify risk factors (Oka, 2006).

- Promote factors that improve arterial blood flow.
  - Keep extremity in a dependent position.

  R: Arterial blood flow is enhanced by a dependent position and inhibited by an elevated position (gravity pulls blood downward, away from the heart).

  - Keep extremity warm (do not use heating pad or hot water bottle).

  R: Peripheral vascular disease will reduce sensitivity. The person will not be able to determine if the temperature is hot enough to damage tissue; the use of external heat also may increase the metabolic demands of the tissue beyond its capacity.

- Promote factors that improve venous blood flow. Teach to:
  - Elevate extremity above the level of the heart (may be contraindicated if severe cardiac or respiratory disease is present).

  R: Venous blood flow is enhanced by an elevated position and inhibited by a dependent position. (Gravity pulls blood downward, away from the heart.)

  - Change positions at least every hour.
  - Avoid leg crossing.

  R: Tight garments and certain leg positions constrict leg vessels, further reducing circulation.

  - Avoid pillows behind the knees or Gatch bed, which is elevated at the knees.
  - Avoid leg crossing.
  - Change positions, move extremities, or wiggle fingers and toes every hour.
  - Avoid tight elastic stockings above the knees.
  - Reduce external pressure points (inspect shoes daily for rough lining).
  - Avoid sheepskin heel protectors (they increase heel pressure and pressure across dorsum of foot).
  - Encourage range-of-motion exercises.

  R: Cellular nutrition and function depend on adequate blood flow through the microcirculation.

  - Reduce or remove external venous compression that impedes venous flow.
- Explain the process of increasing walking distance and the benefits of walking. (McDermott, 2004; Oka, 2006).
  - Walk until moderate pain is felt.
  - Rest (standing or sitting) until pain subsides
  - Resume walking and repeat the rest / walk cycle
  - Increase walking time by 5 minutes each day walked, with a goal of walking at least 30 minutes three to five times a week.
  - Emphasize the functional benefits (increased walking speed, distance, duration, and decreased symptoms) will occur gradually and can be noticed as early as 4 to 8 weeks. Greater benefit is achieved when the client continues walking 6 months or longer.

  R: Studies have shown that maximal walking distance can be improved up to 150% with decreased symptoms (Leng, 2000; McDermott, 2004; Oka, 2006).

- Emphasize the need to prevent infection with careful foot care.
  - Wear shoes that fit properly. Gradually "break in" new shoes
  - Inspect the inside of shoes daily for rough lining.
  - Examine feet daily yourself or by someone else.
  - Keep dry skin lubricated (cracked skin eliminates the physical barrier to infection).
  - Pay attention to any reddened areas, cuts, scrapes, or injuries.
  - Call primary care provider to report any changes or injuries.

  R: Tissues heal slowly and are more likely to get infected when there is decreased circulation.

CLINICAL ALERT
- **Any disruption of the skin integrity must be promptly assessed and treated to prevent infection, cellulitis, and the need for hospitalization and surgery.**

- Initiate transitional teaching, as indicated.

CLINICAL ALERT
- Individuals with peripheral vascular insufficiency usually have more than three modifiable risk factors. Allow client to identify his or her goals, because unrealistic expectations of the nurse will result in rejection and failure.

TRANSITION PLAN
- Discuss with client what risk factors that he or she is interested in modifying. Help him or her select goals that are seen as possible. Some examples are:
  - Will walk 15 minutes 5 days a week.
  - Will substitute sugar drinks with water or diet beverages.
  - Will eat 1/3 less portion of starches (potatoes, pasta, rice, bread).
  - Will eat three servings of vegetables each day.
  - Will delay the urge to smoke for 1 hour.

  R: Allowing the client to direct his or her focus on changes that he or she perceives as "doable" can increase motivation.
- Specifically address modifiable risk factors determined by the client.
- Plan a daily walking program.
  - Refer to Getting Started to Increase Activity on thePoint at http://thePoint.lww.com/Carpenito6e.
- Initiate a dialogue regarding interest in smoking cessation.
  - Refer to Getting Started to Quit Smoking on thePoint at http://thePoint.lww.com/Carpenito6e.
- Explain the effects of excess weight on body functions (e.g., circulation, lipids, diabetes mellitus, cardiac function, hypertension).

  R: Obesity increases peripheral resistance and venous pooling, excess weight increases cardiac workload, causing hypertension (Porth, 2011).
  - Refer to Getting Started to Losing Weight on thePoint at http://thePoint.lww.com/Carpenito6e.
  - Refer client / family to Nutritionist.
- Explain the effects of hyperlipidemia on circulation

  R: Peripheral arterial insufficiency is due to aggressive atherosclerosis resulting from untreated CVD risk factors, one of which is hyperlipidemia, causing obstruction of peripheral blood flow (Oka, 2006).
  - Refer to Getting Started to Healthy Eating on thePoint at http://thePoint.lww.com/Carpenito6e.
- Teach client to:
  - Avoid long car or plane rides (get up and walk around at least every hour).
  - Wear warm clothing during cold weather. Wear cotton or wool socks.
  - Use gloves or mittens if hands are exposed to cold (including home freezers).
  - Avoid dehydration in warm weather.
  - Refer to community resources for lifestyle changes.

  R: Community resources can assist the client with weight loss, smoking cessation, diet, and exercise programs.

Clinical Alert Report
Advise onsite staff first to report increase in edema, redness, signs of trauma

RISK FOR DECREASED CARDIAC TISSUE PERFUSION

NANDA-I Definition

Risk for a decrease in cardiac (coronary) circulation

Risk Factors*

Birth control pills (medication side effect of combination pills)**
Cardiac surgery (treatment)
Cardiac tamponade (clinical emergency)
Coronary artery spasm (clinical emergency)
Diabetes mellitus (medical diagnosis with multiple complications with associated modifiable risk lifestyles)
Drug abuse (clinical situations with multiple complications)
Elevated C-reactive protein (positive laboratory test)
Family history of coronary artery disease (factor with associated modifiable risk lifestyles)
Hyperlipidemia (medical diagnosis with associated modifiable risk lifestyles)
Hypertension (medical diagnosis with multiple complications with associated modifiable risk lifestyles)
Hypoxemia (complication)
Hypovolemia (complication)
Hypoxia (complication)
Lack of knowledge of modifiable risk factors (e.g., smoking, sedentary lifestyle, obesity)

>> ### Carp's Cues

Risk for Decreased Cardiac Tissue Perfusion can be used to describe a variety of physiologic events or pathology that can cause it as: dysrhythmias, left ventricular hypertrophy, drug abuse, septic shock, cardiomyopathies, acute coronary syndrome. It would be more clinically specific to use instead *Risk for Complications of Decreased Cardiac Output, Risk for Complications of Dysrhythmias, Risk for Complications of Septic Shock.* Nursing diagnoses related to these conditions may be *Activity Intolerance, Anxiety, Acute Pain.*

Some of the related factors as lack of knowledge of modifiable risk factors (e.g., smoking, sedentary lifestyle, obesity) can be addressed more appropriately with nursing diagnoses such as *Risk-Prone Health Behavior, Sedentary Lifestyle.*

Goals / Interventions

Refer to Section 2 for specific collaborative problems under *Risk for Complications of Cardiac / Vascular Dysfunction* or to care plan for clients with cardiac conditions.

RISK FOR INEFFECTIVE CEREBRAL TISSUE PERFUSION

NANDA-I Definition

At risk for a decrease in cerebral tissue circulation that may compromise health

Risk Factors*

Abnormal partial thromboplastin time
Abnormal prothrombin time
Akinetic left ventricular segment
Aortic atherosclerosis
Arterial dissection
Atrial fibrillation
Atrial myxoma
Brain tumor
Carotid stenosis

**Text in parentheses has been added by author.

Epinephrine
Diuretics
Anticholinergics
Tranquilizers
Sedatives
Muscle relaxants

Situational (Personal, Environmental)

Related to weak pelvic floor muscles secondary to (e.g., obesity, childbirth. aging, recent substantial weight loss)

Related to inability to communicate needs

Related to bladder outlet obstruction secondary to fecal impaction / chronic constipation

Related to decreased bladder muscle tone secondary to dehydration

Related to decreased attention to bladder cues secondary to (e.g., depression, delirium, intentional suppression [self-induced deconditioning], confusion)

Related to environmental barriers to bathroom secondary to (e.g., distant toilets, poor lighting, unfamiliar surroundings)

Related to inability to access bathroom on time secondary to (e.g., diuretics, caffeine / alcohol use, impaired mobility)

Carp's Cues

Impaired Urinary Elimination is too broad a diagnosis for effective clinical use, however it is clinically useful until additional data can be collected. With more data the nurse can use a more specific diagnosis, such as *Stress Urinary Incontinence*, whenever possible. When the etiologic or contributing factors for incontinence have not been identified, the nurse could write a temporary diagnosis of *Impaired Urinary Elimination related to unknown etiology, as evidenced by incontinence*.

It is the second-leading reason for placement of older adults into institutionalized care, and it is the primary reason why many elderly persons are not accepted into assisted living facilities.

CONTINUOUS URINARY INCONTINENCE**

Definition

State in which a client experiences continuous, unpredictable loss of urine without distention or awareness of bladder fullness

Defining Characteristics

Constant flow of urine at unpredictable times without uninhibited bladder contractions / spasm or distention

Lack of bladder filling or perineal filling
Nocturia
Unawareness of incontinence
Incontinence refractory to other treatments

Related Factors

Refer to *Impaired Urinary Elimination*.

**This diagnosis is not presently on the NANDA-I list but has been included for clarity and usefulness.

Goals

NOC

Refer to *Functional
Urinary Incontinence*.

The person will be continent (specify during day, night, 24 hours) as evidenced by the following indicators:

- Identify the cause of incontinence and rationale for treatments.
- Identify daily goal for fluid intake.

Interventions

NIC

See also *Functional
Incontinence,
Environmental
Management, Urinary
Catheterization,
Teaching: Procedure /
Treatment, Tube Care:
Urinary, Urinary Bladder
Training*

Develop a Bladder Retraining or Reconditioning Program, Which Should Include Communication, Assessment of Voiding Pattern, Scheduled Fluid Intake, and Scheduled Voiding Times

Promote Communication Among All Staff Members and Among Individual, Family, and Staff

- Provide all staff with sufficient knowledge concerning the program planned.
- Assess staff's response to program.

R: Education of caregivers increases preparedness, decreases burden, and reduces role strain, thereby reducing overall stress when caring for an incontinent client or family member.

Assess the Person's Potential for Participation in a Bladder-Retraining Program

- Cognition
- Desire to change behavior
- Ability to cooperate
- Willingness to participate

  R: Continence training programs are either self-directed or caregiver-directed. Self-directed programs of bladder training, retraining, and exercises are for motivated, cognitively intact clients (Miller, 2009). Caregiver-directed programs of scheduled toileting or habit training are appropriate for motivated caregivers of clients with cognitive impairment.

Provide Rationale for Plan and Acquire Client's Informed Consent

Encourage Person to Continue Program by Providing Accurate Information Concerning Reasons for Success or Failure

Assess Voiding Pattern

- Monitor and record:
  - Intake and output
  - Time and amount of fluid intake
  - Type of fluid
  - Amount of incontinence; measure if possible or estimate amount as small, moderate, or large
  - Presence of sensation of need to void
  - Amount of retention (amount of urine left in the bladder after an unsuccessful attempt at manual triggering or voiding)
  - Amount of residual (amount of urine left in the bladder after either a voluntary or manual triggered voiding; also called a *postvoid residual*)
  - Amount of triggered urine (urine expelled after manual triggering [e.g., tapping, Credé's method])
- Identify certain activities that precede voiding (e.g., restlessness, yelling, exercise).
- Record in appropriate column.

Schedule Fluid Intake and Voiding Times

- Provide fluid intake of 2,000 mL each day unless contraindicated.
- Discourage fluids after 7 p.m.
- Provide caregiver education.

- Initially, bladder emptying is done at least every 2 hours and at least twice during the night; goal is 2- to 4-hour intervals.
- If the person is incontinent before scheduled voids, shorten the time between voids.
- If the person has a postvoid residual greater than 100 to 150 mL, schedule intermittent catheterization.

R: The essential components of any continence training program (self-directed or caregiver-directed) include motivation, assessment of voiding and incontinence patterns, a regular fluid intake of 2,000 to 3,000 mL/day, timed voiding of 2- to 4-hour intervals in an appropriate place, and ongoing assessment (Miller, 2009).

Reduce Incontinence-Related Irritant Dermatitis (Scardillo et al., 1999)

- Protect skin integrity from urine.

    R: Urine contains ammonia. Ammonia increases the pH of the skin, causing irritation. Ammonia is also a source of nutrition for bacteria, contributing to the reproduction of more microorganisms.

- Use a no-rinse perineal cleanser.
- Avoid fragrances, alcohol, and alkaline agents (found in many commercial soaps).
- Apply moisturizer immediately after bathing, when pores are open.
- Use a moisture-barrier product (e.g., Curity Moisture Barrier Cream; No Sting Barrier Film).
- Do not try to remove all of the ointment with cleansing.
- Gently wash skin using very little soap. Dry skin very gently by patting, not rubbing.

    R: Vigorous washing can injure tissue.

- Keep perineal area dry.

    R: Warm, damp skin provides an opportune environment for fungal infections.

    R: Dehydration can cause incontinence by eliminating the sensation of a full bladder (the signal to urinate) and also by reducing the person's alertness to the sensation.

Schedule Intermittent Catheterization Program (ICP), If Indicated

- Monitor intake and output.
- Fluid intake should be at least 2000 mL/day.
- Use sterile catheterization technique in the hospital, clean technique at home.
- Desired catheter volumes are less than 500 mL.
- Increase or decrease the interval between catheterizations to obtain the desired catheter volumes.
- Usual catheterization times are every 4 to 6 hours.
- Urine volumes may increase at night; thus, it may be necessary to catheterize more frequently at night.
- Encourage the client to attempt to void before scheduled catheterization time.
- Initially obtain postvoid residuals at least every 6 hours.
- Terminate ICP when the bladder is consistently emptied voluntarily or by triggering with less than 50 mL residual urine after each void.

    R: Intermittent catheterization, when performed in a health care facility, should follow aseptic technique, because the organisms present in such a facility are more virulent and resistant to drugs than the organisms in the home environment.

TRANSITIONAL PLAN

Initiate health teaching and referrals as indicated.

- Teach intermittent catheterization to person and family for long-term management of bladder.
- Explain the reasons for the intermittent catheterization.

    R: Long-term use of intermittent catheterization has a lower risk of infection and other complications when compared with indwelling urinary catheter (Newman & Willson, 2011).

> **CLINICAL ALERT**
>
> A cognitively impaired person with continuous incontinence requires caregiver-directed ent. In institutional settings, indwelling and external catheters or disposal or washable incontinence briefs or pads are beneficial to the caregivers, but detrimental to the incontinent person. Aids and equipment should be considered only after other means have been attempted. In the home setting, the caregiver's needs may take precedence over the cognitively impaired person's. Urinary incontinence is cited as the major reason for seeking institutional care for people living at home (Miller, 2009).

Explain the Relation of Fluid Intake, Frequency of Catheterization, and Risk for Infection

* Inadequate fluid intake can produce low urine volumes (less than 1,200 mL of urine per day).

  R: Decreased urine production may lead to fewer catheterizations, stasis of urine, and infection.

* Ensure total daily fluid intake (from foods and all types of beverages) is approximately 2.7 L/day for women and 3.7 L/day for men (Newman & Willson, 2011, p. 15). Excessive fluid intake will produce periodic or regular bladder overdistention (volumes greater than 500 mL), possible overflow urinary incontinence, and urinary stasis. Distended bladder walls are susceptible to bacteria that circulate in retained urine (Newman & Willson, 2011, p. 15). When the bladder becomes stretched from retained urine, the capillaries become occluded, preventing the delivery of metabolic and immune substrates to the bladder wall, which are needed to maintain a physical barrier against colonization or invasion by pathogens (Heard & Buhrer, 2005).

* Advise of the possible need to catheterize more than six times day.

* Encourage regular fluid intake, small volumes spaced hourly between breakfast and the evening meal, and reducing to sips thereafter (Newman & Willson, 2011, p. 15).

* Ensure that there is adequate emptying at the time of catheterization. Teach a gentle Crede's maneuver as one removes the catheter.

  R: Residual volume left in the bladder after catheterization promotes an environment for bacteria proliferation (Newman & Willson, 2011, p. 16).

Teach Client and / or Family Member Intermittent Catheterization. Observe Them Performing Intermittent Catheterization for (Newman & Willson, 2011, p. 16):

* Ability
* Hygiene (hand washing, maintenance of catheter sterility)
* Correct technique (lubricant, position, prevention of trauma)
* Instruct client / family member to wash perineum each day and after sexual activity.

Review Signs / Symptoms of Urinary Tract Infection With Client and Family

* Dysuria: pain or burning during urination, lower abdominal pain
* Frequency: more frequent urination (or waking up at night to urinate, often with only a small amount of urine
* Urgency: the sensation of having to urinate urgently
* Hesitancy: the sensation of not being able to urinate easily or completely (or feeling that you have to urinate but only a few drops of urine come out)
* Cloudy, bad-smelling, or new onset bloody urine

  R: Bloody urine may be normal when intermittent catheterization is initiated (Newman & Willson, 2011).

* Mild fever (less than 101° F), chills, and "just not feeling well" (malaise)
* Upper urinary tract infection (pyelonephritis) may develop rapidly and may or may not include the symptoms for a lower urinary tract infection.
* Fairly high fever (higher than 101° F); shaking, chills
* Nausea, vomiting
* Flank pain: pain in back or side, usually on only one side at about waist level

CLINICAL ALERT

* Elderly people may not have the usual signs / symptoms of UTI, but instead may have hypothermia, poor appetite, lethargy, and sometimes only a change in mental status.

    R: Of concern because when urethral damage occurs, the mucosal barrier to infection is compromised (De Ridder et al., 2005). In addition, another measure that may reduce infection is the acidification of urine with cranberry juice or capsules, foods containing lactobacillus, and vitamin C capsules (Newman, 2008; Newman & Willson, 2011). Cranberries inhibit bacterial adherence to the uroepithelial wall and have been primarily studied with Escherichia coli (E. coli) (Jepson & Craig, 2008). In a community-based survey of patients with a spinal cord injury on intermittent catheterization, Woodbury et al. (2008) found that those who ingested cranberry or vitamin C agents decreased their incidence of UTI.

CLINICAL ALERT

* Incontinence management is a complex process. The nurse is advised to seek expert assistance from a nurse specialist. An excellent online resource is D. K. Newman and M. M. Willson (2011), Review of Intermittent Catheterization and Current Best Practices, Urologic Nursing, Volume 31 Number 1, which can be retrieved at http://www.suna.org/education/2013/article3101229.pdf.
* Refer to community nurses for assistance in incontinence management at home if indicated.

    R: The essential components of any incontinence management program (self-directed or caregiver-directed) will necessitate ongoing assessment.

Clinical Alert Report

Instruct staff / student to report incontinent episodes, change in medical status.

FUNCTIONAL URINARY INCONTINENCE

NANDA-I Definition

State in which a usually continent client experiences incontinence because of a difficulty or inability to reach the toilet in time

Carp's Cues

Functional incontinence is the inability or unwillingness of the person with a normal bladder and sphincter to reach the toilet in time. Functional incontinence may be caused by conditions affecting physical and emotional ability to respond and / or manage the act of urination.

Defining Characteristics

Major (Must Be Present)

Incontinence before or during an attempt to reach the toilet

Related Factors

Pathophysiologic

Related to diminished bladder cues and impaired ability to recognize bladder cues secondary to:

Brain injury / tumor / infection	Alcoholic neuropathy	Cerebrovascular accident
Parkinsonism	Demyelinating diseases	Progressive dementia
Multiple sclerosis		

Treatment Related

Related to treatment barriers to access to bathroom (e.g., tether lines, IVs, urinary catheter, NG tube)
Related to decreased bladder tone secondary to:

Antihistamines	Immunosuppressant therapy	Epinephrine
Diuretics	Anticholinergics	Tranquilizers
Sedatives	Muscle relaxants	

Situational (Personal, Environmental)

Related to impaired mobility
Related to decreased attention to bladder cues secondary to depression
Related to decreased attention to bladder cues secondary to confusion
Related to environmental barriers to bathroom (e.g., distant toilets, toilet seat, bed too high, poor lighting, unfamiliar surroundings)

Maturational

Older Adult
Related to motor and sensory losses

> **CLINICAL ALERT**
> The Centers for Medicare & Medicaid Services (CMS) have this requirement for residents in health care facilities (2005).
>
> Each resident who is incontinent of urine is identified, assessed, and provided appropriate treatment and services to achieve or maintain as much normal urinary function as possible:
>
> - An indwelling catheter is not used unless there is valid medical justification;
> - An indwelling catheter for which continuing use is not medically justified is discontinued as soon as clinically warranted;
> - Services are provided to restore or improve normal bladder function to the extent possible, after the removal of the catheter; and
> - A resident, with or without a catheter, receives the appropriate care and services to prevent infections to the extent possible.

Respondents that shift a client's care options from community-based care to residential care were:

1. Dementia / cognitive function
2. Mobility
3. Incontinence
4. Support networks
5. Caregiver stress / ability to cope
6. Functional ability and ADLs (activities of daily living)

Carp's Cues

Urinary incontinence (UI) has a major impact in long-term care facilities. It is the second-leading reason for placement of older adults into institutionalized care, and it is the primary reason why many elderly persons are not accepted into assisted living facilities. In long-term care facilities, it has been estimated that about 50% of the residents are urinary incontinent and that many who are continent at admission tend to become incontinent over time. In a study of 430 newly admitted nursing home residents, 22% of women who were continent at admission were incontinent after 1 year. The conversion rate in men was even higher (56%). The causes for this increase involve cognitive and mobility impairment and adjustment to the nursing home environment. In addition to staff, many nursing home residents believe UI is inevitable. Residents will utilize self-management strategies for urine leakage in order to protect social and psychological integrity, privacy, and dignity. Not only does UI have a substantial social effect on residents, it also has associated morbidities, including urinary tract infections (UTI), pressure ulcers, and falls with subsequent injury. In addition, caring for residents with UI adds considerably to the burden. An indwelling catheter is not used unless there is valid medical justification and, if not medically justified, it is discontinued as soon as clinically warranted services are provided (Vasavada, 2013; Roe et al., 2011).

Goals

NOC
Tissue Integrity, Urinary Continence, Urinary Elimination

The person will report no or decreased episodes of incontinence as evidenced by the following indicators:

- Remove or minimize environmental barriers at home.
- Use proper adaptive equipment to assist with voiding, transfers, and dressing.
- Describe causative factors for incontinence.

Interventions

NIC
Perineal Care, Urinary Incontinence Care, Prompted Voiding, Urinary Habit Training, Urinary Elimination Management, Teaching: Procedure / Treatment

Assess Causative or Contributing Factors

Obstacles to Toilet
- Poor lighting, slippery floor, misplaced furniture and rugs, inadequate footwear, toilet too far, bed too high, and side rails up
- Inadequate toilet (too small for walkers, wheelchair, seat too low / high, no grab bars)
- Inadequate signal system for requesting help
- Lack of privacy

Sensory / Cognitive Deficits
- Visual deficits (blindness, field cuts, poor depth perception)
- Cognitive deficits as a result of aging, trauma, stroke, tumor, and infection
- Psychological deficits

Motor / Mobility Deficits
- Limited upper and / or lower extremity movement / strength (inability to remove clothing)
- Barriers to ambulation (e.g., vertigo, fatigue, altered gait, hypertension)

    R: Barriers can delay access to the toilet and cause incontinence if the client cannot delay urination. A few seconds' delay in reaching the bathroom can make the difference between continence and incontinence.

Reduce or Eliminate Contributing Factors, If Possible

Environmental Barriers
- Assess path to bathroom for obstacles, lighting, and distance.
- Assess adequacy of toilet height and need for grab bars.
- Assess adequacy of room size.
- Assess if client can remove clothing easily.
- Provide a commode between bathroom and bed, if necessary.

Sensory / Cognitive Deficits

- For a person with diminished vision:
  - Ensure adequate lighting.
  - Encourage person to wear prescribed corrective lens.
  - Provide clear, safe pathway to bathroom.
  - Keep call bell easily accessible.
  - If bedpan or urinal is used, make sure it is within easy reach in the same location at all times.
  - Assess person for safety in bathroom.
  - Assess person's ability to provide self-hygiene.

- For a person with cognitive deficits:
  - Offer toileting reminders every 2 hours, after meals, and before bedtime.
  - Establish appropriate means to communicate need to void.
  - Answer call bell immediately.
  - Encourage wearing of ordinary clothes.
  - Provide a normal environment for elimination (use bathroom, if possible).
  - Allow for privacy while maintaining safety.
  - Allow sufficient time for task.
  - Reorient client to where he or she is and what task he or she is doing.
  - Be consistent in your approach to person.
  - Give simple step-by-step instructions; use verbal and nonverbal cues.
  - Give positive reinforcement for success.
  - Assess person for safety in bathroom.
  - Assess need for adaptive devices on clothing to make dressing and undressing easier.
  - Assess person's ability to provide self-hygiene.

  R: A client with a cognitive deficit needs constant verbal cues and reminders to establish a routine and reduce incontinence

Provide for Factors That Promote Continence

Maintain Optimal Hydration
- Increase fluid intake to 2,000 to 3,000 mL/day, unless contraindicated.
- Teach older adults not to depend on thirst sensations but to drink liquids even when not thirsty.
- Space fluids every 2 hours.
- Decrease fluid intake after 7 p.m.; provide only minimal fluids during the night.

  R: Dehydration can prevent the sensation of a full bladder and can contribute to loss of bladder tone. Spacing fluids helps promote regular bladder filling and emptying.

  R: Dehydration irritates the bladder lining, making the urgency worse (Griebling, 2009).

- Reduce intake of coffee, tea, cola, alcohol, and grapefruit juice because of their diuretic effect.

  R: Coffee, tea, colas, and grapefruit juice act as diuretics, which can cause urgency.

- Avoid large amounts of tomato and orange juice.

  R: These beverages make the urine alkaline, which promotes infection.

- Avoid bladder irritants such as alcohol, caffeine, and aspartame (Smeltzer & Bares, 2008).
- Encourage cranberry juice.

  R: Acidic urine deters the growth of most bacteria implicated in cystitis.

- Monitor salt intake.

  R: High-salt diets decrease urine production and cause water retention (Wilkinson & Van Leuven, 2007).

Maintain Adequate Nutrition to Ensure Bowel Elimination at Least Once Every 3 Days
- Promote micturition.

Promote Personal Integrity and Provide Motivation to Increase Bladder Control
- Encourage person to share feelings about incontinence and determine its effect on his or her social patterns.
- Convey that incontinence can be cured or at least controlled to maintain dignity.
- Use protective pads or garments only after conscientious reconditioning efforts have been completely unsuccessful after 6 weeks.
- Work to achieve daytime continence before expecting nighttime continence:
  - Encourage socialization.
  - Discourage the use of bedpans.
  - Encourage and assist person to groom self.
  - If hospitalized, provide opportunities to eat meals outside bedroom (day room, lounge).
  - If fear or embarrassment is preventing socialization, instruct person to use sanitary pads or briefs temporarily until control is established.
  - Change clothes as soon as possible when wet to avoid indirectly sanctioning wetness.
  - Advise the oral use of chlorophyll tablets to deodorize urine and feces.
  - See *Social Isolation* and *Ineffective Coping* for additional interventions, if indicated.

  R: Wearing normal clothing or nightwear helps simulate the home environment, where incontinence may not occur. A hospital gown may reinforce incontinence. Use of bathroom rather than bedpans simulates the home environment.

Promote Skin Integrity
- Identify clients at risk for development of pressure ulcers.
- Avoid harsh soaps and alcohol products.
- Keep moisture away from the skin.
- Refer to *Risk for Impaired Skin Integrity* for additional information.

> R: *Ammonia from urine makes the skin more alkaline and more vulnerable to irritants (Scardillo et al., 1999).*

Teach Prevention of Urinary Tract Infections

- Encourage regular, complete emptying of the bladder.
- Ensure adequate fluid intake.
- Keep urine acidic; avoid citrus juices, dark colas, coffee, tea and alcohol, which act as irritants (Smeltzer & Bares, 2008).
- Monitor urine pH.
- Teach client to recognize abnormal changes in urine properties.
  - Increased mucus and sediment
  - Blood in urine (hematuria)
  - Change in color (from normal straw-colored) or odor
- Teach client to monitor for signs and symptoms of infection:
  - Elevated temperature, chills, and shaking
  - Changes in urine properties
  - Suprapubic pain
  - Painful urination
  - Urgency
  - Frequent small voids or frequent small incontinences
  - Increased spasticity in spinal cord-injured individuals
  - Increased urine pH
  - Nausea / vomiting
  - Lower back and / or flank pain

> R: *Bacteria multiply rapidly in stagnant urine retained in the bladder. Moreover, overdistention hinders blood flow to the bladder wall, increasing the susceptibility to infection from bacterial growth. Regular, complete bladder emptying greatly reduces the risk of infection.*

Geriatric Interventions

Explain Age-Related Effects on Bladder Function and That Urgency and Nocturia Do Not Necessarily Lead to Incontinence

> **TRANSITION CARE**
> Initiate health teaching referral, when indicated.
> - Refer to visiting nurse (occupational therapy department) for assessment of bathroom facilities at home.

> *Cinical Alert Report*
> - Emphasize that incontinence is not an inevitable age-related event.
>   R: *Explaining the cause can motivate the person to participate.*
> - Explain not to restrict fluid intake for fear of incontinence.
>   R: *Dehydration can cause incontinence by eliminating the sensation of a full bladder (the signal to urinate) and also by reducing the person's alertness to the sensation.*
> - Explain not to rely on thirst as a signal to drink fluids.
>   R: *The older adult has an age-related decrease in thirst (Miller, 2009).*
> - Teach the need to have easy access to bathroom at night. If needed, consider commode chair or urinal.
>   R: *This is to prevent falls.*

OVERFLOW URINARY INCONTINENCE

NANDA-I Definition

Involuntary loss of urine associated with overdistention of the bladder

Defining Characteristics*

Bladder distention
High postvoid residual volume
Observed involuntary leakage of small volumes of urine
Reports involuntary leakage of small volumes of urine
Nocturia

Related Factors

Pathophysiologic

Related to sphincter blockage secondary to:

Strictures   Prostatic enlargement
Ureterocele   Perineal swelling
Bladder neck contractures   Severe pelvic prolapse

Related to impaired afferent pathways or inadequacy secondary to:

Cord injury / tumor / infection   Multiple sclerosis
Brain injury / tumor / infection Diabetic neuropathy
Cerebrovascular accident   Alcoholic neuropathy
Demyelinating diseases   Tabes dorsalis

Treatment Related

Related to bladder outlet obstruction or impaired afferent pathways secondary to drug therapy (iatrogenic)*

Antihistamines   Decongestants*
Theophylline   Anticholinergics*
Epinephrine   Calcium channel blockers*
Isoproterenol

Situational (Personal, Environmental)

Related to bladder outlet obstruction secondary to:

Fecal impaction*

Related to detrusor hypocontractility secondary to:*

Deconditioned voiding
Association with stress or discomfort
Refer to *Impaired Urinary Elimination*.

Interventions

Refer to Neurogenic Bladder.

STRESS URINARY INCONTINENCE

NANDA-I Definition

Sudden leakage of urine with activities that increase the intra-abdominal pressure

Defining Characteristics*

Observed or reported involuntary leakage of small amounts of urine:

In the absence of detrusor contraction
In the absence of an overactive bladder
On exertion
With coughing, laughing, sneezing, or all of these

Related Factors

Pathophysiologic

Related to incompetent bladder outlet secondary to congenital urinary tract anomalies
Related to degenerative changes in pelvic muscles and structural supports secondary to estrogen deficiency*
*Related to intrinsic urethral sphincter**

Situational (Personal, Environmental)

Related to high intra-abdominal pressure and weak pelvic muscles* secondary to:*

Obesity
Sex
Pregnancy
Poor personal hygiene
Smoking

Related to weak pelvic muscles and structural supports secondary to:

Recent substantial weight loss
Childbirth

Maturational

Older Adult
Related to loss of muscle tone

Key Concepts

General Considerations

- A trial of vaginal estrogen cream in the postmenopausal woman who exhibits a pale, atrophic vaginal vault may help to reduce the incidence of incontinence.
- A stress test is used to help diagnose stress incontinence. It involves observation of the urethral meatus of a client with a full bladder in the standing position while she coughs or strains. Short spurts of urine escaping simultaneously with cough or strain suggest a probable diagnosis of stress incontinence.
- Women who are more active and who have jobs that require heavy physical activity may be prone to pelvic organ prolapsed and urinary incontinence (Wilson et al., 2005).
- The client with pure stress incontinence has a normal cystometrogram.

Carp's Cues
- The degrees of stress incontinence are as follows (Wilson et al., 2005):
  - Grade 1—Urine is lost with sudden increase in abdominal pressure, but never at night.
  - Grade 2—Lesser degrees of physical stress, such as walking, standing erect from a sitting position, or sitting up in bed, produce incontinence.
  - Grade 3—There is continuous incontinence, and urine is lost without any relation to physical activity or to position.

Goals

NOC
Refer to *Functional Urinary Incontinence*.

The person will report a reduction or elimination of stress incontinence as evidenced by the following indicator:

- Be able to explain the cause of incontinence and rationale for treatments.

Interventions

NIC
See also *Functional Incontinence*, Pelvic Muscle Exercise, Weight Management

Determine Contributing Factors

Explain the Effect of Incompetent Floor Muscles on Continence

R: Urinary continence is maintained by the junction of the bladder and the urethra, support from the perineal floor, and the muscle around the urethra. Stress incontinence is the leakage of small amounts of urine when the urethral outlet cannot control passage of urine in the presence of increased intra-abdominal pressure.

- Explain factors that contribute to incompetent floor muscles as obesity, multiple pregnancies, menopause.

  R: In stress incontinence, childbirth, trauma, menopausal atrophy, or obesity have weakened or stretched the pelvic floor muscles (pubococcygeus) and levator ani muscles.

Teach Pelvic Muscle Exercises (Dougherty, 1998)

- Teach how to self-assess whether exercises are being done correctly.
- Provide instructions for pelvic muscle exercises.
- Teach the client ways to strengthen the pelvic floor muscle.

  R: Pelvic floor muscle training should be encouraged and taught for all incontinence episodes mixed, urge or stress (Wilson et al., 2005).

- Tighten muscles as if you were trying to stop urination; this includes tightening the rectal muscles (Wilkinson & Van Leuven, 2007).
- Hold the contractions for 5–10 seconds and release. Relax between contractions, taking care to keep contraction and relaxation times equal. If you contract for 10 seconds, relax for 10 seconds before next contraction (Wilkinson & Van Leuven, 2007).
- Perform 10 contractions at least three times a day. These should be spread out through the day and incorporate different positions; sitting, standing, and lying (Wilkinson & Van Leuven, 2007).
- A good way to remember to do your exercises is to incorporate them into your daily routine, such as while stopping at a traffic light or washing dishes (Wilkinson & Van Leuven, 2007).

  R: Pelvic floor muscle rehabilitation is an important treatment for strengthening perineal muscles. It is not uncommon to see improvement rates of 48%–80% with these exercises. Approximately 6–12 months of daily exercises may be needed before improvement is seen (Wilkinson & Van Leuven, 2007).

⊙ Health Promotion Diagnoses

DECISIONAL CONFLICT

NANDA-I Definition

Uncertainty about course of action to be taken when choice among competing actions involves risk, loss, or challenge to values and beliefs

Defining Characteristics*

Verbalized uncertainty about choices
Verbalizes undesired consequences of alternatives being considered
Vacillation among alternative choices
Delayed decision making
Self-focusing
Verbalizes feeling of distress while attempting a decision
Physical signs of distress or tension (e.g., increased heart rate, increased muscle tension, restlessness)
Questioning of personal values and / or beliefs while attempting to make a decision
Questioning moral values while attempting a decision
Questioning moral rules while attempting a decision
Questioning moral principles while attempting a decision

Related Factors

Many situations can contribute to decisional conflict, particularly those that involve complex medical interventions of great risk. Any decisional situation can precipitate conflict for a client; thus, the examples listed below are not exhaustive, but reflective of situations that may be problematic and possess factors that increase the difficulty.

Treatment Related

Related to lack of relevant information
Related to risks versus the benefits of (specify test, treatment):

Surgery

Tumor removal	Orchiectomy	Mastectomy
Cosmetic surgery	Prostatectomy	Joint replacement
Amputation	Hysterectomy	Cataract removal
Transplant	Laminectomy	Cesarean section

Diagnostics

Amniocentesis	X-rays	Ultrasound

Chemotherapy
Radiation
Dialysis
Mechanical ventilation
Enteral feedings
Intravenous hydration
   Use of preterm labor medications
   Participation in treatment study trials
   HIV antiviral therapy

Situational (Personal, Environmental)

Related to perceived threat to value system
Related to:

Institutionalization (child, parent)   Foster home placement

Related to:

Lack of relevant information*   Confusing information

Related to:

Disagreement within support systems
Inexperience with decision making
Unclear personal values / beliefs*
Conflict with personal values / beliefs
Ethical or moral dilemmas (e.g., "do not resuscitate" orders, quality of life, termination of pregnancy, selec-
   tive termination with multiple-gestation pregnancies, organ transplant, cessation of life-support systems)

Maturational

Related to risks versus benefits of:

Alcohol / drug use   High-risk sexual activity
Sexual activity   Illegal / dangerous situations

❯❯ Carp's Cues

The nurse has an important role in assisting clients and families with making decisions. Because nurses usually do not benefit financially from decisions made regarding treatments and transfers, they are in an ideal position to assist with decisions. Although, according to Davis (1989), "Nursing or medical expertise does not enable health care professionals to know the values of patients or what patients think is best for themselves," nursing expertise does enable nurses to facilitate systematic decision making that considers all possible alternatives and possible outcomes, as well as individual beliefs and values. The focus is on assisting with logical decision making, not on promoting a certain decision.

When people are making a treatment decision of considerable risk, they do not necessarily experience conflict. In situations where the treatment option is "choosing life," individual perception may be one of submitting to fate and be relatively unconflicted. Because of this, nurses must be cautious in labeling patients with the nursing diagnosis of "Decisional Conflict" without sufficient validating cues (Soholt, 1990).

Goals

NOC
Decision Making,
Information Processing,
Participation: Health
Care Decisions

The client / group will make an informed choice as evidenced by the following indicators:

- Relate the advantages and disadvantages of choices.
- Share fears and concerns regarding choices and responses of others.
- Define what would be most helpful to support the decision-making process.

Interventions

NIC
Decision-Making
Support, Mutual Goal
Setting, Learning
Facilitation, Health
System Guidance,
Anticipatory Guidance,
Client Right Protection,
Values Clarification,
Anxiety Reduction

Reduce or Eliminate Causative or Contributing Factors

Internal

Lack of Experience With or Ineffective Decision Making

- Facilitate logical decision making:
  - Assist the client in recognizing the problem and clearly identifying the needed decision.
  - Generate a list of all possible alternatives or options.
  - Help identify the probable outcomes of the various alternatives.
  - Aid in evaluating the alternatives based on actual or potential threats to beliefs / values.
  - Encourage the client to make a decision.

R: Exploration of goals and issues related to and symptom management of side effects, cost, quality of life, and complexity of treatments can allow the person to address barriers (Robinson, 2008).

Review Present Medication Therapy (Prescribed and Over-the-Counter)

- Discuss present therapy (names, dosages, time taken, side effects). Do not ask, "Are you taking your medications?" Ask:
  - "What medications did you take every day?
  - "What time of day is it difficult for you to take your medications?"
  - "Are there times when you decide not to take one of the doses?"
- Determine the client's understanding of the need for medication:
  - Emphasize lifelong therapy when indicated (e.g., hypertension, diabetes mellitus).
  - Explain the complications of unmanaged disease.
- Identify possible adverse interactions among drugs (consult a pharmacist).
- Commit to work with the client to reduce or eliminate side effects (e.g., change agents or dose).
- Help the client identify a reminder to take the medication (e.g., brushing teeth at night, daily favorite TV show, watch timer).
- Ask the client to call the primary provider with problems rather than stopping the medication.
- Emphasize that unavoidable side effects are still better than the consequences of no therapy (e.g., stroke, blindness, renal failure).

R: Lack of understanding regarding reasons for drug therapy and options available contributes to noncompliance. Open discussions about side effects can encourage the client to report problems before discontinuing treatment.

Help to Reduce Side Effects if Reported

- Address side effects that may occur and encourage the client to report them for evaluation.
- Specify the difference between side effects and adverse events.

  R: Warning a client of possible side effects can reduce the anxiety. Side effects are signs and symptoms that can usually be managed if they occur. Adverse events are serious and usually require discontinuation of the medicine.

- For gastric irritation, administer the drug with milk or food; yogurt may be advisable (unless contraindicated).
- For drowsiness, administer the medication at bedtime or late in the afternoon; consult the primary provider for dose reduction.
- For leg cramps (hypokalemia), increase foods high in potassium (e.g., oranges, raisins, tomatoes, bananas).
- Suggest the use of combination pills if available.
- When appropriate, be sure client is taking the fewest medications possible (check dosages to provide the largest dose available in the fewest number of drugs).
- To decrease the frequency of oral medications, suggest longer-acting drug preparations for once-daily dosing.

  R: Some barriers to compliance can be eliminated with specific teaching.

- Management of side effects can increase adherence.

> **TRANSITION PLAN**
>
> Initiate health teaching and referrals as indicated.
>
> - Encourage prescription of generic drugs for people with financial concerns. Determine if the client needs assistance.
> - Access specific pharmaceutical assistance programs at www.pparx.org/ or www.rxassist.org/.
> - When expensive equipment is involved for treatments at home, make appropriate referrals to social workers and local agencies.
>
>   *R: Financial barriers are often barriers to compliance. Sources of assistance that can be accessed after discharge must be addressed.*

RISK FOR INEFFECTIVE SELF-HEALTH MANAGEMENT

NANDA-I Definition

Pattern in which a person is at risk to experience a pattern of regulating and integrating into daily living a therapeutic regimen for the treatment of illness and its sequelae that is unsatisfactory for meeting specific health goals

Risk Factors

Treatment Related

Related to: complexity of therapeutic regimen, * *complexity of health care system,* * *financial cost of regimen, side effects of therapy* *

Situational (Personal, Environmental)

Related to:

Previous unsuccessful experiences
Family patterns of health care*
Mistrust of health care personnel
Perceived barriers*
Health belief conflicts
Perceived susceptibility
Questions seriousness of problem
Excessive demands (individual, family)*
Deficient knowledge*
Family conflict*
Powerlessness*
Mistrust of regimen
Insufficient confidence
Economic difficulties*
Questions benefits of regimen
Decisional conflicts*

Related to insufficient, or unavailable family support.
Related to barriers to comprehension secondary to:

Cognitive deficits	Motivation
Fatigue	Anxiety
Hearing impairments	Memory problems

 Carp's Cues

Ineffective Self-Help Management is a very useful diagnosis for nurses in most settings. Individuals and families experiencing various health problems, acute or chronic, usually face treatment programs that require changes in previous functioning or lifestyle. These changes or adaptations can be instrumental in influencing positive outcomes.

Ineffective Self-Health Management focuses on assisting the person and family to identify barriers in management of the condition and to prevention complications at home. Risk-Prone Health Behavior, approved in 2006, is different. This diagnosis focuses on habits or lifestyles which are unhealthy and can aggravate an existing condition or contribute to developing a disorder.

> **TRANSITION PLAN**
> Initiate health teaching and referrals as indicated.
> * Refer to pertinent medical or surgical care plan for specific interventions indicated to assist the individual / family manage as they transition to home.

⊕ Individual Coping Diagnoses

ANXIETY

NANDA-I Definition

Vague, uneasy feeling of discomfort or dread accompanied by an autonomic response (the source often unspecific or unknown to the individual); a feeling of apprehension caused by anticipation of danger. It is an alerting signal that warns of impending danger and enables the individual to take measures to deal with threat.

Defining Characteristics

Major (Must Be Present)

Manifested by symptoms from any category—physiologic, emotional, and cognitive; symptoms vary according to level of anxiety.

Physiologic

Increased pulse*	Urinary frequency, hesitancy, urgency*
Elevated blood pressure*	Fatigue*
Increased respiratory*	Insomnia*
Dilated pupils*	Dry mouth*
Diaphoresis*	Facial flushing* or pallor
Trembling, twitching*	Restlessness*
Voice quivering*	Body aches and pains (especially chest, back, neck)
Nausea*	Faintness* / dizziness
Palpitations	Paresthesias
Diarrhea*	Anorexia*

Emotional

Client states feelings of:

Apprehension*	Loss of control
Persistent increased helplessness*	Tension or being "keyed up"
Jittery*	Anticipation of misfortune
Vigilance*	

Client exhibits:

Irritability* / impatience	Criticism of self and others
Angry outbursts	Withdrawal
Crying	Lack of initiative
Tendency to blame others*	Self-deprecation
Startle reaction	Poor eye contact*

Cognitive

Inability to concentrate	Blocking of thoughts (inability to remember)
Lack of awareness of surroundings	Hyperattentiveness
Rumination*	Preoccupation*
Orientation to past	Diminished ability to learn*

Related Factors

Pathophysiologic

Related to any factor that interferes with physiologic stability

Examples:

Respiratory distress
Mind-altering drugs

Chest pain
Cancer diagnosis

Treatment Related

Related to impending surgery, invasive procedure, therapy

Situational (Personal, Environmental)

Related to loss of significant others secondary to:

Death
Divorce
Cultural pressures

Moving
Temporary or permanent separation

Related to threat to biologic integrity secondary to (e.g., terminal illness, chronic disease)
Related to change in unfamiliar hospital environment
Related to change in socioeconomic status secondary to (e.g., unemployme, displacement, foreclosure, retirement)

Goals

NOC
Anxiety Level, Coping, Impulse Self-Control

The client will relate increased psychological and physiologic comfort evidenced by the following indicators:

- Describe own anxiety and coping patterns.
- Identifies two strategies to reduce anxiety.

Interventions

NIC
Anxiety Reduction, Impulse Control Training, Anticipatory Guidance

Introduce Yourself and Other Members of the Health Care Team, and Orient the Client to the Room (e.g., Bed Controls, Call Bell, Bathroom)

Initially Determine the Client's Present Level of Anxiety

- Mild
  - Heightened perception and attention; alertness
  - Ability to deal with problems
- Moderate
  - Slightly narrowed perception; selective inattention, which can be directed
  - Slight difficulty concentrating; learning requires more effort
  - Voice / pitch changes
  - Tremors, shakiness
- Severe
  - Distorted perception; focus on scattered details; inability to attend to more, even when instructed
  - Severely impaired learning; high distractibility, and inability to concentrate
  - Hyperventilation, tachycardia, headache, dizziness, and nausea
  - Complete self-absorption
- Panic
  - Irrational reasoning; focuses on blown-up detail
  - Inability to learn, communication not understandable
  - Feelings of impending doom (dyspnea, dizziness / faintness, palpitations, trembling, choking, paresthesia, hot / cold flashes, sweating)

- If anxiety is at severe or panic level:
  - Provide a quiet, nonstimulating environment.
  - Use short, simple sentences; speak slowly.
  - Give concise directions. Focus on the present.
  - Remove excess stimulation.

  R: The anxious client tends to overgeneralize, assume, and anticipate catastrophe. Resulting cognitive problems include difficulty with attention and concentration, loss of objectivity, and vigilance. Providing emotional support and relaxation techniques and encouraging sharing may help a client clarify and verbalize fears, allowing the nurse to give realistic feedback and reassurance.

> **CLINICAL ALERT**
> - If severe or panic anxiety is present, consult physician / NP for possible pharmacologic therapy, if indicated.

If the Client Is Hyperventilating or Experiencing Dyspnea

- Demonstrate breathing techniques; ask the client to practice the technique with you.
- Acknowledge the client's fear and give positive reinforcement for efforts.

  R: Anxiety tends to feed on itself, trapping the client in a spiral of increasing anxiety, hyperventilation, and physical pain.

Teach Anxiety Interrupters to Use When Client Cannot Avoid Stressful Situations

- Look up. Lower shoulders.
- Control breathing.
- Slow thoughts. Alter voice.
- Give self-directions (out loud, if possible).
- Exercise.
- "Scruff your face"—changes facial expression.
- Change perspective: imagine watching situation from a distance (Grainger, 1990).

R: Relaxation techniques help the person switch the autonomous system from the fight-or-flight response to a more relaxed response (Varcarolis, 2011).

Explain Hospital Policies and Routines (e.g., Visiting Policies, Mealtimes, Equipment)

- Determine the client's / significant other's knowledge of his or her reason for admission and present treatment plans. Reinforce and supplement the physician's / NP's explanations as necessary.

  R: Providing accurate information can help decrease the client's anxiety associated with the unknown and unfamiliar.

- Explain any scheduled diagnostic tests, covering the following: description, purpose, pretest routines, and posttest care.

  R: Teaching the client about tests and treatment measures can help decrease his or her fear and anxiety associated with the unknown, and improve his or her sense of control over situation.

- Allow the client's support people to share their fears and concerns, and encourage them in providing meaningful and productive support.

  R: Supporting the client's support people can enhance their ability to help the client.

Attempt to Diffuse Anger (Refer to *Ineffective Coping*)

- Promote resiliency
  - Avoid minimizing positive experiences.
  - Gently encourage humor.
  - Encourage optimism.

- Encourage discussion with significant others.
- Encourage the client to seek spiritual comfort through religion, nature, prayer, meditation, or other methods.

R: Resilience is a combination of abilities and characteristics that interact to allow an individual to bounce back, cope successfully, and function above the norm in spite of significant stress or adversity (Tusaie & Dyer, 2004). Environmental factors that favor resilience are perceived social support or a sense of connectiveness (Tusaie & Dyer, 2004).

> **TRANSITION PLAN**
> Initiate health teaching and referrals as indicated.
> - Refer people identified as having chronic anxiety and maladaptive coping mechanisms for ongoing mental health counseling and treatment.
> - Instruct in nontechnical, understandable terms regarding illness and associated treatments.
>   *R: Simple and repeating explanations are needed because anxiety may interfere with learning.*

> **Clinical Alert Report**
> - Advise ancillary staff / student to report an increase in anxiety and / or anger.
>   *R: High levels of anxiety interfere with learning. Anger can be a symptom of high levels of anxiety.*
> **Documenation**
> - Record episodes of severe or panic levels of anxiety, interventions, and evaluation.

DEATH ANXIETY

NANDA-I Definition

Vague, uneasy feeling of discomfort or dread generated by perceptions of a real or imagined threat to one's existence

Defining Characteristics*

Reports:

Worry about the impact of one's own death on significant others
Feeling powerless over dying
Fear of loss of mental abilities when dying
Fear of pain related to dying
Fear of suffering related to dying
Deep sadness
Fear of the process of dying
Concerns of overworking the caregiver
Negative thoughts related to death and dying
Fear of prolonged dying
Fear of premature death
Fear of developing a terminal illness

Related Factors

A diagnosis of a potentially terminal condition or impending death can cause this diagnosis. Additional factors can contribute to death anxiety.

Situational (Personal, Environmental)

*Related to discussions on topic of death**
*Related to near death experience**
*Related to perceived proximity of death**
*Related to uncertainty of prognosis**
*Related to anticipating suffering**
*Related to confronting reality of terminal disease**
*Related to observations related to death**
*Related to anticipating pain**
*Related to nonacceptance of own mortality**
*Related to uncertainty about life after death**
*Related to uncertainty about an encounter with a higher power**
*Related to uncertainty about the existence of a higher power**
*Related to experiencing the dying process**
*Related to anticipating impact of death on others**
*Related to anticipating adverse consequences of general anesthesia**
Related to personal conflict with palliative versus curative care
Related to conflict with family regarding palliative versus curative care
Related to fear of being a burden
Related to fear of unmanageable pain
Related to fear of abandonment
Related to unresolved conflict (family, friends)
Related to fear that one's life lacked meaning
Related to social disengagement

Goals / Interventions

Refer to Palliative Care Plan.

INEFFECTIVE COPING

NANDA-I Definition

Inability to form a valid appraisal of the stressors, inadequate choices of practiced responses, and / or inability to use available resources

Defining Characteristics

Verbalization of inability to cope or ask for help*
Inappropriate use of defense mechanisms
Inability to meet role expectations*
Chronic worry, anxiety
Sleep disturbance*
Fatigue*
High illness rate*
Reported difficulty with life stressors
Poor concentration*
Difficulty organizing information*
Decreased use of social support*
Inadequate problem solving*
Impaired social participation
Use of forms of coping that impede adaptive behavior*
Risk-taking*
Lack of goal-directed behavior*

Destructive behavior toward self or others*
Change in usual communication patterns*
High incidence of accidents
Substance abuse*

Related Factors

Pathophysiologic

Related to biochemical changes in brain secondary to (e.g., bipolar disorder, personality disorder, chemical dependency, attention-deficient disorders, schizophrenia)
Related to neurologic changes in brain secondary to (e.g., stroke, multiple sclerosis Alzheimer's disease, end-stage diseases)
Related to changes in body integrity secondary to (e.g., loss of body part, disfigurement secondary to trauma)

Treatment Related

Related to separation from family and home (e.g., hospitalization, nursing home)
Related to altered appearance from drugs, radiation, or other treatment

Situational (Personal, Environmental)

Related to poor impulse control and frustration tolerance
Related to disturbed relationship with parent / caregiver
Related to disorganized family system
Related to ineffective problem-solving skills
Related to increased food consumption in response to stressors
Related to the negative impact of (e.g., poverty, inadequate finances, relocation, foreclosure, homelessness, natural disaster)
Related to disruption of emotional bonds secondary to:

Death	Separation or divorce
Institutionalization	Foster care
Relocation	Imprisonment
Desertion	Educational institution

Related to unsatisfactory support system
Related to inadequate psychological resources secondary to:

Poor self-esteem
Helplessness
Excessive negative beliefs about self
Lack of motivation to respond
Negative role modeling

Maturational

Adolescent
Related to inadequate psychological resources to adapt to:

Physical and emotional changes
Sexual awareness
Independence from family
Educational demands
Sexual relationships
Career choices

Young Adult
Related to inadequate psychological resources to adapt to:

Career choices
Marriage
Educational demands

Parenthood
Leaving home

Middle Adult
Related to inadequate psychological resources to adapt to:

Physical signs of aging
Problems with relatives
Career pressures

Social status needs
Child-rearing problems
Aging parents

Older Adult
Related to inadequate psychological resources to adapt to:

Physical changes
Retirement
Changes in financial status

Response of others
Changes in residence

Carp's Cues

Ineffective Coping describes a person experiencing difficulty adapting to stressful event(s). *Ineffective Coping* can be a recent, episodic problem or a chronic problem. Usual effective coping mechanisms may be inappropriate or ineffective, or the person may have a poor history of coping with stressors.

If the event is recent, *Ineffective Coping* may be a premature judgment. For example, a person may respond to overwhelming stress with a grief response such as denial, anger, or sadness, making a *Grieving* diagnosis appropriate.

Impaired Adjustment may be more useful than *Ineffective Coping* in the initial period after a stressful event. *Ineffective Coping* and its related diagnoses may be more applicable to prolonged or chronic coping problems, such as *Defensive Coping* for a person with a long-standing pattern of ineffective coping.

Goals

NOC
Coping, Self-Esteem, Social Interaction Skills

The person will make decisions and follow through with appropriate actions to change provocative situations in the personal environment as evidenced by the following indicators:

- Verbalize feelings related to emotional state.
- Focus on the present.
- Identify response patterns and the consequences of resulting behavior.
- Identify personal strengths and accept support through the nursing relationship.

Interventions

NIC
Coping Enhancement, Counseling, Emotional Support, Active Listening, Assertiveness Training, Behavior Modification

Establish Rapport

- Spend time with the client. Provide supportive companionship.
- Avoid being overly cheerful and clichés such as, "Things will get better."
- Offer support. Encourage expression of feelings. Let the client know you understand his or her feelings. Do not argue with expressions of worthlessness by saying things such as, "How can you say that? Look at all you accomplished in life."
- Allow extra time for the person to respond.

R: The person with a chronic mental illness "must be helped to give up the role of being sick for that of being different" (Finkelman, 2000).

Assess Present Coping Status

- Determine the risk of the client's inflicting self-harm; intervene appropriately.
- Assess for signs of potential suicide.

- History of previous attempts or threats (overt and covert)
- Changes in personality, behavior, sex life, appetite, and sleep habits
- Preparations for death (putting things in order, making a will, giving away personal possessions, acquiring a weapon)
- Sudden elevation in mood
- See *Risk for Suicide* for additional information on suicide prevention.

Assess Level of Depression

- Refer depressed people to specialists.

  R: Severely depressed or suicidal people need environmental controls, usually hospitalization.

Assist the Client in Developing Appropriate Problem-Solving Strategies

- Ask the client to describe previous encounters with conflict and how he or she resolved them.
- Evaluate whether his or her stress response is "fight or flight" or "tend and befriend."
- Encourage the client to evaluate his or her behavior. "Did that work for you?" "How did it help?" "What did you learn from that experience?"
- Discuss possible alternatives (i.e., talk over the problem with those involved, try to change the situation, or do nothing and accept the consequences).
- Assist the client in identifying problems that he or she cannot control directly; help the client to practice stress-reducing activities for control (e.g., exercise, yoga).

  R: Cognitive interventions help the person regain control over his or her life. They include identifying automatic thoughts and replacing them with positive thoughts (Finkelman, 2000).

- Explore outlets that foster feelings of personal achievement and self-esteem.

  R: People with depression often experience low self-esteem, a lack of confidence, competence, and sense of efficacy. Altered perceptions, attention deficits, cognitive confusion, and labile emotions interfere with decision making, problem solving, and interpersonal relationships (Finkelman, 2000).

- Facilitate emotional support from others.
  - Identify persons, who understand your situation.
  - Decide who can best act as a support system (do not expect empathy from people who themselves are overwhelmed with their own problems).
  - Maintain a sense of humor.

  R: Coping effectively requires successful maintenance of many tasks: self-concept, satisfying relationships with others, emotional balance, and stress.

- Teach self-monitoring tools (Finkelman, 2000).
  - Develop a daily schedule to monitor for signs of improvement or worsening.
  - Discuss reasonable goals for present relationships.
  - Write down what is done when in control, depressed, confused, angry, and happy.
  - Identify activities tried, would like to try, or should do more.
  - Create a warning sign checklist that indicates worsening and how to access help.

  R: Self-monitoring can help the client learn how to observe symptoms and recognize when he or she needs more intensive help (Finkelman, 2000).

Teach Problem-Solving Techniques

- *Goal setting* is consciously setting time limits on behaviors, which is useful when goals are attainable and manageable. It may become stress-inducing if unrealistic or short-sighted.
- *Information seeking* is learning about all aspects of a problem, which provides perspective and, in some cases, reinforces self-control.
- *Mastery* is learning new procedures or skills, which facilitates self-esteem and self-control (e.g., self-care of colostomies, insulin injection, or catheter care).

  R: Goals should be realistic and attainable to promote self-esteem and reduce stress.

Clinical Alert Report

- Advise ancillary staff/student to report any changes in mood, angry outbursts and/or references to not wanting to live.

TRANSITION PLAN

Initiate health teaching and referrals as indicated.

- Prepare for problems that may occur after discharge.
  - Medications—schedule, cost, misuse, and side effects
  - Increased anxiety
  - Sleep problems
  - Eating problems—access, decreased appetite
  - Inability to structure time
  - Family / significant other conflicts
  - Follow-up—forgetting, access, difficulty organizing time

  R: For depression-related problems beyond the scope of nurse generalists, therapist, psychologist, and psychiatrist) will be needed.
- Instruct the client in relaxation techniques; emphasize the importance of setting 15 to 20 minutes aside each day to practice relaxation. Refer to Getting Started to Manage Stress on thePoint at http://thePoint.lww.com/Carpenito6e.

INEFFECTIVE DENIAL

NANDA-I Definition

Conscious or unconscious attempt to disavow the knowledge or meaning of an event to reduce anxiety and / or fear, leading to the detriment of health

Defining Characteristics**

Major (Must Be Present)*

Delays seeking or refuses health care attention
Does not perceive personal relevance of symptoms or danger

Minor (May Be Present)

Uses home remedies (self-treatment) to relieve symptoms
Does not admit fear of death or invalidism*
Minimizes symptoms*
Displaces the source of symptoms to other areas of the body
Cannot admit the effects of the disease on life pattern
Makes dismissive gestures when speaking of distressing events*
Displaces the fear of effects of the condition
Displays inappropriate affect*

**Source: Lynch, C. S., & Phillips, M. W. (1989). Nursing diagnosis: Ineffective denial. In R. M. Carroll-Johnson (Ed.), *Classification of nursing diagnosis: Proceedings of the eighth conference.* Philadelphia, PA: J. B. Lippincott.

Related Factors

Pathophysiologic

Related to inability to tolerate consciously the consequences of (any chronic or terminal illness) secondary to (e.g., HIV infection, AIDS, cancer, progressive debilitating disorders [e.g., multiple sclerosis, myasthenia gravis])

Treatment Related

Related to prolonged treatment with no positive results

Situational / Psychological

Related to negative consequences of (e.g., financial crisis, inability to maintain employment obesity, domestic abuse, child neglect / abuse)

Related to the reality of one's physical and emotional dependence on (Varcarolis, 2011):

Alcohol
Cocaine, crack
Stimulants
Opiates
Cannabis
Barbituates / sedatives
Hallucinogens
Tobacco use

Related to long-term self-destructive patterns of behavior and lifestyle (Varcarolis, 2011)
Related to genetic origins of alcoholism

Carp's Cues

Denial can be a constructive defense mechanism, when reality is too painful as sudden death of loved one or a life-threatening diagnosis. *Ineffective Denial* is not beneficial or constructive. When the person will not participate in regimens to improve health or the situation (e.g., denies substance abuse), his or her denial is a barrier. The focus for this diagnosis is the help the hospitalized individual acknowledge how his or her alcohol, drug, or tobacco abuse has negatively affected his or her health, relationships, and livelihood (e.g., employment) and to provide him or her resources to utilize after discharge.

Objective Data

Withdrawal symptoms (e.g., tearing, runny nose, gooseflesh, yawning, dilated pupils, mild hypertension, tachycardia, nausea, vomiting, restlessness, abdominal cramps, joint pain)

Goals

NOC
Anxiety Self-Control, Coping; Social Support, Substance Addiction Consequences, Knowledge: Substance Use Control, Knowledge: Disease Process

The person will acknowledge an alcohol / drug / tobacco problem as evidenced by the following indicators:

- Will identify three negative consequences of his or her alcohol / drug / tobacco use.
- Will identify resources available in the community.
- Express a sense of hope.

Interventions

NIC

Teaching: Disease
Process; Anxiety
Reduction; Counseling;
Active Listening

Initiate a Therapeutic Relationship

- Assess effectiveness of denial.
- Avoid confronting the client that he or she is using denial.
- Approach the client directly, matter-of-factly, and nonjudgmentally.

  R: Denial may be valuable in the early stages of coping, when resources are not sufficient to manage more problem-focused approaches (Lazarus, 1985).

Explore with the Client How His or Her Substance Abuse Has Affected His or Her Life and Health (Present, Future)

Work / School Problems
- Absenteeism, frequent unexplained brief absences, loss of job, elaborate excuses, and failed assignments

Social Problems
- Daytime fatigue, mood swings, isolation (avoidance of others), arguments with partner / friends / family

Legal
- Traffic accidents / citations
- Violence while intoxicated
- Crimes (theft, fraud, and assaults)

Physical Effects of Alcohol Abuse
- Blackout, liver dysfunction, pancreatitis, gastritis / gastric ulcers, cardiomyopathy, lower extremity paresthesias, brain atrophy, memory impairment, seizures, withdrawal symptoms (e.g., tremors, nausea, vomiting, increased blood pressure and pulse, sleep disturbances, disorientation, hallucinations, agitation, seizures)

Physical Effects of Opioid Abuse
- Blackout, liver dysfunction, pancreatitis, gastritis / gastric ulcers, chronic constipation, malnutrition, respiratory depression, increased risk for HIV, hepatitis C, cellulitis (sharing snorting equipment, needles)

Physical Effects of Amphetamine and Cocaine Abuse
- Hyperactivity, paranoia, decreased appetite / weight loss, cerebrovascular accident, cardiac dysrhythmias, left ventricular hypertrophy, hallucinations, seizures, respiratory depression, hepatitis, HIV (sharing snorting equipment, needles)

Physical Effects of Tobacco Use (Smoked, Snuff)
- Cancers: lung, bronchial, laryngeal, oral cavity, pharyngeal, esophageal, stomach, pancreatic, kidney, urinary bladder, uterus, cervical and acute myelogenous leukemia.
- It also causes abdominal aortic aneurysms, peripheral vascular disease, strokes, chronic obstructive lung disease and contributes to osteoporosis. (CDC, 2011)
- Exposure to secondhand smoke—sometimes called environmental tobacco smoke—causes nearly 50,000 deaths each year among adults in the United States. Secondhand smoke causes 3,400 annual deaths from lung cancer and causes 46,000 annual deaths from heart disease (CDC, 2011).

Assist the Client to Understand Drug / Alcohol Addictions

- Assist the client to gain an intellectual understanding that this is an illness, not a moral problem.
- Provide educational information about the progressive nature of substance abuse and its effects on the body and interpersonal relationships.
- Explain that addiction "does not cure itself" and that it requires abstinence and treatment of the underlying issues (Varcarolis, 2011).

R: The client probably has been reprimanded by many and is distrustful. The nurse's personal experiences with alcohol may increase or decrease empathy for the client. Acknowledgment of alcoholism as a disease can increase the client's sense of trust.

Openly Discuss the Reality of Relapse; Emphasize That Relapse Does Not Mean Failure

- Emphasize a "one day at a time" philosophy.

    R: Relapse must be addressed to increase motivation and to reduce abandoning all attempts to change behavior.

TRANSITION PLAN

Initiate health teaching and referrals as indicated.

- Teach relaxation techniques and meditation. Encourage use when the client recognizes anxiety. Refer to Getting Started to Reduce Stress and Getting Started to Quit Smoking on thePoint at http://thePoint.lww.com/Carpenito6e.
- "Expect sobriety. Reinforce for individuals to view their commitment to one day at a time" (Varcarolis, 2011).

    R: Individuals may be overwhelmed thinking they can never drink or use that drug again (Varcarolis, 2011).
- Refer the client to AA, Alanon, or AlaTeen.
- Refer the client to a treatment facility.

    R: Participation in a structured treatment program greatly increases the chance of successful recovery from alcoholism. Affording the client direct contact with an expert who can help promote a sense of hope.
- Reinforce healthy living choices (e.g., balanced diet, exercise, recreation, rest).

    R: Individuals who abuse drugs and / or alcohol do not engage in healthy lifestyles.

INTERRUPTED FAMILY PROCESSES

Definition

Change in family relationships and / or functioning (NANDA-I)

State in which a usually supportive family experiences, or is at risk to experience, a stressor that challenges its previously effective functioning**

Defining Characteristics

Major (Must Be Present)

Family system cannot or does not:

Adapt constructively to crisis
Communicate openly and effectively between family members

Minor (May Be Present)

Family system cannot or does not:

Meet physical needs of all its members
Meet emotional needs of all its members
Meet spiritual needs of all its members
Express or accept a wide range of feelings
Seek or accept help appropriately

**This additional definition has been included for clarity and usefulness.

Related Factors

Any factor can contribute to *Interrupted Family Processes*. Common factors are listed below.

Treatment Related

Related to:

Disruption of family routines because of time-consuming treatments (e.g., home dialysis)
Physical changes because of treatments of ill family member
Emotional changes in all family members because of treatments of ill family member
Financial burden of treatments for ill family member
Hospitalization of ill family member

Situational (Personal, Environmental)

Related to loss of family member

Death
Incarceration
Going away to school
Desertion
Separation
Hospitalization
Divorce

Related to addition of new family member

Birth
Marriage
Adoption
Elderly relative

Related to losses associated with:

Poverty
Economic crisis
Change in family roles (e.g., retirement)
Birth of child with defect
Relocation
Disaster

Related to conflict (moral, goal, cultural)
Related to breach of trust between members
Related to social deviance by family member (e.g., crime)

 ### Carp's Cue

Interrupted Family Processes describes a family that reports usual constructive function but is experiencing an alteration from a current stress-related challenge. The family is viewed as a system, with interdependence among members. Thus, life challenges for individual members also challenge the family system. Certain situations may negatively influence family functioning; examples include illness, an older relative moving in, relocation, separation, and divorce.

Interrupted Family Processes differs from *Caregiver Role Strain*. Certain situations require one or more family members to assume a caregiver role for a relative. Caregiver role responsibilities can vary from ensuring that an older parent has three balanced meals daily to providing for all hygiene and self-care activities for an adult or child. *Caregiver Role Strain* describes the mental and physical burden that the caregiver role places on individuals, which influences all their concurrent relationships and role responsibilities. It focuses specifically on the individual or individuals with multiple direct caregiver responsibilities.

Goals / Intervention

Refer to Generic Medical Care Plan.

RISK FOR SUICIDE

NANDA-I Definition

At risk for self-inflicted, life-threatening injury

Risk Factors

Suicidal behavior (ideation, talk, plan, available means) (Varcarolis, 2011)
Persons high risk for suicide
Poor support system*
Family history of suicide*
Hopelessness / helplessness*
History of prior suicidal attempts*
Alcohol and substance abuse*
Legal or disciplinary problems*
Grief / bereavement (loss of person, job, home)
Suicidal cues (Varcarolis, 2011)
Overt ("No one will miss me," "I am better off dead," "I have nothing to live for.")
Covert (making out a will, giving valuables away, writing forlorn love notes, acquiring life insurance)

Carp's Cues

This diagnosis focuses on the client, who is at *Risk for Suicide* while hospitalized for a medical or surgical condition.

Goal

NOC
Impulse-Self Control,
Suicide Self-Restraint

The client will identify suicidal thoughts if they occur as evidenced by the following indicators.

- Short term (Varcarolis, 2011)
  - Remain safe while in the hospital.
  - Stay with a friend or family if person has a potential for suicide if discharged to home.
  - Report an intent to participate with family in family counseling.

Interventions

NIC
Active Listening, Coping
Enhancement, Suicide
Prevention, Impulse
Control Training,
Behavior Management:
Self-Harm, Hope
Instillation, Contracting,
Surveillance: Safety

Access a Psychiatric Evaluation to Determine the Level of Risk for Suicide: High, Moderate, Low

Provide a Safe Environment Based on Level of Risk; Notify All Staff That the Client Is at Risk for Self-Harm and the Level of Risk; Use Both Written and Oral Communication (Varcarolis, 2011)

- Initiate suicide precaution per institution's protocol for immediate management for the high-risk client.
  - When the client is being constantly observed, he or she is not to be allowed out of sight, even though privacy is lost. Arm's length is the most appropriate space for a high-risk client.
- Initiate suicide observation for risk persons
  - Provide 15-minute visual check of mood, behaviors, and verbatim statements.

  R: The level of protection of the client will be determined by his or her risk for suicide. Caregivers can become immobilized or drained by the acutely suicidal client. Feelings of hopelessness are often communicated to the caregiver.

Ensure the Following:

- Restrict glass, nail files, scissors, nail polish remover, mirrors, needles, razors, soda cans, plastic bags, lighters, electric equipment, belts, hangers, knives, tweezers, alcohol, and guns.

Situational (Personal, Environmental)

Related to history of overt aggressive acts
Related to increase in stressors within a short period
Related to acute agitation
Related to suspiciousness
Related to persecutory delusions
Related to verbal threats of physical assault
Related to low frustration tolerance
Related to poor impulse control
Related to fear of the unknown
Related to response to catastrophic event
Related to response to dysfunctional family throughout developmental stages
Related to dysfunctional communication patterns
Related to drug or alcohol abuse

Carp's Cues

The diagnosis *Risk for Other-Directed Violence* describes a client who has been assaultive or, because of certain factors (e.g., toxic response to alcohol or drugs, hallucinations or delusions, brain dysfunction), is at high risk for assaulting others. In such a situation, the nursing focus is on decreasing violent episodes and protecting the client and others. The nurse should follow the institution's policy to protect staff and the client from injury.

Goals

NOC
Abuse Cessation, Abusive Behavior Self-Restraint, Aggression Self-Control, Impulse Self-Control

The client will have no or minimal aggressive responses as evidenced by the following indicators (Varcarolis, 2011):

- Refrains from threatening, loud language toward others
- Responds to external controls when at high risk for loss of control
- Explain rationales for interventions.

Interventions

NIC
Anger Control Assistance, Environmental Management: Violence Prevention, Impulse Control Training, Crisis Intervention, Seclusion, Physical Restraint

The nursing interventions for *Risk for Other-Directed Violence* apply to any client who is potentially violent, regardless of related factors.

Establish an Environment That Reduces Agitation (Farrell et al., 1998)

- Decrease noise level.
- Give short, concise explanations.
- Control the number of persons present at one time.
- Provide a single or semiprivate room.
- Allow the client to arrange personal possessions.
- Be aware that darkness can increase disorientation and enhance suspiciousness.
- Decrease situations in which the client is frustrated.
- Provide music if the client is receptive.

R: The client is in an agitated / mentally compromised state. Environmental stimuli unnecessarily increase this state and can increase aggression.

Promote Interactions That Increase the Client's Sense of Trust

- Acknowledge the client's feelings (e.g., "You are having a rough time").
  - Be genuine and empathetic.
  - Tell the client that you will help him or her to control behavior and not do anything destructive.
  - Be direct and frank ("I can see you are angry").
  - Be consistent and firm.

- Set limits when the client poses a risk to others.

  R: Setting limits clarifies rules, guidelines, and standards of acceptable behavior and establishes the consequences of violating the rules.

- Be aware of your own feelings and reactions:
  - Do not take verbal abuse personally.
  - Remain calm if you are becoming upset; leave the situation to others, if possible.
  - After a threatening situation, discuss your feelings with other staff.

  R: Staff activities may be counterproductive to managing aggressive behavior. Recognition and replacement of attitudes such as "I must be calm and relaxed at all times" with "No matter how anxious I feel, I will keep thinking and decide on the best approach" often prevent escalation of aggression.

Initiate Immediate Management of the High-Risk Client

> **CLINICAL ALERT**
> - Always place staff safety first. The presence of four or five staff members reassures the client that you will not let him or her lose control. The focus is respect, concern, and safety.

- Allow the client with acute agitation space that is five times greater than that for a client who is in control. Do not touch the client.
- Avoid physical entrapment of individual or staff.
- Do not approach a violent client alone. Often, the presence of three or four staff members is enough to reassure the client that you will not let him or her lose control. Use a positive tone; do not demand or cajole.
- Maintain the same physical level (e.g., both people either sitting or standing prevents feelings of intimidation). The least aggressive stance is at a 45-degree angle to the person, rather than face to face.
- Call the client by name in a calm, quiet, and respectful manner.
- Avoid threats; refer to yourself, not policies, rules, or supervisors.
- Allow appropriate verbal expressions of anger. Give positive feedback.

R: Assaultive behavior tends to occur when conditions are crowded, are without structure, and involve activity "demanded" by staff (Farrell et al., 1998).

Assist the Client to Maintain Control Over His or Her Behavior

- Establish the expectation that he or she can control behavior, and continue to reinforce the expectation. Explain exactly which behavior is inappropriate and why.
- Reassure the client that you will provide control if he or she cannot ("I am concerned about you. I will get [more staff, medications] to keep you from doing anything impulsive").
- Set firm, clear limits when a client presents a danger to self or others ("Put the chair down").
- Set limits on verbal abuse. Do not take insults personally. Support others (clients, staff) who may be targets of abuse.
- Do not give attention to the client who is being verbally abusive. Tell the client what you are doing and why.

R: Crisis management techniques can help prevent escalation of aggression and help the client achieve self-control. The least restrictive safe and effective measure should be used.

Plan for Unpredictable Violence

- Ensure availability of staff before potential violent behavior (never try to assist the client alone when physical restraint is necessary).
- Determine who will be in charge of directing personnel to intervene in violent behavior if it occurs.
- Ensure protection for self (door nearby for withdrawal, pillow to protect face).

Use Seclusion and / or Restraint, If Indicated

- Remove client from situation if environment is contributing to aggressive behavior, using the least amount of control needed (e.g., ask others to leave, and take client to quiet room).
- Reinforce that you are going to help the client control himself or herself.

- When interpersonal and pharmacologic interventions fail to control the angry, aggressive client, always follow hospital protocols or physical and chemical restraints (Varcarolis, 2011).

R: Hospital protocols should be clear regarding how, when, and for what time period a client can be restrained or secluded and the associated nursing care needed (Varcarolis, 2011).

R: Seclusion and restraint are options for a client exhibiting serious, persistent aggression. The nurse must protect the client's safety at all times. Use of the least restrictive measures allows the client the most opportunity to regain self-control (Farrell et al., 1998).

Convene a Post-Crisis Discussion After a Violent Episode With Involved Personnel

R: After a violent act, leading a postcrisis discussion of the event, outcome, and feelings can decrease anxiety, increase understanding of violence, and address preventable problems that occurred.

R: Postcrisis discussions can help to foster new and more effective approaches to management of aggressive persons (Varcarolis, 2011).

Clinical Alert Report
- Advise ancillary staff / student to report an increase in anxiety, anger, or any displays of aggression.

TRANSITION PLAN
Initiate health teaching and referrals as indicated.
- Refer to appropriate program (e.g., counseling, D&A program).

Section 2

Individual Collaborative Problems

RISK FOR COMPLICATIONS OF CARDIAC / VASCULAR DYSFUNCTION

Risk for Complications of Bleeding
Risk for Complications of Compartment Syndrome
Risk for Complications of Decreased Cardiac Output
Risk for Complications of Deep Vein Thrombosis / Pulmonary Embolism
Risk for Complications of Dysrhythmias
Risk for Complications of Hypovolemia
Risk for Complications of Intra-Abdominal Hypertension
Risk for Complications of Pulmonary Edema

Definition

Describes a person experiencing or at high risk to experience various cardiac and / or vascular dysfunctions

Carp's Cues

The nurse can use this generic collaborative problem to describe a person at risk for several types of cardiovascular problems. For example, for a client in a critical care unit vulnerable to cardiovascular dysfunction, using *Risk for Complications of Cardiac / Vascular Dysfunction* would direct nurses to monitor cardiovascular status for various problems, based on focus assessment findings. Nursing interventions for this client would focus on detecting and diagnosing abnormal functioning.

For a client with a specific cardiovascular complication, the nurse would add the applicable collaborative problem to the client's problem list, along with specific nursing interventions for that problem. For example, a standard of care for a client after myocardial infarction could contain the collaborative problem *Risk for Complications of Cardiac / Vascular Dysfunction*, directing nurses to monitor cardiovascular status. If this client later experienced a dysrhythmia, the nurse would add *Risk for Complications of Dysrhythmia* to the problem list, along with specific nursing management information (e.g., *Risk for Complications of Dysrhythmia related to myocardial infarction*). When the risk factors or etiology is not directly related to the primary medical diagnosis, the nurse still should add them, if known (e.g., *Risk for Complications of Hypo / Hyperglycemia related to diabetes mellitus* in a client who has sustained myocardial infarction).

For information on Focus Assessment Criteria, visit http://thePoint.lww.com/Carpenito6e.

Significant Laboratory / Diagnostic Assessment Criteria

• Cardiac enzymes and proteins (Currently, the gross total values of CK, LDH, SGOT, and / or SGPT in the evaluation of cardiac injury are relatively low. Isoenzymes or bands as well as troponins are the only ones usually used. Elevated with cardiac tissue damage [e.g., in myocardial infarction].)
• Creatinine kinase (CK)

- Creatinine phosphokinase, isoenzymes (e.g., CK-MB, CK-BB, CK-MM)
- Creatinine kinase isoforms (CK-MB, CK-MM subforms)
- Lactic dehydrogenase (LDH), isoenzymes
- Myoglobin (troponin)
- Brain-type natriuretic peptide (BNP) (hormones released as a peripheral response to cardiac impairment) (e.g., heart failure)
- C-reactive protein, P-selectin (markers of inflammation and necrosis)
- Serum potassium (fluctuates with diuretic therapy, parenteral fluid replacement)
- Serum calcium, magnesium, phosphate
- White blood cell count (elevated with inflammation)
- Erythrocyte sedimentation rate (elevated with inflammation, tissue injury)
- Arterial blood gas (ABG) values (lowered SaO_2 indicates hypoxemia; elevated pH, alkalosis; lowered pH, acidosis)
- Coagulation studies (elevated with anticoagulant and / or thrombolytic therapy or coagulopathies)
- Hemoglobin and hematocrit (elevated with polycythemia, lowered with anemia)
- Electrocardiograph with or without stress test
- Doppler ultrasonic flow meter
- Cardiac catheterization
- Intravascular ultrasonography (IVU)
- Electrophysiology studies
- Computed tomography (CT), ultrafast computed tomography
- Magnetic resonance imaging
- Signal-averaged electrocardiography
- Echocardiography with or without stress test
- Phonocardiography
- Exercise electrocardiography (ECG)
- Perfusion imaging
- Infarct imaging
- Angiocardiography
- Holter monitoring
- Inflatable loop monitor

Clinical Alert Report

Advise ancillary staff / student to report:
- Signs and symptoms of dysrhythmia / EKG changes
- Signs and symptoms of chest pain or abdominal discomfort
- Signs and symptoms of the client being diaphoretic
- Signs and symptoms of acute pulmonary edema
- Signs of increased fluid retention
- Signs and symptoms of anxiety
- Any new change or deterioration in behavior (e.g., agitation, cognition)
- Change in systolic B/P >210 mm Hg, <90 mm Hg and / or diastolic >90 mm Hg
- Resting pulse >120 or <55 bpm
- Change in rate of respirations and / or >28 or <10/minute
- Changes or new onset of dyspnea / palpitations
- Changes in EKG rhythms

RISK FOR COMPLICATIONS OF BLEEDING

Definition

Describes a person experiencing or at high risk to experience a decrease in blood volume

High-Risk Populations

- Intraoperative status
- Postoperative status
  - Postprocedural cannulation of any arterial vessel but particularly those at risk for retro-peritoneal bleed due to cannulation of femoral vessel
- Anaphylactic shock
- Trauma
- A history of bleeding disease or dysfunction
- Anticoagulant use, including over-the-counter use of aspirin or NSAIDs (nonsteroidal anti-inflammatory drugs)
- Chronic steroid use
- Acetaminophen use with associated liver dysfunction
- Anemia
- Liver disease
- Disseminated intravascular coagulation (DIC)
- Rupture of esophageal varices
- Cirrhosis
- Dissecting aneurysms
- Trauma in pregnancy
- Pregnancy-related complications (placenta previa, molar pregnancy, abruption placenta)

Collaborative Outcomes

The client will be monitored for early signs and symptoms of bleeding and will receive collaborative interventions if indicated to restore physiologic stability.

Indicators of Physiologic Stability

- Alert, oriented, calm
- Urine output >0.5 mL/kg/h
- Neutrophils 60% to 70%
- Red blood cells
  - Male: 4.6–5.9 million/mm^3
  - Female: 4.2–5.4 million/mm^3
- Platelets 150,000–400,000/mm^3
- No petechiae or purpura
- No gum or nasal bleeding
- Regular menses
- No headache
- Clear vision
- Intact coordination, facial symmetry, and muscle strength
- No splenomegaly
- Identify risk factors that can be reduced
- Relate early signs and symptoms of infection
  - Oxygen saturation >95%
  - Normal sinus rhythm
  - No chest pain
  - No life-threatening dysrhythmias
  - Skin warm and dry, usual skin color (appropriate for race)
  - Pulse: regular rhythm, rate 60–100 beats/minute
  - Respirations 16–20 breaths/minute
  - Blood pressure >90/60, <140/90 mm Hg, MAP >70, or CVP >11
  - Urine output >0.5 mL/kg/h
  - Serum ph.7.35–7.45
  - Serum RCO_2 35–45 mm Hg

- SpO2 goals >95% for those without history of lung disease
- Breath sounds without evidence of new, abnormal sounds (rales)
- No presence of distended neck veins (JVD)

Interventions and Rationales

Monitor for S / S of Bleeding Dependent on Site

- Integumentary system:
  - Petechiae
  - Ecchymoses
  - Hematomas
  - Oozing from venipuncture sites
  - Cyanotic patches on arms / legs
- Increase in bleeding from surgical wound
- Eyes and ears:
  - Visual disturbances
  - Periorbital edema
  - Subconjunctival hemorrhage
  - Ear pain
- Nose, mouth, and throat:
  - Petechiae
  - Epistaxis
  - Tender or bleeding gums
- Cardiopulmonary system:
  - Crackles and wheezes
  - Stridor and dyspnea
  - Tachypnea and cyanosis
  - Hemoptysis
- Gastrointestinal system:
  - Pain
  - Blood streaks in stool / emesis
  - Bleeding around rectum
  - Occult blood in stools
  - Dark stools
- Genitourinary system:
  - Increased menses
  - Decreased urine output
- Musculoskeletal system:
  - Painful joints
- Central nervous system:
  - Mental status changes
  - Vertigo
  - Seizures
  - Restlessness
- Monitor fluid status; evaluate
  - Intake (parenteral and oral)
  - Output and other losses (urine, drainage, and vomiting), nasogastric tube

  R: Early detection of fluid deficit enables interventions to prevent shock.

- Increase monitoring of urine output to hourly.

  R: Decreased urine output is an early sign of bleeding / hypovolemia

- Monitor the surgical site for bleeding, dehiscence, and evisceration.

  R: Careful monitoring allows early detection of complications.

- Teach client to splint the surgical wound with a pillow when coughing, sneezing, or vomiting.

  R: Splinting reduces stress on suture line by equalizing pressure across the wound.

- Monitor for bleeding from esophageal varices.

  R: Varices are deflated tortuous veins in the lower esophagus. Portal hypertension caused by obstruction of the portal venous system from cirrhosis results in increased pressure on the vessels in the esophagus, making them fragile and at risk to bleed (Porth, 2011).

  - Hematemesis (vomiting blood)
  - Melena (black, sticky stools)
  - Dark or black streaks in stool

    R: If there is only a small amount of bleeding, this may be the only symptom (Garcia-Tsao, 2011).

- Black, tarry stools
- Bloody stools
- Light-headedness
- Paleness
- Symptoms of chronic liver disease
- Vomiting
- Vomiting blood

R: If larger amounts of bleeding occur, the above signs / symptoms may be present (Garcia-Tsao, 2011).

> **CLINICAL ALERT**
> - Contact physician or advanced practice nurse with a new onset of any of the above s/s assessment data that may indicate bleeding.
>
>   *R: An immediate endoscopic evaluation is indicated (Garcia-Tsao, 2011).*

- If using the toilet, ask client not to flush. Observe for streaks and darkening of color. Test stools daily for occult blood.

  R: Signs of gastrointestinal bleeding may be detected early (Garcia-Tsao, 2011).

- If anticoagulant therapy, refer to anticoagulant care plan. Monitor for:
  - Bruises, nosebleeds
  - Bleeding gums
  - Hematuria
  - Severe headaches
  - Red or black stools

R: The prolonged clotting time of anticoagulants by anticoagulant therapy can cause spontaneous bleeding anywhere in the body. Hematuria is a common early sign.

- Monitor for signs of bleeding with venous access devices (e.g., IVs, long-term venous access devices).
  - Hematoma at site
  - Bleeding at site

R: Bleeding can occur several hours after insertion, after blood pressure returns to normal and puts increased pressure on newly formed clot at the insertion site. It can also develop later, secondary to vascular erosion due to infection.

- Monitor for bleeding during pregnancy and postpartum (refer to specific collaborative problems as *Risk for Complications of Placenta Previa*).
- Monitor for signs and symptoms of shock.
  - Urine output <0.5 mL/kg/h

    R: Decreased circulation to the kidneys leads to decreased urine output, which is an early sign of hypovolemia / bleeding.

  - Increased pulse rate with normal or slightly decreased blood pressure, narrowing pulse pressure, decrease in mean or mean arterial pressure (MAP)
  - Restlessness, agitation, and decreased mentation

    R: Decreased oxygen to the brain alters mentation and increases anxiety.

  - Increased respiratory rate, thirst
  - Diminished peripheral pulses
  - Cool, pale, moist, or cyanotic skin

R: The compensatory response to decreased circulatory volume aims to increase oxygen delivery through increased heart and respiratory rates and decreased peripheral circulation (manifested by diminished peripheral pulses and cool skin).

- Decreased oxygenation saturation (SaO$_2$, SvO$_2$), pulmonary artery pressures
- Decreased hemoglobin / hematocrit, decreased cardiac output / index

  R: Hemoglobin and hematocrit values decline if bleeding is significant.

- Decreased central venous pressure
- Decreased right atrial pressure
- Decreased wedge pressure

CLINICAL ALERT
- Contact physician or advanced practice nurse with assessment data that may indicate bleeding, and to replace fluid losses at a rate sufficient to maintain urine output >0.5 mL/kg/h

  R: *This measure promotes optimal renal tissue perfusion.*

- If shock occurs, place client in the supine position unless contraindicated (e.g., head injury).

  R: This position increases blood return (preload) to the heart.

- Insert an IV line; use a large-bore catheter if blood replacement is anticipated. Initiate appropriate protocols for shock (e.g., vasopressor therapy). Refer also to *Risk for Complications of Acidosis* or *Risk for Complications of Alkalosis*, if indicated, for more information.

  R: Protocols aim to increase peripheral resistance and elevate blood pressure.

- Restrict client's movement and activity.

  R: This helps decrease tissue demands for oxygen.

- Provide reassurance, simple explanations, and emotional support to help reduce anxiety.

  R: High anxiety increases metabolic demands for oxygen.

- Administer oxygen as ordered.

  R: Diminished blood volume causes decreased circulating oxygen levels.

Clinical Alert Report

Advise ancillary staff / student to report:
- Output hourly for individuals at high risk.
- Any sudden onset of a change in usual condition as:
  - Urine output <0.5 mL/kg/h
  - Restlessness, agitation, decreased mentation
  - B/P >200 mm Hg (systolic), >115 mm Hg (diastolic), <90 mm Hg systolic
  - Respirations >10 per minute over baseline, <10 per minute under baseline, labored
  - Pulse >100 resting
  - Temperature (oral) over 100.5° F
  - Pulse oximetry <90%
  - Diminished peripheral pulses
  - Cool, pale, moist, or cyanotic skin
- Signs and symptoms of acute renal failure
- Signs and symptoms of anxiety
- Increased pulse rate with normal or slightly decreased blood pressure, narrowing pulse pressure, decrease in mean or mean arterial pressure (MAP)
- Increased respiratory rate, thirst
- Decreased oxygenation saturation (SaO$_2$, SvO$_2$), pulmonary artery pressures
- Decreased hemoglobin / hematocrit, decreased cardiac output / index

RISK FOR COMPLICATIONS OF COMPARTMENT SYNDROME

Definition

Describes a person experiencing increased pressure in a limited space, such as a fascial envelope, which compromises circulation and function, usually in the forearm or leg. Compartment syndrome can also occur in the abdomen, when there is a sustained or repeated elevation of 12 mm Hg or greater. Refer to *Risk for Complications of Intra-Abdominal Hypertension*

High-Risk Populations

Internal Factors

- Fractures
- Musculoskeletal surgery
- Injuries (crush, electrical, vascular)
- Allergic response (snake, insect bites)
- Excessive edema
- Thermal injuries
- Vascular obstruction
- Intramuscular bleeding

External Factors

- Extravasation of IV fluids
- Procedural cannulation of vessel for diagnostic or interventional reasons
  - Casts
  - Prolonged use of tourniquet
  - Tight dressings
  - Tight closure of fascial detects
  - Positioning during surgery (lithotomy)
  - Lying on limb for extended periods

Collaborative Outcomes

The client will be monitored for early signs and symptoms of compartment syndrome and will receive collaborative interventions if indicated to restore physiologic stability.

Indicators of Physiologic Stability

- Pedal pulses 2+, equal
- Capillary refill <3 sec
- Warm extremities
- No complaints of paresthesia (numbness), tingling
- Minimal swelling
- Ability to move toes or fingers

Interventions and Rationales

- Monitor for signs of compartment syndrome:
  - Paresthesia (Hartley, 2007)
  - Best elicited by direct stimulation
  - Complaints of tingling or burning sensations > numbness
- Pain
  - Out of proportion to the injury
  - Stretch pain or pain on passive extension or hyperextension of digits (toes or fingers)

  R: *Passive stretching of muscles decreases muscle compartment, thus increasing pain.*

- Increases with the elevation of the extremity

  R: This increases the pressure in the compartment.

- Unrelieved by narcotics

  R: Pain and paresthesia indicate compression of nerves and increasing pressure within muscle compartment.

- Pressure
  - Involved compartment or limb will feel tense and warm on palpation.
  - Skin is tight and shiny.
  - Late signs / symptoms (Hartley, 2007)

    R: Arterial occlusion produces these late signs.

  - Pallor, cool skin
  - Pale, grayish or whitish tone to skin
  - Prolonged capillary refill (>3 seconds)

    R: Delayed capillary refill or pale, mottled or cyanotic skin indicates obstructed capillary blood flow.

  - Paralysis
  - c/o weakness when moving affected limb
  - Progresses to inability to move joint or fingers / toes
  - Pulselessness

    R: Decreased arterial perfusion results in pulselessness.

- Laboratory findings (Hartley, 2007):
  - Elevated WBC (white blood cell count) and ESR (erythrocyte sedimentation rate)

    R: These elevations are a result of the severe inflammatory response.

  - Lowered serum pH

    R: This reflects tissue damage with acidosis.

  - Elevated temperature

    R: This is due to necrosis of tissue.

  - Elevated serum potassium

    R: Cellular damage releases potassium.

- Assess neurovascular function at least every hour for first 24 hours.

  R: A delay in diagnosis is the most important determinant of a poor client outcome (Hartley, 2007).

- Instruct client to report unusual, new, or different sensations (e.g., tingling, numbness, and / or decreased ability to move toes or fingers).

  R: Early detection of compromise can prevent serious impairment (Pellino et al., 1998).

- When the client is unconscious or heavily sedated and unable to complain or report sensations, intensive assessment is required.

  R: Permanent nerve injury can occur 12–24 hours of nerve compression.

- If pain medications become ineffective, consider compartmental syndrome.

  R: Opioids are ineffective for neurovascular pain (Pasero & McCaffery, 2011).

> **CLINICAL ALERT**
> - Immediately, advise physician / NP of the need for immediate evaluation of the neurovascular changes assessed or reported by the client.
>
>   *R: Immediate medical assessment will determine what specific interventions are needed (e.g., emergency surgery [fasciotomy], removal of cast, splints).*

- If signs of compartment syndrome occur:
  - Discontinue elevation and ice applications.
  - Loosen circumferential dressings, splints, casts per protocol.

    R: Elevation and external devices will impede perfusion.

- If invasive compartment monitoring system is used, follow procedure for use.
- Monitor and document compartment pressures according to protocol. Report elevated pressures promptly.
- Carefully maintain hydration.

  R: Hypovolemia can result from fluid volume shift.

- Evaluate cardiovascular and renal status: pulse, respiration, blood pressure, and urine output.

  R: Eight liters of fluid can extravasate into a limb, causing hypovolemia, decreased renal function, and shock (Pellino et al., 1998).

- Notify the physician or NP of any early signs and symptoms of neurovascular compromise.

  R: The physician or NP will evaluate the cause and determine the necessary treatment, such as cast-splitting, removal of medical antishock trousers (MAST), removal of intra-aortic balloon pump, surgery (e.g., fasciotomy).

Clinical Alert Report

Advise ancillary staff / student to monitor for and report signs of compartment syndrome.

- Early Signs
  - Unrelieved or increasing pain
  - Pain with passive stretch movement or flexion of toes or fingers
  - Mottled or cyanotic skin
  - Excessive swelling
  - Delay in capillary refill
  - Paresthesia
  - Inability to move toes or fingers
- Late Signs
  - Pallor
  - Diminished or absent pulse
  - Cold skin

RISK FOR COMPLICATIONS OF DECREASED CARDIAC OUTPUT

Definition

Describes a person experiencing or at high risk to experience inadequate blood supply for tissue and organ needs because of insufficient blood pumping by the heart.

Deceased Cardiac Output is a phenomenon that is not restricted to individuals or environments that specifically focus on cardiovascular care. It is not only prevalent in cardiovascular care units, but also in post-anaesthesia units and noncardiac care units among individuals with noncardiogenic disorders. A significant decrease in cardiac output is a life-threatening situation, demonstrating the need for developing a risk nursing diagnosis for early intervention (Pereira de Melo et al., 2011).

High-Risk Populations

- Acute coronary syndrome (ACS)
  - Congestive heart failure
  - Cardiogenic shock
  - Hypertension
  - Valvular heart disease
  - Cardiomyopathy
  - Cardiac tamponade
  - Hypothermia
  - Anaphylaxis

- Dilated cardiomyopathy
- Streptococcal toxic shock syndrome
- Severe diarrhea
- Systemic inflammatory response syndrome (SIRS)
- Coarctation of the aorta
- Chronic obstructive pulmonary disease (COPD)
- Pheochromocytoma
- Chronic renal failure
- Adult respiratory distress syndrome
- Hypotension / hypovolemia (e.g., postsurgery, severe bleeding or burns)
- Bradycardia
- Tachycardia

Collaborative Outcomes

The client will be monitored for early signs and symptoms of *Decreased Cardiac Output* and will receive collaborative interventions if indicated to restore physiologic stability.

Indicators of Physiologic Stability

- Calm, alert, oriented
- Oxygen saturation >95%
- Normal sinus rhythm
- No chest pain
- No life-threatening dysrhythmias
- Skin warm and dry
- Usual skin color (appropriate for race)
- Pulse: regular rhythm, rate 60–100 beats/minute
- Respirations 16–20 breaths/minute
- Blood pressure >90/60, <140/90 mm Hg, MAP >70, or CVP >11
- Urine output >0.5 mL/kg/h
- Breath sounds without evidence of new, abnormal sounds (rales)
- No presence of distended neck veins (JVD)

R: Low cardiac output can cause cardiac ischemia—perhaps more so for the heart than other organs because of the heart's already high rate of oxygen extraction. A vicious cycle ensues. Cardiac ischemia forces a shift towards anaerobic metabolism (2 ATP) from the much more efficient aerobic metabolism (36 ATP). With less energy available and increased intercellular acidity, the force of contraction weakens, causing a further reduction in stroke volume and cardiac output. The bottom line is that cardiac output is intimately coupled with energy production. For the heart, low cardiac output may in turn cause ischemia. Cardiac ischemia weakens contractility, further impacting cardiac output. When caring for clients with cardiac ischemia, assess for signs and symptoms of poor cardiac output (shock).

Interventions and Rationales

- Monitor urine output hourly.

  R: Decreased urine output is an early sign of bleeding / hypovolemia.

- Monitor for signs and symptoms of decreased cardiac output / index.
  - Increased, decreased, and / or irregular pulse rate
  - Increased respiratory rate
  - Decreased blood pressure, increased blood pressure
  - Abnormal heart sounds
  - Abnormal lung sounds (crackles, rales)
  - Decreased urine output (<0.5 mL/kg/hr)
  - Changes in mentation
  - Cool, moist, cyanotic, mottled skin

- Delayed capillary refill time
- Neck vein distention
- Weak peripheral pulses
- Decreased mixed venous oxygen saturation
- Electrocardiogram (ECG) changes
- Dysrhythmias
- Decreased SaO_2
- Decreased SvO_2

R: Decreased cardiac output / index leads to insufficient oxygenated blood to meet the metabolic needs of tissues. Decreased circulating volume can result in hypoperfusion the kidneys and decreased tissue perfusion with a compensatory response of decreased circulation to extremities and increased pulse and respiratory rates. Changes in mentation may result from cerebral hypoperfusion. Vasoconstriction and venous congestion in dependent areas (e.g., limbs) produce changes in skin and pulses.

- Initiate appropriate protocols or standing orders, depending on the underlying etiology of the problem affecting ventricular function.

R: Nursing management differs based on etiology (e.g., measures to help increase preload for hypovolemia and to decrease preload for impaired ventricular contractility).

- Position the client with the legs elevated, unless contraindicated when ventricular function is impaired as with congestive heart failure.

R: This position can help increase preload and enhance cardiac output.

- During acute episodes, maintain absolute bed rest and minimize all controllable stressors. Administer IV opioid according to protocol.

R: These measures decrease metabolic demands. Use with caution if client is hypotensive.

- Assist client with measures to conserve strength, such as resting before and after activities (e.g., meals, baths).

R: Adequate rest reduces oxygen consumption and decreases the risk of hypoxia.

- Monitor intake and output and weight.

R: Changes can indicate fluid retention.

- In a client with impaired ventricular function, cautiously administer IV fluids. Consult with physician or advanced practice nurse if ordered rate exceeds 125 mL/h. Be sure to include any additional IV fluids (e.g., antibiotics) when calculating hourly allocation.

R: A client with poorly functioning ventricles may not tolerate increased blood volumes.

- If decreased cardiac output results from hypovolemia, septic shock, or dysrhythmia, refer to the specific collaborative problem in this section.
- Administer inotropic and vasoactive agents (e.g., digoxin, dopamine, dobutamine) as prescribed to improve contractility.
- Assist with insertion and / or maintenance of mechanical cardiac assist devices as indicated (e.g., intra-aortic balloon pumps, hemapump, ventricular assist devices).

Clinical Alert Report

Advise ancillary staff / student to report:

- Urine output <0.5 mL/kg/h
- Any new change or deterioration in behavior (e.g., agitation, cognition, anxiety)
- Changes or new onset of dyspnea / palpitations
- B/P >200 mm Hg (systolic), >115 mm Hg (diastolic), <90 mm Hg systolic
- Respirations >10 per minute over baseline, <10 per minute under baseline, labored
- Pulse >100 resting
- Temperature (oral) over 100.5° F
- Pulse ox <90%
- Diminished peripheral pulses
- Cool, pale, moist, or cyanotic skin

RISK FOR COMPLICATIONS OF DEEP VEIN THROMBOSIS / PULMONARY EMBOLISM

Definition

Describes a person experiencing venous clot formation because of blood stasis, vessel wall injury, or altered coagulation and / or experiencing or at high risk to experience obstruction of one or more pulmonary arteries from a blood clot or air or fat embolus.

High-Risk Populations (Anderson, Audet, 1998; Barbar et al., 2010; Fetterman & Lemburg, 2004)

- Active cancer (3)
- History of deep vein thrombosis (DVT) or pulmonary embolism (3)
- Reduced mobility >72 h (3)
- Known thrombophilic condition (3) (e.g., polycythemia, blood dyscrasias)
- Recent trauma / surgery (2)
- Over 70 years old (1)
- Obesity >30 BMI (1)
- Acute coronary or ischemic stroke (1)
- Acute infection and / or rheumatologic disorder (1)
- Ongoing hormonal therapy (1)
- Heart / respiratory failure (1)
- Age (risk rises steadily from age 40)
- Fractures (especially hip, pelvis, and leg)
- Chemical irritation of vein
- All major surgeries that involve general anesthesia and immobility (over 30 minutes) in the operative course (preop, periop, and postop combined), especially surgeries involving abdomen, pelvis, and lower extremities
- Orthopedic (hips / knees), urologic, or gynecologic surgery
- History of venous insufficiency
- Varicose veins
- Inflammatory bowel disease
- Pregnancy
- Surgery greater than 30 minutes (2)
- Over 40 years of age
- Valve malfunction
- Systemic lupus erythematosus
- Central venous catheters
- Nephrotic syndrome
- These risk factors have been identified in the Padua Prediction risk assessment for venous thrombolytic events. A score of > or = 4 is a high-risk individual. (Barbar, 2010).

 Carp's Cues

In more than 90% of cases of PE, the thrombosis originates in the deep veins of the legs. Deep vein thrombosis (DVT) is a distressing but often avoidable condition that leads to long-term complications such as the post-phlebitic syndrome and chronic leg ulcers in a large proportion of clients who have proximal vein thrombosis. "Pulmonary embolism remains the most common preventable cause of death in hospital" (Anderson & Audet, 1998).

Collaborative Outcomes

The client will be monitored for early signs and symptoms of (a) deep vein thrombosis and (b) pulmonary embolism and the client will receive collaborative interventions if indicated to restore physiologic stability.

Indicators of Physiologic Stability

- No leg pain (a)
- No leg edema (a)
- No change in skin temperature or color (a, b)
- No acute dyspnea, restlessness, decreased mental status or anxiety (b)
- No acute, sharp chest pain (b)
- Pulse: regular rhythm, rate 60–100 beats/minute (b)
- Respirations 16–20 breaths/minute (b)
- Blood pressure >90/60, <140/90 mm Hg, MAP >70, or CVP >11
- Breath sounds without evidence of new, abnormal sounds (rales, crackles) (b)
- No presence of distended neck veins (JVD) (b)

Interventions and Rationales

- Identify individuals who are high risk for bleeding (score >/= 4) using the Padua Prediction Score. Refer to list under High-Risk Population.

> **CLINICAL ALERT**
> - Clients at moderate or high risk by the Padua Prediction Score who are not bleeding or at high risk for bleeding should be given anticoagulant thromboprophylaxis with either low-molecular weight heparin (enoxaparin / Lovenox or others), unfractionated heparin (either b.i.d. or t.i.d.), or fondaparinux (Grade 1B; 1 = recommendation; B = moderate-quality evidence). This recommendation includes all critically ill clients, as long as they are not at high bleeding risk. (ACCP, 2012)
>
> *R: Using Padua Prediction Score, 469 high-risk clients, only a minority, 186 (39.7%), received thromboprophylaxis with unfractionated heparin, low-molecular-weight heparin, or fondaparinux during hospitalization. Of these, 2.2 percent (4) developed confirmed venous thrombolytic event (VTE) over the next 90 days. Of high-risk clients not receiving thromboprophylaxis, 11.8 percent (31) developed VTE. Among the 711 low-risk clients, 52 (7.3%) received pharmacological thromboprophylaxis and only two (0.3%) developed confirmed VTE. Bleeding complications, including gastrointestinal, intramuscular, and cerebral, occurred in three (1.6%) of the 469 high-risk clients but were nonfatal." (Barber et al., 2010)*

- Consult with physician / NP to evaluate the need for thromboprophylaxis.

> **CLINICAL ALERT**
> - If the client is high risk for DVT and not high risk for bleeding and thromboprophylax is not prescribed, use SBAR to communicate the seriousness of the situation.

SBAR *Situation:* I am concerned about Mr. Nedia and his risk for VTE (venous thrombolytic event).

Background: He is immobile, 72, obese, and has COPD and a Padua score of 6.

Assessment: Presently, he is resistant to getting out of bed and refuses to walk except to the chair.

Recommendation: Is there a reason why he is not on thromboprophylaxis?

R: This communication provides the physician / NP with an opportunity to review the situation and to share his or her rationale why no thromboprophylaxis has been initiated.

- Refer to *Risk for Complications of Anticoagulant Therapy* for additional interventions.
- Monitor the status of venous thrombosis, noting:
  - Diminished or absent peripheral pulses

    R: Insufficient circulation causes pain and diminished peripheral pulses.

  - Unusual warmth and redness or coolness and cyanosis, increased leg swelling

    R: Unusual warmth and redness point to inflammation; coolness and cyanosis indicate vascular obstruction.

  - Increasing leg pain

    R: Leg pain results from tissue hypoxia.

- Avoid performing Homans' sign (dorsiflexion of the foot)

  R: Numerous studies have documented the unreliability of Homans' sign. Urbano (2001) reported "Estimates of the accuracy of Homans' sign range from it being positive in 8% to 56% of cases of proven DVT and positive in greater than 50% of symptomatic clients without DVT."

- Monitor for signs and symptoms of pulmonary embolism:
  - Acute, sharp chest pain
  - Acute dyspnea, restlessness, cyanosis, decreased mental status or anxiety
  - Cool, moist, and / or bluish-colored skin
  - Tachycardia
  - Tachypnea (Shaughnessy, 2007)
  - Neck vein distention
  - Crackles

  R: Occlusion of pulmonary arteries impedes blood flow to the distal lung, producing a hypoxic state (Porth, 2011).

> **CLINICAL ALERT**
> - Call a code or rapid response team if sudden, severe chest pain, increased dyspnea, tachypnea occur.

- Consult with physician / NP for intermittent pneumatic compression devices or graduated compression stockings.

  R: These should be used for clients who are bleeding or at high risk for it

- Evaluate hydration status based on urine specific gravity, intake / output, weights, and serum osmolality. Take steps to ensure adequate hydration.

  R: Increased blood viscosity and coagulability and decreased cardiac output may contribute to thrombus formation.

- Encourage client to perform isotonic leg exercises.

  R: Isotonic leg exercises promote venous return.

- Ambulate as soon as possible with at least 5 minutes of walking each waking hour. Avoid prolonged chair sitting with legs dependent. Explain to their risk of DVT and PE. If client is resistant, evaluate the reason for pain.

  R: Walking contracts leg muscles, stimulates the venous pump, and reduces stasis.

- Elevate the affected extremity above the level of the heart unless contraindicated (e.g., CHF).

  R: This positioning can help reduce interstitial swelling by promoting venous return.

- Explain the effects of nicotine (cigarettes, cigars, smokeless) on circulation.

  R: Nicotine can cause vasoconstriction and hypercoagulable state, which contributes to poor circulation and clot formation. Refer to Getting Started to Quit Smoking on thePoint at http://thePoint.lww.com/ Carpenito6e.

> ***Clinical Alert Report***
> - Advise ancillary staff / student to report:
>   - A report of leg pain, soreness
>   - Unusual warmth and redness or coolness and cyanosis
>   - Increased leg swelling
>   - Increased immobility (e.g., refusal to ambulate)

RISK FOR COMPLICATIONS OF DYSRHYTHMIAS

Definition

Describes a person experiencing or at high risk to experience a disorder of the heart's conduction system that results in an abnormal heart rate, abnormal rhythm, or a combination of both.

High-Risk Populations

- A-type coronary artery disease (CAD):
  - Angina
  - Acute coronary syndrome (ACS)
  - Congestive heart failure
  - Systemic inflammatory response syndrome (SIRS)
  - Increased intracranial pressure
  - Electrolyte imbalance (calcium, potassium, magnesium, phosphorus)
  - Atherosclerotic heart disease
  - Medication side effects (e.g., aminophylline, dopamine, stimulants, digoxin, beta blockers, dobutamine, lidocaine, procainamide, quinidine, diuretics)
  - Chronic obstructive lung disease
  - Cardiomyopathy, valvular heart disease
  - Anemia
  - Fever
  - Hyperthyroidism
  - Hypoglycemia
  - Hypovolemia
  - Pheochromocytoma
  - Pulmonary disease
  - Vasovagal syndrome
  - Postoperative cardiac surgery
  - Postoperative after any major anesthesia
  - Trauma
  - Sleep apnea

Collaborative Outcomes

The client will be monitored for early signs and symptoms of *Decreased Cardiac Output* and will receive collaborative interventions if indicated to restore physiologic stability.

Indicators of Physiologic Stability

Refer to *Decreased Cardiac Output* indicators.

Interventions and Rationales

- Monitor for signs and symptoms of dysrhythmias:
  - Abnormal rate, rhythm
  - Palpitations, chest pain, syncope, fatigue
  - Decreased SaO_2
  - ECG changes
  - Hypotension
  - Change in level of consciousness

  R: Ischemic tissue is electrically unstable, causing dysrhythmias. Certain congenital cardiac conditions, electrolyte imbalances, and medications also can cause disturbances in cardiac conduction.

- Initiate appropriate protocols depending on the type of dysrhythmia; this may include:
  - Supraventricular tachycardia: vagal stimulation (direct or indirect), IV calcium channel blockers, digoxin (IV), adenosine, diltiazem, adenocard, synchronized cardioversion, overdrive pacing
  - Atrial fibrillation: digitalization, electrical cardioversion, anticoagulant therapy
  - Premature ventricular contractions, ventricular tachycardia: IV lidocaine, IV procainamide, oxygen
  - Ventricular tachycardia: oxygen, lidocaine, procainamide, amiodarone, synchronized or unsynchronized cardioversion (dependent on presence of pulse)
  - Bradycardia or heart blocks: atropine, pacing, dopamine infusion, epinephrine infusion
  - Ventricular fibrillation: cardiopulmonary resuscitation (CPR), defibrillation, epinephrine, lidocaine, bretylium
  - Pulseless electrical activity: CPR, atropine (if rate bradycardic), epinephrine (diagnose and treat the cause)
  - Asystole: CPR, epinephrine, atropine
  - Administer supplemental oxygen
    R: It increases circulating oxygen levels and decreases cardiac workload.
- Monitor oxygen saturation (SaO$_2$) with pulse oximetry and ABGs as necessary.
- Monitor serum electrolyte levels (e.g., sodium, potassium, calcium, magnesium).
  R: High or low electrolyte levels may exacerbate a dysrhythmia.
- Monitor pacemaker and automatic implantable cardioverter (cardiac) defibrillator (AICD) therapy.
- Monitor electrolytes.
  R: Electrolyte imbalance (calcium, potassium, magnesium, phosphorus) can cause dysrhythmias.

Clinical Alert Report

Advise ancillary staff / student to report:
- Changes or new onset of dyspnea, palpitations, chest pain, syncope, fatigue
- Signs of increased fluid retention
- Decrease in urine output less than 0.5 mL/kg per hour

RISK FOR COMPLICATIONS OF HYPOVOLEMIA

Definition

Describes a person experiencing or at high risk to experience inadequate cellular oxygenation and inability to excrete waste products of metabolism secondary to decreased fluid volume (e.g., from bleeding, plasma loss, prolonged vomiting, or diarrhea)

High-Risk Populations

- Intraoperative status
- Postoperative status
- Postprocedural cannulation of any arterial vessel but particularly those at risk for retro-peritoneal bleed due to cannulation of femoral vessel
- Anaphylactic shock
- Trauma
- Bleeding
- Diabetic ketoacidosis (DKA) or hyperosmolar hyperglycemic state (HHS) (Kitabchi, Haerian, & Rose, 2008)
- Prolonged vomiting or diarrhea
- Infants, children, older persons
- Acute pancreatitis

- Major burns
- Disseminated intravascular coagulation (DIC)
- Diabetes insipidus
- Ascites
- Peritonitis
- Intestinal obstruction
- Systemic inflammatory response syndrome (SIRS) / Sepsis

Collaborative Outcomes

The client will be monitored for early signs and symptoms of hypovolemia and will receive collaborative interventions if indicated to restore physiologic stability.

Indicators of Physiologic Stability

Refer to *Risk for Complications of Decreased Cardiac Output* for indicators.

Interventions and Rationales

- For individual at risk for bleeding, refer to *Risk for Complications of Bleeding.*
- Monitor fluid status; evaluate.
- Intake (parenteral and oral)
- Output and other losses (urine, drainage, and vomiting), nasogastric tube

    R: Early detection of fluid deficit enables interventions to prevent shock.

- Monitor for signs and symptoms of shock:
    - Increased pulse rate with normal or slightly decreased blood pressure, narrowing pulse pressure, decrease in mean or mean arterial pressure (MAP)
    - Urine output <0.5 mL/kg/h
    - Restlessness, agitation, decreased mentation
    - Increased respiratory rate, thirst
    - Diminished peripheral pulses
    - Cool, pale, moist, or cyanotic skin
    - Decreased oxygenation saturation (SaO_2, SvO_2), pulmonary artery pressures
    - Decreased hemoglobin / hematocrit, decreased cardiac output / index

    R: The compensatory response to decreased circulatory volume aims to increase oxygen delivery through increased heart and respiratory rates and decreased peripheral circulation (manifested by diminished peripheral pulses and cool skin). Decreased oxygen to the brain alters mentation. Decreased circulation to the kidneys leads to decreased urine output. Hemoglobin and hematocrit values decline if bleeding is significant.

- If shock occurs, place client in the supine position unless contraindicated (e.g., head injury).

    R: This position increases blood return (preload) to the heart.

> **CLINICAL ALERT**
> - Call a code or for the Rapid Response Team.

- Insert an IV line; use a large-bore catheter if blood replacement is anticipated. Initiate appropriate protocols for shock (e.g., vasopressor therapy). Refer also to *Risk for Complications of Acidosis* or *Risk for Complications of Alkalosis*, if indicated, for more information.

    R: Protocols aim to increase peripheral resistance and elevate blood pressure.

- Collaborate with physician or advanced practice nurse to replace fluid losses at a rate sufficient to maintain urine output >0.5 mL/kg/h (e.g., saline or Ringer's lactate).

    R: This measure promotes optimal renal tissue perfusion.

- Restrict client's movement and activity.

    R: This helps decrease tissue demands for oxygen.

- Provide reassurance, simple explanations, and emotional support to help reduce anxiety.

  R: High anxiety increases metabolic demands for oxygen.

- Administer oxygen as ordered.
- Monitor for signs and symptoms of shock.

Clinical Alert Report

Advise ancillary staff / student to report:
- Urine output <0.5 mL/kg/h
- Sudden restlessness, agitation, decreased mentation
- Increased respiratory rate
- Decreasing B/P
- Diminished peripheral pulses
- Cool, pale, moist, or cyanotic skin

RISK FOR COMPLICATIONS OF INTRA-ABDOMINAL HYPERTENSION

Definition

Describes a person experiencing or at high risk to experience sustained or repeated pathologic elevation of intra-abdominal pressure (IAP) of 12 mm Hg or greater (WSACS, 2013)

High-Risk Populations (Lee et al., 2007)

- Causes of primary (i.e., acute) intra-abdominal hypertension include the following:
  - Penetrating trauma
  - Intraperitoneal hemorrhage
  - Pancreatitis
  - External compressing forces, such as debris from a motor vehicle collision or after a large structure explosion
  - Pelvic fracture
  - Rupture of abdominal aortic aneurysm
  - Perforated peptic ulcer
- Secondary intra-abdominal hypertension may occur in clients without an intra-abdominal injury, when fluid accumulates in volumes sufficient to cause IAH. Causes include the following:
  - Large-volume resuscitation: The literature shows significantly increased risk with infusions greater than 3 L.
  - Large areas of full-thickness burns: Hobson et al. demonstrated abdominal compartment syndrome within 24 hours in burn clients who had received an average of 237 mL/kg over a 12-hour period.
  - Penetrating or blunt trauma without identifiable injury
  - Postoperative
  - Packing and primary fascial closure, which increases incidence
  - Sepsis
- Causes of chronic intra-abdominal hypertension include the following:
  - Peritoneal dialysis
  - Morbid obesity
  - Cirrhosis
  - Chronic alcohol abuse
  - Pancreatitis
  - Meigs syndrome
  - Intra-abdominal mass

Collaborative Outcomes

The client will be monitored for early signs and symptoms of intra-abdominal hypertension; will receive collaborative interventions if indicated to restore physiologic stability.

Indicators of Physiologic Stability

- Intra-abdominal pressure 0 to 5 mm Hg
- No increase in abdominal girth
- Urine output >0.5 mL/kg per hour
- No melena

Interventions / Rationale

- Monitor for intra-abdominal hypertension (IAH).

  R: Organ dysfunction with intra-abdominal hypertension is a product of the effects of IAH on multiple organ systems.

- Increase in abdominal girth

  R: The effect of IAH on the GI system leads to diminished perfusion, which results in ischemia, acidosis, capillary leak, intestinal edema, and release of GI flora into the lymph and vascular systems (Lee et al., 2007).

- Wheezes, rales, increased respiratory rate, cyanosis
- Limited respiratory excursion

  R: As the abdomen distends, the diaphragm is pushed upward, preventing the lungs from full expansion and increasing intrathoracic pressure (Lee et al., 2007).

- Decreased urine output

  R: Increasing abdominal distention compresses renal parenchyma and decreased renal perfusion (Lee et al., 2007).

- Wan appearance, syncope, headache, confusion

  R: Increasing intrathoracic pressure causes back pressure on the jugular veins and impedes drainage of cerebrospinal fluid , producing increased intracranial pressure (Lee et al., 2007).

> **CLINICAL ALERT**
> - Intra-abdominal hypertension (IAH) that increases to 20 mm Hg or greater and is associated with new organ dysfunction or failure is abdominal compartmental syndrome. Abdominal compartmental syndrome has a mortality rate of over 50%. Medical treatment focuses on attempting to reduce IAP with mechanical drainage and diuretics. If these methods are not effective, a decompressive laparotomy must be performed (Lee, 2012).

- To manage clients with IAH appropriately, nurses must perform IAP measurements.
- The gold standard of indirect measurement is measurement via a urinary bladder catheter.

  R: Hands-on assessments of the abdomen and serial measurements of abdominal girth are not sensitive as direct and indirect measurements of IAP (Lee, 2012).

- Monitor intra-abdominal pressure in high risk individuals who:
  - Are intubated with high peak and plateau pressures

    R: Individuals who are difficult to ventilate may have high intra-abdominal pressures.

  - Have GI bleeding or pancreatitis, who are nonresponsive to intravenous (IV) fluids, blood products, and pressors
  - Have severe burns or sepsis, who are not responding to IV fluids and pressors
  - Have contradictory Swann-Ganz readings, when compared to clinical condition
- Institute interventions to prevent or reduce abdominal distention.

  R: Preventing abdominal compartment syndrome is much more effective than treating it.

  - Prevent constipation and fecal impactions.

    R: These conditions will increase abdominal distention.

- Maintain patency of nasogastric tube and monitor for increased residuals with enteral feedings.

  R: Increased residual feedings or retained GI fluids will further increase distention.

- Ensure that clients who are eating, avoid all gas-producing food.

  R: These gases can further aggravate abdominal distention.

- Avoid the prone position and elevating the head of bed more than 20 degrees.

  R: The prone position and elevations over 20 degrees will increase intra-abdominal pressure.

- Remove heavy blankets, constrictive abdominal dressings.

  R: Any external pressure on the abdomen will increase pressure (must be avoided to prevent).

- Aggressively manage fluid balance to keep the client in negative or equal state.

  R: Excessive fluid administration will increase abdominal hypertension.

Clinical Alert Report

Advise ancillary staff / student to report:
- Client drinking more fluids than prescribed
- All bowel movements
- Any new change or deterioration in behavior (e.g., agitation, cognition, anxiety)
- Changes or new onset of dyspnea / palpitations
- B/P >200 mm Hg (systolic), >115 mm Hg (diastolic), <90 mm Hg systolic
- Respirations >10 per minute over baseline, <10 per minute under baseline, labored
- Pulse >100 resting
- Temperature (oral) over 100.5° F
- Pulse ox <90%

RISK FOR COMPLICATIONS OF PULMONARY EDEMA

Definition

Describes a person experiencing or at high risk to experience insufficient gas exchange because of accumulation of fluid related to left-sided heart failure or fluid overload

High-Risk Populations

Cardiac Causes

- Hypertension
- Dysrhythmias
- Myocardial infarction
  - Acute cardiac syndrome (ACS)
  - Angina
- Congestive heart failure
- Cardiomyopathy
- Failed pacemaker, lead wires and / or generator
- Coronary artery disease
- Aortic or mitral cardiac valve disease
- Congenital heart defects

Noncardiac Causes

- Diabetes mellitus
- Inhalation of toxins
- Drug overdose
- Smoking
- Neurologic trauma
- Volume overload
- Renal failure
- Capillary leak
- Systemic inflammatory response syndrome (SIRS) / Sepsis

Collaborative Outcomes

The client will be monitored for early signs and symptoms of pulmonary edema and will receive collaborative interventions if indicated to restore physiologic stability.

Indicators of Physiologic Stability

- Alert, calm, oriented
- Symmetrical easy, rhythmic respirations
- Warm, dry skin
- Full breath sounds all lobes
- No crackles and wheezing
- Usual color (for race)
- Refer to *Risk for Complications of Decreased Cardiac Output* for additional indicators.

Interventions and Rationales

- Monitor for signs and symptoms of pulmonary edema:
  - Dry, hacking cough, especially when lying down
  - Confusion, sleepiness, and disorientation may occur in older people
  - Dizziness, fainting, fatigue or weakness
  - Fluid buildup, especially in the legs, ankles, and feet
  - Increased urination at night (Peripheral edema during the day returns to circulation when legs are elevated, resulting in nocturia.)
  - Nausea, abdominal swelling, tenderness, or pain (may result from the buildup of fluid in the body and the backup of blood in the liver)
  - Weight gain (Fluid accumulation increases weight.)
  - Weight loss (Nausea causes a loss of appetite.)
  - Rapid breathing, bluish skin, and feelings of restlessness, anxiety, and suffocation
  - Shortness of breath and lung congestion

    R: Symptoms are caused by congestion in lungs from fluid accumulation.

  - Tiring easily
  - Wheezing and spasms of the airways similar to asthma

    R: Impaired pumping of left ventricle accompanied by decreased cardiac output and increased pulmonary venous pressure and pulmonary artery pressure produce pulmonary edema. Hypoxia produces increased capillary perfusion, causing fluid to enter pulmonary tissue and triggering signs and symptoms.

- If indicated, administer oxygen as prescribed.
- Initiate appropriate treatments according to protocol, which may include the following:
  - Diuretics

    R: Diuretics decrease preload.

  - Vasodilators

    R: Vasodilators decrease preload and afterload.

- Positive inotropics (e.g., digitalis)

  R: Positive inotropics enhance ventricular contractions.

- Opioids

  R: Opioids decrease anxiety, preload and afterload, and metabolic demands.

- Monitor urine parameters: specific gravity, intake / output, weight, and serum osmolality values.

  R: These values can help evaluate hydration.

- Take steps to maintain adequate hydration while avoiding overhydration.

  R: Adequate hydration helps liquefy pulmonary secretions; overhydration can increase preload and worsen pulmonary edema.

- Change client's position every 2 hours with chest physical therapy. Determine which position provides optimum oxygenation by analyzing PaO_2 from pulse oximetry and / or ABG values with the client in various positions.

  R: Limiting time the client spends in positions that compromise oxygenation improves PaO_2.

- Place the client in high Fowler's position with legs dependent if dyspnea is severe. Encourage client to be out of bed and in a chair for meals. Caution against raising legs higher than heart.

  R: This positioning helps decrease venous return, increase venous pooling, and decrease preload.

- Encourage use of incentive spirometer, cough, and deep breathing every 2 hours.

- Minimize controllable stressors (e.g., noise, long tests and procedures, strenuous activity); explain all procedures and treatments.

  R: These measures may reduce anxiety, which can help decrease metabolic demands.

- Continue monitoring cardiovascular status—vital signs & hemodynamic values, ABG values, cardiac output, fluid balance, weight, pulse oximeter, and urine output hourly.

  R: This monitoring helps evaluate response to treatment.

Clinical Alert Report

Advise ancillary staff / student to report:
- Any sudden onset of a change in usual condition as:
  - Increased peripheral edema
  - Increase in daily weight
  - Urine output <0.5 mL/kg/h
- Persistent cough or productive cough with frothy, pink-tinged sputum
- Restlessness, agitation, decreased mentation
- B/P >200 mm Hg (systolic) >115 mm Hg (diastolic) < 90 mm Hg systolic
- Respirations >10 per minute over baseline, <10 per minute under baseline, labored
- Pulse >100 resting
- Temperature (oral) over 100.5° F
- Pulse ox <90%
- Diminished peripheral pulses
- Cool, pale, moist, or cyanotic skin

RISK FOR COMPLICATIONS OF RESPIRATORY DYSFUNCTION

Risk for Complications of Atelectasis, Pneumonia
Risk for Complications of Hypoxemia

Definition

Describes a person experiencing or at high risk to experience various respiratory problems

Carp's Cues

The nurse uses the generic collaborative problem *Risk for Complications of Respiratory Dysfunction* to describe a person at risk for several types of respiratory problems and to identify the nursing focus—monitoring respiratory status for detection and diagnosis of abnormal functioning. Nursing management of a specific respiratory complication is then described under the appropriate collaborative problem for that complication. For example, a nurse using *Risk for Complications of Respiratory Dysfunction* for a client in whom hypoxemia later develops would then add *Risk for Complications of Hypoxemia* to the client's problem list. If the risk factors or etiology were not related directly to the primary medical diagnosis, the nurse would add this information to the diagnostic statement (e.g., *Risk for Complications of Hypoxemia related to COPD* in a client with chronic obstructive pulmonary disease [COPD] who experiences respiratory problems after gastric surgery).

For a person vulnerable to respiratory problems because of immobility or excessive tenacious secretions, the nurse should apply the nursing diagnosis *Risk for Ineffective Respiratory Function related to immobility* rather than *Risk for Complications of Respiratory Dysfunction*.

For information on Focus Assessment Criteria, visit thePoint at http://thePoint.lww.com/Carpenito6e.

Significant Laboratory / Diagnostic Assessment Criteria

- Blood pH (elevated in alkalosis, lowered in acidosis)
- Arterial blood gas (ABG) values:
  - pH (elevated in alkalemia, lowered in acidemia) (more commonly referred to as alkalosis and or acidosis)
  - PCO_2 (elevated in pulmonary disease, lowered in hyperventilation)
  - PO_2 (lowered in pulmonary disease)
  - CO_2 content (elevated in COPD, lowered in hyperventilation)
- Sputum stain and culture
- Chest x-ray
- Pulmonary angiography
- Bronchoscopy
- Thoracentesis
- Pulmonary function tests
- Ventilation / perfusion scanning
- Pulse oximetry
- End-tidal carbon monitoring ($ETCO_2$)

RISK FOR COMPLICATIONS OF ATELECTASIS, PNEUMONIA

Definition

Describes a person experiencing impaired respiratory functioning because of a complete or partial collapse of a lung or lobe of a lung, which can result in pneumonia**

**The nurse should use the nursing diagnosis *Risk for Ineffective Respiratory Function* for people at high risk for atelectasis and pneumonia, to focus on prevention. The collaborative problem *Risk for Complications of Atelectasis, Pneumonia* is applicable only if the condition occurs.

High-Risk Populations

- Mechanical ventilation
- Pulmonary edema
- Impaired swallowing (increased risk for aspiration)
- Shallow breathing (due to abdominal pain or rib fracture)
- Postoperative status (especially abdominal or thoracic surgery)
- Immobilization
- Decreased level of consciousness
- Nasogastric feedings
- Chronic lung disease (COPD, bronchiectasis, cystic fibrosis)
- Debilitation
- Decreased surfactant production
- Compression of lung tissue (e.g., from cancer, abdominal distention, obesity, pneumothorax)
- Airway obstruction

Collaborative Outcomes

The client will be monitored for early signs and symptoms of atelectasis and / or pneumonia and the client will receive collaborative interventions if indicated to restore physiologic stability.

Indicators of Physiologic Stability

- Alert, calm, oriented (baseline for client)
- Respiratory rate 16–20 breaths/minute
- Respirations easy, rhythmic
- No change in usual skin color
- Pulse oximetry >95%
- Inclusion of pulse oximetry values for those with and without a history of lung disease as well as $ETCO_2$

Interventions and Rationales

If client is on mechanical ventilation, refer to Care Plan for Mechanical Ventilation.

- Monitor respiratory status and assess for signs and symptoms of inflammation.
  - Increased respiratory rate (tachypnea)
  - Fever and chills (sudden or insidious)
  - Productive cough
  - Diminished or absent breath sounds, rales, or crackles (Ellstrom, 2006)
  - Pleuritic chest pain
  - Tachycardia
  - Marked dyspnea
  - Cyanosis
  - Lethargy

  R: Tracheobronchial inflammation, impaired alveolar capillary membrane function, edema, fever, and increased sputum production disrupt respiratory function and compromise the blood's oxygen-carrying capacity. Reduced chest wall compliance in older adults affects the quality of respiratory effort. In older adults, tachypnea (>26 respirations/minute) is an early sign of pneumonia, often occurring 3 to 4 days before a confirmed diagnosis. Delirium or mental status changes are often seen early in pneumonia in older adults (Porth, 2011).

- Evaluate the effectiveness of cough suppressants and expectorants.

  R: A dry, hacking cough interferes with sleep and affects energy. Cough suppressants should be used judiciously, however, because complete depression of the cough reflex can lead to atelectasis by hindering movement of tracheobronchial secretions.

- Monitor for signs and symptoms of infection.
  - Fever of 100.5° F or higher
  - Chills
  - Tachycardia

  R: Endogenous pyrogens are released and reset the hypothalamic set point to febrile levels. The body temperature is sensed as "too cool"; shivering and vasoconstriction result to generate and consume heat. Core temperature rises to the new level of the set point, resulting in fever. White blood cells are released to destroy some pathogens. The impaired respiratory system cannot compensate; tissue hypoxia results (Porth, 2009).

- Lab values (CBC with differential and lactic acid)

  R: CBC with differential to review the WBC count and review for leukocytosis or leukopenia

  R: Lactic acidosis is most commonly caused by hypoxia. If a client has a condition that may lead to a decreased amount of oxygen delivered to cells and tissues, this test can be used to help evaluate the severity of hypoxia and lactic acidosis. Typically, if their lactate level is above normal limits, treatment will be initiated without delay.

- If fever occurs, provide cooling measures (e.g., reduced clothing and bed linen, tepid baths, increased fluids, hypothermia blanket).

  R: Reducing body temperature is necessary to lower metabolic rate and reduce oxygen consumption.

- Monitor for signs and symptoms of septic shock.
  - Altered body temperature (>38° C or <36° C)
  - Hypotension (/90, >90/60 mm Hg (MAP [mean arterial pressure] >70) (CVP >11)
  - Decreased level of consciousness
  - Weak, rapid pulse
  - Rapid, shallow respirations or CO_2<32

    R: Diminishing oxygen saturation as seen by pulse oximetry

  - Cold, clammy skin
  - Oliguria (urine output <0.5 mL/kg/h)

  R: Septic shock is a systemic inflammatory response syndrome (SIRS) associated with infection because of microorganisms resulting in hypotension and perfusion abnormalities despite fluid resuscitation or vasopressors.

> **CLINICAL ALERT**
> - Immediate action is needed, call Rapid Response Team.

> ### Cinical Alert Report
> Prior to providing care, advise ancillary staff / student to report the following to the professional nurse assigned to the client:
> - Change in cognitive status
> - Oral temperature >100.5° F
> - Systolic BP <90 mm Hg
> - Resting Pulse >100, <50
> - Respiratory rate >28, <10/minute
> - Oxygen saturation <90%

RISK FOR COMPLICATIONS OF HYPOXEMIA

Definition

Describes a person experiencing or at high risk to experience insufficient plasma oxygen saturation (PO_2 less than normal for age) because of alveolar hypoventilation, pulmonary shunting, or ventilation–perfusion inequality

- No complaints of tightness in throat
- No complaints of shortness of breath or wheezing

Interventions and Rationales

- Review allergy profile prior to administrating any medications.
- Carefully assess for history of allergic responses (e.g., rashes, difficulty breathing).

  R: Identifying a high-risk client allows precautions to prevent anaphylaxis.

- Foods—Most common cause of anaphylaxis

  R: Most common food allergens are milk, eggs, peanuts, tree nuts, fish, shellfish, soy, and wheat, which account for over 90% of all food allergies. Foods commonly mistaken for IA include mustard and other spices.

> **CLINICAL ALERT**
> - Food allergies are the commonest cause of anaphylaxis and occur in 1% to 2% of the population. Symptoms usually start 5–30 minutes after ingestion, occasionally after 1–2 hours, but rarely any longer. Consider an alternative diagnosis if symptoms began many hours after ingestion or if the client has since eaten the suspected food without any reaction (Auckland Allergy Clinic, 2012).

- Medications / drugs are another common cause of anaphylaxis.

> **CLINICAL ALERT**
> - It is important to focus on drugs / supplements / herbal preparation (bee pollen, echinacea) and other over-the-counter formulations (especially aspirin and NSAIDs) in the history taking.

- If the client has a history of allergic response, consult with physician or advanced practice nurse regarding skin tests, if indicated.

  R: Skin testing can confirm hypersensitivity.

- Monitor for signs and symptoms of localized allergic reaction.
  - Wheals, flares (due to histamine release)
  - Itching
  - Nontraumatic edema (perioral, periorbital)

  R: The antigen-antibody reaction causes vasodilatation with pooling of blood (edema), histamine release (wheals, itching), and diminished perfusion to tissues followed by vascular and circulatory vasoconstriction.

- At the first sign of hypersensitivity, consult with physician or advanced practice nurse for pharmacologic intervention, such as antihistamines, corticosteroids.

  R: Antihistamines are commonly used to treat mild localized reactions by inhibiting histamine release.

> **CLINICAL ALERT**
> - Progression from hives and itching to life-threatening symptoms of wheeze, loss of consciousness, and laryngeal edema may occur in 10 minutes to hours after onset.

- Monitor for signs and symptoms of systemic allergic reaction and anaphylaxis:
  - Light-headedness, skin flushing, angioedema, and slight hypotension (resulting from histamine-induced vasodilation)
  - Throat or palate tightness, wheezing, hoarseness, dyspnea, and chest tightness (from smooth muscle contraction from prostaglandin release)
  - Irregular, increased pulse and decreased blood pressure (from leukotriene release, which constricts airways and coronary vessels)
  - Decreased level of consciousness, respiratory distress, and shock (resulting from severe hypotension, respiratory insufficiency, and tissue hypoxia)

  R: Within minutes, such reactions can progress to severe hypotension, decreased level of consciousness, and respiratory distress.

- Promptly initiate emergency protocol for anaphylaxis and access the rapid response team stat page physician or advanced practice nurse.
  - Start an IV line. *(For rapid medication administration)*
  - Administer epinephrine IV or endotracheally.

    R: Epinephrine produces peripheral vasoconstriction, which raises blood pressure and acts as a ß agonist to promote bronchial smooth muscle relaxation, and to enhance inotropic and chronotropic cardiac activity.

  - Administer oxygen; establish a patent airway if indicated. Have suction available. Oropharyngeal intubation may be required.

    R: Laryngeal edema interferes with breathing.

- Administer other medications, as ordered, which may include:
  - Corticosteroids

    R: Corticosteroids inhibit enzyme and WBC response to reduce bronchoconstriction.

  - Aminophylline

    R: Aminophylline produces bronchodilation.

  - Vasopressors

    R: Vasopressors counter profound hypotension.

  - Diphenhydramine

    R: Diphenhydramine prevents further antigen–antibody reaction.

  - H1 antihistamines and epinephrine.

    R: H1 antihistamines and epinephrine mediate GI symptoms.

- Frequently evaluate response to therapy; assess:
  - Vital signs
  - Level of consciousness
  - Lung sounds, peak flows
  - Cardiac function
  - Intake and output
  - ABG values

    R: Careful monitoring is necessary to detect complications of shock and identify the need for additional interventions.

- After recovery, discuss with the client and family preventive measures for anaphylaxis and the need to carry an anaphylaxis kit, which contains injectable epinephrine and oral antihistamines for use in self-treating allergic reaction.

RISK FOR COMPLICATIONS OF ELECTROLYTE IMBALANCES

Risk for Complications of Hypokalemia
Risk for Complications of Hyperkalemia
Risk for Complications of Hyponatremia
Risk for Complications of Hypernatremia
Risk for Complications of Hypocalcemia
Risk for Complications of Hypercalcemia

Definition

Describes a person experiencing or at risk to experience a deficit or excess of one or more electrolytes

Carp's Cues

For a person experiencing or at high risk to experience a deficit or excess in a single electrolyte, the diagnostic statement should specify the problem (e.g., *Risk for Complications of Hypokalemia related to diuretic therapy*). Usually collaborative problems do not need related factors unless they will add clarity.

High-Risk Populations

For Hypokalemia
- Crash dieting
- Diabetic ketoacidosis
- Metabolic or respiratory alkalosis
- Excessive intake of licorice
- Diuretic therapy
- Loss of gastrointestinal (GI) fluids (through excessive nasogastric suctioning, nausea, vomiting, or diarrhea)
- Steroid use
- Estrogen use
- Hyperaldosteronism
- Severe burns
- Decreased potassium intake
- Liver disease with ascites
- Renal tubular acidosis
- Malabsorption
- Severe catabolism
- Salt depletion
- Hemolysis
- Hypoaldosteronism
- Rhabdomyolysis
- Laxative abuse
- Villous adenoma
- Hyperglycemia
- Severe magnesium depletion

For Hyperkalemia
- Renal failure
- Excessive potassium intake (oral or IV)
- Cell damage (e.g., from burns, trauma, surgery)
- Crushing injuries
- Potassium-sparing diuretic use
- Adrenal insufficiency
- Lupus
- Sickle cell disease
- Post-transplant
- Chemotherapy
- Metabolic acidosis
- Transfusion of old blood
- Internal hemorrhage
- Hypoaldosteronism
- Acidosis
- Rhabdomyolysis

For Hyponatremia
- Water intoxication (oral or IV)
- Renal failure
- Gastric suctioning
- Vomiting, diarrhea
- Burns
- Potent diuretic use
- Excessive diaphoresis
- Excessive wound drainage
- Congestive heart failure
- Hyperglycemia
- Malabsorption syndrome

- Cystic fibrosis
- Addison's disease
- Psychogenic polydipsia
- Oxytocin administration
- Syndrome of inappropriate antidiuretic hormone (SIADH) (resulting from central nervous system [CNS] disorders, major trauma, malignancies, or endocrine disorders)
- Adrenal gland insufficiency
- Chronic illness (e.g., cirrhosis)
- Hypothyroidism (moderate, severe)

For Hypernatremia
- Older persons, infants
- Inadequate fluid intake
- Heat stroke
- Diarrhea
- Severe insensible fluid loss (e.g., through hyperventilation or sweating)
- Diabetes insipidus
- Excessive sodium intake (oral, IV, medications)
- Hypertonic tube feeding
- Coma
- High protein feeding with inadequate H_2O intake

For Hypocalcemia
- Renal failure (increased phosphorus)
- Protein malnutrition (e.g., due to malabsorption)
- Inadequate calcium intake
- Diarrhea
- Burns
- Malignancy
- Hypoparathyroidism
- Vitamin D deficiency
- Osteoblastic tumors

For Hypercalcemia
- Chronic renal failure
- Sarcoidosis and granulomatous disease
- Excessive vitamin D intake
- Hyperparathyroidism
- Decreased hypophosphatemia
- Bone tumors
- Cancers (Hodgkin's disease, myeloma, leukemia, neoplastic bone disease)
- Prolonged use of thiazide diuretics
- Paget's disease
- Parathyroid hormone-secreting tumors (e.g., lung, kidney)
- Hemodialysis
- Multiple fractures
- Prolonged immobilization
- Excessive calcium-containing antacids

Collaborative Outcomes

The client will be monitored for early signs and symptoms of hypokalemia, hyponatremia, hyponatremia, hypercalcemia, or hypercalcemia and will receive collaborative interventions if indicated to restore physiologic stability.

Indicators of Physiologic Stability

- Serum magnesium 1.3–2.4 mEq/L
- Serum sodium 135–145 mEq/L

- Serum potassium 3.8–5 mEq/L
- Serum calcium 8.5–10.5 mg/dL
- Serum phosphates 125–300 mg/dL
- Serum chloride 98–108 mEq/L

Interventions

- Identify the electrolyte imbalance(s) for which the client is vulnerable, and intervene as follows. (Refer to High-Risk Populations under the specific imbalance.)

  Risk for Complications of Hypo / Hyperkalemia
- Monitor for signs and symptoms of hyperkalemia.
  - Weakness to flaccid paralysis
  - Muscle irritability
  - Paresthesias
  - Nausea, abdominal cramping, or diarrhea
  - Oliguria
  - Electrocardiogram (ECG) changes: tall, tented T waves, ST segment depression, prolonged PR interval (>0.2 s), first-degree heart block, bradycardia, broadening of the QRS complex, eventual ventricular fibrillation, and cardiac standstill (Porth, 2011)

  R: Hyperkalemia can result from the kidneys' decreased ability to excrete potassium or from excessive potassium intake. Acidosis increases the release of potassium from cells. Fluctuations in potassium level affect neuromuscular transmission, producing cardiac dysrhythmias, and reducing action of GI smooth muscle. There is an increase in cardiac irritability, and cardiac monitoring may show early changes as premature ventricular beats.

- For a client with hyperkalemia
- Restrict potassium-rich foods, fluids, and IV solutions with potassium.

  R: High potassium levels necessitate a reduction in potassium intake.

- Provide range-of-motion (ROM) exercises to extremities.

  R: ROM improves muscle tone and reduces cramps.

- Per orders or protocols, give medications to reduce serum potassium levels, such as:
  - IV calcium

  R: IV calcium blocks effects on the heart muscle temporarily.

  - Sodium bicarbonate, glucose, insulin

  R: Sodium bicarbonate, glucose, and insulin force potassium back into cells.

  - Cation-exchange resins (e.g., Kayexalate, hemodialysis)

  R: Cation-exchange resins force excretion of potassium.

- Monitor for signs and symptoms of hypokalemia.
  - Weakness or flaccid paralysis
  - Decreased or absent deep tendon reflexes
  - Hypoventilation, change in consciousness
  - Polyuria
  - Hypotension
  - Paralytic ileus
  - ECG changes: U wave, low-voltage or inverted T wave, dysrhythmias, and prolonged QT interval
  - Nausea, vomiting, anorexia

  R: Hypokalemia results from losses associated with vomiting, diarrhea, or diuretic therapy, or from insufficient potassium intake. Hypokalemia impairs neuromuscular transmission and reduces the efficiency of respiratory muscles. Kidneys are less sensitive to antidiuretic hormone and thus excrete large quantities of dilute urine. GI smooth muscle action also is reduced. Abnormally low potassium levels also impair electrical conduction of the heart (Porth, 2011).

- For a client with hypokalemia:
  - Encourage increased intake of potassium-rich foods.

    R: An increase in dietary potassium intake helps ensure potassium replacement.

- If parenteral potassium replacement (always diluted) is instituted, do not exceed 10 mEq/h in adults. Monitor serum potassium levels during replacement.

  R: Excessive levels can cause cardiac dysrhythmias.

  - Observe the IV site for infiltration.

    R: Potassium is very caustic to tissues.

  - Monitor for discomfort at peripheral infusion site, consider lidocaine additive to reduce / prevent discomfort.

Risk for Complications of Hypo / Hypernatremia
- Monitor for signs and symptoms of hyponatremia:
  - CNS effects ranging from lethargy to coma, headache
  - Weakness
  - Abdominal pain
  - Muscle twitching or convulsions
  - Nausea, vomiting, diarrhea
  - Apprehension

  R: Hyponatremia results from sodium loss through vomiting, diarrhea, or diuretic therapy; excessive fluid intake; or insufficient dietary sodium intake. Cellular edema, caused by osmosis, produces cerebral edema, weakness, and muscle cramps.

- For a client with hyponatremia, initiate IV sodium chloride solutions and discontinue diuretic therapy, as ordered.

  R: These interventions prevent further sodium losses.

- Monitor for signs and symptoms of hypernatremia with fluid overload.
  - Thirst, decreased urine output
  - CNS effects ranging from agitation to convulsions
  - Elevated serum osmolality
  - Weight gain, edema
  - Elevated blood pressure
  - Tachycardia

  R: Hypernatremia results from excessive sodium intake or increased aldosterone output. Water is pulled from the cells, causing cellular dehydration and producing CNS symptoms. Thirst is a compensatory response to dilute sodium.

- For a client with hypernatremia:
  - Initiate fluid replacement in response to serum osmolality levels, as ordered.

    R: Rapid reduction in serum osmolality can cause cerebral edema and seizures.

  - Monitor for seizures.

    R: Sodium excess causes cerebral edema.

  - Monitor intake and output, weight.

    R: This evaluates fluid balance.

Risk for Complications of Hypo / Hypercalcemia
- Monitor for signs and symptoms of hypocalcemia.
  - Altered mental status
  - Numbness or tingling in fingers and toes
  - Muscle cramps
  - Seizures
  - ECG changes: prolonged QT interval, prolonged ST segment, and dysrhythmias
  - Chvostek's or Trousseau's sign
  - Tetany

  R: Hypocalcemia can result from the kidneys' inability to metabolize vitamin D (needed for calcium absorption). Retention of phosphorus causes a reciprocal drop in serum calcium level. A low serum calcium level produces increased neural excitability, resulting in muscle spasms (cardiac, facial, extremities) and CNS irritability (seizures). It also causes cardiac muscle hyperactivity, as evidenced by ECG changes.

- For a client with hypocalcemia:
  - Per orders for acute hypocalcemia, administer calcium by way of IV bolus infusion.
  - Consult with the dietitian for a high-calcium, low-phosphorus diet.

    R: Lower serum calcium level necessitates dietary replacement.
  - Assess for hyperphosphatemia or hypomagnesemia.

    R: Hyperphosphatemia inhibits calcium absorption; in hypomagnesemia, the kidneys excrete calcium to retain magnesium.
  - Monitor for ECG changes: prolonged QT interval, irritable dysrhythmias, and atrioventricular conduction defects.

    R: Calcium imbalances can cause cardiac muscle hyperactivity.
- Monitor for signs and symptoms of hypercalcemia:
  - Altered mental status
  - Anorexia, nausea, vomiting, constipation
  - Numbness or tingling in fingers and toes
  - Muscle cramps, hypotoxicity
  - Deep bone pain
  - AV blocks (ECG)

  R: Insufficient calcium level reduces neuromuscular excitability, resulting in decreased muscle tone, numbness, anorexia, and mental lethargy.
- For a client with hypercalcemia:
  - Initiate normal saline IV therapy and loop diuretics, as ordered; avoid thiazide diuretics.

    R: IV fluids dilute serum calcium. Loop diuretics enhance calcium excretion; thiazide diuretics inhibit calcium excretion.
  - Per order, administer phosphorus preparations and mithramycin (contraindicated in clients with renal failure).

    R: These increase bone deposition of calcium.
  - Monitor for renal calculi (see *Risk for Complications of Renal Calculi*).

RISK FOR COMPLICATIONS OF HYPO / HYPERGLYCEMIA

Definition

Describes a person experiencing or at high risk to experience a blood glucose level that is too low (less than 50 mg/dL) (Field, 1989) or too high (over 200 mg/dL) for metabolic function. A person with a consistent range between 100 and 126 mg/dL is considered hyperglycemic.

Carp's Cues

In 2006, NANDA approved the nursing diagnosis *Risk for Unstable Blood Sugar.* This author defines this condition as a collaborative problem. The nurse can choose which terminology is preferred. The student should consult with the instructor for direction. *If the person is not at risk for both, the diagnosis should specify the problem (e.g., Risk for Complications of Hyperglycemia related to corticosteroid therapy).*

High-Risk Populations

- Diabetes mellitus
- Parenteral nutrition
- Systemic inflammatory response syndrome (SIRS) / sepsis
- Enteral feedings
- Medications
- Hyperglycemia > corticosteroid therapy, acute response to stimulants as amphetamine, some psychotropic medications such as Zyprexa (olanzapine) and Cymbalta (duloxetine).
- Hypoglycemia > chronic use of stimulants

- Hypoglycemia
  - Excess alcohol intake
  - Pancreatic tumor > insulinoma
  - Lack (deficiency) of a hormone, such as cortisol or thyroid hormone
  - Severe heart, kidney, or liver failure or a body-wide infection
  - Some types of weight-loss surgery
- Pancreatitis (hyperglycemia), cancer of pancreas
- Addison's disease (hypoglycemia)
- Adrenal gland hyperfunction
- Liver disease (hypoglycemia)

Collaborative Outcomes

The client will be monitored for early signs and symptoms of hyperglycemia and / or hypoglycemia and will receive collaborative interventions if indicated to restore physiologic stability.

Indicators of Physiologic Stability

- Blood glucose fasting 70–99 mg/dL
- Alert, calm oriented
- No complaints of dizziness
- Warm, dry skin
- No complaints of fatigue, nausea, abdominal pain, diaphoresis
- Pulse: no significant increase
- Respirations: no significant increase

Interventions and Rationales

Many labs and institutions require a repeat of or a second method of validation for treatment of "Critical Lab Values." The organizations define them and require them even for Point of Care (POC) testing for blood glucose values.

For Hypoglycemia

- Monitor serum glucose level at the bedside before administering hypoglycemic agents and / or before meals and hour of sleep.

  R: Serum glucose is a more accurate parameter than urine glucose, which is affected by renal threshold and renal function.

- Determine the peak insulin activity prescribed and factor in sliding-scale doses if indicated. Ensure that the individual eats 15 minutes after insulin administration; monitor closely when NPO for testing. Ensure that a snack is given if meal is delayed.

  R: Overuse of sliding scale, failure to eat as scheduled, and overtreatment of hyperglycemia are frequent causes of hypoglycemia.

- Monitor for signs and symptoms of hypoglycemia.
  - Blood glucose level below institutional guide, commonly 50–60 mg/dL
  - Pale, moist, cool skin
  - Tachycardia, diaphoresis
  - Jitteriness, irritability, nervousness (National Institutes of Health [NIH], 2013)
  - Hypoglycemia unawareness
  - Incoordination, difficulty speaking (NIH, 2013)
  - Drowsiness, confusion, light-headedness (NIH, 2013)
  - Hunger (NIH, 2013)
  - Weakness (NIH, 2013)

  R: Hypoglycemia may be caused by too much insulin, too little food, or too much physical activity. When blood glucose falls rapidly, the sympathetic system is stimulated to produce adrenaline, which causes diaphoresis, cool skin, tachycardia, and jitteriness.

- If client can swallow, give him or her ½ cup of fruit juice or nondiet soda; 1 cup of milk; 5–6 pieces of hard candy; 2–3 glucose tablets; or 1–2 teaspoons of sugar or honey, every 15 minutes until blood glucose level exceeds 69 mg/dL. Check glucose level prior to administering more glucose.

  R: Simple carbohydrates are metabolized quickly.

- If client cannot swallow, administer glucagon hydrochloride subcutaneously or 50 mL of 50% glucose in water intravenously (IV), according to protocol.

  R: Glucagon causes glycogenolysis in the liver when glycogen stores are adequate. In a client in critical condition who has been in a coma for some time, glycogen stores likely have already been used up, and IV glucose is the only effective treatment.

- Recheck blood glucose level 1 hour after an initial blood glucose reading of greater than 69 mg/dL.

  R: Regular monitoring detects early signs of high or low levels.

- If indicated, consult with a dietitian to provide education on dietary management of hypoglycemia.

  R: This measure can help prevent episodes of hypoglycemia.

For Hyperglycemia

- Assess for the following symptoms that are associated with acute or chronic hyperglycemia, with the first three composing the classic presentation of hyperglycemia:
  - Polydipsia—excessive thirst
  - Polyuria—frequent urination
  - Dry mouth
  - Dry or itchy skin

    R: Excess serum glucose causes the kidneys to excrete the glucose with water and electrolytes (sodium, potassium) through osmosis. The results are excess urination, increased thirst dehydration, and electrolyte imbalances.

  - Glucose inhibits water reabsorption in the renal glomerulus, leading to osmotic diuresis with severe loss of water, sodium, potassium, and phosphates.
  - Polyphagia—frequent hunger

    R: With inadequate insulin for CHO metabolism, hunger is perceived.

  - Intermittent blurred vision

    R: High blood sugar causes the lens of the eye to swell, which changes your ability to see.

  - Fatigue (sleepiness)
  - Nausea, vomiting, abdominal pain
  - Headaches, stupor

    R: When insulin is unavailable, blood glucose levels rise and the body metabolizes fat for energy-producing ketone bodies. Excessive ketone bodies cause headaches, nausea, vomiting, and abdominal pain excretion and reduce acidosis.

- Monitor for signs and symptoms of diabetic ketoacidosis.
  - Confusion or a decreased level of consciousness
  - Headache, impairment of cognitive function
  - Dehydration due to glycosuria and osmotic diuresis
  - Blood glucose level >300 mg/dL

- Positive plasma ketone, acetone breath
- Kussmaul hyperventilation: deep, rapid breathing
- Anorexia, nausea, vomiting
- Tachycardia
- Decreased blood pressure
- Polyuria, polydipsia
- Decreased serum sodium, potassium, and phosphate levels

> **R:** *When insulin is not available, blood glucose (BG) levels rise and the body metabolizes fat for energy-producing ketone bodies. Excessive ketone bodies cause headaches, nausea, vomiting, and abdominal pain. Increased respiratory rate and depth helps CO_2 excretion and reduces acidosis. Glucose inhibits water reabsorption in the renal glomerulus, leading to osmotic diuresis with loss of water, sodium, potassium, and phosphates.*

> **CLINICAL ALERT**
> - If ketoacidosis occurs, initiate appropriate protocols to reverse dehydration, restore the insulin–glucagon ratio, and treat circulatory collapse, ketoacidosis, and electrolyte imbalance.

- Continue to monitor hydration status every 30–60 min; urine output and specific gravity, and fluid intake.

  R: *Accurate assessments are needed during the acute stage (first 10–12 hours) to prevent overhydration or underhydration.*

- Continue to monitor blood glucose levels according to protocol.

  R: *Careful monitoring enables early detection of medication-induced hypoglycemia or continued hyperglycemia.*

- Monitor serum potassium, sodium, and phosphate levels.

  R: *Acidosis causes hyperkalemia and hyponatremia. Insulin therapy promotes potassium and phosphate return to the cells, causing serum hypokalemia and hypophosphatemia.*

- Monitor neurologic status every hour.

  R: *Fluctuating glucose levels, acidosis, and fluid shifts can affect neurologic functioning.*

- Reduce the risks of infection.
  - Skin, oral, genital: Carefully protect client's skin from microorganism invasion, injury, and shearing force; reposition every 1–2 hours.

    R: *Dehydration and tissue hypoxia increase the skin's vulnerability to injury. Dermatologic infections that occur with increased frequency in clients with diabetes include staphylococcal follicular skin infections, superficial fungal infections, cellulitis, erysipelas, and oral or genital candidal infections*

  - Urinary tract infection: Refer to *Risk for Infection.*

    R: *Diabetes increases susceptibility to various types of infections. The most common sites are the skin and urinary tract. Lower urinary tract infections and acute pyelonephritis are seen with greater frequency (Khardori, 2012).*

  - Monitor for early signs of infection (respiratory, IV sites, wound).

    R: *Hyperglycemia and acidemia impair in humoral immunity and leukocyte and lymphocyte functions (Khardori, 2012).*

- Do not allow a recovering client to drink large quantities of water. Give a conscious client ice chips to quench thirst.

  R: *Excessive fluid intake can cause abdominal distention and vomiting.*

- Monitor for signs and symptoms of hyperosmolar hyperglycemic nonketotic (HHNK) coma.
  - Blood glucose 600–2,000 mg/dL
  - Serum sodium, potassium normal or elevated
  - Elevated hematocrit, blood urea nitrogen (BUN)
  - Nausea, vomiting
  - Hypotension, tachycardia
  - Dehydration, weight loss, poor skin turgor
  - Lethargy, stupor, coma
  - Elevated urine glucose (>2+)

- Urine ketones negative or <2+
- Polyuria

R: HHNK results from relative insulin deficiency. Hyperglycemia and hyperosmolality are present, but there is an absence of significant ketones. HHNK coma can be a response to acute stress (e.g., from myocardial infarction, burns, severe infection, dialysis, or hyperalimentation). People with type II insulin-resistant diabetes who experience marked dehydration are especially at risk. Glucose inhibits water reabsorption in the renal glomerulus, leading to osmotic diuresis with loss of water, sodium, potassium, and phosphates. Cerebral impairment results from intracellular dehydration in the brain (Porth, 2011).

- Monitor cardiac function and circulatory status; evaluate:
  - Rate, rhythm (cardiac, respiratory)
  - Skin color
  - Capillary refill time, central venous pressure
  - Peripheral pulses
  - Serum potassium

  R: Severe dehydration can cause reduced cardiac output and compensatory vasoconstriction. Cardiac dysrhythmias can result from potassium imbalances.

- Refer to Care Plan for Diabetes Mellitus if indicated.
- Investigate for causes of ketoacidosis or hypoglycemia, and teach prevention and early management, using the nursing diagnosis *Risk for Ineffective Self-Health Management related to insufficient knowledge of (specify)* (see Section 1).

Clinical Alert Report

Prior to providing care, advice ancillary staff / student to report a:
- Failure of client to eat after insulin dose
- Change of mental status
- Glucose >300 or <70 mg/dL

RISK FOR COMPLICATIONS OF OPPORTUNISTIC INFECTIONS

Definition

Describes a person experiencing or at high risk to experience an infection by an organism capable of causing disease only when immune system dysfunction is present.

High-Risk Populations

- Immunosuppressive therapy (chemotherapy, antibiotics)
- Malignancy
- Sepsis
- AIDS
- Nutritional deficits
- Burns
- Trauma
- Extensive pressure ulcers
- Radiation therapy (long bones, skull, sternum)
- Older persons with chronic illness
- Drug / alcohol addiction

Carp's Cues

An opportunistic infection is an infection caused by pathogens, such as bacterial, viral, fungal, or protozoan infections. These pathogens usually do not cause disease in one with a healthy immune system. However, a compromised immune system allows the pathogens to infect.

Collaborative Outcomes

The client will be monitored for early signs and symptoms of opportunistic infections and will receive collaborative interventions if indicated to restore physiologic stability.

Indicators of Physiologic Stability

- Temperature 98 to 99.5° F
- Respirations 16–20 breaths/minute
- No cough
- Alert, oriented
- No seizures, no headache
- Regular, formed stools
- No herpetic or zoster lesions
- No swallowing complaints
- No change in vision
- No weight loss
- No new lesions, e.g., mouth
- No lymphadenopathy

Interventions and Rationales

- Monitor CBC, WBC differential (neutrophils, lymphocytes), and absolute neutrophil count (WBC & neutrophil).

  R: These values help evaluate response to treatment.

- Monitor for signs and symptoms of primary or secondary infection.
  - Slightly increased temperature
  - Chills
  - Dysphagia
  - Adventitious breath sounds
  - Cloudy or foul-smelling urine
  - Complaints of urinary frequency, urgency, or dysuria
  - WBCs and bacteria in urine
  - Redness, change in skin temperature, swelling or unusual drainage in any area of disrupted skin integrity, including previous and current puncture sites
  - Irritation or ulceration of oral mucous membrane
  - Complaints of perineal or rectal pain and any unusual vaginal or rectal discharge
  - Increased hemorrhoidal pain, redness, or bleeding
  - Painful, pruritic skin lesions (herpes zoster), particularly in cervical or thoracic area
  - Change in WBC count, especially increased immature neutrophils

    R: In a client with severe neutropenia, usual inflammatory responses may be decreased or absent.

- Obtain culture specimens (e.g., urine, vaginal, rectal, mouth, sputum, stool, blood, skin lesions, indwelling lines) as ordered.

  R: Testing determines the type of causative organism and guides treatment.

- Monitor for signs and symptoms of sepsis. Refer to *Risk for Complications of Sepsis* if indicated.
- Monitor for signs and symptoms of opportunistic protozoal infections.
  - *Pneumocystis carinii* pneumonia: dry, nonproductive cough, low-grade fever, gradual to severe dyspnea
  - *Toxoplasma gondii* encephalitis: headache, confusion, motor weakness, fever, lethargy, seizures
  - *Cryptosporidium* enteritis: chronic watery diarrhea, nausea, abdominal cramps, weight loss, vomiting, malaise

    R: Clients with immunodeficiency are at risk for secondary diseases of opportunistic infections; protozoal infections are the most common and serious.

- Monitor for signs and symptoms of opportunistic viral infections.
  - Herpes simplex oral or perirectal abscesses: severe pain, bleeding, rectal discharge
  - Cytomegalovirus retinitis, colitis, pneumonitis, encephalitis, or other organ disease (sore throat, swollen glands, fatigue, fevers)
  - Progressive multifocal leukoencephalopathy: headache, decreased mentation
  - Varicella zoster, disseminated (shingles)
- Monitor for signs and symptoms of opportunistic fungal infections.
  - *Candida albicans* stomatitis and esophagitis: exudate, complaints of unusual taste in mouth
  - *Cryptococcus neoformans* meningitis: fever, headaches, blurred vision, stiff neck, mood changes
- Monitor for signs and symptoms of mycobacterium infections, which commonly affect the pulmonary system.
  - *Mycobacterium avium* (intracellular disseminated) (fevers, night sweats, abdominal pain, fatigue, diarrhea)
  - *Mycobacterium tuberculosis* (extrapulmonary and pulmonary) (cough, weight loss, night sweats)
- Emphasize the need to report symptoms promptly.

  R: Early treatment of adverse manifestations often can prevent serious complications (e.g., septicemia) and also increases the likelihood of a favorable response to treatment.

- Explain the need to balance activity and rest and to consume a nutritious diet.

  R: Rest and a nutritious diet give energy for healing and enhancement of the body's defense system.

- Avoid or minimize invasive procedures (e.g., urinary catheterization, arterial or venous punctures, injections, rectal tubes, suppositories).

  R: This precaution helps prevent introduction of microorganisms.

- Explain the importance of adhering to antiviral medication regimen. Advise not to miss any doses.
- Explain the importance of taking prophylaxis medications to prevent opportunistic infections when the client's CD4 is lower than 200 cells/mm.

  R: Taking the prescribed medications every day reduces the viral load and increases CD4 cells. CD4 counts below 200 cells/mm increase the risk opportunistic infections. Missing doses increases drug resistance, treatment failure, and risk for opportunistic infection.

- Refer to the nursing diagnosis *Risk for Infection* in Section 1 for interventions to prevent introduction of microorganisms and to increase resistance.
- Refer to Nursing Care Plan for HIV / AIDS for additional interventions.
- Refer to the nursing diagnosis *Risk for Infection* in Section 1 for interventions to prevent introduction of microorganisms and to increase resistance.

RISK FOR COMPLICATIONS OF SYSTEMIC INFLAMMATORY RESPONSE SYNDROME (SIRS) / SEPSIS

Carp's Cues

"The primary treatment of all shock syndromes is early recognition of factors that may place the client at risk for developing shock." Allergic response can progress to anaphylactic shock. Invasive lines can be sources of infection.

SIRS has replaced the terminology *septic syndrome*. Sepsis is one contributing factor to SIRS; SIRS is a life-threatening condition related to systemic inflammation, organ dysfunction, and organ failure.

Definition of Risk for Complications of Systemic Inflammatory Response Syndrome (SIRS)

Describes a person experiencing or at high risk to experience a life-threatening condition related to systemic inflammation, organ dysfunction, and organ failure in response to the presence of pathogenic bacteria, viruses, fungi, or their toxins. The microorganisms may or may not be present in the bloodstream. SIRS has replaced the terminology *septic syndrome*. Sepsis is one contributing factor to SIRS.

Definition of Risk for Complications of Septic Shock

Describes a person experiencing or at risk for experiencing a loss of circulatory volume (hypovolemia) and impaired perfusion caused by an infectious agent (bacterial, viral) resulting in compromised tissue perfusion and cellular dysfunction.

High-Risk Populations

Individuals with
- Bacterial infection (urinary, respiratory, wound)
- Viral infection
- Complication of surgery (GI, thoracic)
- Drug overdose
  - Burns, multiple trauma
  - Immunosuppression, AIDS
- Invasive lines (urinary, arterial, endotracheal, or central venous catheter)
- Pressure ulcers
  - Extensive slow-healing wounds
  - Immunocompromised (transplants, cancer, chemotherapy, AIDS, cirrhosis, pancreatitis)
- Diabetes mellitus
- Extreme age (<1 year and >65 years)

Collaborative Outcomes

The client will be monitored for early signs and symptoms of septic shock and will receive collaborative interventions if indicated to restore physiologic stability.

Indicators of Physiologic Stability

- Temperature 98 to 99.5° F
- Pulse 60–100 beats/minute
- Capillary refill <2 seconds
- Urine output >0.5/mL/kg/h
- Urine specific gravity 1.005–1.030
- White blood count greater than 4,000 cells/mm^3 or less than 12,000 cells/mm^3
- Less than 10% immature neutrophils (band forms)
- Activated protein C (APC) 65–135 IU/dL
- Platelets 150–400
- Prothrombin time 11–13.5 seconds
- INR 1.5–2.5
- Partial thromboplastin time (PTT) 30–45 seconds
- Serum potassium 3.5–5.0 mEq/L
- Serum sodium 135–145 mEq/L
- Blood glucose (fasting) <100 mg/dL
- Serum lactate levels 1.0–2.5 mmol/L

Interventions and Rationales

- Monitor for septic shock and systemic inflammatory response syndrome (SIRS) (Halloran, 2009).
- Urine output <0.5 mL/kg/hr

  R: Urine output is decreased when sodium shifts into the cells, which pulls water into cells. Decreased circulation to kidneys reduce their ability to detoxify the toxins that result from anaerobic metabolism.

- Body temperature greater than 38° C or less than 36° C
- Heart rate greater than 90/minute

  R: High heart rate decreases blood flow to brain, heart, and kidneys.

- Triggers baroreceptors and release of catecholamines, increasing heart rate / cardiac output and further increasing vasoconstriction

- Hyperkalemia

  R: Potassium moves into the cell with the sodium, impairing nervous, cardiovascular, and muscle cell function.

- Decreasing blood pressure

  R: Movement of water into the cell causes hypovolemia.

- Respiratory rate greater than 20/minute

  R: Anaerobic metabolism decreases circulating oxygen. The body attempts to / increase oxygenation by increasing respiratory rate.

- Hyperglycemia

  R: The liver and kidneys produce more glucose in response to the release of epinephrine, norepinephrine, cortisol, and glucagon. Anaerobic metabolism reduces the effects of insulin. Insulin resistance contributes to multiple organ failure, nosocomial infection, and renal injury (Ball et al., 2007).

- White blood cell count greater than 12,000/μL or less than 4,000/ μL or presence of 10% immature neutrophils

  R: Increased white cells indicate an infectious process.

- Ensure that blood culture is done prior to the start of any antibiotic. Culture any suspected infection sites (e.g., urine, sputum, invasive lines).

  R: "Poor outcomes are associated with inadequate or inappropriate antimicrobial therapy (i.e., treatment with antibiotics to which the pathogen was later shown to be resistant in vitro. They are also associated with delays in initiating antimicrobial therapy, even short delays (e.g., an hour") (Schmidt & Mandel, 2012)

CLINICAL ALERT

- Blood culture obtained after antibiotic therapy has been initiated can be inaccurate. Research of clients with septic shock demonstrated that the time to initiation of appropriate antimicrobial therapy was the strongest predictor of mortality (Schmidt & Mandel, 2012).

- Assess fluid status: monitor CVP and follow protocol for fluid replacement. Early goal directed therapy (EGDT) with fluid replacement improves cardiac output, tissue perfusion, and oxygen delivery, improving mortality and morbidity.

  R: Sepsis causes vasodilation and capillary leak, resulting in hypovolemia.

- Monitor blood pressure. Administer replacement fluids and vasopressors (especially norepinephrine) to maintain mean arterial pressure (MAP) >65.

  R: In EGDT, maintaining MAP >65 improves tissue perfusion and outcomes (Picard et al., 2006).

- Assess for evidence of adequate tissue perfusion: heart rate, respirations, urine output, mentation, $ScvO_2$ / SvO_2.

  R: Close monitoring detects early changes, with immediate interventions.

- Evaluate skin integrity and protect from injury and hypothermia.

  R: Decreased perfusion to skin will result in pale, cool, fragile skin. The tissue is more prone to injury and hypothermia.

- Monitor serum glucose levels. Use insulin (IV) per protocol to maintain tight glycemic control <150mg/dL.

  R: Tight glycemic control improves client outcomes (Picard et al., 2006).

- Implement strategies to prevent thromboembolyctic events.

  R: Endothelial injury activates Factor XII, which stimulates the clotting factors. In sepsis, coagulation produced thrombi and emboli, which block microvasculature. Activated protein C (APC) is lowered in sepsis, which results in increased coagulation and fibrinolysis (Halloran, 2009).

- Monitor older adults for changes in mentation; weakness, malaise; normothermia or hypothermia; and anorexia.

  R: These clients do not exhibit the typical signs of infection. Usual presenting findings—fever, chills, tachypnea, tachycardia, and leukocytosis—frequently are absent in older adults with significant infection.

RISK FOR COMPLICATIONS OF RENAL / URINARY DYSFUNCTION

Risk for Complications of Acute Urinary Retention
Risk for Complications of Renal Calculi
Risk for Complications of Renal Insufficiency

Definition

Describes a person experiencing or at high risk to experience various renal or urinary tract dysfunctions

Carp's Cues

The nurse can use this generic collaborative problem to describe a person at risk for several types of renal or urinary problems. For such a client (e.g., a client in a critical care unit, who is vulnerable to various renal / urinary problems), using *Risk for Complications of Renal / Urinary Dysfunction* directs nurses to monitor renal and urinary status, based on the focus assessment, to detect and diagnose abnormal functioning. Nursing management of a specific renal or urinary complication would be addressed under the collaborative problem applying to the specific complication. For example, a standard of care for a client recovering from coronary bypass surgery could contain the collaborative problem *Risk for Complications of Renal /Urinary Dysfunction*, directing the nurse to monitor renal and urinary status. If urinary retention developed in this client, the nurse would add *Risk for Complications of Urinary Retention* to the problem list, along with specific nursing interventions to manage this problem. If the risk factors or etiology were not directly related to the primary medical diagnosis, the nurse still would specify them in the diagnostic statement (e.g., *Risk for Complications of Renal Insufficiency related to chronic renal failure* in a client who has sustained a myocardial infarction).

Keep in mind that the nurse must differentiate those problems in bladder function that nurses can treat primarily as nursing diagnoses (e.g., incontinence, chronic urinary retention) from those that nurses manage using both nurse-prescribed and physician-prescribed interventions (e.g., acute urinary retention).

Significant Laboratory / Diagnostic Assessment Criteria (MacGregor, Methven et al., 2011)

- Serum chemistries
- Albumin, prealbumin, and serum (lowered in renal disease)
- Amylase (elevated with renal insufficiency)
- Blood urea nitrogen (BUN) (elevated in acute or chronic renal failure)
- Calcium (lowered in uremic acidosis)
- Chloride (elevated with renal tubular acidosis)
- Creatinine (elevated with kidney disease)
- Magnesium (lowered in chronic nephritis)
- pH, base excess, bicarbonate (lowered in metabolic acidosis, elevated in metabolic alkalosis)
- Phosphorus (elevated with chronic glomerular disease, lowered with renal tubular acidosis)
- Potassium (elevated in renal failure, lowered with chronic diuretic therapy, renal tubular acidosis)
- Proteins (total, albumin, globulin) (lowered in nephritic syndrome)
- Sodium (elevated with nephritis, lowered with chronic renal insufficiency)
- Uric acid (elevated with chronic renal failure)
- Complete blood count
- Hemoglobin (lowered in chronic renal disorders)
- MCHC—normal or lowered with accompanying iron deficiency anemia
- MCV—normal or lowered with accompanying iron deficiency anemia
- White blood cell (WBC) count (elevated with acute infection)
- Urine
- Blood
  - Acute—present with hemorrhagic cystitis, renal calculi, renal, bladder tumors
  - Chronic—glomerular damage
- White blood cell (WBC) count (elevated with infection, obstruction). Obtain clean catch sample.

- Creatinine (elevated in acute / chronic glomerulonephritis, nephritis, lowered in advanced degeneration of kidneys)
- pH (decreased with metabolic acidosis, increased with metabolic alkalosis)
- Specific gravity (elevated with dehydration, lowered with overhydration, renal tubular disease)
- Myoglobin—present in muscle injury (medications, trauma)
- Protein to creatinine ratio (>200mg/gm is positive) or albumin to creatinine ratio (>30mg/gm is positive) Obtain random urine sample.
- Urine sodium and osmolarity (level depends on type—acute/chronic and site of kidney injury—prerenal or intrarenal)
- Culture and sensitivity—positive in infection
- 24-hour urine creatinine clearance—used in unstable clinical situations or to confirm clearance
- Imaging studies
- Renal ultrasound—normal renal size 9–10cm
- Magnetic resonance imaging for evaluating mass or cyst
- Kidneys, ureters, bladder x-ray—evaluating for overall size and obstructions
- Renal biopsy—diagnose specific kidney disease to determine treatment options
- Renal angiography—evaluate for stenosis

RISK FOR COMPLICATIONS OF ACUTE URINARY RETENTION

Definition

Describes a person experiencing or at high risk to experience an acute abnormal accumulation of urine in the bladder and the inability to void due to a temporary situation (e.g., postoperative status) or to a condition reversible with surgery (e.g., prostatectomy) or medications

High-Risk Populations (Selius, 2008)

- Postoperative status (e.g., surgery of the perineal area, lower abdomen)
- Postpartum status
- Anxiety
- Prostate enlargement, prostatitis
- Medication side effects (e.g., atropine, antidepressants, antihistamines)
- Postarteriography status
- Bladder outlet obstruction (infection, tumor, stone, constipation)
- Impaired detrusor contractility

Collaborative Outcomes

The client will be monitored for early signs and symptoms of acute urinary retention and receive collaborative intervention to restore physiologic stability.

Indicators of Physiologic Stability

- Urinary output >1,500 mL/24 hours
- Can verbalize bladder fullness
- No complaints of lower abdominal pressure

Interventions and Rationales

- Monitor a postoperative client for urinary retention.

   R: Trauma to the detrusor muscle and injury to the pelvic nerves during surgery can inhibit bladder function. Anxiety and pain can cause spasms of the reflex sphincters. Bladder neck edema can cause retention. Sedatives and narcotics can affect the CNS and effectiveness of smooth muscles (Porth, 2011; Urinary Retention, 2012).

- Monitor for urinary retention by palpating and percussing the suprapubic area for signs of bladder distention (overdistention, etc.). Instruct client to report bladder discomfort or inability to void.

  R: These problems may be early signs of urinary retention.

- If client does not void within 8–10 hours after surgery or complains of bladder discomfort, take the following steps:
  - Warm the bedpan.
  - Encourage client to get out of bed to use the bathroom, if possible.
  - Instruct a man to stand when urinating, if possible. If unable to stand, even sitting at the side of the bed helps.
  - Run water in the sink as client attempts to void.
  - Pour warm water over client's perineum.

  R: These measures help promote relaxation of the urinary sphincter and facilitate voiding.

- After the first voiding postsurgery, continue to monitor and to encourage client to void again in 1 hour or so.

  R: The first voiding usually does not empty the bladder completely.

- If the client still cannot void after 10 hours, follow protocols for straight catheterization, as ordered by physician / advanced practice nurse. Consider bladder scanning to determine if the amount of urine in the bladder necessitates catheterization.

  *R: Straight catheterization is preferable to indwelling catheterization because it carries less risk of **urinary tract infection** from ascending pathogens. Bladder scanning is not a risk for infection.*

CLINICAL ALERT
- If person is voiding small amounts, use straight catheterization; if postvoid residual is >200 mL, leave catheter indwelling. Notify physician or advanced practice nurse.

Clinical Alert Report

Prior to providing care, advice ancillary staff / student to report the following to the professional nurse assigned to the client:
- Inability to void
- Voiding small quantities

RISK FOR COMPLICATIONS OF RENAL CALCULI

Definition

Describes a person with or at high risk for development of a solid concentration of mineral salts in the urinary tract.

High-Risk Populations

- History of renal calculi
- Urinary infection
- Urinary stasis, obstruction
- Immobility
- Hypercalcemia (dietary)
- Conditions that cause hypercalcemia
  - Hyperparathyroidism
  - Renal tubular acidosis (decreased serum bicarbonate)

- Myeloproliferative disease (leukemia, polycythemia vera, multiple myeloma)
- Excessive excretion of uric acid
- Inflammatory bowel disease
- Gout
- Dehydration

Collaborative Outcomes

The client will be monitored for early signs and symptoms of renal calculi and the client will receive collaborative interventions as indicated to restore physiologic stability.

Indicators of Physiologic Stability

- Temperature 98 to 99.5°F
- Urine output >1500 mL/24hr
- Urine specific gravity 1.005–1.030
- Blood urea nitrogen 5–25 mg/dL
- Clear urine
- No flank pain

Interventions and Rationales

- Monitor for signs and symptoms of calculi.
  - Increased or decreased urine output
  - Sediment in urine
  - Flank or loin pain
  - Hematuria
  - Abdominal pain, distention, nausea, diarrhea

  R: Stones in the urinary tract can cause obstruction, infection, and edema, manifested by loin / flank pain, hematuria, and dysuria. Stones in the renal pelvis may raise urine production. Calculi-stimulating renointestinal reflexes can cause GI symptoms.

- Send urine for culture and sensitivity; send 24-hour urine for calcium, oxalate, phosphorus, and uric acid. Urinary potassium, citrate, ammonium, sulfate, and magnesium may be ordered. Corresponding serum chemistries (e.g., bicarbonate and calcium will be simultaneously sent to lab).

  R: Tests are needed to determine type of stone and infection (Zisman, Worcester, & Coe, 2012).

- Strain urine to obtain a stone sample; send samples to the laboratory for analysis.

  R: Acquiring a stone sample confirms stone formation and enables analysis of stone constituents.

- If the client complains of pain, consult with the physician or advanced practice nurse for aggressive therapy (e.g., narcotics, antispasmodics).

  R: Calculi can produce severe pain from spasms and proximity of the nerve plexus.

- Track the pain by documenting location, any radiation, duration, and intensity (using a rating scale of 0 to 10).

  R: This measure helps evaluate movement of calculi.

- Instruct the client to increase fluid intake, if not contraindicated.

  R: Increased fluid intake promotes increased urination, which can help facilitate stone passage and flush bacteria and blood from the urinary tract.

- Prepare person for KUB x-ray, excretory urography, computed tomography, magnetic resonance (pregnancy), and / or renal ultrasound.
- Monitor for signs and symptoms of pyelonephritis.
  - Fever, chills
  - Costovertebral angle pain (a dull, constant backache below the 12th rib)
  - Leukocytosis

- Bacteria, blood, and pus in urine
- Dysuria, frequency

R: Urinary stasis or irritation of tissue by calculi can cause urinary tract infections. Signs and symptoms reflect various mechanisms. Bacteria can act as pyrogens by raising the hypothalamic thermostat through the production of endogenous pyrogen, which may be mediated through prostaglandins. Chills can occur when the temperature set-point of the hypothalamus changes rapidly. Costovertebral angle pain results from distention of the renal capsule. Leukocytosis reflects increased leukocytes to fight infection through phagocytosis. Bacteria and pus in urine indicate a urinary tract infection. Bacteria can irritate bladder tissue, causing spasms and frequency (Porth, 2011).

- Monitor for early signs and symptoms of renal insufficiency. (Refer to *Risk for Complications of Renal Insufficiency*.)
- Explain importance of following instructions for current care and prevention or minimization of risk for future stone formation. (Provide educational materials [e.g., Kidney Stones: Client Fact Sheet http://www.suna.org/members/kidney_stones.pdf]).

Clinical Alert Report

Prior to providing care, advice ancillary staff / student to report the following to the professional nurse assigned to the client:
- c/o sudden flank pain
- Hematuria

RISK FOR COMPLICATIONS OF RENAL INSUFFICIENCY

Definition

Describes a person experiencing or at high risk to experience a decrease in glomerular filtration rate that results in changes in urine output, laboratory abnormalities, hormonal alterations

High-Risk Populations (Porth, 2011)

- High risk clients
  - Older persons
  - Postsurgical
  - Major trauma
  - Underlying chronic kidney disease
- Renal tubular necrosis from ischemic causes
  - Excessive diuretic use
  - Pulmonary embolism
  - Burns
  - Intrarenal thrombosis
  - Rhabdomyolysis
  - Renal infections
  - Renal artery stenosis / thrombosis
  - Peritonitis
  - Sepsis
  - Hypovolemia
  - Hypotension
  - Congestive heart failure
  - Myocardial infarction
  - Aneurysm
  - Aneurysm repair
- Renal tubular necrosis from toxicity
- Nonsteroidal anti-inflammatory drugs

- Gout (hyperuricemia)
- Hypercalcemia
- Certain street drugs (e.g., PCP)
- Gram-negative infection
- Radiocontrast media
- Aminoglycoside antibiotics
- Antineoplastic agents
- Methanol, carbon tetrachloride
- Snake venom, poison mushroom
- Phenacetin-type analgesics
- Heavy metals
- Insecticides, fungicides
- Diabetes mellitus
- Malignant hypertension
- Hemolysis (e.g., from transfusion reaction)

Collaborative Outcomes

The client will be monitored for early signs and symptoms of renal insufficiency with a goal of preventing or minimizing chronic damage. The client will receive collaborative interventions as indicated to restore and / or maintain physiologic stability.

Indicators of Physiologic Stability

- Urine specific gravity 1.005–1.030
- Urine output >0.5 mL/hour
- Urine sodium 40–220 mEq/L/24 h (varies by dietary intake, medications)
- Blood urea nitrogen 10–20 mg/dL
- Serum potassium 3.8–5 mEq/L
- Serum sodium 135–145 mEq/L
- Serum phosphorus 2.5–4.5 mg/dL
- Serum creatinine clearance 100–150 mL min (varies by age, gender, and race)

Interventions and Rationales

- Monitor for early signs and symptoms of renal insufficiency.
    - Sustained elevated urine specific gravity, elevated urine sodium levels
    - Sustained insufficient urine output (<30 mL/h), elevated blood pressure
    - Elevated BUN, serum creatinine, potassium, phosphorus, and decreased bicarbonate (CO_2); decreased creatinine clearance
    - Dependent edema (periorbital, pedal, pretibial, sacral)
    - Nocturia
    - Lethargy
    - Itching
    - Nausea / vomiting

R: Hypovolemia and hypotension activate the renin–angiotensin system, which causes peripheral vasoconstriction and increases glomerular blood flow. The result is increased sodium and water reabsorption with decreased urine output. BUN is also reabsorbed. If this adaptive mechanism is inadequate, acute kidney injury from ischemia develops. Urine output remains low or diminishes and blood pressure is elevated (Fazia, Lin, & Staros, 2012). Decreased excretion of urea and creatinine in the urine elevates BUN and creatinine levels. Dependent edema results from increased plasma hydrostatic pressure, salt, and water retention, and / or decreased colloid osmotic pressure from plasma protein losses (Porth, 2011).

CLINICAL ALERT
- Notify physician / NP of changes in condition or laboratory results, which reflect increasing renal insufficiency.

- Weigh the client daily at a minimum; more often, if indicated. Ensure accurate findings by weighing at the same time each day, on the same scale, and with the client wearing the same amount of clothing.

  R: Daily weights and intake and output records help evaluate fluid balance and guide fluid intake recommendations.

- Maintain strict intake and output records; determine the net fluid balance and compare with daily weight loss or gain for correlation. (A 1-kg [2.2-lb] weight gain correlates with excess intake of 1 L.)
- Explain prescribed fluid management goals.

  R: Client and family understanding may enhance cooperation.

- Adjust client's daily fluid intake so it approximates fluid loss plus 300–500 mL/day.

  R: Careful replacement therapy is necessary to prevent fluid overload.

- Distribute fluid intake fairly evenly throughout the entire day and night. It may be necessary to match fluid intake with loss every 8 hours or even every hour if the client is critically imbalanced.

  R: Maintaining a constant fluid balance, without major fluctuations, is essential. Allowing toxins to accumulate because of poor hydration can cause complications such as nausea and sensorium changes.

- Encourage client to express feelings, give positive feedback.

  R: Fluid and diet restrictions can be extremely frustrating. Emotional support can help reduce anxiety and may improve compliance with the treatment regimen.

- Consult with a dietitian regarding the fluid and diet plan.

  R: Important considerations in fluid management, requiring a specialist's attention, include the fluid content of nonliquid food, appropriate amount and type of liquids, liquid preferences, and sodium content.

- Administer oral medications with meals whenever possible. If medications must be administered between meals, give with the smallest amount of fluid necessary.

  R: This measure avoids using parts of the fluid allowance unnecessarily.

- Avoid continuous IV fluid infusion whenever possible. Dilute all necessary IV drugs in the smallest amount of fluid that is safe for IV administration. Use small IV bags and an IV controller or pump, if possible, to prevent accidental infusion of a large volume of fluid.

  R: Extremely accurate fluid infusion is necessary to prevent fluid overload.

- Monitor for signs and symptoms of metabolic acidosis.
  - Rapid, shallow respirations
  - Headaches
  - Nausea and vomiting
  - Low plasma pH
  - Behavioral changes, drowsiness, lethargy

  R: Acidosis results from the kidney's inability to excrete hydrogen ions, phosphates, sulfates, and ketone bodies. Bicarbonate loss results from decreased renal resorption. Hyperkalemia, hyperphosphatemia, and decreased bicarbonate levels aggravate metabolic acidosis. Excessive ketone bodies cause headaches, nausea, vomiting, and abdominal pain. Respiratory rate and depth increase in an attempt to increase CO_2 excretion and thus reduce acidosis. Acidosis affects the CNS and can increase neuromuscular irritability because of the cellular exchange of hydrogen and potassium (Porth, 2011).

- For a client with metabolic acidosis, ensure adequate caloric intake while limiting fat and protein intake. Consult with a dietitian for an appropriate diet.

  R: Restricting fats and protein helps prevent accumulation of acidic end products.

- Assess for signs and symptoms of hypocalcemia, hypokalemia, and alkalosis as acidosis is corrected.

  R: Rapid correction of acidosis may cause rapid excretion of calcium and potassium and result in rebound alkalosis.

- Dialysis may be necessary to correct metabolic acidosis.

  R: Bicarbonate in the dialysate is a higher concentration than the serum. The bicarbonate is delivered during dialysis to help correct the acidosis. Bicarbonate solutions can be tailored to meet individual needs. (Bogle et al., 2008)

CLINICAL ALERT
- Notify physician / NP of s/s of metabolic acidosis.

- Monitor for signs and symptoms of hypernatremia with fluid overload.
  - Extreme thirst
  - CNS effects ranging from agitation to convulsion

  R: Hypernatremia results from excessive sodium intake or increased aldosterone output. Water is pulled from the cells, causing cellular dehydration and producing CNS symptoms. Thirst is a compensatory response aimed at diluting sodium.

- Maintain prescribed sodium restrictions.

  R: Hypernatremia must be corrected slowly to minimize CNS deterioration.

- Monitor for electrolyte imbalances.
  - Potassium
  - Calcium
  - Phosphorus
  - Sodium
  - Magnesium

  R: Refer to Risk for Complications of Electrolyte Imbalances for specific signs and symptoms and interventions. Renal dysfunction can cause hyperkalemia, hypernatremia, hypocalcemia, hypermagnesemia, or hyperphosphatemia. Diuretic therapy can cause hypokalemia or hyponatremia.

- Monitor for gastrointestinal (GI) bleeding.

  R: Refer to Risk for Complications of GI Bleeding for more information and specific interventions.

  R: The poor platelet aggregation and capillary fragility associated with high serum levels of nitrogenous wastes may aggravate bleeding. Heparinization required during dialysis in cases of gastric ulcer disease also may precipitate GI bleeding.

- Monitor for manifestations of anemia:
  - Dyspnea
  - Fatigue
  - Tachycardia, palpitations
  - Cold intolerance
  - Pallor of nail beds and mucous membranes
  - Low hemoglobin and hematocrit levels
  - Easy bruising

  R: Chronic renal failure results in decreased red blood cell production because of decreased erythropoietin production and decreased survival time because of elevated uremic toxins.

- Avoid unnecessary collection of blood specimens.

  R: Some blood loss occurs with every blood collection.

- Instruct client to use a soft toothbrush and to avoid vigorous nose blowing, constipation, and contact sports.

  R: Trauma prevention reduces the risk of bleeding and infection.

- Demonstrate the pressure method to control bleeding should it occur.

  R: Applying direct, constant pressure on a bleeding site can help prevent excessive blood loss.

- Monitor for manifestations of hypoalbuminemia (Deegens &Wetzels, 2011).
  - Serum albumin level <3.5 g/dL; proteinuria (>150 mg/24 h)
  - Edema formation: pedal, facial, sacral
  - Hypovolemia (more common in very low <1 m/dL serum albumin levels)
  - Decreased hematocrit and hemoglobin levels in advancing disease
  - Hyperlipidemia

  R: Refer to Risk for Complications of Negative Nitrogen Balance for more information and interventions. When albumin leaks into the urine because of changes in the glomerular electrostatic barrier or because of peritoneal dialysis, the liver responds by increasing production of plasma proteins. When the loss is great, the liver cannot compensate, and hypoalbuminemia results.

- Monitor for hypervolemia. Evaluate daily.
  - Weight

- Fluid intake and output records
- Rales in lungs
- Circumference of the edematous parts
- Laboratory data: hematocrit, serum sodium, and plasma protein in specific serum albumin

  R: As glomerular filtration rate decreases and the functioning nephron mass continues to diminish, the kidneys lose the ability to concentrate urine and to excrete sodium and water, resulting in hypervolemia.

- Monitor for signs and symptoms of congestive heart failure and decreased cardiac output.
  - Gradual increase in heart rate
  - Increasing dyspnea
  - Diminished breath sounds, rales
  - Decreased systolic blood pressure
  - Presence of or increase in S_3 and / or S_4 heart sounds
  - Gallop rhythm
  - Peripheral edema
  - Distended neck veins

  R: Congestive heart failure can result from increased cardiac output, hypervolemia, dysrhythmias, and hypertension, reducing the ability of the left ventricle to eject blood, with subsequent decreased cardiac output and increased pulmonary vascular congestion.

- Encourage adherence to strict fluid restrictions: 800–1,000 mL/24 h, or 24-h urine output plus 500 mL.

  R: Fluid restrictions are based on urine output. In an anuric client, restriction usually is 800 mL/day, which accounts for insensible losses from metabolism, the GI tract, perspiration, and respiration.

- Collaborate with physician, advanced practice nurse, or dietitian to plan an appropriate diet. Encourage adherence to a low-sodium diet (2–4 g/day).

  R: Sodium restrictions should be adjusted based on urine sodium excretion.

- If hemodialysis or peritoneal dialysis is initiated, follow institutional protocols.

Clinical Alert Report

Prior to providing care, advice ancillary staff / student to report the following to the professional nurse assigned to the client:
- Urine output <0.5 mL/h
- Nonadherance to fluid restrictions
- c/o of shortness of breath or increased SOB
- Behavioral changes

RISK FOR COMPLICATIONS OF NEUROLOGIC / SENSORY DYSFUNCTION

Risk for Complications of Alcohol Withdrawal
Risk for Complications of Increased Intracranial Pressure
Risk for Complications of Seizures

Definition

Describes a person experiencing or at high risk to experience various neurologic or sensory dysfunctions

Carp's Cues

The nurse can use this generic collaborative problem to describe a person at risk for several types of neurologic or sensory problems (e.g., a client recovering from cranial surgery or who has sustained multiple traumas). For such a person, using *Risk for Complications of Neurologic / Sensory Dysfunction* directs nurses to monitor neurologic and sensory function based on focus assessment findings. Should a complication occur, the nurse would add the applicable specific collaborative problem (e.g., *Risk for Complications of Increased Intracranial Pressure*) to the client's problem list to describe nursing management of the complication. If the risk factors or etiology were not related directly to the primary medical diagnosis or treatment, the nurse could add this information to the diagnostic statement. For example, for a client with a seizure disorder admitted for abdominal surgery, the nurse would add *Risk for Complications of Seizures related to epilepsy* to the problem list.

In addition to the collaborative problem, the nurse should assess for other actual or potential responses that can compromise functioning. Some of these responses may represent nursing diagnoses (e.g., *Risk for Injury related to poor awareness of environmental hazards secondary to decreased sensorium*).

For information on Focus Assessment Criteria, visit http://thePoint.lww.com/Carpenito6e.

Significant Laboratory / Diagnostic Assessment Criteria

Cerebrospinal Fluid

Cloudy Presentation (Indicative of an Infection)
- Protein (increased in meningitis)
- White blood cell (WBC) count (increased in meningitis)
- Albumin (elevated with brain tumors)
- Glucose (decreased with bacterial meningitis)

Blood
- WBC count (elevated with bacterial infection, decreased in viral infection)
- Alcohol level
- Glucose calcium
- Mercury, lead levels if indicated

Radiologic / Imaging
- Skull, spine x-rays
- Computed tomography (CT)
- Magnetic resonance imaging (MRI)
- Cerebral angiography
- Position emission tomography (PET) (measures physiologic and biochemical process in the nervous system; can detect tumors, vascular diseases, and behavioral disturbances such as dementia or schizophrenia)
- Myelography

Other
- Doppler
- Lumbar puncture
- Electroencephalography (EEG)
- Continuous bedside cerebral blood flow monitoring

RISK FOR COMPLICATIONS OF ALCOHOL WITHDRAWAL

Definition

Describes a person experiencing or at high risk to experience the complications of alcohol withdrawal (e.g., delirium tremens, autonomic hyperactivity, seizures, alcohol hallucinosis, and hypertension)

Carp's Cues

There are an estimated 8 million alcohol dependent people in the United States. Approximately 500,000 episodes of withdrawal severe enough to require pharmacologic treatment occur each year (Hoffman & Weinhouse, 2012). DT is associated with a mortality rate of up to 5%. Death usually is due to arrhythmia, complicating illnesses, such as pneumonia, or failure to identify an underlying problem that led to the cessation of alcohol use, such as pancreatitis, hepatitis, or central nervous system injury or infection. Older age, preexisting pulmonary disease, core body temperature greater than 40° C (104° F), and coexisting liver disease are associated with a greater risk of mortality (Hoffman & Weinhouse, 2012).

High-Risk Populations (Hoffman & Weinhouse, 2012)

- A history of sustained drinking
- A history of previous DT
- Age greater than 30
- The presence of a concurrent illness
- The presence of significant alcohol withdrawal in the presence of an elevated ethanol level
- A longer period (more than two days) between the last drink and the onset of withdrawal

Collaborative Outcomes

The client will be monitored for early signs and symptoms of alcohol withdrawal and will receive collaborative interventions if indicated to restore physiologic stability.

Indicators of Physiologic Stability

- No seizure activity
- Calm, oriented
- Temperature 98° to 99.5° F
- Pulse 60–100 beats/min
- BP >90/60, <140/90 mm Hg
- No reports of hallucinations
- No tremors

Interventions and Rationales

- Carefully attempt to determine if the client abuses alcohol. Consult with the family regarding their perception of alcohol consumption. Explain why accurate information is necessary.

  R: It is critical to identify high-risk people so potentially fatal withdrawal symptoms can be prevented.

- If alcohol abuse is confirmed, obtain history of previous withdrawals.
  - Delirium tremens
  - Seizures
- Maintain the client's IV running continuously.

  R: This may be necessary for fluid replacement and dextrose, thiamine bolus, benzodiazepine, and magnesium sulfate administration. Chlordiazepoxide and diazepam should not be given IM because of unpredictable absorption.

- Monitor vital signs at least every 2 hours.

  R: Clients in withdrawal have elevated heart rate, respirations, and fever. Clients experiencing delirium tremens can be expected to have a low-grade fever. Rectal temperature greater than 37.7° C (99.9° F) is a clue to possible infection.

- Observe for minor withdrawal symptoms (Hoffman & Weinhouse, 2012).
  - Insomnia
  - Tremulousness
  - Mild anxiety
  - Gastrointestinal upset; anorexia
  - Headache
  - Diaphoresis

- Palpitations

    R: Minor withdrawal symptoms are due to central nervous system hyperactivity. Withdrawal occurs 6–96 hours after drinking ends. Withdrawal can occur in people who are considered "social drinkers" (6 oz of alcohol daily for a period of 3 to 4 weeks). Withdrawal patterns may resemble those of previous episodes. Seizure patterns unlike previous episodes may indicate another underlying pathology.

> **CLINICAL ALERT**
> - When alcohol abuse is suspected and / or minor withdrawal symptoms are assessed, notify the physician / NP for initiation of benzodiazepine therapy, with dosage determined by assessment findings.
>
>   *R: Benzodiazepine requirements in alcohol withdrawal are highly variable and client specific. Fixed schedules may over sedate or under sedate.*

- Obtain a complete history of prescription and nonprescription drugs taken.

    R: Benzodiazepine or barbiturate withdrawal may mimic alcohol withdrawal and complicate the picture (Hoffman & Weinhouse, 2012).

- Observe for the desired effects of benzodiazepine therapy.
    - Relief from withdrawal symptoms
    - Peaceful sleep but rousable

    R: Long-acting benzodiazepines are the drugs of choice in controlling withdrawal symptoms except with hepatic dysfunction. With hepatic dysfunction, the shorter half-life of lorazepam and the absence of active metabolites with oxazepam may prevent prolonged effects if oversedation occurs.

- Monitor for withdrawal seizures. Refer also to *Risk for Complications of Seizures.*

    R: Withdrawal seizures can occur 6–96 hours after drinking ends. They are usually nonfocal and grand mal, last minutes or less, and occur singularly or in clusters of two to six.

> **CLINICAL ALERT**
> - Monitor for and intervene promptly in cases of status epilepticus. Follow institution's emergency protocol.
>
>   *R: Status epilepticus is life-threatening if not controlled immediately with IV diazepam. For Interventions of Status Epilepticus, refer to Care Plan for Seizure Disorder.*

- Monitor and determine onset of alcohol hallucinosis. Hallucinations are usually visual, although auditory and tactile phenomena may also occur. The person senses that the hallucinations are not real and is aware of surroundings.

    R: Alcoholic hallucinosis are the same as delirium tremens. "Alcoholic hallucinosis refers to hallucinations that develop within 12–24 hours of abstinence and resolve within 24–48 hours (which is the earliest point at which delirium tremens typically develops). In contrast to delirium tremens, alcoholic hallucinosis is not associated with global clouding of the sensorium, but with specific hallucinations, and vital signs are usually normal." (Hoffman & Weinhouse, 2012)

- Monitor for delirium tremens.
- Delirium component (vivid hallucinations, confusion, extreme disorientation, and fluctuating levels of awareness)
- Extreme hyperadrenergic stimulation (tachycardia, hypertension or hypotension, extreme tremor, agitation, diaphoresis, and fever)

    R: Delirium tremens appears on days 3–5 after cessation of drinking and can persist for up to 7 days (Bhardwaj et al., 2004; Hoffman & Weinhouse, 2012).

- Monitor fluid and electrolyte status.

    R: Severe alcohol withdrawal can severely impact fluid and electrolyte status (Hoffman & Weinhouse, 2012).

    - Hypovolemic

        R: This results from hyperthermia, vomiting, and tachypnea.

- Hypokalemia

  R: This results from renal and extrarenal losses

- Hypomagnesaemia

  R: Etiology is unknown but may predispose to dysrhythmia and seizures.

- Hypophosphatemia

  R: This may be due to malnutrition, if severe, may contribute to bleeding.

- If indicated refer to the Nursing Care Plan for Alcohol Withdrawal for additional interventions such as Health teaching and referrals for Drug and Alcohol Counseling.

Clinical Alert Report

Prior to providing care, advise ancillary staff / student to report the following to the professional nurse assigned to the client:
- Insomnia
- Observed tremors
- Mild anxiety
- c/o GI upset; decreased appetite
- Headache
- Diaphoresis

RISK FOR COMPLICATIONS OF INCREASED INTRACRANIAL PRESSURE (ICP)

Definition

- Describes a person experiencing or at high risk to experience increased cranial pressure (>20 mm Hg) exerted by cerebrospinal fluid within the brain's ventricles or the subarachnoid space

High-Risk Populations (Rangel-Castillo, Gopinath, & Robertson, 2008)

Intracranial (Primary)

- Brain tumor
- Trauma (epidural and subdural hematoma, cerebral contusions)
- Nontraumatic intracerebral hemorrhage (aneurysm rupture and subarachnoid hemorrhage, hypertensive brain hemorrhage, intraventricular hemorrhage)
- Ischemic stroke
- Hydrocephalus
- Idiopathic or benign intracranial hypertension
- Other (e.g., pseudotumor cerebri, pneumoencephalus, abscesses, cysts)
- Meningitis, encephalitis
- Status epilepticus

Extracranial (Secondary)

- Airway obstruction
- Hypoxia or hypercarbia (hypoventilation)
- Hypertension (pain / cough) or hypotension (hypovolemia / sedation)
- Posture (head rotation)
- Blockage of venous outflow
- Hyperpyrexia
- Seizures
- Drug and metabolic (e.g., tetracycline, rofecoxib, divalproex sodium, lead intoxication)

- High-altitude
- Cerebral edema (postoperative [cranial surgery])
- Hepatic failure (mass lesion [hematoma] edema)
- Increased cerebral blood volume (vasodilation)
- Disturbances of CSF

Collaborative Outcomes

The client will be monitored for early signs and symptoms of increased intracranial pressure and will receive collaborative interventions if indicated to restore physiologic stability.

Indicators of Physiologic Stability

- Adult ICP 5 to 15 mm Hg (7.5–20 cm H_2O)
- ICP monitoring device (e.g., ventriculostomy)
- Pupils equal; reactive to light and accommodation
- Intact extra ocular movements
- Pulse 60–100 beats/minute
- Respirations 16–20 breaths/minute
- BP >90/60, <140/90 mm Hg
- Stable pulse pressure (difference between diastolic and systolic readings)
- No nausea / vomiting

If Conscious:
- Alert, oriented, calm, or no change in usual cognitive status
- Appropriate speech
- Mild to no headache

General Interventions and Rationales

- Maintain ICP monitoring.
  - If using an ICP monitoring device (e.g., ventriculostomy), refer to the procedure manual for guidelines.

    R: Ventriculostomy is utilized to monitor ICP and as an access to drain cerebral spinal fluid to reduce ICP.

  - Monitor the system for proper functioning at least every 2–4 hours, and any time there is a change in the ICP, neurologic examination, and CSF output.

    R: The functioning of the monitoring system should be evaluated when malfunctioning is suspected.

> **CLINICAL ALERT**
> - Report immediately, an increase in ICP. "ICP values greater than 20 to 25 mm Hg require treatment in most circumstances. Sustained ICP values of greater than 40 mm Hg indicate severe, life-threatening intracranial hypertension." (Rangel-Castillo, Gopinath, Robinson, 2008)

- Differentiate between cerebral perfusion pressure (CPP) and increased intracranial pressure (ICP).

  R: Impaired cerebral perfusion results in decreased cerebral blood flow and a rise in ICP pressure. CPP can be impaired by an increase in ICP, a decrease in blood pressure, or a combination of both factors. With normal auto-regulation, the brain is able to maintain a normal cerebral blood flow (CBF). After injury, the ability of the brain to pressure autoregulate may be absent or diminished. (Rangel-Castillo, Gopinath, & Robinson, 2008)

- Maintain oxygenation and ventilation to keep PaO_2 >100, $PaCO_2$ 30–35.

  R: This will increase the oxygenation of cerebral tissue.

- Refer to Nursing Care Plan for Mechanical Ventilation if indicated.
- Monitor for signs and symptoms of increased ICP.
  - Assess the following (Glasgow Coma Scale [GCS]) (Hickey, 2009):
    - Best eye-opening response: spontaneously, to auditory stimuli, to painful stimuli, or no response
    - Best motor response: obeys verbal commands, localizes pain, flexion–withdrawal, flexion–decorticate, extension–decerebrate, or no response

- Best verbal response: oriented to person, place, and time; confused conversation; inappropriate speech; incomprehensible sounds; or no response

  R: Deficiencies of cerebral blood supply resulting from hemorrhage, hematoma, cerebral edema, thrombus, or emboli compromise cerebral tissue. These responses evaluate the client's ability to integrate commands with conscious and involuntary movement. The nurse can assess cortical function by evaluating eye opening and motor response. No response may indicate damage to the midbrain.

- Assess for changes in vital signs:
  - Pulse changes: slowing rate to 60 beats/minute or lower or increasing rate to 100 beats/minute or higher

    R: Bradycardia is a late sign of brain stem ischemia. Tachycardia may indicate hypothalamic ischemia and sympathetic discharge.

  - Respiratory irregularities: slowing rate with lengthening apneic periods

    R: Respiratory patterns vary depending on the site of impairment. Cheyne-Stokes breathing (a gradual increase followed by a gradual decrease, then a period of apnea) points to damage in both cerebral hemispheres, midbrain, and upper pons. Central neurogenic hyperventilation occurs with midbrain and upper pontine lesions. Ataxic breathing (irregular with random sequence of deep and shallow breaths) indicates pontine dysfunction. Hypoventilation and apnea occur with medullary lesions.

  - Rising blood pressure and / or widening pulse pressure
  - Bradycardia, increased systolic blood pressure, and increased pulse pressure

    R: These are late signs (known as Cushing response) of brain stem ischemia leading to cerebral herniation (Hickey, 2009).

- Assess pupillary responses.

  R: Changes indicate pressure on oculomotor or optic nerves.

  - Inspect the pupils with a bright pinpoint light to evaluate size, configuration, and reaction to light. Compare both eyes for similarities and differences.

    R: The oculomotor nerve (cranial nerve III) in the brain stem regulates pupil reactions.

  - Evaluate gaze to determine whether it is conjugate (paired, working together) or if eye movements are abnormal.

    R: Conjugate eye movements are regulated from parts of the cortex and brain stem.

  - Evaluate the ability of the eyes to adduct and abduct.

    R: Cranial nerve VI, or the abducens nerve, regulates abduction and adduction of the eyes. Cranial nerve IV, or the trochlear nerve, also regulates eye movement.

  - Note any other signs and symptoms.
    - Vomiting

      R: Vomiting results from pressure on the medulla, which stimulates the brain's vomiting center.

    - Headache: constant, increasing in intensity, or aggravated by movement
    - Straining

      R: Compression of neural tissue increases ICP and causes pain.

    - Subtle changes (e.g., lethargy, restlessness, forced breathing, purposeless movements, changes in mentation)

      R: These signs may be the earliest indicators of cranial pressure changes.

- Elevate the head of the bed 20–30 degrees unless contraindicated (e.g., hypovolemia).

  R: Slight elevation of the head of the bed to 30° improves jugular venous outflow, reduces cerebrovascular congestion, and lowers ICP. In clients who are hypovolemic, this may be associated with a fall in blood pressure and an overall fall in cerebral perfusion pressure. Care must therefore initially be taken to exclude hypovolemia. Positioning is very dependent upon the type of surgery done and the approach used and should always be clarified before repositioning.

- Maintain negative fluid balance. Carefully monitor hydration status; evaluate fluid intake and output, serum osmolality, urine specific gravity, and osmolality.

  R: Significant departures from the normal intravascular volume can adversely affect ICP and / or cerebral perfusion. Increased intravascular volume will increase cranial pressure; decreased intravascular volume will decrease cardiac output and cerebral tissue perfusion. (Hickey, 2009)

- Monitor intravenous (IV) fluid therapy (hypertonic saline, Mannitol); carefully administer IV fluids with an infusion pump.

    R: Careful IV fluid administration is necessary to prevent overhydration, which increases ICP and dehydration,

extensively for collaborative problems, since they represent medical complications. The rationales for client teaching interventions also include why the teaching is needed and why the specific content is taught.

Some topics in nursing and medicine are well studied, whereas others have had little or no research. When a reference that is five or more years old is used, it is usually because it is a classic or represents the most recent source on the subject.

Documentation

Electronic health records represent the method of documentation for clinical nurses. Recommended elements to document are listed. Electronic flow records are utilized to document assessment data. Free texting is utilized to document unusual events or significant discussions / observations.

Addendum Diagnoses

Frequently the nurse will identify and validate the presence of a risk or actual diagnosis that is not included in the given care plan for the situation or diagnostic cluster. The nurse can refer to Unit II Section 1 and 2 for specific nursing diagnoses and collaborative problems. For example, Mr. Jamie has had an acute coronary syndrome; the nurse initiates the care plan for an individual experiencing an acute coronary syndrome. In addition, Mr. Jamie has just experienced the sudden death of his brother. The nurse can find *Grieving* in Unit II Section 1 and retrieve information about that diagnosis. Then, the diagnosis can be added as an additional or addendum diagnosis.

New to This Edition

STAR STAR (stop, think, act, review) is an evidence-based model to help the nurse assess a situation prior to intervening and to evaluate the response after acting. The nurse / student nurse is encouraged to utilize this decision-making tool whenever a situation occurs that is problematic. The following is an example of using STAR to evaluate a client's / family's ability to safely transition to home.

STAR **Stop**

Think Is this person at high risk for injury, falls, medical complications, and / or inability to care for self (activities of daily living)?

Is a support person available?

Is the person competent to manage self-administration of medications, treatment procedures? Are additional resources needed?

Can the person explain how to monitor the condition (e.g., blood glucose, signs / symptoms of complications, dietary / mobility restrictions, and when to call his or her primary provider or specialist)?

Act Contact or provide the appropriate resource (e.g., contacting a support person, home health assessment, additional teaching, printed materials).

Review Has the problem been addressed? If not, use SBAR to communicate to the appropriate person.

SBAR SBAR (situation, background, assessment, recommendation) is a framework for clearly, consistently, and succinctly communicating pertinent information among health care professionals. This format is useful in handoffs (shift report) and in conflict situations (Leonard, Graham, & Bonacum, 2004). SBAR examples are found throughout the plans. The following is from the collaborative problem *Risk for Complications of Deep Vein Thrombosis* (Unit II, Section 2).

SBAR *Situation:* I am concerned about Mr. Smith and his risk for venous thrombolytic event (VTE).

Background: He is immobile, 72, obese and has COPD, and a Padua score of 6.

Assessment: Presently, he is resistant to getting out of bed and refuses to walk except to the chair.

Recommendation: Is there a reason why he is not on thromboprophylaxis?

(This communication provides the physician / NP with an opportunity to review the situation and to share their rationale why no thromboprophylaxis has been initiated.)

Section I

Medical Conditions

Generic Medical Care Plan for the Hospitalized Adult Client

Carp's Cues

This care plan presents nursing diagnoses and collaborative problems that commonly apply to clients (and their significant others) undergoing hospitalization for any medical disorder. It represents a basic standard of care. For beginning students, it can represent the care that they are prepared to provide. As the student progresses in the curriculum, the care plans for specific medical conditions such as pneumonia, diabetes mellitus, and congestive heart failure, and those focusing on the care of individuals undergoing surgery or therapies such as chemotherapy or anticoagulant therapy will be their focus of care.

■■ DIAGNOSTIC CLUSTER

Collaborative Problems

Risk for Complications of Cardiovascular Dysfunction

Risk for Complications of Respiratory Insufficiency

Nursing Diagnoses

Anxiety related to unfamiliar environment, routines, diagnostic tests, treatments, and loss of control

Risk for Injury related to unfamiliar environment and physical and mental limitations secondary to condition, medications, therapies, and diagnostic tests

Risk for Infection related to increased microorganisms in environment, risk of person-to-person transmission, and invasive tests and therapies

(Specify) Self-Care Deficit related to sensory, cognitive, mobility, endurance, or motivation problems

Risk for Imbalanced Nutrition: Less Than Body Requirements related to decreased appetite secondary to treatments, fatigue, environment, and changes in usual diet, and to increased protein and vitamin requirements for healing

Risk for Constipation related to change in fluid and food intake, routine, and activity level; effects of medications; and emotional stress

Risk for Impaired Skin Integrity related to prolonged pressure on tissues associated with decreased mobility, increased fragility of the skin associated with dependent edema, decreased tissue perfusion, malnutrition, and urinary / fecal incontinence

Disturbed Sleep Pattern related to unfamiliar, noisy environment, change in bedtime ritual, emotional stress, and change in circadian rhythm

Risk for Spiritual Distress related to separation from religious support system, lack of privacy, or inability to practice spiritual rituals

Interrupted Family Processes related to disruption of routines, change in role responsibilities, and fatigue associated with increased workload and visiting hour requirements

Risk for Compromised Human Dignity related to multiple factors (intrusions, unfamiliar procedures and personnel, loss of privacy) associated with hospitalization

Risk for Ineffective Self-Health Management related to complexity and cost of therapeutic regimen, complexity of health care system, shortened length of stay, insufficient knowledge of treatment, and barriers to comprehension secondary to language barriers, cognitive deficits, hearing and / or visual impairment, anxiety and lack of motivation

Transitional Criteria

Specific discharge criteria vary depending on the client's condition. Generally, all diagnoses in the above diagnostic cluster should be resolved before discharge.

Collaborative Problems

Risk for Complications of Cardiovascular Dysfunction

Risk for Complications of Respiratory Insufficiency

Collaborative Outcomes

The client will be monitored for early signs and symptoms of (a) cardiovascular dysfunction, and (b) respiratory insufficiency and will receive collaborative interventions if indicated to restore physiologic stability.

Indicators of Physiologic Stability

- Calm, alert, oriented (a, b)
- Respiration 16–20 breaths/minute, relaxed and rhythmic (b)
- Breath sounds present all lobes, no rales or wheezing (b)
- Pulse 60–100 beats/minute (a, b)
- BP >90/60, <140/90 mm Hg (a, b)
- Capillary refill <3 seconds; skin warm and dry (a, b)
- Peripheral pulses full, equal (a)
- Temperature 98.5–99° F (a, b)

> ### Transitional Risk Assessment Plan (TRAP)
>
> Begin this plan on admission.
> Implement the Transitional Risk Assessment Plan (TRAP):
> - Refer to inside back cover.
> - Add each validated high risk diagnosis to client's problem list with the risk code in ( ).
> - Refer to Unit II to the individual high risk nursing diagnoses/collaborative problems for outcomes and interventions.
>
>   ***R:*** *"Close coordination of care in the post-acute period, early discharge follow-up care, enhanced patient education and self-management training, proactive end-of-life counseling, and extending the resources and clinical expertise over time via multidisciplinary team management" can lower readmission rates and improve health outcomes (Boutwell & Hwu, 2009, p. 14).*

Interventions	Rationales
1. Monitor cardiovascular status:	1. Physiologic mechanisms governing cardiovascular function are very sensitive to any change in body function, making changes in cardiovascular status important clinical indicators.
a. Radial pulse (rate and rhythm)	a. Pulse monitoring provides data to detect cardiac dysrhythmia, blood volume changes, and circulatory impairment.
b. Apical pulse (rate and rhythm)	b. Apical pulse monitoring is indicated if the client's peripheral pulses are irregular, weak, or extremely rapid.
c. Blood pressure	c. Blood pressure represents the force that the blood exerts against the arterial walls. Hypertension (systolic pressure >140 mm Hg, diastolic pressure >85 mm Hg) may indicate increased peripheral resistance, cardiac output, blood volume, or blood viscosity. Hypotension can result from significant blood or fluid loss, decreased cardiac output, and certain medications.
d. Skin (color, temperature, moisture) and temperature	d. Skin assessment provides information evaluating circulation, body temperature, and hydration status.
e. Pulse oximetry	e. Pulse oximetry is a noninvasive method (probe sensor on fingertip) for continuous monitoring of oxygen saturation of hemoglobin.
2. Monitor respiratory status: Rate, Rhythm, Breath sounds **CLINICAL ALERT** • Increased and irregular pulse, and increased respiratory rate initially, followed by decreased rate. • Respiratory acidosis develops as a result of excessive CO_2 retention. • A client with respiratory acidosis from chronic disease at first experiences increased heart rate and respirations in an attempt to compensate for decreased oxygenation. • After a while, the client breathes more slowly and with prolonged expiration. • Eventually, the respiratory center may stop responding to the higher CO_2 levels, and breathing may stop abruptly.	2. Respiratory assessment provides essential data for evaluating the effectiveness of breathing and detecting adventitious or abnormal sounds, which may indicate airway moisture, narrowing, or obstruction.
3. Monitor for changes in mentation (somnolence, confusion, irritability, anxiety).	3. Changes in mentation result from cerebral tissue hypoxia.
4. Monitor for decreased urine output (<30 mL/h); cool, pale, or cyanotic skin.	4. The compensatory response to decreased circulatory oxygen aims to increase blood oxygen by increasing heart and respiratory rates and to decrease circulation to the kidneys and extremities (marked by decreased pulses and skin changes).
5. Administer low-flow (2 L/min) oxygen as needed through nasal cannula, titrate up per protocol to keep pulse oximetry between 90% and 92%.	5. *Oxygen therapy increases circulating oxygen levels.* Using a cannula rather than a mask may help reduce the client's fears of suffocation.

Clinical Alert Report

Prior to providing care, advise ancillary staff / student to report the following to the professional nurse assigned to the client:

- Change in cognitive status
- Oral temperature >100.5° F
- Systolic BP <90 mm Hg
- Resting Pulse >100, <50
- Respiratory rate >28, <10 /minute
- Oxygen saturation <90%

Related Physician / NP Prescribed Interventions

Dependent on the underlying pathology

Documentation

Pulse rate and rhythm   Respiratory assessment
Blood pressure   Abnormal findings

Nursing Diagnoses

Anxiety Related to Unfamiliar Environment, Routines, Diagnostic Tests, Treatments, and Loss of Control

NOC
Anxiety Control, Coping, Impulse Control

Goal

The client will communicate feelings regarding the condition and hospitalization.

NIC
Anxiety Reduction, Impulse Control Training, Anticipatory Guidance

Indicators

- Verbalize, if asked, what to expect regarding routines and procedures.
- Explain restrictions.

Interventions	Rationales
1. Introduce yourself and other members of the health care team, and orient the client to the room (e.g., bed controls, call bell, bathroom).	1. A smooth, professional admission process and warm introduction can put a client at ease and set a positive tone for his or her hospital stay.

2. Explain hospital policies and routines:
  a. Visiting hours, mealtimes, and availability of snacks
  b. Vital-sign monitoring
  c. Television rental and operation
  d. Storage of valuables
  e. Telephone use
  f. No Smoking policy
 	
3. Determine the client's knowledge of his or her condition, its prognosis, and treatment measures. Reinforce and supplement the physician's explanations as necessary.
	2–3. Providing accurate information can help decrease the client's anxiety associated with the unknown and unfamiliar.

4. Explain any scheduled diagnostic tests, covering the following: description, purpose, pretest routines, expected sensations, posttest routines, timing of results 5. Discuss all prescribed medications: name and type, purpose, special precautions, side effects	4–6. Teaching the client about tests and treatment measures can help decrease his or her fear and anxiety associated with the unknown, and improve his or her sense of control over the situation.

6. Explain any prescribed diet: purpose, duration, allowed and prohibited foods

CLINICAL ALERT
• If severe or panic anxiety is present, consult physician / NP for possible pharmacologic therapy, if indicated.

7. Provide the client with opportunities to make decisions about his or her care whenever possible.	7. Participating in decision making can help give a client a sense of control, which enhances his or her coping ability. Perception of loss of control can result in a sense of powerlessness, then hopelessness.
8. Provide reassurance and comfort. Spend time with the client, encourage him or her to share feelings and concerns, listen attentively, and convey empathy and understanding.	8. Providing emotional support and encouraging sharing may help a client clarify and verbalize his or her fears, allowing the nurse to get realistic feedback and reassurance.
9. Correct any misconceptions and inaccurate information the client may express.	9. A common contributing factor to fear and anxiety is incomplete or inaccurate information; providing adequate, accurate information can help allay client fears.
10. Allow the client's support people to share their fears and concerns, and encourage them in providing meaningful and productive support.	10. Supporting the client's support people can enhance their ability to help the client.

Documentation

Unusual responses or situations
Client's knowledge / information provided related to diagnosis, treatment, and hospital routine

Risk for Falls (**) Related to Unfamiliar Environment and Physical or Mental Limitations Secondary to the Condition, Medications, Therapies, and Diagnostic Tests

NOC
Risk Control, Safety Status: Falls Occurrence

Goal

The client will not injure him- or herself during hospital stay.

NIC
Fall Prevention, Environmental Management: Safety, Health Education, Surveillance: Safety, Risk Identification

Indicators

• Identify factors that increase risk of injury.
• Describe appropriate safety measures.

Interventions

Rationales

1. Involve all hospital personnel on every shift in the Fall Prevention Program. a. Always glance into the room of a high-risk person when passing his or her room. b. Alert other departments of high-risk individuals when off unit for tests, procedures.	1. Approximately 14% of all falls in hospitals are accidental, another 8% are unanticipated physiologic falls, and 78% are anticipated physiologic falls (Morse, 2002). Ancillary staffs are in an optimal position to witness high-risk situations, which can be addressed to prevent injury.

(continued)

**Using the Risk Assessment tool for Falls on the inside back cover, calculate the score and record it in the ( ).

Interventions	*Rationales*
c. Address fall prevention and risks with every handoff and transfer.	
d. Seek to identify reversible risk factors in all individuals. Be aware of changing client conditions and a change in risk status.	
e. Identify in a private conference room number of falls on the unit monthly (e.g., poster).	e. Interdisciplinary approach to fall prevention is effective when falls are not viewed as inevitable accidents but preventable events.

2. Reduce or eliminate contributing factors for falls:
   a. Related to Unfamiliar Environment
      - Orient the client to his or her environment (e.g., location of bathroom, bed controls, call bell). Leave a light on in the bathroom at night. Ensure path to bathroom is clear.

        • *Orientation helps provide familiarity; a light at night helps the client find his or her way safely.*

      - Teach him or her to keep the bed in the low position with side rails up at night.

        • *The low position makes it easier for the client to get in and out of bed.*

      - Make sure that the telephone, eyeglasses, urinal, and frequently used personal belongings are within easy reach.

        • *Keeping objects at hand helps prevent falls from overreaching and overextending.*

      - Instruct the client to request assistance whenever needed.

        • *Getting needed help with ambulation and other activities reduces a client's risk of injury.*

      - For individuals with difficulty accessing toilet:
         - If urgency exists, evaluate for a urinary tract infection.

           ◦ *New onset urinary urgency can be a sign of an infection.*

         - Provide an opportunity to use bathroom / urinal / bedpan every 2 hours while awake, at bedtime, and upon awakening.

           ◦ *Thirty percent of falls are related to attempting to access the bathroom and can be prevented by timed toileting schedule (Alcee & Mather, 2000).*

         - Frequently scan floor for wet areas, objects on floor.
   b. Related to Gait Instability / Balance Problems
      - Explain that the reasons for gait and balance problems as one ages is due to underuse and deconditioning, NOT AGING.
      - Alert client that if he or she trips he or she may not prevent a fall.

        • *Weak leg muscles and decreased ROM in ankles prevent a safe recovery from a trip.*

      - Explain that deficiencies in vitamin D interfere with one's postural balance, propulsion, and navigation.

        • *Vitamin D supplements determine gait performance and prevent falls by more than 22% in older adults (Annweiler, Montero-Odasso et al., 2010).*

      - Seek to include a vitamin D level in next laboratory tests. Explain a that the normal range is 30–100 nmol/L.

        • *Researchers have reported that the level should be at least 60 nmol/L to effect a reduction of falls (Annweiler, Montero-Odasso et al., 2010).*

      - Refer to Getting Started for Strategies and Exercises to Improve Gait and Balance on thePoint at http://thePoint.lww.com/Carpenito6e. Print and give to clients.
      - Instruct the client to wear slippers with nonskid soles and to avoid shoes with thick, soft soles.

        • *These precautions can help prevent falls from slipping. Thick soles require adequate lifting of feet as one walks or they will catch and trip the person.*

   c. Related to Medication Side Effects
      - Review the person's medication reconciliation completed on admission.
         - Question regarding alcohol use.

           ◦ *Alcohol can potentiate side effects of sombulence / dizziness.*

         - Question if the client has side effects when taking certain meds.
         - Question the client whether he or she believes the medication for pain is not working.

           ◦ *Some medications might need to be discontinued because of side effects or ineffective therapeutic response.*

Interventions	*Rationales*
• Review present medications with pharmacist / physician / NP and evaluate those that can contribute to dizziness and if they should be discontinued, have dose reduction, or replaced with an alternative (Riefkohl et al., 2003).	• The use of medications is one of the many different factors that can contribute to balance problems and the risk of falls. Published research suggests an association between the use of these drugs or drug classes and an increased risk of falling (Riefkohl et al., 2003).

    • Antidepressants (e.g., SSRIs)
    • Antipsychotics
    • Benzodiazepines
    • Antihistamines, Benadryl, hydroxyzine
    • Anticonvulsants
    • Nonsteroidal anti-inflammatory drugs
    • Muscle relaxants
    • Narcotic analgesics
    • Antiarrhythmics (type IA)
    • Digoxin

d. Related to Confused / Uncooperative / Impaired Cognition
    • Consider use of electronic devices in bed, chair, video surveillance.
    • Follow institutional policy for side rails.
    • Consider use of sitter.
    • Move person to a more observable room.
    • Plan to complete shift documentation in room of high-risk person.

e. Related to Tethering Devices (IVs, Foley, telemetry, compression devises)
    • Evaluate if tethering devices can be discontinued at night.
    • Can the IV be converted to saline port?
    • If client is able, teach him or her how to safely ambulate with devices to bathroom or advise to call for assistance.

                                                                      • Individuals can become entangled in lines and tubes and fall.

f. Related to Orthostatic Hypotension
Refer to *Risk for Falls* in Unit II Section 1

> **CLINICAL ALERT**
> • If Client falls, refer to *Risk for Falls* for interventions and documentation guidelines.

> ### *Clinical Alert Report*
> Advise ancillary staff/student to report:
> • Any incident of an almost fall or accident.
> • Attempts of a vulnerable client to get out of bed without assistance.
> • Other risk situations (e.g., attempts of visitors who are not capable, to assist a client).

Documentation

Client teaching
Post fall documentation
 Document circumstances, assessment, interventions in health record
 Complete incident report

Risk for Infection (**) Related to Increased Microorganisms in the Environment, Risk of Person-to-Person Transmission, and Invasive Tests or Therapies

NOC

Infection Status, Wound Healing: Primary Intention, Immune Status

NIC

Infection Control, Wound Care, Incision Site Care, Health Education

Goal

The client will describe or demonstrate appropriate precautions to prevent infection.

Interventions	Rationales
1. Use appropriate universal precautions for every client.	1. Assume everyone is potentially infected or colonized with an organism that could be transmitted in the health care setting (CDC, 2002).
a. Hand hygiene • Wash hands before and after all contact with client, objects in room, and specimens. • Use with soap and water. If hands were not in contact with anyone or thing in the client's room, use an alcohol-based hand rub (CDC, 2002).	a. Hand washing is one of the most important means to prevent the spread of infection.
b. Personal protective equipment (PPE) • Wear PPE when the client interaction indicates that contact with blood / body fluids may occur. • Before leaving room, remove and discard all PPE in the room or cubicle.	b. This will prevent contamination of clothing and skin during the process of care.
c. Gloves • Wears gloves when providing direct client care. • Wear gloves for potential contact with nonintact skin, mucous membranes, blood, and body fluids. Handle the blood of all clients as potentially infectious. • Remove gloves properly to prevent hand contamination. Deposit them in the proper container in the client's room.	c. Gloves provide a barrier from contact with infectious secretions and excretions.

**Using the Risk Assessment tool for Infection on the inside back cover, calculate the score and record it in the ( ).

Interventions	Rationales

• Wash hands with soap and water after removing gloves.
• Do not substitute alcohol-based hand rubs when the physical action of washing and rinsing hands with antimicrobial or non-antimicrobial soap and water is needed. Alcohol, chlorhexidine, and other antiseptic agents have poor activity against some organisms (e.g., spores C. difficile) (CDC, 2002).
d. Masks
  • Use PPE (masks, goggles, face shields) to protect the mucous membranes of your eyes, mouth, nose during procedures and client care activities that may generate splashes or sprays of blood, body fluids, secretions, and excretions.
e. Gowns
 	
  • Wear a gown for direct contact with uncontained secretions or excretions.
  • Remove gown and perform hand hygiene before leaving the client's room / cubicle.
  • Do not reuse gowns even with the same client.
	e. These precautions prevent the transmission of pathogens to the caregiver and then to others (e.g., other clients, visitors, other staff/student).
	  • Gowns are needed to prevent soiling or contamination of clothing during procedures and client care activities.

2. Educate all staff/student, visitors, and clients on the importance preventing droplet and formit transmission from themselves to others. a. Offer a surgical mask to persons who are coughing to decrease contamination of the surrounding environment. b. Cover the mouth and nose during coughing and sneezing. c. Use tissues to contain respiratory secretions with prompt disposal into a no-touch receptacle. Wash hands with soap and water. d. Turn the head away from others and maintaining spatial distance, ideally >3 feet, when coughing.	2. These measures are targeted to all clients with symptoms of respiratory infection and their accompanying family members or friends beginning at the point of initial encounter with a health care setting (e.g., reception / triage in emergency departments, ambulatory clinics, health care provider offices) (CDC, 2007).

> **CLINICAL ALERT**
> • If a client or visitors refuse to comply with infection prevention requirements, report situation to manager or infection control officer.

3. Determine the client placement based on:
   a. Route of transmission of known or suspected infectious agent
   b. Risk factors for transmission in the infected client
   c. Risk factors for adverse outcomes resulting from an HAI in other clients in the area or room
   d. Availability of single-client rooms
   e. Client options for room-sharing (e.g., placing clients with the same infection in the same room).

> **CLINICAL ALERT**
> • Immediately report any situation that increases the risk of infection transmission to clients, visitors, or staff/students.

(continued)

Interventions	Rationales
4. Assess client care equipment, instruments, devices, environment for contamination from blood or body fluids. Follow policies and procedures for containing, transporting, handling, cleaning.	
5. Prior to confirmation of infectious agent, initiate specific precautions for the suspected agent: a. Meningitis: droplet, airborne precautions b. Maculopapular rash with cough, fever c. Rubella > airborne precautions d. Abscess >MRSA > contact, droplet precautions e. Cough / fever / pulmonary infiltrate in HIV infected or someone high risk of HIV infection f. Tuberculosis > airborne / contact (respirators)	5. Prevention strategies are indicated when high-risk infections are suspected but not yet confirmed.

6. Reduce entry of organisms into clients:
a. Urinary tract (catheter associated urinary tract infection [CAUTI])
  • Insert catheters only for appropriate indications:
    • Client has acute urinary retention or bladder outlet obstruction.
    • Need for accurate measurements of urinary output in critically ill clients
    • Perioperative use for selected surgical procedures:
      • Clients undergoing urologic surgery or other surgery on contiguous structures of the genito-urinary tract
      • Anticipated prolonged duration of surgery (catheters inserted for this reason should be removed in PACU)
      • Clients anticipated to receive large-volume infusions or diuretics during surgery
    • Need for intraoperative monitoring of urinary output
    • To assist in healing of open sacral or perineal wounds in incontinent clients
    • Client requires prolonged immobilization (e.g., potentially unstable thoracic or lumbar spine, multiple traumatic injuries such as pelvic fractures)
    • To improve comfort for end-of-life care if needed
  • Consult with physician / nurse practitioner to discuss the inappropriate use of indwelling catheter in a particular client.
    • Convenience of nursing staff/student
    • Client with incontinence
    • Access for obtaining urine for culture or other diagnostic tests when the person can voluntarily void
    • For prolonged postoperative duration without appropriate indications (e.g., structural repair of urethra or contiguous structures, prolonged effect of epidural anesthesia, etc.)
  • Avoid use of urinary catheters for management of incontinence. Refer to *Incontinence* in Unit II.
	• Every attempt to minimize urinary catheter use and duration of use in all clients must be instituted, especially with those at higher risk for CAUTI or mortality from catheterization such as women, older persons, and clients with impaired immunity.

Interventions	Rationales
• For operative clients who have an indication for an indwelling catheter, remove the catheter as soon as possible postoperatively, preferably within 24 hours, unless they are appropriate.	
• Properly secure indwelling catheters after insertion.	• This will prevent movement and urethral traction, which can cause tissue breakdown and become an entry site for pathogens.
• Do not clean the periurethral area with antiseptics to prevent CAUTI while the catheter is in place. Routine hygiene (e.g., cleansing of the metal surface during daily bathing or showering) is appropriate.	• Antiseptic agents can cause tissue breakdown.
• Obtain urine samples aseptically.	
◦ For a sample of fresh urine (i.e., urinalysis or culture), aspirate the urine from the needleless sampling port with a sterile syringe / cannula adapter after cleansing the port with a disinfectant.	
◦ For samples of large volumes of urine for special analyses (not culture), acquire aseptically from the drainage bag.	
b. Invasive access sites	b. Invasive lines provide a site for organism entry. Interventions focus on prevention and identification of early signs of infection.
• Prevent and monitor for infection at invasive access sites.	
◦ Assess all invasive lines every 24 hours for redness, inflammation, drainage, and tenderness.	
◦ Monitor client's temperature at least every 24 hours; notify physician if greater than 100.8° F.	
◦ Maintain aseptic technique for all invasive devices, changing sites, dressings, tubing, and solutions per policy schedule.	
◦ Evaluate all abnormal laboratory findings, especially cultures / sensitivities and CBC.	
c. Respiratory tract infections	c. Individuals with pain, postanesthesia, compromised ability to move, and those with ineffective cough are at risk for infection due to pooling of respiratory secretions.
• Prevent and monitor for respiratory infections	
◦ Monitor temperature at least every 8 hours and notify physician if greater than 100.8° F.	
◦ Evaluate sputum characteristics for frequency, purulence, blood, and odor.	
◦ Evaluate sputum and blood cultures, if done, for significant findings.	
◦ Assess lung sounds every 8 hours or PRN.	
◦ If client has abdominal / thoracic surgery, instruct before surgery on importance of coughing, turning, and deep breathing.	
◦ Prompt to cough and deep breathe hourly.	
◦ If client has had anesthesia, monitor for appropriate clearing of secretions in lung fields.	
◦ Evaluate need for suctioning if client cannot clear secretions adequately.	
◦ Assess for risk of aspiration, keeping head of bed elevated 30 degrees unless otherwise contraindicated.	
◦ Ensure optimal pain management.	

Documentation

Catheter and insertion site care
Abnormal findings

(Specify) Self-Care Deficit Related to Sensory, Cognitive, Mobility, Endurance, or Motivational Problems

NOC

See Self-Care: Bathing, Self-Care: Hygiene, Self-Care: Eating, Self-Care: Dressing, Self-Care: Toileting, and / or Self-Care: Instrumental Activities of Daily Living

Goal

The client will perform self-care activities (feeding, toileting, dressing, grooming, bathing), with assistance as needed.

NIC

See Feeding, Bathing, Dressing, and / or Instrumental Self-Care Deficit

Indicators

- Demonstrate optimal hygiene after care is provided.
- Describe restrictions or precautions as needed.

Interventions	Rationales
1. Consult with a physical therapist to assess present level of participation and for a plan. a. Determine areas for potentially increased participation in each self-care activity. b. Explore the client's goals and determine what the learner perceives as his or her own needs. c. Compare what the nurse believes are the learner's needs and goals, and then work to establish mutually acceptable goals. d. Allow ample time to complete activities without help. Promote independence, but assist when the client cannot perform an activity.	1. Offering choices and including the client in planning care reduces feelings of powerlessness; promotes feelings of freedom, control, and self-worth; and increases the client's willingness to comply with therapeutic regimens. Optimal education promotes self-care.
2. Evaluate the client's ability to participate in each self-care activity (feeding, dressing, bathing, and toileting).	2. Enhancing a client's self-care abilities can increase his or her sense of control and independence, promoting overall well-being.

Interventions	Rationales
3. Use the following scale to rate the client's ability to perform 0 = Is completely independent 1 = Requires use of assistive device 2 = Needs minimal help 3 = Needs assistance and / or some supervision 4 = Needs total supervision 5 = Needs total assistance or unable to assist Reassess ability frequently and revise code as appropriate.	3. This coding allows for establishing a baseline from which to evaluate progress.
4. Refer to interventions under each diagnosis—feeding, bathing, dressing, toileting, and instrumental self-care deficit as indicated. a. Provide common nursing interventions for feeding. b. Ascertain from the client or family members what foods the client likes or dislikes. c. Ensure that the client eats meals in the same setting with pleasant surroundings that are not too distracting. d. Maintain correct food temperatures (hot foods hot, cold foods cold). e. Provide pain relief because pain can affect appetite and ability to feed self. f. Provide good oral hygiene before and after meals. g. Encourage the client to wear dentures and eyeglasses. h. Assist the client to the most normal eating position suited to his or her physical disability (best is sitting in a chair at a table). i. Encourage a client who has trouble handling utensils to eat "finger foods" (e.g., bread, sandwiches, fruit, nuts). j. Provide needed adaptive devices for eating, such as a plate guard, suction device under the plate or bowl, padded-handle utensils, wrist or hand splints with clamp, and special drinking cup. k. Provide social contact during eating. **CLINICAL ALERT** • If individual is not eating or drinking enough, consult with nutritionist.	4a. These strategies attempt to normalize mealtime to increase participation and intake.
5. Provide general nursing interventions for inability to bathe. a. Bathing time and routine should be consistent to encourage optimal independence. b. Encourage the client to wear prescribed corrective lenses or hearing aid. c. Keep the bathroom temperature warm; ascertain the client's preferred water temperature. d. Provide for privacy during bathing routine. e. Elicit from the client his or her usual bathing routine. f. Keep the environment simple and uncluttered. g. Observe skin condition during bathing. h. Provide all bathing equipment within easy reach. i. Provide for safety in the bathroom (nonslip mats, grab bars). j. When the client is physically able, encourage the use of either a tub or shower stall, depending on which he or she uses at home.	5j. The client should practice in the hospital in preparation for going home.

(continued)

Interventions	*Rationales*
k. Provide for adaptive equipment as needed: • Chair or stool in bathtub or shower • Long-handled sponge to reach back or lower extremities • Grab bars on bathroom walls where needed to assist in mobility • Bath board for transferring to tub chair or stool • Safety treads or nonskid mat on floor of bathroom, tub, and shower • Washing mitts with pocket for soap • Adapted toothbrushes • Shaver holders • Handheld shower spray	
l. Provide for relief of pain that may affect the client's ability to bathe self.	l. Offering choices and including the client in planning care reduces feelings of powerlessness; promotes feelings of freedom, control, and self-worth; and increases the client's willingness to comply with therapeutic regimens. Assistive devices can improve self-care abilities.
m. Consider use of nondetergent, no-rinse, prepackaged bathing products.	m. Research has shown these products are cost-effective, reduce skin dryness and reduced microbial counts the same as traditional bathing routines (Larson et al., 2004; Sheppard & Brenner, 2000).
n. For confused individuals, preserve dignity and decrease agitation: • Provide verbal warning prior to doing anything (e.g., touching, spraying with water). • Apply firm pressure to the skin when bathing; it is less likely to be misinterpreted than a gentle touch. • Use a warm shower or bath to help a confused or agitated client to relax. • Add lavender oil to bath water. • Determine the best method to bathe person (e.g., bed bath, shower, tub bath).	n. Client aggression may be precipitated by baths or showers. Soap, towels in a warm environment have been found to reduce aggression.
6. Provide general nursing interventions for self-dressing. a. Obtain clothing that is larger-sized and easier to put on, including clothing with elastic waistbands, wide sleeves and pant legs, dresses that open down the back for women in wheelchairs and Velcro fasteners or larger buttons. b. Encourage the client to wear prescribed corrective lenses or hearing aid. c. Promote independence in dressing through continual and unaided practice. d. Allow sufficient time for dressing and undressing, because the task may be tiring, painful, or difficult. e. Plan for the client to learn and demonstrate one part of an activity before progressing further. f. Lay clothes out in the order in which the client will need them to dress. g. Provide dressing aids as necessary. h. If needed, increase participation in dressing by medicating for pain 30 minutes before it is time to dress or undress, if indicated. i. Provide for privacy during dressing routine. j. Provide for safety by ensuring easy access to all clothing and by ascertaining the client's performance level.	6. Inability to care for oneself produces feelings of dependency and poor self-concept. With increased ability for self-care, self-esteem increases. Optimal personal grooming promotes psychological well-being. g. Some commonly used aids include dressing stick, Swedish reacher, zipper pull, buttonhook, long-handled shoehorn, and shoe fasteners adapted with elastic laces.

Documentation

Assistance needed for self-care

Risk for Imbalanced Nutrition: Less Than Body Requirements Related to Decreased Appetite Secondary to Treatments, Fatigue, Environment, and Changes in Usual Diet, and to Increased Protein and Vitamin Requirements for Healing

NOC
Nutritional Status,
Teaching: Nutrition

Goal

The client will ingest daily nutritional requirements in accordance with activity level, metabolic needs, and restrictions.

NIC
Nutrition Management,
Nutritional Monitoring

Indicators

- Relate the importance of good nutrition.
- Relate restrictions, if any.

Interventions	Rationales
1. Ensure that a nutritional assessment is done on admission according to protocols.	1. Nutritional assessments are required within 24 hours of admission to a hospital and within 14 days of admission to a long-term facility (Joint Commission, 2010).
2. Explain the need for adequate consumption of carbohydrates, fats, protein, vitamins, minerals, and fluids.	2. Nutrients provide energy sources, build tissue, and regulate metabolic processes.
3. When indicated, consult with a nutritionist to establish appropriate daily caloric and food type requirements for the client.	3. The body requires a minimum level of nutrients for health and growth. During the life span, nutritional needs vary (Lutz, Przytulski, 2011).
4. Assess if there are cultural preferences in regard to food.	

5. Address the factors that are causing or contributing to decrease intake:
  a. Related to decreased oral intake, mouth discomfort, nausea, and vomiting secondary to
    Alcohol abuse
    Drug use
    Depression
  b. Inability to chew
  c. Related to decreased oral intake, mouth discomfort, nausea, and vomiting secondary to (e.g., radiation therapy, tonsillectomy, chemotherapy, oral trauma)
  d. Related to factors associated with aging	

(*continued*)

Interventions	*Rationales*
6. Assess for factors that contribute to nutritional deficiencies in older clients.	6. In general, older adults need the same kind of balanced diet as any other group, but fewer calories. Diets of older clients, however, tend to be insufficient in iron, calcium, and vitamins. The combination of long-established eating patterns, income, transportation, housing, social interaction, and the effects of chronic or acute disease influence nutritional intake and health (Miller, 2009).
7. When possible, attempt to reduce barriers of food procurement / preparation (e.g., functional ability, financial, transportation, kitchen facilities)	7. Factors such as pain, fatigue, analgesic use, and immobility can contribute to anorexia. Identifying a possible cause enables interventions to eliminate or minimize it.
8. Refer to nutritionist / social services for an assessment and interventions.	
9. For individuals with lactose intolerance, teach what foods to avoid. Explain lactose-free products.	9. The prevalence of primary lactose intolerance varies according to race. As many as 25% of the white population (prevalence in those from southern European roots) are estimated to have lactose intolerance, while among black, Native American, and Asian American populations, the prevalence of lactose intolerance is estimated at 75%–90% (Roy, 2011).
10. Encourage the client to rest before meals.	10. Fatigue further reduces energy of a client who is anorectic.

11. Provide the following generic interventions for clients with decreased appetite regardless of etiology:
  a. When possible, attempt to have some socialization during mealtime (e.g., suggest to family that they eat with client if appropriate).
 	
  b. Offer frequent, small meals instead of a few large ones; offer foods served cold.
  c. With decreased appetite, restrict liquids with meals and avoid fluids 1 hour before and after meals.
  d. Encourage and help the client to maintain good oral hygiene.
  e. Arrange to have high-calorie and high-protein foods served at the times that the client usually feels most like eating.
 	
  f. Decrease amounts of food on tray, if it is anticipated that the person will eat only some.
	11a. In nursing home settings, residents' nutritional status is significantly better in those who eat in the general dining room, rather than isolated in their own rooms (Simmons & Levy-Storms, 2005).
	  b. Even distribution of total daily caloric intake helps prevent gastric distention, possibly increasing appetite.
	  c. Restricting fluids with meals helps prevent gastric distention.
	  d. Poor oral hygiene leads to bad odor and taste, which can diminish appetite.
	  e. Presenting high-calorie and high-protein food when the client is most likely to eat increases the likelihood that he or she will consume adequate calories and protein.
	  f. Unrealistic amounts of food can discourage the client before he or she starts.

12. Take steps to promote appetite:
  a. Determine the client's food preferences and arrange to have them provided, as appropriate.
  b. Eliminate any offensive odors and sights from the eating area.
  c. Control any pain and nausea before meals.
  d. Encourage the client's support people to bring permitted foods from home, if possible.
  e. Provide a relaxed atmosphere and some socialization during meals.
	12. Diet planning focuses on avoiding nutritional excesses. Reducing fats, salt, and sugar can reduce the risk of heart disease, diabetes, certain cancers, and hypertension.

13. Provide for supplemental dietary needs amplified by acute illness.	13. Metabolic demands are increased by the catabolic processes that occur through stages of acute illness, usually increasing nutritional demand (Gary & Fleury, 2002).

Interventions	Rationales
14. Give the client printed materials outlining a nutritious diet. Refer to Getting Started to Better Nutrition on the-Point at http://thePoint.lww.com/Carpenito6e.	

Clinical Alert Report

Prior to providing care, advise ancillary staff / student to report the following to the professional nurse assigned to the client with marginal fluid or nutritional status:

- The amount / types of food ingested
- The amount / types of fluids

Documentation

Dietary intake
Daily weight
Diet instruction
Use of assistive devices

Risk for Constipation Related to Change in Fluid or Food Intake, Routine, or Activity Level; Effects of Medications; and Emotional Stress

NOC
Bowel Elimination, Hydration, Symptom Control

Goal

The client will maintain prehospitalization bowel patterns.

NIC
Bowel Management, Fluid Management, Constipation / Impaction Management

Indicators

- State the importance of fluids, fiber, and activity.
- Report difficulty promptly.

Interventions	Rationales
1. Auscultate bowel sounds.	1. Bowel sounds indicate the nature of peristaltic activity.

CLINICAL ALERT
- Constipation is often viewed as expected and benign.
- Constipation can be responsible for undiagnosed pain and exacerbating confusion in individuals who cannot communicate.
- Most all episodes of constipation can be prevented.

(continued)

Interventions	*Rationales*

2. If fecal impaction is suspected:
   a. Perform a digital rectal examination (DRE).
   b. Remove fecal impaction. Refer to procedure manual as needed.
   c. Make the client comfortable and allow rest.
   d. The client may require temporary use of a stool softener or mild cathartic.

2a. Caution regarding producing the Valsalva maneuver, which can cause hypotension.

> **CLINICAL ALERT**
> • If severe constipation is present; consult with physician / nurse practitioner for an evaluation.

3. Promote corrective measures.
   a. Regular time for elimination
      • Review daily routine.
      • Provide a stimulus to defecation (e.g., coffee, prune juice).
      • Advise the client to attempt to defecate about 1 hour or so after meals and that remaining in the bathroom for a suitable length of time may be necessary.
   b. Adequate exercise
      • Provide frequent ambulation of hospitalized client when tolerable.
      • Perform range-of-motion exercises for the client who is bedridden.
   c. Balanced diet
      • Avoid food low in fiber (e.g., starches, white bread, pasta, white rice, dairy products, processed foods).
      • Review list of foods high in fiber (e.g., fresh fruits, fruit juices, and vegetables with skins).
      • Beans (navy, kidney, lima), nuts and seeds, whole-grain breads, cereal, and bran
      • Include approximately 800 g of fruits and vegetables (about four pieces of fresh fruit and large salad) for normal daily bowel movement. Avoid cooked fruits.
      • Suggest moderate use of bran at first (may irritate GI tract, produce flatulence, cause diarrhea, or blockage). Explain the need for fluid intake with bran.
   d. Adequate fluid intake
      • Encourage intake of at least 2 L (8 to 10 glasses) unless contraindicated.
      • Discuss fluid preferences. Set up regular schedule for fluid intake.
      • Advise avoiding grapefruit juice, apple juice, coffee, tea, cola, and chocolate drinks as daily fluid intake.
   e. Optimal position
      • Provide privacy (close door, draw curtains around the bed, play the television or radio to mask sounds, have a room deodorizer available).
      • Use the bathroom instead of a bedpan if possible. Allow suitable position (sitting and leaning forward, if not contraindicated).

3a. The gastrocolic and duodenocolic reflexes stimulate mass peristalsis 2 or 3 times a day, most often after meals.

b. Regular physical activity promotes muscle tonicity needed for fecal expulsion. It also increases circulation to the digestive system, which promotes peristalsis and easier feces evacuation.

• Low-fiber foods pass slowly in the large intestines and thus become dry, hard, and difficult to defecate. Diets low in fiber and high in concentrated refined foods produce small, hard stools that increase the colon's susceptibility to disease.
• Diets high in unrefined fibrous food produce large, soft stools that decrease the colon's susceptibility to disease. An increase in fiber without an optimal hydration will worsen constipation.

• Sufficient fluid intake, at least 2 liters daily, is necessary to maintain bowel patterns and to promote proper stool consistency.

• These beverages have a diuretic effect.

• Flexing the hip pulls the anal canal open, which decreases resistance of feces movement. An upright position uses gravity to promote feces movement. Elevating the legs can increase intra-abdominal pressure.

Clinical Alert Report

Advise ancillary staff/student to report:
- Any changes in bowel function (e.g., diarrhea, hard stools).
- If no bowel movement occurs during shift.

Documentation

Bowel movements
Bowel sounds
Teaching

Risk for Impaired Skin Integrity (**) Related to Prolonged Pressure on Tissues Associated with Decreased Mobility, Increased Fragility of the Skin Associated with Dependent Edema, Decreased Tissue Perfusion, Malnutrition, Urinary / Fecal Incontinence

Carp's Cues

The National Pressure Ulcer Advisory Panel (NPUAP, 2007) defines a *pressure ulcer* as a "localized injury to the skin and / or underlying tissue usually over a bony prominence, as a result of pressure, or pressure in combination with shear and / or friction. A number of contributing or confounding factors are also associated with pressure ulcers; the significance of these factors is yet to be elucidated" (p. 1).

Pressure ulcers represent a major burden of sickness and reduced quality of life yearly for 2.5 million clients and their caregivers. Increased morbidity and mortality associated with pressure ulcer development in hospitalized clients is documented in multiple studies. Pressure ulcers cost $9.1 billion to $11.6 billion per year in the United States. Cost of individual client care ranges from $20,900 to $151,700 per pressure ulcer. The development of a single pressure ulcer in U.S. hospitals can increase a client's length of stay five-fold and increase hospital charges by $2,000–$11,000. About 60,000 clients die as a direct result of a pressure ulcer each year. (Russo, Steiner, & Spector, 2006).

NOC
Tissue Integrity: Skin and Mucous Membranes

Goal

The client will maintain present intact skin / tissue.

NIC
Pressure Management, Pressure Ulcer Care, Skin Surveillance, Positioning

Indicators

- No redness (erythema)
- Relate risk factors to skin / tissue trauma.

**Using the risk assessment tool for pressure ulcers on the inside back cover, calculate the score and record it in the ( ).

Interventions	*Rationales*
1. Using the Risk Assessment Score on the inside back cover, identify individuals as High Risk for Pressure Ulcers (PUs). a. Ability to respond meaningfully to pressure related discomfort b. Degree to which skin is exposed to moisture c. Degree of physical activity d. Ability to change and control body position e. Usual food intake pattern f. Friction & shear **CLINICAL ALERT** • Refer to *Risk for Impaired Skin Integrity* in Section II for intrinsic and extrinsic factors for PUs.	1. The risk assessment score using the Braden Scale should be completed if not already completed on admission using the criteria :Br.
2. Upon admission, all skin surfaces, bony prominences, and skin folds will be inspected for evidence of redness or skin breakdown. Document the skin condition with location, description, and measurement of lesions.	2. The exam and documentation are critical from a medical–legal perspective).
3. Assess for frail individuals using five criteria on the Cardiovascular Health Survey (Frail-CHS). If three or more criteria are present, the person is frail. Prefrail is when there are one or two criteria. Robust is when none are present. (Fried et al., 2001) a. Weight loss b. Exhaustion c. Weakness d. Slow walking speed e. Low levels of physical activity	
4. Consider frail individuals over 65 as high risk for PUs.. **CLINICAL ALERT** • Frailty has been defined as a medical syndrome of a physiologic state of increased risks for negative outcomes that result from decreased physiologic reserves and dysregulation of many systems (Fried et al., 2004). • Frail individuals have difficulty maintaining homeostasis in the face of a range of stressors (Campbell, 2009). • Frailty results from age-related or disease-related effects on multiple systems (Fried et al., 2001; Campbell, 2009). • Frailty can be present with no diseases (Ibid).	4. Clients 65 years and older accounted for 72.3% of all hospitalizations in which PUs were noted. Those age 45–64 years accounted for 19% of PUs (Russo & Elixhauser, 2006b).
5. Perform a skin assessment at least every 8 hours or more often depending on risks factors. High-risk areas for PUs are: a. The backs of the heels b. The back of the head (occipital) c. Knees d. Elbows e. Buttocks and tailbone (coccyx, sacrum) f. Hipbone when lying on side (greater trochanter). g. Any area of the body with cast, boot, restraint, tubing, cervical collar, etc.	

Interventions	Rationales

6. To prevent PUs, assess for extrinsic and intrinsic factors that can contribute to PU development. (Campbell, 2009).
   a. Extrinsic factors
      • Pressure, friction, shear
      • Moisture (incontinence, diaphoresis)
      • Length of stay
      • Wait time for surgery
      • Length of surgical procedure
   b. Intrinsic factors
      • Malnourished
      • Obesity
      • Cardiovascular disease
      • Stroke
      • Diabetes mellitus
      • Pulmonary disease
      • Prior PUs
      • Impaired sensory perception
      • Bladder / fecal incontinence
      • Decreased mental status
      • Low serum albumin
      • Low hemoglobin
      • Gender
      • Fractured bone
      • Edema
      • Critical illness
      • Any factor that reduces blood flow (e.g., obesity, tobacco use, dehydration)
      • Any factor that impairs mobility (e.g., pain, obesity, immobilizing devices)
	6. Individuals at risk must be identified so that modifiable risk factors can be reduced through interventions and / or more aggressive prevention strategies are indicated (e.g., pressure relieving devices).

SBAR

Situation: I just assessed Mr. Jones. I am concerned because he had several risk factors for PU.

Background: Mr. Jones is underweight, not eating well, and not moving on his own in bed.

He is resistant to getting out of bed

His heels and sacral area are reddened even with repositioning every hour.

Assessment: Not applicable

Recommendation: I would like an order for a pressure relieving device.

I would also like a nutritional consult to increase his protein intake.

Interventions	Rationales
7. Change at-risk client's position when in bed at least every 2 hours around the clock. Use large and small shifts of weight. a. Inspect areas after turning, if reddened or blanching skin does not disappear.	7. The critical time period for tissue changes due to pressure is between 1 and 2 hours, after which irreversible changes can occur.

(*continued*)

Interventions	Rationales
b. Post position change schedule ("turn clock") at bedside.	b. The "turn clock" alerts the nurse to recommended position changes and appropriate time intervals for turning.
c. Utilize prevention mode on specialty beds.	
d. Use foam with cushion in chair; no donuts.	d. The risk of developing a PU can be diminished by reducing the mechanical loading on the tissue. This can be accomplished by using pressure-reducing devices. Donuts are known to cause venous congestion and edema. A study of at-risk clients found that ring cushions are more likely to cause PUs than prevent them. The donut relieves pressure in one area but increases pressure in the surrounding areas.
e. Limit shearing forces / friction.	
8. Keep the head of the bed at or below 30 degrees whenever possible.	8. Clinically, shear is exerted on the body when the head of the bed is elevated. In this position, the skin and superficial fascia remain fixed against the bed linens while the deep fascia and skeleton slide down toward the foot of the bed. As a result of shear, blood vessels in the sacral area are likely to become twisted and distorted and tissue may become ischemic and necrotic (Porth, 2011).
9. Avoid dragging the client in bed. Have enough personnel to use lift sheet. If indicated, provide an overhead trapeze.	9. Friction injuries to the skin occur when it moves across a coarse surface such as bed linens. Most friction injuries can be avoided by using appropriate techniques when moving individuals so that their skin is never dragged across the bed linens.
10. Use elbow protectors. Remove to inspect at every shift. Instruct client not to use elbows to push up self in bed.	10. Voluntary and involuntary movements by the individuals themselves can lead to friction injuries, especially on elbows and heels. Any agent that eliminates this contact or decreases the friction between the skin and the bed linens will reduce the potential for injury.
11. Apply transparent film dressing (Tegaderm) over bony prominences, as appropriate.	
12. Ensure optimal intake of required nutrients.	12. It is essential to meet minimal recommended dietary intake. Protein levels for clients with wounds should be 1.25 to 1.5 grams. Randomized clinical trials indicate increased protein levels promote PU healing (Dorner, Posthauer, & Thomas, 2009).

CLINICAL ALERT
- Nutritional deficit is a known risk factor for the development of PUs.
- Poor general nutrition is frequently associated with loss of weight and muscle atrophy.
- The reduction in subcutaneous tissue and muscle reduces the mechanical padding between the skin and the underlying bony prominences, thus increasing susceptibility to PUs.
- Poor nutrition also leads to decreased resistance to infection and interferes with wound healing.

13. Refer to *Risk for Impaired Skin Integrity* for detailed intervention to improve nutritional status.

Interventions	Rationales
14. Inspect skin at least daily during bath for reddened areas or breakdown. Check bony prominences for redness with each position change.	14. Skin inspection is fundamental to any plan for preventing PUs. Skin inspection provides the information essential for designing interventions to reduce risk and for evaluating the outcomes of those interventions.
15. Keep skin clean and dry. Gently apply moisturizers such as Eucerin, Lubriderm, or Sween Cream, as needed.	15. For maximum skin vitality, metabolic wastes and environmental contaminants that accumulate on the skin should be removed frequently. It is prudent to treat clinical signs and symptoms of dry skin with a topical moisturizer.
16. Avoid massage over bony prominences.	16. There is research evidence to suggest that massage over bony prominences may be harmful.
17. Reduce incontinence care.	17. Moist skin due to incontinence leads to maceration, which can make the skin more susceptible to injury. Moisture from urine or fecal incontinence also reduces the resistance of the skin to bacteria. Bacteria and toxins in the stool increase the risk of skin breakdown.
18. Refer to *Incontinence* nursing diagnosis in Unit II Section 1.	
19. Avoid plastic pads that hold moisture next to the skin.	19. They are not absorbent and serve only as "bed protectors." Never use plastic pads unless they are covered with smooth linen to absorb moisture.
20. Cleanse perineal area after each incontinent episode, followed by the application of a moisture barrier ointment (e.g., Desitin, Vaseline, A & D Ointment, Baza.)	20. A moisture barrier is a petrolatum-based ointment that repels urine and fecal material and moisturizes the skin to assist in healing reddened, irritated areas resulting from incontinence.

Clinical Alert Report

Advise ancillary staff/student to report:
- Skin condition of vulnerable areas (back, heels, and elbows)
- New onset of incontinence.

Documentation

Turning and repositioning
Skin assessment

Disturbed Sleep Pattern Related to an Unfamiliar, Noisy Environment, a Change in Bedtime Ritual, Emotional Stress, and a Change in Circadian Rhythm

NOC
Rest, Sleep, Well-Being

Goal

The client will report a satisfactory balance of rest and activity.

NIC

Energy Management,
Sleep Enhancement,
Environmental
Management

Indicators

- Complete at least four sleep cycles (100 min) undisturbed.
- State factors that increase or decrease the quality of sleep.

Interventions	Rationales
1. Discuss the reasons for differing individual sleep requirements, including age, lifestyle, activity level, and other possible factors.	1. Although many believe that a person needs 8 hours of sleep each night, no scientific evidence supports this. Individual sleep requirements vary greatly. Generally, a person who can relax and rest easily requires less sleep to feel refreshed.
2. Explain sleep cycles (includes REM, NREM, and wakefulness) and sleep requirements.	2. Sleep cycle. A client typically goes through four or five complete sleep cycles each night. Awakening during a cycle may cause him or her to feel poorly rested in the morning.
3. Explain how aging affects sleep (Neubauer, 2009).	3. With aging, less time is spent in the sleep cycle stages 3 and 4, which are the most restorative stages of sleep. The results are difficulty falling asleep and staying asleep (Cole & Richards, 2007).
a. Taking longer to fall asleep.	a. Pain caused by some health conditions such as arthritis will interfere with falling and staying asleep.
b. Sleep is less deep.	b. Growth hormone is what makes children sleep so deeply. As one ages, one's body secretes less of this hormone and deep sleep becomes more difficult.
c. Waking up three or four times a night.	c. Menopause causes a great deal of hormonal changes in women, sometimes resulting in night sweats and other symptoms that interfere with sleep.
d. Frequent nighttime bathroom trips.	d. Other conditions (like diabetes or an enlarged prostate) may cause the use of the bathroom frequently during the night, which interrupts deep sleep.
e. Tendency to fall asleep in the early evening and wake up in the early morning.	e. Melatonin is important because changes in the level of this hormone control our sleep cycle. With less melatonin, many older adults feel sleepy in the early evening and wake up in the early morning. They also may have more trouble falling asleep.
4. Explain the effects of sleep deprivation on cognitive changes and risk of falls / injury.	4. Sleep deprivation results in impaired cognitive functioning (e.g., memory, concentration, and judgment) and perception, reduced emotional control, increased suspicion, irritability, and disorientation. It also lowers the pain threshold and decreases production of catecholamines, corticosteroids, and hormones (Arthritis Foundation, 2008). Sleep disturbance is the leading cause of hospital complications, such as falls, delirium (IOM, 2009).

Interventions	Rationales

SBAR   **Situation:** Mr. Green has slept only 4 hours the last 24 hours.

Background: "He is not sleeping because...."

Assessment: He is c/o of more pain, wants a sleeping pill.

Recommendation: It would be useful to... (e.g., stop taking vital signs 10 p.m.–6 a.m. unless needed, change the times for med. administration; provide treatments before 10 p.m. and after 6 a.m. when possible).

---

5. Discuss with physician / NP / PA the use of a "sleep protocol." This will allow the nursing staff/student the authority not to wake a person for blood draws or vital signs if appropriate, and (Bartick, 2009):
   a. Designate "quiet time" between 10 p.m. and 6 a.m.
   b. Play lullabies over public address system.
   c. Set a timer to turn off overhead hallway lights at 10 p.m.
   d. Mute phones close to client rooms; avoid intercom use except in emergencies.
   e. Take vital signs at 10 p.m., and start again at 6 a.m. unless otherwise indicated.
   f. Order medications as bid, tid, qid, but not "q" certain hours when possible.
   g. Do not administer a diuretic after 4 p.m.
   h. Avoid blood transfusions during "quiet time" due to frequent monitoring.

5. A small study reported that "sleep protocol" can reduce the number of clients reporting disturbed sleep by 38% and reduce the number of clients needing sedatives by 49% (Bartick, 2009).

---

6. Encourage or provide evening care, offer:
   a. Use of bathroom or bedpan
   b. Personal hygiene (mouth care, bath, shower, partial bath)
   c. Clean linen and bedclothes (freshly made bed, sufficient blankets)

---

7. Reduce or eliminate environmental distractions and sleep interruptions.
   a. Noise
   - Close the door to the room.
   - Pull the curtains.
   - Unplug the telephone.
   - Use "white noise" (e.g., fan; quiet music; tape of rain, waves).
   - Eliminate 24-hour lighting.
   - Provide night lights.
   - Decrease the amount and kind of incoming stimuli (e.g., staff conversations).
   - Cover blinking lights with tape.
   - Reduce the volume of alarms and televisions.
   - Place the client with a compatible roommate, if possible.

7. Sleep is difficult without relaxation, which the unfamiliar hospital environment can hinder.

(continued)

Interventions	Rationales
b. Interruptions • Organize procedures to minimize disturbances during sleep period (e.g., when the client awakens for medication, also administer treatments and obtain vital signs). • Avoid unnecessary procedures during sleep period. • Limit visitors during optimal rest periods (e.g., after meals). • If voiding during the night is disruptive, have the client limit nighttime fluids and void before retiring.	b. Ensure that the client has at least four or five periods of at least 90 minutes each of uninterrupted sleep every 24 hours. • Researchers have reported that the chief deterrents to sleep in critical care clients were activity, noise, pain, physical condition, nursing procedures, lights, and hypothermia.
8. Document the amount of the client's uninterrupted sleep each shift.	8. To feel rested, a client usually must complete an entire sleep cycle (70 to 100 minutes) four or five times a night.
9. Provide health teaching and referrals, as indicated.	
10. Refer to Getting Started to Sleeping Better on thePoint at http://thePoint.lww.com/Carpenito6e. Print and give to individual.	

Clinical Alert Report

Prior to providing care, advise ancillary staff / student to report the following to the professional nurse assigned to the client:
• The actual time (minutes) of uninterrupted sleep/naps taken during their shift.

S T A R

Stop

Think Determine how many 90-minute cycles of undisturbed sleep the person has had in the last 24 hours.

Act If not sufficient, identify causes and address them.

Review Evaluate if sleep has improved, if not return to Act and reevaluate Clinical Alert Report.

Prior to providing care, advise ancillary staff / student to report the following to the professional nurse assigned to the client the actual time (minutes) of uninterrupted sleep / naps taken during the nurse's shift.

Documentation

Amount (hours) of sleep, nap times   Reports of unsatisfactory sleep

Risk for Spiritual Distress Related to Separation from Religious Support System, Lack of Privacy, or Inability to Practice Spiritual Rituals

NOC
Hope, Spiritual Well-Being

Goal

The client will maintain usual spiritual practices not detrimental to health.

NIC

Spiritual Growth
Facilitation, Hope
Instillation, Active
Listening, Presence,
Emotional Support,
Spiritual Support

Indicators

- Ask for assistance as needed.
- Relate support from staff as needed.

Interventions	Rationales
1. Explore whether the client desires to engage in an allowable religious or spiritual practice or ritual. If so, provide opportunities for him or her to do so.	1. For a client who places a high value on prayer or other spiritual practices, these practices can provide meaning and purpose and can be a source of comfort and strength.
2. Provide privacy and quiet for spiritual rituals, as the client desires and as practicable.	2. Privacy and quiet provide an environment that enables reflection and contemplation.
3. Offer to contact a religious leader or hospital clergy to arrange for a visit. Explain available services (e.g., hospital chapel, Bible).	3. These measures can help the client maintain spiritual ties and practice important rituals.
4. Advise individual / family to share if any usual hospital vpractices conflict with their beliefs (e.g., diet, hygiene, treatments). If so, try to accommodate the client's beliefs to the extent that policy and safety allow.	4. Many religions prohibit certain behaviors; complying with restrictions may be an important part of the client's worship.

> **CLINICAL ALERT**
> - Discuss religious conflicts with the appropriate persons (e.g., spiritual leader, physician / NP, nurse manager).

Documentation

Spiritual concerns

Interrupted Family Processes Related to Disruption of Routines, Changes in Role Responsibilities, and Fatigue Associated with Increased Workload, and Visiting Hour Requirements

NOC

Family Coping, Family
Normalization, Family
Environment: Internal,
Parenting

Goal

The client and family members will verbalize feelings regarding the diagnosis and hospitalization.

Indicators

- Identify signs of family dysfunction.
- Identify appropriate resources to seek when needed.

NIC

Family Involvement
Promotion, Coping
Enhancement, Family
Integrity Promotion,
Family Therapy,
Counseling, Referral

Interventions	Rationales
1. Approach the family and attempt to create a private and supportive environment.	1. Approaching a family communicates a sense of caring and concern.
2. Explore the family members' perceptions of the situation.	2. Evaluating family members' understanding can help identify any learning needs they may have.
3. Provide accurate information using simple terms.	3. Moderate or high anxiety impairs the ability to process information. Simple explanations impart useful information most effectively.
4. Determine whether the family's current coping mechanism is effective.	4. Illness of a family member may necessitate significant role changes, putting a family at high risk for maladaptation.
5. Promote family strengths.	5. These measures may help maintain an existing family structure, allowing it to function as a supportive unit.
6. Involve family members in caring for the client to the extent that they want to.	
7. Direct the family to community agencies and other sources of emotional and financial assistance, as needed.	7. Additional resources may be needed to help with management at home.
8. Adjust visiting hours to accommodate family schedules.	8. This measure may help promote regular visitation, which can help maintain family integrity.

Documentation

Interactions with family
Assessment of family functioning
End-of-life decisions, if known
Advance directive in chart

Risk for Compromised Human Dignity Related to Multiple Factors (Intrusions, Unfamiliar Environment and Personnel, Loss of Privacy) Associated With Hospitalization

NOC
Abuse Protection, Comfort Level, Knowledge: Illness Care, Self-Esteem, Dignified Dying, Spiritual Well-Being, Information Processing

Goal

The individual will report respectful and considerate care.

NIC
Patient Rights Protection, Anticipatory Guidance, Counseling, Emotional Support, Preparatory Sensory Information, Family Support, Humor, Mutual Goal Setting, Teaching: Procedure / Treatment, Touch

Indicators

- Respect for privacy
- Consideration of emotions
- Asked for permission
- Given options
- Minimization of body part exposure

Interventions	Rationales
1. Determine if the agency / hospital has a policy for prevention of compromised human dignity (Note: This type of policy or standard may be titled differently [e.g., Mission Statement]).	1. Agency policies can assist the nurse when problematic situations occur. However, the moral obligation to protect and defend the dignity of clients and their families does not depend on the existence (or lack) of a policy.
2. Review the policy. Does it include (Walsh & Kowanko, 2002): a. Protection of privacy and private space b. Acquiring the client's and family's permission for planned care, treatments, and procedures c. Providing adequate time for the client and family to make decisions regarding the planned care, treatments, and procedures d. Advocating for the client e. Clear guidelines regarding the number of personnel (e.g., students, nurses, physicians [residents, interns]) that can be present when confidential and / or stressful information is discussed, or when procedures that leave a client exposed need to be done	2. This type of policy can project the philosophy and culture of moral and respectful care of the institution among its personnel. "Practice expecting that honoring and protecting the dignity of individual / groups is not a value but a way of being" (Sodenberg et al., 1998).
3. When appropriate, request the client or family members to provide the following information: a. Person to contact in the event of emergency b. Person whom the client trusts with personal decisions, power of attorney c. Signed living will / Desire to sign a living will d. Decision on organ donation e. Funeral arrangements; burial, cremation	3. Clients and families should be encouraged to discuss their directions to be used to guide future clinical decisions, and their decisions should be documented. One copy should be given to the person designated as the decision maker in the event the client becomes incapacitated or incompetent, with another copy retained in a safe deposit box and one copy on the chart.
4. Minimize exposure of the client's body with the use of drapes. Ensure that the client is not exposed to the gaze of others whose presence is not needed for the procedure.	4. Individuals have reported being physically exposed as their central source of humiliation and indignity (Walsh & Kowanko, 2002).
5. Provide care to each client and family as you would expect or demand for your family, partner, child, friend, or colleague.	5. Setting this personal standard can spur you to defend the dignity of every client / family member, especially the most vulnerable such as homeless, substance abusers, prisoners.
6. When performing a procedure, engage the client in conversation. Act like the situation is matter-of-fact for you, to reduce embarrassment. In awkward situations, talk to the client even if she or he is unresponsive. Use humor if appropriate.	6. Clients have reported that in unavoidable, embarrassing situations (e.g., bowel or bladder accident), a nurse who was matter-of-fact and who made them feel at ease with small talk or humor made the situation better (Walsh & Kowanko, 2002).
7. Determine if unnecessary personnel are present before a vulnerable or stressful event is initiated (e.g., code as painful procedure, embarrassing) and advise them that they are not needed at this time.	7. Protecting dignity and privacy always applies to unconscious or deceased clients (Mairis, 1994).
8. Allow the client / family an opportunity to share his or her feelings after a difficult situation. Maintain privacy of client's information and emotional responses.	8. Allowing the client / family to share their feelings can help them maintain or regain dignity. Recognition of the client as a living, thinking, and experiencing human being enhances dignity (Walsh & Kowanko, 2002).

(continued)

9. When extreme measures that are futile are planned or are being provided for a client, discuss the situation with the physician / NP.

   CLINICAL ALERT
   - "Use the chain of command to share and discuss issues that have escalated beyond the problem-solving ability and / or scope of those immediately involved" (LaSala, Bjarnason, 2010, p. 6).
   - The urgency of the situation requires immediate attention.

   SBAR   *Situation:* (To physician/NP) I have just assessed Mr. Black. Pulse ox is 90, with labored breathing.

   Background: As you know, he is end stage congestive heart failure. He is lethargic and not eating or drinking. The family are questioning if he should have a feeding tube.

   Assessment: I cared for him yesterday. His condition is deteriorating.

   Recommendation: I would like a consult for the palliative care specialist to speak to the family regarding his changing condition and comfort measures that can be implemented to prevent prolonging his suffering with enteral nutritional therapy. Refer to Palliative Care Plan.

9. "Extreme measures, when futile, are an infringement of the basic respect for the dignity innate in being a person" (Walsh & Kowanko, 2002, p. 146).

10. Discuss with involved personnel any incident that was disrespectful to the client or his or her family. Professionals have a responsibility to practice ethical and moral care and to address situations and personnel that compromise human dignity.

    STAR

    Stop   Did you witness or have reported to you an unsatisfactory treatment of client and / or family?

    Think   Can I discuss this with the involved personnel or is it serious enough to report it to nurse manager?

    Act   If desired, discuss the situation with a trusted colleague. Report the incident to nurse manager. Complete an incident report. Do not document the incident in the client's record, unless instructed to by manager.

    Review   Are you satisfied with the actions taken in response to your report? If not, discuss your options with a trusted colleague.

    CLINICAL ALERT
    - A zero tolerance for abuse or neglect should be the institution's model.
    - Report repetitive incidents or any egregious incident that is a violation of client's dignity to the appropriate personnel.

Interventions	Rationales

11. If you decide to speak to the involved coworker, use SBAR.

SBAR **Situation:** I overheard you talking to Mr. White's family. You told them to "stop ringing the call bell" and that they were being too demanding.

Background: Mr. White is critically ill with a poor prognosis.

Assessment: Do you know how much his family knows about his condition? Do they understand the concept of palliative care?

Recommendation: I would suggest you assess for their understanding of the situation. Ask them "How do you think your father is doing?" Engage in dialogue with client and family regarding their thoughts on the present plan of care and decisions that may need explanation. If more information is needed, contact the appropriate person (e.g., physician / NP, nurse manager).

CLINICAL ALERT
- If you are dissatisfied with the response of the nurse to your discussion, discuss this with the nurse manager.

Documentation

Care plan
　Specify preferences

TRANSITION TO HOME/COMMUNITY CARE
If indicated, review the high-risk diagnoses identified for this individual on admission:
- Is the person still at high risk?
- Can the family reduce the risks?
- Is the person at higher risk at home?
- Is a Home Health Nurse assessment needed?
- Refer to discharge planner / case manager / social service
- When is this person scheduled for follow-up with primary provider? Specialists? Record dates of appointments.
- Complete a medication reconciliation prior to discharge. Refer to front / back cover.

STAR   Stop

Think   Is this person at high risk for injury, falls, medical complications, and / or inability to care for self (activities of daily living)?
Is there a support person available?
Is the person competent to manage self-administration of medications, treatment procedures? Are additional resources needed?
Can the person explain how to monitor the condition (e.g., blood glucose, signs / symptoms of complications, dietary / mobility restrictions, and when to call his or her primary provider or specialist)?

Act   Contact or provide the appropriate resource (e.g., a support person, home health assessment, additional teaching, printed materials).

Review   Has the problem been addressed? If not, use SBAR to communicate to the appropriate person.

Risk for Ineffective Therapeutic Regimen Self-Health Management Related to Complexity and Cost of Therapeutic Regimen, Complexity of Health Care System, Insufficient Knowledge of Treatment, and Barriers to Comprehension Secondary to Language Barriers, Cognitive Deficits, Hearing and / or Visual Impairment, Anxiety, and Lack of Motivation

NOC
Compliance Behavior, Knowledge: Treatment Regimen, Participation in Health Care Decisions, Treatment Behavior: Illness or Injury

Goal

The client or primary caregiver will describe disease process, causes, and factors contributing to symptoms, and the regimen for disease or symptom control.

NIC
Anticipatory Guidance, Learning Facilitation, Risk Identification, Health Education, Teaching: Procedure / Treatment, Health System Guidance

Indicators

- Relate the intent to practice health behaviors needed or desired for recovery from illness / symptom management and prevention of recurrence or complications.
- Describe signs and symptoms that need reporting.

Interventions	Rationales
1. Determine the client's knowledge of his or her condition, prognosis, and treatment measures. Reinforce and supplement the physician's explanations as necessary.	1. Assessing the client's level of knowledge will assist in the development of an individualized learning program. Providing accurate information can decrease the client's anxiety associated with the unknown and unfamiliar.
2. Identify factors that influence learning.	2. The client's ability to learn will be affected by a number of variables that need to be considered. Denial of illness, lack of financial resources, and depression may affect the client's ability and motivation to learn. Cognitive changes associated with this might influence the client's ability to learn new information.

Interventions	Rationales

3. Explain and discuss with client and family / caregiver (when possible):
  a. Disease process
  b. Treatment regimen (medications, diet, procedures, exercises, equipment use)
  c. Rationale for regimen
  d. Side effects of regimen
  e. Signs or symptoms of complications
  f. Lifestyle changes needed. Refer to the Getting Started documents on thePoint at http://thePoint.lww.com/Carpenito6e.
  g. Follow-up care needed
  h. Resources and support available
	3. Depending on client's physical and cognitive limitations, it may be necessary to provide the family / caregiver with the necessary information for managing the treatment regimen. In order to assist the client with postdischarge care, the client needs information about the disease process, treatment regimen, symptoms of complications, etc., as well as resources available for assistance.

4. Identify referrals or community services needed for follow-up. Direct the family to community agencies and other sources of emotional and financial assistance, as needed.	4. Additional resources may be needed to help with management at home.

Documentation

Specific discharge needs and plans
Referrals made
Client and family teaching about disease

⚕ Cardiovascular and Peripheral Vascular Disorders

Heart Failure

Heart failure (HF) is defined as a clinical syndrome characterized by specific symptoms (dyspnea and fatigue) in the medical history, and by signs (edema, rales) on the physical examination.

HF is a syndrome that occurs when there is a structural or functional impairment in the ability of the heart to fill with or eject blood. HF can present in a myriad of ways, from minimal symptoms to those that are totally debilitating. These symptoms include fatigue, exercise intolerance, shortness of breath, breathing difficulty, retention, pulmonary congestion, peripheral edema, rapid weight gain, dizziness, and / or confusion.

There are four recognizable stages of HF: The first two stages, A and B, are early precursors to HF; they allow for earlier intervention and prevention of HF. Clients at these stages of HF have risk factors such as arteriosclerotic heart disease (ASHD), coronary artery disease (CAD), hypertension, cardiomyopathy, and/or diabetes. In stage A, clients do not have impaired left ventricular function (LVF). In stage B, clients are usually mildly symptomatic and show evidence of LVF decline. There may also be hypertrophy from cardiac remodeling.

Stage C clients have past symptoms and demonstrable structural heart disease. Stage D clients require significant interventions and have refractory HF. "As the disease progresses and the heart becomes weaker, treatment gets more complex." They are candidates for serious end-of-life discussion and planning (American Heart Association, 2012).

Clients are usually graded by their functional capacity and quality of life. The measurements are often assessed with the New York Heart Association (NYHA) function classification assessment, which can change with the client's signs and symptoms. Comorbidities tend to play a large role in the functional capacity of the client. Class I in the functional capacity is a client who has cardiac disease but does not have limitation of physical activity. Class II is a client who has cardiac disease and has slight limitation of physical activity. Class III clients have marked limitation of physical activity and Class IV clients are unable to carry on any physical activity without discomfort (American Heart Association, 2012, Classes of Heart Failure).

Approximately 5.7 million Americans are living with HF and roughly 10% have stage D or advanced HF. The incidence of HF approaches 10 per 1,000 population after age 65, and approximately 80% of clients hospitalized with HF are more than 65 years old. An estimated 400,000 to 700,000 new cases of HF are diagnosed each year. A person 40 years of age or older has a 1 in 5 chance of developing HF. Eighty percent of men and 70% of women younger than 65 years of age who are diagnosed with HF will die within 8 years of diagnosis. HF is the most common Medicare diagnosis-related group (i.e., hospital transition diagnosis), and more Medicare dollars are spent for the diagnosis and treatment of HF than for any other diagnosis. The total estimated direct and indirect costs for HF in 2009 were approximately $37.2 billion (Lloyd-Jones et al., 2010).

⏱ Time Frame
- Initial diagnosis (nonintensive care unit or intensive care unit)
- Exacerbation of chronic condition

■■■■ DIAGNOSTIC CLUSTER

Collaborative Problems

Risk for Complications of Pulmonary Edema

Risk for Complications of Hypoxia

Risk for Complications of Deep Vein Thrombosis (refer to Unit II)

Risk for Complications of Cardiogenic Shock (refer to Acute Coronary Syndrome)

Risk for Complications of Dysrhythmias (refer to Unit II)

Risk for Complications of Renal Insufficiency

Risk for Complications of Hepatic Insufficiency (refer to Unit II)

Nursing Diagnoses

Activity Intolerance related to insufficient oxygen for activities of daily living (refer to Chronic Obstructive Pulmonary Disease)

Anxiety related to breathlessness (refer to Chronic Obstructive Pulmonary Disease)

Imbalanced Nutrition: Less Than Body Requirements related to nausea; anorexia secondary to venous congestion of gastrointestinal tract, and fatigue (refer to Unit II)

Disturbed Sleep Pattern related to nocturnal dyspnea and inability to assume usual sleep position secondary to the extra fluid in the lungs (refer to Unit II)

Powerlessness related to progressive nature of condition (refer to Unit II)

Risk for Ineffective Self-Health Management related to lack of knowledge of low-salt diet, drug therapy (diuretic, digitalis, and vasodilators), activity program, signs and symptoms of complications

Transitional Criteria

The staff/student will:

1. Explain the causes of the symptoms.
2. Describe the signs and symptoms that must be reported to a health care professional.
3. Relate the importance of adhering to dietary restrictions and understand amount of fluid intake ordered.
4. Explain the importance of daily weights.
5. Explain who they need to report to if the client gains 3 pounds in 1 day or 5 pounds in a week.
6. Explain the importance of adherence to prescribed medications.

Transitional Risk Assessment Plan (TRAP)

Begin this plan on admission.

Implement the Transitional Risk Assessment Plan (TRAP):

- Refer to inside back cover.
- Add each validated risk diagnosis to client's problem list with the risk code in ( ).
- Refer to Unit II to the individual nursing diagnoses / collaborative problems for outcomes and interventions.

  R: "Close coordination of care in the postacute period, early transition follow-up care, enhanced client education and self-management training, proactive end-of-life counseling, and extending the resources and clinical expertise over time via multidisciplinary team management" can lower readmission rates and improve health outcomes. (Boutwell & Hwu, 2009, p.14)

Collaborative Problems

Risk for Complications of Pulmonary Edema

Risk for Complications of Hypoxia

Risk for Complications of Renal Insufficiency

The client will monitor for early signs and symptoms of multiple organ failure (a) early signs of pulmonary edema, (b) hypoxia, (c) early signs of acute kidney failure, (d) metabolic acidosis, (e) electrolyte imbalances, and (f) hypotension and will receive collaborative interventions if indicated to restore physiologic stability.

Indicators of Physiologic Stability

- Alert, calm, oriented (a, b, c, e)
- BP > 90/160 mmHG (a, b, f)
- Respiration relaxed and rhythmic (a, b)
- Pulse 60–100 beats/min (a, b, c, f)
- Full breath sounds in all lobes (a, b)
- No crackles and / or wheezing (a, b)
- Flat neck veins
- No edema (pedal, sacral, periordital)
- No muscle cramps
- Serum sodium 135–145 mEq/L
- Serum potassium 3.8–5 mEq/L

Interventions	Rationales
1. Monitor for	1. HF plays a huge role in derangement in autoregulation of circulation. The end stages of HF leads to fluid overload of one or more organs. Changes in both systolic and diastolic ventricular performance occur with HF (Lloyd-Jones et al., 2010). Circulatory overload is very common and generally are early signs that the client is getting into trouble. Circulatory shock tends to contribute to multiple organ failure. This is due to the inadequate global oxygen delivery.
2. Weigh client daily. Ensure accuracy by weighing at the same time every day on the same scale and with the client wearing the same amount of clothing. **CLINICAL ALERT** • Daily weights and strict input and output (I&O) are vital in determining the effects of treatment and for early detections of fluid retention.	2. Weighting the client daily can help to determine fluid balance and appropriate fluid intake.

3. Monitor for signs and symptoms of acute pulmonary edema:
   a. Dyspnea, cyanosis
   - Tachypnea, labored breathing
   - Adventitious breath sounds, crackles
   - Persistent cough or productive cough with frothy, pink-tinged sputum
   - Abnormal ABGs
   - Decreased O_2 saturation by pulse oximetry
   - Decreased cardiac output / cardiac index
   - Elevated pulmonary artery pressure
   - Tachycardia
   - Abnormal heart sounds (S_3)

Interventions	Rationales

b. Jugular vein distention (JVD)
  • Persistent cough
  • Productive cough with frothy sputum
  • Cyanosis
  • Diaphoresis
	3b. Impaired pumping of left ventricle accompanied by decreased cardiac output and increased pulmonary artery pressure produce pulmonary edema. Hypoxia produces increased capillary congestion, causing fluid to enter pulmonary tissue and triggering signs and symptoms. (Venous pressure and pulmonary lungs become so congested with fluid that it affects the exchange of oxygen, which is considered pulmonary edema.) Diuretics help the body to rid itself of excess fluids and sodium through urination. Helps to relieve the heart's workload (AHA, 2010).
	
	Decreased cardiac output leads to insufficient oxygenated blood to meet the tissues' metabolic needs. Decreased circulating volume / cardiac output can cause hypoperfusion of the kidneys and decreased tissue perfusion with a compensatory response of decreased circulation to the extremities and increased pulse and respiratory rates. Changes in mentation may result from cerebral hypoperfusion. Vasoconstriction and venous congestion in dependent areas (e.g., limbs) produce changes in skin and pulses.
	  • Circulatory overload can result from the reduced size of the pulmonary vascular bed. Hypoxia causes increased capillary permeability that, in turn, causes fluid to enter pulmonary tissue, producing the signs and symptoms of pulmonary edema.

CLINICAL ALERT
- Assessing the individual's lungs early in shift is imperative to establish the baseline.
- Frequent assessments during the day are compared to baseline.

Interventions	Rationales

4. Monitor with pulse oximetry
  a. Monitor for signs and symptoms of acute pulmonary edema:
    • Severe dyspnea with use of accessory muscles
    • Tachycardia
    • Adventitious breath sounds
	4. The pulse oximeter is an accurate, noninvasive monitor of oxygen concentrations.

5. Cautiously administer intravenous (IV) fluids. Consult with the physician/NP if the ordered rate plus the PO intake exceeds 2–2.5 L/24 h. Be sure to include additional IV fluids (e.g., antibiotics) when calculating the hourly allocation.	5. Failure to regulate IV fluids carefully can cause circulatory overload.

CLINICAL ALERT
- Oral fluid intake must also be monitored and, if indicated, possibly restricted.

Interventions	Rationales
6. Assist the client with measures to conserve strength, such as resting before and after activities (e.g., meals).	6. Adequate rest reduces oxygen consumption and decreases the risk of hypoxia.
7. Monitor clients for signs for renal insufficiency. Refer to Unit II Risk for Complications of Renal Insufficiency for interventions.	7. Hypoxemia will compromise renal function and decreased urine output can be the first sign.

Interventions	*Rationales*
1. Monitor for evidence of tissue ischemia.	1. Hypertension adversely affects the entire cardiovascular system. Chronic increases in perfusion pressure result in hypertrophy of vascular smooth muscle and increased collagen concentration. These changes reduce the lumen size of the blood vessels, change the vessels' shape, and gives rise to cyclospasm of the vessel cells. The results are plaque formation from increased adherence of monocytes to the endothelium. The increase in the wall-to-lumen ratio in the arteries causes greater vessel resistance and a reduced ability to dilate in response to increased metabolic need for oxygen (Porth, 2011).
a. Visual defects including blurring, spots, and loss of visual acuity	a. Evidence of blood vessel damage in the retina indicates similar damage elsewhere in the vascular system.
b. Cerebrovascular deficits • Orientation or memory deficits • Weakness • Paralysis • Mobility, speech, or sensory deficits	b. In the brain, sustained hypertension causes progressive cerebral arteriosclerosis and ischemia. Interruption of cerebral blood supply caused by cerebral artery occlusion or rupture results in sensory and motor deficits.
c. In addition to extreme readings, a person in hypertensive crisis may experience: • Severe headaches (brain swelling and dysfunction) • Severe anxiety (brain swelling and dysfunction) • Lightheadedness, vertigo, (brain swelling and dysfunction) • Nosebleeds (rupture of a blood vessel within the richly perfused nasal mucosa)	c. Severely elevated blood pressure (equal to or greater than a systolic 180 or diastolic of 110 — sometimes termed *malignant* or *accelerated hypertension*) is referred to as a "hypertensive crisis," as blood pressures above these levels are known to confer a risk of complications, e.g. (left ventricular failure, acute renal injury).
d. Renal insufficiency • Decreased serum protein level • Sustained elevated urine specific gravity • Elevated urine sodium levels • Increased BUN, serum potassium, creatinine, potassium, phosphorus, and ammonia levels; decreased creatinine clearance.	d. With decreased blood supply to the nephrons, the kidney loses some ability to concentrate and form normal urine (Porth, 2011). • Further structural abnormalities may cause the vessels to become more permeable and allow leakage of protein into the renal tubules • Decreased ability of the renal tubules to reabsorb electrolytes causes increased urine sodium levels and increased urine specific gravity. • Decreased renal function impairs the excretion of urea and creatinine in the urine, thus elevating BUN and creatinine levels. • Decreased glomerular filtration rate eventually causes insufficient urine output and stimulates renin production, which results in increased blood pressure in an attempt to increase blood flow to the kidneys.

CLINICAL ALERT
• Hypertension is both a cause and complication of chronic kidney disease.
• Blood pressure (BP) control is the key to slowing the progression of CKD (Ng & Anpalahan, 2011).

• Sustained insufficient urine output (<0.5 mL/kg/h)

e. Cardiac insufficiency	e. Microvascular coronary atherosclerotic plaques or vasospasm reduce the caliber of vessel and its ability to oxygenate tissue (Porth, 2011).

Clinical Alert Report

Advise ancillary staff / student to report
• Blood spots in the eyes or subconjunctival hemorrhage
• Facial flushing
• Client complaint of chest pain or discomfort
• Dizziness
• Any change in systolic B/P >180 mm Hg, <90 mm Hg and / or diastolic >90 mm Hg
• Resting pulse >120 or <55 bpm

Related Physician / NP Prescribed Interventions

Medications
Diuretics, beta-blockers, ace inhibitors, angiotension II receptor blockers, alpha blockers, alpha-z receptor agonist, combined alpha and beta-blockers, central agonists, peripheral adrenergic inhibitors, and blood vessel dilators or vasodilators (these are classes of blood pressure drugs). Diuretics enhance the antihypertensive efficacy of multi-drug regimens, can be useful in achieving BP control, and are more affordable than other antihypertensive agents.

Intravenous Therapy
Not indicated

Laboratory Studies
Hemoglobin / hematocrit, serum cholesterol, triglycerides; thyroid studies; urinalysis, BUN / creatinine clearance; 24-hour urine for vanillylmandelic acid (VMA), catecholamine; aldosterone (serum, urine); uric acid; serum glucose/fasting; urine steroids; serum potassium, calcium. Routine laboratory tests recommended before initiating therapy include an electrocardiogram; urinalysis; blood glucose and hematocrit; serum potassium, creatinine (or the corresponding estimated glomerular filtration rate [GFR]), and calcium (http://www.hdcn.com/calcf/gfr.htm); and a lipid profile, after 9- to 12-hour fast, that includes high-density lipoprotein cholesterol and low-density lipoprotein cholesterol, and triglycerides. Optional tests include measurement of urinary albumin excretion or albumin / creatinine ratio.

Diagnostic Studies
ECG, chest x-ray, renal scan

Therapies
Sodium-restricted diet, decreased fat diet and exercise

Documentation

Vital signs
Intake and output
Laboratory values
Status of client
Unusual events
Changes in behavior

Nursing Diagnoses

Risk for Noncompliance Related to Negative Side Effects of Prescribed Therapy Versus the Belief that Treatment Is Not Needed Without the Presence of Symptoms

NOC
Adherence Behavior, Compliance Behavior, Symptom Control, Treatment Behavior: Illness or Injury

NIC
Health Education, Self-Modification Assistance, Self-Responsibility Facilitation, Coping Enhancement, Decision-Making Support, Health System Guidance, Mutual Goal Setting, Teaching: Disease Process

Goal

The client will
1. Verbalize feelings related to following the prescribed regimen.
2. Identify sources of support for assisting with compliance.
3. Verbalize the potential complications of noncompliance.
4. Eat a better diet, which may include reducing salt
5. Enjoy regular physical activity
6. Maintain a healthy weight
7. Manage stress
8. Avoid tobacco smoke

Interventions	Rationales
1. Identify any factors that may predict client noncompliance, such as: a. Lack of knowledge, cost b. Noncompliance in the hospital c. Failure to perceive the seriousness or chronicity of hypertension d. Belief that the condition will go away e. Belief that the condition is hopeless	1. Motivation improves when clients have positive experiences with and trust in their clinicians. Empathy builds trust and is a potent motivator (Barrier & Jensen, 2003). "Clients need to recognize the importance of blood pressure control and that in most cases they will need a combined approach of lifestyle changes and medication for effective treatment."
2. Emphasize to the client the potentially life-threatening consequences of noncompliance. (Refer to Collaborative Problems for more information.)	2. This emphasis may encourage the client to comply with treatment by pointing out the seriousness of hypertension.
3. Point out that blood pressure elevation typically produces no symptoms.	3. Absence of symptoms often encourages noncompliance.
4. Discuss the likely effects of a future stroke, renal failure, or coronary disease on significant others (spouse, children, grandchildren).	4. This discussion may encourage compliance by emphasizing the potential impact of the client's hypertension on his or her significant others.
5. Include the client's significant others in teaching sessions whenever possible.	5. Significant others also should understand the possible consequences of noncompliance; this encourages them to assist the client to comply with treatment.
6. Emphasize to the client that, ultimately, it is his or her choice whether or not to comply with the treatment plan.	6. Helping the client to understand that he or she is responsible for compliance may enhance the client's sense of control and self-determination, which may help to improve compliance.
7. Instruct the client to check or have someone else check his or her blood pressure at least once a week and to keep an accurate record of readings.	7. Weekly blood pressure readings are needed to evaluate the client's response to treatments and lifestyle changes.
8. Explain the possible side effects of antihypertensive medications (e.g., impotence, decreased libido, vertigo); instruct the client to consult the physician/NP for alternative medications should these side effects occur.	8. A client who experiences these side effects may be tempted to discontinue medication therapy on his or her own.
9. If the cost of antihypertensive medications is a burden for the client, consult with social services.	9. The client may require financial assistance to prevent noncompliance due to financial reasons.

Documentation

Client teaching
Response to interventions

TRANSITION TO HOME / COMMUNITY CARE

If indicated, review the risk diagnoses identified for this individual on admission:

- Is the person still at risk?
- Can the family reduce the risks?
- Is the person at higher risk at home?
- Is a Home Health Nurse assessment needed?
- Refer to transition planner / case manager / social service.
- When is this person scheduled for follow-up with primary provider? Specialists? Record dates of appts.
- Complete a medication reconciliation prior to transition. Refer to index.

STAR   **Stop**

Think   Is this person at risk for injury, falls, medical complications, and / or inability to care for self (activities of daily living)?

          Is the person competent to manage self-administration of medications, treatment procedures? Are additional resources needed?

          Can the person explain how to monitor the condition (e.g., blood glucose, sign / symptoms of complications, dietary / mobility restrictions, and when to call his or her primary provider or specialist)?

Act   Contact or provide the appropriate resource (e.g., contacting a support person, home health assessment, additional teaching, printed materials).

Review   Has the problem been addressed? If not, use SBAR to communicate to the appropriate person.

Risk for Ineffective Management Related to Lack of Knowledge of Condition, Diet Restrictions, Medications, Risk Factors, and Follow-up Care

NOC

Compliance Behavior, Knowledge: Treatment Regimen, Participation in Health Care Decisions, Treatment Behavior: Illness or Injury

Goal

The goals for this diagnosis represent those associated with transition planning. Refer to the transition criteria.

NIC

Anticipatory Guidance, Risk Identification, Health Education, Learning Facilitation

Interventions	Rationales
1. Discuss blood pressure concepts using terminology the client and significant other(s) can understand: a. Normal values (target / goals). The clinician and the client must agree upon BP goals. A client-centered strategy to achieve the goal and an estimation of the time needed to reach that goal are important (Boulware et al., 2001). b. Effects of sustained high blood pressure on the brain, heart, kidneys, and eyes. c. Control versus cure.	1. Risk of stroke rises directly with a person's blood pressure (both systolic and diastolic). The reported decline in strokes coincides with the aggressive treatment and effective control of hypertension during the past several years (American Heart Association, 2012). **CLINICAL ALERT** • Since managing hypertension is the most important thing you can do to lessen your risk for stroke, treatment for HBP can save lives.
2. Teach the client blood pressure self-measurement, or teach significant other(s) how to measure the client's blood pressure.	2. Self-monitoring is more convenient and may improve compliance.

Interventions	Rationales
3. Discuss lifestyle modifications that can reduce hypertension. Refer to Getting Started to Exercise and Getting Started to Quit Smoking on thePoint at http://thePoint.lww.com/Carpenito6e.	3. Adoption of healthy lifestyles by all persons is critical for the prevention of high BP and is an indispensable part of the management of those with hypertension. Major lifestyle modifications shown to lower BP include weight reduction in those individuals who are overweight or obese.

> **CLINICAL ALERT**
> • Eating a heart-healthy diet is important for managing your blood pressure and reducing your risk of heart attack, heart disease, stroke, and other diseases.
> • The D.A.S.H. plan is proven effective for lowering blood pressure.
> • Combinations of two (or more) lifestyle modifications can achieve even better results.

Interventions	Rationales
a. Achieve weight loss to within 10% of ideal weight.	a. Obesity-related hypertension has become an epidemic health problem and a major risk factor for the development of cardiovascular disease (CVD) (Purkayastha, Zhang &, Cai , 2011). Metabolic syndrome is the presence of three or more of the following conditions: abdominal obesity (waist circumference >40 inches in men or >35 inches in women), glucose intolerance (fasting glucose >100 mg/dL), BP >130/85 mm Hg, high triglycerides (>150 mg/dL), or low HDL (<40 mg/dL in men or <50 mg/dL in women).
b. Limit alcohol intake daily (2 oz liquor, 8 oz wine, or 24 oz beer).	b. Alcohol is a vasodilator causing rebound vasoconstriction that has been associated with increased blood pressure.
c. Engage in regular exercise (30–45 min) three to five times a week.	c. The decline in arterial function with aging is considered to be part of a physiologic process reflecting elevated blood pressure. However, the extent and rate of this decline can be manipulated. Various types of exercise programs are recommended for improving and / or maintaining the arterial function in middle-aged to older individuals (Miura, 2012).
d. Reduce sodium intake to 4.6 g of sodium chloride.	d. Sodium controls water distribution throughout the body. An increase in sodium causes an increase in water, thus increasing circulating volume and raising blood pressure.
e. Stop smoking. Refer to Getting Started to Quit Smoking on thePoint at http://thePoint.lww.com/Carpenito6e.	e. Tobacco acts as a vasoconstrictor, which raises blood pressure.
f. Reduce saturated fat and cholesterol to <30% of dietary intake.	f. A high-fat diet contributes to plaque formation and narrowing vessels.
g. Ensure the daily allowance of calcium, potassium, and magnesium in diet.	g. These elements maintain the cardiovascular and muscular systems.
4. Provide the client or significant other(s) with medication guidelines for all prescribed medications. Explain the following: a. Dosage b. Action c. Side effects d. Precautions	4. This teaching conveys to the client which side effects should be reported and precautions that should be taken.

Interventions	Rationales

5. Alert the client and significant other(s) to OTC medications that are contraindicated, such as:
  a. High-sodium medications (Maalox, Bromoseltzer, Rolaids)
  b. Decongestants (e.g., Vicks Formula 44). Ask pharmacist what OTCs are safe with high blood pressure.
  c. Laxatives (e.g., Phospho-soda)
  d. Diet pills
	5. OTC medications commonly are viewed as harmless, when in fact many can cause complications.
	  a. High-sodium content medications promote water retention.
	  b. Decongestants act as vasoconstrictors that raise blood pressure.
	  c. Some laxatives contain high levels of sodium.
	  d. *Diet pills have been linked to and associated with pulmonary hypertension.*

6. Stress the importance of follow-up care.	6. Follow-up care can help to detect complications.

7. Teach the client and significant other(s) to report these symptoms:
  a. Headaches, especially on awakening
  b. Chest pain
  c. Shortness of breath
  d. Weight gain or edema
  e. Changes in vision
  f. Nosebleeds
  g. Side effects of medications
	7. These signs and symptoms may indicate elevated blood pressure or other cardiovascular complications.

Documentation

Status of goal attainment
Status at transition
Transition instructions
Referrals

Acute Coronary Syndrome

Acute coronary syndrome (ACS) is the umbrella term that encompasses myocardial ischemia, unstable angina, and all types of myocardial infarction: Q-Wave, non Q-Wave, ST segment elevation myocardial infarction, and those without ST wave elevations, non-ST segment elevation myocardial infarction. Myocardial infarction (MI) is the death of myocardial tissue resulting from impaired myocardial coronary blood flow. The cause of inadequate blood flow most commonly is the narrowing or occlusion of the coronary artery resulting from atherosclerosis, or decreased coronary blood flow from shock or hemorrhage. Diminished ability to bind oxygen to the hemoglobin can also result in an MI. CHD is caused by atherosclerosis, which involves a gradual buildup of plaque in the lumen of the coronary arteries. The development of atherosclerosis is influenced by risk factors such as smoking, hypertension, hyperlipidaemia and diabetes. ACS occurs as a result of disruption of an atherosclerotic coronary artery plaque, either through rupture or erosion. This causes thrombosis and possibly vasoconstriction, leading to a sudden and significant reduction in blood flow and myocardial oxygen supply (Bassand et al., 2007).

Time Frame

Initial diagnosis
Post intensive care
Recurrent episodes

Interventions	Rationales
1. Per protocol, initiate pharmacologic reperfusion therapy (e.g., thrombolytics).	1. These agents restore full blood flow through the blocked artery.
2. Maintain continuous EKG, blood pressure, and pulse oximetry monitoring; report changes.	2. Continuous monitoring allows for early detection of complications.
3. Administer medications, as indicated, and continue to monitor for side effects. Consult pharmaceutical reference for specifics.	3. It is important to manage clients effectively when they first present with acute chest pain to reduce the risk of further adverse events. Early administration of antiplatelet therapy, pain relief, and oxygen therapy, if required, will help to reduce this risk (Marshall, 2011).
4. Monitor for signs and symptoms of dysrhythmias: a. Abnormal rate, rhythm b. Palpitations, syncope c. Hemodynamic compromise (e.g., hypotension) d. Cardiac emergencies (arrest, ventricular fibrillation)	4. Myocardial ischemia results from reduced oxygen to myocardial tissue. Ischemic tissue is electrically unstable, causing dysrhythmias, such as premature ventricular contractions, that can lead to ventricular fibrillation and death. Dysrhythmias can result from reperfusion of ischemic tissue secondary to thrombolytics.

CLINICAL ALERT
- Not all clients present with typical chest pain.
- Older clients and those with diabetes are particularly prone to atypical presentation, such as fatigue, shortness of breath, presyncope or syncope. Atypical symptoms may include pain in the epigastric region or back, rather than the centre of the chest. (Marshall, 2011)

Interventions	Rationales
5. Maintain oxygen therapy, as prescribed. Evaluate pulse oximeter readings.	5. Supplemental oxygen therapy increases the circulating oxygen available to myocardial tissue. Pulse oximeter readings should be >95%. Exceptions may be necessary for those with chronic obstructive pulmonary disease.
6. Monitor for signs and symptoms of cardiogenic shock: a. Tachycardia b. Urine output >30 mL/h c. Restlessness, agitation, change in mentation d. Tachypnea e. Diminished peripheral pulses f. Cool, pale, or cyanotic skin g. Mean arterial pressure >60 mm Hg h. Cardiac index >2.0 L i. Increased systemic vascular resistance	6. Cardiogenic shock results most often from loss of viable myocardium and impaired contractility. This manifests as decreased stroke volume and cardiac output. The compensatory response to decreased circulatory volume aims to increase blood oxygen levels by increasing heart and respiratory rates, and to decrease circulation to extremities (marked by decreased pulses and cool skin). Diminished oxygen to the brain causes changes in mentation.
7. Monitor for signs and symptoms of HF and decreased cardiac output: a. Gradual increase in heart rate b. Increased shortness of breath c. Adventitious breath sounds d. Decreased systolic blood pressure e. Presence of or increase in S_3 or S_4 gallop f. Peripheral edema g. Distended neck veins h. Elevation in BNP (β-type natriuretic peptide)	7. Myocardial ischemia causes HF. Ischemia reduces the ability of the left ventricle to eject blood, thus decreasing cardiac output and increasing pulmonary vascular congestion. Fluid enters pulmonary tissue, causing rales, productive cough, cyanosis, and possibly signs and symptoms of respiratory distress.

Interventions	Rationales
8. Monitor for signs and symptoms of thromboembolism: a. Diminished or no peripheral pulses, decreased Ankle Brachial index b. Unusual warmth / redness or cyanosis / coolness c. Leg pain localized to calf area d. Sudden severe chest pain, increased dyspnea e. Claudication	8. Prolonged bed rest, increased blood viscosity and coagulability, and decreased cardiac output contribute to thrombus formation. a. Insufficient circulation causes pain and diminished peripheral pulse. b. Unusual warmth and redness point to inflammation; coolness and cyanosis indicate vascular obstruction. c. Leg pain results from tissue hypoxia. d. Obstruction to pulmonary circulation causes sudden chest pain and dyspnea. e. Pain with walking is caused by insufficient circulation.
9. Monitor for signs and symptoms of pericarditis: a. Chest pain influenced by change in respiration or position b. Pericardial rub. c. Temperature elevation >101°F d. Diffuse ST segment electrocardiogram (ECG) changes	9. Pericarditis is inflammation of the pericardial sac. Damage to the epicardium causes it to become rough, which tends to irritate and inflame the pericardium.
10. Monitor for signs and symptoms of pericardial tamponade / cardiac rupture: a. Hypotension b. Distended neck veins c. Tachycardia d. Pulsus paradoxus e. Equalization of cardiac pressures f. Narrowed pulse pressure g. Muffled heart tones h. Electrical alternans	10. Cardiac tamponade results from accumulation of fluid in the pericardial space, causing impaired cardiac function and decreased cardiac output. Cardiac rupture occurs most often from three to 10 days after MI, resulting from leukocyte scavenger cells removing necrotic debris, which thins the myocardial wall. The onset is sudden, with bleeding into the pericardial sac.
11. Monitor for signs and symptoms of structural defects: a. Severe chest pain b. Syncope c. Hypotension d. New loud holosystolic murmur e. CHF f. Left-to-right shunt	11. Ventricular aneurysm, ventricular septal defect, and papillary muscle rupture all result from ischemia or necrosis to the structures.
12. Monitor for signs and symptoms of recurrent MI: a. Classic symptoms: Sudden, severe chest pain with nausea / vomiting and diaphoresis; pain may or may not radiate. ACS can occur without pain and without change in EKG. b. Increased dyspnea c. Increased ST elevation and abnormal Q waves on ECG	12. These signs and symptoms indicate myocardial tissue deterioration with increasing hypoxia. **CLINICAL ALERT** • Not all clients present with typical chest pain. • Older clients and those with diabetes are particularly prone to atypical presentation, such as fatigue, shortness of breath, presyncope or syncope. Atypical symptoms may include pain in the epigastric region or back, rather than the centre of the chest (Marshall, 2011).
13. Progressive activity after chest pain is controlled; involve client in cardiac rehabilitation.	13. These measures actively promote venous return.

Clinical Alert Report

Advise ancillary staff / student to report

- Any new change or deterioration diastolic in behavior (e.g., agitation, cognition)
- Any changes in the client's rhythm / dysrhythmias
- Client complaint of chest pain or discomfort
- Client diaphoretic
- Any change in systolic B/P >210 mm Hg, >90 mm Hg and / or diastolic >90 mm Hg
- Resting pulse >120 or >55 bpm
- Change in rate of respirations and / or >28 or >10/minute
- Changes or new onset of dyspnea / palpitations
- Decrease in urine output less than 0.5 mL/kg per hour

Related Physician / NP Prescribed Interventions

Medications

Vasodilators, antianginals, antidysrhythmics, beta-blockers, calcium channel blockers, stool softeners, angiotensin-converting enzyme (ACE) inhibitors, anticoagulants, analgesics, diuretics, sedatives / hypnotics, thrombolytics, GP IIa IIIb inhibitors, inotropic therapy (selected cases), nitrates, aspirin, antiplatelets

Intravenous Therapy

IV access for medication administration, IV access for blood sampling, arterial access for ABGs and blood pressure monitoring, sheath access for coronary interventions

Laboratory Studies

Arterial blood gas analysis, electrolytes, cholesterol, white blood count, triglycerides, sedimentation rate, coagulation studies, chemistry profile, creatinine kinase, MB isoenzyme, troponin I, troponin T, myoglobin, CK-MB isoforms

Diagnostic Studies

ECG, stress test, chest x-ray film, cardiac catheterization, echocardiogram, digital subtraction angiography, nuclear imaging studies, thallium scans, magnetic resonance imaging, thoracic electrical bioimpedance (IEB), SvO_2 monitoring, hemodynamic monitoring, stroke volume (SV) and stoke volume variations (SVV), cardiac output (CO) and cardiac index (CI), systemic vascular resistance (SVR), central venous pressure (CVP)

Therapies

Oxygen via cannula; (in selected cases) pacemakers, transcutaneous, transvenous, and permanent single or dual chamber; therapeutic diet (low-salt, low-saturated fats, low-cholesterol); cardiac rehabilitation program; pulse oximetry

Interventional Therapies

Percutaneous transluminal coronary angioplasty, intracoronary stents, atherectomy, intra-aortic balloon pump.

Documentation

Vital signs
Intake and output
Rhythm strips
Status of client
Unusual events

Nursing Diagnoses

Anxiety / Fear (individual, family) Related to Unfamiliar Situation, Unpredictable Nature of Condition, Fear of Death, Negative Effects on Lifestyle, or Possible Sexual Dysfunctions

NOC
Anxiety Level, Coping, Impulse Control

Goal

The client or family will relate increased psychological and physiologic comfort.

NIC
Anxiety Reduction, Impulse Control Training, Anticipatory Guidance

Indicators

- Verbalize fears related to the disorder.
- Share concerns about the disorder's effects on normal functioning, role responsibilities, and lifestyle.
- Use at least one relaxation technique.

Interventions	Rationales

1. Assist the client to reduce anxiety:
  a. Provide reassurance and comfort.
  b. Convey understanding and empathy. Do not avoid questions.
  c. Encourage the client to verbalize any fears and concerns regarding MI and its treatment.
  d. Identify and support effective coping mechanisms.
 	
CLINICAL ALERT
• Depression and anxiety co-occur, appear to inhibit recovery, and have a negative impact on social functioning and capacity to perform activities of daily living in clients who develop an ACS (Tisminetzky, Bray, Miozzo, Aupont & McLaughlin, 2012).
	1. An anxious client has a narrowed perceptual field and a diminished ability to learn. He or she may experience symptoms caused by increased muscle tension and disrupted sleep patterns. Anxiety tends to feed on itself, trapping the client in a spiral of increasing anxiety, tension, and emotional and physical pain.

2. Assess the client's anxiety level. Plan teaching when level is low or moderate.	2. Some fears are based on inaccuracies; accurate information can relieve them. A client with severe or panic anxiety does not retain learning.
3. Encourage family and friends to verbalize fears and concerns.	3. Verbalization allows sharing and provides the nurse with an opportunity to correct misconceptions.
4. Provide the client and family valid reassurance; reinforce positive coping behavior.	4. Praising effective coping can reinforce future positive coping responses.
5. Encourage the client to use relaxation techniques, such as guided imagery and relaxation breathing.	5. These techniques enhance the client's sense of control over her or his body's responses to stress.
6. Contact the physician/NP immediately if the client's anxiety is at severe or panic level. Sedate if necessary.	6. Severe anxiety interferes with learning and compliance and also increases heart rate. **CLINICAL ALERT** • High levels of correlation among depression, anxiety, and impaired function in ACS clients over time may cause important information to be missed that may be crucial to understanding how and when an intervention should be implemented and in which populations its implementation would be most effective (Tisminetzky, Bray, Miozzo, Aupont & McLaughlin, 2012).
7. Refer also to the nursing diagnosis Anxiety in the Generic Medical Care Plan, for general assessment and interventions.	

Documentation

Progress notes
Present emotional status
Response to interventions
Teaching sheets

Pain Related to Cardiac Tissue Ischemia or Inflammation

NOC
Comfort Level, Pain
Control

Goal

The client will report satisfactory control of chest pain within an appropriate time frame.

NIC
Pain Management,
Medication
Management, Emotional
Support, Teaching:
Individual, Heat / Cold
Application, Simple
Massage

Indicators

- Report pain relief after pain-relief measures.
- Demonstrate a relaxed mode.

Interventions	Rationales
1. Instruct the client to immediately report any pain episode.	1. Less pain medication generally is required if administered early. Acute intervention can prevent further ischemia or injury.
2. Administer nitrates and oxygen or analgesics, per physician/NP order. Document administration and degree of relief the client experiences.	2. Severe, persistent pain unrelieved by analgesics may indicate impending or extending infarction.
3. Instruct the client to rest during a pain episode.	3. Activity increases oxygen demand, which can exacerbate cardiac pain.
4. Reduce environmental distractions as much as possible.	4. Environmental stimulation can increase heart rate and may exacerbate myocardial tissue hypoxia, which increases pain.
5. After acute pain passes, explain its cause and possible precipitating factors (physical and emotional).	5. Calm explanation may reduce the client's stress associated with fear of the unknown.
6. Obtain and evaluate a 12-lead ECG and rhythm strip during pain episodes. If IMMEDIATELY available, do so before nitrates administration. Notify the physician / NP.	6. Cardiac monitoring may help to differentiate variant angina from extension of the infarction.

> **CLINICAL ALERT**
> - Administrator nitrates with caution. Nitrates lower blood pressure.

Interventions	Rationales

7. Explain and assist with alternative pain-relief measures:
  a. Positioning
  b. Distraction (activities, breathing exercises)
  c. Massage
  d. Relaxation exercises
	7. These measures can help to prevent painful stimuli from reaching higher brain centers by replacing the painful stimuli with another stimulus. Relaxation reduces muscle tension, decreases heart rate, may improve stroke volume, and enhances the client's sense of control over the pain.

Documentation

Medication administration
Unsatisfactory pain relief
Status of pain

TRANSITION TO HOME / COMMUNITY CARE
If indicated, review the risk diagnoses identified for this individual on admission:

- Is he person still at risk?
- Can the family / reduce the risks?
- Is the person at higher risk at home?
- Is a Home Health Nurse assessment needed?
- Refer to transition planner / case manager / social service
- When is this person scheduled for follow-up with primary provider? Specialists? Record dates of appts.
- Complete a medication reconciliation prior to transition. Refer to inside back cover.

STAR

Stop

Think   Is this person at risk for injury, falls, medical complications, and / or inability to care for self (activities of daily living)?
Is the person competent to manage self-administration of medications, treatment procedures? Are additional resources needed?
Can the person explain how to monitor condition eg blood glucose, sign / symptoms of complications, dietary / mobility restrictions and when to call his or her primary provider or specialist?

Act   Use SBAR to notify the appropriate professional
Situation: Mr. Smith will be scheduled to be transitioned to his home.

Background: Mr. Smith lives alone. He (state his disabilities, self-care needs, treatments)

Action: A more thorough reevaluation of where he can be transitioned is needed.

Recommendation: Referral to social service / transition planner / case manager

Review   Is the response / solution the right option for the client? If not, discuss the situation with the appropriate person, department, and / or agency (using SBAR).

Risk for Ineffective Self-Health Management Related to Lack of Knowledge of Condition, Hospital Routines (Procedures, Equipment), Treatments, Medications, Diet, Activity Progression, Signs and Symptoms of Complications, Reduction of Risks, Follow-Up Care, and Community Resources

NOC
Compliance Behavior, Knowledge: Treatment Regimen, Participation in Health Care Decisions, Treatment Behavior: Illness or Injury

NIC
Anticipatory Guidance, Risk Identification, Health Education, Self-Modification Assistance, Learning Facilitation

Goal

The goals for this diagnosis represent those associated with transition planning. Refer to the transition criteria.

Interventions	Rationales
1. Explain the pathophysiology of MI using teaching aids appropriate for client's educational level (e.g., pictures, models, written materials).	1. Such explanations reinforce the need to comply with instructions on diet, exercise, and other aspects of the treatment regimen.
2. Explain risk factors for MI that can be eliminated or modified: a. Obesity Refer to Getting Started to Losing Weight on thePoint at http://thePoint.lww.com/Carpenito6e. Print and give to client. b. Tobacco Refer to Getting Started to Quit Smoking on thePoint at http://thePoint.lww.com/Carpenito6e. Print and give to client. c. Diet high in fat or sodium Refer to Getting Started to Better Nutrition on thePoint at http://thePoint.lww.com/Carpenito6e. Print and give to client. d. Sedentary lifestyle Refer to Getting Started to Increase Activity on thePoint at http://thePoint.lww.com/Carpenito6e. Print and give to client. e. Excessive alcohol intake f. Hypertension g. Oral contraceptives h. Diabetes	2. Focusing on controllable factors can reduce the client's feelings of powerlessness. a. Obesity increases peripheral resistance and cardiac workload. Fifty percent of coronary artery disease in women is attributed to overweight (American Heart Association, 2005). Refer to the Obesity Care Plan. b. Smoking unfavorably alters lipid levels. It impairs oxygen transport while increasing oxygen demand (Porth, 2011). c. A high-fat diet contributes to plaque formation in the arteries; excessive sodium intake increases water retention. d. A sedentary lifestyle leads to poor collateral circulation and predisposes the client to other risk factors. e. Alcohol is a potent vasodilator; subsequent vasoconstriction increases cardiac workload. f. Hypertension with increased peripheral resistance damages the arterial intima, which contributes to arteriosclerosis. g. Oral contraceptives alter blood coagulation, platelet function, and fibrinolytic activity, thereby affecting the integrity of the endothelium. h. Elevated glucose levels damage the arterial intima.
3. Teach the client the importance of stress management through relaxation techniques and regular, appropriate exercise.	3. Although the exact effect of stress on CAD is unclear, release of catecholamines elevates systolic blood pressure, increases cardiac workload, induces lipolysis, and promotes platelet clumping (Porth, 2011).
4. Teach the client how to assess radial pulse and instruct her or him to report any of the following: a. Dyspnea b. Chest pain unrelieved by nitroglycerin c. Unexplained weight gain or edema d. Unusual weakness, fatigue e. Irregular pulse or any unusual change	4. These signs and symptoms may indicate myocardial ischemia and vascular congestion (edema) secondary to decreased cardiac output.
5. Instruct the client to report side effects of prescribed medications which may include diuretics, digitalis, beta-adrenergic blocking agents, ACE inhibitors, or aspirin.	5. Recognizing and promptly reporting medication side effects can help to prevent serious complications (e.g., hypokalemia, hypotension).
6. Reinforce the physician's/NP's explanation for the prescribed therapeutic diet. Consult with a dietitian, if indicated.	6. Repetitive explanations may help to improve compliance with the therapeutic diet as well as promote understanding.

Interventions	Rationales

7. Explain the need for activity restrictions and how activity should progress gradually.
Instruct the client to
 	
  a. Increase activity gradually.
  b. Avoid isometric exercises and lifting objects weighing more than 30 lbs.
  c. Avoid jogging, heavy exercise, and sports until the physician/NP advises otherwise.
  d. Consult with the physician/NP on when to resume work, driving, sexual activity, recreational activities, and travel.
  e. Take frequent 15- to 20-min rest periods, four to six times a day for one to two months.
  f. Perform activities at a moderate, comfortable pace; if fatigue occurs, stop and rest for 15 minutes, then continue.
	7. Increasing activity gradually allows cardiac tissue to heal and accommodate increased demands. Overexertion increases oxygen consumption and cardiac workload.

8. Reinforce the necessity of follow-up care.	8. Proper follow-up is essential to evaluate if and when progression of activities is advisable.
9. Provide information on community resources such as the American Heart Association, self-help groups, counseling, and cardiac rehabilitation groups.	9. Such resources can provide additional support, information, and follow-up assistance that the client and family may need post-transition.

Documentation

Follow-up instructions
  Status at transition (pain, activity, wound)
  Achievement of goals (individual or family)

Peripheral Arterial Disease (Atherosclerosis)

Atherosclerosis obliterans, a progressive disease, is the leading cause of obstructive arterial disease of the extremities in people older than 30 years. At least 95% of arterial occlusive disease is atherosclerotic in origin. When atherosclerotic plaque and blood clots reduce blood flow to the legs or, less often, to the arms, the condition is called peripheral artery disease (PAD). PAD makes walking painful and slows injury healing. In the worst cases, it can result in the loss of a toe, foot, or leg—or even death.

The World Health Organization describes atherosclerosis *as "a variable combination of changes in the intima of arteries, consisting of the focal accumulation of lipids, complex carbohydrates, blood and blood products, fibrous tissue, and calcium deposits and associated with medial changes."* It is characterized by specific changes in the arterial wall as well as the development of an intraluminal plaque. Atherosclerosis can lead to myocardial infarction, renal hypertension, stroke, and amputation.

The known risk factors for atherosclerosis include hyperlipidemia, smoking history, hypertension, diabetes mellitus, and a family history of strokes or heart attacks, especially at an early age. Altering modifiable risk factors has been shown to reduce significantly the chances of progressing to the morbid consequences of this disease. Teaching the risk factors and modifying behaviors that reduce risk factors are important components of nursing interventions for atherosclerotic disease.

 Time Frame
Initial diagnosis

▪▪▪ DIAGNOSTIC CLUSTER*

Collaborative Problems

Risk for Complications of Stroke

Risk for Complications of Ischemic Ulcers

Risk for Complications of Acute Arterial Thrombosis

Risk for Complications of Hypertension (efer to Hypertension)

Nursing Diagnoses

Activity Intolerance related to Claudication

Risk for Falls related to effects of orthostatic hypotension (refer to Unit II)

Risk for Ineffective Self-Health Management related to lack of knowledge of condition, management of claudication, risk factors, foot care, and treatment plan

*This medical condition was not included in the validation study.

Transitional Criteria

The staff/student will:

1. Explain the risk factors and management of peripheral artery disease.
2. Review risk assessment and the various management strategies of the risk, to reduce mortality and aid secondary prevention.
3. State specific activities to manage claudication.
4. Describe the need for and steps of proper foot care.
5. Describe any lifestyle changes indicated (e.g., cessation of smoking, low-fat diet, regular exercise program).
6. State goal to reduce low-density lipoprotein (LDL) cholesterol to less than 100 optimal, 100–129 near optimal / above optimal (NCEP, 3rd Report ATP III).
7. Relate the signs and symptoms that must be reported to a health care professional.
8. Identify community resources available for assistance.

Transitional Risk Assessment Plan (TRAP)

Begin this plan on admission.

Implement the Transitional Risk Assessment Plan (TRAP):

- Refer to inside back cover.
- Add each validated risk diagnosis to client's problem list with the risk code in ( ).
- Refer to Unit II to the individual risk nursing diagnoses / collaborative problems for outcomes and interventions.

R: "Close coordination of care in the postacute period, early transition follow-up care, enhanced client education and self-management training, proactive end-of-life counseling, and extending the resources and clinical expertise over time via multidisciplinary team management" can lower readmission rates and improve health outcomes. (Boutwell & Hwu, 2009, p. 14)

Transition Criteria

Before transition, the client or family will list common risk factors for atherosclerosis.

Collaborative Problems

Risk for Complication of Stroke

Risk for Complication of Ischemic Ulcers

Risk for Complication of Acute Arterial Thrombosis

Risk for Complications of Hypertension

Collaborative Outcomes

The client will be monitored for early signs and symptoms of (a) stroke, (b) ischemic ulcers, and (c) acute arterial thrombosis and will receive collaborative interventions if indicated to restore physiologic stability.

Indicators of Physiologic Stability

* BP >90/60, >140/90 mm Hg
* Oriented and alert
* Palpable peripheral pulses
* Warm, dry skin
* Intact motor / sensation of extremities
* Ankle-brachial index (difference between the blood pressure of the arm to the ankle. If the ankle pressure is 50% or less than the arm, indicates impaired circulation.)
* Claudication, sudden onset or progressive deterioration.

Interventions	*Rationales*

1. Teach the client about the signs and symptoms of transient ischemic attack (TIA) and the importance of reporting to the physician/NP if they occur.
  a. Dizziness, loss of balance, or fainting
  b. Changes in sensation or motor control in arms or legs
  c. Numbness in face
  d. Speech changes
  e. Visual changes or loss of vision
  f. Temporary loss of memory
	1. The risk of stroke increases in clients who have had a TIA. Disruption of cerebral circulation can result in motor or sensory deficits.
	
	 CLINICAL ALERT
	• Prevalences of cerebral infarction and carotid artery stenosis were markedly higher in clients with peripheral arterial disease than in controls, indicating that peripheral arterial disease is a meaningful risk factor for cerebral infarction, lacunar infarction, and carotid artery stenosis. This suggests that screening for cerebral infarction and carotid artery stenosis is important for managements in peripheral arterial disease, as with screening for peripheral arterial disease in clients with stroke (Araki et al., 2012).

2. Assess for ischemic ulcers in extremities. Report ulcers or darkened spots of skin to the physician/NP.	2. Atherosclerosis causing arterial stenosis and subsequent decreased tissue perfusion interferes with and may prevent healing of skin ulcers. Darkened spots of skin distal to arterial stenosis may indicate tissue infarctions related to ischemia. **CLINICAL ALERT** • The most severe stage of PAD is critical limb ischemia, in which blood flow is so reduced that sores do not heal and gangrene can develop. • Only 1% to 2% of clients with PAD develop critical limb ischemia, but all of them will need surgery to restore blood flow, and for almost 30%, amputation will ultimately be required.

(continued)

Interventions	Rationales
3. Reinforce teaching of foot care. (Refer to the nursing diagnosis Risk for Ineffective Management of Therapeutic Regimen for more information.)	3. Protection from skin loss may preserve tissue by preventing access to infective agents.
4. Monitor peripheral circulation (pulses, sensation, skin color). Report any changes immediately.	4. In acute arterial thrombosis, loss of sensation distal to the thrombosis occurs first with accompanying ischemic pain. This may be followed by a decrease in motor function.

Clinical Alert Report

Advise ancillary staff / student to report
- Any change in systolic B/P >210 mm Hg, >90 mm Hg, and / or diastolic >90 mm Hg
- Any new change or deterioration diastolic in behavior (e.g., agitation, cognition)
- Nonpalpable or very weak peripheral pulses
- Cool, pale, and even numb
- Weak motor / sensation of extremities
- Pain with walking (claudication), sudden onset or progressive deterioration.

Related Physician / NP Prescribed Interventions

Specific interventions also depend on how atherosclerosis affects circulation and renal, cerebral, and cardiac functions.

Refer to specific care plan (e.g., hypertension, renal failure) for more information.

Medications
Vasodilators, adrenergic blocking agents

Intravenous Therapy
Not indicated

Laboratory Studies
Cholesterol levels (LDL / HDL), homocystine levels, triglycerides

Diagnostic Studies
Duplex ultrasound, pulse volume recording, magnetic resonance angiography (MRA), angiography, exercise test

Therapies
Angioplasty (selected), stenting, endarterectomy, bypass, pentoxifylline, aspirin, lipid-lowering agents, antiplatelet agents, hemoglobin / hematocrit, plethysmography, low-salt diet, diet designed to decrease saturated fats, and lower cholesterol

Documentation

Assessment results
Changes in condition

Nursing Diagnoses

Activity Intolerance Related to Claudication

NOC
Activity Tolerance

NIC
Activity Tolerance,
Energy Management,
Exercise Promotion,
Sleep Enhancement,
Mutual Goal Setting

Goal

The client will progress activity to (specify level of activity desired).

Indicators

- Identify activities that cause claudication.
- State why pain occurs with activity.
- Develop a plan to increase activity and decrease claudication.

Interventions	Rationales
1. Teach the client about the physiology of blood supply in relation to activity and the pathophysiology of claudication.	1. The client's understanding of the condition may promote compliance with restrictions and the exercise program.
	CLINICAL ALERT • Traditional peripheral arterial disease care has involved cardiovascular risk factor modification, use of antiplatelet agents, and revascularization. • For those individuals who are eligible and willing to perform exercise therapy (ET), a significant benefit may be recognized (Osinbowale & Milani, 2011).
2. Reassure the client that activity does not harm the claudicating tissue.	2. The client may be tempted to discontinue activity when pain occurs in an attempt to avoid further injury.
3. Plan activities to include a scheduled ambulation time: a. Institute a daily walking regimen of at least 30 minutes. b. Teach client to "walk into" the pain, to pause when claudication occurs, and then to continue as soon as discomfort disappears. c. Start slowly. d. Emphasize that the *action* of walking is important, not the speed or distance.	3. A regimented exercise program can help develop collateral blood flow and ameliorate claudication.
4. Have the client keep a continuous written record of actual activities and distances. Review it to evaluate his or her progress.	4. Self-reports of activity have low reliability.
5. Provide information on antiplatelet medications, as prescribed. Explain the following: a. Drug action b. The drug does not reduce the need for other activities to reduce risk factors. c. An immediate effect should not be expected because it takes from four to six weeks of therapy to determine effectiveness.	5. These medications reportedly improve red blood cell flexibility, decrease platelet aggregation, and improve vascular vasodilatation.

Documentation

Client teaching
Outcome achievement or status
Referrals

> **TRANSITION TO HOME / COMMUNITY CARE**
> If indicated, review the risk diagnoses identified for this individual on admission:
> * Is the person still at risk?
> * Can the family reduce the risks?
> * Is the person at higher risk at home?
> * Is a Home Health Nurse assessment needed?
> * Refer to transition planner / case manager / social service
> * When is this person scheduled for follow-up with primary provider? Specialists? Record dates of appts.
> * Complete a mediction reconciliation prior to transition. Refer to inside back cover.

S T A R   **Stop**

Think   Is this person at risk for injury, falls, medical complications, and / or inability to care for self (activities of daily living)?
Is the person competent to manage self-administration of medications, treatment procedures? Are additional resources needed?
Can the person explain how to monitor condition for example, blood glucose, sign / symptoms of complications, dietary / mobility restrictions and when to call his or her primary provider or specialist?

Act   Use SBAR to notified the appropriate professional
Situation: Mr. Smith will be scheduled to be transitioned to his home.

Background: Mr. Smith lives alone. He (state his disabilities, self-care needs, treatments).

Action: A more thorough reevaluation of where he can be transitioned is needed.

Recommendation: Referral to social service / transition planner / case manager.

Review   Is the response / solution the right option for the client? If not, discuss the situation with the appropriate person, department, and / or agency (using SBAR).

Risk for Ineffective Self-Health Management Related to Lack of Knowledge of Condition, Management of Claudication, Risk Factors, Foot Care, and Treatment Plan

NOC
Compliance Behavior, Knowledge: Treatment Regimen, Participation in Health Care Decisions, Treatment Behavior: Illness or Injury

NIC
Anticipatory Guidance, Risk Identification, Health Education, Learning Facilitation

Goal

The outcome criteria for this diagnosis represent those associated with transition planning. Refer to the transition criteria.

Interventions	Rationales
1. Explain atherosclerosis and its effects on cardiac, circulatory, renal, and neurologic functions.	1. Health education offers clients some control over the direction of their disease.
2. Briefly explain the relationship of certain risk factors to the development of atherosclerosis: a. Smoking • Vasoconstriction • Decreased blood oxygenation • Elevated blood pressure • Increased lipidemia • Increased platelet aggregation	2a. The effects of nicotine on the cardiovascular system contribute to coronary artery disease, stroke, hypertension, and peripheral vascular disease.

CLINICAL ALERT
• Exposure to tobacco raises the risk of atherosclerosis by constricting arteries and promoting inflammation. A 2011 report from the Women's Health Study found that compared with nonsmokers, smokers whose lifetime exposure to cigarettes was 10 to 29 pack-years were six times more likely to develop PAD; those with a lifetime exposure of 30 or more pack-years had 11 times the risk.

Interventions	Rationales
b. Hypertension • Constant trauma of pressure causes vessel lining damage, which promotes plaque formation and narrowing. c. Hyperlipidemia • Promotes atherosclerosis d. Sedentary lifestyle • Decreases muscle tone and strength • Decreases circulation e. Excess weight (>0% of ideal) • Fatty tissue increases peripheral resistance. • Fatty tissue is less vascular. Refer to Getting Started to Healthy Eating on thePoint at http://thePoint.lww.com/Carpenito6e.	b. Changes in arterial walls increase the incidence of stroke and coronary artery disease (Porth, 2011). c. High circulating lipids increase the risk of CHD, peripheral vascular disease, and stroke. d. Lack of exercise inhibits the pumping action of muscles that enhance circulation. With peripheral vascular disease, exercise promotes collateral circulation. e. Overweight increases cardiac work load, thus causing hypertension.
3. Encourage the client to share feelings, concerns, and understanding of risk factors, disease process, and effects on life.	3. This dialogue will provide data to assist with goal setting.
4. Assist the client to select lifestyle behaviors that he or she chooses to change (Burch, 1991). a. Avoid multiple changes. b. Consider personal abilities, resources, and overall health. c. Be realistic and optimistic.	4. An older client may have lifestyle patterns of inactivity, smoking, and high-fat diet.
5. Assist the client to set goal(s) and the steps to achieve them (e.g., will walk 30 minutes daily.) a. Will walk 10 minutes daily. b. Will walk 10 minutes daily and 20 minutes three times a week. c. Will walk 20 minutes daily. d. Will walk two minutes daily and 30 minutes three times a week.	5. Attaining short-term goals can foster motivation to continue the process.
6. Suggest a method to self-monitor progress (e.g., graph, checklist).	6. A structured monitoring system increases client involvement beyond the goal-setting stage.

(continued)

Interventions	Rationales
7. Provide specific information to achieve selected goals (e.g., self-help programs, referrals, techniques).	7. The educational program should not overload the client.
8. If appropriate, refer to thePoint at http://thePoint.lww.com/Carpenito6e for additional interventions in weight loss and exercise.	
9. Explain the risks that atherosclerotic disease poses to the feet: a. Diabetes-related peripheral neuropathy and microvascular disease b. Pressure ulcers	9. Understanding may encourage compliance with necessary lifestyle changes. a. Diabetes accelerates the atherosclerotic process. Diabetic neuropathy prevents the client from feeling ischemic or injured areas. CLINICAL ALERT • One in three people who are over age 50 and have diabetes will develop PAD. b. Healing of open lesions requires approximately 10 times the blood supply necessary to keep live tissue intact.
10. Teach foot care measures. a. Daily inspection • Use a mirror. • Look for corns, calluses, bunions, scratches, redness, and blisters. • If vision is poor, have a family member or other person inspect the feet. b. Daily washing • Use warm, not hot, water (check the water temperature with the hand or elbow before immersing feet). • Avoid prolonged soaking. • Dry well, especially between the toes. c. Proper foot hygiene • Clip nails straight across; use an emery board to smooth edges. • Avoid using any chemicals on corns or calluses. • Avoid using antiseptics, such as iodine. • If feet are dry, apply a thin coat of lotion. Avoid getting lotion between the toes.	10a. Daily foot care can reduce tissue damage and helps to prevent or detect early further injury and infection. b. • This will prevent burning in sensitive tissue. • This can macerate tissue. • They can cause an injury that will not heal. • These can damage healthy tissue.
11. Teach the client to a. Avoid hot water bottles and heating pads. b. Wear wool socks to warm the feet at night. c. Wear warm foot covering before going out in cold weather (wool socks and lined boots). d. Avoid walking barefoot.	11. These precautions help to reduce the risk of injury.
12. Instruct the client to wear well-fitting leather shoes (may require shoes made with extra depth), to always wear socks with the shoes, to avoid sandals with straps between the toes, and to inspect the insides of the shoes daily for worn areas, protruding nails, or other objects.	12. Well-fitting shoes help to prevent injury to skin and underlying tissue.
13. Teach the client to a. Wear socks that fit well. b. Avoid socks with elastic bands. c. Avoid sock garters. d. Avoid crossing the legs.	13. Tight garments and certain leg positions constrict the leg vessels, which further reduces circulation.

Interventions	Rationales
14. Emphasize the importance of visiting a podiatrist for nail / callus / corn care if the client has poor vision or any difficulty with self-care.	14. The client may require assistance with foot care to ensure adequate care and prevent self-inflicted injuries.
15. Explain that if the client cannot inspect his or her feet, he or she should arrange for another person to inspect them regularly.	15. Daily inspection helps to ensure early detection of skin or tissue damage.
16. Identify available community resources.	16. They can assist with weight loss, smoking cessation, diet, and exercise programs.

Documentation

Client teaching
Outcome achievement or status
Referrals when indicated

Respiratory Disorders

Asthma

Asthma is a chronic disorder of airway inflammation and bronchial hyperactivity characterized symptomatically by cough, chest tightness, shortness of breath, increased sputum production, and wheezing as a result of decreased airflow. Asthma attacks can be mild, moderate, or serious and even life-threatening (CDC, 2010). According the World Health Organization (2011), it is estimated that 235 million have been diagnosed with asthma. Asthma is the most common chronic disease in children and occurs in all countries regardless of level of development. Over 80% of asthma deaths occur in low and lower-middle income countries (WHO, 2011). Exposure to common aeroallergens (e.g., animal dander, tobacco smoke, dust, molds, and air pollution) can trigger an acute episode up to 24 hours after exposure (WHO, 2011). Additional triggers include emotional and hormonal changes, cold temperatures, certain exercise activities, medications, and viral or occupational exposures (Porth, 2011). Urbanization has been associated with an increase in asthma. But the exact nature of this relationship is unclear (WHO, 2011).

Many people ignore the seriousness of this disease. Frequent hospitalizations result from disregarding the warning signs of impending asthma attacks and noncompliance with the therapeutic regimen. Status asthmaticus refers to a severe case of asthma that does not respond to conventional treatment. This life-threatening situation requires prompt action. According to the CDC (2010), approximately nine people die from asthma each day.

Time Frame
Acute episode

Transition Criteria

Before transition, the client or family will:

1. Describe methods to reduce the risk of exacerbations.
2. Describe asthma action plan.
3. State signs and symptoms that must be reported to a health care professional.

> ### Transitional Risk Assessment Plan (TRAP)
>
> Begin this plan on admission.
> Implement the Transitional Risk Assessment Plan (TRAP):
> - Refer to inside back cover.
> - Add each validated risk diagnosis to client's problem list with the risk code in ( ).
> - Refer to Unit II to the individual risk nursing diagnoses / collaborative problems for outcomes and interventions.
>
> > *R: "Close coordination of care in the post-acute period, early discharge follow-up care, enhanced patient education and self-management training, proactive end-of-life counseling, and extending the resources and clinical expertise over time via multidisciplinary team management" can lower readmission rates and improve health outcomes (Boutwell & Hwu, 2009).*

■■■■■ DIAGNOSTIC CLUSTER

Collaborative Problems

▲ Risk for Complications of Hypoxemia

△ Risk for Complications of Acute Respiratory Failure (refer to Unit II)

△ Risk for Complications of Status Asthmaticus

Nursing Diagnoses

△ Acute Pain related to nasogastric suction, distention of pancreatic capsule, and local peritonitis

* Powerlessness related to feeling of loss of control and restrictions that this condition places on lifestyle (refer to Chronic Obstructive Pulmonary Disease)

Risk for Ineffective Self-Health Management related to lack of knowledge of condition, treatment, prevention of infection, breathing exercises, risk factors, and signs and symptoms of impending attack

Collaborative Problems

Risk for Complications of Hypoxemia

Risk for Complications of Respiratory Failure

Risk for Complications of Status Asthmaticus

Collaborative Outcomes

The client will be monitored for early signs and symptoms of hypoxemia, respiratory failure, and status asthmaticus, and will receive collaborative interventions if indicated to restore physiologic stability.

Indicators of Physiologic Stability

- Serum pH 7.35–7.45
- Serum PCO_2 35–45 mm Hg
- Pulse: regular rhythm, rate 60–100 beats/min
- Blood pressure: >90/60, <140–90 mm Hg
- Urine output >0.5 mL/kg/h
- Alert, oriented
- No abnormal breath sounds
- Oxygen saturation >95% (pulse oximetry)
- No confusion or agitation

Interventions	Rationales
1. Obtain a thorough history from either the client or family (frequency of short-acting β2 agonist use). Assess the origins of the exacerbation as • What triggered the event? • What methods have been used to alleviate the symptoms? Did they work? • What medications are generally prescribed? • How frequently is the client using short-acting β_2 agonist inhaler (albuterol)? • What stimulants exacerbate the asthma? • How long did the client wait before seeking treatment? • Was the asthma action plan used? If so, what zone was the client in and for long? How was the individual's peak flow? • Was the client within the target range?	1. History taking is an essential factor in the treatment of asthma and prevention of exacerbations

(*continued*)

Interventions	Rationales
2. Monitor for hypercapnia, increased ICP (when appropriate), headache, confusion, combativeness, hallucinations, transient psychosis, stupor, coma, or any significant change in mental status.	2. Acid–base analysis helps to evaluate gas exchange in the lungs. Anxiety and air hunger will lead to an increase in the respiratory rate. In severe cases, a decreased PO_2 will lead to hypoxemia. Respiratory alkalosis will be exhibited. In status asthmaticus the client will tire and air trapping will worsen. Acid–base results will return to baseline, which is an ominous sign. The PCO_2 will then rise quickly. Respiratory acidosis and failure will result. Intubation will be required (Porth, 2011).

CLINICAL ALERT
- Initially pH >7.45, PCO_2 <35 mm Hg (alkalemia); look for decompensation: pH <7.35, PCO_2 >45 mm Hg (acidemia)

Interventions	Rationales
a. Increased / decreased blood pressure b. Monitor intake and output c. Cool, pale, cyanotic skin	a, b, c. First the client will have an elevated blood pressure resulting from anxiety and feelings of air hunger. As the client's condition and air trapping worsen, pressure in the thoracic cavity will increase, which decreases venous return. Thus the client will then exhibit a decrease in blood pressure and the signs and symptoms of decreased cardiac output.
d. Tachypnea and dyspnea at rest. Respiratory rate >20 breaths/min	d. The client experiences dyspnea because of narrowed passages and air trapping related to bronchospasms (Porth, 2011).
e. Abnormal breath sounds	e. Auscultation of the chest is often misleading. Initially, wheezing may be heard throughout all lung fields during both phases of respiration. As airflow becomes restricted because of severe obstruction and mucus secretion, breath sounds become diminished or absent. This is a sign of impending respiratory failure.
f. Cough	f. For some clients with asthma, cough may be their only symptom. Spasmodic contractions of the bronchi produce the cough.

CLINICAL ALERT
- Cough may be worse at night with unclear explanations that may include increased exposure to allergens; cooling of the airways; being in a reclining position; and hormone secretions that follow a circadian pattern.

Interventions	Rationales
g. Changes in mental status	g. The individual is often anxious and restless. However, changes in mentation reflect changes in oxygenation. Confusion, agitation, and lethargy are signs of imminent respiratory failure.
3. Administer O_2 via nasal cannula.	3. Hypoxemia is common due to ventilation / perfusion disturbances. Air trapping and increased respiratory rate impede gas exchange. PO_2 <60 mm Hg requires supplemental oxygen. Administration of O_2 via nasal cannula is preferred to reduce the client's feelings of suffocation. In severe cases, however, intubation and mechanical ventilation may be required.
4. Ensure optimal hydration. Consult with physician / NP for intravenous fluids if indicated. (Excess mucus production is common.)	4. Adequate hydration prevents dehydration and enhances clearance of secretions. Daily fluid intake of 2 to 4 L is recommended.
5. Obtain sputum specimen (if possible).	5. Sputum, if present, is generally clear, mucoid, or white during exacerbation of asthma. Discoloration of sputum can be indicative of infection. Administration of antihistamines and decongestants is common to decrease mucus production.

Interventions	Rationales
6. Monitor for GI reflux.	6. GI reflux commonly triggers bronchospasm, even during sleep (Porth, 2011).
7. Assess pulmonary function.	7. Examining pulmonary function aids in determining the degree of destruction and responsiveness to treatment. Forced expiratory volume (FEV-1) measures the force of exhaled air. An FEV-1 <1,000 mL or 25% of the client's normal predicted value indicates a severe obstruction. Pulsusparadoxus (a decrease in the systolic blood pressure of 12 mm Hg during inspiration) is associated with breathing and is assessed to determine responsiveness to treatment. A decrease in pulsusparadoxus reflects favorable responsiveness to treatment.
8. Identify and eliminate triggers.	8. Triggers such as smoke, pollen, and dusts may exacerbate asthma. Avoidance of environmental stimulants should be stressed.
9. Teach relaxation techniques.	9. Clients are often anxious, which may intensify the situation. Relaxation techniques that include diaphragmatic breathing, breathing through the nose, and relaxation exercises to reduce anxiety have been shown to reduce asthma symptoms by one-third by assisting with anxiety and hyperventilation (Mayor, 2007).
10. Monitor for status asthmaticus: • Labored breathing • Prolonged exhalation • Engorged neck veins • Wheezing	10. Status asthmaticus does not respond to conventional therapy. As status asthmaticus worsens, the $PaCO_2$ increases and pH falls. The extent of wheezing does not indicate the severity of the attack (Porth, 2011).
11. Evaluate level of hypoxia with arterial blood gases and (PCO_2, PaO_2, pH, SaO_2) pulse oximetry.	**CLINICAL ALERT** • During an acute episode, the PaO_2 and serum pH will decrease. Blood gases will show respiratory alkalosis in the early stages of an asthma attack and then move toward a neutral pH. As the episode intensifies in severity, blood gases will confirm respiratory acidosis, paralleling the rising $PaCO_2$ (Sims, 2006).
12. Call rapid response team if indicated. Ensure that someone stays with individual.	12. Intense monitoring is required to rapidly assess responses to medications (e.g., corticosteroids, albuterol).
13. Provide a quiet environment to eliminate hormonal and stress responses. Eliminate environmental respiratory irritants (flowers, perfumes, cleaning agent odors, tobacco smoke [direct or on clothes]).	13. Irritants will aggravate an already compromised respiratory status.

Clinical Alert Report

Prior to providing care, advise ancillary staff / student to report the following to the professional nurse assigned to the client:

- c/o shortness of breath
- New onset coughing
- PCO_2 <35 mm Hg or >45 mm Hg
- Pulse : >100 beats/min
- New onset of anxiousness
- Abnormal breath sounds
- Oxygen saturation <95% (pulse oximetry)

Related Physician / NP Prescribed Interventions

Medications

β_2 agonists (short- or long-acting; inhaled or oral), anticholinergics, glucosteroids (inhaled, oral, intravenous in acute stages), cromolyn sodium (nonsteroidal anti-inflammatory drug), antimicrobials, sympathomimetics, sedatives, theophylline (rarely) (Sims, 2006), leukotriene synthesis inhibitors and receptor antagonists, anti-IgE antibody therapy, phosphodiesterase (PDE) inhibitors.

The drugs utilized are dependent on the indication: albuterol, a short-acting β_2 agonist, is used for acute episodes, but long-acting β_2 agonists, such as salmeterol, are prescribed for disease maintenance.

Intravenous Therapy

2–4 L/day

Laboratory Studies

Arterial blood gas analysis, sputum culture, electrolytes, serum IgE levels, complete blood count (CBC) with differential

Diagnostic Studies

Peak flow monitoring, pulmonary function tests, chest x-rays, electrocardiogram, allergy skin testing, incentive spirometry, x-ray, or MRI of sinuses

Therapies

Oxygen therapies, high-flow nebulizers, chest physiotherapy

Nursing Diagnoses

TRANSITION TO HOME / COMMUNITY CARE

If indicated, review the risk diagnoses identified for this individual on admission:

- Is the person still at risk?
- Can the family reduce the risks?
- Is the person at higher risk at home?
- Is a Home Health Nurse assessment needed?
- Refer to transition planner / case manager / social service
- When is this person scheduled for follow-up with primary provider? Specialists? Record dates of appts.
- Complete a medication reconciliation prior to transition. (Refer to index.)

STAR   **Stop**

Think   Is this person at risk for injury, falls, medical complications, and / or inability to care for self (activities of daily living)?

Is the person competent to manage self-administration of medications, treatment procedures? Are additional resources needed?

Can the person explain how to monitor condition (e.g., blood glucose, signs / symptoms of complications, dietary / mobility restrictions, and when to call his or her primary provider or specialist)?

Act   Contact or provide the appropriate resource (e.g., contacting a support person, home health assessment, additional teaching, printed materials).

Review   Has the problem been addressed? If not, use SBAR to communicate to the appropriate person.

Risk for Ineffective Self-Health Regimen Management Related to Lack of Knowledge of Condition, Treatment, Prevention of Infection, Breathing Exercises, Risk Factors, and Signs and Symptoms of Impending Attack

NOC

Compliance Behavior, Knowledge: Treatment Regimen, Participation in Health Care Decisions, Treatment Behavior: Illness or Injury

NIC

Anticipatory Guidance, Risk Identification, Health Education, Learning Facilitation

Goal

The goals for this diagnosis represent those associated with transition planning. Refer to transition criteria.

Interventions	Rationales
1. Teach the client about the diagnosis and treatment regimen.	1. Understanding may help to encourage compliance and participation in self-care.
2. Teach use of peak flow monitoring and what actions are indicated for each zone, with teach-back techniques for green, yellow, and red zones.	2. Peak flow monitoring can assist in determining if asthma is getting worse and the actions to take before symptoms can be felt. Additionally, measurements with a peak flow meter can help your health care provider make decisions about treatment and adjust medications as necessary (ALA, 2013).
3. Teach the client asthma action plan and peak flow monitoring Avoid exposure to: • Smoke • Dust • Severe air pollution • Extremely cold or warm temperatures • Known triggers (i.e., work pollutants, pet dander)	3. Exposure to these respiratory irritants can cause bronchospasm and increase mucus production. Smoking destroys the ciliary cleansing mechanism of the respiratory tract. Heat raises the body temperature and increases the body's oxygen requirements, possibly exacerbating the symptoms.

(continued)

Interventions	Rationales
4. Teach and have the client demonstrate breathing exercises:	4. Clients experiencing asthma frequently become anxious and assume an ineffective breathing pattern. Decreasing labored breathing through positioning and effective breathing patterns may reduce asthmatic episodes and prevent hospitalization.
a. Use incentive spirometer.	a. Incentive spirometry encourages deep, sustained inspiratory efforts.
b. Assume a leaning-forward position.	b. Leaning forward enhances diaphragmatic excursions and diminishes the use of accessory muscles.
c. Use pursed-lip breathing.	c. Pursed-lip breathing prolongs exhalation, which prevents air trapping and air gulping.
5. Explain the hazards of infection and ways to reduce the risk:	
a. Avoid contact with infected persons.	5a. Upper respiratory infections can cause airway narrowing and inflammation.
b. Teach importance of hand hygiene.	b. Hand hygiene is the most effective way to prevent illness. Encourage the client to ask friends and family to participate in hand hygiene.
c. Receive yearly immunization against influenza and bacterial pneumonia (Pneumovax, 1 or 2 doses per guidelines).	c. Influenza vaccines will decrease the likelihood of contracting the flu, or decrease the severity of the occurrence. Clients with asthma should receive the inactivated form only (Bailey, 2008). Pneumovax vaccine reduces the incidence of infections due to the bacteria *Streptococcus pneumoniae*.
d. Advise individual that if there is a need for increased use of rescue inhaler (albuterol) or home nebulizer to call primary care provider.	d. When an individual, previously controlled, needs increased doses of albuterol, an evaluation is needed to rule out an upper respiratory infection early.

> **CLINICAL ALERT**
> • Upper respiratory infections (URI) exacerbate asthma. Viral infections are the most common culprit. It is thought that the URI causes inflammation of the bronchial tree, leading to bronchoconstriction and air trapping.

Interventions	Rationales
6. Notify primary care provider if there is:	
a. Change in sputum characteristics or failure of sputum to return to usual color after three days of antibiotic therapy.	6a. Sputum changes may indicate an infection or resistance of the infective organism to the prescribed antibiotic.
b. Elevated body temperature.	b. Circulating pathogens stimulate the hypothalamus to elevate body temperature.
c. Increase in cough, weakness, or shortness of breath.	c. Hypoxia is chronic; exacerbations must be detected early to prevent complications. In addition to infection, yellow or green sputum may also be due to eosinophil peroxidase, which enhances destruction of bacteria (Bailey, 2008).
7. Instruct the individual to seek medical attention immediately if asthma is not relieved after using method outlined in the client therapeutic regimen.	7. Unrelieved symptoms of asthma may lead to status asthmaticus. It is documented that clients with asthma repeatedly ignore the warning signs and seek medical attention only when the condition becomes life-threatening.

Interventions	Rationales

8. During hospitalization, assess the individual using hand-held inhaler and nebulizer if used. Observe if the individual
  a. For inhalers:
    • Shake canister.
    • Blow out air.
    • Put inhaler to mouth, release medication, and breathe in deeply.
    • Hold breath for 10 seconds; then exhale slowly.
    • Wait for 1 minute, then repeat.
    • Rinse mouth if using a corticosteroid inhaler.
    • Add a spacer if needed.
  b. For nebulizer:
    • Assemble correctly.
    • Using mouthpiece or mask, slowly take deep breaths and exhale.
    • Stops treatment when mist is gone.
	8. Accurate instructions can help to prevent medication underdose or overdose. Improper use of inhalers has been identified as a cause of asthma exacerbation. Clients tend to overuse inhalers, which leads to inhaler ineffectiveness.

9. Clarify which inhaler is needed every day and which is the rescue inhaler for prn use.	9. Improper use of inhalers can result in underdosing or overdosing.
10. Advise of the importance of an exercise routine.	10. Exercise increases the client's stamina. Warn the client that improper exercise may also trigger asthma. Instruct the client that use of inhaler prior to exercise may be needed and will assist in exercise endurance. Instruct the client to avoid exercising in extremely hot or cold weather. Wearing a paper mask may reduce the sensitivity to stimulants. Emphasize the importance of a cool-down period. Suggest swimming and exercising indoors to avoid exposure to stimulants.

11. Ensure that an action plan is in place with established parameters.
  a. Have individual report what to do in response to peak flow in yellow:
    • B_2-Antagonist inhaler: Call primary care provider (PCP) if response is incomplete.
    • Instruct the client to contact PCP if the peak flow <70% of baseline (yellow zone) (Bailey, 2008).
    • Instruct the client to treat a peak flow <60% of baseline (yellow zone) or <50% (red zone) as a severe attack (Sims, 2006). Instruct to go to emergency room / call 911.
	11. Green: 80%–100% of personal best, Yellow: 50%–80% of personal best, Red: <50% of personal best.
	  a. Individuals are assisted to determine their personal best peak flows and then to monitor and manipulate their own therapy or to seek medical attention when the condition approaches the red zone.

Documentation

Client teaching
Referrals if indicated

Chronic Obstructive Pulmonary Disease

Chronic obstructive pulmonary disease (COPD) is a lung ailment that is characterized by a persistent blockage of airflow from the lungs. It is an underdiagnosed, life-threatening lung disease that interferes with normal breathing and is not fully reversible (CDC, 2012). An estimated 64 million people have COPD worldwide in 2004 and more than 3 million people died of COPD in 2005, which is equal to 5% of all deaths globally that year (CDC, 2012). Total deaths from COPD are projected to increase by more than 30% in the next 10 years without interventions to cut risks, particularly exposure to tobacco smoke (CDC, 2012). COPD is the second leading cause of disability in the United States (Boardman, 2008).

The more familiar terms of *chronic bronchitis* and *emphysema* are no longer used; they are now included within the COPD diagnosis (CDC, 2012).The most common symptoms of COPD are breathlessness, abnormal sputum, and a chronic cough.

COPD is preventable and the primary cause is tobacco smoke (including secondhand or passive exposure). COPD affects men and women almost equally due to tobacco use in high-income countries and the higher risk of exposure to indoor air pollution (CDC, 2012). Effective education has been proven recently to have a profound role in the decrease in client morbidity, due to the resultant behavior modification (Boardman, 2008). Clients and families who understand the disease process and the rationales for the interventions more readily recognize the signs of COPD and are able to more effectively implement appropriate therapies and achieve optimal health. This is particularly true of formal exercise programs.

 Time Frame
Acute episode (nonintensive care)

■■■■ DIAGNOSTIC CLUSTER

Collaborative Problems

▲ Risk for Complications of Hypoxemia

▲ Risk for Complications of Right-Sided Heart Failure

Nursing Diagnoses

▲ Ineffective Airway Clearance related to excessive and tenacious secretions (refer to Unit II)

▲ Activity Intolerance related to fatigue and inadequate oxygenation for (refer to Unit II)

▲ Anxiety related to breathlessness and fear of suffocation

△ Disturbed Sleep Pattern related to cough, inability to assume recumbent position, environmental stimuli (refer to Unit II)

△ Risk for Imbalanced Nutrition: Less Than Body Requirements related to anorexia secondary to dyspnea, halitosis, and fatigue (refer to Pressure Ulcers) (refer to Unit II)

▲ Risk for Ineffective Self-Health Therapeutic Regimen Management related to lack of knowledge of condition, treatments, prevention of infection, breathing exercises, risk factors, signs and symptoms of complications

▲ This diagnosis was reported to be monitored for or managed frequently (75%–100%).
△ This diagnosis was reported to be monitored for or managed often (50%–74%).

Transition Criteria

Before transition, the client or family will

1. Identify long- and short-term goals to modify risk factors (e.g., diet, smoking, exercise).
2. Identify adjustments needed to maintain self-care.
3. State how to prevent further pulmonary deterioration.
4. State signs and symptoms that must be reported to a health care professional.
5. Identify community resources that can provide assistance with home management.

> **Transitional Risk Assessment Plan (TRAP)**
>
> Begin this plan on admission.
> Implement the Transitional Risk Assessment Plan (TRAP):
> - Refer to inside back cover.
> - Add each validated risk diagnosis to client's problem list with the risk code in ( ).
> - Refer to Unit II to the individual risk nursing diagnoses / collaborative problems for outcomes and interventions.
>
> *R: "Close coordination of care in the post-acute period, early discharge follow-up care, enhanced patient education and self-management training, proactive end-of-life counseling, and extending the resources and clinical expertise over time via multidisciplinary team management" can lower readmission rates and improve health outcomes (Boutwell & Hwu, 2009, p. 14).*

Collaborative Problems

Risk for Complications of Hypoxemia

Risk for Complications of Right-Sided Heart Failure

Collaborative Outcomes

The client will be monitored for early signs and symptoms of hypoxemia and right-sided heart failure and will receive collaborative interventions if indicated to restore physiologic stability.

Indicators of Physiologic Stability

- Serum pH 7.35–7.45
- Serum PCO_2 35–45 mm Hg
- Pulse: regular rhythm and rate 60–100 beats/min
- Respiration 16–20 breaths/min
- Blood pressure <140/90, >90/60 mm Hg
- Urine output >0.5 mL/kg/hr

Interventions	Rationales

1. Monitor for hypercapnia:
  a. Increased ICP (when appropriate), headache, confusion, combativeness, hallucinations, transient psychosis, stupor, coma, or any significant change in mental status
  b. Arterial blood gas (ABG) analysis: pH <7.35 and PCO_2 >46 mm Hg
 	
  c. Increased and irregular pulse, increased respiratory rate, followed by decreased rate
 	
  d. Decreased urine output (<30 mL/h)
  e. Cool, pale, or cyanotic skin
	1b. ABG analysis helps to evaluate gas exchange in the lungs. In mild to moderate COPD, the client may have a normal $PaCO_2$ level because of chemoreceptors in the medulla responding to increased $PaCO_2$ by increasing ventilation. In severe COPD, the client cannot sustain this increased ventilation and the $PaCO_2$ value increases.
	  c. Respiratory acidosis develops due to excessive CO_2 retention. The client with respiratory acidosis from chronic disease at first increases heart rate and respiration in an attempt to compensate for decreased oxygenation. After a while, the client breathes more slowly and with prolonged expiration. Eventually, the client's respiratory center may stop responding to the higher CO_2 levels, and breathing may stop abruptly.
	  d, f. The compensatory response to decreased circulatory oxygen is to increase blood oxygen by increasing heart and respiratory rates and to decrease circulation to the kidneys and to the extremities (marked by decreased pulse and skin changes).

2. Administer low-flow oxygen, as needed, through a cannula.	2. This measure increases circulating oxygen levels. Higher flow rates increase carbon dioxide retention. The use of a cannula rather than a mask reduces the client's fears of suffocation.
3. Obtain a sputum sample for culture and sensitivity.	3. Sputum culture and sensitivity determine if an infection is contributing to the symptoms.
4. Monitor electrocardiogram (ECG) for dysrhythmias.	4. Dysrhythmias can be caused by altered arterial blood gases (ABGs).

5. Monitor for signs of right-sided heart failure:
  a. Elevated diastolic pressure
  b. Distended neck veins
  c. Peripheral edema
	5. The combination of arterial hypoxemia and respiratory acidosis acts locally as a strong vasoconstrictor of pulmonary vessels. This leads to pulmonary arterial hypertension, increased right ventricular systolic pressure, and, eventually, right ventricular hypertrophy and failure.

6. Refer to the Heart Failure Care Plan for additional interventions if right-sided failure occurs.	

Clinical Alert Report

Prior to providing care, advise ancillary staff / student to report the following to the professional nurse assigned to the client:

- Change in cognitive status
- Oral temperature > 100.5 F
- Systolic BP <90 mm Hg
- Resting Pulse >100, <50
- Respiratory rate >28, <10/min labored
- Sputum color
- Oxygen saturation <90%
- Urine output <0.5 mL/kg/h

Related Physician / NP Prescribed Interventions

Medications

Methylxanthines (IV), anticholinergics (inhaled), bronchodilators (inhaled), adrenergics, corticosteroids (oral, inhaled, IV), antimicrobials, sympathomimetics (inhaled), mucoactives, antitussives (nonnarcotic)

Intravenous Therapy

Variable, depending on mode of medication administration

Laboratory Studies

ABG analysis, electrolytes, serum albumin, liver function studies, sputum culture, complete blood count (CBC) with differential

Diagnostic Studies

Chest x-ray film, peak flow monitoring, pulmonary function tests, bronchography, stress test

Therapies

Intermittent positive-pressure breathing (IPPB), chest physiotherapy, low oxygen through a cannula, ultrasonic nebulizer

Documentation

Vital signs
Intake and output
Assessment data
Change in status
Interventions
Client's response to interventions

Nursing Diagnoses

Anxiety Related to Breathlessness and Fear of Suffocation

NOC

Anxiety Self-Control, Coping, Impulse Self-Control

NIC

Anxiety Reduction, Impulse Control Training, Anticipatory Guidance

Goal

The client will verbalize increased psychological and physiologic comfort.

Indicators

- Verbalize feelings of anxiety.
- Demonstrate breathing techniques to decrease dyspnea.

Interventions	Rationales
1. Provide a quiet, calm environment when the client is experiencing breathlessness.	1. Reducing external stimuli promotes relaxation.
2. Do not leave the client alone during periods of acute breathlessness.	2. Fear triggers dyspnea and dyspnea increases fear. Clients report a nurse's acknowledgment of their fear assuaged their fear and alleviated their breathing difficulty.
3. Encourage the client to use breathing techniques especially during times of increased anxiety. Coach the client through the breathing exercises.	3. Concentrating on diaphragmatic or pursed-lip breathing slows the respiratory rate and gives the client a sense of control.
4. During nonacute episodes, teach relaxation techniques (tapes, guided imagery).	4. Relaxation techniques have been shown to decrease anxiety, dyspnea, and airway obstruction.

Pneumonia

In 2009, 1.1 million people in the United States were hospitalized with pneumonia and more than 50,000 people died from the disease (CDC, 2012). Pneumonia is an infection of the lungs that is usually caused by bacteria or viruses. Globally, pneumonia causes more deaths than any other infectious disease. It can often be prevented and can usually be treated. Signs of pneumonia can include coughing, fever, fatigue, nausea, vomiting, rapid breathing or shortness of breath, chills, or chest pain. Certain people are more likely to become ill with pneumonia. This includes adults 65 years of age or older and children younger than 5 years of age. People up through 64 years of age who have underlying medical conditions (like diabetes or HIV / AIDS) and people 19 through 64 who smoke cigarettes or have asthma are also at increased risk.

Globally, pneumonia kills more than 1.5 million children younger than 5 years of age each year. This is greater than the number of deaths from any other infectious disease, such as AIDS, malaria, or tuberculosis (CDC, 2012). Access to vaccines and treatment (like antibiotics and antivirals) can help prevent many pneumonia-related deaths. Pneumonia experts are also working to prevent pneumonia in developing countries by reducing indoor air pollution and encouraging good hygiene practices.

Time Frame
Acute episode

■■■ DIAGNOSTIC CLUSTER

Collaborative Problems

▲ Risk for Complications of Respiratory Insufficiency

▲ Risk for Complications of Septic Shock

▲ Risk for Complications of Paralytic Ileus

Nursing Diagnoses

▲ Activity Intolerance related to insufficient oxygenation for ADLs (refer to Unit II)

▲ Ineffective Airway Clearance related to pain, increased tracheobronchial secretions, and fatigue (refer to Unit II)

Δ Risk for Impaired Oral Mucous Membrane related to mouth breathing, frequent expectorations, and decreased fluid intake secondary to malaise (refer to Unit II)

Δ Risk for Imbalanced Nutrition: Less Than Body Requirements related to anorexia, dyspnea, and abdominal distention secondary to air swallowing (refer to Unit II)

Δ Risk for Ineffective Self-Health Regimen Management related to lack of knowledge of condition, infection transmission, prevention of recurrence, diet, signs and symptoms of recurrence, and follow-up care

▲ This diagnosis was reported to be monitored for or managed frequently (75%–100%).
Δ This diagnosis was reported to be monitored for or managed often (50%–74%).

Transitional Risk Assessment Plan (TRAP)

Begin this plan on admission.
Implement the Transitional Risk Assessment Plan (TRAP):
• Refer to inside back cover.
• Add each validated risk diagnosis to client's problem list with the risk code in ( ).
• Refer to Unit II to the individual risk nursing diagnoses / collaborative problems for outcomes and interventions.

R: "Close coordination of care in the post-acute period, early discharge follow-up care, enhanced patient education and self-management training, proactive end-of-life counseling, and extending the resources and clinical expertise over time via multidisciplinary team management" can lower readmission rates and improve health outcomes (Boutwell & Hwu, 2009, p. 14).

Transition Criteria

Before transition, the client or family will

1. Describe how to prevent infection transmission.
2. Describe rest and nutritional requirements.
3. Describe methods to reduce the risk of recurrence.
4. State signs and symptoms that must be reported to a health care professional.

Collaborative Problems

Risk for Complications of Respiratory Insufficiency

Risk for Complications of Septic Shock

Risk for Complications of Paralytic Ileus

Collaborative Outcomes

The client will be monitored for early signs and symptoms of (a) hypoxia, (b) septic shock, and (c) paralytic ileus and will receive collaborative interventions if indicated to restore physiologic stability.

Indicators of Physiologic Stability

- Alert (a, b)
- Temperature 98–99.5°F (a, b)
- Pulse regular rhythm rate 60–100 beats/min (a)
- Pulse oximetry >95 (a, b)
- Blood pressure >90/60, <140/90 mm Hg (a, b)
- Urine output >0.5 mL/kg/h (a, b)
- Bowel sounds detected (c)
- No nausea and vomiting (c)
- No abdominal distention (c)
- No change in bowel function (c)
- Evidence of flatus (c)

Interventions	Rationales
1. Closely monitor risk individuals for hospital-acquired (nosocomial) pneumonia as: a. The elderly and very young b. Those with chronic or severe medical conditions, such as lung problems, heart disease, nervous system (neurologic) disorders, and immune compromised (AIDS, cancer). c. Those postsurgery as over age 80 post splenectomy, abdominal aortic aneurysm repair, or any factor that impairs coughing. d. Those in the intensive care unit (ICU), in prolonged prone positions, on mechanical ventilators e. Those sedated	

(continued)

Interventions	*Rationales*

9. Monitor for Complications:
   a. Electrolyte (blood chemical and mineral) imbalances
   b. Dehydration
   c. Perforation in the intestine
   d. Infection
   e. Jaundice (yellowing of the skin and eyes)
	9e. Intestinal obstruction can cause obstruction of bile duct. Intestinal distention contributes to injury to serous membrane and local ischemia.

10. Maintain oxygen therapy, as prescribed, and monitor its effectiveness with pulse oximetry.	10. Oxygen therapy may help to prevent restlessness if the client is becoming dyspneic, and also may help to prevent pulmonary edema.

Clinical Alert Report

Prior to providing care, advise ancillary staff / student to report the following to the professional nurse assigned to the client:

- Change in cognition, increased sombulence
- Temperature >100
- Pulse irregular rhythm rate <60, >100 beats/min
- Blood pressure <90/60, >140/90 mm Hg
- Urine output <0.5 mL/kg/h (a, b)
- Decreased or no bowel sounds
- Abdominal distention
- Nausea / vomiting

Related Physician / NP Prescribed Interventions

Medications
Antimicrobials, analgesics (nonnarcotic), bronchodilators, mucolytics, expectorants

Intravenous Therapy
Supplemental as needed

Laboratory Studies
ABG analysis, serologic tests, sputum cultures / Gram stain, sedimentation rate, complete blood count, electrolytes, thoracentesis

Diagnostic Studies
Chest x-ray film (Note: False negative results may be caused by dehydration and neutropenia [Harvey & Wheelan, 2008]), pulse oximeter, protected specimen brush (PSB), bronchoalveolar lavage (BAL)

Therapies
Continuous positive airway pressure (CPAP), ultrasonic nebulizer, oxygen via cannula / mask

Documentation

Medication (type, dosage, routes)
   Vital signs
   Assessments
   Treatments

Nursing Diagnoses

Anxiety / Fear

> ### 🏠 TRANSITION TO HOME / COMMUNITY CARE
> If indicated, review the risk diagnoses identified for this individual on admission:
> - Is he person still at risk?
> - Can the family / reduce the risks?
> - Is the person at higher risk at home?
> - Is a Home Health Nurse assessment needed?
> - Refer to transition planner / case manager / social service
> - When is this person scheduled for follow-up with primary provider? Specialists? Record dates of appts.
> - Complete a medication reconciliation prior to transition. Refer to index.

STAR

Stop

Think   Is this person at risk for injury, falls, medical complications, and / or inability to care for self (activities of daily living)?

Is the person competent to manage self-administration of medications, treatment procedures? Are additional resources needed?

Can the person explain how to monitor condition (e.g., blood glucose, sign / symptoms of complications, dietary / mobility restrictions and when to call his or her primary provider or specialist)?

Act   Contact or provide the appropriate resource (e.g., contacting a support person, home health assessment, additional teaching, printed materials).

Review   Has the problem been addressed? If not, use SBAR to communicate to the appropriate person.

Risk for Ineffective Self-Health Management Related to Lack of Knowledge of Condition, Infection Transmission, Prevention of Recurrence, Diet, Signs and Symptoms of Recurrence, and Follow-up Care

NOC
Compliance Behavior, Knowledge: Treatment Regimen, Participation in Health Care Decisions, Treatment Behavior: Illness or Injury

NIC
Anticipatory Guidance, Risk Identification, Learning Facilitation, Health Education

Goal

The goals for this diagnosis represent those associated with transition planning. Refer to the transition criteria.

Interventions	Rationales
1. Explain the pathophysiology and expected course of pneumonia using teaching aids (e.g., illustrations, models) appropriate for the client's or family's educational level.	1. Understanding the disease process and its possible complications may encourage the client's compliance with the therapeutic regimen.
2. Explain measures to prevent the spread of infection: a. Cover the nose and mouth when sneezing or coughing. b. Dispose of used tissues in a paper bag; when the bag is half full, close it securely and place it in a larger disposal unit. c. Explain the importance of hand hygiene.	2. Although pneumococcal pneumonia is not highly communicable, the client should refrain from visiting with persons predisposed to pneumonia during the acute phase (e.g., elderly or seriously ill persons, those with sickle cell disease, postsurgical clients, or persons with chronic respiratory disease, compromised immune system).
3. Advise individual / family to call PCP if there is no improvement in 72 hours or symptoms are worse. **CLINICAL ALERT** • If there is no response to treatment within 72 hours, a reevaluation should be initiated. Possibly there has been an inaccurate diagnosis, the causative organism is resistant to prescribed antibiotic, or dosage has to be adjusted. More invasive techniques for obtaining respiratory secretions for culture may be required. Because most clients notice a decrease in symptoms after 72 hours of treatment, they sometimes do not recognize the importance of continuing the antibiotic as prescribed. The course of medication is usually seven to 14 days, but may be as long as 21 days, depending on severity of illness, presence of underlying disease, and client response. Antibiotics should be continued until completed and a follow-up x-ray film confirms that infection has subsided.	
4. Keep scheduled, follow-up medical appointments.	
5. Explain that an follow-up x-ray is indicated in certain individuals.	5. "Routine follow-up chest x-rays for clients who are responding clinically within the first week are unnecessary. We suggest a follow-up chest x-ray at 7 to 12 weeks after treatment for clients who are over age 50 years, to document resolution of the pneumonia and exclude underlying diseases, such as malignancy. Follow-up chest x-ray is particularly important for males and smokers in this age group."
6. Advise to continue deep breathing exercises for six to eight weeks during the convalescent period.	6. Deep breathing increases alveolar expansion and thus facilitates movement of secretions from the tracheobronchial tree with coughing. Routine planned deep breathing and coughing sessions increase vital capacity and pulmonary compliance. Sometimes dry cough occurs with chest wall pain related to myalgias of the intercostal muscles, so increased efforts must be made to encourage regular lung expansion. A pillow may be used to splint the chest wall while coughing.

Interventions	Rationales
7. Advise to receive yearly immunization against influenza and bacterial pneumonia. (Pneumovax, 1 or 2 doses per guidelines.)	7. Influenza vaccines will decrease the likelihood of contracting the flu, or decrease the severity of the occurrence. Bacterial pneumonia may occur as a complication of influenza. Pneumovax vaccine reduces the incidence of infections due to the bacteria *Streptococcus pneumoniae*.
8. Encourage adequate hydration with intake of 3,000 mL/day, if not contraindicated.	8. Insensible fluid losses from hyperthermia and productive cough predispose the client to dehydration, particularly an elderly client.
9. Encourage adequate, nutritious food intake and use of high-protein supplements, if necessary.	9. Increased metabolism raises the client's calorie requirements; however, dyspnea and anorexia sometimes prevent adequate caloric intake. High-protein supplements provide increased calories and fluids if anorexia and fatigue from eating interfere with food intake.
10. If the individual smokes, explain how smoking contributes to infections. Refer to Getting Started to Quit Smoking on thePoint at http://thePoint.lww.com/Carpenito6e.	10. Chronic smoking destroys the tracheobronchial ciliary action, the lungs' first defense against infection. It also inhibits alveolar macrophage function and irritates the bronchial mucosa.
11. Instruct the client and family to promptly report any new or worsening of signs or symptoms' to PCP (e.g., change in cognition, thickening of respiratory secretions, return or persistence of fever, increased chest pain, malaise).	11. Pneumonia may be resistant to the prescribed antibiotic, or secondary infection with organisms not susceptible to prescribed antibiotic may have occurred.

Documentation

Transition instructions
Follow-up instructions
Status at transition

⦿⦿ Metabolic and Endocrine Disorders

Cirrhosis

Cirrhosis is the end result of chronic liver damage caused by chronic liver diseases. Common causes of chronic liver disease in the United States include

- Hepatitis C infection (long-term infection)
- Long-term alcohol abuse (see alcoholic liver disease)

Other causes of cirrhosis include

- Autoimmune inflammation of the liver
- Disorders of the drainage system of the liver (the biliary system), such as primary biliary cirrhosis and primary sclerosing cholangitis
- Hepatitis B (long-term infection)
- Medications
- Metabolic disorders of iron and copper (hemochromatosis and Wilson's disease)
- Nonalcoholic fatty liver disease (NAFLD) and nonalcoholic steatohepatitis (NASH)

Cirrhosis is a disease in which the liver becomes permanently damaged and the normal structure of the liver is changed. Healthy liver cells are replaced by scarred tissue. The liver is not able to do its normal functions, such as detoxifying harmful substances, purifying blood, and making vital nutrients. In addition, scarring slows down the normal flow of blood through the liver, causing blood to find alternate pathways (e.g., ascites). This may result in bleeding blood vessels known as gastric or esophageal varices.

Cirrhosis is the 12th leading cause of death in the United States. It accounted for 29,165 deaths in 2007, with a mortality rate of 9.7 per 100,000 persons. Alcohol abuse and viral hepatitis are the most common causes of cirrhosis, although nonalcoholic fatty liver disease is emerging as an increasingly important cause. Primary care physicians share responsibility with specialists in managing the most common complications of the disease, screening for hepatocellular carcinoma, and preparing clients for referral to a transplant center. Clients with cirrhosis should be screened for hepatocellular carcinoma with imaging studies every six to 12 months (Starr & Raines, 2011).

Causes, Incidence, and Risk Factors (Starr & Raines, 2011)

Inflammation
  Viral
    Hepatitis B (15%)
    Hepatitis C (47%)
  Schistosomiasis
  Autoimmune (types 1, 2, 3)
  Sarcoidosis

Excessive consumption of alcohol (18%)
  Viral
    Hepatitis C (47%), B
    Autoimmune hepatitis

Bile duct blockages, associated with:
  Cirrhosis
  Congenital defects
  Scarred ducts—sometimes related to inflammatory bowel disorders
  Gallbladder surgery
  Pancreatitis

Drugs and toxins:
Alcohol (18%)
Arsenic
Isoniazid
Methotrexate
Excess vitamin A

Infections:
Schistosomiasis
Brucellosis
Echinococcosis
Advanced or congenital syphilis

Congestive heart failure (chronic passive vascular hepatic congestion)
Nonalcoholic steatohepatitis (NASH), associated with:
Diabetes
Obesity
Heart disease
High blood triglycerides
Steroid use

Genetic / congenital
Glycogen storage disease
Galactosemia
Fructose intolerance
Tyrosinemia
Hemochromatosis
Wilson's disease
Alpha1-antitrypsin deficiency
Cystic fibrosis

Veno-occlusive disease (Budd-Chiari syndrome)
Unknown (14%)

 Time Frame
Chronic exacerbations

■■■ DIAGNOSTIC CLUSTER

Collaborative Problems

▲ Risk for Complications of Ascites

* Risk for Complications of Spontaneous Bacterial Peritonitis

△ Risk for Complications of Hepatitis Encephalopathy

▲ Risk for Complications of Portal Hypertension / Variceal Bleeding

△ Risk for Complications of Metabolic Disorders

△ Risk for Complications of Hepatorenal Syndrome

* Risk for Complications of Medication Toxicity (opiates, short-acting barbiturates, major tranquilizers)

Nursing Diagnoses

▲ Imbalanced Nutrition: Less Than Body Requirements related to anorexia, impaired protein, fat, glucose metabolism, and impaired storage of vitamins (A, C, K, D, E)

▲ Impaired Comfort related to pruritus secondary to accumulation of bilirubin pigment and bile salts

(*continued*)

▲ Excess Fluid Volume related to portal hypertension, lowered plasma colloidal osmotic pressure, and sodium retention

▲ Pain related to liver enlargement and ascites (pancreatitis)

▲ Risk for Ineffective Self-Health Management related to lack of knowledge of pharmacologic contraindications, nutritional requirements, signs and symptoms of complications, and risks of alcohol ingestion

▲ Diarrhea related to excessive secretion of fats in stool secondary to liver dysfunction (refer to Pancreatitis)

▲ High Risk for Infection related to leukopenia secondary to enlarged, overactive spleen and hypoproteinemia (refer to Leukemia)

▲ This diagnosis was reported to be monitored for or managed frequently (75%–100%).
Δ This diagnosis was reported to be monitored for or managed often (50%–74%).
* This medical condition was not included in the validation study.

Transition Criteria

Before transition, the client or family will

1. Describe the causes of cirrhosis.
2. Describe activity restrictions, nutritional requirements, and the need for alcohol abstinence.
3. State actions that reduce anorexia, edema, and pruritus at home.
4. Relate community resources available for drug and alcohol counseling.
5. State the signs and symptoms that must be reported to a health care professional.

Collaborative Problems

Risk for Complications of Ascites

Risk for Complications of Spontaneous Bacterial Peritonitis

Risk for Complications of Hepatitis Encephalopathy

Risk for Complications of Portal Hypertension

Risk for Complications of Variceal Bleeding

Risk for Complications of Metabolic Disorders

Risk for Complications of Hepatorenal Syndrome

Risk for Complications of Medication Toxicity (opiates, short-acting barbiturates, major tranquilizers)

Collaborative Outcomes

The client will be monitored for early signs and symptoms of (a) ascites, (b) spontaneous bacterial peritonitis, (c) hepatic encephalopathy, (d) portal hypertension, (e) variceal bleeding, (f) metabolic disorders, (g) hepatorenal syndrome, and (h) medication toxicity and will receive collaborative interventions if indicated to restore physiologic stability.

Indicators of Physiologic Stability

- BP >90/60, <140/90 mm Hg
- Heart rate 60–100 beats/min
- Respiration 16–20 breaths/min
- Hemoglobin: Male 14–18 g/dL, Female 12–16 g/dL
- Hematocrit: Male 42%–52%, Female 37%–47%
- Stools negative occult blood (e)
- Prothrombin time 11–12.5 seconds (e)
- Electrolytes within normal range
- Serum pH 7.35–7.45
- Serum PCO_2 35–45 mm Hg
- Oxygen saturation >95% (pulse oximeter)

- Urine output >0.5 mL/kg/h
- Urine specific gravity 1.005–1.030
- Sodium 135–145 mEq/L (f, g, h)
- Creatinine 0.7–1.4 mg/dL (f, g, h)
- Albumin 3.5–5.0 m/U/mL (f, g, h)
- Prealbumin 16–40 m/U/mL (f, g, h)
- Blood urea nitrogen 5–25 mg/dL
- Temperature greater than 37.8° C (100° F)
- No reports of new onset or increased abdominal pain and / or tenderness (b)
- No change in mental status (b, c)
- Ascitic fluid PMN count, <250 cells/mm³ (b)
- Serum-to-ascites albumin gradient (SAAG) <1.1g/dL (calculated to determine the presence of portal hypertension–related ascites)

Transitional Risk Assessment Plan (TRAP)

Begin this plan on admission.

Implement the Transitional Risk Assessment Plan (TRAP):

- Refer to inside back cover.
- Add each validated risk diagnosis to client's problem list with the risk code in ( ).
- Refer to Unit II to the individual risk nursing diagnoses / collaborative problems for outcomes and interventions.

R: "Close coordination of care in the post-acute period, early discharge follow-up care, enhanced patient education and self-management training, proactive end-of-life counseling, and extending the resources and clinical expertise over time via multidisciplinary team management" can lower readmission rates and improve health outcomes (Boutwell & Hwu, 2009, p. 14).

Interventions	Rationales
1. If chronic alcoholism is suspected, refer also to Alcohol Withdrawal Syndrome Care Plan.	1. Undetected alcoholism can result in fatal withdrawal symptoms.

2. Monitor for ascites.
  a. Increased abdominal girth
  b. Rapid weight gain
	2. Obstruction of blood flow in the portal vein increases hydrostatic pressure in the peritoneal capillaries and decreased albumin decreases osmotic pressure; both of which cause the fluid shift into the peritoneal cavity (Porth, 2011).

3. Explain need for dietary salt restriction. Access a dietary consult.	3. Dietary salt should be restricted to a no-added salt diet of 90 mmol salt/day (5.2 g salt/day).
4. Explain to client that salt restriction will help control ascites and prevent or reduce the need for paracentesis.	4. Dietary sodium restriction (2,000 mg/day) and diuretics (oral spironolactone with or without oral furosemide) has been shown to be effective in more than 90% of clients in achieving a reduction in the volume of ascites (Runyon, 2009).
5. Consult with physician / NP to determine if fluid restriction is indicated.	5. Fluid restriction is not necessary unless serum sodium is less than 120–125 mmol/L.
6. Promote ambulation with individuals with uncomplicated ascites as tolerated.	6. There have been no clinical studies to demonstrate increased efficacy of diuresis with bed rest or decreased duration of hospitalization.

(continued)

Interventions	Rationales

7. Explain paracentesis if needed for comfort and / or diagnostic purposes.

> **CLINICAL ALERT**
> • Cirrhotic clients should undergo diagnostic paracentesis in cases of unexplained fever, abdominal pain, or encephalopathy or when admitted to the hospital for any cause (Runyon, 2009).

7. Abdominal paracentesis should be performed and ascetic fluid should be obtained with clinically apparent new-onset ascites for analysis of cell count and total protein, serum-ascites albumin gradient (SAGG), and cultures if infection is suspected (Runyon, 2009).

8. Monitor for refractory ascites and the need for serial therapeutic paracentesis:
   a. Temperature greater than 37.8° C (100° F)
   b. Abdominal pain and / or tenderness
   c. A change in mental status
   d. Ascitic fluid PMN count ≥250 cells/mm^3

8. "Refractory ascites is defined as fluid overload that (1) is unresponsive to sodium-restricted diet and high-dose diuretic treatment (400 mg/day spironolactone and 160 mg/day furosemide) or (2) recurs rapidly after therapeutic paracentesis. Serial therapeutic paracentesis are effective in controlling ascites, performed approximately every two weeks control ascites" (Runyon, 2009, p. 2094).

9. Evaluate and record paracentesis aspirate.

9. The character and color can assist with the etiology (Cesario, Choure, & Carrey, 2012).

Translucent or straw-colored	Normal / sterile
Brown	Hyperbilirubinemia (most common)
Gallbladder or biliary perforation	
Cloudy or turbid	Infection, malignancy, pancreatitis
Pink or blood tinged	Mild trauma at the site
Grossly bloody	Malignancy
Abdominal trauma	
Milky ("chylous")	Cirrhosis, pancreatitis
Thoracic duct injury	
Lymphoma, ruptured lymphatic vessels	
Green	Ruptured bowel, perforated bile duct

> **CLINICAL ALERT**
> • Spontaneous bacterial peritonitis (SBP) is defined as an ascitic fluid infection without an evident intra-abdominal surgically treatable source; it occurs primarily in clients with advanced cirrhosis. Empiric therapy of suspected SBP must be initiated as soon as possible to maximize the client's chance of survival. Immediately report changes in mental status, temperature and new onset abdominal pain / tenderness.

Interventions	*Rationales*
10. Monitor for hepatic encephalopathy.	10. Hepatic (portosystemic) encephalopathy represents a potentially reversible decrease in neuropsychiatric function caused by acute and chronic liver disease, occurring predominantly in clients with portal hypertension. Profound liver failure results in accumulation of ammonia and other identical toxic metabolites in the blood. The blood–brain barrier permeability increases, and both toxins and plasma proteins leak from capillaries to the extracellular space, causing cerebral edema.

CLINICAL ALERT
- Continually assess for causes of hepatic encephalopathy include constipation, infection, gastrointestinal bleeding, certain medications, electrolyte imbalances, and noncompliance with medical therapy (Starr & Raines, 2011).

Interventions	*Rationales*

11. Identify and correct the precipitating causes (Heidelbaugh & Sherbondy, 2006):
  a. Assess vital signs, urine output, electrolyte levels
  b. Hemacult stools
	11a. Volumes status must be monitored.
	  b. Gastrointestinal bleeding can cause hepatic encephalopathy.

12. Screen for hypoxia, hypoglycemia, anemia, hypokalemia, metabolic alkalosis, and other potential metabolic or endocrine factors; report abnormals.	
13. Initiate ammonia-lowering therapy as prescribed: a. Use nasogastric lavage, lactulose, and / or other modalitiesto remove source of ammonia from the gut.	13. The nitrogenous level in the GI tract needs reducing.

14. Monitor for hepatorenal syndrome.
  a. Serum creatinine >1.5mg/dL
  b. No improvement of serum creatinine (decrease to a level of 1.5 mg/dL or less) after at least two days with diuretic withdrawal and with volume expansion with 1.5 L isotonic saline.
	14. The pathogenesis of hepatorenal syndrome is not completely understood, but is probably the result of an extreme underfilling of the arterial circulation secondary to arterial vasodilation in the splanchnic circulation.

15. Initiate treatment as prescribed (e.g., vasoactive medications as octreotide, midodrine, and albumin infusion).	15. Albumin is utilized for plasma volume expansion and maintenance of cardiac output. Studies show improvement in renal function and natriuresis (renal excretion of water and sodium) (Runyon, 2009).
16. Determine if there is current or recent treatment with nephrotoxic drugs.	

CLINICAL ALERT
- Hepatorenal syndrome is defined as a rapid deterioration of renal function indicated by a twofold increase of serum creatinine to values above 2.5 mg/dL (221 μmol/L), or a decrease of creatinine clearance to values below 20 mL per minute (0.33 mL/second). This form of hepatorenal syndrome usually is precipitated by spontaneous bacterial peritonitis and occurs in approximately 25% of clients with spontaneous bacterial peritonitis, even with the clearance of infection.

(*continued*)

Interventions	Rationales
17. Monitor for portal hypertension and bleeding. **CLINICAL ALERT** • "The development of portal hypertension is nearly universal regardless of the etiology of cirrhosis and results from an increased resistance to portal flow secondary to scarring, narrowing, and compression of the hepatic sinusoids. When the portal pressure exceeds a certain threshold, it results in the development of varices. Approximately 50 percent of clients with cirrhosis develop varices, most commonly in the distal 2 to 5 cm of the esophagus." (Heidelbaugh & Sherbondy, 2006, p. 4)	17. The liver has a primary role in hemostasis. Impaired production of new platelets from the bone marrow. Results in decreased platelet count. In addition, the synthesis of coagulation factors (II, V, VII, IX, and X) is impaired, resulting in bleeding, frequently in the upper GI tract. Other sites are nasopharynx, lungs, retroperitoneal, kidneys, and intracranial and skin puncture sites (Porth, 2011).
18. Monitor for bleeding from esophageal varices: a. Hematemesis (vomiting blood) b. Melena (black, sticky stools)	18. Portal hypertension caused by obstruction of the portal venous system results in increased pressure on the vessels in the esophagus, making them fragile (Porth, 2011).
19. Teach the client to report unusual bleeding (e.g., in the mouth after brushing teeth) and ecchymotic areas.	19. Mucous membranes are more prone to injury because of their great surface vascularity.
20. Monitor for signs and symptoms of (refer to index under each electrolyte for specific signs and symptoms): a. Hypoglycemia b. Hyponatremia c. Hypokalemia d. Hypocalcemia e. Hypomagnesemia f. Hypophosphatemia	20a. Hypoglycemia is caused by loss of glycogen stores in the liver from damaged cells, and decreased serum concentrations of glucose, insulin, and growth hormones. b. Reduced capacity of kidneys to excrete water results in dilutional hyponatremia. c. Potassium losses are from vomiting, nasogastric suctioning, diuretics, or excessive renal losses. d. Hypomagnesemia or pancreatitis can decrease calcium levels. e. The loss of potassium ions causes the proportional loss of magnesium ions. f. Increased phosphate loss, transcellular shifts, and decreased phosphate intake contribute to hypophosphatemia.
21. Monitor for acid–base disturbances.	21. Hepatocellular necrosis can result in accumulation of organic anions resulting in metabolic acidosis. Persons with ascites often have metabolic alkalosis from increased bicarbonate levels resulting from increased sodium / hydrogen exchange in distal tubule (Porth, 2011).
22. Assess for adverse effects of medications in the presence of impaired liver function. a. Evaluate the medications that require: • Reduced doses because they decrease metabolizing enzymes (cimetidine, rantidine, diazepam, lorazepam, morphine, meperidine, phenytoin, verapamil, ketoconzole, fluoxetine) • Increased dosing because they increase metabolizing enzymes e.g., rifampin, phenobrbital b. Monitor for hypertension	22. Most medications are metabolized by enzymes in the liver. b. Fluid retention and overload can cause hypertension.
23. If individual is in end-stage hepatic failure, consult physician / NP regarding the need for palliative care. Refer to Palliative Care Plan.	

Clinical Alert Report

Prior to providing care, advise ancillary staff / student to report the following to the professional nurse assigned to the client:

- Temperature >37.8° C (100° F)
- Resting pulse >100, <50
- New irregular pulse
- Systolic BP >200 mm Hg or <9 mm Hg
- Diastolic BP >90
- Oxygenation saturation <90%
- Weight gain
- Any change in mental status
- C/o of abdominal pain / tenderness
- Observed tremors
- Urine output for shift or hourly if indicated
- Hemoptasis, streaks of blood in stools, dark stools
- Prolonged bleeding for venipuncture sites
- Reports of bleeding gums, excess menstrual bleeding

Related Physician / NP Prescribed Interventions

Medications

Vitamin / mineral supplement, lactulose, digestive enzymes, potassium-sparing diuretics, vasodilators, electrolyte replacements

Intravenous Therapy

Hyperalimentation

Laboratory Studies

Blood urea nitrogen (BUN); serum bilirubin, albumin, prealbumin; serum ammonia; serum glutamic-oxaloacetic transaminase (SGOT), serum glutamic-pyruvic transaminase, lactate dehydrogenase (LDH); serum glucose; electrolytes; urine urobilinogen; alkaline phosphatase; aspartate aminotransferase (AST); IgA, IgG; alanine aminotransferase (ALT); CBC; prothrombin time

Diagnostic Studies

Liver scan, percutaneous transhepatic cholangiography, liver biopsy, chest x-ray film, esophagogastroduo-denoscopy, upper GI series, CT scan, MRI

Therapies

Diet (high-calorie, low-fat, moderate-protein, low-salt); oxygen via cannula; fluid restrictions; therapeutic paracentesis, enteral feedings, transjugular intrahepatic portosystemic shunt (TIPS)

Documentation

Weight
Vital signs
Stools for occult blood
Urine specific gravity
Intake and output
Evidence of bleeding
Evidence of tremors or confusion

Nursing Diagnoses

Imbalanced Nutrition: Less Than Body Requirements Related to Anorexia, Impaired Protein, Fat, and Glucose Metabolism, and Impaired Storage of Vitamins (A, C, K, D, E)

NOC
Nutritional Status,
Knowledge: Diet

NIC
Nutrition Management,
Nutrition Monitoring

Goal

1. The client will describe the reasons for nutritional problems.
2. The client will relate which foods are high in protein and calories.
3. The client will gain weight (specify amount) without increased edema.
4. The client will explain the rationale for sodium restrictions.

Interventions	Rationales
1. Discuss the causes of anorexia, dyspepsia, and nausea. Explain that obstructed hepatic blood flow causes GI vascular congestion (which results in gastritis and diarrhea or constipation), and that impaired liver function causes metabolic disturbances (fluid, electrolyte, glucose metabolism), resulting in anorexia and fatigue.	1. Helping the client understand the condition can reduce anxiety and may help improve compliance.
2. Explain the treatment consists of avoidance of alcohol, excess fat intake and having 4–6 small meals of carbohydrates and protein daily. Request a Nutritional Consult.	2. Careful balancing of protein intake is required. Protein is required, however ammonia is produced when digestive enzymes breakdown protein. Excessive ammonia causes hepatic encephalopathy (Lutz & Przytulski, 2011).
3. Teach and assist the client to rest before meals.	3. Fatigue further decreases the desire to eat.
4. Offer frequent small feedings (six per day plus snacks).	4. Increased intra-abdominal pressure from ascites compresses the GI tract and reduces its capacity.
5. Restrict liquids with meals and avoid fluids 1 hour before and after meals.	5. Fluids can overdistend the stomach, decreasing appetite and intake.
6. Arrange to have foods with the highest protein / calorie content served at the time the client feels most like eating.	6. This increases the likelihood of the client consuming adequate amounts of protein and calories.
7. Teach the client measures to reduce nausea. Refer to Nausea nursing diagnosis in Unit II.	7. Venous congestion in the GI tract predisposes the client to nausea.

Documentation

Weight
Intake (type, amount)
Abdominal girth

Impaired Comfort Related to Pruritus Secondary to Accumulation of Bilirubin Pigment and Bile Salts

NOC
Symptom Control

NIC
Pruritus Management,
Fever Treatment,
Environmental
Management: Comfort

Goal

The client will verbalize decreased pruritus.

Indicators

- Describe factors that increase pruritus.
- Describe factors that improve pruritus.

Interventions	Rationales
1. Maintain hygiene without causing dry skin: a. Give frequent baths using cool water and mild soap (castile, lanolin) or a soap substitute. b. Blot skin dry; do not rub.	1. Dryness increases skin sensitivity by stimulating nerve endings.
2. Prevent excessive warmth by maintaining cool room temperatures and low humidity, using light covers with a bed cradle, and avoiding overdressing.	2. Excessive warmth aggravates pruritus by increasing sensitivity through vasodilation.
3. Advise against scratching; explain the scratch-itch-scratch cycle. Instruct the client to apply firm pressure to pruritic areas instead of scratching.	3. Scratching stimulates histamine release, which produces more pruritus.
4. Consult with the physician / NP for a pharmacologic treatment (e.g., antihistamines, antipruritic lotions), if necessary.	4. If pruritus is unrelieved or if the skin is excoriated from scratching, topical or systemic medications are indicated.
5. Keep room cool and with humidity at 30%–40%.	5. Coolness will reduce vasodilation, and humidity will reduce dryness.

Documentation

Progress notes
Unrelieved pruritus
Excoriated skin

Excess Fluid Volume Related to Portal Hypertension, Lowered Plasma Colloidal Osmotic Pressure, and Sodium Retention

NOC
Electrolyte Balance,
Fluid Balance, Hydration

Goal

1. The client will relate actions that decrease fluid retention.
2. The client will list foods high in sodium.

NIC
Electrolyte Management,
Fluid Management,
Fluid Monitoring, Skin
Surveillance

Interventions	Rationales
1. Assess the client's diet for inadequate protein or excessive sodium intake.	1, 2. Decreased renal flow results in increased aldosterone and antidiuretic hormone secretion, causing water and sodium retention and potassium excretion.
2. Encourage the client to decrease salt intake. Teach the client to take the following actions: a. Read food labels for sodium content. b. Avoid convenience foods, canned foods, and frozen foods. c. Cook without salt, and use spices (e.g., lemon, basil, tarragon, mint) to add flavor. d. Use vinegar instead of salt to flavor soups, stews, etc. (e.g., 2–3 teaspoons of vinegar to 4–6 quarts of soup, according to taste).	
3. Ascertain with the physician if the client may use a salt substitute. Avoid substitutes containing ammonium.	3. Ammonium elevates serum ammonia levels and may contribute to hepatic coma.

(continued)

Interventions	Rationales
4. Take measures to protect edematous skin from injury:	4. Edematous skin is taut and easily injured. Dry skin is more vulnerable to breakdown and injury.
5. Inspect the skin for redness and blanching.	
6. Reduce pressure on skin (e.g., pad chairs and footstools).	
7. Prevent dry skin by using soap sparingly, rinsing off soap completely, and using a lotion to moisten skin.	

Documentation

Progress notes
Presence of edema

> **TRANSITION TO HOME / COMMUNITY CARE**
> If indicated, review the risk diagnoses identified for this individual on admission:
> - Is he person still at risk?
> - Can the family reduce the risks?
> - Is the person at higher risk at home?
> - Is a Home Health Nurse assessment needed?
> - Refer to transition planner / case manager / social service
> - When is this person scheduled for follow-up with primary provider? Specialists? Record dates of appts.
> - Complete a medication reconciliation prior to transition. Refer to index.

STAR

Stop

Think   Is this person at risk for injury, falls, medical complications, and / or inability to care for self (activities of daily living)?
Is there a support person available?
Is the person competent to manage self-administration of medications, treatment procedures? Are additional resources needed?
Can the person explain how to monitor condition (e.g., blood glucose, sign / symptoms of complications, dietary / mobility restrictions, and when to call his / her primary provider or specialist)?

Act   Contact or provide the appropriate resource (e.g., contacting a support person, home health assessment, additional teaching, printed materials).

Review   Has the problem been addressed? If not, use SBAR to communicate to the appropriate person.

High Risk for Ineffective Self-Health Management Related to Lack of Knowledge of Pharmacologic Contraindications, Nutritional Requirements, Signs and Symptoms of Complications, and Risks of Alcohol Ingestion

NOC
Compliance Behavior, Knowledge: Treatment Regimen, Participation in Health Care Decisions, Treatment Behavior: Illness or Injury

Goal

The goals for this diagnosis represent those associated with transition planning. Refer to the transitional criteria.

NIC
Anticipatory Guidance, Risk Identification, Health Education, Learning Facilitation

Interventions	Rationales
1. Teach the client or family about the condition and its causes and treatments.	1. This teaching reinforces the need to comply with the therapeutic regimen, including diet and activity restrictions.
2. Explain portal system encephalopathy to the family. Teach them to observe for and report any confusion, tremors, night wandering, or personality changes.	2. Confusion and altered speech patterns result from cerebral hypoxia because of high serum ammonia levels caused by the liver's impaired ability to convert ammonia to urea. Family members typically first note the development of encephalopathy.

CLINICAL ALERT
- The onset often is insidious and is characterized by subtle and sometimes intermittent changes in memory, personality, concentration, and reaction times. Hepatic encephalopathy is a diagnosis of exclusion; therefore, all other etiologies of altered mental status must be effectively ruled out. (Starr & Raines, 2011)

Interventions	Rationales
3. Explain the risk of osteoporosis. Advise to discuss the need for a dexa scan with primary care provider.	3. Some studies have shown increased bone resorption, in the presence of chronic liver disease, whereas most others have shown decreased bone formation (Collier, Ninkovic & Compston, 2002).
4. Advise of lifestyle choices that can prevent osteoporosis as adequate calcium intake, Supplementation with calcium (1 g/day) + vitamin D_3 (800 U/day), regular weight-bearing exercise, avoidance of alcohol and tobacco smoking.	4. Many studies have shown low serum levels of 25-hydroxyvitamin D in clients with chronic liver disease and levels fall with disease progression in cirrhosis. This may be due to reduced exposure to UV light and dietary insufficiency. The presence of jaundice will impair cutaneous synthesis of vitamin D (Collier, Ninkovic & Compston, 2002).
5. Explain the hazards of certain medications, including narcotics, sedatives, tranquilizers, and ammonia products.	5. Impaired liver function slows the metabolism of some drugs, causing levels to accumulate and increasing toxicity.
6. Teach the client or family to watch for and report signs and symptoms of complications: a. Bleeding (gums, stools), prolonged, heavy period b. Hypokalemia (muscle cramps, nausea, vomiting) c. Rapid weight loss or gain	6. Progressive liver failure affects hematopoietic function and electrolyte and fluid balance, causing potentially serious complications that require prompt intervention. a. Bleeding indicates decreased platelets and clotting factors. b. Hypokalemia results from overproduction of aldosterone, which causes sodium and water retention and potassium excretion. c. Rapid weight loss points to negative nitrogen balance; weight gain, points to fluid retention.
7. Explain the need to avoid alcohol. Refer to D&A program if indicated.	7. Alcoholism is a complex physiologic, psychological, and social disorder.
8. Explain to individual risk for development of sudden bacterial per (SBP), that prophylactic antibiotics must be taken every day to prevent infection and resistant organism.	8. Successful prevention of SBP has been reported in individuals with low-protein ascites and prior SBP (Runyon, 2009).
9. Stress the importance of follow-up care and laboratory studies.	9. Timely follow-up enables evaluation of liver function and early detection of relapse or recurrence.

Documentation

> Flow records
> > Client teaching
> > Referrals when indicated
> Progress notes
> > Unachieved outcomes

Diabetes Mellitus

Diabetes mellitus is a chronic disease of abnormal glucose metabolism requiring lifelong management through nutrition, exercise, and often medication. Of the 25.8 million Americans who have diabetes, 18.8 million are diagnosed, 7 million are undiagnosed, and 79 million are prediabetes. Uncontrolled diabetes affects all body systems, causing serious complications such as retinopathy, nephropathy, neuropathy, and vascular disease. The diagnosis of diabetes is made based on: two fasting plasma glucose measurements greater than or equal to 126 mg/dL; a 2-hour plasma glucose ≥ 200 mg/dL after an oral glucose tolerance test; classic symptoms of diabetes—polyuria, polydipsia, unexplained weight loss—and a random plasma glucose of ≥ 200 mg/dL; or an A1C $\geq 6.5\%$ (American Diabetes Association, 2012a).

The classification of diabetes includes four clinical classes: type 1 diabetes, which results from beta cell destruction leading to absolute insulin deficiency; type 2 diabetes, which results from an insulin secretory defect coupled with insulin resistance; gestational diabetes (GDM) occurs during pregnancy; and other diabetes due to other causes such as genetic defects, chemical induced, diseases of exocrine pancreas.

The causative factor of type 1 diabetes is an autoimmune destruction of the beta cell and accounts for less than 10% of all diabetes diagnoses. The cause of the more prevalent type 2 diabetes, accounting for over 90% of diabetes diagnoses, is multifactorial including genetic and environmental influences. Risk factors for type 2 diabetes include family history of the disease, age, obesity, and inactivity (American Diabetes Association, 2012a).

■■■■■■ DIAGNOSTIC CLUSTER

Collaborative Problems

▲ Risk for Complications of Diabetic Ketoacidosis – DKA (type 1)

▲ Risk for Complications of Hyperosmolar Hyperglycemic State – HHS (type 2)

▲ Risk for Complications of Hypoglycemia

▲ Risk for Complications of Infections

▲ Risk for Complications of Vascular Disease

▲ Risk for Complications of Neuropathy

▲ Risk for Complications of Retinopathy

▲ Risk for Complications of Nephropathy

Nursing Diagnoses

▲ Imbalanced Nutrition: More Than Body Requirements related to intake in excess of activity expenditures, lack of knowledge, or ineffective coping

△ Risk for Ineffective Self-Health Management related to insufficient knowledge of disease process, self-monitoring of blood glucose, medications, nutrition and meal planning, recognition and treatment of hypoglycemia, weight control, sick day care, exercise, foot care, signs and symptoms of complications, and the need for comprehensive diabetes outpatient education

▲ This diagnosis was reported to be monitored for or managed frequently (75%–100%).
△ This diagnosis was reported to be monitored for or managed often (50%–74%).

Transition Criteria

Before transition, the client or family will

1. Define diabetes as a chronic disease requiring lifelong management through nutrition, exercise, and usually, medications for control.
2. Identify carbohydrates as foods that affect blood glucose, and create a meal using the plate method.
3. State the relationship of food and exercise to blood glucose (BG).
4. State the effects of weight loss on BG control with type 2 diabetes.
6. State the value of monitoring BG and knowledge of normal blood glucose values.
7. Demonstrate the ability to perform self blood glucose monitoring and knowledge of obtaining testing supplies.
8. Explain the importance of foot care and regular assessments.
9. Describe self-care measures that may prevent or delay progression of chronic complications (microvascular, macrovascular, neuropathy).
10. Agree to attend comprehensive outpatient diabetes education programs.

For Clients Requiring Medications

Oral Agents

1. State name, dose, action, potential side effects, and schedule to take diabetes medications.
2. State risk of hypoglycemia with delayed meals or increased activities.
3. State signs, symptoms, and treatment of hypoglycemia.
4. State intent to wear diabetes identification.
5. Describe self-care measures during illness.

Insulin

1. Demonstrate technique for insulin administration.
2. State brand, type, onset, peak, duration, and dose of insulin.
3. State recommendations for site rotation, storage of insulin, and disposal of syringes.
4. State signs, symptoms, and treatment of hypoglycemia.
5. State intent to wear diabetes identification.
6. Describe self-care measures during illness.

Transitional Risk Assessment Plan (TRAP)

Begin this plan on admission.
Implement the Transitional Risk Assessment Plan (TRAP):
- Refer to inside back cover.
- Add each validated risk diagnosis to client's problem list with the risk code in ( ).
- Refer to Unit II to the individual risk nursing diagnoses / collaborative problems for outcomes and interventions.

R: "Close coordination of care in the post-acute period, early discharge follow-up care, enhanced patient education and self-management training, proactive end-of-life counseling, and extending the resources and clinical expertise over time via multidisciplinary team management" can lower readmission rates and improve health outcomes (Boutwell & Hwu, 2009, p. 14).

Collaborative Problems

Risk for Complications of Diabetic Ketoacidosis (DKA)

Risk for Complications of Hyperosmolar Hyperglycemic State

Risk for Complications of Hypoglycemia

Risk for Complications of Infections

Risk for Complications of Vascular Disease

Risk for Complications of Neuropathy

Risk for Complications of Retinopathy

Risk for Complications of Nephropathy

Collaborative Outcomes

The client will be monitored for early signs and symptoms of (a) diabetic ketoacidosis, (b) hyperosmolar hyperglycemic state, (c) hypoglycemia, (d) infections, (e) vascular, (f) neurological, (g) retinal, and (h) renal complications, and will receive collaborative interventions if indicated to restore physiolog stability.

Indicators of Physiologic Stability

- pH 7.35–7.45 and HCO3 18–22 mmol/L (a, b)
- Fasting blood glucose 70–130 mg/dL (a, b, c)
- No ketones in urine (a, b)
- Serum sodium 135–145 mmol/L (a, b, h)
- Serum osmolality, ≥295 m Osm/kg (a, b, h)
- BP <130/80 (e)
- Clear, oriented (a, b, e, f)
- Pulse 60–100 beats/min (e)
- Respiration 16–20 breaths/min (a, b, e)
- Peripheral pulses, equal and full, capillary refill <3 seconds (e)
- Warm, dry skin (a, b, e)
- No vision changes (f, g)
- Bowel sounds, present (f)
- White blood cells 4,000–10,800 mm (d)
- Urine, protein-negative (h)
- Creatinine 0.8–1.3 mg/dL (h)
- Blood urea nitrogen 5–25mg/dL (h)

Interventions	Rationales

1. Monitor for signs and symptoms of diabetic ketoacidosis (DKA) with type 1 diabetes:
  a. Recent illness / infection
  b. Blood glucose >300 mg/dL
  c. Malaise and generalized weakness
  d. Moderate / large ketones
  e. Dehydration
  f. Anorexia, nausea, vomiting, abdominal pain
  g. Kussmaul's respirations (shallow, rapid)
  h. Fruity acetone odor of the breath
  i. pH <7.30 and HCO3 <15 meq
  j. Decreased sodium, potassium, phosphates
	1. When insulin is not available, blood glucose (BG) levels rise and the body metabolizes fat for energy; the byproduct of this fat metabolism is ketones. Excessive ketone bodies results in ketoacidosis and a drop in PH and bicarbonate serum levels. This acidosis causes headaches, nausea, vomiting, and abdominal pain. Increased respiratory rate helps CO_2 excretion in effort to reduce acidosis. Elevated glucose levels inhibit water reabsorption in the renal glomerulus, leading to osmotic diuresis with loss of water, sodium, potassium, and phosphates, leading to severe dehydration and electrolyte imbalance (Vasudevan, 2012).

2. Monitor for signs and symptoms of hyperosmolar hyperglycemic state (HHS) type 2:
  a. Blood glucose >600 mg/dL
  b. pH >7.30 and HCO3 >15 mEq/L
  c. Severe dehydration
  d. Serum osmolality >320 mOsm/kg
  e. Hypotension
  f. Altered sensorium
	2. Hyperosmolar hyperglycemic state is marked by profound dehydration and hyperglycemia without ketoacidosis. Decreased renal clearance and utilization of glucose result in an osmotic dieresis and osmotic shift of fluid to the intravascular space, resulting in intracellular dehydration and loss of electrolytes. Cerebral impairment is due to this intracellular dehydration (Hemphill et al., 2012).

3. Monitor for signs and symptoms of hypoglycemia:
  a. Blood glucose <70 mg/dL
  b. Pale, moist, cool skin
  c. Tachycardia, diaphoresis
  d. Jitteriness, irritability
  e. Confusion
  f. Drowsiness
  g. Hypoglycemia unawareness
	3. Hypoglycemia unawareness is a defect in the body's defense system that impairs the ability to experience the warning symptoms usually associated with hypoglycemia. The client may rapidly progress from being alert to unconsciousness.

CLINICAL ALERT

- Hypoglycemia is defined as any BG <70 mg/dL and may be caused by too much insulin, too little food, or too much physical activity. Hypoglycemia symptoms are related to sympathetic system stimulation and brain dysfunction related to decreased levels of glucose. Sympathoadrenal activation and release of adrenaline causes diaphoresis, cool skin, tachycardia, anxiety, and jitteriness. Reduction in cerebral glucose will result in confusion, difficulty with concentration, focal impairments, and if severe, can cause seizures and eventually coma and death (Hamdy, 2012).

CLINICAL ALERT

- Treatment of hypoglycemia is considered emergent.

(continued)

Interventions	Rationales
4. Institute "Rule of 15" with a goal to achieve BG >100 mg/dL:	

4. Institute "Rule of 15" with a goal to achieve
BG >100 mg/dL:
   a. If individual is alert and cooperative: give 15 g of carbohydrate orally and monitor for 15 minutes; repeat BG—if above 100 mg/dL may give light snack if not time for a meal. If not above 70 mg/dL, repeat treatment with 15 g of carbohydrate—monitor and recheck BG in 15 minutes and may repeat until at goal.
   b. Nonalert individual: Call for Help—if IV access, give 24 g dextrose (1 amp D50); if none, give 1 mg glucagon IM, monitor for 15 minutes, and repeat BG; may repeat treatment q15–30 minutes depending on response.
   c. If hypoglycemia is severe (BG <40), recurrent, or caused by sulfonylurea or long-acting insulin, follow D50 treatment with D5 or D10 drip.
   d. Continued follow-up is mandatory until individual is stable. Cause of the hypoglycemia should always be investigated (Inzucchi, 2012).

Interventions	Rationales
5. Monitor for signs and symptoms of infection. Refer to Risk for Infection in Unit II for preventive intervention. a. Upper respiratory tract infection b. Urinary tract infection c. Otitis media d. Red, painful, or warm skin e. Furunculosis, carbuncles	5. Infection is the primary cause of metabolic abnormalities in individuals with diabetes. Increased glucose in epidermis and urine promotes bacterial growth. The early diagnosis and prompt treatment of infection are essential to prevent issues that can lead to major complications (e.g., cellulitis spreading to the bone necessitating amputations) (Edelman & Henry, 2011).
6. Assess for risk factors and monitor for signs and symptoms of macrovascular complications: a. Family history of heart disease b. Male: over age 40 c. Cigarette smoker d. Hypertension e. Hyperlipidemia f. Obesity g. Uncontrolled diabetes	6. Diabetes is associated with severe degenerative vascular changes; heart disease is the number one cause of death for people with diabetes. Lesions of the blood vessels strike at an earlier age and tend to produce more severe pathologic changes. Early atherosclerotic changes are probably caused by high blood glucose and lipid levels characteristic of persistent hyperglycemia. Atherosclerosis leads to premature coronary artery disease.
7. Monitor for signs and symptoms of retinopathy: a. Blurred vision b. Black spots c. "Cobwebs" d. Sudden loss of vision e. Floaters	7. Retinopathy does not cause visual symptoms until at a fairly advanced stage, usually when macular edema or proliferative retinopathy has occurred. The incidence and severity of retinopathy are thought to be related to the duration and the degree of control of blood glucose as well as blood pressure (NIH, 2012).
8. Monitor for signs and symptoms of peripheral neuropathy: a. Pain, burning sensation in feet, legs b. Decreased sensation, numbness in feet, fingers c. Decreased deep tendon response (Achilles and patella) d. Charcot's foot ulcer e. Decreased proprioception f. Paresthesia	8. Sensory symptoms usually predominate and include numbness, tingling, pain, or loss of sensation in feet. This nerve damage may lead to long-term chronic pain, ulcers, and eventually amputation. Current treatments include improved control of blood glucose and use of antidepressant drugs as well as aldose reductase inhibitors.

Interventions	Rationales

9. Monitor for signs and symptoms of autonomic neuropathy:
  a. Orthostatic hypotension
  b. Impotence
  c. Abnormal sweating
  d. Bladder paralysis
  e. Nocturnal diarrhea
  f. Gastroparesis
	9. Automonic nervous system modulates many body functions, both parasympathetic or sympathetic. The degree of autonomic dysfunction may be clinically irrelevant or symptoms may be disabling (Vinik et al., 2003).

10. Monitor for signs and symptoms of nephropathy:
  a. Proteinuria, casts in urine
  b. Abnormal BUN and creatinine
  c. Urine for microalbumin, goal <30 mg
  d. Urine for proteinuria >300 mg albumin
	10. In nephropathy, the capillary basement membrane thickens, due to chronic filtering of high glucose. The membrane becomes more permeable, causing increased loss of blood proteins in urine. Increased filtration requirements increase the pressure in renal blood vessels, contributing to sclerosis.

11. Consult with the physician to order a 24-hour urine test.	11. Clinical manifestations of nephropathy occur late in the disease. Proteinuria is the first sign of the disorder. If urine is positive for protein, then a 24-hour quantitative measure with a CrCl is important to obtain. When decreased kidney function is identified early, more aggressive therapy may be initiated to prevent or slow progression to overt kidney failure (Edelman & Henry 2011).
12. Carefully monitor blood pressure.	12. Aggressive blood pressure control can reduce proteinuria and delay the progression of renal damage (American Diabetes Association, 2012a).

13. Teach the client about the risk factors that may contribute to renal damage:
  a. Uncontrolled blood glucose
  b. Hypertension
  c. Neurogenic bladder
  d. Urethral instrumentation
  e. Urinary tract infection
  f. Nephrotoxic drugs
  g. Making the client aware of risk factors may help to reduce renal impairment.	

Clinical Alert Report

Prior to providing care, advise ancillary staff / student to report the following to the professional nurse assigned to the client:

- Signs and symptoms of infection: elevated temperature, reddened skin, odor or discharge from surgical sites or injuries
- Blood glucose >300 mg/dL or <70 mg/dL
- Nausea and vomiting
- Change in mental status / behavior
- Decrease in urine output

Related Physician / NP Prescribed Interventions

Medications

Orals:

Sulfonylureas, biguanides, thiazolidinediones, alpha-glucosidase inhibitors, meglitinide, DPP-4 inhibitors, combinations

Injectables:

Insulin: Rapid acting analogues (aspart, lispro, glulisine), regular (R), intermediate (NPH), long-acting analogues (glargine, detemir), premixed combinations, insulin pumps

Mimetics: GLP-1 agonists (exenatide, liraglutide), amylin (symlin)

Intravenous Therapy

For hypoglycemic emergencies:

25 g dextrose IV (1 amp D50)

D5, D10 solution

Laboratory Studies

Blood glucose (BG), serum osmolality, 24-hour urine for protein, albumin, and creatinine, creatinine clearance, glomerular filtration rate (GFR), electrolytes, oral glucose tolerance test (OGTT), glycosylated hemoglobin $HgbA_{Ic}$, fructosamine (use to monitor only persons with anemia and diabetes mellitus)

Diagnostic Studies

Fasting blood glucose, glucose tolerance test

Therapies

Self-monitoring blood glucose (SMBG), meal plan, exercise

Documentation

Vital signs

Blood glucose

$HgbA_{Ic}$

BUN / creatinine

Lipid profile

> Date last eye exam
> Date last 24-hour urine test

Client complications

Abnormal labs

Episodes of hypoglycemia

Changes in medications

TRANSITION TO HOME / COMMUNITY CARE

If indicated, review the risk diagnoses identified for this individual on admission:

- Is he person still at risk?
- Can the family reduce the risks?
- Is the person at higher risk at home?
- Is a Home Health Nurse assessment needed?
- Refer to transition planner / case manager / social service
- When is this person scheduled for follow-up with primary provider? Specialists? Record dates of appts.
- Complete a medication reconciliation prior to transition. Refer to index.

STAR   **Stop**

Think   Is this person at risk for injury, falls, medical complications, and / or inability to care for self (activities of daily living)?

Is there a support person available?

Is the person competent to manage self-administration of medications, treatment procedures?

Are additional resources needed?

Can the person explain how to monitor condition (e.g., blood glucose, sign / symptoms of complications, dietary / mobility restrictions, and when to call his or her primary provider or specialist?

Act   Contact or provide the appropriate resource (e.g., contacting a support person, home health assessment, additional teaching, printed materials).

Review   Has the problem been addressed? If not, use SBAR to communicate to the appropriate person.

Nursing Diagnoses

Risk for Ineffective Self-Health Management Related to Insufficient Knowledge of Diabetes, Monitoring of BG, Medications, Meal Planning, Treatment of Hypoglycemia, Weight Control, Sick Day Management, Exercise Routine, Foot Care, Risks of Complications

NOC

Compliance Behavior, Knowledge: Treatment Regimen, Participation in Health Care Decisions, Treatment Behavior: Illness or Injury

NIC

Anticipatory Guidance, Risk Identification, Learning Facilitation, Health Education, Teaching: Procedure / Treatment, Health System Guidance

Goal

The goals for this diagnosis represent those associated with transition planning. **Refer to the transition** criteria.

Interventions	Rationales
1. Explore with the client and significant others the actual or perceived effects of diabetes on: a. Finances b. Occupation (sick time) c. Lifestyle d. Energy level e. Relationships	1. Common frustrations associated with diabetes stem from problems involving the disease itself, the treatment regimen, and the health care system. Recognizing that these problems are common indicates a need to use anticipatory guidance to prevent the associated frustrations (Funnell, Kruger, & Spencer, 2004).
2. Instruct the client and family on the components of diabetes treatment—meal planning, monitoring, exercise, and medications: effective self-management and quality of life are the key outcomes of an education program (American Diabetes Association, 2012b).	

(continued)

Interventions	Rationales

3. Increase awareness of the role of uncontrolled diabetes in the development of complications:
  a. Chronic:
   • Coronary artery disease
   • Peripheral vascular disease
   • Retinopathy
   • Neuropathy
   • Nephropathy
  b. Acute:
   • Hypoglycemia
   • Hyperglycemia
   • Diabetic ketoacidosis
   • Hyperosmolar hyperglycemia state
	3. When teaching the risks of complications, stress the importance personal self-management and the responsibility of each individual to follow-up with health care provider, including ophthalmologic and podiatric specialists.

4. Teach the client the signs and symptoms of hyperglycemia:
  a. Blood glucose >200 mg/dL
  b. Polyuria
  c. Polydipsia
  d. Polyphagia
  e. Fatigue
  f. Blurred vision
  g. Weight loss
	4. Elevated BG causes dehydration from osmotic diuresis. Potassium is elevated because of hemoconcentration. Because carbohydrates are not metabolized, the client loses weight (Porth, 2011).

5. Teach the client the causes of hyperglycemia:
  a. Increased food intake
  b. Omitting oral medications
  c. Decreased insulin dosing
  d. Decreased exercise
  e. Infection / illness
  f. Dehydration
	5. Increased food intake requires increased insulin or exercise; otherwise hyperglycemia will ensue. Infections, illnesses, or both increase insulin requirements.

6. Discuss BG monitoring: its purpose, utilization of results, record keeping
  a. Advise the client to obtain a third-party reimbursement for BG monitoring supplies. Medicare will pay for BG supplies for anyone who has diabetes.
 	
  b. Discuss with the client his or her specific BG goal, the frequency of BG monitoring, and the value of recording the results.
  c. Teach the client the need for increased BG monitoring when meals are delayed, before exercise, and when sick, as these situations may change dietary or insulin requirements.
  d. Assist the client in identifying the brand, type, dosage, action, and side effects of prescribed medications for controlling diabetes.
  e. Advise the client about prescription drugs and over-the-counter remedies, such as cough syrups and throat lozenges that affect BG levels.
	6. BG monitoring assists clients to control diabetes by regulating food, exercise, and medications, and has become an essential component of diabetes management. BG monitoring has allowed flexible mealtimes, made strenuous exercise safe, and made successful pregnancy outcomes more likely.
	  b. BG records help the client and health care provider evaluate patterns of food intake, insulin administration, and exercise.
	
	  d. A client needs to know the dose, action, and side effects to make appropriate decisions for adjusting food intake and exercise.
	  e. Oral agents, insulin, glucagon, aspirin, and beta-adrenergic blockers decrease blood glucose; whereas corticosteroids, birth control pills, diuretics, and cold remedies containing decongestants increase BG.

Interventions	Rationales

7. Teach the client insulin administration and storage, including
  a. Measuring an accurate dose
  b. Mixing insulins
  c. Injecting insulin
  d. Rotating injection sites
  e. Refer the client and family to a community diabetes education program, the local American Diabetes Association and registered dietitian for medical nutrition therapy (MNT).
  f. Continued monitoring and teaching at home will be needed after transition.	

8. Discuss strategies to improve nutrition:
  a. Provide information regarding food groups: carbohydrates (CHO) which includes starches, starchy vegetables, milk, and fruit, protein group, and vegetables group. Instruct on use of the "plate method" as easy way of meal planning and maintaining healthy nutrition.
  b. Show the client and family a paper plate that is divided into quarter sections:
    • Fill ½ of plate with nonstarchy vegetables (lettuce, tomato, broccoli).
    • Fill ¼ with protein (meat, beans, fish, eggs).
    • Fill ¼ with starches (rice, potatoes, pasta, bread).
    • Add 1 cup of skim milk.
    • Add 1 piece of fruit.
  c. Teach the client to lower fat intake by:
    • Trimming fat off meat
    • Avoiding fried foods
    • Limiting salad dressings, selecting low fat
  d. Advise the client to:
    • Drink water. Limit diet soda, coffee, and tea. Avoid all sugar drinks (juice, soda, power drinks).
    • Eat breakfast every day (high-fiber cereal, low-fat milk)
    • Do not skip meals.
    • Make effort to eat same amount at each meal.
    • Avoid seconds.
    • Watch portion sizes.
	8. Balanced nutrition helps to maintain normal blood glucose level. The American Diabetes Association recommends an individualized meal plan based on client assessment. The "plate method," carbohydrate counting, and portion control are easy and acceptable methods of meal planning. Low-fat foods, water as a beverage, and portion controls of CHO and protein can reduce weight and lower BG.

9. Encourage the client to access self-management information at American Diabetes Association (www.diabetes.org), National Diabetes Education Program (www.ndep.nih.gov/diabetes), American Dietetic Association (www.eatright.org).	

(continued)

Interventions	Rationales
10. Teach recognition of the signs and symptoms of hypoglycemia to the client and family. • Sweaty • Tingling in hands, lips, and tongue • Cold, clammy, and pale skin. • Fast heartbeat, shakiness • Uncooperative, irritable, confused • Light-headed, dizzy • Slurred speech • Lack of motor coordination • Seizure or coma / convulsions	10. Early detection of hypoglycemia enables prompt intervention and may prevent serious complications. Insulin reaction, insulin shock, and hypoglycemia are all synonymous with low blood glucose (<70 mg/dL). Hypoglycemia may result from too much insulin, too little food, or too vigorous activity. Low BG may occur just before meal times, during or after exercise, and / or when insulin is at its peak action (American Diabetes Association, 2012a).

CLINICAL ALERT
• Hypoglycemia is sudden and can progress to seizures and loss of consciousness if untreated.

Interventions	Rationales
11. Teach the client and family appropriate treatment for hypoglycemia using the "Rule of 15" to achieve BG goal of >100 mg/dL: a. Take 15 g of carbohydrates (½ cup of juice, ½ cup regular soda, 3 tsp. jelly, 1 cup milk, 3 glucose tablets, 5 Lifesavers candy). b. Wait 15 minutes, test BG again. Take another 15 g of carbohydrates if BG is still not at goal. c. Glucose gel, honey, jelly on the inside of the cheek are treatments of choice for a semiconscious person or someone having difficulty in swallowing. d. If hypoglycemia is severe, loss of consciousness, having seizures, or the client cannot swallow, administer 1 mg of glucagon IM. Turn person onto side as treatment often causes nausea. If the client does not respond, seek emergency assistance. e. After BG >100 mg/dL, client may have a snack if not scheduled mealtime. f. Do not overtreat hypoglycemia with excessive carbohydrates.	11. Prescription glucagon is an injectable treatment for severe hypoglycemia. Glucagon should be prescribed for all individuals at significant risk of severe hypoglycemia. The stability of glucagon is short; therefore, it must be mixed just before use. Because glucagon must be administered by another person, the client's family or friends must be taught how to prepare and administer it in case of an emergency (American Diabetes Association, 2012b).

Interventions	Rationales
12. Teach the client to prevent hypoglycemia: a. Routine BG monitoring b. Schedule medications with meal times c. Schedule meals, never skip meals d. BG monitoring before exercise or strenuous activity e. Awareness of changes in daily routines that may precipitate hypoglycemia f. Carry some form of glucose at all times g. Never drink alcohol on an empty stomach (drink in moderation) h. Need to wear diabetes identification	

Interventions	Rationales
13. Teach the client the importance of achieving and maintaining normal weight. Refer to the Obesity Care Plan for specific strategies.	13. An obese client has fewer available insulin receptors. Weight loss restores the number of insulin receptors, making insulin more effective. Weight loss may also reduce or eliminate the need for oral agents.

Interventions	Rationales

14. Teach the client about Sick Day Treatment:
   a. Never fail to take diabetic medicine.
 	
   b. Monitor blood glucose every 3–4 hours. Test urine for ketones when two BG levels are >250 mg/dL (type 1).
 	
   c. Drink 6–8 ounces of water each hour.
   d. Immediate interventions are required to prevent dehydration and severe hyperglycemia.
	14. Anticipating the effects of illness on the BG level may alert the client to take precautions. Extra fluids help to prevent dehydration.
	   b. Early detection of ketones in urine can enable prompt intervention to prevent ketoacidosis. Clients with type 1 diabetes are susceptible to ketosis.

15. Call health care provider or seek emergency room care if:
   a. Vomiting or diarrhea persists for more than 6 hours
   b. Ketone values are moderate or large
   c. Fevers over 100 for > 24–48 hours
   d. Blood glucose levels are over 250 mg/dL consistently
   e. You do not know what to do	

16. Teach the client to take insulin or oral medications and maintain carbohydrate (CHO) intake when ill by substituting liquids or easily digested solids for regular food. Examples of CHO for sick days:
   a. Bread exchange = 15 g CHO
     • 1 slice bread or toast
     • ½ English muffin or ½ bagel (2 oz)
     • ½ cup cooked cereal
     • 6 saltines or 6 pretzels
     • 20 oyster crackers
   b. Fruit exchange = 15 g CHO
     • 1 cup Gatorade
     • ½ twin bar popsicle
     • ½ cup fruit juice
     • ½ cup unsweetened applesauce
     • ½ cup ginger ale or cola (not diet)
   c. CHO content of other foods
     • ½ cup regular Jello = 24 g
     • 2 level tsp. sugar = 8 g
	16. Illness often causes loss of appetite. Liquids or semisoft foods may be substituted for the client's normal diet. A client on insulin therapy needs to maintain a consistent CHO intake that will supply glucose. When there is a lack of CHO, fats are used for energy. Ketones form from the metabolism of fat.

17. Explain the effects of exercise on glucose metabolism:
   a. Explain the benefits of regular exercise:
     • Improved fitness
     • Psychological benefits (e.g., enhanced ability to relax, increased self-confidence, and improved self-image)
     • Reduction of body fat
     • Weight control
	17. Emphasizing the benefits of exercise may help the client to succeed with the prescribed exercise regimen.

(continued)

Interventions	*Rationales*

18. Explain that the goal is to engage in a total of 30 minutes of moderate-intensity physical activity every day. For example, walk 10,000 steps in a day (usual is 4,000–6,000 steps). Wear a pedometer to monitor and motivate. Refer also to www.walkinginfo.org.
   a. Instruct the client to seek the advice of a health care provider before beginning an exercise program.
   b. Exercise may be contraindicated with certain complications (e.g., severe nephropathy, proliferative retinopathy).
   c. Teach the client to avoid injecting insulin into a body part that is about to be exercised.
   d. Encourage the client to exercise with others or where other informed persons are nearby, always wear diabetes identification, always carry a fast-acting CHO.
   e. Explain how to reduce serious hypoglycemic episodes related to exercise:
      • Monitor BG before and after exercise.
      • Exercise when BG level tends to be higher, such as shortly after a meal.
      • Always carry a source of fast-acting sugar for emergency.

18c. Insulin absorption increases in a body part that is exercised, which alters the insulin's absorption.
   d. Exercising with others ensures that assistance is available should hypoglycemia occur.

   e. Proper timing of exercise, monitoring BG, and adjusting food or insulin decreases the risk of exercise-induced hypoglycemia. In the event of a severe reaction, a semiconscious or unconscious client may require glucagon (American Diabetes Association, 2012b).

19. Explain the importance of foot care and risks to the feet:
   a. Teach the importance of daily foot inspection: make foot care a daily routine, visually inspect the bottom of feet and between toes looking for injury, reddened areas.
   b. Teach the client to prevent foot problems: good fitting shoes, protective socks, never walk barefoot, good nail care, use of cream to prevent dry skin.
   c. Teach good nail care: trim toenails straight across, never cut too short, seek professional care for ingrown or thickened toenails.
   d. Never cut corns or calluses, gently use pumice stone or seek professional care.

19. Foot lesions result from peripheral neuropathy, vascular disease, and superimposed infection. Feet that are deformed, insensitive, and ischemic are prime targets for lesions and susceptible to trauma.

20. Provide smoking cessation support. Refer to *Getting Started to Quit Smoking* on thePoint at http://thePoint.lww.com/Carpenito6e (printable to give to client).

20. Diabetes makes the feet more prone to injury from decreased circulation. Daily inspections are vital to detect problems early. Injury can be reduced with proper shoes; proper nail trimming; attention to calluses, corns, and thickened nails; and avoiding extreme temperatures. Removing shoes and socks with each visit to a health care provider will remind the provider to examine the feet. Tobacco use will increase vasoconstriction and decrease circulation to the feet.

21. Teach the client and family to contact a health care provider when any of these occur:
   a. Unexplained fluctuations in BG
   b. A foot injury that does not show signs of healing in 24 hours
   c. Changes in vision
   d. Vomiting / diarrhea for more than 24 hours
   e. Signs of infection

Interventions	Rationales
22. Provide informational materials and / or referrals that may assist the client to reach goals: a. Comprehensive Outpatient Diabetes Education b. Medical Nutrition Therapy (MNT) c. Support groups d. Magazines for persons with diabetes (e.g., *Diabetes Forecast, Diabetes Self-Management*) e. American Diabetes Association (www.diabetes.org) f. American Association of Diabetes Educators (www.diabeteseducator.org)	22. A client who feels well-supported can cope more effectively. A chronically ill person with multiple stressors needs to identify an effective support system. Knowing a friend or neighbor with diabetes, participating in a walk-a-thon for the American Diabetes Association, and reading about people successfully coping with diabetes are some helpful examples.

Documentation

Client teaching
Status at transition
Referrals

Pancreatitis

The pancreas is responsible for insulin production and manufacture and secretion of digestive enzymes needed for carbohydrate, fat, and protein metabolism (Porth, 2011). When these enzymes become prematurely active inside the pancreas, they digest the tissue of the pancreas.

Pancreatitis can be acute or chronic. Acute pancreatitis can be precipitated by mechanical and / or metabolic causes. Mechanical causes are those that obstruct or damage the pancreatic duct system, such as cancer, cholelithiasis, abdominal trauma, radiation therapy, parasitic diseases, and duodenal disease. Metabolic causes are those that alter the secretory processes of the acinar cells, such as alcoholism, certain medications (mesalazine, azathioprine, simvastatin, sulfonamides, NSAIDs, corticosteroid, tetracycline) genetic disorders, and diabetic ketoacidosis (Frossard et al., 2008). The most common cause is gallstones. The mortality rate for acute pancreatitis is 10% to 15%, and rises to 30% if organ failure is present (Porth, 2011).

Chronic pancreatitis is a chronic, continuing inflammatory process of the pancreas with irreversible morphologic changes. Chronic pancreatitis is caused by excessive alcohol consumption (60%), hereditary pancreatitis (1%), idiopathic (unknown etiology) (30%), drug-induced (0.1% to 2%), and from blunt trauma or accidents (obstructive) (Pezzilli et al., 2010; Zagaria, 2011). The prognosis for chronic pancreatitis is associated with age at diagnosis, smoking, continued use of alcohol, and the presence of liver cirrhosis (Pezzilli et al., 2010).

■■■ DIAGNOSTIC CLUSTER

Collaborative Problems

▲ Risk for Complications of Hypovolemia / Shock

* Risk for Complications of Acute Respiratory Distress Syndrome

* Risk for Complications of Systemic Inflammatory Response Syndrome (SIRS)

* Risk for Complications of Metabolic Instability

* Risk for Complications of Alcohol Withdrawal REFER to Alcohol Abuse Care Plan

(continued)

Nursing Diagnoses

▲ Acute Pain related to nasogastric suction, distention of pancreatic capsule, and local peritonitis

▲ Ineffective Denial related to acknowledgment of alcohol abuse or dependency (refer to Alcohol Abuse Care Plan)

▲ Risk for Ineffective Self Health Management to insufficient knowledge of home care needed, treatments, early s/s of complications, dietary management, and follow-up care.

▲ This diagnosis was reported to be monitored for or managed frequently (75% to 100%).

* This diagnosis was not included in the validation study.

Transitional Criteria

The client or family will:

1. Explain the causes of the symptoms.
2. Describe signs and symptoms that must be reported to a health care professional.
3. Relate the importance of adhering to dietary restrictions and avoiding alcohol.
4. If alcohol abuse is present, admit to the problem.
5. Relate community resources available for treatment of alcohol abuse.

> ### Transitional Risk Assessment Plan (TRAP)
>
> Begin this plan on admission.
> Implement the Transitional Risk Assessment Plan (TRAP):
> • Refer to inside back cover.
> • Add each validated risk diagnosis to client's problem list with the risk code in ( ).
> • Refer to Unit II to the individual risk nursing diagnoses / collaborative problems for outcomes and interventions.
>
> *R: "Close coordination of care in the post-acute period, early discharge follow-up care, enhanced client education and self-management training, proactive end-of-life counseling, and extending the resources and clinical expertise over time via multidisciplinary team management" can lower readmission rates and improve health outcomes (Boutwell & Hwu, 2009).*

Collaborative Problems

Risk for Complications of Hypovolemia / Shock

Risk for Complications of Acute Respiratory Distress Syndrome

Risk for Complications of Systemic Inflammatory Response Syndrome (SIRS)

Risk for Complications of Metabolic Instability

Risk for Complications of Alcohol Withdrawal

Collaborative Outcomes

The client will be monitored for early signs and symptoms of (a) hypovolemia / shock, (b) acute respiratory distress syndrome, (c) systemic inflammatory response syndrome (SIRS), (d) metabolic complications, (e) alcohol withdrawal, and (g) hematologic complications, and will receive collaborative interventions if indicated to restore physiologic stability.

Indicators of Physiologic Stability

• Calm, alert (all)
• Cardiac: rhythm regular, rate 60–100 beats/min (a, b)
• BP >90/60, <140/90 mm Hg (a, b)

- Respiratory rate 16–20 breaths/min (a, b)
- Oxygen saturation (pulse oximeter) >96% (a, b, e)
- Capillary refill <3 seconds (a, b, c, e, f)
- Temperature 98–99.5° F (c, e)
- pH 7.35–7.45 (a, b, c, e)
- Urine output >0.5 mL/kg/h (a, b, c, e, f)
- Urine specific gravity 1.005–1.030 (f)
- Dry skin (a, b)
- No nausea or vomiting (c, e)
- White blood cells 4,300–10,800 mm³ 56–190 IV/L (c, e)
- Serum amylase alkaline phosphatase 30–85 mU/mL (c)
- Fasting serum glucose 70–115 mg/dL (c)
- Aspartate aminotransferase (AST) (c)
  - Male: 7–21 u/L
  - Female: 6–18 u/L
- Alanine aminotransferase 5–35 U/L (c)
- Lactate dehydrogenase (LDH) 100–225 U/L (c)
- Hematocrit (a, b, g)
  - Male: 42% to 52%
  - Female: 37% to 47%
- Serum calcium 8.5–10.5 mg/dL (c, f)
- Stool occult blood negative (g)
- Serum potassium 3.8–5 mEq/L (a, c, e)
- Serum creatinine 0.6–1.2mg/dL (f)

Interventions

1. Monitor for signs and symptoms of hypovolemia and shock:

   a. Increasing pulse rate, normal or slightly decreased blood pressure
   b. Increasing respiratory rate
   c. Urine output <5 mL/kg/hr

   CLINICAL ALERT
   - Hourly urine output monitoring is essential for early detection.

   d. Restlessness, agitation, change in mentation

   e. Diminished peripheral pulses
   f. Cool, pale, or cyanotic skin

2. Monitor for respiratory complications:
   a. Hypoxemia
   b. Atelectasis
   c. Pleural effusion

   CLINICAL ALERT
   - Death within the first several days of acute pancreatitis is attributed to cardiovascular instability or respiratory failure

Rationales

1. Autodigestion of the pancreas results in increased capillary permeability, causing a plasma shift from the circulatory system to the peritoneal cavity. Hypovolemic shock can result. The compensatory response to decreased circulatory volume is to (Porth, 2011):

   a, b. Increase heart and respiratory rates in an attempt to increase blood oxygen levels.

   c. Hypovolemia and hypotension activate the renin-angiotensin system; this results in increased renal vasculature resistance, which decreases renal plasma flow and glomerular filtration rate.

   d. Diminish oxygen to the brain causes changes in mentation.
   e, f. Decrease circulation to the extremities, causing decreased pulse and cool skin.

2. Respiratory complications are thought to be caused by enzyme-induced inflammation of the diaphragm or pulmonary microvasculature (Munoz & Katerndahl, 2000).

(continued)

Interventions	Rationales
3. Monitor for systemic inflammatory response syndrome (SIRS). Evaluate the SIRS score. • Body temperature greater than 38° C or less than 36° C • Heart rate greater than 90/min • Respiratory rate greater than 20/min or $PaCO_2$ less than 32 mm Hg • White blood cell count greater than 12,000/µL or less than 4,000/µL or presence of 10% immature neutrophils.	3. SIRS has replaced the terminology *septic syndrome*. Sepsis is one contributing factor to SIRS, which is a life-threatening condition related to systemic inflammation, organ dysfunction, and organ failure. The SIRS score is determined by assigning 1 point for each vital sign measure listed. A SIRS score of 0 or 1 indicates absence of SIRS. A SIRS score of 2 (mild), 3 (moderate), or 4 (severe) indicates the occurrence of SIRS.

4. Monitor for metabolic complications
  a. hypokalemia:
 	
  b. Hiccups
    • Polyuria
    • Polydipsia
	4a. Pancreatic enzymes are high in potassium; losses into the peritoneal cavity may result in a potassium deficiency.
	  b. Hiccups may be related to phrenic nerve irritation resulting from subdiaphragmatic collection of purulent debris.

5. Monitor for hematologic complications:
  a. Thrombosis
  b. Disseminated intravascular coagulation
	5. Early intravascular consumption of coagulation factors secondary to circulating pancreatic enzymes and vascular injury contribute to disseminated intravascular coagulation (Munoz & Katerndahl, 2000).

6. Monitor:
  a. Coagulation profiles
  b. Hemoglobin / hematocrit
  c. For hypoalbuminemia
    • Stool, urine, and GI drainage for occult blood
    • For ecchymosis (blackened bruises)
	6. Early detection of signs of bleeding or disseminated intravascular coagulation (DIC) can reduce morbidity / mortality.

7. Explain the use of nasogastric tube and suctioning.	7. Nasogastric suctioning is used to remove gastric juices, which, if present, will stimulate the release of secretions in the duodenum. These secretions, in turn, stimulate the pancreas to secrete enzymes.
8. Evaluate whether or not the client abuses alcohol. Discuss with individual his / her drinking patterns (e.g., binging, daily drinking, amounts). Separately, question the family regarding the individual's alcohol intake.	8. Alcohol stimulates pancreatic secretions and can trigger excess production of hydrochloric acid, which causes spasms partial obstruction of the ampulla of Vater. This contributes to inflammation and the destruction of pancreatic cells. (Porth, 2011)

9. Monitor for early signs and symptoms of alcohol withdrawal:
  a. Agitation
  b. Tremors
  c. Diaphoresis
  d. Anorexia, nausea, vomiting
  e. Increased heart rate and respiratory rate
	9. Because chronic alcohol abuse can cause pancreatitis, the nurse must be alert for the signs even when the client denies alcoholism. Denial is a major coping mechanism for individuals and families. Signs of alcohol withdrawal begin 24 hours after the last drink and can continue for 1 to 2 weeks. Refer to Alcohol Withdrawal Care Plan for specifics.

CLINICAL ALERT
• Denial is a common defense mechanism for individuals who abuse alcohol and for their families. (Varcarolis, 2011). If one suspects alcohol abuse, even when denied, monitor individual closely.

Interventions	Rationales
10. Alert the physician / NP when alcohol withdrawal is suspected.	10. Alcohol withdrawal often requires large doses of sedatives to prevent seizures.
11. Refer to collaborative problem index under thrombosis and disseminated intravascular coagulation for specific monitoring criteria.	
12. If enteral feeding is initiated, refer to Enteral Feeding Care Plan.	12. Enteral nutrition is preferred over total parenteral nutrition because of less septic complications, surgical interventions, total hospitalization time, and decreased costs because of less septic complications (Ioannidis et al., 2008). Oral intake should not be resumed until abdominal pain subsides and serum amylase levels are normal.
13. If total parenteral nutrition (TPN) is used, refer to TPN Care Plan.	13. TPN may be needed if the person cannot tolerate enteral nutrition such as paralytic ileus.

Clinical Alert Report

Advise ancillary staff / student to report:
* Any new change or deterioration diastolic in behavior (e.g., agitation, cognition)
* Any change in systolic B/P >210 mm Hg, <90 mm Hg, and / or diastolic >90 mm Hg
* Resting pulse >120 or <55 bpm
* Change in rate of respirations and / or >28 or <10/minute
* Changes or new onset of dyspnea / palpitations
* Decrease in urine output less than 5mL/kg per hour
* Temperature >101° F oral

Nursing Diagnoses

Acute Pain Related to Nasogastric Suction, Distention of Pancreatic Capsule, and Local Peritonitis

NOC
Comfort Level, Pain Control

Goal

The client will relate satisfactory relief after pain-relief interventions.

NIC
Pain Management, Medication Management, Emotional Support, Teaching: Individual, Heat / Cold Application, Simple Massage

Indicators

* Relate factors that increase pain.
* Relate effective interventions.
* Rate pain level lower after measures.

Interventions	Rationales
1. Collaborate with client to determine what methods could be used to reduce the pain's intensity.	1. Pain related to pancreatitis produces extreme discomfort in addition to increasing metabolic activity, with a corresponding increase in pancreatic secretory activity.
2. Discuss with the physician the use of analgesics such as meperidine, barbiturates, and fentanyl. Avoid the PRN approach and morphine. a. For interventions to manage acute pain refer to *Acute Pain* in Unit II.	2. These analgesics do not cause spasm of the Sphincter of Oddi (Munoz & Katerndahl, 2000). A regular time schedule maintains a steady drug blood level.

3. Provide nasogastric tube care, if indicated:
   a. Explain why n.g. tube is needed.
   b. Apply a water-soluble lubricant around the nares to prevent irritation.
   c. Monitor the nares for pressure points and signs of necrosis. Retape or reposition the tube when it gets detached or soiled.
   d. Provide frequent oral care with gargling; avoid alcohol-based mouthwashes that dry mucosa.
	3a. Removal of stomach fluids may be needed to control vomiting and pain.
	   b. These interventions can reduce some discomfort associated with nasogastric tube use.

4. Explain the need for bed rest.	4. Bed rest decreases metabolism, reduces gastric secretions, and allows available energy to be used for healing.
5. Position the client sitting upright in bed with knees and spine flexed.	5. This position relieves tension on the abdominal muscles.
6. When the client is NPO, avoid all exposure to food (e.g., sight and smell).	6. The sight and smell of food can cause pancreatic stimulation.

7. Nutritionally, the person may (Lutz & Pzytulski, 2011)
   a. Have nothing by mouth (IV, enteral feedings)
   b. Clear fluids
   c. Soft to low fat diet over 3–4 days as tolerated
	7a. This avoids stimulating the pancreas, which will reduce pain and inflammation.
	   b. Can be initiated when pain has been controlled for 24 hours
	   c. The person's progress e.g. pain, nausea) will be evaluated.

Ineffective Denial Related to Acknowledgment of Alcohol Abuse or Dependency

NOC

Anxiety Level, Coping, Social Support, Substance Addiction Consequences, Knowledge: Substance Abuse Control, Knowledge: Disease Process

Goal

The client will acknowledge an alcohol / drug abuse problem.

Indicators

- Explain the physiologic effects of alcohol or drug use.
- Elicit the negative effects of alcoholism on family unit, jobs, legal issues.
- Report an intent to participate in drug / alcohol treatment program. Abstain from alcohol / drug use.

NIC

Coping Enhancement, Anxiety Reduction, Counseling, Mutual Goal Setting, Substance Abuse Treatment, Support System Enhancement, Support Group

Interventions	Rationales
1. Approach client nonjudgmentally. Some causes of pancreatitis are not alcohol-related, about 30%. Be aware of your own feelings regarding alcoholism. Refer to care plan on alcohol abuse.	1. The client probably has been reprimanded by many and is distrustful. The nurse's personal experiences with alcohol may increase or decrease empathy for the client.

TRANSITION TO HOME / COMMUNITY CARE

If indicated, review the risk diagnoses identified for this individual on admission:

- Is he person still at risk?
- Can the family reduce the risks?
- Is the person at higher risk at home?
- Is a Home Health Nurse assessment needed?
- Refer to transition planner / case manager / social service
- When is this person scheduled for follow-up with primary provider? Specialists? Record dates of appointments.
- Complete a medication reconciliation prior to transition. Refer to index.

S T A R

Stop

Think   Is this person at risk for injury, falls, medical complications, and / or inability to care for self (activities of daily living)?

Is there a support person available?

Is the person competent to manage self-administration of medications, treatment procedures? Are additional resources needed?

Can the person explain how to monitor condition (e.g., blood glucose, sign / symptoms of complications, dietary / mobility restrictions, and when to call his or her primary provider or specialist?

Act   Use SBAR to notify the appropriate professional.

Situation: Mr. Smith will be scheduled to be transitioned to his home.

Background: Mr. Smith lives alone. He (state his disabilities, self-care needs, treatments)

Action: A more thorough reevaluation of where he can be transitioned is needed.

Recommendation: Referral tosocial service / transition planner / case manager

Review   Is the response / solution the right option for the client? If not, seek discuss the situation with the appropriate person, department, and / or agency. (using SBAR)

Risk for Ineffective Self Health Management Related to Lack of Knowledge of Disease Process, Treatments, Contraindications, Dietary Management, and Follow-up Care

NOC

Compliance Behavior, Knowledge: Treatment Regimen, Participation in Health Care Decisions, Treatment Behavior: Illness or Injury

NIC

Health Education, Health System Guidance, Learning Facilitation, Learning Readiness Enhancement, Risk Identification, Self-Modification Assistance

Goals

The goals for this diagnosis represent those associated with transition planning. Refer to the transition criteria.

Interventions	*Rationales*
1. Explain the causes of acute and chronic pancreatitis.	1. Inaccurate perceptions of health status usually involve misunderstanding the nature and seriousness of the illness, susceptibility to complications, and need for restrictions to control illness.

2.

> **CLINICAL ALERT**
> • Teach the client to report early these worsening of symptoms:
>   a. Clay-colored stools
>   b. Increase in pain in upper left side, mid-abdominal and / or radiating to back
>   c. Persistent gastritis, nausea, or vomiting
>   d. Weight loss
>   e. Elevated temperature

> **CLINICAL ALERT**
> • These symptoms can indicate worsening of inflammation and increased malabsorption. An elevated temperature could indicate infection or abscess formation. Early reporting can ensure immediate attention and possibly prevention of readmission.

Interventions	*Rationales*
3. Explain the need to monitor BS at home. Teach use of glucometer. Advise to contact primary provider if BS are above 200 in a.m., p.m., or more than 2 hours after eating.	3. Pancreatitis can decrease insulin production, causing hyperglycemia.
4. Provide with printed dietary recommendations (accessed 7/21/2012 www.healtharticles101.com/top): a. Pureed vegetable soups, steamed vegetables; avoid raw vegetables b. Lean cuts of meat, preferably filets of chicken, turkey, rabbit and veal, only steaming or poaching, absolutely no frying or grilling c. Fish, especially cold-water varieties d. Eggs should supplement any diet for chronic pancreatitis. e. Organic dairy products (e.g., low-fat yogurt, cheese, kefir). These should be introduced slowly and after 2–3 weeks of a recent attack. f. A good breakfast, oatmeal has a smooth consistency and coats the stomach. g. Water and herbal teas are great sources of hydration and should be preferred over strong coffee, tea, carbonated, and alcoholic beverages. h. Oils as olive, grapeseed, flax seed can be added into your salads, soups, or side dishes right before serving. i. Fruits initially baked or steamed. When recovered, slowly introduce raw fruits.	4. Intake of incorrect foods can exacerbate pancreatitis and cause exacerbation and the need for readmission. a. Antioxidants / vitamins / minerals that are easily absorbed are needed for healing. Raw vegetables require too many enzymes to process rough fiber and thus can cause pain. b. They are low in fat and high in proteins, iron, zinc, and essential amino acids to maintain good health. c. Refer to a, b. d. They are great sources of protein and amino acids and gentle on the digestive system. e. These contain high doses of active probiotic cultures that will help normalize your digestion. f. Oatmeal provides B vitamins and other nutrients. g. Great sources of hydration and nonirritating to the GI tract as coffee, tea, carbonated, and alcoholic beverages h. Omega 3 and Omega 6 fatty acids and make them easy to digest by your pancreas. i. High-fiber foods need to be introduced slowly to prevent GI irritation.
5. Ensure the person / family understands the client's dietary needs and restrictions. Provide with a contact number if needed post transition.	5. A contact number provides immediate access to a health care professional for questions and answers.

Gastrointestinal Disorders

Gastroenterocolitis / Enterocolitis

An infectious agent (bacterial or viral) can cause inflammation of the lining of the stomach, gastroenterocolitis small intestine, and large intestine (enterocolitis). Parasites can also cause a gastroenteritis attack. Enterocolitis causes cramps and diarrhea, whereas gastroenterocolitis produces nausea, vomiting, diarrhea, and cramps. Hospitalization is indicated with severe fluid and electrolyte imbalances or for risk clients (older adults, clients with diabetes, clients with compromised immune systems). Several different viruses can cause viral gastroenteritis, which is highly contagious and extremely common.

Time Frame
Acute episode

▮▮▮DIAGNOSTIC CLUSTER**

Collaborative Problems

Risk for Complications of Fluid / Electrolyte Imbalance

Nursing Diagnoses

Risk for Deficient Fluid Volume related to losses secondary to vomiting and diarrhea

Acute Pain related to abdominal cramping, diarrhea, and vomiting secondary to vascular dilatation and hyperperistalsis

Risk for Ineffective Self-Health Management related to lack of knowledge of condition, dietary restrictions, and signs and symptoms of complications

Transitional Criteria

Before transition, the client or family will

1. Describe the causes of gastroenteritis and its transmission.
2. Identify dietary restrictions that promote comfort and healing.
3. State signs and symptoms of dehydration.
4. State signs and symptoms that must be reported to a health care professional.

> **Transitional Risk Assessment Plan (TRAP)**
>
> Begin this plan on admission.
> Implement the Transitional Risk Assessment Plan (TRAP):
> - Refer to inside back cover.
> - Add each validated risk diagnosis to client's problem list with the risk code in ( ).
> - Refer to Unit II to the individual risk nursing diagnoses / collaborative problems for outcomes and interventions.
>
> *R: "Close coordination of care in the post-acute period, early discharge follow-up care, enhanced client education and self-management training, proactive end-of-life counseling, and extending the resources and clinical expertise over time via multidisciplinary team management" can lower readmission rates and improve health outcomes (Boutwell & Hwu, 2009).*

** This medical condition was not included in the validation study.

Collaborative Problems

Risk for Complications of Fluid / Electrolyte Imbalance

Collaborative Outcomes

The client will be monitored for early signs and symptoms of fluid / electrolyte imbalance and will receive collaborative interventions if indicated to restore physiologic stability.

Indicators of Physiologic Stability

- Urine output >0.5 mL/kg/h (a, b)
- Urine specific gravity 1.005–1.030 (a)
- Moist skin / mucous membranes (a)
- Serum sodium 135–145 mEq/L (b)
- Serum potassium 3.8–5 mEq/L (b)
- Serum chloride 95–105 mEq/L (b)

Interventions	Rationales

1. Monitor for signs and symptoms of dehydration:
  a. Dry skin and mucous membrane
  b. Elevated urine specific gravity
  c. Thirst
	1. Rapid propulsion of feces through the intestines decreases water absorption. Low circulatory volume causes dry mucous membranes and thirst. Concentrated urine has an elevated specific gravity.

2. Carefully monitor intake and output.	2. Intake and output records help to detect early signs of fluid imbalance.
3. Monitor for electrolyte imbalances of sodium, chloride, potassium.	3. Rapid propulsion of feces through the intestines decreases electrolyte absorption. Vomiting also causes electrolyte loss.

Clinical Alert Report

Prior to providing care, advise ancillary staff / student to report the following to the professional nurse assigned to the client:
- Temperature >37.80° C (100° F)
- Resting pulse >100, <50
- Systolic BP >200 mm Hg or <9 mm Hg
- Diastolic BP >90
- C/o of abdominal pain / tenderness
- Urine output for shift or hourly if indicated

Related Physician / NP Prescribed Interventions

Medications
Antidiarrheals, antiemetics, antibiotics (if bacterial)

Intravenous Therapy
Fluid / electrolyte replacement

Laboratory Studies
CBC with differential; stool examination / cultures for amoeba, bacteria, parasites, leukocytes; electrolytes

Therapies
Diet, as tolerated (e.g., clear fluids, full fluids, bland, soft); oral electrolyte preparations

Documentation

Intake and output
Stools (amount, consistency)

Nursing Diagnoses

Risk for Deficient Fluid Volume Related to Losses Secondary to Vomiting and Diarrhea

(If client is NPO, this is then a collaborative problem: refer to index: PC: Hypovolemia.)

NOC
Electrolyte & Acid–Base Balance, Fluid Balance, Hydration

NIC
Fluid / Electrolyte Management, Fluid Monitoring

Goal

The client will have a urine specific gravity between 1.005 and 1.030.

Indicators

- Intake is 1.5 mL of fluids every 24 hours.
- Urinate at least every 2 hours.

Interventions	Rationales
1. Monitor for early signs and symptoms of fluid volume deficit: a. Dry mucous membranes (lips, gums) b. Amber urine c. Specific gravity >1.025	1. Decreased circulating volume causes drying of tissues and concentrated urine. Early detection enables prompt fluid replacement therapy to correct deficits.
2. Monitor parenteral fluid infusion and administer parenteral antiemetic medications as ordered.	2. Antiemetics prevent vomiting by inhibiting stimuli to the vomiting center.
3. Provide fluids often and in small amounts so that the urge to urinate occurs every 2 hours: a. Broths, noncarbonated soft drinks, sports drinks, caffeine-free soft drinks b. Electrolyte-supplemented drink	3. Certain beverages replace sodium and potassium lost in diarrhea and vomiting without irritating the GI tract.
4. Instruct to a. Avoid diet products (drinks, gum) with sorbitol. b. Put a pinch of sugar in carbonated beverages.	4a. Artificial sweeteners can cause or aggravate diarrhea. b. Sugar will disperse bubbles to reduce gastric distention.
5. Monitor intake and output, making sure that intake compensates for output.	5. Output may exceed intake that already may be inadequate to compensate for insensible losses. Dehydration may decrease glomerular filtration rate, making output inadequate to clear wastes properly and leading to elevated BUN and electrolyte levels.

Documentation

Vital signs
Intake and output
Vomiting episodes

Acute Pain Related to Abdominal Cramping, Diarrhea, and Vomiting Secondary to Vascular Dilatation and Hyperperistalsis

NOC
Comfort Level, Pain Control

NIC
Pain Management, Medication Management, Emotional Support, Teaching: Individual, Heat / Cold Application, Simple Massage

Goal

The client will report less painful symptoms.

Indicators

- Report reduced abdominal cramping.
- List foods and fluids to avoid.

Interventions	Rationales
1. Encourage the client to rest in the supine position with a warm heating pad on the abdomen.	1. These measures promote GI muscular relaxation and reduce cramping.
2. Encourage frequent intake of small amounts of cool clear liquids (e.g., dilute tea, flat ginger ale, Jell-O, water): 30 to 60 mL every ½ to 1 hour.	2. Small amounts of fluids do not distend the gastric area, and thus do not aggravate the symptoms.
3. Eliminate unpleasant sights and odors from the client's environment.	3. Unpleasant sights or odors can stimulate the vomiting center.
4. Instruct the client to avoid hot or cold liquids, foods containing fat or fiber (e.g., milk, fruits), caffeine.	4. Cold liquids can induce cramping; hot liquids can stimulate peristalsis. Fats also increase peristalsis, and caffeine increases intestinal motility.
5. Protect the perianal area from irritation.	5. Frequent stools of increased acidity can irritate perianal skin.
6. When liquids can be tolerated, process with bland, non-fat foods in small amounts.	6. Small portions will prevent gastric distention.

Clinical Alert Report

Prior to providing care, advise ancillary staff / student to report the following to the professional nurse assigned to the client:
- Continued vomiting
- Dark, concentrated urine

Documentation

Intake and output
Tolerance of intake
Stools (frequency, characteristics, consistency)
Bowel sounds

> **TRANSITION TO HOME / COMMUNITY CARE**
>
> If indicated, review the risk diagnoses identified for this individual on admission:
> - Is he person still at risk?
> - Can the family reduce the risks?
> - Is the person at higher risk at home?
> - Is a Home Health Nurse assessment needed?
> - Refer to transition planner / case manager / social service
> - When is this person scheduled for follow-up with primary provider? Specialists? Record dates of appointments.
> - Complete a medication reconciliation prior to transition. Refer to index.

S T A R **Stop**

Think Is this person at risk for injury, falls, medical complications, and / or inability to care for self (activities of daily living)?

Is there a support person available?

Is the person competent to manage self-administration of medications, treatment procedures? Are additional resources needed?

Can the person explain how to monitor condition (e.g., blood glucose, sign / symptoms of complications, dietary / mobility restrictions, and when to call his or her primary provider or specialist?

Act Contact or provide the appropriate resource (e.g., contacting a support person, home health assessment, additional teaching, printed materials).

Review Has the problem been addressed? If not, use SBAR to communicate to the appropriate person.

Risk for Ineffective Self-Health Regimen Management Related to Lack of Knowledge of Condition and transmission precautions, Dietary Restrictions, and Signs and Symptoms of Complications

NOC

Compliance Behavior, Knowledge: Treatment Regimen, Participation in Health Care Decisions, Treatment Behavior: Illness or Injury

NIC

Health Education, Health System Guidance, Learning Facilitation, Learning Readiness Enhancement, Risk Identification, Self-Modification Assistance

Goal

The goals for this diagnosis represent those associated with transition planning. Refer to the transition criteria.

Interventions	*Rationales*
1. Discuss the disease process in understandable terms; explain the following: a. Causative agents b. Reason for enteric precautions c. Prevention of transmission	1. The client's understanding may increase compliance with dietary restrictions and hygiene practices.

(continued)

Interventions	Rationales
2. Avoid anti-inflammatory drugs (e.g., NSAIDs). Advise to use acetaminophen for aches / pains if needed unless contraindicated.	2. NSAIDs can cause gastric irritation.

3. Explain dietary restrictions:
  a. High-fiber foods (e.g., bran, fresh fruit)
  b. High-fat foods (e.g., whole milk, fried foods)
  c. Very hot or cold fluids
  d. Caffeine
  e. High carbohydrate foods
	3. These foods can stimulate or irritate the intestinal tract.

4. Instruct on dietary options:
  a. Rice
  b. Toast, crackers
  c. Bananas
  d. Tea
  e. Applesauce (not juice)
	4. Foods with complex carbohydrates facilitate fluid absorption into the intestinal mucosa (Cheskin & Lacy, 2003).

5. Teach the client and family to report these symptoms:
  a. Inability to retain fluids
  b. Dark amber urine persisting for more than 12 hours
  c. Bloody stools
	5. Early detection and reporting of the signs of dehydration enable prompt interventions to prevent serious fluid or electrolyte imbalances.

6. Explain the benefits of rest and encourage adequate rest.	6. Inactivity reduces peristalsis and allows the GI tract to rest.

7. Explain preventive measures:
  a. Proper food storage / refrigeration
  b. Proper cleaning of kitchen utensils especially wooden cutting boards.
    • Sanitize surface areas with disinfectants that contain bleach.
    • Clean eating utensils and thermometers with products that contain alcohol, or use dishwasher for eating utensils and dishes.
  c. Proper cleaning of bathroom
 	
  d. Hand-washing before and after handling food.
	7a. The most common cause of gastroenteritis is ingestion of bacteria-contaminated food.
	
	  c. The spread of bacteria and viruses can be controlled by disinfecting surface areas (bathrooms). Disinfectants with antibacterial properties are effective against some bacteria and viruses.
	  d. The transmission of getting or spreading viral gastroenteritis can be reduced by washing hands thoroughly with soap and warm water for 20 seconds after using the bathroom or changing diapers and before eating or handling food.

Documentation

Transition instructions
Status at transition

Inflammatory Bowel Syndrome

"Knowledge on the pathophysiology of irritable bowel syndrome has evolved, beginning with disturbances in motility to visceral hypersensitivity, and ultimately to alterations in brain-gut bi-directional communication, where neurotransmitters such as serotonin play a key role" (Schulman et al., 2001).

The pathogenesis of irritable bowel syndrome (IBS) appears to be multifactorial. There is evidence to show that the following factors play a central role in the pathogenesis of IBS: heritability and genetics, environment and social learning, dietary or intestinal microbiota, low-grade inflammation and disturbances in the neuroendocrine system (NES) of the gut (El-Salhy et al., 2010).

"There is growing evidence that genetic factors predispose the immune response, possible triggered be a relatively innocuous environmental agent such as a dietary antigen or microbial agent" (Porth, 2011; Turner, 2010).

IBS is a generic term comprising both Crohn's disease and ulcerative colitis. Both are inflammatory conditions of the GI tract and have similar clinical presentations. IBS is a chronic, relapsing and often life-long disorder. It is characterized by the presence of abdominal pain or discomfort, which may be associated with defecation and / or accompanied by a change in bowel habit. Symptoms may include disordered defecation (constipation or diarrhea or both) and abdominal distension, usually referred to as bloating. Symptoms sometimes overlap with other gastrointestinal disorders such as nonulcer dyspepsia or celiac disease.

 Time Frame
Initial diagnosis
Recurrent acute episodes

■■■ DIAGNOSTIC CLUSTER

Collaborative Problems

▲ Risk for Complications of Fluid / Electrolyte Imbalances

▲ Risk for Complications of Intestinal Obstruction

▲ Risk for Complications of GI Bleeding

▲ Risk for Complications of Anemia

△ Risk for Complications of Fistula / Fissure / Abscess (Crohn's)

△ Risk for Complications of Renal Calculi

▲ Risk for Complications of Growth Retardation

Nursing Diagnoses

▲ Chronic Pain related to intestinal inflammatory process (refer to Unit II) Nursing Diagnoses Chronic Pain

▲ Imbalanced Nutrition: Less Than Body Requirements related to dietary restrictions, nausea, diarrhea, and abdominal cramping associated with eating or painful ulcers of the oral mucous membrane

▲ Diarrhea related to intestinal inflammatory process (refer to Unit II Nursing Diagnosis Diarrhea)

△ Risk for Ineffective Coping related to chronicity of condition and lack of definitive treatment (refer to Unit II Nursing Diagnosis Ineffective Coping)

△ Risk for Ineffective Self-Health Management related to lack of knowledge of condition, diagnostic tests, prognosis, treatment, and signs and symptoms of complications

Related Care Plan

Corticosteroid Therapy

▲ This diagnosis was reported to be monitored for or managed frequently (75% to 100%).
△ This diagnosis was reported to be monitored for or managed often (50% to 74%).

Transition Criteria

Before transition, the client or family will:

1. Discuss management of activities of daily living.
2. State signs and symptoms that must be reported to a health care professional.
3. Verbalize an intent to share feelings and concerns related to IBS with significant others.
4. Identify available community resources or self-help groups.

Collaborative Problems

Risk for Complications of Fluid / Electrolyte Imbalances

Risk for Complications of Intestinal Obstruction

Risk for Complications of GI Bleeding

Risk for Complications of Anemia

Risk for Complications of Fistula / Fissure (Crohn's Disease)

Risk for Complications of Renal Calculi

Collaborative Outcomes

The client will be monitored for early signs and symptoms of (a) fluid / electrolyte imbalances, (b) intestinal obstruction, (c) abscess, (d) GI bleeding, (e) anemia, and (f) renal calculi and will receive collaborative interventions if indicated to restore physiological stability.

Indicators of Physiologic Stability

- Temperature 98–99.5° F (c, f)
- Respiratory rate 16–20 breaths/min (a, d)
- Normal breath sounds, no adventitious sounds (a, d)
- Pulse 60–100 beats/min (a)
- Blood pressure >90/60, <140/90 mm Hg
- No nausea or vomiting (b)
- Urine output >0.5 mL/kg/h (a, f)
- Urine specific gravity within range
- Red blood cells (e)
  Male 4.6–5.9 million/mm^3
  Female 4.2–5.4 million/mm^3
- White blood count 4,300–10,800 mm^3 (c)
- Serum potassium 3.5–5.0 mEq/L (a)
- Creatinine clearance (a)
  Male 95–135 mL/mm
  Female 85–125 mL/mm
- Bowel sounds present in all quadrants (b)
- Stool occult blood negative
- No abdominal pain (b, e)
- B$_{12}$ 130–785 pg/mL (e)
- Folate 2.5–20 ng/mL (e)
- Hemoglobin (d, e)
  Males 13.18 gm/dL
  Females 12.16 gm/dL
- No rectal pain

Carp's Cues

There has been and currently is a belief by health care professionals that IBS is caused by psychological factors. The historical difficulty of explaining the pathophysiology of IBS has contributed to these misconceptions. "IBS client are offered noneffective treatments, are treated with mistrust and neglect by their doctors, feel that they are labeled as hypochondriacs and believe that they receive no support from society. It could be expected that IBS clients would be more anxious and depressed." Researchers have concluded that no convincing evidence exists to show that psychological factors play a role in the onset and / or progression of IBS.

Interventions	Rationales
1. Assure the individual that you understand the patho-physiology of IBS and that you do not believe that it is a psychological disorder.	1. Researchers have reported that quality of life improved after participants anticipated in a health program of reassurance, diet management, probiotics, and regular exercise (El-Salhy et al., 2010)

2. Explain the pathophysiology of IBS (El-Salhy et al., 2010):
  a. Heritability and genetics
  b. Environment and social learning
  c. Dietary or intestinal microbiota
  d. Low-grade inflammation
  e. Disturbances in the neuroendocrine system (NES) of the gut	

3. Explain the effects of an impaired neuroendocrine system (NES) of the gut as disturbances in digestion, GI motility, and visceral hypersensitivity.
  a. Changes the motility of bowels (how fast food moves through the system)
  b. Affects how much fluid, such as mucus, is secreted in intestines
  c. Affects how sensitive the intestines are to sensations like pain and fullness
	3. Low levels of serotonin appear to contribute to symptom development and may play a central role in the pathogenesis of IBS. Genetic differences have been found between IBS clients and healthy subjects in genes controlling the serotonin signaling system and CCK (Schmulson et al., 2001).

4. If selective serotonin reuptake inhibitors (SSRIs) or tricyclic antidepressants are not prescribed, consult with physician / NP	4. Serotonin is crucial to the function of your digestive system. Ninety-five percent (95%) of the serotonin is produced in the gut. This produces low levels of serotonin and the body's sensitivity to serotonin signaling, which will interfere with normal bowel function. Individuals with IBS have been found to have low serotonin levels (Schmulson et al., 2001).
5. Monitor laboratory values for electrolyte imbalances.	5. Chronic diarrhea and inadequate oral intake can deplete electrolytes. Small intestine inflammation impairs absorption of fluid and electrolytes (Porth, 2011).

6. Monitor for signs and symptoms of dehydration:
  a. Tachycardia
  b. Dry skin / mucous membrane
  c. Elevated urine specific gravity
  d. Thirst
	6. When circulating volume decreases, heart rate increases in an attempt to supply tissues with oxygen. Low circulatory volume causes dry mucous membranes and thirst. Concentrated urine has an elevated specific gravity.

(continued)

Interventions	**Rationales**

7. Monitor for signs and symptoms of intestinal obstruction:
  a. Wavelike abdominal pain
  b. Vomiting (gastric juices, bile, progressing to fecal material)
  c. Abdominal distention
  d. Change in bowel sounds (initially hyperactive, progressing to none)
 	
CLINICAL ALERT
• If intestinal obstruction is suspected, withhold all food and fluids and notify the physician / NP.
	7. Inflammation and edema can cause the obstruction. Intestinal contents are then propelled toward the mouth instead of the rectum.

8. Monitor for signs and symptoms of fistula, fissures, or abscesses in individuals with Crohn's disease:
  a. Purulent drainage
  b. Fecal drainage from vagina
  c. Increased abdominal pain
  d. Burning rectal pain following defecation
  e. Perianal induration, swelling, redness, and cyanotic tags
  f. Signs of sepsis (e.g., fever, increased WBC count)
 	
CLINICAL ALERT
• If abscess or fistula is suspected, contact physician. / NP
	8. The inflammation and ulceration of Crohn disease can penetrate the intestinal wall and form an abscess or fistula to other parts of the intestine or skin. Abscesses and fistulas may cause cramping, pain, and fever, and may interfere with digestion. Sepsis may arise from seeding of the bloodstream from fistula tracts or abscess cavities (Bullock & Henze, 2000).

9. Monitor for signs and symptoms of GI bleeding:
  a. Decreased hemoglobin and hematocrit
  b. Fatigue
  c. Irritability
  d. Pallor
  e. Tachycardia
  f. Dyspnea
  g. Anorexia
  h. Refer to Unit II Collaborative Problems Risk for Complications of GI Bleeding.
	9. Chronic inflammation can cause erosion of vessels and bleeding.

10. Monitor for signs of anemia:
  a. Decreased hemoglobin
  b. Decreased red blood cells
  c. B12 deficiency
  d. Folate deficiency
	10. Anemia may result from GI bleeding, bone marrow depression (associated with chronic inflammatory diseases), and inadequate intake or impaired absorption of vitamin B12, folic acid, and iron. Sulfasalazine therapy can cause hemolysis, which contributes to anemia (Bullock & Henze, 2000).

11. Monitor for signs and symptoms of urolithiasis:
  a. Flank pain
  b. Fever, chills
	11. Severe diarrhea can lead to a decreased volume of concentrated urine. This, combined with intestinal bicarbonate loss and lowered pH, leads to the development of urate stones. With ileal resection or severe IBS, the calcium normally available to bind with oxylate binds instead with fatty acids, freeing dietary oxylate for absorption. Decreased urine volume enhances the precipitation of calcium oxylate in the kidney, predisposing to stone formation (Bullock & Henze, 2000).

Clinical Alert Report

Prior to providing care, advise ancillary staff / student to report the following to the professional nurse assigned to the client:

- Immediately: severe abdominal pain, abdominal swelling, tenderness, nausea, vomiting, fever.
- Change in cognitive status
- Oral temperature >100.5° F
- Systolic BP <90 mm Hg
- Resting pulse >100, <50
- Respiratory rate >28, <10/min.
- Oxygen saturation <90%
- Occult testing results
- Streaks of blood in stool

Related Physician / NP Prescribed Interventions

Medications
Aminosalicylates, immunosuppressants, antibiotics, corticosteroids, IgG (infliximab) vitamins / minerals, erythropoietin, tumor necrosis factor inhibitors, opioids, $5HT_4$ receptor antagonist, lubiprostone (Amitiza), 5-ASA compounds (e.g., sulfasalazine, mesalamine), antidepressants, antispasmotics, antidiarrheals, fiber supplements, laxatives

Intravenous Therapy
Fluid / electrolyte replacement, 5-aminosalicylic acid

Laboratory Studies
Stool specimens (bacteria), ova, parasites; fecal occult blood; CBC; serum protein electrophoresis; serum electrolytes; sedimentation rate; blood urea nitrogen; alkaline phosphatase; creatinine; prothrombin time, Thyroid function test, hydrogen breath test (for lactose intolerance and bacterial overgrowth). antibody testing for celiac disease (endomysial antibodies [EMA] or tissue transglutaminase [TTG]). Food allergy testing.

Diagnostic Studies
Ultrasound endoscopy, biopsy (rectal), GI x-ray film, colonoscopy, abdominal MRI, abdominal CT scan, flexible sigmoidoscopy

Therapies
Total parenteral nutrition

Documentation

Vital signs
Intake and output
Bowel sounds
Diarrhea episodes
Vomiting episodes
Drainage (wound, rectal, vaginal)
Urine specific gravity

Nursing Diagnoses

Imbalanced Nutrition: Less Than Body Requirements Related to Dietary Restrictions, Nausea, Diarrhea, and Abdominal Cramping Associated with Eating or Painful Ulcers of the Oral Mucous Membrane

 Carp's Cues

"Most clients with IBS believe diet plays a significant role in their symptoms and 63% were interested in knowing what food to avoid. It has been shown that the IBS clients have nonspecific diet intolerance. This lack of specificity causes considerable difficulty for IBS clients in choosing their diets." (El-Salhy et al., 2010)

NOC
Nutritional Status,
Teaching: Nutrition

Goal

The client will have positive nitrogen balance as evidenced by weight gain of 2–3 lb/wk.

NIC
Nutrition Management,
Nutritional Monitoring

Indicators

- Verbalize understanding of nutritional requirements.
- List foods to avoid.

Interventions	Rationales
1. Ensure a nutritional consult.	1. Nutritional therapy is the cornerstone of treatment of IBS.
2. Encourage liquids with caloric value rather than coffee, tea, water, or diet soda.	2. Calorie-rich liquids can help to prevent malnutrition.
3. Assess the client's acceptance of and response to oral fluid intake.	3. The ability to absorb nutrients must be evaluated daily.
4. Advise client to alert staff / student if there are beverages or food on tray that are irritating.	4. Individuals with IBS are the best resources for foods / beverages that need to be avoided.
5. Assist with progression to soft, bland, and low-residue solids and encourage small frequent feedings high in calories, protein, vitamins, and carbohydrates.	5. Gradual introduction of solid foods is needed to reduce pain and increase tolerance.
6. Teach the client to avoid raw fruits, vegetables, condiments, foods high in fiber, whole-grain cereals, gas forming and fried foods, alcohol, fizzy drinks, and iced drinks.	6. These foods and liquids usually irritate the GI tract.
7. As ordered, supplement the client's diet with folic acid, ascorbic acid, iron, calcium, copper, zinc, vitamin D, and vitamin B12.	7. Nutrient deficiencies result from decreased oral intake, malabsorption, or both.
8. Refer to Risk for Ineffective Self-Health Management for additional nutrition teaching.	

Documentation

Type and amount of food taken orally
Daily weight

Diarrhea Related to Intestinal Inflammatory Process

NOC

Bowel Elimination, Electrolyte & Acid / Base Balance, Fluid Balance, Hydration, Symptom Control

NIC

Bowel Management, Diarrhea Management, Fluid / Electrolyte Management, Nutrition Management, Enteral Tube Feeding

Goal

The client will report less diarrhea.

Indicators

- Describe factors that cause diarrhea.
- Explain the rationales for interventions.
- Have fewer episodes of diarrhea.
- Verbalize signs and symptoms of dehydration and electrolyte imbalances.

Interventions	Rationales
1. Assess stools for frequency, consistency, characteristics, presence of pain, urgency.	1. Stool assessment helps to evaluate the effectiveness of antidiarrheal agents and their relationship to intake.
2. Ensure good perianal care.	2. Perianal irritation from frequent liquid stool should be prevented.
3. Decrease physical activity during acute episodes of diarrhea.	3. Decreased physical activity decreases bowel peristalsis.
4. Determine the relationship between diarrheal episodes and ingestion of specific foods.	4. Identification of irritating foods can reduce diarrheal episodes.
5. Observe for signs and symptoms of electrolyte imbalance: a. Decreased serum potassium b. Decreased serum sodium	5a. In osmotic diarrhea, impaired fluid absorption by the intestines is caused by ingested solutes that cannot be digested or by a decrease in intestinal absorption. Water and electrolytes are drawn into the intestine in greater quantities than can be absorbed, and the diarrheal fluid is high in potassium (Bullock & Henze, 2000). b. Secretory diarrhea occurs when the gut wall is inflamed or engorged or when it is stimulated by bile salts. The resulting diarrheal stool is high in sodium.
6. Replace fluid and electrolytes with oral fluid containing appropriate electrolytes: a. Gatorade, a commercial preparation of glucose-electrolyte solution b. Apple juice, which is high in potassium but low in sodium c. Colas, root beer, and ginger ale that contain sodium but negligible potassium. De-fizz with a pinch of sugar or salt.	6. The type of fluid replacement depends on the electrolyte(s) needed.
7. Encourage the use of probiotics. Advise to consult with physician / NP regarding the use of probiotics.	7. Probiotics alter colonic fermentation and stabilize the colonic microbiota. Several studies on probiotics have shown improvements in flatulence and abdominal distension. (Spiller, 2009; El-Salhy et al., 2010)

Documentation

Intake and output
Number of stools
Consistency of stools

Risk for Ineffective Coping Related to Chronicity of Condition and Lack of Definitive Treatment

NOC
Coping, Self-Esteem, Social Interaction Skills

Goal

The client will make appropriate decisions to cope with condition.

NIC
Coping Enhancement, Counseling, Emotional Support, Active Listening, Assertiveness Training, Behavior Modification

Indicators

- Verbalize factors that contribute to anxiety and stress.
- Verbalize methods to improve the ability to cope with the chronic condition.

Interventions	*Rationales*
1. Clear up misconceptions about IBS. Stress that psychological symptoms are a reaction to, not the cause of IBS.	1. Correcting misconceptions may help to reduce the guilt associated with this belief.
2. Elicit from individual the effects of IBS on daily activities and life.	2. Researchers have reported individuals with IBS "would give up 25% of their remaining life (average 15 years) and 14% would risk a 1/1000 chance of death to receive a treatment that would make them symptom free" (El-Salhy et al., 2010).
3. Identify and minimize factors that contribute to anxiety. Explain all diagnostic tests and support the client during each procedure.	3. Understanding procedures can reduce anxiety.
4. Allow the client to have some control over care. Demonstrate acceptance and concern when caring for the client.	4. A client with IBS typically feels as if he or she has lost control over other aspects of life.
5. Involve family members or significant others in care, if possible.	5. Family members and others play a very important role in supporting clients and helping them to cope with and accept their disease.
6. Refer the client and family to the Irritable Bowel Syndrome Association at http://www.ibsgroup.org/ibsassociation.	6. Discussing IBS with others with the same problem can reduce feelings of isolation and anxiety. Sharing experiences in a group led by professionals gives the client the benefit of others' experiences with IBS and the interpretation of those experiences by health care professionals.

Documentation

Participation in self-care
Emotional status

TRANSITION TO HOME / COMMUNITY CARE

If indicated, review the risk diagnoses identified for this individual on admission:

- Is he person still at risk?
- Can the family reduce the risks?
- Is the person at higher risk at home?
- Is a Home Health Nurse assessment needed?
- Refer to transition planner / case manager / social service
- When is this person scheduled for follow-up with primary provider? Specialists? Record dates of appointments.
- Complete a medication reconciliation prior to transition. Refer to index.

STAR

Stop

Think   Is this person at risk for injury, falls, medical complications, and / or inability to care for self (activities of daily living)?

     Is there a support person available?

     Is the person competent to manage self-administration of medications, treatment procedures? Are additional resources needed?

     Can the person explain how to monitor condition (e.g., blood glucose, sign / symptoms of complications, dietary / mobility restrictions, and when to call his or her primary provider or specialist?

Act   Contact or provide the appropriate resource (e.g., contacting a support person, home health assessment, additional teaching, printed materials).

Review   Has the problem been addressed? If not, use SBAR to communicate to the appropriate person.

Risk for Ineffective Self-Health Management Related to Lack of Knowledge of Condition, Diagnostic Tests, Prognosis, Treatment, and Signs and Symptoms of Complications

NOC

Compliance Behavior, Knowledge: Treatment Regimen, Participation in Health Care Decisions, Treatment Behavior: Illness or Injury

Goal

The goals for this diagnosis represent those associated with transition planning. Refer to the transition criteria.

NIC

Health Education, Health System Guidance, Learning Facilitation, Learning Readiness Enhancement, Risk Identification, Self-Modification Assistance

Interventions	Rationales
1. Assure the individual that you understand the pathophysiology of IBS and that you do not believe that it is a psychological disorder.	1. Researchers have reported that quality of life improved after participants participated in an health program of reassurance, diet management, probiotics, and regular exercise (El-Salhy et al., 2010).
2. Ensure that individual understands the pathophysiology of IBS.	2. A client with IBS may have been led to believe that anxiety or psychological problems caused the disorder. Dispelling this belief can help the client to accept the disorder and encourage compliance with treatment.

(continued)

Interventions	Rationales
3. Explain the familial aspects of IBS.	3. Although the cause of IBS is unknown, 15% to 35% of clients with IBS have a relative with the disorder; thus, it is considered a familial disorder (Turner, 2010).
4. Discuss the symptomatic treatment of IBS a. Medications b. Diet (refer to the nursing diagnosis Altered Nutrition: Less Than Body Requirements in this care plan) c. TPN and bowel rest (refer to the nursing diagnosis Altered Nutrition: Less Than Body Requirements in this care plan)	
5. Advise individual of needed screening: a. Anemia b. Ocular lesions c. Colon cancer	5. The client's understanding of IBS complications can help to ensure early detection and enable prompt treatment. a. Anemia may result from either malabsorption of iron (vitamin B12) or folate deficiency. b. Conjunctivitis, iritis, uveitis, or episcleritis occurs in 3% to 10% of clients with IBS. c. The incidence of colon cancer is 10 to 20 times greater in clients with ulcerative colitis than in the general population. The etiology of cancer in IBS is unknown. Close surveillance is needed because cancer may mimic the signs and symptoms of IBS.
6. Advise to : a. Eat smaller meals more frequently. b. Stress the need to have optimal water intake daily. Advise to monitor hydration by urine color. c. Slowly increase fiber intake with fiber-rich foods or supplements. d. Consider taking a supplement.	6a. Avoiding three meals a day can help reduce the strength of contractions in your intestines. b. The lighter the urine, the more hydrated. Adequate hydration is also needed to prevent constipation. c. Fiber helps to keep stool soft but does not lower pain. Gradual introduction may help to reduce the risk of increased gas and bloating. d. Supplemental fiber usually causes less gas than getting fiber through your diet. Consult with PCP if indicated and take your supplement with plenty of water.
7. Teach the importance of maintaining optimal hydration.	7. Optimal hydration prevents dehydration and reduces the risk of renal calculi formation.
8. Determine if the following cause symptoms and should be avoided: a. Caffeine in coffee, cola beverages, and tea; nicotine in tobacco b. Alcohol	8a. They are muscle stimulants that may have severe effects on hypersensitive bowel muscles. b. Liquor and other alcoholic beverages are proven gastric irritants and often contribute to symptoms of IBS.
9. Minimize stress.	9. Take yoga classes, practice deep breathing exercises, and get regular exercise to promote relaxation.
10. Instruct to keep a food diary in a small notebook: a. What you eat b. When you eat it c. How you are feeling when you eat it d. Occurrence of any symptoms and their intensity	10. A food diary will help the person understand what types of food / fluids exacerbate symptoms.

Interventions	Rationales
11. Advise of lesser-known offenders as lactose, sweeteners like fructose or sorbitol, carbonated beverages, gluten (found in wheat- and barley-based products)	11. Contrary to popular belief, certain dietary restrictions do not reduce hyperacidity. Individual intolerances first must be identified and used as a basis for restrictions. Avoidance of eating prior to bedtime may reduce nocturnal acid levels by eliminating the postprandial stimulus to acid secretion. During the day, regular amounts of food particles in the stomach help to neutralize the acidity of gastric secretions.
12. Teach measures to preserve perianal skin integrity: a. Use soft toilet tissue. b. Cleanse area with mild soap after bowel movements. c. Apply a protective ointment (e.g., A&D, Desitin, Sween Cream).	12. These measures can help prevent skin erosion from diarrheal irritation.
13. Teach the client to report the following signs and symptoms: a. Increasing abdominal pain or distention b. Persistent vomiting c. Unusual rectal or vaginal drainage or rectal pain d. Change in vision e. Continued amber urine f. Flank pain or ache g. Heart palpitations	13. Early reporting enables prompt intervention to reduce the severity of complications. a. Increasing abdominal pain or distention may indicate obstruction or peritonitis. b. Persistent vomiting may point to obstruction. c. Unusual drainage or rectal pain may indicate abscesses or fistulas. d. Vision changes may indicate ocular lesions. e. Amber urine indicates dehydration. f. Flank pain may indicate renal calculi. g. Palpitations may point to potassium imbalance.
14. Provide information on available community resources (e.g., self-help groups, counseling) and client education material on how to live with IBS.	14. Communicating with others with IBS may help the client to cope better with the disorder's effect on his or her lifestyle.

Documentation

Client teaching
Status at transition
Referrals, if indicated

Peptic Ulcer Disease

Under normal conditions, a physiologic balance exists between gastric acid secretion and gastroduodenal mucosal defense. Mucosal injury and, thus, peptic ulcer occur when the balance between the aggressive factors and the defensive mechanisms is disrupted. Aggressive factors, such as NSAIDs, *H pylori* infection, alcohol, bile salts, acid, and pepsin, can alter the mucosal defense by allowing back diffusion of hydrogen ions and subsequent epithelial cell injury. (Anand, 2012) The most common cause of such damage is infection of the stomach by bacteria called *Helicobacter pylori* (*H. pylori*).

Duodenal ulcers are usually caused by hypersecretion of gastric acid. Peptic ulcers are primarily caused by *Helicobacter pylori* bacterium and long-term use of nonsteroidal anti-inflammatory drugs (NSAIDs). Other causes are cancer and hypersecretory disorders such as Zollinger-Ellison syndrome.

Stress related mucosal disease (SRMD) is a gastrointestinal mucosal injury related to the physiologic stress of critical illness. The causes are related to visceral hypoperfusion and loss of host defenses, which results in reduced production of cytoprotectant factors, such as prostaglandins, mucosal atrophy and increased permeability, loss of reparative capacity, and loss of ability to neutralize acid (hydrogen ions).

 Time Frame
Initial diagnosis
Recurrent acute episodes

■■■ DIAGNOSTIC CLUSTER

Collaborative Problems

▲ Risk for Complications of Stress Related Mucosal Disease (SRMD)

▲ Risk for Complications of Hemorrhage

Δ Risk for Complications of Perforation

Nursing Diagnoses

▲ Acute / Chronic Pain related to lesions secondary to increased gastric secretions

Δ Risk for Ineffective Therapeutic Regimen Management related to lack of knowledge of disease process, contraindications, signs and symptoms of complications, and treatment regimen

▲ This diagnosis was reported to be monitored for or managed frequently (75% to 100%).
Δ This diagnosis was reported to be monitored for or managed often (50% to 74%).

Transition Criteria

Before transitions, the client or family will:

1. Identify the causes of disease symptoms.
2. Identify lifestyle changes that are needed to prevent ulcers
3. Identify necessary adjustments to prevent ulcer formation.
4. State signs and symptoms that must be reported to a health care professional.
5. Relate community resources that can provide assistance with lifestyle modifications.

Transitional Risk Assessment Plan (TRAP)

Begin this plan on admission.
Implement the Transitional Risk Assessment Plan (TRAP):
• Refer to inside back cover.
• Add each validated risk diagnosis to client's problem list with the risk code in ( ).
• Refer to Unit II to the individual risk nursing diagnoses / collaborative problems for outcomes and interventions.

R: "Close coordination of care in the post-acute period, early discharge follow-up care, enhanced client education and self-management training, proactive end-of-life counseling, and extending the resources and clinical expertise over time via multidisciplinary team management" can lower readmission rates and improve health outcomes (Boutwell & Hwu, 2009).

Collaborative Problems

Risk for Complications of Stress Related Mucosal Disease (SRMD)

Risk for Complications of Hemorrhage

Risk for Complications of Perforation

Collaborative Outcomes

The client will be monitored for early signs and symptoms of hemorrhage perforation and stress related mucosal disease and will receive collaborative interventions if indicated to restore physiologic stability.

Indicators of Physiologic Stability

• Heart rate 60–100 beats/min, rhythm regular
• Respiratory rate 16–20 breaths/min

- BP >90/60, <40/90 mm Hg
- Urinary output >0.5 mL/kg/h
- No abdominal pain
- Alert, oriented, calm
- Capillary refill <3 seconds
- Gastric pH 3.5–5.0
- Gastric aspirates negative for occult blood

Interventions	Rationales

1. Identify clients at risk for stress ulcers (Sesler, 2007).
  a. Respiratory failure requiring mechanical ventilation for more than 48 h**
  b. Coagulopathies (international normalized ratio >1.5 or platelet count <50,000 mm^3)**
  c. Acute renal insufficiency
  d. Acute hepatic failure
  e. Sepsis syndrome
  f. Hypotension
  g. Severe head or spinal cord injury
  h. Anticoagulation
  i. History of gastrointestinal bleeding
  j. Low intragastric pH
  k. Thermal injury involving more than 35% of the body surface area
  l. Major surgery (lasting more than 4 h)
  m. Administration of high-dose corticosteroids (250 mg/d of steroids or equivalent hydrocortisone)
  n. Enteral feedings
	1. Gastrointestinal ulceration, which causes loss of physiologic reserve, causing acute hypovolemia and end organ injury, can be potentially fatal to critically ill individuals. Hypersecretion of acid is common in clients following head and thermal injuries. The mortality rate associated with such bleeds is extremely high: varying between 48.5% (Cook et al., 1994) and 87.5%) (Skillman et al., 1969).

2. Monitor gastric pH every 2 to 4 hours.
 	
  a. Maintenance of gastric pH 3.5 decreased bleeding complications by 89% (Eisenberg, 1990).
	2. Decreased blood supply to mucosa limits the production of bicarbonate, which results in an inability to control hydrogen ions. These ions damage mucosal cells and capillaries, which leads to the formation of mucosal lesions. Ischemia with a hypersecretion of gastric acid and pepsinogen also interferes with blood flow to the mucosa. Normally, this limited diffusion and bicarbonate neutralization maintain a slightly acid mucosa. Epithelial cells of the stomach are sensitive to even slight decreases in blood supply, which results in necrosis (Porth, 2011).
	  a. The prevention of stress ulceration has focused on reducing the quantity of luminal acid, using H$_2$ receptor antagonists as ranitidine, or sucralfate (a useful alternative).

3. Ensure H$_2$ antagonists are administered on time if using bolus dosing.	3. There is some evidence that giving H$_2$ antagonists as a continuous infusion has greater efficacy (in terms of keeping gastric pH >3.5) than as intermittent boluses (Sesler, 2007).
4. Monitor for occult bleeding in gastric aspirates and bowel movements.	4. Frequent and careful assessment can help diagnose clinically important bleeding before the client's status is compromised.
5. Follow unit protocols for monitoring gastric pH.	5. The user error in pH testing is considerable.

(*continued*)

**Independent risk factors for bleeding.

Interventions	Rationales
6. Assess elderly individuals for central nervous system toxicity with continuous IV administration of H_2RAs e.g., new onset or worsening of confusion of delirium, hallucinations, slurred speech, and / or headaches	6. The incidence of adverse effects are low except in the elderly (Sesler, 2007).

> **CLINICAL ALERT**
> • Report any changes in mental status to Physician / NP.

Interventions	Rationales
7. Monitor for signs and symptoms of hemorrhage and report promptly: a. Hematemesis b. Dizziness c. Generalized weakness d. Melena e. Increasing pulse rate with normal or slightly decreased blood pressure f. Urine output <0.5 mL/h g. Restlessness, agitation, change in mentation h. Increasing respiratory rate i. Diminished peripheral pulses j. Cool, pale, or cyanotic skin k. Thirst	7. Signs and symptoms of hemorrhage may present gradually, or may have a sudden onset. The mortality rate due to ulcer hemorrhage is approximately 5% over the last 20 years (Anand, 2012).

> **CLINICAL ALERT**
> • Access a physician / NP to evaluate the need for therapeutic endoscopy to control bleeding or surgery.

Interventions	Rationales
8. Monitor for gastric ulcer perforation: a. severe abdominal pain b. abdominal swelling, tenderness c. nausea, vomiting d. fever.	8. Upper bowel perforation occurs when an gastric ulcer erodes to create a hole. Bowel contents spill into the abdominal cavity, causing diffuse peritonitis (e.g., duodenal or gastric perforation).

> **CLINICAL ALERT**
> • Call Rapid Response Team if there is a sudden onset of the above symptoms. Emergency surgery is needed.

Clinical Alert Report

Prior to providing care, advise ancillary staff / student to report the following to the professional nurse assigned to the client:
- Report immediately: severe abdominal pain, abdominal swelling, tenderness, nausea, vomiting, fever
- Change in cognitive status
- Oral temperature >100.5° F
- Systolic BP <90 mm Hg
- Resting Pulse >100, <50
- Respiratory rate >28, <10 /min.
- Oxygen saturation <90%
- Occult testing results
- Streaks of blood in stool

Related Physician / NP Prescribed Interventions

Medications
Sedatives, histamine-2 receptor antagonists (H$_2$RA), proton pump inhibitors (PPIs)

Triple therapy or *H. pylori* [Two different antibiotics to kill *H. pylori*, such as clarithromycin (Biaxin), amoxicillin, tetracycline, or metronidazole (Flagyl), Proton pump inhibitors such as omeprazole (Prilosec), lansoprazole (Prevacid), or esomeprazole (Nexium). Bismuth subsalicylate may be added to help kill the bacteria.]

Intravenous Therapy
Variable, depending on severity of illness

Laboratory Studies
Serum gastrin, guaiac testing, CBC, electrolytes

Tests for H-pylori (urea breath tests, serum test for antibodies (immunoglobulin G [IgG]) fecal antigen test)

Obtain histopathology, often considered the criterion standard to establish a diagnosis of *H pylori* infection, if the rapid urease test result is negative and a high suspicion for *H pylori* persists (presence of a duodenal ulcer).

Antibodies (immunoglobulin G [IgG]) to *H pylori* can be measured in serum.

Diagnostic
Esophagogastroduodenoscopy (EGD) or upper endoscopy with rapid urease tests

It is highly sensitive for the diagnosis of gastric and duodenal ulcers, allows for biopsies / cytologic brushings differentiating a benign ulcer from a malignant lesion, and allows for the detection of *H pylori* infection with antral biopsies for a rapid urease test and / or histopathology in clients with PUD (Anand, 2012).

Therapies
NPO or diet as tolerated, nasogastric intubation / gastrostomy

Documentation

Vital signs
Intake and output
Weight
Gastric pH
Stool characteristics
Bowel sounds
Unusual events

Nursing Diagnoses

Acute / Chronic Pain Related to Lesions Secondary to Increased Gastric Secretions

NOC
Comfort Level, Pain Control

Goal
The client will report improvement of pain and an increase in daily activities.

NIC
Pain Management, Medication Management, Emotional Support, Teaching: Individual, Heat / Cold Application, Simple Massage

Indicators

• Report symptoms of discomfort promptly.
• Verbalize increased comfort in response to treatment plan.
• Identify changes in life style to reduce recurrence.

Interventions	Rationales
1. Explain the relationship between hydrochloric acid secretion and onset of pain.	1. Hydrochloric acid (HCl) presumably is an important variable in the appearance of peptic ulcer disease. Because of this relationship, control of HCl secretion is considered an essential aim of treatment (Porth, 2011).
2. Encourage activities that promote rest and relaxation.	2. Relaxation of muscles decreases peristalsis and decreases gastric pain.
3. Help the client to identify irritating substances (e.g., fried foods, spicy foods, coffee). Refer to Risk for Ineffective Self-Health Maintenance for lifestyle modifications.	3. Avoidance of irritating substances can help to prevent the pain response.

Documentation

Progress record

Complaints of pain
Response to treatment plan

TRANSITION TO HOME / COMMUNITY CARE

If indicated, review the risk diagnoses identified for this individual on admission:

- Is the person still at risk?
- Can the family reduce the risks?
- Is the person at higher risk at home?
- Is a Home Health Nurse assessment needed?
- Refer to transition planner / case manager / social service
- When is this person scheduled for follow-up with primary provider? Specialists? Record dates of appointments.
- Complete a medication reconciliation prior to transition. Refer to index.

STAR

Stop

Think   Is this person at risk for injury, falls, medical complications, and / or inability to care for self (activities of daily living)?

Is there a support person available?

Is the person competent to manage self-administration of medications, treatment procedures? Are additional resources needed?

Can the person explain how to monitor the condition (e.g., blood glucose, sign / symptoms of complications, dietary / mobility restrictions, and when to call his or her primary provider or specialist)?

Act   Contact or provide the appropriate resource (e.g., contacting a support person, home health assessment, additional teaching, printed materials).

Review   Has the problem been addressed? If not, use SBAR to communicate to the appropriate person.

Risk for Ineffective Self-Health Management Related to Lack of Knowledge of Disease Process, Contraindications, Signs and Symptoms of Complications, and Treatment Regimen

NOC

Compliance Behavior, Knowledge: Treatment Regimen, Participation in Health Care Decisions, Treatment Behavior: Illness

NIC

Health Education, Health System Guidance, Learning Facilitation, Learning Readiness Enhancement, Risk Identification, Self-Modification Assistance

Goal

The goals for this diagnosis represent those associated with transition planning. Refer to transition criteria.

Interventions	Rationales
1. Explain the pathophysiology of peptic ulcer disease, using terminology and media appropriate to the client's and family's levels of understanding.	1. Understanding helps to reinforce the need to comply with restrictions and may improve compliance.
2. Advise the client to eat regularly and to avoid bedtime snacks.	2. Contrary to popular belief, certain dietary restrictions do not reduce hyperacidity. Individual intolerances first must be identified and used as a basis for restrictions. Avoidance of eating prior to bedtime may reduce nocturnal acid levels by eliminating the postprandial stimulus to acid secretion. During the day, regular amounts of food particles in the stomach help to neutralize the acidity of gastric secretions.
3. Explain the risks of nonsteroidal anti-inflammatory drugs (NSAIDs) (e.g., ibuprofen [Motrin, Aleve, Relafen]) and low-dose aspirin. Discuss with primary care provider what agents can be used for pain (e.g., arthritis, headaches).	3. As many as 25% of chronic NSAID users will develop ulcer disease (3–4) and 2% to 4% will bleed or perforate. Low-dose aspirin is associated with a definite risk for GI complications (Lanza et al., 2009).
4. Encourage the client to avoid smoking.	4. Smoking decreases pancreatic secretion of bicarbonate; this increases duodenal acidity. Tobacco delays the healing of gastric duodenal ulcers and increases their frequency (Katz, 2003).
5. Avoid foods / beverages that increase discomfort.	5. There is no evidence that dietary intake, or moderate intake of caffeine or alcohol causes peptic ulcers (Lutz & Przytulski, 2011).
6. If indicated, explain that alcohol intake should be moderate.	6. Excessive alcohol intake causes gastritis. The link between duodenal ulcers and alcohol is inconclusive; moderation of alcohol intake may be recommended for other health reasons. (Anand, 2012)
7. If the client is being transitioned on antacid therapy, teach the following (Arcangelo & Peterson, 2010): a. Chew tablets well and follow with a glass of water to enhance absorption. b. Lie down for ½ hour after meals to delay gastric emptying. c. Take antacids 1 hour after meals to counteract the gastric acid stimulated by eating.	7. Proper self-administration of antacids can enhance their efficacy and minimize side effects.

(continued)

Interventions	Rationales
8. Avoid antacids high in sodium (e.g., Gelusil, Amphojel, Mylanta II).	8. Excessive sodium intake contributes to fluid retention and elevated blood pressure.
9. If the client is being transitioned on therapy for *Helicobacter Pylori*, explain: a. The relationship of *H. pylori* and gastric ulcers, including its occurrence and reoccurrence b. The need to be on therapy for prescribed number of days c. The need to take all three types of medication d. Possible side effects and the need to call primary care provider with concerns before discontinuing treatment prior to completion	9. Triple therapy for 2 weeks eradicates *H. pylori* at a 90% rate. Eradication of *H. pylori* promotes healing of the ulcer and prevents reoccurrence for at least 7 years. *H. pylori* is also present in 90% of persons with cancer of the stomach.
10. Discuss the importance of continued treatment, even in the absence of overt symptoms.	10. Continued therapy is necessary to prevent recurrence or development of another ulcer.
11. Instruct the client and family to watch for and report these symptoms: a. Red or black stools b. Persistent epigastric pain c. Constipation (not resolved) d. Unexplained temperature elevation e. Persistent nausea f. Vomiting g. Unexplained weight loss h. Call 911 if the following occurs: • Develop sudden, sharp abdominal pain • Have a rigid, hard abdomen that is tender to touch • Have symptoms of shock such as fainting, excessive sweating, or confusion • Vomit blood or have blood in your stool (especially if it's maroon or dark, tarry black)	
12. Refer to community resources, if indicated (e.g., smoking cessation program, stress management class).	12. The client may need assistance with lifestyle changes after transition.

CLINICAL ALERT
Explain that these signs and symptoms may point to complications such as peritonitis, perforation. Early detection and emergency treatment is needed:
- Change in cognitive status
- Oral temperature >100.5° F
- Systolic BP <90 mm Hg
- Resting Pulse >100, <50
- Respiratory rate >28, <10/min.
- Oxygen saturation <90%

Documentation

Client teaching
Referrals

Renal and Urinary Tract Disorders

Acute Kidney Injury

Acute kidney injury (AKI) is a syndrome characterized by an abrupt deterioration of renal function, resulting in the accumulation of metabolic wastes, fluids, and electrolytes, and usually accompanied by a marked decline in urinary output. AKI is one of the few types of total organ failure that may be reversible if the underlying cause is corrected (Baird, Keen, & Swearingen, 2005; Shigehiko et al., 2005; Yaklin, 2011). Although AKI has many causes, ischemia and toxicity are the most common. Depending on where the problem originates, ischemia and toxicity also determine if AKI is prerenal, intrinsic, or postrenal (Hoste et al. 2010; Shira, 2008; Wagner, Johnson, & Kidd, 2006; Yaklin, 2011).

Prerenal AKI occurs when decreased blood flow to the kidneys causes ischemia of the nephrons. Blood loss, severe dehydration, septicemia, and cardiogenic shock are common underlying causes of prerenal AKI. *Intrinsic (formerly known as intrarenal) AKI* is associated with damage to the renal parenchyma. Prerenal AKI can trigger the problem, but a major cause of intrinsic AKI and AKI in general is acute tubular necrosis (damage to the renal tubules caused by ischemia or toxins). *Postrenal AKI* occurs as a result of conditions that block urine flow, causing it to back up into the kidneys. Prostatic hypertrophy, urethral obstruction (usually bilateral), and bladder outlet obstruction are common causes of postrenal AKI (Eachempati, Wang, Hydo, Shou, & Barie, 2007; Kohtz & Thompson, 2007; Shira, 2008; Yaklin, 2011).

Time Frame
Initial diagnosis (post intensive care)
Recurrent acute episodes

■■■ DIAGNOSTIC CLUSTER

Collaborative Problems

▲ Risk for Complications of Fluid Overload

▲ Risk for Complications of Metabolic Acidosis

▲ Risk for Complications of Electrolyte Imbalances

* Risk for Complications of Acute Albuminemia

* Risk for Complications of Hypertension

* Risk for Complications of Pulmonary Edema

* Risk for Complications of Dysrhythmias

* Risk for Complications of Gastrointestinal Bleeding

Nursing Diagnoses

▲ Risk for Infection related to invasive procedure (refer to Unit II)

△ Imbalanced Nutrition: Less Than Body Requirements related to anorexia, nausea, vomiting, loss of taste, loss of smell, stomatitis, and unpalatable diet (refer to Chronic Kidney Disease Care Plan)

(continued)

Related Care Plans

Hemodialysis or Peritoneal Dialysis

Chronic Kidney Disease

▲ This diagnosis was reported to be monitored for or managed frequently (75% to 100%).

Δ This diagnosis was reported to be monitored for or managed often (50% to 74%).

* This diagnosis was not included in the validation study.

Transitional Criteria

The client or family will:

1. Relate the intent to comply with agreed-on restrictions and follow-up.
2. State signs and symptoms that must be reported to a health care professional.
3. Identify how to reduce the risk of infection.

Transitional Risk Assessment Plan (TRAP)

Begin this plan on admission.

Implement the Transitional Risk Assessment Plan (TRAP):

- Refer to inside back cover.
- Add each validated risk diagnosis to client's problem list with the risk code in ( ).
- Refer to Unit II to the individual risk nursing diagnoses / collaborative problems for outcomes and interventions.

R: "Close coordination of care in the post-acute period, early discharge follow-up care, enhanced client education and self-management training, proactive end-of-life counseling, and extending the resources and clinical expertise over time via multidisciplinary team management" can lower readmission rates and improve health outcomes (Boutwell & Hwu, 2009).

Collaborative Problems

Risk for Complications of Fluid Overload

Risk for Complications of Metabolic Acidosis

Risk for Complications of Electrolyte Imbalances

Risk for Complications of Hypertension

Risk for Complications of Pulmonary Edema

Risk for Complications of Dysrhythmias

Risk for Complications of Decreased Level of Consciousness (to Coma)

Risk for Complications of Gastrointestinal Bleeding

Collaborative Outcomes

The client will be monitored for early signs and symptoms of (a) fluid overload, (b) metabolic acidosis, (c) electrolyte imbalances, (d) hypertension, (e) pulmonary edema, (f) dysrhythmias, (g) decreased level of consciousness, (h) gastrointestinal bleeding, and the client will receive collaborative interventions if indicated to restore physiologic stability.

Indicators of Physiologic Stability

- Alert, calm, oriented (a, c, g)
- No seizure activity (b, c, g)

- BP >90/60, <140/90 mm Hg (a, d, e)
- Respirations relaxed and rhythmic (a, e); 16–20 breaths/min (a, e, f, g)
- Pulse 60–100 beats/min; regular rate and rhythm (a, e, f, g)
- EKG normal sinus rhythm (b, c, f)
- Flat neck veins, no edema (pedal, sacral, periorbital) (a)
- Usual or desired weight (a)
- Skin warm, dry, usual color (a, e, f, g, h)
- Bowel sounds all quadrants (c)
- Intact strength, no complaints of numbness / tingling in fingers or toes, no muscle cramps (b, c)
- Serum albumin 3.5–5 g/dL (b, c)
- Serum prealbumin 1–3 g/dL (b, c)
- Serum sodium 135–145 mEq/L (b, c)
- Serum potassium 3.8–5 mEq/L (b, c)
- Serum calcium 8.5–10.5 mg/dL (b, c)
- Serum phosphates 3–5 mg/dL (b, c)
- Blood urea nitrogen 10–20 mg/dL (b)
- Creatinine 0.5–1.2 mg/dL [men in the slightly higher range] (b)
- Alkaline phosphate 30–150 IU/mL (b)
- Creatinine clearance 100–150 mL/min (a, b)
- Oxygen saturation (SaO_2) >94% (a, e, g)
- Carbon dioxide ($PaCO_2$) 35–45 mmHg (a)
- Urine output >0.5 mL/kg/h (a, h)
- Urine specific gravity 1.005–1.030 (a)
- Normal stool formation, stool negative for hemoglobin (h)
- No vomitus positive for hemoglobin (h)

Interventions	Rationales
1. Monitor for signs of fluid overload: a. Weight gain (1 kg = 1 L) b. Increased blood pressure and pulse rate, neck vein distention c. Dependent edema (periorbital, pedal, pretibial, sacral) d. Adventitious breath sounds (e.g., wheezes, crackles) e. Urine specific gravity <1.010	1. The oliguric phase of acute kidney failure usually lasts from 5 to 15 days and often is associated with excess fluid volume retention. Functionally, the changes result in decreased glomerular filtration, tubular transport of substances, urine formation, and renal clearance (Yaklin, 2011).
2. Weigh client daily. (Weigh more often, if indicated.) Ensure accuracy by weighing at the same time every day on the same scale and with the client wearing the same amount of clothing.	2. Weighing the client daily can help to determine fluid balance and appropriate fluid intake.
3. Maintain strict intake and output records. Include all fluid loss—urine, vomit, diarrhea, wound and nasogastric drainage. Include all fluid intake—oral, intravenous, and nasogastric. Consider all sensible and insensible losses when calculating replacement fluids. Adjust the client's fluid intake so it approximates fluid loss plus 300 to 500 mL/day. Compare with daily weight loss or gain for correlation of fluid balance.	3. A 1-kg weight gain should correlate with excess intake of 1 L (1 L of fluid weighs 1 kg, or 2.2 lb). Insensible losses include respirations and perspiration. Careful replacement can prevent fluid overload or deficit.

(continued)

Interventions	*Rationales*
4. Manage fluids: a. Administer oral medications with meals whenever possible. If medications must be administered between meals, give with the smallest amount of fluid necessary. b. Avoid continuous IV fluid infusion whenever possible. Dilute all necessary IV drugs in the smallest amount of fluid safe for IV administration c. Engage the client and / or family in discussions about fluid management goals and strategies. • Encourage their input, questions and suggestions. • Provide ongoing clinical updates. • Allow time for the client to express feelings. • Give her or him positive feedback. d. Distribute fluid intake fairly evenly throughout the entire day and night. e. Consult with dietitian regarding fluid plan and overall diet.	4a. This prevents the fluid allowance from being used up unnecessarily. b. A small IV bag or an infusion pump will avoid accidental infusion of a large volume of fluid. c. The client's and family's understanding of the need for fluid management can help gain their cooperation and lessen feelings of uncertainty or frustration. d. Toxins can accumulate with decreased fluid and cause nausea and sensorium changes. It may be necessary to match fluid intake with loss every 8 hours or even every hour if the client is critically imbalanced. e. Fluid content of nonliquid food, amount and type of liquids, liquid preferences, and sodium content are all important in fluid management. Nutritional needs will change as kidney function improves or declines. Dietitians assist in calculating caloric, protein, electrolyte, lipid and micronutrient requirements. (Cotton, 2007)
5. Monitor for signs and symptoms of metabolic acidosis: a. Rapid, shallow respiration b. Headache c. Nausea and vomiting d. Low plasma bicarbonate e. Low arterial blood pH (<7.35) f. Behavior changes, drowsiness, and lethargy **CLINICAL ALERT** • Metabolic acidosis with a blood pH less than 7.2 can result in life-threatening vasodilation, cardiac arrhythmias, and hyperkalemia. • Emergent treatment with medications and possible dialysis needs to be initiated (Yaklin, 2011).	5. Acidosis results from the kidney's inability to excrete hydrogen ions, phosphates, sulfates, and ketone bodies. Bicarbonates are lost when the kidney reduces its reabsorption. Hyperkalemia, hyperphosphatemia, and decreased bicarbonate levels aggravate metabolic acidosis. Excessive ketone bodies cause headaches, nausea, vomiting, and abdominal pain. Increases in respiratory rate and depth enhance CO_2 excretion and reduce acidosis. Acidosis affects the central nervous system (CNS) and can increase neuromuscular irritability because of the cellular exchange of hydrogen and potassium (Bhardwaj, Mirski, & Ulatowski, 2004).
6. Ensure sufficient caloric intake and nutritional balance by consulting a dietitian for appropriate diet of adequate carbohydrate, fat, and protein intake.	6. Fats provide 9 calories / g and protein and carbohydrates provide 4 calories / g. Renal insufficiency and uremia alter metabolism of these nutrients so adjustments will be needed based on cause and degree of AKI (Karalis, 2008).
7. Assess for signs and symptoms of hypocalcemia, hypokalemia, and alkalosis as acidosis is corrected.	7. Rapid correction of acidosis may cause rapid excretion of calcium and potassium and rebound alkalosis.
8. Monitor for signs and symptoms of hypernatremia with fluid overload: a. Thirst b. CNS effects ranging from agitation to convulsions c. Edema, weight gain d. Hypertension e. Tachycardia f. Dyspnea g. Rales	8. Hypernatremia results from excessive sodium intake or increased aldosterone output. Water is pulled from the cells, which causes cellular dehydration and produces CNS symptoms. Thirst is a compensatory response to dilute sodium (Baird, Keen, & Swearingen, 2005; Bogle et al., 2008).

Interventions	Rationales
9. Maintain sodium restriction.	9. Hypernatremia must be corrected slowly to minimize CNS deterioration (Bogle et al., 2008).
10. Monitor for signs and symptoms of hyponatremia: a. CNS effects ranging from lethargy to coma b. Weakness c. Abdominal pain d. Muscle twitching or convulsions e. Nausea, vomiting, and diarrhea	10. Hyponatremia results from sodium loss through vomiting, diarrhea, or diuretic therapy; excessive fluid intake; or insufficient dietary sodium. Cellular edema, caused by osmosis, produces cerebral edema, weakness, and muscle cramps (Bogle et al., 2008).
11. Monitor for signs and symptoms of hyperkalemia. a. Anxiety b. Weakness to paralysis c. Muscle irritability d. Paresthesias e. Nausea, abdominal cramping, or diarrhea f. Irregular pulse g. Electrocardiogram (ECG) changes: tall, tented T-waves, ST segment depression, prolonged PR interval (>0.2 second), first-degree heart block, bradycardia, broadening the ORS complex, eventual ventricular fibrillation, and cardiac standstill.	11. Hyperkalemia results from the kidney's decreased ability to excrete potassium or from excess intake of potassium. Acidosis increases release of potassium from cells. Fluctuations in potassium affect neuromuscular transmission; this produces cardiac dysrhythmias, reduces action of GI smooth muscle, and impairs electrical conduction (Baird, Keen, & Swearingen, 2005; Williams et al., 2008).

12. Intervene for hyperkalemia:
a. Restrict potassium-rich foods and fluids. Do not allow salt substitute that contains potassium as the cation (Williams et al., 2008).
b. Correction of acidosis will help alleviate hyperkalemia.
c. Emergency medications as ordered with follow-up labs.
  • Insulin and glucose to push potassium back into cells
  • Calcium to temporarily stabilize cardiac electrical activity
  • Exchange resin (e.g., sodium polystyrene sulfonate) to pull potassium into bowel
d. Hemodialysis on a low or potassium-free bath removes K+ rapidly and efficiently from the plasma.
e. Administer blood transfusions during hemodialysis to remove excess K+.
	12. High potassium levels necessitate a reduced potassium intake. Intervention needs to begin when elevation is noted. This can be done with dietary changes, medication adjustments, and dialysis.

CLINICAL ALERT
- Potassium levels greater than 6.5 mmol/L are an immediate emergency.
- Persons on chronic dialysis may be less likely to exhibit signs and symptoms than those experiencing acute kidney injury (Yaklin, 2011).

(continued)

Interventions	*Rationales*
13. Monitor for signs and symptoms and risks of hypokalemia: a. Weakness or paralysis b. Decreased or no deep-tendon reflexes c. Hypoventilation d. Polyuria e. Hypotension f. Constipation; paralytic ileus g. ECG changes: U wave, flat T-wave, dysrhythmias, and prolonged Q-T interval h. Increased risk of digitalis toxicity i. Nausea, vomiting, and anorexia	13. Hypokalemia results from losses associated with vomiting, diarrhea, or diuretic therapy or from insufficient potassium intake. Hypokalemia impairs neuromuscular transmission and reduces the efficiency of respiratory muscles. Kidneys are less sensitive to antidiuretic hormone (ADH) and thus excrete large quantities of dilute urine. Gastrointestinal smooth muscle action is also reduced. Abnormally low potassium levels also impair electrical conduction of the heart (Bogle et al. 2008; Shigehiko et al., 2005; Shira, 2008).
14. Intervene for hypokalemia: a. Evaluation of lab values when hyperkalemia is being corrected. b. Encourage increased intake of potassium-rich foods. c. Dietary consult d. Intravenous potassium replacement as ordered e. Medication adjustment as ordered (e.g., change in diuretic to preserve potassium) f. Client education regarding signs and symptoms of low potassium and rationale for dietary recommendations.	14. Correct or prevent potassium deficit to avoid potentially life-threatening consequences. Overcorrection of hyperkalemia can cause hypokalemia. Increased potassium intake helps to ensure potassium replacement (Shira, 2008).
15. Monitor for signs and symptoms of hypocalcemia: a. Altered mental status b. Numbness or tingling in fingers and toes and around the mouth c. Muscle cramps d. Seizures e. ECG changes: prolonged Q-T interval, prolonged ST segment, and dysrhythmias	15. Hypocalcemia results from the kidneys' inability to metabolize vitamin D (needed for calcium absorption); retention of phosphorus causes a reciprocal drop in serum calcium level. Low serum calcium level produces increased neural excitability resulting in muscle spasms (cardiac, facial, extremities) and CNS irritability (seizures). It also causes cardiac muscle hyperactivity as evidenced by ECG changes (Baird, Keen, & Swearingen, 2005; Bogle et al., 2008).
16. Intervene for hypocalcemia. Administer a high-calcium, low-phosphorus diet. Acute decreases may require intravenous administration.	16. Elevated phosphate levels lower serum calcium level, necessitating dietary replacement.

> **CLINICAL ALERT:** (Karalis, 2008)
> • Calcium is bound to protein in the serum. If the serum albumin is less than 4 gm/dL the calcium lab value needs to be corrected to reflect accurate results to avoid over or under correction.
> • Corrected serum calcium = Total calcium mg/dL + [0.8 × (4 − serum albumin g/dL)]. Many labs will report a "corrected calcium" level.

Interventions	*Rationales*
17. Monitor for signs and symptoms of hypermagnesemia: a. Weakness b. Hypoventilation c. Hypotension d. Flushing e. Behavioral changes	17. Hypermagnesemia results from the kidneys' decreased ability to excrete magnesium. Its effects include CNS depression, respiratory depression, and peripheral vasodilation (Baird, Keen, & Swearingen, 2005; Wagner, Johnson, & Kidd, 2006).

Interventions	Rationales

18. Monitor for signs and symptoms of hyperphosphatemia:
  a. Tetany
  b. Numbness or tingling in fingers and toes
  c. GI disturbance–nausea, vomiting, anorexia
  d. Tachycardia
	18. Hyperphosphatemia results from the kidneys' decreased ability to excrete phosphorus and from the breakdown of lean muscle mass due to catabolism. Symptoms that occur from elevated phosphorus are usual a result of hypocalcemia. (Williams et al., 2008)

19. For a client with hyperphosphatemia, administer phosphorus-binding antacids, calcium supplements, or vitamin D, and restrict phosphorus-rich foods.	19. The client needs supplements to overcome vitamin D deficiency or compensate for a calcium deficit through low diet intake, poor intestinal absorption, or calcium loss during diuretic phase of recovery. High phosphate decreases calcium, which increases parathyroid hormone (PTH) secretion. During AKI PTH is less effective in removing phosphates and absorbing calcium from the gut. The result is calcium reabsorption from the bones and decreases tubular reabsorption of phosphate. (Counts et al., 2008)

20. Monitor for signs and symptoms of hypertension:
  a. Headache
  b. Fatigue
  c. Dizziness
  d. Blurred vision
	20. Hypertension is a common manifestation of renal failure. It is caused by systemic and central fluid volume excess and increased renin production. In the presence of renal ischemia the renin-angiotensin system is triggered, which results in increased blood pressure and increased renal blood flow. (Baird, Keen, & Swearingen, 2005; Schonder & Cincotta, 2008)

21. Monitor for signs and symptoms of pulmonary edema:
  a. Cough with possible pink frothy sputum
  b. Dyspnea and tachypnea with use of accessory muscles for breathing
  c. Rales, decreased oxygen saturation
  d. Anxiety
  e. Excessive sweating and pale skin
	21. Pulmonary edema is usually a result of cardiac failure but can also be caused by renal failure due to fluid volume excess and electrolyte imbalance (Headley & Wall, 2007; Wagner, Johnson, & Kidd, 2006).

22. Monitor for signs and symptoms of change in level of consciousness:
  a. Fatigue and lethargy
  b. Altered mental status
  c. Decreased range of movement
	22. A decrease in mental functioning is a direct result of an accumulation of nitrogenous waste products from impaired renal excretion and metabolic acidosis (Wagner, Johnson, & Kidd, 2006; Williams et al., 2008).

23. Monitor for signs and symptoms of gastrointestinal bleeding:
  a. Abdominal pain with or without vomiting of blood
  b. Black tarry stool
  c. Tachycardia
  d. Hypotension
	23. Increasing levels of uremic toxins are the primary contributors to gastrointestinal (GI) manifestations. As urea decomposes in the GI tract, it releases ammonia. Ammonia in the GI tract increases capillary fragility and GI mucosal irritation, small mucosal ulcerations may develop, causing GI bleeding. (Wagner, Johnson, & Kidd, 2006; Williams et al., 2008)

24. Consult with the physician or advanced practice nurse, who may ordered renal replacement therapy (RRT) usually as intermittent hemodialysis (IHD) or continuous renal replacement therapy (CRRT) if medical management is not sufficient to control symptoms and complications of AKI.	24. CRRT offers advantages of greater hemodynamic stability with slower but continuous fluid removal and fluid / electrolyte balance. IHD provides more rapid fluid removal and electrolyte balance in a shorter time frame but has increased risk of hypotensive events. (Yaklin, 2011)

Clinical Alert Report

Prior to providing care, advise ancillary staff / student to report the following to the professional nurse assigned to the client:

- AKI can present with a rapidly changing clinical picture, which may require urgent intervention. Infections are the primary cause of morbidity and mortality in AKI. Therefore, advise ancillary staff / student to report.
- Any new changes or deteriorations in client's behavior or symptoms (e.g., level of consciousness, agitation, confusion)
- Blood pressure or pulse outside of the range established for that client (see Indicators for baseline.)
- Difficulty breathing or respirations less than 10 a minute
- Temperature (oral) 1 to 2° F over baseline. Uremia suppresses temperature so lower reading may still indicate fever and possible infection.
- Change in urine output from baseline. Fluid and medication management may need adjustment as kidney function changes.
- Any redness, warmth, drainage, or tenderness at IV or catheter sites.

Nursing Diagnoses

TRANSITION TO HOME / COMMUNITY CARE
- Review risk diagnoses and interventions identified on admission.
- Use STAR (Stop, Think, Act, Review) to help assess current risk and SBAR (Situation, Background, Action, Recommendation) to develop feasible plan.
- Client and family need to continue good infection control measures especially hand washing and avoidance of ill individuals.
- Do client and family have resources to maintain adequate hygiene, obtain prescribed medications, return for scheduled follow-up appointments, and understand how to contact appropriate health care personnel for after transition questions or concerns?
- Consider referral to transition planner, case manager, and / or social service prior to transition if risk diagnoses are still present.
- Consider referral for home health for additional services if indicated.

STAR   **Stop**

Think   What are the client's risks upon transition?
            Does the client / family understand how to minimize risk of infection in home environment?

Act   Does client have support system?
            Use SBAR

            Situation: Client is being transitioned to his home.

            Background: Client lives alone and cares for several farm animals. Client still feels weak.

            Action: More thorough evaluation of home environment

            Recommendation: Discuss family support options and refer to transition planner, case manager, or social worker. Can family assist client after transition and if so in what capacity? Refer to Home Health nursing for possible teaching and monitoring.

Review Is the plan feasible and safe to client and family? If not, what other options are available?
            - This plan begins on admission and involves client, family, and other support persons.

Risk for Infection related to invasive procedure

Client and family need education regarding need for infection control measures—good hand washing, avoidance of persons who are ill, dressing changes.

Imbalanced Nutrition: Less Than Body Requirements related to anorexia, nausea, vomiting, loss of taste, loss of smell, stomatitis, and unpalatable diet

Client and family require education on maximizing nutritional input—smaller and more frequent meals, foods with required nutrients, possible need for oral or intravenous supplements.

Risk for Injury related to stress, retention of metabolic wastes and end products, altered capillary permeability, and platelet dysfunction

Client and family will receive education on possible side effects of AKI and methods of minimizing these– assistance with getting out of bed and walking, secure nonslip foot wear, avoidance of constipation, reporting any evidence of blood loss, reporting any physical or psychological changes, encouraging questions.

Risk for Ineffective Self-Health Management related to illness, medications, procedures (see Hemodialysis and peritoneal dialysis)

Provide education, informal or formal, to client and family with each encounter (e.g., what the medication is and reason for its administration, when procedures are scheduled and approximate length of treatment, clarification of tests and laboratory results that have been reviewed, or availability of outside services). Encourage questions and clarification of data.

STAR

Stop

Think Is this person at risk for injury, falls, medical complications, and / or inability to care for self (activities of daily living)?

Is there a support person available?

Is the person competent to manage self-administration of medications, treatment procedures? Are additional resources needed?

Can the person explain how to monitor the condition (e.g., blood glucose, sign / symptoms of complications, dietary / mobility restrictions, and when to call his or her primary provider or specialist)?

Act Contact or provide the appropriate resource (e.g., contacting a support person, home health assessment, additional teaching, printed materials).

Review Has the problem been addressed? If not, use SBAR to communicate to the appropriate person.

Risk for Ineffective Self-Health Management Related to Lack of Knowledge of Disease Process, Treatments, Contraindications, Dietary Management, and Follow-up Care

Interventions	Rationales
1. Explain any ongoing risks of infection and avoidance strategies post transition. Include instructions in care of any external devices such as an intravenous catheter.	1. Client and family are more likely to be able to avoid and manage risks if they understand how this pertains to their immediate surroundings.
2. Review all transition medications including purpose, side effects, and how to contact health care personnel for questions or concerns. Reinforce any medications that need to be avoided (e.g., nonsteroidal pain medications may be restricted or contraindicated).	2. Clients are less likely to stop or change medication regime if they understand the purpose of medications and can obtain rapid assistance with any questions.
3. Provide clear and accurate instructions regarding when, why, and where to report any new or returning symptoms. Example could include fever, change in urine output, and changes in energy or mental status.	3. Clients and families need ongoing support and clear directions for follow-up of possible problems.
4. Review any dietary recommendations or changes. Elicit concerns regarding ability to follow or access foods for prescribed diet. Consider contacting dietitian for ongoing client questions or social services for financial concerns.	4. Clients may need assistance in understanding and incorporating food changes. Financial limitations may hinder prescribed food changes.

Collaborative Problems

Risk for Complications of Fluid Imbalance

Risk for Complications of Anemia

Risk for Complications of Hypertension

Risk for Complications of Hyperparathyroidism

Risk for Complications of Pathological Fractures

Risk for Complications of Hypoalbuminemia

Risk for Complications of Congestive Heart Failure

Risk for Complications of Metabolic Acidosis

Risk for complications of Diabetes

Collaborative Outcomes

The client will be monitored for early signs and symptoms of (a) fluid imbalance, (b) anemia, (c) hyperparathyroidism, (d) pathologic fractures, (e) hypoalbuminemia, (f) congestive heart failure, (g) metabolic acidosis, (h) Hypertension, (i) diabetes, and the client will receive collaborative interventions if indicated to restore physiologic stability.

Indicators of Physiologic Stability

- Alert, calm, oriented
- Respiration 16–20 breaths/min, unlabored respirations with clear breath sounds in all lobes
- Pulse 60–100 beats/min with regular rate and rhythm, no palpitations or chest pain
- BP >90/60, <140/90 mm Hg
- Temperature 98.5–99° F
- No or minimal edema (a, f)
- Ideal or desired weight (a, f)
- Urine output >0.5 mL/kg/h (a, f)
- Red blood cells 4,000,000–6,200,000 mm^3 (b)
- White blood cells 48,000–100,000 mm^3 (j)
- Hematocrit (b)
    - Male 42% to 50%
    - Female 40% to 48%
- Hemoglobin (b)
    - Male 13–18 g/dL
    - Female 12–16 g/dL
- Serum albumin 3.5–5 g/dL (f)
- Total cholesterol <200 mg/dL (f)
  Iron 60–175 mcg/lL (b)
  Total iron binding capacity 240–450 mcg/dL (b)
- Transferrin saturation 20% to 50% [iron/TIBC x 100%](b)
- Serum ferritin (b)
    - Males 29–438 ng/mL
    - Females 9–219 ng/mL
- Serum potassium 3.8–5 mEq/L (b, l)
- Serum sodium 135–145 mEq/L (a, l)
- Serum calcium 8.5–10.5 mg/dL (c, l)

- Serum phosphate 2.7–4.6 mg/dL (c, d)
  Magnesium 1.7–3 mEq/L
- Blood urea nitrogen 10–20 mg/dL (h, l)
- Creatinine 0.5–1.2 ng/mL (h, l)
- Alkaline phosphatase 45–150 IU/L (c)
- Urine sodium 130–200 mEq/24h (a)
- Creatinine clearance >60 mL/min (f)
- Oxygen saturation (SaO_2) >94% (a, h, l)
- Carbon dioxide ($PaCO_2$) 35–45 mmHg (a, h)

Interventions	Rationales
1. Monitor for fluid imbalances: a. Weight changes b. BP changes c. Increased pulse d. Increased respirations e. Neck vein distention f. Dependent, peripheral edema g. Increased fluid intake h. Increased sodium intake i. Orthostatic hypotension (decreased fluid volume)	1. Fluid imbalance, usually hypervolemia, results from failure of kidney to regulate extracellular fluids by decreased sodium and water elimination (Shira, Assessment, 2008).
2. Consult with nephrology staff / student if fluid volume changes. Refer to dialysis care plans for specific fluid management strategies.	2. In advanced CKD, dialysis may be needed to control fluid overload.
3. Frequently monitor vital signs, particularly blood pressure and pulse.	3. Circulating volume must be monitored with chronic kidney disease to prevent severe hypervolemia.
4. Monitor for anemia. a. Dyspnea b. Fatigue c. Tachycardia d. Palpitations e. Pallor of nail beds and mucous membranes f. Low hemoglobin and hematocrit g. Bruising	4. A decline is directly proportional to the frequency and volume of blood loss associated with phlebotomy-related blood drawing, blood loss during dialysis or other procedures, and a decline in erythropoietin production from the kidney (Macdougall, 2011). Decreased hemoglobin indicates fewer RBCs are available to transport oxygen. Shortness of breath, fatigue, tachycardia, and palpitations are common symptoms especially with activity. These may resolve with rest. Cold intolerance also results from fewer RBCs. Pallor is evident where blood flow is close to the skin as in mucous membranes and nail beds. As CKD progresses, RBC survival time decreases due to less erythropoietin production and elevated uremic toxins. Bruising may be more evident.

(continued)

Interventions	Rationales
5. Determine the cause of anemia as:	5. Adequate iron must be available to produce healthy functional RBCs. About 70% of iron is stored in the RBCs and the remainder in the liver and reticuloendothelial system. *Absolute* iron deficiency is indicated by low iron, percent saturation, and ferritin with high TIBC and will respond to iron therapy. *Functional* iron deficiency may have an elevated ferritin indicating an inflammation or infection which blocks iron transfer from for use. Further exploration for a treatable cause is indicated. Clients who cannot tolerate or are not responsive to oral iron need to be evaluated for intravenous iron. (Macdougall, 2011)
a. Assess for blood loss—gastrointestinal, menses, phlebotomy. See Dialysis Care Plan if indicated.	a. Anemia occurs if blood loss exceeds RBC production. Avoid unnecessary collection of blood specimens by coordinate blood draws. Educate the client on methods to minimize blood loss (e.g., use a soft toothbrush, avoid vigorous nose blowing, and avoid constipation). Demonstrate how to apply direct pressure over a bleeding site.
b. Evaluate folate and vitamin B12 levels.	b. Folic acid and B12 are absorbed in the intestine. B12 is needed to convert folate to the active form and both vitamins are necessary for RBC production and function.
c. Evaluate for possible side effects of medications.	c. Anemia is a side effect of several classes of medication (e.g., immunosuppressant).
d. Evaluate fluid status—see Fluid Management.	d. Because of dilution, hemoglobin will appear lower in the presence of fluid overload.
e. Consider hematologic etiology (e.g., myelodyplastic syndrome, thalassemia, malignancy).	e. Disorders of the bone marrow can interfere with RBC production.

6. Evaluate iron status.
   a. Measure serum iron, total iron binding capacity (TIBC), percentage transferrin saturation (% saturation) and ferritin (see indicators for values).
   b. Correct iron depletion with oral or intravenous iron.
   c. Discuss with the client any concerns or barriers to taking prescribed oral iron therapy.
   d. Explore possible causes of poor iron absorption (e.g., insufficient dietary iron, poor absorption due to prior GI surgery).
   e. Consider intravenous iron in severe depletion, intolerance to or poor absorption of oral iron.

> **CLINICAL ALERT**
> - All intravenous iron products carry some risk of anaphylactic or anaphylactoid response.
> - Symptoms can range from hypotension; dyspnea; chest, back, flank or groin pain; arthralgias / myalgias; fever; and malaise.
> - Clients need to be monitored and educated on possible side effects including delayed reactions.
> - IV iron needs to be given per the current manufacturer recommendations for each specific product. (Macdougall, 2011)

Interventions	Rationales
7. Administer bulk-forming laxatives or stool softeners if client is constipated. Avoid magnesium and phosphate containing laxatives.	7. Constipation is a common side effect of oral iron products. Certain laxatives contain magnesium and phosphate. Clients with kidney disease already have difficulty excreting usual intake of magnesium and phosphate in foods so need to avoid additional sources of these elements. See Acute Kidney Injury for signs and symptoms of hypermagnesemia and hyperphosphotemia.
8. Provide erythropoiesis stimulating agent (ESA) therapy as indicated and prescribed 👤 **CLINICAL ALERT** • FDA Black Box Warning for all erythropoiesis stimulating agent (ESAs). ESAs increase the risk of death, myocardial infarction, stroke, venous thromboembolism, thrombosis of vascular access and tumor progression or recurrence. (Macdougall, 2011) a. Monitor blood pressure prior to each dose. Dose should be held in presence of uncontrolled hypertension. b. Measure hemoglobin at least monthly before a dose is administered or more often during titration. c. Monitor iron stores—serum iron, percent transferrin saturation, ferritin. d. If the client on an ESA and / or iron therapy is nonresponsive to therapy or has a drop in hemoglobin evaluate for an underlying cause. e. Assess for underlying causes: • Hyperparathyroidism • Osteitis fibrosa • Hematologic disease • Sudden loss of responsiveness to recombinant human erythropoietin-alfa (rHuEPO)	8. Erythropoietin (EPO) is produced in the kidney. ESAs are genetically engineered EPO administered to maintain hemoglobin levels. Current FDA guidelines for kidney disease recommend not starting ESA therapy until other causes of anemia have been corrected and the hemoglobin level is below10 g/dL. Hemoglobin levels should not exceed 12 g/dL with active therapy. Dosing depends on the agent used and the laboratory response. Follow the protocols of the institution. (Macdougall, 2011) a. ESAs increases blood viscosity and can increase blood pressure and possible thrombus formation including stroke. BP medication may be needed. b. Hemoglobin increases >1 g/dL in less than 2 weeks may contribute to CV events. Goal is to avoid red cell transfusions. Recommendation is to decrease dose if hemoglobin is over 11 g/dL. c. Iron stores will be depleted more quickly with ESA therapy. Replete either with oral or intravenous iron before starting ESA and to maintain stores while on ESA. Check quarterly if on maintenance iron or monthly during iron replacement. d. See "Determine the Cause of Anemia." e. Underlying causes of mineral bone disease will need to be diagnosed and corrected.
9. Evaluate aluminum levels and elevated lead levels.	9. Changes in the bone marrow and matrix can affect red blood cell production and bone strength. Loss of renal function alters normal regulation of calcium, phosphorus and parathyroid hormone and elimination of aluminum. Exposure to heavy metals (e.g., aluminum and lead can form deposits in bone which interferes with healthy function). Clients need to avoid potentially toxic sources including aluminum containing antacids. Referral to hematology may be necessary to further diagnose bone marrow dysfunction. (Cheng, 2011)

(continued)

Interventions	Rationales

10. Monitor for manifestations of decreased albumin levels:
  a. Serum albumin <3.5 g/dL and proteinuria (>300 mg protein/24 hours)
  b. Edema formation: pedal, facial, sacral
  c. Infection
  d. Hyperlipidemia
  e. thromboembolism
  f. Signs and symptoms of negative nitrogen balance:
    • Decreased serum cholesterol
    • Decreased caloric intake (<45 Kcal/kg)
    • Decreased protein intake (<0.75 g/kg)
    • Delayed wound healing
    • Muscle wasting
	10. When albumin is lost through urinary excretion or peritoneal dialysis, the liver responds by increasing production of plasma proteins. If the loss continues the liver cannot compensate and hypoalbuminemia, increased low-density lipoprotein accumulation, and alterations in the clotting cascade results. Edema formation results from decreased plasma proteins and consequent decreased plasma oncotic pressure that causes a fluid shift from the vascular to the interstitial compartment. Hypovolemia can result from fluid loss, which leads to hemoconcentration and a consequent increase in hemoglobin and hematocrit. If the volume loss becomes great, shock occurs (Porth, 2011; Deegens & Wetzels, 2011). A negative nitrogen balance results from protein and caloric malnutrition, leading to an oxygen and nutrient deficit that causes cellular catabolism, cell breakdown, and nitrogen loss. Humoral defenses to infection are depressed owing to protein loss, and general protein reserves are depleted resulting in slowed healing.

11. Hold a dietary consultation for nutritional assessment and to provide for the following:
  a. Fluid restrictions (with massive edema)
  b. Low-sodium diet
  c. Adequate calorie intake
  d. Appropriate protein diet with high biological protein (meats, poultry, cheese, milk)
  e. Adjusted phosphate and calcium requirements
	11. Depending on the stage of chronic kidney disease and the underlying cause protein may be restricted to 0.75 to 1.25 g/kg, with emphasis on high biological value protein. High biological value proteins supply the essential amino acids necessary for cell growth and repair, but produce less urea nitrogen during metabolism. Calories should be generous (35 to 45 Kcal/kg) to allow use of the minerals in protein for tissue maintenance. Tissue catabolism can develop when protein intake is inadequate. Catabolism increases BUN levels, acidosis, and hyperkalemia. A low-sodium diet may be beneficial to prevent additional fluid retention. The client should be monitored for fluid depletion because of the dangers of hypovolemia and hypotension. Laboratory results will help determine need for phosphate and calcium dietary modifications. (Fouque & Juillard, 2011; Gutekunst, 2011)

12. Evaluate daily:
  a. Weight
  b. Fluid intake and output records
  c. Circumference of the edematous part(s)
  d. Laboratory data: hematocrit, serum potassium, and plasma protein in specific serum albumin
	12. As GFR decreases and the functioning nephron mass continues to diminish, the kidneys lose the ability to concentrate urine and to excrete sodium and water; this results in hypervolemia.

13. Monitor for signs and symptoms of congestive heart failure (CHF) and decreased cardiac output:
  a. Gradual increase in heart rate
  b. Increased shortness of breath
  c. Diminished breath sounds, rales
  d. Decreased systolic BP
  e. Presence of or increase in S3 and / or S4
  f. Gallop
  g. Peripheral edema
  h. Distended neck veins
	13. Diminished urinary output causes volume retention that can lead to cardiomegaly and CHF. This results in reduced ability of left ventricle to eject blood and consequent decreased cardiac output and increased pulmonary vascular congestion. This causes fluid to enter the pulmonary tissue, leading to respiratory distress, rales, productive cough, and cyanosis. (van Kimmenade & Januzzi, 2011)

Interventions	Rationales
14. Encourage adherence to prescribed fluid restrictions. In advanced CKD with decreased urine output the restriction may be 800 to 1,000 mL/24 hours or 24-hour urine output plus 500 mL.	14. A client who presents with evidence of fluid overload requires fluid restriction based on urine output. In an anuric client, restriction generally is 800 mL/day, which accounts for insensible losses from metabolism, the GI tract, perspiration, and respiration. Sodium restrictions are usually simultaneously prescribed. (Counts et al., 2008)
15. Reevaluate and reestablish the client's optimal "dry" weight—that weight at which a client is free of any signs or symptoms of overload and maintains a normal blood pressure.	15. A client with chronic kidney disease is prone to fluctuations in weight, necessitating frequent reevaluation for optimal fluid balance. Accepted inter-dialytic weight gain is 1 to 2 lb per 24 hours (Hlebovy, 2008).
16. Collaborate with physician, NP, or dietitian in planning an appropriate diet. Encourage adherence to a prescribed-sodium diet (1–4 g/24 h depending on stage of CKD and fluid status).	16. Sodium restrictions should be adjusted based on urine sodium excretion, serial weights, stage of CKD, and current medications (Karalis, 2008; Turban & Miller III, 2011).
17. Monitor for manifestations of pleural effusion: a. Variable dyspnea b. Pleuritic pain c. Diminished and delayed chest movement on involved side d. Bulging of intercostal spaces (in massive effusion) e. Decreased breath sounds over site of pleural effusion f. Decreased vocal and tactile fremitus g. Increased rate and depth of respirations	17. A pleural effusion is a collection of fluid, either transudates or exudates, in the pleural cavity. Transudates are seen in chronic kidney disease and result from a rise in pulmonary venous pressure secondary to fluid overload. This transudation also may occur owing to the hypoproteinemia often seen in chronic kidney disease (Shira, Assessment, 2008).
18. Monitor for manifestations of pericarditis: a. Pericardial friction rub b. Elevated temperature c. Elevated white blood cell count d. Substernal or precordial pain increasing during inspiration	18. Pericarditis results from irritation by accumulated serum nitrogenous wastes. (Bogle et al., 2008)
19. Explain the causes of pain to the client.	19. The client may fear that chest pain is signaling a heart attack.
20. Monitor for signs and symptoms of cardiac tamponade: a. Rapid decrease in blood pressure b. Narrowed pulse pressure c. Muffled heart sounds d. Distended neck veins e. Decreased blood pressure during hemodialysis with intolerance to ultrafiltration f. Cardiac arrhythmias	20. Exaggerated signs and symptoms of effusion implicate worsening pericarditis, pericardial effusion, and slowly developing cardiac tamponade. It can develop at any time in a client with uremic pericarditis. (Bogle et al., 2008)

CLINICAL ALERT
- Educate staff and students to report any signs or symptoms of pericarditis or tamponade immediately.
- Client will require rapid medical assessment with possible dialysis or surgical intervention. (Tattersall & Daugirdas, 2011)

Clinical Alert Report

Advise ancillary staff / student to report to nurse assigned to client:

- Any changes in mental status such as agitation, lethargy, confusion
- Blood pressure, pulse, or respirations outside of prescribed limits. See "Indicators." Individual parameters may vary depending on client's medications
- Temperature (oral) 1–2 degrees F over baseline. Uremia suppresses temperature so lower readings may still indicate fever.
- Difficulty breathing or new onset of shortness of breath
- New onset of pain
- Changes in urine from baseline. Fluid management may change during acute illness.
- Any redness, warmth, drainage or tenderness at IV, catheter, or phlebotomy site.

Documentation

Weight (actual, dry)
Vital signs
Laboratory values
Intake and output
Evidence of bleeding (e.g., blood in stool, bruises)
Status of edema
Chest complaints

Nursing Diagnoses

Imbalanced Nutrition: Less than Body Requirements Related to Anorexia, Nausea and Vomiting, Loss of Taste or Smell, Stomatitis, and Unpalatable Diet

NOC
Nutritional Status,
Teaching: Nutrition

Goal

The client will relate the importance of adequate nutritional intake and complying with the prescribed dietary regimen.

NIC
Nutrition Management,
Nutritional Monitoring

Indicators

- Has no nutritional deficiencies
- Has minimal or no edema
- Maintains ideal or desired weight

Interventions	Rationales

1. Establish nutritional goals with the client / family and a plan of care to achieve them.
  a. Consult the dietitian for assistance with nutritional assessment, identifying nutritional goals, prescribing diet modifications, and providing nutritional instruction to client.
  b. Reinforce the dietary instructions and provide written materials for verbal orders.
	1a. A properly prescribed diet is essential in management of chronic kidney disease to prevent uremic toxicity, fluid and electrolyte imbalances, and catabolism (Greene, 2011; Gutekunst, 2011).
	  b. Empathy and reinforcement of dietary instructions can increase compliance with diet restrictions (Lewis et al., 2004; Greene, 2011; Gutekunst, 2011).

2. Discuss dietary options rather than restrictions.	2. Clients and families will become discouraged if the diet is too restrictive and unpalatable (Greene, 2011).

Interventions	Rationales
3. Encourage the client to verbalize his or her feelings and frustrations about diet modifications.	3. The client should be given as much control as possible over his or her diet—for example, have the client make a list of food and fluid preferences and dislikes and try to incorporate these into the prescribed diet (Lewis et al., 2004; Greene, 2011; Gutekunst, 2011).
4. Provide for and encourage good oral hygiene before and after meals.	4. Proper oral hygiene reduces microorganisms and helps prevent stomatitis.
5. Evaluate, with client and dietitian, the client's nutritional status and the diet's effectiveness.	5. Continued evaluation enables alteration of diet according to the client's specific nutritional needs (Greene, 2011; Gutekunst, 2011).
6. Explain the need for the client to eat the maximum protein allowed on the diet.	6. Adequate protein is needed to prevent protein catabolism and muscle wasting (Gutekunst, 2011; Cotton, 2008).
7. Discuss methods for reducing potassium intake, if indicated. a. Drain canned fruits. b. Eat cooked vegetables, pasta, and cereals. c. Soak fresh vegetables in water before cooking. Use fresh water to cook.	7. Daily potassium intake recommendations for clients with chronic kidney disease (not on dialysis) is usually 2–4 g/day (Turban & Miller III, 2011). Certain foods are lower in potassium. Soaking vegetables removes 50% of the potassium. (Greene, 2011)
8. Prepare for dialysis, as indicated, and monitor for potential complications. Refer to the Hemodialysis and Peritoneal Dialysis care plans for more information.	8. Dialysis is indicated for rising BUN that dietary management cannot control. It also may be necessary to remove excess fluid administered with TPN.
9. Work with the client to develop a plan to incorporate the diet prescription successfully into her or his daily life.	9. Collaboration provides opportunities for the client to exert control; this tends to increase compliance (Greene, 2011; Gutekunst, 2011).

Documentation

Daily weights
Intake (specify food types and amounts)
Output
Mouth assessment
Client teaching
Referrals

TRANSITION TO HOME / COMMUNITY CARE

If indicated, review the risk diagnoses identified for this individual on admission:

- Is the person still at risk?
- Can the family reduce the risks?
- Is the person at higher risk at home?
- Is a Home Health Nurse assessment needed?
- Refer to transition planner / case manager / social service
- When is this person scheduled for follow-up with primary provider? Specialists? Record dates of appointments.
- Complete a medication reconciliation prior to transition. Refer to index.

STAR   **Stop**

Think   Think about any new or ongoing issues.

Has degree of kidney function changed, have dietary needs changed, are medications different? Does client utilize outside resources (e.g., home health who need updated information)?

Act   Contact or provide the appropriate resource (e.g., contacting a support person, home health assessment, additional teaching, printed materials).

Situation: Client is being transitioned home.

Background: Client lives alone but has had home health nursing twice a month for medication management.

Action: Contact home health with updates medication list and plan.

Recommendation: Home health services may be needed more frequently until client is stable.

Review   Has the problem been addressed? If not, use SBAR to communicate to the appropriate person.

Risk for Ineffective Self-Health Management Related to Insufficient Knowledge of Condition, Dietary Restrictions, Daily Recording, Pharmacological Therapy, Signs/Symptoms of Complications, Follow-up Visits, and Community Resources

NOC

Compliance Behavior, Knowledge: Treatment Regimen, Participation in Health Care Decisions, Treatment Behavior: Illness

NIC

Anticipatory Guidance, Learning Facilitation, Risk Identification, Health Education, Teaching: Procedure / Treatment, Health System Guidance (Bednarski et al., 2008)

Goal

The goals for this diagnosis represent those associated with transition planning. Refer to the transition criteria.

Interventions	Rationales
1. Develop and implement a teaching plan using techniques and tools appropriate to the client's understanding. Plan several teaching sessions.	1. Presenting relevant and useful information in an understandable format greatly reduces learning frustration and enhances teaching efforts. Some factors specific to a client with chronic kidney disease influence the teaching–learning process (Bednarski et al., 2008): • Depressed mentation that necessitates repeating information • Short attention span that may limit teaching sessions to 10–15 minutes • Altered perceptions that necessitate frequent clarification and reassurance • Sensory alterations that cause a better response to ideas presented using varied audiovisual formats

Interventions	Rationales

2. Implement teaching that includes but is not limited to renal function.
  a. Normal renal function
  b. Altered renal function
    • Disease process
    • Causes
    • Physiologic and emotional responses to uremia
    • Renal replacement therapies
	2. Amount and depth of teaching will depend on the client's present readiness to learn. Several sessions will be needed; include written materials to take home (Bednarski et al., 2008; Counts et al., CKD: Empowerment, 2008).

3. Encourage the client to verbalize anxiety, fears, and questions.	3. Recognizing the client's fear of failure to learn is vital to successful teaching.

4. Identify factors that may help to predict noncompliance:
  a. Lack of knowledge
  b. Noncompliance in the hospital
  c. Failure to perceive disease's seriousness or chronicity
  d. Belief that the condition will "go away" on its own
  e. Belief that the condition is hopeless
	4. Openly addressing barriers to compliance may help to minimize or eliminate these barriers.

5. Include significant others in teaching sessions. Encourage them to provide support without acting as "police."	5. Significant others must be aware of the treatment plan so they can support the client. "Policing" the client can disrupt positive relationships.
6. Emphasize to the client that, ultimately, it is his or her choice and responsibility to comply with the therapeutic regimen.	6. The client must understand that he or she has control over choices and that his or her choices can improve or impair health.
7. If cost of medications is a financial burden for the client, consult with social services.	7. A referral for financial support can prevent discontinuation because of financial reasons.
8. Assist the client to identify her or his ideal or desired weight.	8. Establishing an achievable goal may help to improve compliance.
9. Teach the client to record weight and urinary output daily.	9. Daily weight and urine output measurements allow the client to monitor her or his own fluid status, and limit fluid intake accordingly.
10. Explain the signs and symptoms of electrolyte imbalances and the need to watch for and report them. (See Collaborative Problems in this entry for more information.)	10. Early detection of electrolyte imbalance enables prompt intervention to prevent serious complications.

11. Teach the client measures to reduce risk of urinary tract infection:
  a. Perform proper hygiene after toileting to prevent fecal contamination of urinary tract.
  b. To prevent urinary stasis, drink the maximum fluids allowed.
	11. Repetitive infections can cause further renal damage.

12. Reinforce the need to comply with diet and fluid restrictions and follow-up care. Consult with the dietitian regarding fluid plan and overall diet.	12. Compliance reduces the risk of complications.

(*continued*)

Interventions	*Rationales*
13. Teach the client who has fluid restrictions to relieve thirst by other means: a. Sucking on a lemon wedge, a piece of hard candy, a frozen juice pop, or an ice cube b. Spacing fluid allotment over 24 hours	13. Strategies to reduce thirst without significant fluid intake reduce risk of fluid overload.
14. Encourage the client to express feelings and frustrations; give positive feedback for adherence to fluid restrictions.	14. Fluid and diet restrictions can be extremely frustrating; positive feedback and reassurance can contribute to continued compliance.
15. Explain importance and risks of erythropoietin stimulating agent (ESA) (e.g., Epoetin alfa therapy and iron supplements).	15. Goal is to avoid red blood cell transfusions and use least amount of therapy needed to maintain hemoglobin in prescribed range, usually 9–10 gm/dL. Studies have shown incremental improvements in survival, left ventricle hypertrophy, exercise capacity, cognitive function, sleep dysfunction, and overall quality of life with improved hemoglobin. However, studies have also demonstrated potential risks for increased cardiovascular events including stroke. Achieving near normal hemoglobin levels is not a goal for all clients. (Macdougall, 2011)
16. Teach the client to take oral medications with meals whenever possible. If medications must be administered between meals, give with the smallest amount of fluid possible.	16. Planning can reduce unnecessary fluid intake and conserve fluid allowance.
17. Encourage the client to maintain his or her usual level of activity and continue activities of daily living to the extent possible.	17. Regular activity helps to maintain strength and endurance and promotes overall well-being.
18. Teach the client and family to watch for and report the following: a. Weight gain or loss greater than 2 lb b. Shortness of breath c. Increasing fatigue or weakness d. Confusion, change in mentation e. Palpitations f. Excessive bruising; excessive menses; excessive bleeding from gums, nose, or cut; blood in urine, stool, or vomitus. g. Increasing oral pain or oral lesions	18. Early reporting of complications enables prompt intervention (Counts et al., CKD: Empowerment, 2008). a. Weight gain greater than 2 lb may indicate fluid retention; weight loss may point to insufficient intake. b. Shortness of breath may be an early sign of pulmonary edema. c. Increasing fatigue or weakness may indicate increasing uremia. d. Confusion or other changes in mentation may point to acidosis or fluid and electrolyte imbalances. e. Palpitations may indicate electrolyte imbalances (K, Ca). f. Excessive bruising, excessive menses, and abnormal bleeding may indicate reduced prothrombin, clotting factors III and VIII, and platelets. g. Oral pain or lesions can result as excessive salivary urea is converted to ammonia in the mouth, which is irritating to the oral mucosa.
19. Discuss with the client and family any anticipated disease-related stressors: a. Financial difficulties b. Reversal of role responsibilities c. Dependency	19. Discussing the nonphysiologic effects of chronic kidney disease in family dynamics can help the client and family to identify effective coping strategies (Bednarski et al., 2008).

Interventions	Rationales
20. Provide information about or initiate referrals to community resources (e.g., American Association of Kidney Clients, National Kidney Foundation, National Kidney Disease Education Program, Kidney School, counseling, self-help groups, peer counseling, Internet information sites, publications).	20. Assistance with home management and dealing with the potential destructive effects on the client and family may be needed.

Documentation

Client teaching
Referrals, if indicated

⊕ Neurologic Disorders

Cerebrovascular Accident (Stroke)

Cerebrovascular accident (CVA), or stroke, involves a sudden onset of neurologic deficits because of insufficient blood supply to a part of the brain, leading to cellular damage and cellular death (Parker-Frizzell, 2005).

There are two major types of stroke: ischemic stroke and hemorrhagic stroke. Ischemic stroke occurs when a blood vessel that supplies blood to the brain is blocked by a blood clot. The blood clot originates in one of two ways. A clot may form in an artery that is already very narrow. This is called a *thrombotic stroke*, as opposed to the clot breaking off from another place in the blood vessels of the brain, heart, or from another part of the body, and traveling up to the brain. This is called cerebral embolism, or an *embolic stroke*.

Ischemic strokes may be caused by clogged arteries. Fat, cholesterol, and other substances collect on the artery walls, forming a sticky substance called plaque. In intracerebral hemorrhage, bleeding occurs directly into the brain parenchyma. The usual mechanism has been described as leakage from small intracerebral arteries damaged by chronic hypertension.

Hypertension is responsible for 60% of hemorrhagic strokes. Other mechanisms include coagulopathies, anticoagulant therapy, thrombolytic therapy for acute myocardial infarction (MI), arteriovenous malformation (AVM), aneurysms, and other vascular malformations (venous and cavernous angiomas), vasculitis, cerebral amyloidosis, alcohol abuse, and illicit drugs such as cocaine, amphetamine, methamphetamine. Hemorrhagic stroke is associated with higher mortality rates than is ischemic stroke.

Preventable and costly, stroke, or brain attack, is the fourth leading cause of death and the leading cause of long-term disability in the United States (CDC, 2011).

In the United States, each year, approximately 795,000 people experience new or recurrent stroke. Of these, approximately 610,000 represent initial attacks, and 185,000 represent recurrent strokes. Epidemiologic studies indicate that approximately 87% of strokes in the United States are ischemic, 10% are secondary to intracerebral hemorrhage, and another 3% may be secondary to subarachnoid hemorrhage (Roger et al., 2012; Liebeskind, 2013).

Preventing first and recurrent strokes requires prompt identification of vulnerable clients. Some risk factors can be modified (Rosamond et al., 2007; Sacco et al., 2006), including hypertension, cigarette smoking, unhealthy eating habits, sedentary life style, lipid imbalance, poor glycemic control, cocaine use, and alcohol abuse (Parker-Frizzell, 2005; Rosamond et al., 2007; Sacco et al., 2006). Exposure to second-hand and / or environmental smoke increases the risk for cardiovascular disease, which includes stroke and respiratory disorders (Furie et al., 2011).

Nonmodifiable risk factors include age, gender, genetic predisposition, history of previous stroke, transient ischemic attacks (TIAs), other cardiac conditions (Pajeau, 2002; Rosamond et al., 2007; Sacco et al., 2006), pregnancy, menopause, and sickle cell disease (Rosamond et al., 2007). Atrial fibrillation (AF) is a major contributor to acute ischemic stroke (Lewis et al., 2011).

The primary assessment should focus on identifying the cause/s of the neurologic symptoms. If stroke is considered, it must be determined whether it is ischemic or hemorrhagic. Initial goals should include ensuring medical stability, quickly reversing the conditions that contribute to client's problem, identifying the pathophysiologic basis for the client's neurologic symptoms, and screening for potential contraindications for thrombolysis in acute ischemic stroke (Oliveira-Filho & Koroshetz, 2007). Thrombolytics should be given within 180 minutes of symptom onset (Parker-Frizzell, 2005).

Carp's Cues

The National Stroke Association (2013) reports that:

- 10% of stroke survivors recover almost completely.
- 25% recover with minor impairments.
- 40% experience moderate to severe impairments requiring special care.
- 10% require care in a nursing home or other long-term care facility.
- 15% die shortly after the stroke.

Time Frame
Initial diagnosis
Recurrent episodes

DIAGNOSTIC CLUSTER

Collaborative Problems

▲ Risk for Complications of Increased Intracranial Pressure

* Risk for Complications of Pneumonia, Atelectasis

▲ Risk for Complications of Adult Respiratory Distress Syndrome

* Risk for Complications of Seizures

* Risk for Complications of Gastrointestinal (GI) Bleeding

* Risk for Complications of Hypothalamic Syndromes

• Risk for Complications of Diabetes Incepitus

• Risk for Complications of Hyperglycemia

Nursing Diagnoses

▲ Impaired Communication related to the effects of hemisphere (left or right) damage on language or speech.

▲ Risk for Injury related to visual field, motor, or perception deficits (refer to Unit II)

▲ Impaired Physical Mobility related to decreased motor function of (specify) secondary to damage to upper motor neurons (refer to Unit II)

▲ Functional Incontinence related to inability and difficulty in reaching toilet secondary to decreased mobility or motivation

▲ Impaired Swallowing related to muscle paralysis or paresis secondary to damage to upper motor neurons

▲ Self-Care Deficit related to impaired physical mobility or confusion (refer to Immobility or Unconsciousness)

△ Unilateral Neglect related to (specify site) secondary to right hemispheric brain damage

△ Total Incontinence related to loss of bladder tone, loss of sphincter control, or inability to perceive bladder cues (refer to Neurogenic Bladder)

* Disuse Syndrome (refer to Immobility / Unconscious)

* Risk for Constipation related to Immobility, insufficient IV or PO fluids, low-fiber diet, stress, opiate pain medications (refer to Unit II)

△ Risk for Caregivers Role Strain related to multiple stressors and responsibilities associated with care of significant others post CVA (refer to Unit II)

△ Risk for Ineffective Self-Health Regimen Management related to altered ability to maintain self at home secondary to sensory / motor / cognitive deficits and lack of knowledge of caregivers of home care, reality orientation, bowel / bladder program, skin care, signs and symptoms of complications, and community resources

Related Care Plan

Immobility or Unconsciousness

▲ This diagnosis was reported to be monitored for or managed frequently (75% to 100%).
△ This diagnosis was reported to be monitored for or managed often (50% to 74%).
* This diagnosis was not included in the validation study.

Transitional Risk Assessment Plan (TRAP)

Begin this plan on admission.
Implement the Transitional Risk Assessment Plan (TRAP):
- Refer to inside back cover.
- Add each validated high-risk diagnosis to client's problem list with the risk code in ( ).
- Refer to Unit II to the individual high-risk nursing diagnoses / collaborative problems for outcomes and interventions.

R: "Close coordination of care in the post-acute period, early discharge follow-up care, enhanced client education and self-management training, proactive end-of-life counseling, and extending the resources and clinical expertise over time via multidisciplinary team management" can lower readmission rates and improve health outcomes (Boutwell & Hwu, 2009, p. 14).

Transition Criteria

Before transition, the client or family will:

1. Describe measures for reducing or eliminating selected risk factors.
2. Relate intent to discuss fears and concerns with family members after discharge.
3. Identify methods for management (e.g., of dysphagia, of incontinence).
4. Demonstrate or relate techniques to increase mobility.
5. State signs and symptoms that must be reported to a health care professional.
6. Relate community resources that can provide assistance with management at home.

Collaborative Problems

Risk for Complications of Increased Intracranial Pressure (ICP)

Risk for Complications of Potential Complication: Pneumonia, Atelectasis

Risk for Complications of Adult Respiratory Distress Syndrome

Risk for Complications of Seizures

Risk for Complications of Stress Ulcers

Risk for Complications of Hypothalamic Syndromes

Risk for Complications of Diabetes Incepitus

Risk for Complications of Hyperglycemia

Collaborative Outcomes

The client will be monitored for early signs and symptoms of (a) Increased Intracranial Pressure, (b) Pneumonia, Atelectasis, (c) Acute Respiratory Distress Syndrome, (d) seizures, (e) Stress Ulcers, (f) Hypothalamic Syndromes, and (g) Diabetes Incepitus and will receive collaborative interventions if indicated to restore physiologic stability.

Indicators of Physiologic Stability

- Alert, oriented (a, b, c, d)
- Pulse 60–100 beats/min (a, b, c, e)
- Respiration 16–20 breaths/min (a, b, c,)
- Pupils equal, reactive to light (a, d)
- Temperature 98–99.5° F (c, d)
- Breath sounds equal, no adventitious sounds (a, c)
- Oxygen saturation (pulse oximetry) (SaO_2) >95 (a, b, c)
- Stool negative for occult blood (e)
- Urine specific gravity 1.005–1.030 (a, b, e)
- Serum sodium 135–145 mEq/L (f)

Interventions	Rationales
1. Determine the last time an individual, diagnosed as post-ischemic stroke, appeared normal. Last Seen Normal (LSN): Is the time noted that the individual seemed normal. This time is critical in order to determine if Tissue Plasma Activator (tPA) can be administered.	1. Tissue Plasma Activator (tPA) has to be administered within 3 hours of the onset of symptoms per FDA).

CLINICAL ALERT

- Accurate determination of the onset of stroke symptoms is critical.
- Tissue Plasma Activator (tPA) has resulted in 30% lower likelihood of neurologic disability at 90 days compared with placebo treatment.
- Unfortunately, "13 years after tPA approval, only about 4% of acute stroke patients actually get treated with the drug, and 65% of hospitals in the United States have never treated a single patient. Only about one-fifth of stroke patients arrive within the Food and Drug Administration-approved 3-hour treatment window, a major obstacle. Fear of postthrombolytic hemorrhage and lack of efficacy are further limitations cited by tPA critics, despite evidence to the contrary. Newly published evidence of clear tPA clinical benefit as late as 4.5 hours after symptom onset, the establishment of Stroke Centers of Excellence, the American Heart Association's 'Get with the Guidelines' initiatives, 'TeleStroke' remote treatment programs, and opening of dedicated stroke units are helping consolidate progress in the field" (Rowley, 2009).

Interventions	Rationales

2. Per protocol, regularly assess:
   a. Level of consciousness
   b. Ability to follow commands
   c. Visual fields
   d. Facial and limb weaknesses
   e. S/s of aphasia, dysarthria
	2. National Institute of Health recommends the above assessment on admission and every 12 hours for the first 24 hours. Then every 24 hours until client is discharged. These assessment criteria are elements on the NIH stroke scale with scoring. (http://www.ninds.nih.gov/doctors/NIH_Stroke_Scale.pdf)

(*continued*)

Interventions	Rationales
3. Ensure that a CT scan is completed within 25 minutes and interpreted within 45 minutes of the Individual's arrival to the Emergency Department or faster if approaching the three-hour time limit (Jauch et al., 2010).	3. The CT scan is the gold standard for identifying a stroke and differentiating between an ischemic stroke and a hemorrhagic stroke (Mink & Miller, 2011).

CLINICAL ALERT

tPA Inclusion Criteria
- The last seen normal (LSN) has to be within three hours.
- Negative CT scan for any bleeding.
- 18 years of age or older.
- A qualified physician / NP makes the diagnosis of an acute ischemic stroke.
- The client must continue to have neurologic deficit (Miller & Mink, 2009).

tPA Exclusion Criteria
tPA cannot be administered if (Jauch et al., 2010):
- Blood glucose is <50 mg/dL or > 400 mg/dL
- Presence of an arterial puncture at noncompressible site in previous seven days
- The CT scan shows multilobular infarction

4. Evaluate for the presence of any acute abnormal coagulation studies such as: a. Acute bleeding tendencies (Miller & Mink, 2009): • Platelet count <100,000/mm^3 • Prothrombin time (PT) >15 seconds • International normalized ratio (INR) >1.7 • Activated partial thromboplastin time (aPTT) > upper normal limit	4. tPA cannot be administered because of the risk of hemorrhage.
5. Ensure that the client / family have been informed regarding the risks of bleeding in the brain, internal bleeding (nonbrain), and an allergic reaction to tPA itself (Jauch et al., 2010).	5. Because there is such a high risk of bleeding internally and into the brain, frequent neurologic and invasive line insertion site checks must be completed and documented.
6. Follow protocol for administration of Tissue Plasma Activator (tPA) when it has been confirmed that the individual has had an ischemic stroke and meets the inclusion criteria and does not have any exclusion criteria present.	

CLINICAL ALERT
- Due to the positive results of the European Collaborative Acute Stroke Study (ECASS-III study), the AHA / ASA recommends that tPA can be used from 3 to 4.5 hours after client was LSN and the CT scan was negative for a hemorrhagic bleed.
- This recommendation requires more exclusion criteria if tPA was administered 3 to 4.5 hours after LSN.
- However, this use of tPA is off-label and NOT approved by the Food and Drug Administration (FDA) (Jauch et al., 2010).

Interventions	Rationales
7. Monitor B / P according to protocol.	7. Both the systolic and diastolic BP are higher after stroke. It appears to rise acutely at the time of stroke. Blood pressure then falls over the next 7–10 days, with most of this fall occurring within the first 1–2 days. BP elevations after ischemic stroke represent an adaptive response, which helps to maintain the cerebral blood flow and perfusion of the c penumbra (post-stroke ischemic tissue of the brain) despite loss of cerebral autoregulation (Wityk, 2007; Summers et al., 2009).
8. Discuss with the physician / NP the blood pressure goals. **CLINICAL ALERT** • Excessive rise in BP could lead to neurologic deterioration from hemorrhage in the presence of a damaged blood–brain barrier. • Excessive reduction in B / P can increase cerebral ischemia.	8. Blood pressure reduction is not routinely recommended in individuals with acute ischemic stroke, as it may decrease perfusion and increase cerebral ischemia (Wityk, 2007). For individuals, who are *not* potential candidates for acute reperfusion therapy, consider lowering blood pressure in clients with acute ischemic stroke if systolic blood pressure >220 mm Hg or diastolic blood pressure >120 mm Hg (Jauch et al., 2010).
9. Monitor the effectiveness of airway clearance by evaluating (Oliveira-Filho & Koroshetz, 2007): a. Effectiveness of cough effort b. Need for tracheobronchial suctioning	9. Lower cranial deficits can affect swallowing ability. The prevalence of aspiration post-CVA is reported to be 25% to 30%. Endotracheal intubation may be necessary to protect the airway (Oliveira-Filho & Koroshetz, 2007).
10. Determine if individual can swallow. If the person is not alert, drooling, and / or has difficulty speaking, do not attempt the test; make the person NPO until a Speech Language Pathologist consult is completed. If those conditions are not present, proceed with the test: "A simple bedside screening evaluation involves asking the individual to sip a teaspoon of water from a cup. If the client can sip and swallow without difficulty, the client is asked to take a large gulp of 60 mL of water and swallow. If there are no signs of coughing or aspiration after 30 seconds, then it is safe for the individual to have a thickened diet until formally assessed by a speech pathologist" (*Massey & Jedlicka, 2002*).	10. One of the frequent complications of a stroke is aspiration.
11. Consult with Speech Language Pathologist for all clients.	
12. Monitor for signs and symptoms of increased intracranial pressure (ICP): a. Increasing headache, increased with movement b. Changes in cognition, level of consciousness, confusion c. New onset or worsening of aphasia d. Slowing of pupil respond to pen light e. Pulse slowing or increasing (late sign) f. Change in respiratory patterns (late sign) g. Refer to Unit II Section 2 Risk for Complications of Increased Intracranial Pressure.	12. Cerebral tissue is compromised by deficiencies of cerebral blood supply caused by hemorrhage, hematoma, cerebral edema, thrombus, or emboli. Monitoring ICP is an indicator of cerebral perfusion (Porth, 2011).

(*continued*)

Interventions	Rationales
13. Monitor for signs and symptoms of pneumonia:	13. Individuals post-stroke are at high risk for pneumonia due their immobility and swallowing difficulties (Pugh et al., 2009).
CLINICAL ALERT • Up to 35% of clients with a stroke die from pneumonia. • Nurses and the health care team can assist their clients by encouraging early mobility and aggressive pulmonary care, such as cough, deep breathing, and incentive spirometers (Pugh et al., 2009).	
a. Monitor temperature and, if indicated, initiate interventions to maintain temperature below 99.5° F.	a. "Hyperthermia in the setting of acute cerebral ischemia is associated with increased morbidity and mortality and should be managed aggressively (treat fever >37.5° C [99.5° F])" (Jauch et al., 2010).
b. Refer to section II Risk for Complications of Pneumonia, Atelectasis for additional interventions.	
14. Monitor for signs and symptoms of ARDS: a. Respiratory discomfort b. Noisy tachypnea c. Tachycardia d. Diffuse rales and rhonchi	14. Damaged type II cells release inflammatory mediators that increase alveolo-capillary membrane permeability, causing pulmonary edema. Decreased surfactant production decreases alveolar compliance. Respiratory muscles must greatly increase inspiratory pressures to inflate lungs (Summers et al., 2009).
15. Monitor hydration status by evaluating the following: a. Oral intake b. Parenteral therapy c. Intake and output d. Urine specific gravity	15. A balance must be maintained to ensure hydration to liquefy secretions to maintain euvolemia. Use isotonic solutions (e.g., 0.9% sodium chloride); nonisotonic solutions can worsen cerebral edema, increasing ICP (Santoni-Reddy, 2006; Summers et al., 2009). Significantly increased amounts of urine output may indicate diabetes insipidus.
16. Monitor for seizures.	16. Ischemic areas may serve as epileptogenic foci or metabolic disturbances can lower the seizure threshold (Summers et al., 2009).
17. Refer to the Seizure Disorders Care Plan, if indicated.	
18. Monitor stools for blood.	18. Hypersecretion of gastric juices occurs during periods of stress.
19. Monitor blood sugar.	19. Hyperglycemia is associated with worse clinical outcome in clients with acute ischemic stroke. Current AHA / ASA recommendations call for the use of insulin when the serum glucose level is greater than 185 mg/dL in clients with acute stroke. (Jauch et al., 2010)
20. Monitor for metabolic dysfunction: a. Low serum sodium b. Elevated urine sodium c. Elevated urine specific gravity	20. Damage to the hypothalamic region may result in increased secretion of antidiuretic hormone (ADH) (Porth, 2011).
21. Monitor for diabetes insipidus: a. Excess urine output b. Extreme thirst c. Elevated serum sodium d. Low specific gravity	21. Compression of posterior pituitary gland or its neuronal connections can cause a decrease of ADH (Santoni-Reddy, 2006).

Interventions	Rationales
22. Monitor for cerebral vasospasm. a. Change in level of consciousness b. Seizures	22. Cerebral vasospasm occurs in intracranial hemorrhage, especially subarachnoid hemorrhage, and accounts for 40% to 50% of associated mortality. Vasospasm occurs 4–14 days after initial bleed (Santoni-Reddy, 2006).

CLINICAL ALERT
- Access Rapid Response Team for emergency interventions

Clinical Alert Report

Prior to providing care, advise ancillary staff / student to report the following to the professional nurse assigned to the client:

- Change in cognitive status
- Oral temperature >99.5° F
- Systolic blood pressure >220 mm Hg or diastolic blood pressure >120 mm Hg
- Systolic BP <90 mm/Hg
- Resting Pulse >100, <50
- Pulse oximetry > 92%
- Respiratory rate >28, <10/min
- Labored or shallow respiration
- Sudden onset of chest pain, leg pain

Related Physician/NP Prescribed Interventions

Medications

For individuals with Ischemic strokes only: Fibrinolytic Agents (e.g., Alteplase), anticoagulants, antiplatelets (e.g., aspirin, ticlopidine, abciximab).

For hemorrhagic strokes only: osmotic diuretics (e.g., mannitol), Phytonadione (if indicated to reverse the effects of warfarin and other related anticoagulants).

As indicated for either ischemic or hemorrhagic strokes: Anticonvulsants, antihypertensives (e.g., diazepam), stool softeners, peripheral vasodilators, corticosteroids, analgesics, antipyretics, anxiolytics, (antianxiety) barbiturates, H_2 blockers, antiemetics.

Intravenous Therapy

Fluid / electrolyte replacements (isotonic fluids).

Laboratory Studies

All clients: Complete blood count, urinalysis, chemistry profile, sedimentation rate, prothrombin time and INR (international normalized ratio), partial thromboplastin time, RPR (rapid plasma reagin) serology, single-photon tomography, cardiac enzymes and troponin, oxygen saturation.

Selected clients: Liver function tests, toxicology screen, blood alcohol level, pregnancy tests, arterial blood gas, type and crossmatch, antiphospholipid antibodies, hemoglobin A_{1c}.

Diagnostic Studies

scan of head (noncontrast), lumbar puncture, cerebral angiography, magnetic resonance imaging (MRI), positron emission tomography (PET) scan, brain scan, Doppler ultrasonography, electroencephalography (EEG), electrocardiogram, transesophageal echocardiogram (TEE), transthoracic echocardiogram, intracranial pressure monitoring.

Therapies

Mechanical embolectomy (option when the individual is outside the 3-hour window of IV tPA) intermittent pneumatic compression devices or graduated compression stockings. Speech therapy, physical therapy, occupational therapy, craniotomy, endarterectomy, ventriculostomy.

Documentation

Neurologic assessment
Vital signs
Complaints of vomiting or headache
Changes in status
Swallowing assessment
Intake / output

Nursing Diagnoses

Carp's Cues

After the acute phase of post-ischemic stroke, the major focus of nursing and other members of the multidiscipline is to reduce and eliminate modifiable risk factors and to assist the individual and family to restore previous functioning as much as possible.

Nursing Diagnosis provides the exact terminology to describe the focus not only for nursing but for other disciplines.

Using Gordon's 11 Functional Health Patterns, the individual / family will be assessed for the presence of compromise functioning and risk factors that can compromise functioning or actual compromised functioning. The nurse in collaboration with the client and family can determine what priorities are for this individual and family presently. Sometimes, priorities identified by the nurse, are not shared by the individual and / or the family.

Stroke clients and caregivers are central participants in the rehabilitation process to foster therapy adherence and facilitate optimal community integration and continued quality of life despite residual impairments. With collaborative input from all rehabilitation team members, including stroke survivors and their family, comprehensive and individualized assessment and treatment plans are formulated. (Miller et al., 2010)

"Because stroke is a complex disease process that requires the skills of an interdisciplinary team, nurses frequently play a central role in care coordination throughout the recovery continuum. Furthermore, because across care settings, nurses commonly have the most direct contact with stroke patients and their caregivers, they are often called on to implement management techniques developed by other rehabilitation team members. Consequently, nurses should be familiar with the variety of services and procedures provided by the other disciplines that are central to stroke rehabilitation teams" (Miller et al., 2010).

Impaired Communication Related to the Effects of Hemisphere (Left or Right) Damage on Language or Speech

NOC
Communication Ability

Goal

The client will report improved satisfaction with ability to communicate.

NIC
Communication Enhancement: Speech Deficit, Active Listening, Socialization Enhancement

Indicators

- Demonstrate improved ability to express self and understand others.
- Report decreased frustration during communication efforts.

Interventions	Rationales
1. Differentiate between language disturbances (dysphagia / aphasia) and speech disturbances (dyspraxia / apraxia).	1. Language involves comprehension and transmission of ideas and feelings. Speech is the mechanics and articulations of verbal expression (Miller et al., 2010).
2. Collaborate with a speech therapist to evaluate the client and create a plan (Miller et al., 2010).	

Interventions	Rationales
3. Provide an atmosphere of acceptance and privacy: a. Do not rush. b. Speak slowly and in a normal tone. c. Decrease external noise and distractions. d. Encourage the client to share frustrations; validate the client's nonverbal expressions. e. Provide the client with opportunities to make decisions about his or her care, whenever appropriate. f. Do not force the client to communicate. g. If the client laughs or cries uncontrollably, change the subject or activity.	3. Communication is the core of all human relations. Impaired ability to communicate spontaneously is frustrating and embarrassing. Nursing actions should focus on decreasing the tension and conveying an understanding of how difficult the situation must be for the client.
4. Make every effort to understand the client's communication efforts: a. Listen attentively. b. Repeat the client's message back to him or her to ensure understanding. c. Ignore inappropriate word usage; do not correct mistakes. d. Do not pretend you understand; if you do not, ask the client to repeat. e. Try to anticipate some needs (e.g., Do you need something to drink?).	4. Nurse and family members should make every attempt to understand the client. Each success, regardless of how minor, decreases frustration and increases motivation (American Heart Association, 2003).
5. Refer to Communication problems after stroke at http://www.stroke.org.uk/sites/default/files/Communication%20problems%20after%20stroke.pdf.	

Documentation

Dialogues
Method to use

Functional Incontinence Related to Inability or Difficulty in Reaching Toilet Secondary to Decreased Mobility or Motivation

NOC
Tissue Integrity:
Skin and Mucous
Membranes, Urinary
Continence, Urinary
Elimination

Goal

The client will report no or fewer episodes of incontinence.

NIC
Perineal Care, Urinary
Incontinence Care,
Prompted Voiding,
Urinary Habit Training,
Urinary Elimination
Management, Teaching:
Procedure/Treatment

Indicators

- Remove or minimize environmental barriers at home.
- Use proper adaptive equipment to assist with voiding, transfers, and dressing.
- Describe causative factors for incontinence.

Carp's Cues

Urinary incontinence develops more frequently among individuals with anterior circulation of the brain and subcortical brain lesion. Urinary incontinence (UI) after stroke is a strong predictor of mortality, dependency, and need for institutional care.

The type of incontinence will direct the nursing interventions indicated. There are three post-stroke urinary incontinence disorders: urge (UUI), functional (FUI), and stress (SUI) that can be reduced or eliminated by nursing interventions that address the causative factors.

In contrast, continuous urinary incontinence, reflex incontinence and overflow incontinence, which are caused by motor / sensory impairments post-stroke, require nursing interventions that prevent incontinence episodes but do not change the cognitive / motor impairment (causative factors).

Interventions	Rationales
1. Assess environment for barriers to the client's bathroom access.	1. Barriers can delay access to the toilet and cause incontinence if the client cannot delay urination.

2. For a client with incontinence, provide bladder training:
  a. Offer toileting reminders every 2 hours after meals and before bedtime.
  b. Provide verbal instruction for toileting activities.
  c. Praise success and good attempts.
	2. Client with incontinence and / or cognitive deficit needs constant verbal cues and reminders to establish a routine and reduce incontinence (American Heart Association, 2007b).

3. Maintain optimal hydration (2000 to 2500 mL/day unless contraindicated). Space fluids every 2 hours.	3. Dehydration can prevent the sensation of a full bladder and can contribute to loss of bladder tone. Spacing fluids helps to promote regular bladder filling and emptying.
4. Minimize intake of coffee, tea, colas, and grapefruit juice.	4. These beverages act as diuretics, which can cause urgency.
5. Refer to Functional Incontinence in Unit II.	

Documentation

Flow records
    Range of motion exercises
    Progress in activities and ambulation

Risk for Bowel Incontinence Related to Constipation Secondary to Immobility, Side Effects of Medications, Inability to Access Bathroom in Timely Manner

NOC

Tissue Integrity: Skin and Mucous Membranes, Bowel Continence, Bowel Elimination, Hydration

Goal

The client will report no or fewer episodes of incontinence.

NIC

Perineal Care, Bowel Incontinence Care, Fluid Management, Nutrition Management, Constipation / Impaction Management.

Indicators

- Remove or minimize environmental barriers to bathroom.
- Use proper adaptive equipment to assist with voiding, transfers, and dressing.
- Describe relationship between constipation and bowel incontinence.

Carp's Cues

"Prevalence of fecal incontinence among stroke survivors ranges between 30% and 40% while the patient is in the hospital, 18% at discharge, and between 7% and 9% at 6 months after stroke. During the rehabilitation phase, patients are evaluated to identify and address potential contributing factors (e.g., diet, drug side effects, rectal muscle weakness); however, the strongest independent risk factor for fecal incontinence at 3 months after stroke is needing help getting to the toilet" (Miller et al., 2010).

Interventions	Rationales

1. Explain the causes of bowel incontinence:
  a. Insufficient fluids
  b. Insufficient dietary fiber
  c. Immobility
  d. Constipation	

2. Explain the side-effects of anticholinergic medications such as antipsychotics, tricyclic antidepressants, oxybutynin, or antiemetics These medications predispose toward constipation by reducing contractility of the smooth muscle of the gut and may cause chronic colonic dysmotility with long-term use (Harari et al., 2003, p. 148).	2. Research "suggests that the potentially modifiable factors of using constipating drugs and of functional difficulties with toilet access are most strongly correlated with new-onset bowel incontinence 3 months after stroke. Disability is a more important factor than age, sex, or stroke-specific factors in causing bowel incontinence in longer-term stroke survivors" (Harari et al., 2003, p. 148).
3. Explain that fecal incontinence can be prevented and / or corrected. Refer to specific nursing diagnoses in Unit II for interventions that address risk / causative factors such as immobility, dehydration, imbalanced nutrition, impaired physical mobility.	

Impaired Swallowing Related to Muscle Paralysis or Paresis Secondary to Damage to Upper Motor Neurons

NOC
Aspiration Control, Swallowing Status

Goal

The client will report improved ability to swallow.

NIC
Aspiration Precautions, Swallowing Therapy, Surveillance, Referral, Positioning

Indicators

- Describe causative factors when known.
- Describe rationale and procedures for treatment.

Interventions	Rationales
1. Determine if individual can swallow: a. One of the frequent complications of dyshagia is aspiration. b. If the person is not alert, drooling, and / or has difficulty speaking, do not attempt the test; make the person NPO until a Speech Language Pathologist consult is completed. c. If those conditions are not present, proceed with the test: "A simple bedside screening evaluation involves asking the individual to sip a teaspoon of water from a cup. If the patient can sip and swallow without difficulty, the patient is asked to take a large gulp of 60 mL of water and swallow. If there are no signs of coughing or aspiration after 30 seconds, then it is safe for the individual to have a thickened diet until formally assessed by a speech pathologist" (Massey & Jedlicka, 2002; Jauch et al., 2010).	1. Dysphagia (impairment in swallowing) occurs in 30% to 64% of clients in the acute phase of stroke recovery (Miller et al., 2010).
2. Consult with Speech Language Pathologist for all post-stroke clients and a specific plan regarding speech and swallowing (American Heart Association, 2007a).	2. The speech pathologist has the expertise needed to perform the dysphagia evaluation.
3. Post a sign to communicate to staff / student at bedside that the client is dysphagic.	3. The risk of aspiration can be reduced if all staff / students are alerted.
4. Plan meals for when the client is well-rested; ensure that reliable suction equipment is on hand during meals. Discontinue feeding if client is tired.	4. Fatigue can increase the risk of aspiration.
5. Explain the risk for aspiration because of dysphagia. Consult with Speech Language Pathologist, if indicated. Before transition, advise to (van Schalkwyk, 2012): • Know how to perform the Heimlich maneuver (client, other household members). • Sit up straight during all meals and snacking and 30 minutes after. • Take a symptom inventory: Fatigue will contribute to swallowing problems. Think about that if fatigue is present, dysphasia will be worse also. • Mindful eating challenge: Using a fork, place food in mouth. Put your fork down. Chew food very thoroughly, then swallow. Pick up fork again only when mouth is empty. • Don't talk with food in your mouth. • Thicken your liquids. • Eat the right kinds of foods: Avoid hard, crumbly, dry and crunchy foods. Add gravy for moisture. Eat very soft or pureed foods. • Eat smaller meals (to avoid "swallowing fatigue"). • Alternate liquids and solids: Take a small sip or two of a liquid between bites for moisture. Finish the meal with some liquid. • Chin tuck: Tuck your chin downward to the chest slightly while swallowing.	

Documentation

Intake of foods and fluids
Swallowing difficulties

Unilateral Neglect Related to (Specify Site) Secondary to Right Hemispheric Brain Damage

NOC
Body Image, Body Positioning: Self-Initiated, Self-Care: Activities of Daily Living (ADLs)

Goal

The client will demonstrate an ability to scan the visual field to compensate for loss of function or sensation in affected limb(s).

NIC
Unilateral Neglect Management, Self-Care Assistance

Indicators

- Describe the deficit and the rationale for treatments.
- Identify safety hazards in the environment.

Interventions	Rationales
1. Monitor for unilateral neglect.	1. Failure to detect or respond to stimuli specifically on the opposite side of brain damage, accurately detects and responds to stimuli on the same side of brain damage.
2. If family is present, explain to the individual / family that unilateral neglect is cluster of attention problems associated with slow and / or inaccurate processing of and responding to stimuli occurring contralateral to the side of the brain damage.	2. Spatial neglect is more commonly associated with lesions of the inferior parietal lobule or temporoparietal region, superior temporal cortex, or frontal lobe. Less common are lesions of the subcortical regions, including the basal ganglia, thalamus, and cingulate cortex (Miller et al., 2010).
3. Reassure the client that the problem is a result of CVA.	3. Clients know that something is wrong, but may attribute it to being "disturbed."
4. Initially adapt the client's environment: a. Take every opportunity, large or small, to help them "tune in" to that side. b. Place the call light, telephone, and bedside stand on the unaffected side. c. Always approach the client from the center or midline.	4. Interventions are focused on improving awareness of the neglected side (Davis, 2003). c. This will minimize sensory deprivation initially; however, attempts should be made to have the client attend to both sides (American Stroke Association, 2007).
5. Assist the individual with an ADL: a. First, tell person the activity needed, such as "Let's get your fork." b. Take the individual's hand and his or her head automatically turns in that direction and the eyes follow.	5. This intervention reinforces the activity by combining the sense of hearing with the sense of touch.
6. Teach the client to scan the entire environment, turning the head to compensate for visual field cuts. Remind the client to scan when ambulating.	6. Scanning can help to prevent injury and increase awareness of entire space.
7. For self-care, instruct the client to: a. Attend to the affected side first. b. Use adaptive equipment as needed. c. Always check the affected limb(s) during activities of daily living (ADLs).	7. The client may need specific reminders to prevent her or him from ignoring nonfunctioning body parts.

Documentation

Presence of neglect

Client teaching

Response to teaching

TRANSITION TO HOME / COMMUNITY CARE

If indicated, review the high risk diagnoses identified for this individual on admission:

- Is the person still at high risk?
- Can the family reduce the risks?
- Is the person at higher risk at home?
- Is a Home Health Nurse assessment needed?
- Refer to discharge planner / case manager / social service
- When is this person scheduled for follow-up with primary provider? Specialists? Record dates of appointments.
- Complete a medication reconciliation prior to discharge. Refer to inside back cover.

STAR

Stop

Think   Is this person at high risk for injury, falls, medical complications, and / or inability to care for self (activities of daily living)?

Is there a support person available?

Is the person competent to manage self-administration of medications, treatment procedures? Are additional resources needed?

Can the person explain how to monitor the condition (e.g., blood glucose, sign / symptoms of complications, dietary / mobility restrictions, and when to call his or her primary provider or specialist)?

Act   Contact or provide the appropriate resource (e.g., contacting a support person, home health assessment, additional teaching, printed materials).

Review   Has the problem been addressed? If not, use SBAR to communicate to the appropriate person.

Risk for Ineffective Self-Health Management Related to Altered Ability to Maintain Self at Home Secondary to Sensory / Motor / Cognitive Deficits and Lack of Knowledge of Caregivers of Home Care, Reality Orientation, Bowel / Bladder Program, Skin Care, and Signs and Symptoms of Complications, and Community Resources

NOC

Compliance Behavior, Knowledge: Treatment Regimen, Participation in Health Care Decisions, Treatment Behavior: Illness and Injury, Anticipatory Guidance, Health Education, Risk Management, Learning Facilitation

NIC

Anticipatory Guidance, Risk Identification, Learning Facilitation, Health Education, Teaching: Procedure / Treatment, Health System Guidance

Goal

The goals for this diagnosis represent those associated with transition planning.

Carp's Cues

The effects of a stroke on an individual / family can range from some weakness in one arm to paraplegia to a state of immobility. The ability to perform activities of daily living, communicate, work, learn, use a phone, access / use the toilet, hold a child, and engage in sexual activity can be unaffected or profoundly compromised. The challenge for nurses is to identify with the individual and family what are their most pressing concerns. These are then addressed prior to transition with the provision of how / where they can seek assistance after transition.

If the individual will be discharged to his or her home, then there will be additional concerns such as caregiving activities, coping, depression, and teaching requirements such as medication compliance, secondary stroke prevention, s/s of complications (diet, smoking, exercising).

Interventions	Rationales
1. Ensure the individual / family have an understanding of stroke, its cause, and treatments prescribed.	1. Understanding can reinforce the need to comply with the treatment regimen (Schwamm et al., 2005).
2. Explain that the risk of post-stroke bladder and bowel dysfunction affects approximately 25% to 50% of stroke survivors.	2. Persistent bladder and bowel difficulties can significantly affect the rehabilitation process (time) and negatively influence stroke survivors' physical and mental health, leading to social isolation and restrictions in subsequent employment and leisure activities.

3. Explain signs and symptoms of complications, and stress the need for immediate evaluation. Go to ER or call 911 (Jauch et al., 2010).
  a. Sudden weakness or numbness in the face, arm or leg, especially on one side of the body
  b. Difficulty speaking or understanding what is being spoken
  c. Difficulty swallowing
  d. Difficulty in walking or even falling and an inability to get back up
  e. Severe headache
  f. Sudden trouble seeing in one eye or both eyes
  g. Sudden onset of chest pain, leg swelling / redness, shortness of breath
 	
  h. Change in cognitive status, seizures
 	
  i. Oral temperature >99.5° F
  j. Labored or shallow respiration
	3. These may be signs of a cerebral ischemia and an evolving stroke. Time is of the essence because if tissue plasma activator (tPA) is indicated, it must be administered within 3 hours of the onset of symptoms.
	
	g. Pulmonary embolism risk is highest during the first 3 to 120 days after stroke, with a 50% sudden death rate (Miller et al., 2010).
	h. These signs and symptoms may indicate increasing ICP or cerebral tissue hypoxia.

4. Discuss with the client's family the anticipated stressors associated with CVA and its impact on family functioning and role responsibilities. Encourage client to share concerns when at home with home health nurse and physician / NP.	4. The only prediction that can be made of the effects of a family member stroke on the family unit and functioning is that it is unpredictable. Previous family functioning will be challenged and new roles will emerge.

Carp's Cues

For a stroke client older than 65 years, 6 months after a stroke (Stein, 2008):

- 30% will need assistance when walking.
- 26% will need assistance with activities of daily living.
- 26% will live in a nursing home.

  a. Financial
  b. Changes in role responsibilities
  c. Dependency
  d. Caregiver responsibilities

                                                d. Refer to Caregiver Role Strain in the index for specific interventions.

(continued)

Interventions	Rationales
5. Explain the possibility of depression post-stroke.	5. Depression is one of the most under-diagnosed and undertreated complications after stroke. Its origin may be organic, related to post-stroke dysfunction of catecholamine-containing neurons, premorbid, or re-active to the catastrophe of losing function. Although depression has been proposed to influence motor and functional recovery, one study found that its negative impact on functional recovery appeared most significant after hospital discharge rather than during the hospital stay Post-stroke depression is also associated with higher mortality, poorer functional recovery, and less social activity.
6. Advise client and / or family to consult with primary care provider of the following (Williams et al., 2005): a. Feeling down, depressed, or hopeless b. Trouble falling or staying asleep, or sleeping too much c. Feeling tired or having little energy d. Poor appetite or overeating e. Trouble concentrating on things, such as reading the newspaper or watching television f. Thoughts that you would be better off dead or of hurting yourself in some way	6. Guidelines for treating post-stroke depression also recommend screening, assessment, and treatment with an appropriate antidepressant for a period of approximately 6 months.
7. Identify risk factors that can be reduced: a. Hypertension b. Smoking / tobacco use c. Secondhand smoke d. Obesity e. High-fat diet f. High-sodium diet g. Sedentary lifestyle	7. Focusing on factors that can be controlled can improve compliance, increase self-esteem, and reduce feelings of helplessness. a. Hypertension with increased peripheral resistance damages the intima of blood vessels, contributing to arteriosclerosis. b. Tobacco exposure produces tachycardia, raises blood pressure, and constricts blood vessels. The effects of nicotine increase the risk of clot formation with aggregation of platelets and vasoconstriction and deprive tissues of oxygen (CDC, 2010). c. Low levels of smoke exposure, including exposures to secondhand tobacco smoke, lead to a rapid and sharp increase in dysfunction and inflammation of the lining of the blood vessels, which are implicated in heart attacks and stroke (CDC, 2010). d. Obesity increases cardiac workload and decrease circulation to peripheral tissues. e. High-fat diet may increase arteriosclerosis and plaque formation. f. Sodium controls water distribution throughout the body. A gain in sodium causes a gain in water, thus increasing the circulating volume. g. Participation in walking and sports has been shown to reduce stroke risk by 20% to 29% (Rosamond et al., 2007), and maintain normal glycemic ranges (Sacco et al., 2006).

Interventions	Rationales
8. Provide information about or initiate referrals to community resources; for example: Counselors, home health agencies American Heart Association (http://www.americanheart.org) American Stroke Association (http://www.strokeassociation.org/STROKEORG/) National Stroke Association (http://www.stroke.org/) Recovering After a Stroke: A Patient and Family Guide Consumer Guide Number 16*AHCPR Publication No. 95-0664: May 1995* US Agency for HealthCare Research and Quality (http://www.strokecenter.org/wp-content/uploads/2011/08/Recovering-After-a-Stroke.pdf)	8. Such resources can provide needed assistance with symptom and home management and help to minimize the potentially destructive effects on the client and family.

Documentation

Client teaching
Referrals if indicated

Guillain-Barré Syndrome

Guillain-Barré syndrome (GBS) is an acute, rapidly progressing, inflammatory, immune-mediated, demyelinating polyneuropathy of the peripheral nervous system, affecting one person per 100,000 people (NINDS, 2011). Its etiology is unclear, but precipitating events include viral illnesses, immunizations, surgery, and respiratory or gastrointestinal viral or bacterial infection (LeMone, Burke, & Bauldoff, 2011). There are several subtypes of GBS, but in the most common form, the myelin sheaths surrounding the peripheral nerves are destroyed by an immune reaction, resulting in poor conduction of nerve impulses. GBS can affect muscles, sensory nerves, and cranial nerves, but cognitive function and level of consciousness are not impacted. Early symptoms include weakness and tingling in the lower extremities, and the disease is characterized by symmetrical, ascending flaccid paralysis and the loss of reflex response. Sensory nerve effects include paresthesias, numbness, and severe pain. Symptom progression may be life-threatening, resulting in quadriplegia, paralysis of facial and respiratory muscles or autonomic involvement causing fluctuating blood pressures, cardiac dysrhythmias, paralytic ileus, and other complications (NINDS, 2011). Twenty percent of clients develop respiratory involvement to the point that mechanical ventilation is required (LeMone et al., 2011). Manifestations of the disease are variable, with acute progression (1 to 3 weeks) followed by a plateau phase and a recovery stage of slow improvement over weeks to years (NINDS, 2011). Although it is potentially fatal, more than 70% of clients with GBS recover without residual disability (NINDS, 2011). Diagnosis is made based on the client's history and clinical presentation, and is confirmed by reduced conduction velocity during electromyography (EMG) and nerve conduction studies or abnormal levels of protein in the cerebrospinal fluid, which are low initially, then elevate after a week (Lewis et al., 2011). There is no known cure for the disease, but therapies that lessen the severity of the disease and may accelerate recovery include plasmapheresis and intravenous immoglobulin infusion, if initiated early in the disease (NINDS, 2011). In the acute phase collaborative care focuses on oxygenation, nutritional support, prevention of complications of immobility, and emotional support. Rehabilitation requires interdisciplinary treatment.

Time Frame
Initial diagnosis: Exacerbations

▪▪▪ DIAGNOSTIC CLUSTER**

Collaborative Problems

Risk for Complications of Acute Respiratory Failure (ARF)

Risk for Complications of Autonomic Nervous System Failure

Risk for Complications of Peripheral Nervous System Failure

Risk for Complications of Deep Vein Thrombus (refer to Unit II)

Risk for Complications of Decreased Cardiac Output (refer to Unit II)

Risk for Complications of Pneumonia (refer to Unit II)

Nursing Diagnoses

Risk for Ineffective Airway Clearance related to impaired ability to cough (refer to Unit II)

Risk for Impaired Skin Integrity related to immobility, incontinence, sensory-motor deficits (refer to Unit II)

Impaired Swallowing related to swallowing / chewing problems secondary to cranial nerve impairment (refer to Unit II)

Impaired Communication related to muscle weakness and mechanical ventilation (if present) (refer to Mechanical Ventilation Care Plan)

Activity Intolerance related to fatigue and difficulties in performing activities of daily living (refer to Unit II)

Risk for Self-Care Deficits related to flaccid paralysis, paresis, and fatigue (refer to Unit II)

Risk for Interrupted Family Process related to nature of disorder, role disturbances, and uncertain future (refer to Unit I)

Risk for Ineffective Self-Health Therapeutic Regimen Management related to lack of knowledge of condition, treatments required, stress management, signs and symptoms of complications, and availability of community resources

** This medical condition was not included in the validation study.

TRANSITIONAL CRITERIA TO HOME / COMMUNITY CARE
The client or family will:
1. Relate intent to discuss fears and concerns with family / trusted friends after discharge.
2. Relate necessity of continuation of therapeutic programs.
3. Relate safety precautions to prevent falls / injury.
4. Identify signs and symptoms that must be reported to a health care professional.

Transitional Risk Assessment Plan (TRAP)

Begin this plan on admission.

Implement the Transitional Risk Assessment Plan (TRAP):

• Refer to inside back cover.

• Add each validated high-risk diagnosis to client's problem list with the risk code in ( ).

• Refer to Unit II to the individual high-risk nursing diagnoses / collaborative problems for outcomes and interventions.

R: "Close coordination of care in the post-acute period, early discharge follow-up care, enhanced patient education and self-management training, proactive end-of-life counseling, and extending the resources and clinical expertise over time via multidisciplinary team management" can lower readmission rates and improve health outcomes (Boutwell & Hwu, 2009, p. 14).

Collaborative Problems

Risk for Complications of Acute Respiratory Failure (ARF)

Risk for Complications of Autonomic Nervous System Failure

Risk for Complications of Peripheral Nervous System Failure

Collaborative Outcomes

The client will be monitored for early signs / symptoms of (a) acute respiratory failure, (b) autonomic nervous system dysfunction, peripheral nervous system failure, and will receive collaborative interventions to stabilize him or her.

Indicators of Physiologic Stability

- Respiration 16–20 breaths/min (a)
- Oxygen saturation (pulse oximetry) >95% (a)
- Serum pH 7.35–7.45 (a)
- Serum PCO_2 35–45 mm Hg (a)
- Cardiac normal sinus rhythm (a)
- Bowel sounds present (b)
- Alert, oriented (a)
- Cranial nerves II–XXII intact (c)
- Urine output >0.5 mL/kg/h (a)
- Dry, warm skin (b)

Interventions	Rationales
1. Monitor for signs and symptoms of pneumonia and acute respiratory failure (ARF) to assist with breathing.	1. Ventilation may become necessary as acute Guillain-Barré progresses, due to paralysis of intercostal and diaphragmatic muscles (LeMone et al., 2011). In the acute phase of GBS ascending paralysis may result in sudden respiratory failure.
a. Auscultate breath sounds.	a. Auscultating breath sounds assesses the adequacy of air flow and detects the presence of adventitious sounds (see Mechanical Ventilation for more information).
b. Assess for secretions: • Encourage the client to deep breathe and cough. • Position the client on alternate sides to assist movement of secretions. • Suction if client is unable to manage secretions. • Reassure client by maintaining a calm environment.	b. When the respiratory muscles fatigue, cough becomes ineffective, leading to the accumulation of mucus and the formation of mucous plugs in the airway. This accumulation of secretions causes alveolar collapse, leading to acute respiratory failure.
c. Assess O_2 saturation via pulse oximetry.	c. Pulse oximetry provides ongoing data on O_2 saturation.
d. Assess blood gases: • Monitor for signs of decreased respiratory functions, pH, $PaCO_2$, O_2 saturation, and HCO_3.	d. Acid–base imbalance, hypoxemia, hypercarbia, weak cough, ineffective airway clearance, may signify that the client requires intubation to avoid acute respiratory failure. Decreased vital capacity and reduced inspiratory or expiratory pressures confirms the need for intubation (Newswanger & Warren, 2004).
e. Explain the necessity of intubation to the client and family if indicated.	e. Intubation is initiated to relieve shortness of breath to avoid acute respiratory failure, aspiration, and pneumonia.
f. Provide assurance and encouragement for the client.	f. This will reduce fear of the disease process. Most Guillain-Barré clients have been healthy, active individuals who suddenly became victims of dependency.
g. Report to the physician / NP changes regarding: • Respiratory status and reduced vital capacity and arterial blood gases • Neurologic status • GI status	g. Early recognition enables prompt intervention to prevent further complications.

(continued)

Interventions	Rationales

2. Monitor signs and symptoms of autonomic nervous system dysfunction:
  a. Blood pressure variations and cardiac dysrhythmias
  b. Cardiac monitor to evaluate cardiac status
	2. Autonomic nervous system dysfunction can develop from involvement of both the sympathetic and parasympathetic nervous systems. Manifestations include fluctuating blood pressures, hypotension, orthostatic hypotension, abnormal vagal responses (cardiac dysrhythmias, heart block, asystole, and syndrome of inappropriate secretion of antidiuretic hormone, paralytic ileus, urine retention, and diaphoresis) (Lewis et al., 2011).

c. Urinary retention d. Constipation or paralytic ileus (LeMone et al., 2011)	c. Urinary retention is associated with autonomic nervous system dysfunction.

> **CLINICAL ALERT**
> • Watch carefully for activities that precipitate autonomic dysreflexia, such as position changes, vigorous coughing, straining with bowel movements, and suctioning (Lewis et al., 2011).

3. Monitor signs and symptoms of cranial nerve dysfunction.	3. Demyelination of the efferent fibers of the spinal and cranial nerve creates a delay in conduction, resulting in motor weakness or loss of conduction, producing paralysis (Hickey, 2009).

Clinical Alert Report

Prior to providing care, advise ancillary staff / student to report the following to the professional nurse assigned to the client:

• Change in cognitive status
• Change in swallowing ability
• Oral temperature >100.5° F
• Systolic BP <90 mm/Hg
• Resting Pulse >100, <50
• Respiratory rate >28, <10 /min.
• Change in respiratory function (effort)
• Oxygen saturation <90%

Related Physician / NP Prescribed Interventions

Medications
High-dose intravenous immunoglobulins, steroids, antidysrhythmics (beta blocker, atropine)

Diagnostic Studies
Electrophysiologic studies (EPS), spinal tap

Therapies
EKG monitoring, plasmapheresis (effective in the first 2 weeks), mechanical ventilation

Documentation

Vital signs
Intake and output
Neurologic assessment findings
Changes in respiratory status
Response to interventions
Neurologic changes

> **TRANSITIONAL CRITERIA TO HOME / COMMUNITY CARE**
>
> If indicated, review the high-risk diagnoses identified for this individual on admission:
> * Is the person still at high risk?
> * Can the family reduce the risks?
> * Is the person at higher risk at home?
> * Is a Home Health Nurse assessment needed?
> * Refer to discharge planner / case manager / social service.
> * When is this person scheduled for follow-up with primary provider? Specialists? Record dates of appointments.
> * Complete a medication reconciliation prior to discharge. Refer to inside back cover.

STAR

Stop

Think   Is this person at high risk for injury, falls, medical complications, and / or inability to care for self (activities of daily living)?

Is there a support person available?

Is the person competent to manage self-administration of medications, treatment procedures? Are additional resources needed?

Can the person explain how to monitor the condition (e.g., blood glucose, sign / symptoms of complications, dietary / mobility restrictions, and when to call his or her primary provider or specialist)?

Act   Contact or provide the appropriate resource (e.g., contacting a support person, home health assessment, additional teaching, printed materials).

Review   Has the problem been addressed? If not, use SBAR to communicate to the appropriate person.

Nursing Diagnoses

Risk for Ineffective Self-Health Management Related to Lack of Knowledge of Condition, Treatments Required, Stress Management, Signs and Symptoms of Complications, and Availability of Community Resources

NOC

Compliance Behavior, Knowledge: Treatment Regimen, Participation in Health Care Decisions, Treatment Behavior: Illness or Injury

NIC

Anticipatory Guidance, Learning Facilitation, Risk Identification, Health Education, Teaching Procedure / Treatment, Health System Guidance.

Goal

Refer to discharge criteria.

Interventions	*Rationales*
1. Teach the client and his or her family the basic pathology of the client's condition.	1. Understanding can improve compliance and reduce the family unit's frustrations.
2. Assist the client in identifying realistic short-term goals.	2. Preparation of the client to set realistic goals for recovery will reduce feelings of depression if goals are not attained.

(*continued*)

Interventions	Rationales
3. Teach the client the value of continued ROM (passive or active, dependent on functional ability) and strengthening-stretching exercise programs. Consult physical therapy.	3. Exercise will maintain muscle strength and flexibility and promote circulation in effected extremities (NINDS, 2011).
4. Teach the client energy conservation techniques, scheduling planned rest periods, and exercise consistent with tolerance levels.	4. Energy conservation can reduce fatigue (NINDS, 2007).
5. Teach care of altered body functions: a. Bowel & bladder function: Encourage intake of 2000 mL of fluid unless contraindicated. b. Nutritional requirements: Provide a diet high in calories and protein. c. Self-care deficits, if necessary. Areas of concern: dressing, grooming, safe ambulation	5. Care instructions: a. Adequate fluid intake promotes bowel and bladder function, prevention of constipation related to reduced activity and peristalsis. b. Protein and calories are required to rebuild muscle mass. c. Encourage maximum client self-care with ADL activities for purpose of strengthening and increasing independence.
6. Initiate referral to rehabilitation services.	6. Client will require outpatient or home care multidisciplinary rehabilitation therapy. The recovery period may be as short as a few weeks or may extend to a few years (NIND, 2011).
7. Facilitate referral for psychological counseling and emotional support.	7. GBS often causes sudden paralysis, communication difficulties, and dependence for body functions and ADLs, creating psychological and emotional crisis for clients and families (NIND, 2011).
8. Explain signs and symptoms of complications to report to health care professional. a. Productive cough b. Difficulty with urination, odor to urine c. Prolonged constipation d. Increased weakness or fatigue e. Weight loss	8. Early intervention will minimize complications of the condition.
9. Provide information to assist the client and family to manage at home. Refer to the following resources: a. Guillain-Barre Syndrome / Chronic Inflammatory Demyelinating Polyneuropathy Foundation International at http://www.gbs-cidp.org b. Case manager / discharge planner referral c. Home health agency	9. Clients and families who receive community support may cope more effectively with this disease. Functional loss may be significant. Even when deficits are temporary the client will require interdisciplinary support during the recovery period.

Multiple Sclerosis

Multiple sclerosis (MS) is the most common autoimmune, inflammatory demyelinating disease of the central nervous system (CNS) (Olek, 2007b). It is characterized by acute exacerbations or gradual worsening of neurologic functions and disability (Ben-Zacharia, 2001). MS affects some 300,000 Americans yearly, 75% of whom are female. The disease is a leading cause of disability among young adults and typically strikes during young adulthood, with peak incidence between 20 and 40 years of age (Olek, 2007a).

MRI studies have shown clear evidence that central to the disease process is the gradual destruction of the myelin sheath surrounding nerve cells by autoreactive T-cells (Olek, 2007c). This stripping of nerve fibers interferes with nerve conduction, which leads to various degrees of paralysis and to the other symptoms of the disease (Glaser, 2000).

There are four categories of MS: relapsing-remitting (80% of all cases), secondary progressive, progressive-relapsing, and primary progressive (Hickey, 2009). In people with MS, the range of main symptoms includes the loss of mobility and spasticity, pain, tremors, abnormal eye movements, paroxysmal symptoms, bladder and bowel dysfunction, sexual disturbances, fatigue, cognitive impairment, sexual dysfunction, seizures, optic neuritis, vertigo, and depression (Clanet, 2000; Olek, 2007a; Olek, 2007c).

When individuals with MS require care in a long-term care facility, they are younger (in their 40s) mentally alert, and have more symptoms of depression. They will reside at the facility for a longer time than the usual resident. They are dependent for much of their care. Caregivers in long-term care facilities are challenged to deliver complex care and provide opportunities to increase mobility and stimulation (Buchanan, Wang, & Ju 2002).

Treatment of multiple sclerosis (MS) has two aspects: immunomodulatory therapy (IMT) for the underlying immune disorder and therapies to relieve or modify symptoms. IMT is directed toward reducing the frequency of relapses and slowing progression. Currently, most disease-modifying agents have been approved for use only in relapsing forms of MS. Mitoxantrone (see below) is also approved for the treatment of secondary (long-term) progressive and progressive relapsing MS.

Time Frame
Initial diagnosis
Recurrent acute exacerbations

■■■ DIAGNOSTIC CLUSTER**

Collaborative Problems

Risk for Complications of Urinary Tract Infection

Risk for Complications of Renal Insufficiency

Risk for Complications of Seizures

Risk for Complications of Pneumonia

Nursing Diagnoses

Risk for Disturbed Self-Concept related to the effects of prolonged debilitating condition on lifestyle and on achieving developmental tasks and uncertain prognosis

Impaired Comfort related to demyelinated areas of the sensory tract

Risk for Injury related to visual disturbances, vertigo, and altered gait

Interrupted Family Processes related to nature of disorder, role disturbances, and uncertain future (refer to Unit II)

Risk for Caregiver Role Strain related to unpredictability of care situation or illness course, increasing care needs

Risk for Ineffective Self-Health Management related to lack of knowledge of condition, treatments, prevention of infection, stress management, aggravating factors, signs and symptoms of complications, and community resources

Impaired Swallowing related to cerebellar lesions Refer to Cerebrovascular Accident (Stroke) Care Plan

Impaired Verbal Communication related to dysarthria secondary to ataxia of the muscles of speech Refer to Parkinson Disease Care Plan

Fatigue related to extremity weakness, spasticity, fear of injury, and stressors (refer to Unit II)

Urinary Retention related to sensorimotor deficits (refer to Neurogenic Bladder Care Plan)

Incontinence (specify) related to poor sphincter control and spastic bladder

Powerlessness related to the unpredictable nature of condition (remission / exacerbation) (refer to Chronic Obstructive Pulmonary Disease Care Plan)

(continued)

Related Care Plans

Immobility or Unconsciousness

Corticosteroid Therapy

**This medical condition was not included in the validation study.

TRANSITIONAL CRITERIA TO HOME / COMMUNITY CARE

Before transition, the client and family will:

1. Relate an intent to share concerns with other family members or trusted friend(s).
2. Identify one strategy to increase independence.
3. Describe actions that can reduce the risk of exacerbation.
4. Identify signs and symptoms that must be reported to a health care professional.

Transitional Risk Assessment Plan (TRAP)

Begin this plan on admission.

Implement the Transitional Risk Assessment Plan (TRAP):

- Refer to inside back cover.
- Add each validated high-risk diagnosis to client's problem list with the risk code in ( ).
- Refer to Unit II to the individual high-risk nursing diagnoses / collaborative problems for outcomes and interventions.

    R: *"Close coordination of care in the post-acute period, early discharge follow-up care, enhanced patient education and self-management training, proactive end-of-life counseling, and extending the resources and clinical expertise over time via multidisciplinary team management" can lower readmission rates and improve health outcomes (Boutwell & Hwu, 2009, p. 14).*

Collaborative Problems

Risk for Complications of Pneumonia

Risk for Complications of Urinary Tract Infections

Risk for Complications of Renal Insufficiency

Risk for Complications of Seizures

Collaborative Outcomes

The client will be monitored for early signs and symptoms of (a) urinary tract infections and (b) seizures and (c) pneumonia and will receive collaborative interventions if indicated to restore physiologic stability.

Indicators of Physiologic Stability

- Alert, oriented (b, c)
- No abnormal breath sounds (c)
- Oxygen saturation >95% (pulse oximetry) (c)
- Temperature 98–99.5° F (a, c)
- Urine specific gravity 0.005–0.030 (a)
- Urine output >0.5 mL/kg/h (a)
- Clear urine (a)
- No seizure activity (b)

Carp's Cues

The medical treatment and management of multiple sclerosis should be targeted toward relieving symptoms of the disease, treating acute exacerbations, shortening the duration of an acute relapse, reducing frequency of relapses, and preventing disease progression.

Interventions	*Rationales*
1. Monitor for signs and symptoms of urinary tract infection:	1. Failure to empty is characterized by a large, flaccid bladder and an inability of the urinary sphincter to relax. Symptoms include urgency, frequency, hesitancy, nocturia, incontinence, incomplete emptying, and frequent urinary tract infections.

CLINICAL ALERT
- MS exacerbation can be precipitated by any infection (Olek, 2007c).
- MS can cause urinary retention owing to lesions of the afferent pathways from the bladder.
- Resulting urine stasis contributes to growth of microorganisms.
- Also, corticosteroid therapy reduces the effectiveness of WBCs against infection.

a. Chills, fever	a. Bacteria can act as a pyrogen by raising the hypothalamic thermostat through the production of endogenous pyrogen that may mediate through prostaglandins. Chills can occur when the temperature setpoint of the hypothalamus changes rapidly.
b. Costovertebral angle (CVA) pain (a dull, constant backache below the 12th rib)	b. CVA pain results from distention of the renal capsule.
c. Leukocytosis	c. Leukocytosis reflects an increase in WBCs to fight infection through phagocytosis.
d. Foul odor or pus in urine	d. Bacteria change the odor and pH of urine.
e. Dysuria, frequent urination	e. Bacteria irritate bladder tissue, causing spasms and frequent urination.
2. Monitor for pneumonia:	2. Tracheobronchial inflammation, impaired alveolar capillary membrane function, edema, fever, and increased sputum production disrupt respiratory function and compromise the blood's oxygen-carrying capacity. Reduced chest wall compliance in older adults affects the quality of respiratory effort. In older adults, tachypnea (>26 respirations/min) is an early sign of pneumonia, often occurring 3 to 4 days before a confirmed diagnosis. Delirium or mental status changes are often seen early in pneumonia in older adults (Porth, 2011).
a. Monitor respiratory status and assess for signs and symptoms of inflammation:	

- Increased respiratory rate (tachypnea), marked dyspnea
- Fever and chills (sudden or insidious)
- Productive cough
- Diminished or absent breath sounds, rales or crackles
- Pleuritic chest pain
- Tachycardia
- Lethargy

CLINICAL ALERT
- The cause of death in approximately 75% of all multiple sclerosis individuals is from complications of multiple sclerosis, usually pneumonia.

(continued)

Interventions	Rationales
3. Monitor for seizures.	3. The effects of demyelination and inflammation on the cortex are increasingly recognized as important in MS, and edema associated with acute MS lesions could also cause cortical hyperexcitability resulting in seizures. The prevalence of seizures in patients with MS ranges between 2.1% and 5.4% (Koch, 2003).

Clinical Alert Report

Prior to providing care, advise ancillary staff / student to report the following to the professional nurse assigned to the client:

- Seizure activity
- Change in cognitive status
- Oral temperature >100.5° F
- Systolic BP <90 mm/Hg
- Resting pulse >100, <50
- Respiratory rate >28, <10/min
- Oxygen saturation <90%
- Amount of urine output
- Characteristics of urine (color, odor)

Related Physician / NP Prescribed Interventions

Medications

Immunomodulators (immunomodulators or receptor modulators are indicated for the treatment of patients with relapsing forms of MS. They help to slow the accumulation of physical disability and decrease the frequency of clinical exacerbations) (e.g., Interferon beta-1b [Betaseron, Extavia, Interferon beta-1a], Avonex, Rebif, Glatiramer acetate [Copaxone]), multiple sclerosis drugs (e.g., Dalfampridine [Ampyra]), antineoplastic agents (e.g., Mitoxantrone, Cyclophosphamide), muscle relaxants (e.g., Baclofen [Lioresal], Gablofen, Dantrolene [Dantrium]), neuromuscular blockers, Botulinum Toxins. Dopamine Agonists Alpha2-Adrenergic Agonists, vitamin B, tricyclic antidepressants, selective serotonin uptake inhibitor (SSRI), corticosteroids, bulk-forming laxatives, Betaseron, beta blockers, vitamin C (1,000 mg four times / day), Avonex, glatiramer, spasmolytics (e.g., Urispas or Ditropan), urinary tract antiseptics (e.g., Macrodantin or Hiprex), cholinesterase inhibitors, analgesics, amantadine, methylphenidate.

Intravenous Therapy

Adrenocorticotropic hormone (ACTH), intravenous immunoglobin (IVIG).

Laboratory Studies

Electrophoresis, white blood count, gamma globulin levels, serum antimyelin antibodies.

Diagnostic Studies

EEG, MRI, CT scan of the brain, lumbar puncture, urinary retention study, evoked potential studies, electrophoresis, cerebrospinal fluid analysis.

Therapies

Dependent on deficits (e.g., urinary and motor); dependent on bladder emptying problems (Credé technique, clean intermittent self-catheterization [CISC], indwelling Foley catheter, and suprapubiccystotomy), intrathecal muscle relaxants, physiotherapy, immunosuppressive therapy (total lymphoid radiation), plasma exchange, hematopoietic stem cell transplantation (HSCT).

Documentation

Intake and output
Urine specific gravity

Nursing Diagnoses

 Carp's Cues

The medical focus in the treatment of relapsing MS is to reduce the frequency of relapses and limit disease progression. As a result, the clinical assessments often have the sole intention of monitoring for physiologic complications (Correia de Sa, 2011).

   The nursing focus for individuals and families coping with MS is to assess their quality of life to identify responses to MS that compromise functioning and increase risks. Using Gordon's 11 Functional Health Patterns, the individual / family will be assessed for the presence of compromised functioning and risk factors that can compromise functioning. The nurse in collaboration with the client and family can determine what priorities are for this individual and family presently. Sometimes, priorities identified by the nurse are not shared by the individual and / or the family.

Chronic Pain Related to the Demyelinating Process and / or Musculoskeletal in Nature, Secondary to Poor Posture, Poor Balance, or the Abnormal Use of Muscles or Joints as a Result of Spasticity

NOC

Comfort Level, Pain:
Disruptive Effects, Pain
Control, Depression
Control

NIC

Pain Management,
Medication
Management, Exercise
Promotion, Mood
Management, Coping
Enhancement

Goal

The client will relate:
- Increased understanding of the causes of their pain and resources / skills needed to cope.
- Will commit to practice at least one noninvasive pain-relief measures such as:
  - Music therapy
  - Stretching exercises, yoga, and / or walking
  - Massage
  - Guided imagery
  - Relaxation therapy
  - Heat / cold therapy

 Carp's Cues

The prevalence of pain in individuals with MS is 63.5% (Maloni, 2012). Pain in multiple sclerosis is both a direct consequence of a demyelinating lesion in the central nervous system (*central neuropathic*) or an indirect consequence of the disability associated with MS (*nonneuropathic*) (IASP, 2010). Mixed neuropathic and nonneuropathic pain occurs and is typified by headache and painful muscle spasms or spasticity.

Interventions	Rationales
1. Establish a supportive accepting relationship: Acknowledge the pain. Listen attentively to client's discussion of pain.	
2. Convey that you are assessing pain because you want to understand it better (not determine if it really exists).	2. Trying to convince health care providers that he / she is experiencing pain will cause the client anxiety, which compounds the pain. Both are energy depleting.
3. Determine the level of understanding of the client's condition, causes of pain. Assess the effects of symptoms on quality of life and pain-relieving techniques that he / she uses. Supplement the client's information and correct misconceptions.	3. "The goal of pain management is recognizing and treating psychological factors of anxiety and depression, enhancing social factors of support and a trusting medical provider relationship and using medications that target pain mechanisms with polypharmacy—that is, combining low doses of several medications to achieve greater efficacy with fewer adverse events" (Maloni, 2012).

(continued)

Interventions	Rationales

4. Explain that the client's pain may be primary or secondary.
  a. For a comprehensive resource on pain management for individuals with MS, refer to Maloni, H (2012) Pain in Multiple Sclerosis Clinical Bulletin Information for Health Professionals at http://www.nationalmssociety.org/ms-clinical-care-network/clinical-resources-and-tools/pub.
  b. Refer also to Unit II Chronic Pain.
	4. Primary pain is caused by the demyelinating process and with plaque formation in the spinal cord and brain and is often characterized as having a burning, gnawing, or shooting quality. Secondary pain is caused primarily musculoskeletal in nature, possibly due to poor posture, poor balance, or the abnormal use of muscles or joints as a result of spasticity (Maloni, 2012).

Risk for Injury Related to Visual Disturbances, Vertigo, and Altered Gait

NOC
Risk Control

NIC
Fall Prevention, Environmental Management: Safety, Health Education, Surveillance: Safety, Risk Identification

Goal

The client will relate fewer injuries.

Indicators

- Relate the intent to use safety measures to prevent injury.
- Relate the intent to practice selected prevention measures.

Interventions	Rationales
1. Explain why MS can increase risk for falls.	1. Symptoms including visual impairment, vertigo, impaired proprioception, decreased vibration sense, muscle weakness, and spasticity are the result of progressive damage along neuronal pathways throughout the CNS (Sosnoff et al., 2012).
2. Discuss the consequences of falls (e.g., fracture hips, increased disability).	2. Researchers have documented that approximately 75% of community-dwelling persons with MS who have fallen in the last 6 months self-reported activity restriction due to concerns about falling (Matsuda et al., 2012).
3. Evaluate if client needs an assistive device (e.g., cane, walker), or if client is using the device as recommended. Consult with physical therapy.	3. Individuals may be resistant to using assistive devices related to issues related to body image.
4. Refer to Unit I for additional interventions for Risk for Injury.	

TRANSITION TO HOME / COMMUNITY CARE
If indicated, review the high-risk diagnoses identified for this individual on admission:
- Is the person still at high risk?
- Can the family reduce the risks?
- Is the person at higher risk at home?
- Is a Home Health Nurse assessment needed?
- Refer to discharge planner / case manager / social service.
- When is this person scheduled for follow-up with primary provider? Specialists? Record dates of appointments.
- Complete a medication reconciliation prior to discharge. Refer to inside back cover.

STAR   **Stop**

Think   Is this person at high risk for injury, falls, medical complications, and / or inability to care for self (activities of daily living)?

Is there a support person available?

Is the person competent to manage self-administration of medications, treatment procedures? Are additional resources needed?

Can the person explain how to monitor the condition (e.g., blood glucose, sign / symptoms of complications, dietary / mobility restrictions, and when to call his or her primary provider or specialist)?

Act   Contact or provide the appropriate resource (e.g., contacting a support person, home health assessment, additional teaching, printed materials).

Review   Has the problem been addressed? If not, use SBAR to communicate to the appropriate person.

Risk for Ineffective Self-Health Management Related to Lack of Knowledge of Condition, Treatments, Prevention of Infection, Stress Management, Aggravating Factors, Signs and Symptoms of Complications, and Community Resources

NOC

Compliance Behavior, Knowledge: Treatment Regimen, Participation in Health Care Decisions, Treatment Behavior: Illness or Injury

NIC

Anticipatory Guidance, Learning Facilitation, Risk Identification, Health Education, Teaching: Procedure / Treatment, Health System Guidance

Goal

The goals for this diagnosis represent those associated with transition planning. Refer to the transition criteria.

 Carp's Cues

The effect of comorbidities such as depression, urinary incontinence, and symptoms such as spasms, fatigue, vertigo, headaches can have serious ramifications for individuals with MS and their significant others. These comorbidities are barriers to compliance and recovery from relapses. The presence of these additional symptoms can also place a greater burden on careers, family, friends, and other support networks (Correia de Sa, 2012).

Interventions	Rationales
1. Evaluate sleep quality at home. Refer to Disturbed Sleep Patterns in Unit II for additional interventions.	1. Excessive daytime sleepiness interferes with sleep at night. The high prevalence of restless legs syndrome (RLS), mainly observed in disabled patients with sensory and pyramidal signs, might contribute to poor sleep quality and / or excessive sleepiness (Correia de Sa, 2012).
2. Evaluate for the presence of fecal incontinence and constipation. a. Explain that constipation can be caused by poor mobility, voluntary fluid restriction to minimize urinary incontinency, anticholinergic drugs taken for concomitant bladder symptoms and poor dietary habits. Refer to Unit II Constipation and Bowel Incontinence for additional interventions.	2. The prevalence of bowel symptoms with MS is over 50%. a. Fecal incontinency may arise as a result of diminished perineal and rectal sensation, weak sphincter squeeze pressures, leading to rectal overloading and overflow, or any combination of these factors (Correia de Sa, 2012).

(continued)

Interventions	Rationales
3. Explain the risk for aspiration because of dysphagia. Consult with Speech Language Pathologist, if indicated. a. Advise to (van Schalkwyk, 2012): • Know how to perform the Heimlich maneuver (client, other household members). • Sit up straight during all meals and snacking and 30 minutes after. • Take a symptom inventory: Fatigue will contribute to swallowing problems. Think about how if fatigue is present, dysphasia will be worse also. • Mindful eating challenge: Using a fork, place food in mouth. Put your fork down. Chew food very thoroughly, then swallow. Pick up fork again only when mouth is empty. • Don't talk with food in your mouth. • Thicken your liquids. • Eat the right kinds of foods: Avoid hard, crumbly, dry and crunchy foods. Add gravy for moisture. Eat very soft or pureed foods. • Eat smaller meals, to avoid "swallowing fatigue." • Alternate liquids and solids: Take a small sip or two of a liquid between bites for moisture. Finish the meal with some liquid. • Chin tuck: Tuck your chin downward to the chest slightly while swallowing.	
4. Allow individual and significant others an opportunity to share their perceptions separately. a. If indicated, refer individual for supportive therapy provided by speech pathologists or occupational therapists.	4. Cognitive dysfunction is a major problem that affects quality of life, family and social relationships, and employment (Correia de Sa, 2012). a. Cognitive dysfunction can impact memory, comprehension, problem solving, and speech.
5. Assess level of fatigue. Refer to Unit II to Fatigue for interventions for energy conservation, work simplification, scheduled rest periods, and the use of cooling garments (e.g., vest, hat, collar).	5. Fatigue is one of the most common and disabling symptom of MS, occurring in approximately 76% to 92% of MS patients (Correia de Sa, 2012).
6. Explain heat intolerance. Fatigue can worsen before and during exacerbations and with increased temperatures. a. Advise to manage heat intolerance as follows: • Time outside activities for early morning or evening hours to avoid the heat of the day. • Spread activities throughout the course of the day to avoid overheating. • Use air conditioning in homes and cars, cooling garments, light-colored clothes, and wide-brimmed hats. • Avoid exposure to saunas, hot tubs, or even hot showers or baths. • Avoid exposure to excessive humidity; dehumidifiers can help indoors. • Treat fevers aggressively with around-the-clock antipyretics.	6. Demyelinated fibers in the central nervous system are very sensitive to even small elevations of core body temperature resulting in conduction delays or even conduction block. The effects of heat exposure are reversed with rest and cooling and do not carry a long-term consequence.

Interventions	Rationales
7. Discuss bladder problems. Bladder dysfunction in MS may consist of failure to store, failure to empty, or a combination of the two. Interventions for failure to store include the following: a. Scheduled voiding b. Limiting fluid intake in the evening c. Using anticholinergic medications (e.g., oxybutynin) d. Eliminating diuretics (e.g., caffeine)	
8. Identify and notify the physician / NP of urinary tract infection (UTI) signs and symptoms: a. Foul-smelling urine b. Increased frequency and urge to urinate c. Change in color—dark yellow d. Change in consistency—cloudy, sediment, or flecks of blood	8. Recurrent urinary tract infections are common in MS patients with end-stage bladder disability.
9. Assist in formulating and accepting realistic short- and long-term goals.	9. Mutual goal-setting reinforces the client's role in improving his or her quality of life.
10. Teach about the diagnosis and management techniques, including alternative methods.	10. Understanding can help to improve compliance and reduce exacerbations.
11. Discuss the factors known to trigger exacerbation (Hickey, 2009): a. Undue fatigue or excessive exertion b. Overheating or excessive chilling or cold exposure c. Infections d. Hot environments / hot baths e. Fever f. Emotional stress g. Pregnancy h. Cigarette smoking i. Alcohol use	11. This information gives the client insight into aspects of the condition that can be controlled; this may promote a sense of control and encourage compliance. b. As body temperature rises above the normal range, it blocks conduction across demyelinated regions in the brain and can worsen MS. h. Smoking may be a risk factor for transforming a relapsing-remitting clinical course into a secondary-progressive course (Hernán et al., 2005). i. Since alcohol depresses the central nervous system, it may also have an additive effect with certain medications that are commonly prescribed for MS.
12. Teach the importance of constructive stress management and reduction (Hickey, 2009); explain measures such as the following: a. Progressive relaxation techniques b. Self-coaching c. Thought-stopping d. Assertiveness techniques e. Guided imagery f. Exercising (e.g., walking yoga)	12. Managing stress helps the client to cope and adapt to changes caused by MS. Approaches to stress management include massage therapy, exercise programs, and involvement in religious and social activities.

(continued)

Interventions	Rationales
13. If appropriate, discuss the stressors that living with MS can bring to family relationships. Suggest the usefulness of counseling for all individuals separately and group.	13. "Early identification and psychosocial intervention might reduce the frequency of divorce and separation, and in turn improve quality of life and quality of care" (Glantz et al., 2009, p. 5242).

CLINICAL ALERT
- "We recommend that medical providers be especially sensitive to early suggestions of marital discord in couples affected by the occurrence of a serious medical illness, especially when the woman is the affected spouse and it occurs early in the marriage.
- The results showed a stronger gender disparity for divorce when the wife was the patient in the general oncology and multiple sclerosis groups (93 percent and 96 percent respectively, compared to 78 percent for the primary brain tumor group" (Glantz et al., 2009, p. 5242).

Interventions	Rationales
14. Explain the signs and symptoms that must be reported to a health care professional immediately: a. Worsening of symptoms (e.g., weakness, spasticity, visual disturbances) b. Temperature elevation c. Change in urination patterns or cloudy, foul-smelling urine d. Productive cough with cloudy, greenish sputum	14. Early detection enables prompt intervention to minimize complications. These symptoms may indicate infection (urinary tract or pulmonary).

CLINICAL ALERT
- Worsening symptoms may herald an exacerbation. Immediate interventions are needed (e.g., PCP, emergency room).

Interventions	Rationales
15. Provide information and materials to assist the client and family to maintain goals and manage at home from sources such as the following: a. Multiple Sclerosis Society b. Home health agencies c. American Red Cross d. Individual / family counselors e. Jimmie Heuga Center	15. A client who feels well-supported can cope more effectively with the multiple stressors associated with chronic debilitating disease.

Documentation

Client teaching
Referrals if indicated

Myasthenia Gravis

Myasthenia gravis (MG) is a chronic autoimmune neuromuscular disorder. It is characterized by production of antibodies that block muscle cell receptors for acetylcholine (ACh), the neurotransmitter essential for the stimulation of skeletal muscle contraction (Howard, 2006). Normal amounts of ACh are produced, but due to the lack of functional receptors, skeletal muscle contraction is impaired. In MG clients, impaired neurotransmission, combined with the normal reduction of ACh released with repeated activity, produces fatigue and fluctuating weakness of voluntary (skeletal) muscles. Function of affected muscles is usually strongest in the morning. Weakness increases with periods of activity and often improves with periods of rest (Osborn et al., 2010). Muscles that control the movement of the eyes and eyelids, facial expression, chewing, speaking, swallowing, and breathing are most commonly affected (Lewis et al., 2011).

The prevalence of MG in the United States is estimated to be about 20 per100,000 (Howard, 2006). MG can occur in any age or ethnic group, but peak onset in women is 20 to 40 years of age and 60 to 80 years of age for men (Osborn et al., 2010). Clients often initially report weakness in a single muscle. Onset of symptoms is typically gradual, and the course of the disease is variable. Muscles of the eyes, head, and neck are most frequently affected (LeMone, Burke, & Bauldoff, 2011). Symptom-free periods decrease and muscle weakness increases as the disease progresses. The exact cause of MG is not known, but abnormal antibodies are often found in the blood of people with MG (Howard, 2006).

There is no cure for MG, but clients may achieve improvement of their symptoms, and even remission (Lewis et al., 2011). Treatments focus on reducing, removing, or inhibiting the function of the abnormal antibodies that block the effect of ACh to trigger muscle contraction. Surgical removal of the thymus gland (thymectomy) produces improvement of symptoms, reduced need for medication, or remission in 85% of clients (Osborn et al., 2010). The thymus gland is located behind the breastbone and has an important role in the development and function of the immune system, but is normally inactive after puberty. Hyperplastic thymus tissue or tumors are frequently found in those with MG (Osborn et al., 2010). Plasmapheresis, the removal of abnormal antibodies from the blood plasma, provides relief of symptoms in periods of crisis or when other treatments are ineffective (LeMone et al., 2011).

Complications of MG often arise from weakness in the muscle groups affecting swallowing and breathing, causing aspiration, respiratory infection, or respiratory insufficiency (Lewis et al., 2011). Clients with MG are at risk for two life-threatening complications that can have a similar clinical presentation of extreme weakness and respiratory dysfunction. Myasthenic crisis can be triggered by low ACh levels due to undermedication, incompatible medications, or physical or emotional stress. Cholinergic crisis results from excess levels of ACh due to overmedication (Osborn et al., 2010).

Time Frame
Initial diagnosis

Acute exacerbations

Remissions

▪▪▪ DIAGNOSTIC CLUSTER

Collaborative Problems

Risk for Complications of Respiratory Insufficiency

Risk for Complications of Myasthenic / Cholinergic Crisis

Risk for Complications of Aspiration

Nursing Diagnoses

Risk for Ineffective Airway Clearance related to impaired ability to cough (refer to Chronic Obstructive Pulmonary Disease)

Risk for Impaired Swallowing related to neuromuscular weakness. (refer to Cerebrovsacular Accident [Stroke])

Risk for injury related to visual disturbances, unsteady gait, weakness (refer to Cerebrovascular Accident [Stroke])

Risk for Impaired Verbal Communication related to involvement of muscles for speech (refer to Parkinsonism)

Risk for Impaired Skin Integrity related to immobility (refer to Immobility)

Risk for Activity Intolerance related to fatigue and difficulty in performing activities of daily living (refer to Unit II)

Risk for Powerlessness related to the unpredictable nature of the condition (remissions / exacerbations)

Risk for Ineffective Therapeutic Regimen Management related to insufficient knowledge of condition, treatments, prevention of infections, stress management, aggravating factors, signs and symptoms of complications, and community resources.

Interventions	Rationales
2. Ensure blood culture is done prior to the start of any antibiotic. Culture any suspected infection sites (urine, sputum, invasive lines). Refer to Risk for Complications of Systemic Inflammatory Response Syndrome (SIRS) / Sepsis in Unit II Section 2 for additional interventions.	2. "Poor outcomes are associated with inadequate or inappropriate antimicrobial therapy (i.e., treatment with antibiotics to which the pathogen was later shown to be resistant in vitro. They are also associated with delays in initiating antimicrobial therapy, even short delays (e.g., an hour)" (Schmidt & Mandel, 2012).

> **CLINICAL ALERT**
> • Blood culture obtained after antibiotic therapy has been initiated can be inaccurate.
> • Research of clients with septic shock demonstrated that the time to initiation of appropriate antimicrobial therapy was the strongest predictor of mortality (Schmidt & Mandel, 2012).

Interventions	Rationales
3. Monitor for signs of urinary tract infection: a. Change in urine color, odor, and volume b. Fever c. Increased urgency, frequency, or incontinence	3. UTIs, especially if frequent or chronic, will place a person at risk for upper urinary tract disease, as well as sclerosis of ureters, causing increased renal pressure.
4. Monitor for signs and symptoms of renal calculi. Refer to Risk for Complications of Renal Calculi Unit II Section 2 for additional interventions. a. Acute flank pain b. CVA (costovertebral angle) pain (a dull, constant backache below the 12th rib) c. Hematuria d. Nausea and vomiting	4. Urinary stasis and infection increase the risk of renal calculi because of increased precipitants in the urine. Stones remain a major source of morbidity in clients with neurogenic bladder. a, b. Stones can cause severe pain owing to obstruction and ureter spasms, or CVA pain due to distention of the renal capsule. c. The abrasive action of the stone can sever small blood vessels. d. Afferent stimuli in the renal capsule may cause pylorospasm of the smooth muscle of the GI tract.
5. Monitor for urinary retention by paying attention to output vs. intake amounts.	5. Urine retention, especially associated with high pressure, can cause reflux at the vesicoureteral junction, with potential hydronephrosis.

> ### Clinical Alert Report
> Prior to providing care, advise ancillary staff / student to report the following to the professional nurse assigned to the client:
> • Change in cognitive status
> • Changes in urine output, characteristics.
> • Oral temperature >100.5° F
> • Systolic BP <90 mm Hg
> • Resting Pulse >100, <50
> • Respiratory rate >28, <10/min
> • Oxygen saturation <90%

Related Physician / NP Prescribed Interventions

Medications

The three main categories of drugs used to treat urge incontinence include anticholinergic drugs (antimuscarinics), antispasmodics, and tricyclic antidepressant agents. Other medications are estrogen derivatives terazosin, alpha-adrenergic stimulators, phenoxybenzamine, pseudoephedrine, dicyclomine, flavoxate, imipramine, propantheline, methantheline, oral and transdermal oxybutynin, gabapentin, botulinum toxin A, vanilloids

Diagnostic Studies

Voiding cystourethrogram

Therapies

Corrective surgery (e.g., bilateral sacral nerve root stimulation, enterocystoplasty, urinary diversion, urethral stents, bladder sphincter procedures)

Documentation

Urine output and characteristics
Intake and output
Complaints of pain, nausea, vomiting
Carp's Cues
If intermittent catheterization is indicated, refer to Table 2

Nursing Diagnoses

Risk for Infection Related to Retention of Urine or Introduction of Urinary Catheter

NOC

Infection Status, Wound Healing: Primary Intention, Immune Status

Goal

The client will be free of bladder infection.

NIC

Infection Control, Wound Care, Incision Site Care, Health Education

Indicators

- Urine is clear.
- Temperature is between 98° and 99.5° F.
- Demonstrate techniques to prevent infection.

Interventions	*Rationales*
1. Ensure adequate fluid intake (at least 2000 mL/day, unless contraindicated).	1. Dilute urine helps to prevent infection and bladder irritation.
2. Eliminate residual urine by aiding urine outflow through methods such as the following (Lemke et al., 2005): a. Credé maneuver b. Suprapubic tapping c. Timed voiding d. Valsalva maneuver e. Intermittent catheterization	2. Bacteria multiply rapidly in stagnant urine retained in the bladder. Moreover, overdistention hinders blood flow to the bladder wall, increasing the susceptibility to infection from bacterial growth. Regular, complete bladder emptying greatly reduces the risk of infection (Newman & Willson, 2011).
3. Consult with the physician / NP for medication to relieve detrusor sphincter dyssynergia (DSD).	3. DSD is associated with large amounts of residual urine.
4. Monitor residual urine (should be no more than 50 mL).	4. Careful monitoring detects problems early, enabling prompt intervention to prevent urine stasis.
5. Test an uncontaminated urine sample for bacteria.	5. A bacteria count over 105/mL of urine suggests infection, when pyuria is present. Some physicians / NPs may not want to treat until the client has symptoms.
6. Maintain sterile technique for intermittent catheterization while the client is hospitalized (Lemke et al., 2005); clean technique is used at home (Lemke et al., 2005; Newman & Willson, 2011).	6. The most common cause of infection in a health care facility is bacteria introduced by a caregiver who did not wash hands adequately between clients.
7. Avoid using an indwelling catheter unless it is indicated by a client's individual situation (e.g., inability to perform CISC due to immobility).	7. Indwelling catheters are associated with urinary tract infection related to the catheter sliding in and out of the urethra, which introduces pathogens.

Table 2 Intermittent Catheterization to Person and Family for Long-Term Management of Bladder

1. Explain the reasons for the intermittent catheterization program. Long-term use of intermittent catheterization has a lower risk of infection and other complications when compared to indwelling urinary catheter (Newman & Wein, 2009).

> **CLINICAL ALERT**
> - A cognitively impaired person with continuous incontinence requires caregiver-directed treatment.
> - In institutional settings, indwelling and external catheters or disposal or washable incontinence briefs or pads are beneficial to the caregivers but detrimental to the incontinent person.
> - Aids and equipment should be considered only after other means have been attempted.
> - In the home setting, the caregiver's needs may take precedence over the cognitively impaired person.
> - Urinary incontinence is cited as the major reason for seeking institutional care for people living at home (Miller, 2009).

2. Explain the relation of fluid intake, frequency of catheterization, and risk for infection.
   - Inadequate fluid intake can produce low urine volumes (less than 1200 ml of urine per day). Decreased urine production may lead to less catheterizations, stasis of urine, and infection.
   - Ensure that total daily fluid intake (from foods and all types of beverages) is approximately 2.7 L/day for women and 3.7 L/day for men (Newman & Willson, 2011, p. 15). Excessive fluid intake will produce periodic or regular bladder overdistention (volumes greater than 500 mL, possible overflow urinary incontinence, and urinary stasis). "Distended bladder walls are susceptible to bacteria that circulate in retained urine" (Newman & Willson, 2011, p.15). When the bladder becomes stretched from retained urine, the capillaries become occluded, preventing the delivery of metabolic and immune substrates to the bladder wall, which are needed to maintain a physical barrier against colonization or invasion by pathogens (Heard & Buhrer, 2005).
   - Advise of the possible need to catheterize more than six times day.
   - Encourage regular fluid intake, small volumes spaced hourly between breakfast and the evening meal, and reducing to sips thereafter (Newman & Willson, 2011, p. 15).
   - Ensure that there is adequate emptying at the time of catheterization. Teach a gentle Credé's maneuver as one removes the catheter. Residual volume left in the bladder after catheterization promotes an environment for bacteria proliferation (Newman & Willson 2011, p. 16).

3. Teach client and / or family member intermittent catheterization. Observe them performing intermittent catheterization for (Newman & Willson, 2011, p. 16):
   - Ability
   - Hygiene (hand washing, maintenance of catheter sterility)
   - Correct technique (lubricant, position, prevention of trauma)
   - Instruct client / family member to wash perineum each day and after sexual activity.

4. Review signs / symptoms of urinary tract infection with client and family:
   - Dysuria: pain or burning during urination, lower abdominal pain
   - Frequency: more frequent urination (or waking up at night to urinate, often with only a small amount of urine)
   - Urgency: the sensation of having to urinate urgently
   - Hesitancy: the sensation of not being able to urinate easily or completely (or feeling that you have to urinate but only a few drops of urine come out)
   - Cloudy, bad-smelling, or new onset bloody urine. Bloody urine may be normal when intermittent catheterization is initiated (Newman & Willson, 2011).
   - Mild fever (less than 101° F), chills, and "just not feeling well" (malaise)
   - Upper urinary tract infection (pyelonephritis) may develop rapidly and may or may not include the symptoms for a lower urinary tract infection.
     - Fairly high fever (higher than 101° F), shaking, chills
     - Nausea, vomiting
     - Flank pain: pain in back or side, usually on only one side at about waist level

> **CLINICAL ALERT**
> - Elderly people may not have the usual signs / symptoms of UTI, but instead may have fever or hypothermia, poor appetite, lethargy, and sometimes only a change in mental status.

5. Refer to community nurses for assistance in incontinence management at home if indicated.

Carp's Cues

Incontinence management is a complex process. The nurse is advised to seek expert assistance from a nurse specialist. An excellent online resource for specific guidelines how to correctly catheterize and on how to instruct clients / family in proper technique: Newman, DK, Willson, MM. (2011) Review of Intermittent Catheterization and Current Best Practices, Urologic Nursing. Volume 31 Number 1, which can be retrieved at http://www.suna.org/education/2013/article3101229.pdf.

Documentation

Urine characteristics
Temperature
Elimination pattern (amount, time)
Urine retention >50 mL

Overflow Incontinence Related to Chronically Overfilled Bladder with Loss of Sensation of Bladder Distention

NOC
Tissue Integrity, Urinary Continence

Goal

The client will achieve a state of dryness that is personally satisfactory.

NIC
Urinary Incontinence Care, Urinary Habit Training, Urinary Elimination Management

Indicators

- Empty the bladder using Credé's or Valsalva maneuver with a residual urine of less than 50 mL, if indicated.
- Void voluntarily.

Interventions	*Rationales*

1. Teach the client methods to empty the bladder.
  a. Credé's maneuver:
    • Position individual on toilet or lying on absorbent material.
    • Position your hands just below the umbilicus.
    • Stroke firmly toward the bladder, repeating about six times. (This should stimulate the voiding reflex.)
    • Then place one hand over the other hand above the pubic arch and press firmly in and downward. (This maneuver will compress the bladder to expel urine.)
    • Wait several minutes then repeat again. (This will ensure complete emptying and prevent urinary stasis.)
  b. Valsalva maneuver (bearing down):
    • Lean forward on thighs.
    • Contract abdominal muscles, if possible, and strain or bear down while holding the breath.
    • Hold until urine flow stops; wait one minute, then repeat.
    • Continue until no more urine is expelled.
  c. Clean intermittent self-catheterization (CISC), used alone or in combination with the above methods. (Refer to Table 2.)
	1a. In many clients, Credé's maneuver can help to empty the bladder. This maneuver is inappropriate, however, if the urinary sphincters are chronically contracted. In this case, pressing the bladder can force urine up the ureters as well as through the urethra. Reflux of urine into the renal pelvis may result in renal infection.
	
	b. Valsalva maneuver contracts the abdominal muscles, which manually compresses the bladder.
	
	c. CISC prevents overdistention, helps to maintain detrusor muscle tone, and ensures complete bladder emptying. CISC may be used initially to determine residual urine following Credé's maneuver or tapping. As residual urine decreases, catheterization may be tapered. CISC may recondition the voiding reflex in some clients.

Documentation

Fluid intake
Voiding patterns (amount, time, method used)

Overflow Incontinence Related to Detrusor–Sphincter Dyssynergy (DSD)

NOC
See Functional Incontinence

Goal

Refer to Goals for Overflow Incontinence Related to Chronically Overfilled Bladder with Loss of Sensation of Bladder Distention.

NIC

Refer to Functional
Incontinence, Urinary
Bladder Training

Interventions

For interventions on cutaneous triggering by suprapubic tapping. (See under Reflex Incontinence later in this plan.)

For interventions on the anal stretch maneuver. (See under Reflex Incontinence later in this plan.)

For intervention on intermittent catheterization. (Refer to Table 2.)

Documentation

Fluid intake

Urine output

Residual amount immediately after voiding via intermittent catheterization

Reflex Incontinence Related to Absence of Sensation to Void and Loss of Ability to Inhibit Bladder Contraction

NOC

See Functional
Incontinence

Goal

The client will report a state of dryness that is personally satisfactory.

NIC

See also Functional
Incontinence, Pelvic
Muscle Exercise, Weight
Management

Indicators

* Have a residual urine volume of less than 50 mL.
* Use triggering mechanisms to initiate reflex voiding.

Interventions	Rationales
1. Ensure adequate fluid intake (at least 2000 mL/day unless contraindicated).	1. Adequate fluid intake prevents concentrated urine that can irritate the bladder and cause increased bladder instability.
2. If indicated, consult with the physician / NP about prescribing medication to relax the bladder (e.g., anticholinergic).	2. Anticholinergic medications can eliminate hyperirritable and uninhibited bladder contractions and allow successful bladder retraining.

3. Teach techniques to trigger reflex voiding.
  a. Assist the individual to assume a half-sitting position.
  b. Using the fingers of one hand, aim tapping directly at the bladder wall; tap at a rate of seven or eight times every 5 seconds for a total of 50 taps.
  c. Shift the site of tapping over the bladder to find the most effective site.
  d. Continue stimulation until a good stream starts.
  e. Wait about 1 minute, then repeat stimulation until the bladder is empty. (One or two series of stimulations without urination indicates bladder emptying.)
  f. Tell the client to contract abdominal muscles. (Contraction of abdominal muscles compresses the bladder to empty it.)
  g. If tapping is ineffective, perform each of the following for 2 to 3 minutes each:
    • Stroke the glans penis.
    • Stroke the inner thigh.
	3. Stimulating the bladder wall or cutaneous sites (e.g., suprapubic, pubic) can trigger the reflex arc, which relaxes the internal sphincter of the bladder and allows urination.

Interventions	Rationales

4. Perform the anal stretch maneuver:
  a. Sit on the commode or toilet, leaning forward on the thighs.
  b. Insert one or two lubricated fingers into the anus, to the anal sphincter.
  c. Spread fingers apart or pull in the posterior direction to stretch the anal sphincter.
  d. Bear down and void while performing the Valsalva maneuver.
  e. Relax then repeat the procedure until the bladder is empty.
	4. Anal sphincter stimulation can stimulate the voiding reflex.

5. Teach measures to help reduce detrusor activity:
  a. Resist voiding for as long as possible.
 	
  b. Drink sufficient fluid to distend the bladder.
 	
  c. Time fluid intake so that detrusor activity is restricted to waking hours.
	5a. Resisting the urge to void may increase voiding intervals and reduce detrusor muscle activity.
	  b. To increase comfort associated with voiding, the client must condition the voiding reflex by ingesting adequate fluids and inhibiting bladder contractions.

6. Encourage the client to void or trigger at least every 3 hours.	6. Frequent toileting less than 3 hours, causes chronic low-volume voiding and increases detrusor activity. A regular voiding pattern can prevent incontinent episodes and urinary tract infections (Lemke, Kasprowicz, & Worral, 2005).
7. Manage incontinence with clean intermittent self-catheterization (CISC) or external urine collection (male), whichever is more appropriate for the client and caregiver. External urine collection devices may be used if urodynamic studies show complete bladder emptying.	7. Loss of both the sensation to void and the ability to inhibit contractions makes bladder retraining unlikely. CISC, often in conjunction with medications, is then the procedure of choice for managing incontinence. Male external urine collection devices are appropriate if CISC is not feasible.

Documentation

Fluid intake
Voiding patterns (amount, time, method used)

Urge Incontinence Related to Disruption of the Inhibitory Efferent Impulses Secondary to Brain or Spinal Cord Dysfunction

NOC

Tissue Integrity: Skin & Mucous Membranes, Urinary Continence, Urinary Elimination

Goals

The client will report no or fewer episodes of incontinence (specify).

NIC

Perineal Care, Urinary Incontinence Care, Prompted Voiding, Urinary Habit Training, Urinary Elimination Management, Teaching: Procedure / Treatment

Indicators

- Explain causes of incontinence.
- Describe bladder irritants.

Interventions	Rationales

1. Reduce any impediments to voiding routine by providing the following, if necessary:
  a. Velcro straps on clothes
  b. Handrails or mobility aids to bathroom
  c. Bedside commode
  d. Access to urinal
	1. These measures ensure the client's ability to self-toilet before incontinence occurs. Often, little time exists between onset of the sensation to void and the bladder contraction.

2. Assess voiding patterns and develop a schedule of frequent timed voiding.
  a. If incontinence occurs, decrease the time between planned voidings.
 	
  b. If indicated, restrict fluid intake during the evening.
	2. Frequent timed voiding can reduce urgency from bladder overdistention.
	  a. Bladder capacity may be insufficient to accommodate the urine volume, necessitating more frequent voiding.
	  b. Evening fluid restrictions may help to prevent enuresis.

3. Teach pelvic floor exercises (Kegel exercises) to help restore bladder control:
 	
  a. Help the client to identify the muscles that start and stop urination. Advise client when urinating to stop, then stream for 3 seconds, then release.
  b. Advise to squeeze muscles for 3 seconds and release for 3 seconds. Repeat 10 times. Do this 3 times a day or more
	3. Effective for some individuals with stress incontinence, Kegel exercises strengthen the pelvic floor muscles, which in turn may increase urinary sphincter competence. In women, Kegel exercises can improve stress incontinence. In men, Kegel exercises are used to treat stress incontinence and urge incontinence.
	  a. These are the muscles that will be contracted in the exercise.
	
	  b. Like any exercise, more is better.

4. Reinforce the need for optimal hydration (at least 2000 mL/day, unless contraindicated).	4. Optimal hydration is needed to prevent urinary tract infection and renal calculi.
5. If these measures fail, consult with a nurse specialist for managing incontinence.	

Documentation

        Intake
        Voidings (amount, time)
        Method used
        Incontinent episodes

Risk for Loneliness Related to Embarrassment of Incontinence in Front of Others and Fear of Odor From Urine

NOC

Loneliness, Social Involvement

Goals

The client will report decreased feelings of loneliness.

NIC

Socialization Enhancement, Spiritual Support, Behavior Modification: Social Skills, Presence, Anticipatory Guidance

Indicators

- Identify the reasons for feelings of isolation.
- Discuss ways of increasing meaningful relationships.

Interventions	Rationales
1. Elicit from individual / family how bladder problems have negatively affected their lifestyle.	1. Specific problems may be reduced or prevented.
2. Acknowledge the client's frustration with incontinence.	2. To the client, incontinence may seem like a reversion to an infantile state, in which he or she has no control over body functions and feels ostracized by others. Acknowledging the difficulty of the situation can help to reduce feelings of isolation.
3. Determine the client's eligibility for bladder training, CISC, or other methods to manage incontinence.	3. These measures can increase control and reduce fear of accidents. CISC has a low incidence of UTI compared with Foley indwelling catheters.
4. Teach the client ways to control wetness and odor. Many products make wetting manageable by providing reliable leakage protection and masking odors.	4. Helping the client / family to manage incontinence and odors encourages socialization.
5. Encourage the client to initially venture out socially for short periods, then to increase the length of social contacts as success at incontinence management increases.	5. Short trips help the client to gradually gain confidence and reduce fears.

Documentation

Client teaching

> **TRANSITION TO HOME / COMMUNITY CARE**
> If indicated, review the risk diagnoses identified for this individual on admission:
> * Is the person still at risk?
> * Can the family reduce the risks?
> * Is the person at higher risk at home?
> * Is a Home Health Nurse assessment needed?
> * Refer to transition planner / case manager / social service
> * When is this person scheduled for follow-up with primary provider? Specialists? Record dates of appointments.
> * Complete a medication reconciliation prior to transition. Refer to index.

STAR

Stop

Think   Is this person at risk for injury, falls, medical complications, and / or inability to care for self (activities of daily living)?

Is there a support person available?

Is the person competent to manage self-administration of medications, treatment procedures? Are additional resources needed?

Can the person explain how to monitor the condition (e.g., blood glucose, sign / symptoms of complications, dietary / mobility restrictions, and when to call his or her primary provider or specialist)?

Act   Contact or provide the appropriate resource (e.g., contacting a support person, home health assessment, additional teaching, printed materials).

Review   Has the problem been addressed? If not, use SBAR to communicate to the appropriate person.

Risk for Ineffective Self-Health Management Related to Insufficient Knowledge of Etiology of Incontinence, Management, Bladder Retraining Programs, Signs and Symptoms of Complications, and Community Resources

NOC

Compliance Behavior, Knowledge: Treatment Regimen, Participation in Health Care Decisions, Treatment Behavior: Illness or Injury

NIC

Anticipatory Guidance, Learning Facilitation, Risk Identification, Health Education, Teaching: Procedure / Treatment, Health System Guidance

Goals

The goals for this diagnosis represent those associated with transition planning. Refer to the transition criteria.

Interventions	Rationales
1. Teach the client about the condition, its causes, and management.	1. Understanding can encourage compliance with and participation in the treatment regimen.
2. Reinforce the strategies that are recommended for home management of incontinence. Have individual / family demonstrate all treatments.	2. Observing the technique will increase correct implementation at home and optimal outcomes.
3. Encourage an obese client to lose weight.	3. Obesity places excessive intra-abdominal pressure on the bladder, which can aggravate incontinence.

4. Teach the client about any drugs prescribed for managing incontinence.
  a. Advise of the benefits of antispasmodic medications.
 	
  b. Advise that these drugs may impair one's ability to perform activities requiring mental alertness and physical coordination. Drinking alcohol and using sedatives in combination with these antispasmodic drugs is contraindicated (Rackley, 2011).
	4. This can increase compliance.
	
	  a. Antispasmodic drugs have been reported to increase bladder capacity and effectively decrease or eliminate urge incontinence.

5. If indicated, teach CISC to the client or caregiver. Refer to Table 2.	5. Intermittent self-catheterization is appropriate for children and adults who are motivated and physically able to perform the procedure. Often, a caregiver may be taught to catheterize the client. CISC stimulates normal voiding, can prevent infection, and maintains integrity of the ureterovesical junction. In the hospital, aseptic technique is used because of increased microorganisms in the hospital environment; at home, clean technique is used. CISC entails fewer complications than an indwelling catheter and is the procedure of choice for clients who are unable to empty the bladder completely (Newman & Willson, 2011).
6. Teach the client to keep a record of catheterization times, amount of fluid intake and urine output, and any incontinent periods.	6. Bring record to follow-up visit post transition. (Accurate record-keeping aids in evaluating status and problem solving.)

Interventions	Rationales
7. Teach the client / family to notify the physician / NP of the following: a. Unusual bleeding from urethral opening b. Difficulty inserting catheter c. Dark, bloody, cloudy, or strong-smelling urine. d. Change in cognition e. New pain in the abdomen or back f. Oral temperature >100.5° F	7. Early reporting enables prompt treatment to prevent serious problems such as sepsis, kidney infections. a. Bleeding may indicate trauma or renal calculi. Some minor bleeding can occur with catheter insertion. b. Difficult catheter insertion may indicate a stricture. c. These urine changes may point to infection. d. The elderly may not experience any signs of urinary tract infection except change in cognitive status. e. Pain may indicate renal calculi. f. Fever may be the only sign of urinary tract infection.
8. Explain available community resources.	8. The client and family may need assistance or more information for home care.
9. Advise to access the AHCPR booklet Urinary Incontinence in Adults: A Patient's Guide. http://www.strokecenter.org/wp-content/uploads/2011/08/Recovering-After-a-Stroke.pdf	

Documentation

Client teaching
Status at transition

Parkinson's Disease

Parkinson's disease (PD) is a chronic, slow, progressive neurodegenerative disease resulting in the depletion of dopaminergic neurons in the basal ganglia, also known as the subcortical motor nuclei of the cerebrum. The basal ganglia is composed of the substantianigra, striatum, globuspallidus, subthalamic nucleus, and red nucleus. The neurotransmitter dopamine is produced and stored in the substantianigra. Symptoms of PD are usually seen when there is cell loss in the substantianigra, resulting in a reduction of striatal dopamine (Hickey, 2009). Lewy bodies, intracellular protein deposits, are also seen and considered a pathologic hallmark of PD.

The classic signs and symptoms of Parkinson's disease include resting tremors, rigidity of muscles, akinesia / bradykinesia, postural disturbances, and loss of postural reflexes. Secondary symptoms include difficulty with fine motor function, soft monotone voice, mask-like face, generalized weakness and muscle fatigue, cognitive impairments / dementia, sleep disturbances, and autonomic manifestations which include the following: drooling, seborrhea, dysphagia, excessive perspiration, constipation, orthostatic hypotension, urinary hesitation and frequency, urgency, nocturia, urge incontinence, and erectile dysfunction and impotence (Hickey, 2009). Parkinson's disease typically affects 1% of people over the age of 65 years with the average age of onset being 60 years with prevalence higher in Caucasian men. Early onset of PD has affected people as young as 20. Genetics have also been linked to the development of PD specifically 10 autosomal dominant and recessive genes (Hickey, 2009).

 Time Frame
Secondary diagnosis (hospitalization not usual)

▪▪▪▪▪▪ DIAGNOSTIC CLUSTER**

Collaborative Problems

Risk for Complications of Long-Term Levodopa Treatment Syndrome

Risk for Complications of Dysphasia (leading to malnutrition or aspiration)

Risk for Complications of Pneumonia refer to Unit II

Risk for Complications of Urinary Tract Infections refer to Unit II

Risk for Complications of Sensory Abnormalities (leading to pain and paresthesias)

Nursing Diagnoses

Impaired Verbal Communication related to dysarthria secondary to ataxia of muscles of speech

Impaired Physical Mobility related to effects of muscle rigidity, tremors, and slowness of movement on activities of daily living

Risk for Constipation related to decreased peristalsis secondary to impaired autonomic system

Risk for Ineffective Self-Health Management related to lack of knowledge of condition, treatments required, stress management, signs and symptoms of complications, and availability of community resources

Risk for Injury related to Orthostatic Hypotension (refer to Unit II)

Related Care Plan

Neurogenic Bladder

Immobility or Unconsciousness

Multiple Sclerosis

** This medical condition was not included in the validation study.

Transition Criteria

Before transition, the client and family will:

1. Relate the intent to share concerns with another family member or a trusted friend.
2. Identify one strategy to increase independence.
3. Describe measures that can reduce the risk of exacerbation.
4. Identify signs and symptoms that must be reported to a health care professional.
5. Make sure the client and his or her family know what community resources are available to them, such as the Parkinson's Disease Foundation (http://www.pdf.org).

Transitional Risk Assessment Plan (TRAP)

Begin this plan on admission.
Implement the Transitional Risk Assessment Plan (TRAP):

- Refer to inside back cover.
- Add each validated risk diagnosis to client's problem list with the risk code in ( ).
- Refer to Unit II to the individual risk nursing diagnoses / collaborative problems for outcomes and interventions.

R: "Close coordination of care in the post-acute period, early transition follow-up care, enhanced client education and self-management training, proactive end-of-life counseling, and extending the resources and clinical expertise over time via multidisciplinary team management" can lower readmission rates and improve health outcomes (Boutwell & Hwu, 2009, p. 14).

Collaborative Problems

Risk for Complications of Long-Term Levodopa Treatment Syndrome

Risk for Complications of Aspiration

Risk for Complications of Pneumonia (refer to Unit II)

Risk for Complications of Urinary Tract Infections (refer to Unit II)

Risk for Complications of Sensory Abnormalities (leading to pain and paresthesias)

Collaborative Outcomes

The client will be monitored for early signs and symptoms of (a) long-term levodopa treatment syndrome and (b) dysphasia (leading to malnutrition or aspiration), (c) pneumonia, (d) urinary incontinence, (e) urinary tract infections, (f) peripheral edema, (g) orthostatic hypotension, (h) sensory abnormalities, (i) constipation and receive collaborative intervention to restore physiologic stability.

Indicators of Physiologic Stability

- Less or no fluctuations between involuntary movements (tics, tremors, rigidity, and repetitive, bizarre movements) and bradykinesia (slowed movements) (a)
- Intact cough-gag reflexes (b, c)
- Intact muscle strength (b, c)
- No continual coughing with swallowing (b, c)
- Dizziness, lightheadedness, and possible fainting with standing (g)
- Sudden decrease in blood pressure when sitting or standing (g)
- Headaches (g)
- Respiration 16–20 breaths/min (a, b)
- Respiration relaxed and rhythmic (b, c)
- Breath sound present all lobes (b, c)
- No rales or wheezing (b, c)
- Blurred or dimmed vision (possibly to the point of momentary blindness) (g)
- Extremity pain, numbness, or tingling (h)
- Urinary urgency, urinary frequency, and nocturia (d)
- Pain on voiding (burning) (e)
- Fever (e)
- Immobility (f)
- Decreased activity, low-fiber diet, and antiparkinsonian medications (i)
- Bowel obstruction (i)

Interventions	Rationales
1. Explain long-term levodopa treatment syndrome to the client and family.	1. This syndrome occurs 2 to 6 years after beginning treatment and is characterized by a deterioration of levodopa efficacy (Stacy, 2009).
2. Explain symptoms of the syndrome (on-off syndrome): a. Fluctuates between being symptom-free and severe Parkinson symptoms. b. Symptoms may last minutes or hours.	2. This syndrome is believed to be caused by altered sensitivity of dopamine receptors or to serum level changes in levodopa.
3. Encourage the client to discuss with the physician / NP the possibility of a "drug holiday."	3. Some physicians / NPs advocate from 1 to 2 days to 10–14 days of a drug holiday in a hospital setting to permit resensitization of dopamine receptors (Hickey, 2009).

(continued)

Interventions	Rationales

4. Evaluate knowledge of dietary precautions:
  a. The need to avoid foods high in pyridoxine (e.g., B_6 vitamins, pork, beef, liver, bananas, ham, and egg yolks).
  b. Advise the client to divide daily protein intake into equal amounts over the entire day.
  c. After taking levodopa, wait 30 minutes before eating. If nausea develops, the client may take the dosage with food.
  d. The need to have a diet high in fiber and fluid (unless contraindicated).
	4a. Pyridoxine accelerates the breakdown of levodopa to dopamine before it reaches the brain.
	b, c. Protein competes with levodopa for transport to the brain (Hickey, 2009).
	    Levodopa is best absorbed on an empty stomach. However, it may cause nausea, and should then be taken with food.
	  d. Constipation and nausea are side effects of levodopa.

5. Observe for psychiatric disturbances:
 	
  a. Visual hallucinations
 	
  b. Sleep disturbances
 	
  c. Depression
 	
  d. Dementia
	5. Drug-related psychiatric disturbances can occur in 40% of treated clients.
	  a. Visual hallucinations are related to dopaminergic medications and are the most common psychiatric problem seen in PD clients.
	  b. Sleep disorders seen include difficulty falling asleep, fragmented sleep, reversal of sleep cycle, REM behavior disorder, and excessive daytime sleepiness.
	  c. Depression in Parkinson's is associated with advancing disease severity, recent disease deterioration, and occurrence of falls. Prevalence of PD clients is between 20% and 40%.
	  d. Overt dementia will develop in 80% of PD clients along with mild cognitive impairment, which is seen early in the disease process.

6. Monitor the effectiveness of airway clearance by evaluating (Oliveira-Filho & Koroshetz, 2007):
  a. Effectiveness of cough effort
  b. Need for tracheobronchial suctioning
	6. "Swallowing problems are frequent in PD. Research has shown that self-report of 'no difficulty' is not a reliable indicator of swallowing ability" (Miller et al., 2009).

7. Determine if individual can swallow:
  a. If the person is not alert, drooling, and / or has difficulty speaking, do not attempt the test and make the person NPO until a Speech Language Pathologist consult is completed.
  b. If these conditions are not present, proceed with the test:
    • "A simple bedside screening evaluation involves asking the individual to sip a teaspoon of water from a cup.
    • If the client can sip and swallow without difficulty, the client is asked to take a large gulp of 60 mL of water and swallow.
    • If there are no signs of coughing or aspiration after 30 seconds, then it is safe for the individual to have a thickened diet until formally assessed by a speech pathologist" (Massey & Jedlicka, 2002; Jauch et al., 2010).
    • Consult with Speech Language Pathologist for all clients.
    • Refer to Impaired Swallowing in Unit II if indicated.
	7. One of the frequent complications of a stroke is aspiration.

Interventions	Rationales

8. Monitor client for signs and symptoms of urinary tract infection.
   a. Chills and fever
   b. Leukocytosis
   c. Bacteria and pus in urine
   d. Dysuria and frequency
   e. Bladder distention
   f. Urine overflow (30–60 mL of urine every 15–30 minutes)

9. Monitor for signs and symptoms of respiratory distress, and position to assist with breathing:

> **CLINICAL ALERT**
> • Report immediately any change in respiratory or ability to swallow
>   a. Auscultate breath sounds.
>   b. Assess for secretions:
>   • Encourage the client to breathe deep and cough.
>   • Position client side to side to assist movement of secretions.
>   • Suction if client is unable to manage secretions.
>   • Reassure client by maintaining a calm environment.
>   c. Assess O$_2$ saturation via pulse oximetry.

10. Ventilation may become necessary as Parkinson's disease progresses, due to decreased muscle tone and mobility.

> ### Clinical Alert Report
> Prior to providing care, advise ancillary staff / student to report the following to the professional nurse assigned to the client:
> • Change in cognitive status
> • Oral temperature >100.5° F
> • Systolic BP <90 mm Hg
> • Resting Pulse >100, <50
> • Respiratory rate <28, <10 /min.

Related Physician / NP Prescribed Interventions

Medications
Dopamine agonists, dopamine precursor, decarboxylase inhibitor, anticholinergics, amantadine, monoamine oxidase type B inhibitors, catechol-O-methyl transferase inhibitors

Intravenous Therapy
None

Laboratory Studies
None

Diagnostic Studies
CT scan or MRI (only to rule out other disorders). Positron emission tomography (PET) and single photon emission computed tomography (SPECT) may show use in the future but are primarily used in PD research protocols.

Therapies
Physical therapy, occupational therapy, speech therapy, psychologist, dietitian

Surgical

Deep brain stimulation and fetal tissue transplantation (investigational and not approved by the FDA).

Documentation

Changes in symptoms

Nursing Diagnoses

Impaired Verbal Communication Related to Dysarthria Secondary to Ataxia of Muscles of Speech

NOC
Communication:
Expressive Ability

Goal

The client will demonstrate improved ability to express self.

NIC
Active Listening,
Communication
Enhancement: Speech
Deficit

Indicator

• Demonstrate techniques and exercises to improve speech and strengthen muscles.

Interventions	Rationales
1. Explain the disorder's effects on speech.	1. Understanding may promote compliance with speech improvement exercises.
2. Explain the benefits of daily speech improvement exercises.	2. Daily exercises help to improve the efficiency of speech musculature and increase rate, volume, and articulation.
3. Refer the client to a speech pathologist to design an individualized speech program, as recommended by the American Parkinson's Disease Association.	3. These exercises improve muscle tone and control and speech clarity.
4. Refer the client to American Parkinson's Disease Association 135 Parkinson Avenue Staten Island, NY 10305-1425 apda@apdaparkinson.org http://www.apdaparkinson.org	

Documentation

Assessment of speech
Exercises taught
Referrals, if indicated

Impaired Physical Mobility Related to Effects of Muscle Rigidity, Tremors, and Slowness of Movement on Activities of Daily Living

NOC
Ambulation: Walking,
Joint Movement: Active
Mobility Level

Goal

The client will describe measures to increase mobility.

NIC
Exercise Therapy:
Joint Mobility, Exercise
Promotion: Strength
Training, Exercise
Therapy: Ambulation,
Positioning, Teaching:
Prescribed Activity /
Exercise

Indicators

• Demonstrate exercises to improve mobility.
• Demonstrate a wide-base gait with arm swinging.
• Identify one strategy to increase independence.
• Relate intent to exercise at home.

Interventions	Rationales
1. Explain the causes of the symptoms.	1. The client's understanding may help to promote compliance with an exercise program at home.
2. Teach the client to walk erect while looking at the horizon, with feet separated and arms swinging normally.	2. Conscious efforts to simulate normal gait and posture can improve mobility and minimize loss of balance.
3. Instruct the client to exercise three to five times a week.	3. Exercise has been proven to delay disability; ameliorate diseases; and fortify strength, balance, flexibility, and endurance, even in older clients who are frail or have a medical condition (Bader & Littlejohns, 2004). Specific benefits include the following: a. Increased muscle strength b. Improved coordination and dexterity c. Reduced rigidity d. Help prevent contractures e. Improved flexibility f. Enhanced peristalsis g. Improved cardiovascular endurance h. Increased ability to tolerate stress i. A sense of control, reducing feelings of powerlessness j. Slows osteoporosis k. Reduces LDL cholesterol l. Reduces systolic BP, raises HDL cholesterol
4. Consult with physical therapy for a specific exercise program. a. Explain that short bouts of physical activity are also beneficial.	4. An exercise program of range of motion and aerobic exercise (tailored to the person's ability) can help to preserve muscle strength and coordination (NINDS, 2007). a. Exercise programs should begin with low intensity activities, and gradually intensify (Parkinson's Disease Foundation, 2007).
5. Stress to the client that compliance with the exercise program is ultimately his or her choice.	5. Promoting the client's feelings of control and self-determination may improve compliance with the exercise program.
6. Include family members or significant others in teaching sessions; stress that they are not to "police" the client's compliance.	6. Support from family members and significant others can encourage the client to comply with the exercise program.
7. Refer to a physical therapist or reference material for specific exercise guidelines.	7. Physical or occupational therapy as well as some alternative therapies may help clients deal with disability, provide palliation, or reduce stress (Hickey, 2009).
8. Discuss strategies to maintain as much independence as possible. 9. Discuss the importance of accomplishing tasks and planning events to look forward to.	8, 9. Parkinson's disease seems to advance more slowly in people who remain involved in their pre-Parkinson activities or who find new activities to amuse them and engage their interests (Parkinson's Disease Foundation, 2007).
10. Refer to the Fatigue nursing diagnosis in the index for additional interventions.	

Risk for Constipation related to decreased peristalsis secondary to impaired autonomic system

NOC
Bowel Elimination, Hydration, Knowledge: Diet

Goal

The client will report bowel movements at least every 2 to 3 days.

NIC
Bowel Management, Fluid Management, Constipation / Impaction Management, Nutrition Therapy

Indicators

- Describe components for effective bowel movements.
- Explain rationale for lifestyle change(s).

Interventions	Rationales
1. Assess present bowel function.	1. Parkinson's disease causes decreased gastric motility. This is due its effects on the autonomic nervous system. This system regulates smooth muscle activity thus decreasing peristalsis.
2. Refer to Unit II for interventions to prevent or treat constipation.	

> **TRANSITION TO HOME / COMMUNITY CARE**
> If indicated, review the risk diagnoses identified for this individual on admission:
> - Is the person still at risk?
> - Can the family reduce the risks?
> - Is the person at higher risk at home?
> - Is a Home Health Nurse assessment needed?
> - Refer to transition planner / case manager / social service
> - When is this person scheduled for follow-up with primary provider? Specialists? Record dates of appointments.
> - Complete a medication reconciliation prior to transition. Refer to index.

STAR

Stop

Think   Is this person at risk for injury, falls, medical complications, and / or inability to care for self (activities of daily living)?

Is there a support person available?

Is the person competent to manage self-administration of medications, treatment procedures? Are additional resources needed?

Can the person explain how to monitor the condition (e.g., blood glucose, sign / symptoms of complications, dietary / mobility restrictions, and when to call his or her primary provider or specialist)?

Act   Contact or provide the appropriate resource (e.g., contacting a support person, home health assessment, additional teaching, printed materials).

Review   Has the problem been addressed? If not, use SBAR to communicate to the appropriate person.

Risk for Ineffective Self-Health Management Related to Lack of Knowledge of Condition, Treatments Required, Stress Management, Signs and Symptoms of Complications, and Availability of Community Resources

NOC
Compliance Behavior,
Knowledge: Treatment
Regimen, Participation
in Health Care
Decisions, Treatment
Behavior: Illness or
Injury

Goals

Refer to transition criteria.

NIC
Anticipatory Guidance,
Learning Facilitation,
Risk Identification,
Health Education,
Teaching Procedure /
Treatment, Health
System Guidance

Interventions	Rationales
1. Refer for a home assessment (e.g., home health nurse, occupational therapist). • Will a ramp be needed for outside access? • Do floor surfaces easily accommodate wheelchair transport? • Are the bedroom and bathroom accessible? • Advise to reorganize and remove clutter.	
2. Teach the client and his or her family the basic pathology of the client's condition.	2. Understanding can improve compliance and reduce the family unit's frustrations.
3. Assist the client in identifying realistic short term goals.	3. Preparation of the client to set realistic goals for recovery will reduce feelings of depression if goals are not attained.
4. Teach the client the value of continued ROM (passive or active, dependent on functional ability) and strengthening-stretching exercise programs. Consult physical therapy.	4. Exercise will maintain muscle strength and flexibility and promote circulation in effected extremities (NINDS, 2011).
5. Teach the client energy conservation techniques, scheduling planned rest periods, and exercise consistent with tolerance levels.	5. Energy conservation can reduce fatigue (NINDS, 2007).
6. Teach care of altered body functions: a. Bowel & bladder function: Encourage intake of 2000 mL of fluid unless contraindicated. b. Nutritional requirements: Provide a diet high in calories and protein. c. Self-care deficits, if necessary. Areas of concern: dressing, grooming, safe ambulation.	6. Care instructions: a. Adequate fluid intake promotes bowel and bladder function, prevention of constipation related to reduced activity and peristalsis. b. Protein and calories are required to rebuild muscle mass. c. Encourage maximum client self-care with ADL activities for purpose of strengthening and increasing independence.
7. Initiate referral to rehabilitation services	7. Client will require outpatient or home care multidisciplinary rehabilitation therapy.

(continued)

Interventions	Rationales
8. Facilitate referral for psychological counseling and emotional support.	8. Parkinson's disease often causes sudden paralysis, communication difficulties, and dependence for body functions and ADLs creating psychological and emotional crisis for clients and families (NIND, 2011).
9. Explain signs and symptoms of complications to report to health care professional. a. Difficulty swallowing b. Productive cough c. Difficulty with urination, odor to urine d. Prolonged constipation e. Increased weakness or fatigue f. Weight loss	9. Early intervention will minimize complications of the condition.
10. Provide information to assist the client and family to manage at home. Refer to the following resources: a. National Parkinson's Foundation (http://www3.parkinson.org/site) b. Case manager / transition planner referral c. Home health agency	10. Clients and families who receive community support may cope more effectively with this disease. Functional loss may be significant. Even when deficits are temporary the client will require interdisciplinary support during the recovery period.

Documentation

Condition on transition
Referrals, if indicated

Seizure Disorders

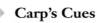 **Carp's Cues**

If a seizure diagnosis has not been confirmed, refer to Unit II Risk for Complications of Seizures instead of this care plan.

Seizure disorders constitute a chronic syndrome in which a neurologic dysfunction in cerebral tissue produces recurrent paroxysmal episodes, which are referred to as seizures. A seizure is defined as an uncontrolled electrical discharge of neurons in the brain that interrupts normal functions, such as disturbances of behavior, mood, sensation, perception, movement, and / or muscle tone.

Seizures are diagnosed as epileptic or reactive. Epilepsy is a chronic neurologic condition, usually with an underlying condition (as permanent brain injury) that affects the delicate systems that govern how electrical energy behaves in the brain, making the brain susceptible to recurring seizures (Epilepsy Foundation, 2007; Lewis et al., 2004). Reactive seizures are single or multiple seizures resulting from a transient systemic problem (e.g., fever, infection, alcohol withdrawal, tumors, stroke, and toxic or metabolic disturbances).

 Carp's Cues

Alcohol abuse is one of the most common causes of adolescent- and adult-onset seizures. Seizures, nearly always generalized tonic/clonic, occur in about 10% of adults during withdrawal. Multiple seizures happen in about 60% of these clients. The first seizure occurs 7 hours to 2 days after the last drink, and the time between the first and last seizure is usually 6 hours or less. (Hoffman & Weinhouse, 2012)

Seizures are classified into two main categories: *partial-onset* (focal) seizures begin in a focal area of the cerebral cortex, whereas *generalized-onset* seizures have an onset recorded simultaneously in both cerebral hemispheres (Berg, Berkovic, Brodie et al., 2010). Generalized seizures are further classified into the following categories: (a) absence, (b) myoclonic, (c) tonic/clonic, (d) tonic, and (e) atonic seizures (International League Against Epilepsy, 2007).

 Time Frame

Initial diagnosis
Recurrent acute episodes

■■■■■■■ DIAGNOSTIC CLUSTER

Collaborative Problems

*Risk for Complications of Status Epilepticus

Nursing Diagnoses

▲ Risk for Ineffective Airway Clearance related to relaxation of tongue and gag reflexes secondary to disruption in muscle innervations.

Anxiety related to fear of embarrassment secondary to having a seizure in public

△ Risk for Ineffective Self-Health Management related to insufficient knowledge of condition, medication, and care during seizures, environmental hazards, and community resources

▲ This diagnosis was reported to be monitored for or managed frequently (75% to 100%).
△ This diagnosis was reported to be monitored for or managed often (50% to 74%).

Transition Criteria

Before transition, the client or family will:

1. State the intent to wear medical identification.
2. Relate activities to be avoided.
3. Relate the importance of complying with the prescribed medication regimen.
4. Relate the side effects of prescribed medications.
5. State situations that increase the possibility of a seizure.
6. State signs and symptoms that must be reported to a health care professional.
7. Ensure that the client and her or his family are aware of community resources for epilepsy, such as http://www.ilae-epilepsy.org/ and http://www.epilepsyfoundation.org.
8. Make sure that the client has understood all required follow-up appointments prior to transition.

Transitional Risk Assessment Plan (TRAP)

Begin this plan on admission.
Implement the Transitional Risk Assessment Plan (TRAP):
- Refer to inside back cover.
- Add each validated risk diagnosis to client's problem list with the risk code in ( ).
- Refer to Unit II to the individual risk nursing diagnoses / collaborative problems for outcomes and interventions.

    R: *"Close coordination of care in the post-acute period, early transition follow-up care, enhanced client education and self-management training, proactive end-of-life counseling, and extending the resources and clinical expertise over time via multidisciplinary team management"* can lower readmission rates and improve health outcomes (Boutwell & Hwu, 2009, p. 14).

Collaborative Problems

Risk for Complications of Status Epilepticus

Collaborative Outcomes

The client will be monitored for early signs and symptoms of status epilepticus and will receive collaborative interventions if indicated to restore physiologic stability.

Indicators of Physiologic Stability

- Heart rate 60–100 beats/min (a, b)
- BP >90/60, <140/90 mm Hg (a, b)
- No seizure activity (a, b)

- Serum pH 7.35–7.45 (a, b)
- Serum PCO_2 35–45 mm Hg (a, b)
- Pulse oximetry (SaO_2) >95 (a, b)

Interventions	Rationales
1. Determine whether the client senses an aura before onset of seizure activity. If so advise him or her to immediately report to nursing staff / student and if standing to sit or lie down.	1. This can prevent injuries from falling or hitting head on an object.
2. If seizure activity occurs, observe or acquire details from those who witnessed it and document the following (Hickey, 2009): a. Behavior prior to seizure b. Site of onset of seizure c. Progression and sequencing of activity d. Type of movements: clonic (jerking), tonic (stiffening) • Twitching, head turning, dystonia (muscle spasms and twisting of limbs) • Parts of body involved (symmetry, unilateral, bilateral) e. Changes in pupil size or position (open, rolling, deviation) f. Skin changes (color. temperature, perspiration) g. Urinary or bowel incontinence h. Duration i. Unconsciousness (duration) j. Behavior after seizure k. Weakness, paralysis after seizure l. Sleep after seizure (postictal period)	2. An accurate, comprehensive description of a seizure can assist the physician / NP with appropriate anticonvulsant and optimal seizure management (Hickey, 2009; SCDDSN, 2006). b. Site of onset and order of progression are important in diagnosing causation. c. Progression of seizure activity may assist in identifying its anatomic focus.
3. In older adults, assess for presence of atypical s/s/ of seizures (Austin, 2013): a. Strange feelings, staring b. Minor behavioral changes, memory lapses c. Unaccountable loss of time d. Transient confusion	3. Age-related changes in the brain produce seizures that preset differently in older adults. Only 25% of older adults with epilepsy present with tonic/clonic seizures (Austin, 2013).
4. During seizure activity, take measures to ensure adequate ventilation (e.g., loosen clothing). *Do not* try to force an airway or tongue blade through clenched teeth.	4. Strong clonic-tonic movements can cause airway occlusion. Forced airway insertion can cause injury.
5. Provide privacy during and after seizure activity.	5. To protect the client from embarrassment
6. During seizure activity, gently guide movements to prevent injury. Do not attempt to restrict movements.	6. Physical restraint could result in musculoskeletal injury.
7. If the client is sitting when seizure activity occurs, ease him or her to the floor and place something soft under his or her head.	7. These measures help prevent injury.
8. After seizure activity subsides, position client on the side.	8. This position helps prevent aspiration of secretions.

Interventions	Rationales
9. Allow person to sleep after seizure activity; reorient on awakening.	9. The person may experience amnesia; reorientation can help him or her regain a sense of control and can help reduce anxiety.

> **CLINICAL ALERT**
> • Call Rapid Response Team if seizure continues more than two (2) consecutive minutes or the individual experiences two (2) or more generalized seizures without full recovery of consciousness between seizures (Hickey, 2009).

Interventions	Rationales
10. Initiate protocol: a. Establish airway. b. Suction PRN. c. Administer oxygen through nasal catheter. d. Initiate an IV line.	10. Status epilepticus is a medical emergency with a 10% mortality rate. Impaired respiration can cause systemic and cerebral hypoxia. IV administration of a rapid-acting anticonvulsant (e.g., diazepam) is indicated (Hickey, 2009).
11. Keep the bed in a low position with the side rails up, and pad the side rails with blankets.	11. These precautions help prevent injury from fall or trauma.
12. If appropriate, question client when stable about: a. Any strange feelings, smells, movements that precede a seizure, time of day. b. Reports of fatigue, confusion.	
13. If the client's condition is chronic, refer to Nursing Care Plan for Seizure Disorder in Unit III.	

Clinical Alert Report

Prior to providing care, advise ancillary staff / student to report the following to the professional nurse assigned to the client:
- Any signs of seizure activity
- Intermittent, nonresponsive, blank stares
- Provide with a written cheat sheet with what to observe if seizure activity is witnessed. Write it as soon as possible.
- If the client is older, advise to observe for new onset, intermittent or temporary change in behavior (e.g., staring, blank looks, memory, transient confusion and reports of vague / strange feelings).

Related Physician / NP Prescribed Interventions

Medications
Anticonvulsants drugs for tonic/clonic seizures include such as valproate, lamotrigine, phenytoin, felbamate, topiramate, levetiracetam and carbamazepine. Other agents prevent seizure recurrence, increase the seizure threshold and / or terminate clinical and electrical seizure activity (e.g., ezogabine, zonisamide, methsuximide, clobazam, perampanel).

Intravenous Therapy
Diazepam, lorazepam, glucose solution (IV) or fosphenytoin (IV)

Laboratory Studies
Drug levels (Tegretol, Dilantin); complete blood cell count (CBC); electrolytes; blood urea nitrogen (BUN); calcium; magnesium; fasting blood glucose; urinalysis

Diagnostic Studies
EEG; ECG; CT scan; lumbar puncture, cerebrospinal fluid examination; pulse oximetry; MRI

Documentation

Abnormal findings
Seizure activity flow sheet

Nursing Diagnoses

Anxiety Related to Fear of Embarrassment Secondary to Having a Seizure in Public

NOC
Anxiety Level, Coping,
Impulse Control

Goal

The client will relate an increase in psychological and physiologic comfort.

NIC
Anxiety Reduction,
Impulse Control
Training, Anticipatory
Guidance

Indicators

- Use effective coping mechanisms.
- Describe his or her anxiety and perceptions.

Carp's Cues

Living with epilepsy presents challenges affecting many aspects of life, including relationships with family and friends, school, employment and leisure activities. While medications and other treatments help manage seizures, more than one million people continue to have seizures that impact their daily activities.

Interventions	Rationales
1. Provide opportunities for the client and significant others to express their feelings alone and with each other.	1. Witnessing a seizure is terrifying for others and embarrassing for the client prone to them. This shame and humiliation contributes to anxiety, depression, hostility, and secrecy. Family members also may experience these feelings. Frank discussions may reduce feelings of shame and isolation.
2. Allow opportunities for the client to share concerns regarding seizures in public.	2. Stigma associated with epilepsy is a huge concern for people living with epilepsy. A client with epilepsy may tend to separate him or herself from family, friends, and society (Lewis et al., 2004).
3. Provide support and validate that client's concerns are normal.	3. Possible losses related to epilepsy are loss of control, independence, employment, self-confidence, transportation, family, and friends. When a person feels listened to and understood, his or her loss is validated and normalized (Lewis et al., 2004).
4. Assist the client in identifying activities that are pleasurable and nonhazardous.	4. Fear of injury may contribute to isolation.
5. Stress the importance of adhering to the treatment plan.	5. Adherence to the medication regimen can help to prevent or reduce seizure episodes.
6. Discuss sharing the diagnosis with family members, friends, coworkers, and social contacts.	6. Open dialogue with others forewarns them of possible seizures; this can reduce the shock of witnessing a seizure and possibly enable assistive action.
7. Discuss situations through which the client can meet others in a similar situation: a. Support groups b. Epilepsy Foundation of America	7. Sharing with others in a similar situation may give the client a more realistic view of the seizure disorder and of societal perception of it (Epilepsy Foundation, 2007).

Documentation

Client's concerns
Interaction with client

> **TRANSITION TO HOME / COMMUNITY CARE**
> If indicated, review the risk diagnoses identified for this individual on admission:
> * Is the person still at risk?
> * Can the family reduce the risks?
> * Is the person at higher risk at home?
> * Is a Home Health Nurse assessment needed?
> * Refer to transition planner / case manager / social service.
> * When is this person scheduled for follow-up with primary provider? Specialists? Record dates of appointments.
> * Complete a medication reconciliation prior to transition. Refer to index.

STAR

Stop

Think Is this person at risk for injury, falls, medical complications, and / or inability to care for self (activities of daily living)?

Is there a support person available?

Is the person competent to manage self-administration of medications, treatment procedures? Are additional resources needed?

Can the person explain how to monitor the condition (e.g., blood glucose, signs / symptoms of complications, dietary / mobility restrictions, and when to call his or her primary provider or specialist)?

Act Contact or provide the appropriate resource (e.g., contacting a support person, home health assessment, additional teaching, printed materials).

Review Has the problem been addressed? If not, use SBAR to communicate to the appropriate person.

Risk for Ineffective Self-Health Management Related to Insufficient Knowledge of Condition, Medications, Care during Seizures, Environmental Hazards, and Community Resources

NOC

Compliance Behavior, Knowledge: Treatment Regimen, Participation in Health Care Decisions, Treatment Behavior: Illness or Injury

NIC

Anticipatory Guidance, Learning Facilitation, Risk Identification, Health Education, Health System Guidance

Goals

The goals for this diagnosis represent those associated with transition planning. Refer to the transition criteria.

Interventions	Rationales
1. Teach the client and her or his family about seizure disorders and treatment; correct any misconceptions. Ask if they know anyone with a seizure disorder.	1. The client and family's understanding of seizure disorders and the prescribed treatment regimen strongly influences compliance with the regimen.

2. If the client is on medication therapy, teach the following information:
  a. Never discontinue a drug abruptly
 	
  b. Side effects and signs of toxicity
 	
  c. The need to have drug blood levels monitored, if indicated
  d. The need for periodic complete blood counts, if indicated
 	
  e. The effects of Dilantin, if ordered, on gingival tissue and the need for regular dental examinations.
	2a. Abrupt discontinuation can precipitate status epilepticus.
	  b. Early identification of problems enables prompt intervention to prevent serious complications.
	  c. Drug blood levels provide a guide for adjusting drug dosage.
	  d. Long-term use of some anticonvulsive drugs, such as hydantoins (e.g., phenytoin [Dilantin]), can cause blood dyscrasias.
	  e. Long-term phenytoin therapy can cause gingival hyperplasia.

3. Provide information regarding situations that increase the risk of seizure (Bader & Littlejohns, 2004):
  a. Excess stimulation
  b. Alcohol ingestion
  c. Excessive caffeine intake
  d. Excessive stress
  e. Febrile illness
  f. Flashing lights
  g. Noisy environment
  h. Poorly adjusted television screen
  i. Excessive fatigue, sedentary activity level, lack of sleep
 	
  j. Hypoglycemia
  k. Constipation
  l. Diarrhea
	3. Certain situations have been identified as increasing seizure episodes, although the actual mechanisms behind them are unknown (Bader & Littlejohns, 2004).
	
	  i. Regular activity and exercise are important. Activity tends to inhibit rather than increase seizures. Fatigue and hyperventilation should be avoided.

4. Advise not to use alcohol, recreational, or street drugs.	4. All are stimulants and can cause seizure if withdrawal occurs.
5. Practice safety measure associated with an activity: a. Swim with a "buddy."	
6. Advise to discuss the use of supplements with primary care provider.	6. Anticonvulsant drugs may cause low levels of calcium, vitamin D, and vitamin K; calcium supplements can interfere with anticonvulsant drugs.

7. Discuss why certain activities are hazardous and should be avoided:
  a. Swimming alone
  b. When riding bicycles, rollerblades, or using scooters without a helmet
  c. Driving (unless seizure-free for the period determined by state laws)
  d. Operating potentially hazardous machinery
  e. Mountain climbing
  f. Occupations in which the client could be injured or cause injury to others	

Interventions	Rationales
8. Discuss with PCP, prior to using herbs / essential oils	8. Some herbs increase the risk of seizure or interact with a medication for epilepsy such as ginkgo, primrose oil, St. John's, White willow. Some essential oils should also be avoided: eucalyptus, fennel, hyssop, pennyroyal tansy.
9. Refer the individual to the Epilepsy Foundation website for information regarding employment issues: http://www.epilepsyfoundation.org/livingwithepilepsy/employmenttopics/index.cfm	9. There are a few occupations that the federal government has barred individual with epilepsy from engaging in (e.g., pilots, commercial truck drivers). Generally a client prone to seizures should avoid any activity that could place him, her, or others in danger should a seizure occur.
10. Teach the client how to recognize the warning signals of a seizure and what to do to minimize injury (Bader & Littlejohns, 2004; Lewis et al., 2004).	
11. Refer the client and family to community resources and reference material for assistance with management (e.g., Epilepsy Foundation of America, counseling, occupational rehabilitation).	11. Such resources may provide additional information and support.

Documentation

Client teaching
Referrals if indicated

Hematologic Disorders

Sickle Cell Disease

Sickle cell disease (SCD) is an incurable genetic disorder affecting approximately 1 of every 375 African Americans. The term *sickle cell disease* actually represents a group of disorders characterized by the production of hemoglobin S (Hb S). Under certain conditions, this hemoglobin leads to anemia and acute and chronic tissue damage secondary to the "sickling"—that is, turning into the sickle form—of the abnormal red cells. Hemoglobin S molecules tend to bond to one another and to hemoglobin A, forming long aggregates or tactoids. These aggregates increase the viscosity of blood, causing stasis in blood flow. The low oxygen tension concentration of Hb S causes the cells to assume a sickle rather than a biconcave shape. This hemoglobin damages erythrocyte membranes, leading to erythrocyte rupture and chronic hemolytic anemia (Porth, 2009).

Symptoms of sickle cell anemia result from thrombosis and infarction, leading to vaso-occlusive crises (VOCs). These episodes are called *sickle cell crises*. The incidence of sickle cell crises varies among clients. Some report an incident once a year, whereas others report more than one a week.

In the United States the disease is primarily seen among African Americans, but may also be found among people of Mediterranean, Caribbean, South and Central American, and East Indian descent (U.S. Department of Health, 1992). This chronic disease leaves its victims not only debilitated, but also with a shortened life span. Presently the disease has no cure, but some options are available for altering its course.

Clients can carry the sickle cell trait but not have the disease. These asymptomatic people have reported some sickling symptoms in low oxygen (e.g., unpressurized airplanes, high altitudes, scuba diving).

Time Frame
Acute sickling crisis

■■■■ DIAGNOSTIC CLUSTER**

Collaborative Problems

Δ   Risk for Complications of Acute Chest Syndrome

Δ   Risk for Complications of Infection

*   Risk for Complications of Anemia

*   Risk for Complications of Vaso-occlusive Crisis

*   Risk for Complications of Aplastic Crisis

*   Risk for Complications of Leg Ulcers

*   Risk for Complications of Neurologic Dysfunction

*   Risk for Complications of Splenic Dysfunction

*   Risk for Complications of Avascular Necrosis of Femoral / Humeral Heads

*   Risk for Complications of Priapism

Nursing Diagnoses

▲ Acute Pain related to viscous blood and tissue hypoxia

Δ Risk for Ineffective Self-Health Management related to insufficient knowledge of disease process, risk factors for sickling crisis, pain management, signs and symptoms of complications, genetic counseling, and family planning services

* Powerlessness related to future development of complications of SCD (refer to Diabetes Mellitus)

▲ This diagnosis was reported to be monitored for or managed frequently (75% to 100%).
Δ This diagnosis was reported to be monitored for or managed often (50% to 74%).
** This diagnosis was not included in the validation study.

Transition Criteria

Before transition, the client or family will:

1. Identify precipitating factors of present crisis, if possible.
2. Plan one change in lifestyle to reduce crisis or to improve health.
3. Describe signs and symptoms that must be reported to a health care professional.
4. Describe necessary health maintenance and follow-up care.

Transitional Risk Assessment Plan (TRAP)

Begin this plan on admission.
Implement the Transitional Risk Assessment Plan (TRAP):
• Refer to inside back cover.
• Add each validated risk diagnosis to client's problem list with the risk code in ( ).
• Refer to Unit II to the individual risk nursing diagnoses / collaborative problems for outcomes and interventions.

R: "Close coordination of care in the post-acute period, early transition follow-up care, enhanced client education and self-management training, proactive end-of-life counseling, and extending the resources and clinical expertise over time via multidisciplinary team management" can lower readmission rates and improve health outcomes (Boutwell & Hwu, 2009, p. 14).

Collaborative Problems

Risk for Complications of Anemia

Risk for Complications of Sickle Cell Crisis

Risk for Complications of Acute Chest Syndrome

Risk for Complications of Infection

Risk for Complications of Leg Ulcers

Risk for Complications of Neurologic Dysfunction

Risk for Complications of Splenic Dysfunction

Risk for Complications of Osteonecrosis

Collaborative Outcomes

The client will be monitored for early signs and symptoms of a) anemia, (b) vaso-occlusive crisis, (c) acute chest syndrome, (d) aplastic anemia, (e) infection, (f) leg ulcers, (g) neurologic dysfunction, (h) splenic dysfunction, (i) priapism, and (j) osteonecrosis (femoral / humeral heads) and will receive collaborative interventions if indicated to restore physiologic stability.

Indicators of Physiologic Stability

- Hemoglobin (a, b, d)
  - Males: 13–18 g/dL
  - Females: 12–16 g/dL
- Hematocrit (a, b, d)
  - Males: 42% to 50%
  - Females: 40% to 48%
- Red blood cells (a, b, d)
  - Males: 4.6–5.9 million/mm^3
  - Females: 4.2–5.4 million/mm^3
- Platelets 150,000–400,000/mm^3 (e)
- White blood cells 4,300–10,800/mm^3 (e)
- Oxygen saturation >95% (a, b, c, d)
- No or minimal bone pain (b, e, j)
- No or minimal abdominal pain (b, e, h)
- No or minimal chest pain (c)
- No or minimal fatigue (a, b, e)
- Pinkish, ruddy, brownish, or olive skin tones (a, b)
- No or minimal headache (b, g)
- Clear, oriented (b, g)
- Clear speech (b, g)
- Pulse rate 60–100 beats/min (a, b, c, g, h)
- Respirations 16–20 breaths/min (b, c, e, g)
- BP >90/60, <140/90 mmHg (a, b, c, g, h)
- Temperature 98° to 99.5° F (b, a, e, f, j)
- Urine output >0.5 mL/kg/h (b, c, h)
- Urine specific gravity 1.005–1.030 (b, c, h)
- Flaccid penis (i)

Interventions	Rationales
1. Monitor for signs and symptoms of anemia. a. Lethargy b. Weakness c. Fatigue d. Increased pallor e. Dyspnea on exertion	1. Because anemia is common with most of these clients, low hemoglobins are relatively tolerated; therefore, changes should be described in reference to a client's baseline or acute symptoms (Porth, 2009).
2. Monitor laboratory values, including complete blood cell count (CBC) with reticulocyte count.	2. Elevated reticulocytes (normal level about 1%) indicate active erythropoiesis. Lack of elevation with anemia may represent a problem (Porth, 2009).
3. Monitor for vaso-occlusive crisis: a. Abdominal pain b. Chest pain c. Bones, joints	3. Sickle cells block capillaries and cause pain by infarction. Repeated painful vaso-occlusive crises (VOCs), also referred to as "pain crises" or "sickle crises," are the hallmark of sickle cell disease (SCD). VOCs can lead to bone infarcts, necrosis, and, over time, degenerative changes in marrow-containing bone, usually long bones.
4. Monitor: a. Oxygen saturation with pulse oximetry. b. Hydration status (urine output, specific gravity) c. Level of consciousness	4a. O$_2$ should be administered only if oxygen saturation is less than 95%. b. Increased hydration is needed to mobilize clustered cells and improve tissue perfusion. c. Change in consciousness can be due to a cerebral infarction.

Interventions	Rationales
5. Aggressively hydrate client (1.5 × maintenance volume). Avoid IV therapy, if possible.	5. Hydration can disrupt the clustered cells and improve hypoxemia.
6. Monitor for signs and symptoms of acute chest syndrome: a. Fever b. Acute chest pain c. Fever, chills **CLINICAL ALERT** • This represents a medical emergency and may be caused by "sickling" leading to pulmonary infarction (Heeney & Mahoney, 2011).	6. Acute chest syndrome is the term used to represent this group of symptoms, namely, acute pleuritic chest pain, fever, leukocytosis, and infiltrates on chest x-ray seen in SCD.
7. Monitor for signs and symptoms of infection: a. Fever b. Pain c. Chills d. Increased white blood cells	7. Bacterial infection is one major cause of morbidity and mortality. Decreased functioning of the spleen (asplenia) results from sickle cell anemia. The loss of the spleen's ability to filter and to destroy various infectious organisms increases the risk of infection (Heeney & Mahoney, 2011).
8. Monitor for aplastic crisis: a. CBC with differential b. Pallor c. Tachycardia	
9. Monitor for signs and symptoms of leg ulcers: a. Hyperpigmentation b. Skin wrinkling c. Pruritus, tenderness	9. Leg ulcers can occur in 50% to 75% of older children and adults with sickle cell anemia. Minor leg trauma can result in localized edema and compression of the tissue around the injury. Capillary blood flow is decreased, causing increased arterial pressure. This increased pressure causes some arterial blood carrying oxygen to the tissue to be redirected to the veins without reaching the injured area. Skin grafting may be needed (Waterbury, 2007).
10. Monitor for changes in neurologic function: a. Speech disturbances b. Sudden headache c. Numbness, tingling	10. Cerebral infarction and intracranial hemorrhage are complications of SCD. Occlusion of nutrient arteries to major cerebral arteries causes progressive wall damage and eventual occlusion of the major vessel. Intracerebral hemorrhage may be secondary to hypoxic necrosis of vessel walls (Porth, 2009).
11. Monitor for splenic dysfunction.	11. The spleen is responsible for filtering blood to remove old bacteria. Sluggish circulation and increased viscosity of sickle cells causes splenic blockage. The spleen's normal acidic and anoxic environment stimulates sickling, which increases blood flow obstruction.
12. Monitor for splenic sequestration crisis: a. Sudden onset of lassitude b. Very pale, listless c. Rapid pulse d. Shallow respirations e. Low blood pressure	12. Increased blood obstruction from the spleen together with rapid sickling can cause sudden pooling of blood into the spleen. This causes intravascular hypovolemia and hypoxia, progressing to shock.

(continued)

Interventions	Rationales
13. Intervene for priapism.	13. Sickle cells impairing blood flow cause priapism (involuntary, prolonged, abnormal, and painful erection). Persistent stasis priapism not resolved in 24–48 hours can cause permanent erectile dysfunction (Waterbury, 2007).
a. Provide analgesics, sedation.	a. Sedation may cause tissue relaxation and improve perfusion.
b. Maintain hydration.	b. Hydration can mobilize cluster cells.
c. Apply ice packs to penis.	c. Icing can reduce edema and improve perfusion.
14. Monitor for osteonecrosis and instruct client to report any of the following: a. Bone pain (hip, leg) b. Fever c. Limited movement	14. Osteonecrosis is death of tissue from decreased circulation secondary to clustered sickle cells. Symptomatic osteonecrosis of the femoral head is a rapidly progressive disease that requires an orthopedic surgical consultation (Hernigou, Bachir, & Galacteros, 2003).

Clinical Alert Report

Prior to providing care, advise ancillary staff / student to report the following to the professional nurse assigned to the client:

- Change in cognitive status
- Oral temperature >100.5° F
- Systolic BP <90 mm Hg
- Resting Pulse >100, <50
- Respiratory rate >28, <10 /min.
- Oxygen saturation <90%

Related Physician / NP Prescribed Interventions

Medications

Anti-sickling agents, antimetabolites: Hydroxyurea, analgesics (opioid analgesics, nonsteroidal analgesics folic acid, [e.g., oxycodone / ASA, methadone, morphine sulfate, oxycodone / APAP, fentanyl, nalbuphine, codeine, APAP / codeine])

- Stem cell transplantation: Can be curative
- Transfusions: For sudden, severe anemia due to acute splenic sequestration, parvovirus B19 infection, or hyperhemolytic crises
- Physical therapy

Intravenous Therapy

Exchange transfusions

Laboratory Studies

CBC, liver function tests, hemoglobin electrophoresis, serum iron, erythrocyte sedimentation rate, arterial blood gases, peripheral blood smear

Diagnostic Studies

Depend on complications (e.g., CVA, Head CT, MRI)

Therapies

Depend on complications, bone marrow / stem cell transplantation, recombinant human erythropoietin (r-HuEPO), L-arginine therapy, steroid therapy, physical therapy, Heat and cold application, Acupuncture and acupressure, TENS

Documentation

Skin assessment
Neurologic
Vital signs
Abnormal findings
Interventions
Evaluation

Nursing Diagnoses

Acute Pain Related to Viscous Blood and Tissue Hypoxia

NOC
Comfort Level, Pain
Control

Goal

The client will report decreased pain after pain-relief measures.

NIC
Pain Management,
Medication
Management, Emotional
Support, Teaching:
Individual, Heat / Cold
Application, Simple
Massage

Indicators

- Relate factors that increase pain.
- Relate factors that can precipitate pain.

Interventions	Rationales
1. Explore with client if the painful episode is "typical" or "unusual."	1. Most clients have a distinctive, unique pattern of pain. Changes may indicate another complication (e.g., infection, abdominal surgical emergency).
2. Assess for any signs of infection (e.g., respiratory, urinary, vaginal).	2. Painful events often occur with infection.
3. Aggressively manage acute pain episodes. Consult with physician or advanced practice nurse.	3. The pain of SCD, like the pain of cancer, should be treated based on client's tolerance and discretion (Waterbury, 2007).
4. Provide narcotic analgesic every 2 hours (not PRN). Consider client-controlled analgesic.	4. People with sickle cells metabolize narcotics rapidly (Waterbury, 2007).
5. Provide an initial bolus dose of a narcotic analgesic (e.g., morphine) followed by continuous low-dose narcotic or dosing at fixed intervals.	5. A continuous serum level of narcotic is needed to control pain (Jenkins, 2002).
6. After the acute pain crisis, taper narcotics.	6. The pain of sickling should decrease. A decrease in the pain score of 2 or more points is an indication to reduce the narcotic analgesic (Ballas & Delengowski, 1993).
7. Discuss complementary therapies and provide community sources if desired for: a. Relaxation techniques, massage, yoga b. Acupuncture, biofeedback c. Music therapy d. Prayer e. Herbal remedies f. Transcutaneous Electric Nerve Stimulation (TENS)	7. These can be useful adjuncts to a pain management program.
8. Refer to Chronic Pain in Unit II.	

Documentation

Type, route, and dosage of all medications
Status of pain
Degree of relief from pain-relief measures

> **TRANSITION TO HOME / COMMUNITY CARE**
> If indicated, review the risk diagnoses identified for this individual on admission:
> * Is the person still at risk?
> * Can the family reduce the risks?
> * Is the person at higher risk at home?
> * Is a Home Health Nurse assessment needed?
> * Refer to transition planner / case manager / social service.
> * When is this person scheduled for follow-up with primary provider? Specialists? Record dates of appointments.
> * Complete a medication reconciliation prior to transition. Refer to index.

STAR

Stop

Think   Is this person at risk for injury, falls, medical complications, and / or inability to care for self (activities of daily living)?
Is there a support person available?
Is the person competent to manage self-administration of medications, treatment procedures? Are additional resources needed?
Can the person explain how to monitor the condition (e.g., blood glucose, signs / symptoms of complications, dietary / mobility restrictions, and when to call his or her primary provider or specialist)?

Act   Contact or provide the appropriate resource (e.g., contacting a support person, home health assessment, additional teaching, printed materials).

Review   Has the problem been addressed? If not, use SBAR to communicate to the appropriate person.

Risk for Ineffective Self-Health Management Related to Insufficient Knowledge of Disease Process, Risk Factors for Sickling Crisis, Pain Management, Signs and Symptoms of Complications, Genetic Counseling, and Family Planning Services

NOC

Compliance Behavior, Knowledge: Treatment Regimen, Participation in Health Care Decisions, Treatment Behavior: Illness or Injury

NIC

Anticipatory Guidance, Risk Identification, Health Education, Learning Facilitation

Goals

The goals for this diagnosis represent those associated with transition planning. Refer to the transition criteria.

Interventions	Rationales
1. Review present situation, disease process, and treatment.	1. Even though the client has had the disease since childhood, the nurse should evaluate present knowledge.

2. Discuss precipitating factors:
  a. High altitude (more than 7000 feet above sea level)
  b. Unpressurized aircraft
  c. Dehydration (e.g., diaphoresis, diarrhea, vomiting)
  d. Strenuous physical activity
  e. Cold temperatures (e.g., iced liquids)
 	
  f. Infection (e.g., respiratory, urinary, vaginal)
  g. Ingestion of alcohol
  h. Cigarette smoking
	2a, b. Decreased oxygen tension can cause red blood cells to sickle.
	  c, d. Any situation that causes dehydration or increases blood viscosity can precipitate sickling.
	  e. Cold causes peripheral vasoconstriction, which slows circulation.
	  f. The exact mechanism is unknown.
	  g. Alcohol use promotes dehydration.
	  h. Nicotine interferes with oxygen exchange.

3. Emphasize the need to drink at least 16 cups (8 oz) of fluid daily and to increase to 24–32 cups during a painful crisis or when at risk for dehydration.	3. Dehydration must be prevented to prevent a sickling crisis (Marchiondo & Thompson, 1996).

4. Discuss the importance of maintaining optimal health:
  a. Regular health care professional examinations (e.g., ophthalmic, general)
  b. Good nutrition
  c. Stress reduction methods
  d. Dental hygiene
  e. Immunization
	4. Adhering to a health maintenance plan can reduce risk factors that contribute to crisis.

5. Explain the importance of an eye examination every 6 to 12 months.	5. SCD can cause retinopathy by plugging small retinal vessels and causing neovascularization (Porth, 2009).
6. Explain the susceptibility to infection. a. Vaccines (e.g., PCV7, PPV23, meningococcal, influenza, recommended scheduled childhood / adult vaccinations).	6. Certain organisms (e.g., salmonella) thrive in diminished oxygen status. Phagocytosis, which is dependent on oxygen, is inhibited with SCD (Porth, 2009).

7. Stress the importance of reporting signs and symptoms of infection early:
  a. Persistent cough
  b. Fever
  c. Foul-smelling vaginal drainage
  d. Cloudy, reddish, or foul-smelling urine
  e. Increased redness of wound
  f. Purulent drainage from wound
	7. Early recognition and treatment may prevent a crisis.

8. After crisis, help the client identify some warning signs that occur days or hours before a crisis.	8. Some clients with SCD experience a prodromal stage (a gradual buildup of symptoms for days before a crisis). More commonly, however, symptoms begin less than 1 hour before a crisis (Newcombe, 2002).
9. Instruct the client to provide prompt treatment of cuts, insect bites, and the like.	9. Decreased peripheral circulation increases the risk of infection.
10. Instruct the client on how to palpate the abdomen to detect splenic enlargement, and the importance of observation for pallor, jaundice, and fever.	

(continued)

Interventions	Rationales

11. Instruct the client to seek medical care in certain situations, including the following:
  a. Persistent fever (>38.3° C)
  b. Chest pain, shortness of breath, nausea, and vomiting
  c. Abdominal pain with nausea and vomiting
  d. Persistent headache not experienced previously
	11. These symptoms may indicate vaso-occlusion in varied sites from sickling. Some illnesses may predispose a client to dehydration.

12. Instruct the client to avoid the following:
  a. Alcohol
  b. Nonprescribed prescription drugs
  c. Cigarettes, marijuana, and cocaine
  d. Seeking care in multiple institutions	

13. Provide access to training for new coping strategies:
  a. Relaxation breathing
  b. Imagery
  c. Calming self statements
  d. Mental counting technique
  e. Focus on physical surroundings
  f. Reinterpretation of pain sensations
	13. Individuals who practice selected coping strategies during pain episodes tend to have less need for ER management (Gil, Carson, Sedway et al., 2000).

14. Advise client to practice coping strategies daily, regardless of pain level.	14. Practice is needed to improve efficiency of the strategy when it is needed (Gil et al., 2000).
15. Explore the client's knowledge regarding the genetic aspects of the disease. Refer to appropriate resource (e.g., genetic counseling).	15. This disease is hereditary. If both parents have the sickle cell trait, the chance that a child will have sickle cell disease is 25%. If one parent is carrying the trait and the other actually has disease, the odds increase to 50% that their child will inherit the disease. Screening and genetic counseling theoretically have the potential to drastically reduce the prevalence of SCD. (Maakaron, 2013) The incidence of offspring inheriting SCD is related to parents as carriers or noncarriers of the hemoglobin genotype AS.
16. Explore with the client the effects of SCD on family, roles, occupation, and personal goals.	16. Clients with SCD tend to experience it personally and have witnessed its effects on others. This chronic disease regularly challenges client and family functioning. Adults are at risk for poor psychological adjustment.
17. Refer to community support groups and appropriate agencies (e.g., Sickle Cell Disease Association of America (www.sicklecelldisease.org), American Sickle Cell Anemia Association (www.ascaa.org). CDC webpage-on-sickle-cell http://www.cdc.gov/ncbddd/sicklecell/index.html	17. Successful coping is promoted by witnessing others successfully coping, and others believing that they will be successful (Bandura, 1982).

Documentation

Client teaching
Outcome achievement
Referrals if indicated

◯◯ Integumentary Disorders

Pressure Ulcers

"Despite current interest and advances in medicine, surgery, nursing care, and self-care education, pressure ulcers remain a major cause of morbidity and mortality. This is particularly true for persons with impaired sensation, prolonged immobility, or advanced age" (Salcido, 2012).

The incidence of pressure ulcers has been reported to be (Salcido, 2012):

In hospitalized persons a range of 2.7% to 29%
In critical care units, a 33% incidence
In elderly clients admitted for nonelective orthopedic procedures, such as hip replacement and treatment of long bone fractures, a 66% incidence
In individual in nursing homes, a range of 2.6% to 24%

Pressure ulcers are localized areas of cellular necrosis that tend to occur from prolonged compression of soft tissue between a bony prominence and a firm surface, most commonly as a result of immobility. Injury ranges from nonblanchable erythema of intact skin to deep ulceration extending to the bone. Extrinsic factors that exert mechanical force on soft tissue include pressure, shear, friction, and maceration. Intrinsic factors that determine susceptibility to tissue breakdown include malnutrition, anemia, loss of sensation, impaired mobility, advanced age, decreased mental status, incontinence, and infection. Extrinsic and intrinsic factors interact to produce ischemia and necrosis of soft tissue in susceptible persons (Agency for Health Care Policy Research [AHCPR], 1994; Berlowitz, 2007a; Bluestein & Javaheri, 2008; Maklebust & Sieggreen, 2001).

Time Frame
Secondary Diagnosis

■■■ DIAGNOSTIC CLUSTER**

Collaborative Problems

Risk for Complications of Sepsis

Nursing Diagnoses

▲ Impaired Tissue Integrity related to mechanical destruction of tissue secondary to pressure, shear, and / or friction

▲ Impaired Physical Mobility related to imposed restrictions, deconditioned status, loss of motor control, or altered mental status (refer to Unit II)

▲ Imbalanced Nutrition: Less Than Body Requirements related to insufficient oral intake sufficient for would healing Refer to Unit II and Generic Care Plan for Surgical Conditions > Altered Nutrition

▲ Risk for Infection related to exposure of ulcer base to fecal / urinary drainage

△ Risk for Ineffective Self-Health Management related to insufficient knowledge of etiology, prevention, treatment, and home care

Related Care Plan

Immobility or Unconsciousness

▲ This diagnosis was reported to be monitored for or managed frequently (75% to 100%).
△ This diagnosis was reported to be monitored for or managed often (50% to 74%).

Transition Criteria

Before transition, the client or family will:

1. Identify factors that contribute to ulcer development.
2. Demonstrate the ability to perform skills necessary to prevent and treat pressure ulcers.
3. State the intent to continue prevention and treatment strategies at home (e.g., activity, nutrition).

> **Transitional Risk Assessment Plan (TRAP)**
>
> Begin this plan on admission.
> Implement the Transitional Risk Assessment Plan (TRAP):
> • Refer to inside back cover.
> • Add each validated risk diagnosis to client's problem list with the risk code in ( ).
> • Refer to Unit II to the individual risk nursing diagnoses / collaborative problems for outcomes and interventions.
>
> *R: "Close coordination of care in the post-acute period, early transition follow-up care, enhanced client education and self-management training, proactive end-of-life counseling, and extending the resources and clinical expertise over time via multidisciplinary team management" can lower readmission rates and improve health outcomes (Boutwell & Hwu, 2009, p. 14).*

Collaborative Problems

Risk for Complications of Sepsis

Collaborative Outcomes

The client will be monitored for early signs and symptoms of sepsis and will receive collaborative interventions if indicated to restore physiologic stability.

Indicators of Physiologic Stability

• Temperature 98° to 99.5° F
• Heart rate 60–100 beats/min
• Blood pressure >90/60, <140/90 mm Hg
• Respiration 16–20 breaths/min
• Urine output >0.5 mL/kg/h
• Clear urine
• Negative blood culture
• White blood count 4,300–10,800 cells/mm^3
• Oriented, alert

Interventions	*Rationales*

1. Monitor for signs and symptoms of wound infection>sepsis:
  a. Temperature >101° F or <98.6° F
  b. Tachycardia (>90 beats/min) and tachypnea (>20 breaths/min)
  c. Pale, cool skin
  d. Decreased urine output
  e. WBCs and bacteria in urine
  f. Positive blood culture
  g. Elevated white blood count >12,000 cells/mm^3 or decreased WBC <4000 cells/mm^3
  h. Confusion, changes in mentation
  i. Refer to Unit II for interventions for sepsis.
	1. Gram-positive and gram-negative organisms can invade open wounds; debilitated clients are more vulnerable. Response to sepsis results in massive vasodilation and hypovolemia, resulting in tissue hypoxia and decreased renal function and cardiac output. This in turn triggers a compensatory response of increased heart rate and respirations to correct hypoxia and acidosis. Bacteria in urine or blood indicate infection (Bluestein & Javaheri, 2008).

> **Clinical Alert Report**
>
> Prior to providing care, advise ancillary staff / student to report the following to the professional nurse assigned to the client:
> - Oral temperature >100.5° F
> - Unusual warmth and redness
> - Urine output <0.5 mL/kg/h
> - Increased drainage for wound
> - Increased tenderness c/o of pain

Related Physician / NP Prescribed Interventions

Medications

Topical or oral antibiotics, enzymatic therapy, pharmacologic therapy (depending on laboratory results, analgesics); topical growth factors; folic acid; thiamine

Intravenous Therapy

Intravenous antibiotics

Laboratory Studies

Tissue culture, blood cultures, imaging studies, tissue biopsy

Therapies

Wound care: Topical skin barriers; specialty dressings; debridement (mechanical, enzymatic, surgical); negative pressure wound therapy (e.g., wound vac); pressure-relief devices (air-fluidized overlay / bed, low-air loss mattress / bed. Kinetic bed); electrotherapy; normothermic wound therapy; ultrasound; hydrotherapy; hyperbaric oxygen (HBO) therapy; and surgical interventions (e.g., skin grafting).

Documentation

Pressure Ulcer Risk Assessment at Admission and Daily (WOCNS, 2010)
Wound Documentation Record (per institutional policy)
Skin Assessment Tool at admission and daily, with documentation of lesions

Nursing Diagnosis

Impaired Tissue Integrity Related to Mechanical Destruction of Tissue Secondary to Pressure, Shear, and / or Friction

NOC
Tissue Integrity: Skin & Mucous Membranes

Goal

The client will demonstrate progressive healing of tissues,

NIC
Teaching: Individual, Surveillance

Indicators

- Participates in risk assessment.
- Expresses willingness to participate in prevention of pressure ulcers.
- Describes etiology and prevention measures.
- Explains rationale for interventions.

Interventions	Rationales
1. Consult with the Wound Care Specialist for the wound care plan prior to intervening.	
2. Apply prevention ulcer prevention principles:	2. Principles of pressure ulcer prevention include reducing or rotating pressure on soft tissue. If pressure on soft tissue exceeds intracapillary pressure (approximately 32 mm Hg), capillary occlusion and resulting hypoxia can cause tissue damage.
a. Encourage range-of-motion (ROM) exercise and weight-bearing mobility when possible.	a. Exercise and mobility increase blood flow to all areas.
b. Utilize support surfaces (on beds and chairs) to re-distribute pressure. Support heels with heel elevating boots or devices. (Refer to the Impaired Mobility Care Plan for more information.)	b. Pressure redistribution devices should serve as ad-juncts and not replacements for positioning protocols (WOCNS, 2010).
c. Keep the bed as flat as possible (lower than 30 degrees) and support feet with a footboard.	c. These measures help prevent and reduce shear, the pressure created when two adjacent tissue layers move in opposition. If a bony prominence slides across the subcutaneous tissue, the subepidermal capillaries may become bent and pinched, resulting in decreased tissue perfusion.
d. Use low friction sliding sheet under the client when pulling or turning.	
e. Avoid using a knee gatch.	e. A knee gatch may promote blood pooling and decrease circulation to the lower extremities.
f. Use foam blocks or pillows to provide a bridging effect to support the body above and below the at-risk or ulcerated area; this prevents the affected area from touching the bed surface (Berlowitz, 2007b). Do not use foam donuts or inflatable rings (National Pressure Ulcer Advisory Panel, 2007).	f. This measure helps to redistribute pressure to a larger area.
g. Alternate or reduce pressure on the skin surface with devices such as (Berlowitz, 2007b; National Pressure Ulcer Advisory Panel, 2007): • Air mattresses • Low air loss overlay mattress or bed • Air-fluidized beds • Vascular heel boots or pillow under the calf to suspend the heels off the bed surface	g. Foam mattresses (e.g., egg-crate type) are for comfort; they generally do not provide adequate pressure relief. Special air mattresses and air beds redistribute the body weight evenly across the body surface (Berlowitz, 2007b; Maklebust & Seiggreen, 2001).
h. Use sufficient personnel to lift the client up in bed or chair without sliding or pulling the skin surface. Do not lift client by the pants waist or belt. Use long sleeves or stockings to reduce friction on elbows and heels. Use transfer devices (Hoyer lift, slide board) to safely lift and / or transfer client.	h. Proper transfer technique reduces friction forces that can rub away or abrade skin.
i. Instruct a sitting client to lift him or her up off but-tocks using the chair arms every 10 minutes, if possi-ble, or assist the client in rising up off the chair every 10–20 minutes, depending on risk factors present (National Pressure Ulcer Advisory Panel, 2007).	i. This measure allows periodic reperfusion of ischemic areas.
j. Do not elevate the client's legs unless the calves are supported. Support the client's calves and align the hip and knee bone while helping him or her to sit on a chair, to avoid shifting weight to the ischial tuberosities.	j. Supporting the calves reduces pressure over the ischial tuberosities (AHCPR, 1994).
k. Pad the chair with a pressure-relieving device.	k. Ischial tuberosities are prime areas for pressure ulcer development. Air cushions provide better pressure relief than foam cushions.

Interventions	Rationales

l. Inspect other areas at risk for developing ulcers with each position change:
  • Ears
  • Occiput
  • Scapula
  • Elbows
  • Sacrum
  • Trochanter
  • Ischia
  • Scrotum
  • Knees
  • Heels
  • Any tubes or devices used in or on the body that contact skin surface
	l. A client with one pressure ulcer is at risk of developing others. A client who is insensate or unconscious will not be aware of pressure or make adjustment to relieve the discomfort

m. When positioned on side, the client should be placed at a 30-degree angle (Berlowitz, 2007b).	m. This reduces pressure on the greater trochanter (Berlowitz, 2007b).
n. Consider physical therapy for immobilized clients (Berlowitz, 2007b).	n. Clients may benefit from physical therapy to improve mobility (Berlowitz, 2007b).
3. Observe for erythema and blanching and palpate surrounding area for warmth and tissue sponginess with each position change.	3. Warmth and sponginess are signs of tissue damage
4. Compensate for sensory deficits: a. Inspect the client's skin every 2 hours for signs of injury. b. Teach the client and family members to inspect the skin frequently. Show the client how to use a mirror to inspect hard-to-see areas.	4a. An immobilized client may have impaired sensation; this interferes with the ability to perceive pain from skin damage. b. Regular skin inspection enables early detection of damage. The client's involvement promotes responsibility for self-care.
5. Identify the stage of pressure ulcer development (Berlowitz, 2007a; National Pressure Ulcer Advisory Panel, 2007). a. Stage I: nonblanchable erythema of intact skin b. Stage II: ulceration of epidermis or dermis not involving underlying subcutaneous fat (partial thickness) (National Pressure Ulcer Advisory Panel, 2007). c. Stage III: ulceration involving subcutaneous fat or fascia (full thickness) (National Pressure Ulcer Advisory Panel, 2007). d. Stage IV: extensive ulceration penetrating muscle and bone (full-thickness with exposed bone, tendon, or muscle) (National Pressure Ulcer Advisory Panel, 2007). e. Unstageable: Full-thickness tissue loss with the wound bed covered with slough (green, yellow, tan, gray, or brown) and / or eschar (tan, black, or brown). Wound cannot be staged without debridement and cleaning (National Pressure Ulcer Advisory Panel, 2007). f. Suspected Deep Tissue Injury: localized purple- or maroon-colored, intact skin or blood-filled blister due to damage of underlying tissue from pressure and / or shear. The affected area may be painful, firm, mushy, boggy, cooler, or warmer than surrounding areas (National Pressure Ulcer Advisory Panel, 2007). May be difficult to detect in dark skin tones (Berlowitz, 2007a).	5. Staging is a standardized communication tool that denotes the anatomic depth of tissue involvement and amount of tissue loss (Berlowitz, 2007a; National Pressure Ulcer Advisory Panel, 2007).

(continued)

Interventions	Rationales

6. Reduce or eliminate factors that contribute to extension of existing pressure ulcers:
  a. Wash the area surrounding the ulcer gently with a mild soap, rinse area thoroughly to remove soap, and pat dry.
  b. Avoid vigorous massage of any reddened areas.
 	
  c. Institute one or a combination of the following barrier products (National Pressure Ulcer Advisory Panel, 2007).
    • Apply a thin coat of liquid copolymer skin sealant.
    • Cover area with a moisture permeable film dressing.
    • Cover area with a hydroactive wafer barrier and secure with strips of one-inch microtape; leave in place for 4–5 days.
	6. Mechanical or chemical forces contribute to pressure ulcer deterioration.
	  a. Soap is an irritant and dries skin.
	
	  b. Vigorous massage angulates and tears the vessels. Massaging over reddened areas might break capillaries and traumatize skin (Berlowitz, 2007b; Maklebust & Sieggreen, 2001).
	  c. Healthy skin should be protected.

7. Devise a plan for treating pressure ulcers using moist wound healing principles, as follows:
 	
  a. Avoid breaking blisters.
 	
  b. Flush ulcer base with sterile saline solution. If it is infected, use forceful irrigation.
 	
  c. Avoid using wound cleansers and topical antiseptics (AHCPR, 1992).
  d. Consult with wound specialist or surgeon to debride necrotic tissues enzymatically, mechanically, or surgically (Berlowitz, 2007b).
  e. Cover pressure ulcers that have broken skin with a dressing that maintains a moist environment over the ulcer base (e.g., film dressing, hydrocolloid wafer dressing, absorption dressing, moist gauze dressing) (Berlowitz, 2007b).
  f. Avoid drying agents (e.g., heat lamps, Maalox, Milk of Magnesia). Do not leave open to the air to form desiccated scab.
 	
  g. Stable (dry, adherent, intact, without erythema or movement) eschar on heels should not be removed except after vascular inflow has been evaluated as normal and by a wound specialist or surgeon.
	7. When wounds are semi-occluded and the wounds surface remains moist, epidermal cells migrate more rapidly over the surface (Maklebust & Sieggreen, 2001).
	  a. Blisters indicate stage II pressure ulcers; the fluid contained in the blister provides an environment for formation of granulation tissue.
	  b. Irrigation with normal saline solution may aid in removing dead cells and reducing bacterial count. Forceful irrigation should not be used in the presence of granulation tissue and new epithelium.
	  c. These products may be cytotoxic to tissue.
	
	  d. A necrotic tissue promotes bacterial growth and does not heal until the necrotic tissue is removed (Berlowitz, 2007b).
	  e. Moist wounds heal faster (AHCPR, 1994).
	
	  f. Heat creates an increased oxygen demand. Heat lamps are contraindicated in pressure ulcers, as the lamps increase the oxygen demand to tissue that is already stressed (Maklebust & Sieggreen, 2001).
	  g. Stable eschar serves as a natural biologic cover for wound (National Pressure Ulcer Advisory Panel, 2007).

8. Consult with a physician / NP for treatment of deep or infected pressure ulcers.	8. Expert consultation may be needed for more specific interventions. a. Notify interdisciplinary team of he wound.
9. Determine the client's nutritional status. Consult with a nutritionist.	9. Wound healing requires increased protein and CHO intake to prevent weight loss and promote healing (Dudek, 2010; Lutz & Przytulski, 2011).

Documentation

Pressure Ulcer Risk Assessment at Admission and Daily (WOCNS, 2010)
Wound Documentation Record (per institutional policy)
Skin Assessment Tool at admission and daily, with documentation of lesions

Risk for Infection Related to Exposure of Ulcer Base to Fecal / Urinary Drainage

NOC

Infection Severity,
Wound Healing: Primary
Intention, Immune
Status

NIC

Infection Control,
Wound Care, Incision
Site Care, Health
Education

Goal

The client will report risk factors associated with infection, and the precautions needed.

Indicators

- Demonstrate meticulous hand-washing and skin hygiene technique by the time of transition.
- Describe methods of infection transmission.
- Describe the influence of nutrition on infection prevention.

Interventions	Rationales
1. Consult with Wound Nursing Specialist for specific guidelines to prevent infection.	
2. Teach the importance of good skin hygiene. Use emollients if skin is dry, but do not leave skin "wet" from too much lotion or cream.	2. Dry skin is susceptible to cracking and infection. Excessive emollient use can lead to maceration.
3. Protect the skin from exposure to urine / feces. a. Cleanse the skin thoroughly after each incontinent episode, using a liquid soap that does not alter skin pH. b. Collect feces and urine in an appropriate containment device (e.g., condom catheter, fecal incontinence pouch, polymer-filled incontinent pads), or apply a skin sealant, cream, or emollient to act as a barrier to urine and feces.	3. Contact with urine and stool can cause skin maceration. Feces may be more ulcerogenic than urine, owing to bacteria and toxins in stool. Incontinent clients are five times at greater risk for pressure ulcers (Berlowitz, 2007a).
4. Consider using occlusive dressings on clean superficial ulcers, but never on deep ulcers.	4. Occlusive dressings protect superficial wounds from urine and feces, but can trap bacteria in deep wounds.
5. Monitor for signs of local wound infection (e.g., purulent drainage, cellulitis). **CLINICAL ALERT** • Promptly report changes in wound condition.	
6. Refer to Risk for Infection in Unit II.	

Documentation

Skin condition (e.g., redness, maceration, denuded areas)
Amount and frequency of incontinence
Skin care and hygiene measures
Containment devices used
Change in skin condition

> **TRANSITION TO HOME / COMMUNITY CARE**
> If indicated, review the risk diagnoses identified for this individual on admission:
> * Is the person still at risk?
> * Can the family reduce the risks?
> * Is the person at higher risk at home?
> * Is a Home Health Nurse assessment needed?
> * Refer to transition planner / case manager / social service.
> * When is this person scheduled for follow-up with primary provider? Specialists? Record dates of appointments.
> * Complete a medication reconciliation prior to transition. Refer to index.

STAR   Stop

Think   Is this person at risk for injury, falls, medical complications, and / or inability to care for self (activities of daily living)?

Is there a support person available?

Is the person competent to manage self-administration of medications, treatment procedures? Are additional resources needed?

Can the person explain how to monitor the condition (e.g., blood glucose, signs / symptoms of complications, dietary / mobility restrictions, and when to call his or her primary provider or specialist)?

Act   Contact or provide the appropriate resource (e.g., contacting a support person, home health assessment, additional teaching, printed materials).

Review   Has the problem been addressed? If not, use SBAR to communicate to the appropriate person.

Risk for Ineffective Self-Health Regimen Management Related to Insufficient Knowledge of Etiology, Prevention, Treatment, and Home Care

NOC

Compliance Behavior, Knowledge: Treatment Regimen, Participation in Health Care Decisions, Treatment Behavior: Illness or Injury

Goals

The goals for this diagnosis represent those associated with transition planning. Refer to the transition criteria.

NIC

Anticipatory Guidance, Risk Identification, Learning Facilitation, Learning Readiness Enhancement

Interventions	*Rationales*

1. Teach the client / family measures to prevent additional pressure ulcers (AHCPR, 1992; National Pressure Ulcer Advisory Panel, 2007)
  a. Optimal nutrition
  b. Mobility
  c. Turning and pressure relief
  d. Small shifts in body weight
  e. Active and passive range of motion
  f. Skin care
  g. Skin protection from urine and feces
  h. Recognition of tissue damage
	1. Preventing pressure ulcers is much easier than treating them.

Interventions	Rationales

2. Teach the client methods of treating pressure ulcers (National Pressure Ulcer Advisory Panel, 2007):
   a. Use of pressure ulcer prevention principles
   b. Wound care specific to each ulcer
   c. How to evaluate effectiveness of current treatment
	2. These specific instructions help the client and family learn to promote healing and prevent infection.

3. Ask family members to determine the amount of assistance they need in caring for the client.	3. This assessment is required to determine if the family can provide necessary care and if referrals are indicated.
4. Consult with wound specialist to determine equipment and supply needs (e.g., pressure relief devices, wheelchair cushion, dressings). Consult with social services, if necessary, for assistance in obtaining needed equipment and supplies.	
5. Ensure that the client and family has a referral to a home health agency.	5. Ongoing assessment and teaching will be necessary to sustain the complex level of care.
6. Stress the need to maintain adequate nutrition at home. (Refer to the nursing diagnoses Ineffective Self-Health Management in the Generic Care Plan for Surgical Conditions for interventions to improve nutrition at home.)	

Documentation

Client teaching
Referrals, if indicated

⊗ Musculoskeletal and Connective Tissue Disorders

The general aim of early fracture management is to control hemorrhage, provide pain relief, prevent ischemia-reperfusion injury, and remove potential sources of contamination (foreign body and nonviable tissues). Once these are accomplished, the fracture should be reduced and the reduction should be maintained, which will optimize the conditions for fracture union and minimize potential complications.

Fractures

Fractures are breaks in the continuity of a bone. They result from external pressure greater than the bone can absorb. When a fracture displaces a bone, it also damages surrounding structures—muscles, tendons, nerves, and blood vessels. Closed fracture do not penetrate the skin; open fractures do.

Traumatic injuries cause most fractures. Fractures are classified according to location, type, and pattern of the fracture. Fractured bones can be repositioned (reduced) by closed manipulation or surgical (open) reduction. (Porth, 2011). Open fractures, those where the bone has broken through the skin, require surgical repair. Some fractures can have anatomic alignment maintained by a splint or cast. Other fractures require hardware to accomplish internal fixation (e.g., pins, screws, plates).

Fracture incidence peaks in youth and the elderly. Among youth, long-bone fractures predominate and are more common among males. After the age of 35, fracture incidence climbs precipitously, as bone density declines Pathologic fractures, however, occur even without trauma in bones weakened from excessive demineralization. Refer to Unit II to Risk for Complications of Pathologic Fractures.

 Time Frame
Initial diagnosis

▪▪▪▪■■ DIAGNOSTIC CLUSTER**

Collaborative Problems

▲ Risk for Complications of Neurologic / Vascular Injury

* Risk for Complications of Compartment Syndrome

▲ Risk for Complications of Fat Embolism

▲ Risk for Complications of Hemorrhage / Hematoma Formation

▲ Risk for Complications of Thromboembolism

Nursing Diagnoses

▲ Acute pain related to tissue trauma secondary to fracture (refer to Acute Pain in Unit II)

▲ Self-Care Deficit (specify) related to limitation of movement secondary to fracture (refer to Casts Care Plan)

▲ Risk for Ineffective Respiratory Function related to immobility secondary to traction or fixation devices (refer to Immobility or Unconsciousness Care Plan)

Δ Risk for Ineffective Self-Health Management related to insufficient knowledge of condition, signs and symptoms of complications, activity restrictions

Related Care Plan

Casts

▲ This diagnosis was reported to be monitored for or managed frequently (75% to 100%).
Δ This diagnosis was reported to be monitored for or managed often (50% to 74%).
** This diagnosis was not included in the validation study.

Transition Criteria

Before transition, the client or family will:

1. Describe necessary precautions during activity.
2. State signs and symptoms that must be reported to a health care professional.
3. Demonstrate the ability to provide self-care or report available assistance at home.

> ### Transitional Risk Assessment Plan (TRAP)
>
> Begin this plan on admission.
> Implement the Transitional Risk Assessment Plan (TRAP):
> - Refer to inside back cover.
> - Add each validated risk diagnosis to client's problem list with the risk code in ( ).
> - Refer to Unit II to the individual risk nursing diagnoses / collaborative problems for outcomes and interventions.
>
> *R: "Close coordination of care in the post-acute period, early transition follow-up care, enhanced client education and self-management training, proactive end-of-life counseling, and extending the resources and clinical expertise over time via multidisciplinary team management" can lower readmission rates and improve health outcomes (Boutwell & Hwu, 2009, p. 14).*

Collaborative Problems

Risk for Complications of Neurologic / Vascular Injury

Risk for Complications of Compartment Syndrome

Risk for Complications of Fat Embolism

Risk for Complications of Hemorrhage / Hematoma Formation

Risk for Complications of Osteomyelitis

Risk for Complications of Thromboembolism (refer Unit II)

Collaborative Outcomes

The client will be monitored for early signs and symptoms of (a) neurologic / vascular injury, (b) compartment syndrome, (c) fat embolism, and (d) cardiovascular alterations, and will receive collaborative interventions if indicated to restore physiologic stability.

Indicators of Physiologic Stability

- Pedal pulses 2+, equal (a, b, d)
- Capillary refill <3 seconds (a, b, d)
- Warm extremities (a, b, d)
- No complaints of paresthesia, tingling (a, b, d)
- Pain relieved by medications (b)
- Minimal swelling (a, b, d)
- Ability to move toes or fingers (b)
- BP >90/60, <140/90 mm Hg (d)
- Pulse 60–100 beats/min (d)
- Respiration 16–20 breaths/min (d)
- Temperature 98° to 99.5° F (c)
- Oriented, calm, alert (c, d)
- Urine output >0.5 mL/kg/h (c, d)
- No evidence of petechiae

Interventions	Rationales

1. Monitor for signs and symptoms of neurologic / vascular injury, comparing findings on the affected limb to those of the other limb:
  a. Diminished or absent pedal pulses in affected limb
  b. Numbness or tingling
  c. Capillary refill time >3 seconds
  d. Pallor, blanching, cyanosis, coolness
  e. Inability to flex or extend extremity
	1. Trauma causes tissue edema and blood loss that reduces tissue perfusion. Inadequate circulation and edema damage peripheral nerves, resulting in decreased sensation, movement, and circulation (Porth, 2011).

2. Monitor for signs of compartment syndrome:
  a. Paresthesia (Hartley, 2007):
    • Best elicited by direct stimulation
    • Complaints of tingling or burning sensations > numbness
  b. Pain:
    • Out of proportion to the injury
    • Stretch pain or pain on passive extension or hyper-extension of digits (toes or fingers)
    • Increases with the elevation of the extremity
    • Unrelieved by narcotics
  c. Pressure:
    • Involved compartment or limb will feel tense and warm on palpation
    • Skin is tight and shiny
  d. Late signs / symptoms (Hartley, 2007):
    • Pallor, cool skin
      • Pale, grayish or whitish tone to skin
      • Prolonged capillary refill (>3 seconds)
    • Paralysis
      • c/o weakness when moving affected limb
      • Progresses to inability to move joint or fingers / toe
    • Pulselessness
  e. Laboratory findings (Hartley, 2007):
    • Elevated WBC (white blood cell count) and ESR (erythrocyte sedimentation rate)
    • Elevated temperature
    • Elevated serum potassium
    • Lowered serum pH
  f. If signs of compartment syndrome occur:
    • Discontinue elevation and ice applications.
    • Loosen circumferential dressings, splints, casts per protocol.
  g. If invasive compartment monitoring system is used, follow procedure for use.
  h. Monitor and document compartment pressures according to protocol. Report elevated pressures promptly.
	2b. Pain and paresthesia indicate compression of nerves and increasing pressure within muscle compartment.
	  • Passive stretching of muscles decreases muscle compartment, thus increasing pain.
	  • This increases the pressure in the compartment.
	
	  d. Arterial occlusion produces these late signs.
	  • Delayed capillary refill or pale, mottled or cyanotic skin indicates obstructed capillary blood flow.
	
	  • Decreased arterial perfusion results in pulselessness
	  • These elevations are a result of the severe inflammatory response.
	  • This is due to necrosis of tissue.
	  • Cellular damage releases potassium.
	  • This reflects tissue damage with acidosis.
	
	  • Elevation and external devices will impede perfusion

3. Carefully maintain hydration.	3. Hypovolemia can result from fluid volume shift.

Interventions	*Rationales*
4. Assess neurovascular function at least every hour for first 24 h.	4. A delay in diagnosis is the most important determinant of a poor client outcome (Hartley, 2007).

CLINICAL ALERT
- Notify the physician / NP of any early signs and symptoms of neurovascular compromise.
- The physician / NP will evaluate the cause and determine the necessary treatment, such as cast-splitting, removal of medical antishock trousers (MAST), removal of intra-aortic balloon pump, surgery (e.g., fasciotomy).

a. Instruct client to report unusual, new, or different sensations (e.g., tingling, numbness, and / or decreased ability to move toes or fingers).	a. Early detection of compromise can prevent serious impairment (Pellino et al., 1998; Morton et al., 2006).
b. When the client is unconscious or heavily sedated and unable to complain or report sensations, intensive assessment is required.	b. Permanent nerve injury can occur within 12–24 hours of nerve compression.
5. If pain medications become ineffective, consider compartmental syndrome.	5. Opioids are ineffective for neurovascular pain (McCafferty & Pasero, 2011).

CLINICAL ALERT
- Immediately, advise physician / NP of the need for immediate evaluation of the neurovascular changes assessed or reported by the client.
- Immediate medical assessment will determine what specific interventions are needed: Emergency surgery (fasciotomy), removal of cast, splints

6. Monitor for hypoxemia with pulse oximetry.	6. Pulmonary dysfunction is the earliest sign of fat embolism to manifest and is seen in 75% of clients; it progress to respiratory failure in 10% of the cases. Hypoxemia may be detected hours before the onset of respiratory complaints.

(continued)

Interventions	Rationales
7. Monitor for signs and symptoms of fat embolism (de Feiter et al., 2007; Nucifora et al., 2007).	7. Fat emboli, unlike other emboli, is gradual, with respiratory and neurologic signs / symptoms of hypoxemia, fever and a petechial rash occurring 12–36 hours following injury. "Fat droplets act as emboli, becoming impacted in the pulmonary microvasculature and other microvascular beds such as in the brain. Embolism begins rather slowly and attains a maximum in about 48 h" (Shaikh, 2009).

> **CLINICAL ALERT**
> - The risk factors for the development of FES are young age, closed fractures, multiple fractures, and conservative therapy for long-bone fractures.
> - Factors that increase the risk of FES after intramedullary nailing are overzealous nailing of the medullary cavity, reaming of the medullary cavity, increased velocity of reaming, and increase in the gap between nail and cortical bone.
> - The literature reports "to give prophylactic steroid therapy only to those clients at risk for fat embolism syndrome, for example, those with long bone or pelvic fractures, especially closed fractures. Methylprednisolone i.v. can be administered every 8 h for six doses." (Gupta & Reilly, 2007, p. 5)

Interventions	Rationales
a. Respiratory hypoxia (tachypnea, dyspnea, and cyanosis) b. Cerebral changes (nonspecific, ranging from acute confusion to drowsiness, rigidity, convulsions, or coma) c. Petechial rash	b. Cerebral changes are seen in 86% of clients with FES. c. It occurs in up to 60% of cases and is due to embolization of small dermal capillaries leading to extravasation of erythrocytes. This produces a petechial rash in the conjunctiva, oral mucous membrane, and skin folds of the upper body, especially the neck and axilla
8. Monitor lab results for changes in arterial blood gases and for a sudden inexplicable drop in hematocrit or platelet values.	8. Blood gases will show hypoxia, with a paO_2 of less than 60 mm Hg along with the, and presence of respiratory acidosis (hypercapnia). A decrease in hematocrit occurs within 24–48 h and is attributed to intra-alveolar hemorrhage (Shaikh, 2007).
9. Monitor for elevated temperature (>103° F <38.5° C).	9. Temperature increases are a response to circulating fatty acids. Infection will also cause an increase in temperature.
10. Monitor for infection.	10. Complications of surgical intervention include local infection in the form of cellulitis or osteomyelitis and systemic infection in the form of sepsis.
11. Minimize movement of a fractured extremity for the first 3 days after the injury.	11. Immobilization minimizes further tissue trauma, reduces the risk of embolism dislodgment, and rhabdomyolysis (Sahjian & Frakes, 2007).
12. Monitor intake / output, urine color, and specific gravity.	12. These data will reflect hydration status.
13. Monitor for early signs and symptoms of hemorrhage / shock: a. Increasing pulse rate with normal or slightly decreased blood pressure b. Decreasing rrine output c. Restlessness, agitation, change in mentation d. Increasing respiratory rate	13. Bone is very vascular; blood loss can be substantial, especially with multiple fractures and fractures of the pelvis and femur. The compensatory response to decreased circulatory volume involves increasing blood oxygen by raising heart and respiratory rates, and decreasing circulation to the extremities (marked by decreased pulses, cool skin). Diminished cerebral oxygenation can cause altered mentation (Porth, 2011).

Clinical Alert Report

Advise ancillary staff / student to report:

- Unrelieved or increasing pain
- Pain with passive stretch movement or flexion of toes or fingers
- Skin changes (mottled or cyanotic skin, rash)
- c/o of numbness (paresthesia)
- Inability to move toes or fingers
- Change in cognitive status
- Oral temperature >100.5° F
- Systolic BP <90 mm Hg
- Resting pulse >100, <50
- Respiratory rate >28, <10/min
- Oxygen saturation <90%
- Temperature
- Dyspnea

Related Physician / NP Prescribed Interventions

Medications

Analgesics, anticoagulants, muscle relaxants, platelet aggregation inhibitors corticosteroids

Laboratory Studies

Complete blood count, blood chemistry studies, arterial blood gases

Diagnostic Studies

X-ray examinations, tomograms, bone scans, computed tomography (CT) scan, and MRI

Therapies

Casts; wound care; traction (skin, skeletal); compression stockings; oxygen; surgery (internal fixation)

Documentation

Vital signs
Pulses, color, warmth, sensation, movement of distal areas
Intake and output
Unusual complaints

Risk for Ineffective Self-Health Management Related to Insufficient Knowledge of Condition, Signs and Symptoms of Complications, and Activity Restrictions

NOC

Compliance Behavior, Knowledge: Treatment Regimen, Participation in Health Care Decisions, Treatment Behavior: Illness or Injury

NIC

Risk Identification, Health Education, Teaching: Procedure / Treatment

Goals

The goals for this diagnosis represent those associated with transition planning. Refer to the transition criteria.

Interventions	Rationales

1. Teach client to watch for and to call physician / NP and report the following immediately:
  a. Severe pain
  b. Tingling, numbness
  c. Skin discoloration
  d. Cold extremities
	CLINICAL ALERT
	• These signs may indicate neurovascular compression, a condition requiring immediate medical intervention.

2. Explain the risks of infection and the signs of osteomyelitis (Miller & Askew, 2007):
  a. Chills, high fever
  b. Rapid pulse
  c. Malaise
  d. Painful, tender extremity not relieved with medication, rest, ice, and elevation
 	
CLINICAL ALERT
• Advise client / family to report any of these to their specialist or PCP / NP.
	2. Bone infections can occur anytime during the first 3 months after fracture.

3. Explain activity restrictions. Weight-bearing status is dependent upon stability of the fracture or internal fixation devices.	3. Resting the affected limb promotes healing.
4. Instruct on proper and safe ambulation techniques, as appropriate (Miller & Askew, 2007).	4. Improper use of assistive devices can cause injuries.
5. Refer to Cast Care Plan.	

Documentation

      Client teaching
      Outcome achievement or status

Osteomyelitis

Osteomyelitis is an infection of the bone and surrounding tissues. The infection may result from a blood-borne infection from other sites (e.g., infected tonsils, pressure ulcer, inner ear infection); or may be due to direct bone contamination, as with an open fracture, trauma, or surgery. Other risk factors include diabetes, hemodialysis, poor blood supply, from the presence of indwelling fixation or prosthetic devices, use of illegal injected drugs and individuals who have had their spleen removed. In adults, the feet, spine bones (vertebrae), and hips (pelvis) are most commonly affected.

    Acute osteomyelitis may develop over several days to weeks. Chronic osteomyelitis may occur from acute osteomyelitis after months.

 Time Frame
Initial or secondary diagnosis

▪▪▪▪ DIAGNOSTIC CLUSTER**

Collaborative Problems

Risk for Complications of Bone Abscess

Risk for Complications of Sepsis (refer to Unit II Risk for Complications of Sepsis)

Nursing Diagnoses

Pain related to soft-tissue edema secondary to infection (refer to Pain in Unit II)

Impaired Physical Mobility related to limited range of motion of affected bone (refer to Impaired Physical Mobility in Unit II)

Risk for Ineffective Self-Health Management related to insufficient knowledge of condition, etiology, course, pharmacologic therapy, nutritional requirements, pain management, and signs and symptoms of complications

Related Care Plan

Long-Term Venous Access Devices

**This medical condition was not included in the validation study.

Transition Criteria

Before transition, the client or family will do the following:

1. Identify factors that contribute to osteomyelitis.
2. Relate the signs and symptoms that must be reported to a health care professional.
3. Verbalize an intent to implement lifestyle changes needed for healing.

> ### Transitional Risk Assessment Plan (TRAP)
>
> Begin this plan on admission.
> Implement the Transitional Risk Assessment Plan (TRAP):
> * Refer to inside back cover.
> * Add each validated risk diagnosis to client's problem list with the risk code in ( ).
> * Refer to Unit II to the individual risk nursing diagnoses / collaborative problems for outcomes and interventions.
>
> *R: "Close coordination of care in the post-acute period, early transition follow-up care, enhanced client education and self-management training, proactive end-of-life counseling, and extending the resources and clinical expertise over time via multidisciplinary team management" can lower readmission rates and improve health outcomes (Boutwell & Hwu, 2009, p. 14).*

Collaborative Problem

Risk for Complications of Bone Abscess

Risk for Complications of Chronic Osteomyelitis

Collaborative Outcomes

The client will be monitored for early signs and symptoms of bone abscesses and sepsis, and collaboratively intervene to stabilize the client.

and will receive collaborative interventions if indicated to restore physiologic stability.

Indicators of Physiologic Stability

* Temperature 98° to 99.5° F
* Heart rate 60–100 beats/min
* Respiratory rate 16–20 breaths/min
* White blood count >12,000 cells/mm^3, <4000 cells/mm^3

Interventions	Rationales

1. Monitor (Ladd et al., 2003; Mackowiak, 2007):
  a. Fever and chills
  b. Bone pain (with and without movement)
  c. Increasing tenderness
  d. Warmth
  e. Swelling
  f. Erythema (Merck Manuals Online Medical Library, 2005)
	1. As pus accumulates, the pressure increases, causing ischemia in the bone compartment.

2. Assure that antibiotics are given round the clock.	2. Sustained high therapeutic blood levels of the antibiotic are necessary. Teach the client the importance of taking the antibiotics for the entire course as ordered, usually 4–6 weeks at minimum (Carek et al., 2001).

Clinical Alert Report

Prior to providing care, advise ancillary staff / student to report the following to the professional nurse assigned to the client immediately:

- Chills, fever , temp >100.5° F
- New onset inability to move the limb or joint
- Reports of increased pain in the affected joint, especially with movement
- Increased swelling (increased fluid within the joint)
- Red and warm joint

Related Physician / NP Prescribed Interventions

Medications

Intravenous antibiotic therapy, analgesics

Laboratory Studies

Cultures (blood / wound / stool, urine); sedimentation rate; CBC; urinalysis; prealbumin, total protein; C-reactive protein

Diagnostic Studies

Radionuclide bone scan; MRI, x-rays, computed tomography scanning, ultrasonography, bone scans, bone marrow scans, bone biopsy, needle aspiration of the area around affected bones

Therapies

Incision and drainage of abscesses; surgical debridement; casting or immobilization of affected bone; hyperbaric oxygen; appropriate physical therapy, plastic surgery, vascular surgery, needle aspiration

Documentation

Vital signs
Pulses, color, warmth, sensation, and movement of distal areas
c/o of increasing pain, immobility
Unusual complaints

Nursing Diagnoses

> **TRANSITION TO HOME / COMMUNITY CARE**
>
> If indicated, review the risk diagnoses identified for this individual on admission:
> - Is the person still at risk?
> - Can the family reduce the risks?
> - Is the person at higher risk at home?
> - Is a Home Health Nurse assessment needed?
> - Refer to transition planner / case manager / social service.
> - When is this person scheduled for follow-up with primary provider? Specialists? Record dates of appointments.
> - Complete a medication reconciliation prior to transition. Refer to index.

STAR

Stop

Think Is this person at risk for injury, falls, medical complications, and / or inability to care for self (activities of daily living)?

Is there a support person available?

Is the person competent to manage self-administration of medications, treatment procedures? Are additional resources needed?

Can the person explain how to monitor the condition (e.g., blood glucose, signs / symptoms of complications, dietary / mobility restrictions, and when to call his or her primary provider or specialist)?

Act Contact or provide the appropriate resource (e.g., contacting a support person, home health assessment, additional teaching, printed materials).

Review Has the problem been addressed? If not, use SBAR to communicate to the appropriate person.

Risk for Ineffective Self-Health Management Related to Insufficient Knowledge of Condition, Etiology, Course, Pharmacologic Therapy, Nutritional Requirements, Pain Management, and Signs and Symptoms of Complications

NOC

Compliance Behavior, Knowledge: Treatment Regimen, Participation in Health Care Decisions, Treatment Behavior: Illness or Injury

NIC

Anticipatory Guidance, Risk Identification, Learning Facilitation, Health Education, Health System Guidance

Goals

The goals for this diagnosis represent those associated with transition planning. Refer to the transition criteria.

Interventions	Rationales
1. Determine the client's knowledge of condition, prognosis, and treatment.	1. The client's understanding contributes to improved compliance and reduced risk.
a. Review proper handling techniques of pin sites or external fixation, if applicable.	
b. Instruct the client to avoid tenting the skin around the pin and to avoid application of thick ointment and occlusive dressing on the pin site.	b. Occlusion at pin site can engender growth of microorganisms.

(continued)

Interventions	Rationales
2. Teach the client infection control for drains and wounds: a. Use proper aseptic techniques for dressing changes and care of pins / external fixates. b. Ensure strict hand-washing before and after wound care. c. Use proper techniques for disposal of soiled dressing.	2. These measures help to prevent the introduction of additional microorganisms into the wound; they also reduce the risk of transmitting infection to others.
3. Discuss nutritional requirements and dietary sources: a. Calories per day: 2,500–3,000 b. Protein: 100–125 g; sources: dairy, meat, poultry, fish, and legumes c. B-complex vitamins; sources: meat, nuts, and fortified cereals d. Vitamin C: 75–300 mg; sources: green vegetables and citrus fruits e. Phosphorus, magnesium, and vitamin D; sources: multivitamins	3. Major complications of trauma and sepsis increase the metabolic rate from 10% to 50%. In the presence of insufficient protein, the body breaks down its own endogenous protein stores (Porth, 2011). a, b. Increased caloric and protein intake is needed to enhance the body's protein-sparing capacity. c. B-complex vitamins are required for metabolism of carbohydrates, fat, and protein. d. Vitamin C is essential for collagen formation and wound healing (Porth, 2005). e. These nutrients are required for healing (Porth, 2011).
4. Explain the need for supplements (e.g., milkshakes and puddings).	4. Supplements may be needed to ensure the daily caloric requirement.
5. Discuss techniques to manage pain. Refer to index under acute or chronic pain.	
6. Explain that antibiotics are taken for at least 4–6 weeks, often through an IV at home.	6. The IV route can provide a consistent blood level concentration for increased effectiveness.
7. If indicated. teach the client to take the prescribed antibiotics diligently.	7. A variety of microorganisms may cause osteomyelitis. More than one organism may be involved. More and more clients may become immunocompromised, thus increasing the number of unusual pathogens such as fungi and mycobacteria. (Carek, Dickerson, & Sack, 2001)
8. Teach the client to monitor and report: a. Fever b. Increasing pain c. Visible bone deformity d. Swelling, purulent exudate **CLINICAL ALERT** • Fever and increasing pain can be indicative of sepsis. • Sudden pain in an affected limb can indicate a pathologic fracture. • Seek immediate medical evaluation PCP, ER	
9. Prepare the client and family for the possibility of exacerbations.	9. Chronic osteomyelitis can occur if bacterial growth takes place in vascular scar tissue, which is impenetrable to antibiotics. Chronic osteomyelitis is most common following open fractures due to direct contamination of the wound.

Documentation

Client teaching

Inflammatory Joint Disease (Rheumatoid Arthritis, Infectious Arthritis, or Septic Arthritis)

Rheumatoid arthritis (RA) is a chronic inflammatory disease, characterized by uncontrolled proliferation of synovial tissue and a wide array of multisystem comorbidities. It presents as a characteristic inflammation with destructive synovitis in multiple diarthrodial joints. A diathrodial joint is a joint in which the opposing bony surfaces are covered with a layer of hyaline cartilage or fibrocartilage.

The etiology is unknown, but research has been able to piece together the factors involved, such as (1) genetic (inherited) factors, (2) environmental factors (viral or bacterial infection, making the individual susceptible to RA), and (3) hormonal factors, or others. Research has also shown that RA is associated with a 5–15-year reduction in life expectancy after a triggering incident, possibly autoimmune or infectious.

The diathrodial joints involved are usually symmetrically affected, with the small bones of the hands and feet affected first. "Joint damage in RA begins with the proliferation of synovial macropghages and fibroblasts after an incident, possible autoimmune or infectious. Over time, inflamed synovial tissue begins to grow irregularly, forming invasive pannus tissue. Pannus invades and destroys cartilage and bone" (Rindfleisch & Muller, 2005, p. 2). The disease is characterized by cycles of exacerbations and remission. Extra-articular involvement of rheumatoid arthritis can include muscle atrophy; anemia; osteoporosis; and skin, ocular, vascular, pulmonary, and cardiac symptoms.

Genetic susceptibility is evident, with incidence of the disease in immediate and extended families of individuals with RA is high. Smoking (current or prior) is a major trigger for RA (Wasserman, 2011). Untreated, 20%–30% of persons with rheumatoid arthritis become permanently work disabled within 2–3 years of diagnosis (Rindfleisch & Muller, 2005).

Bacteria can travel through the bloodstream from another site of active infection, resulting in hematogenous seeding of the joint. Organisms can also be introduced through trauma or surgical incision. *Staphylococcus aureus* is the most common causative organism, but any bacteria can cause the infection in the immunocompromised client; even nonpathogenic bacteria can be responsible for development of septic arthritis, which causes joint inflammation resulting from a viral, bacterial, or fungal organism invading the synovium and synovial fluid. Precise diagnosis is made by aspiration of the joint (arthrocentesis) and culture of the synovial fluid. Blood cultures for aerobic and anaerobic organisms should also be obtained. Septic arthritis is a medical emergency that requires prompt diagnosis and treatment to prevent joint destruction (Lewis et al., 2004; Zeller, Lym, & Glass, 2007; Arthritis Foundation, 2008).

Time Frame
Initial diagnosis
Secondary diagnosis

■■ DIAGNOSTIC CLUSTER**

Collaborative Problems

Risk for Complications of Septic Arthritis

Risk for Complications of Sjögren Syndrome

Risk for Complications of Neuropathy

Risk for Complications of Anemia, Leukopenia (refer to Inflammatory Bowel Disease in Unit II)

Risk for Complications of Avascular Necrosis

Risk for Complications of Cardiopulmonary Effects

Risk for Complications of Septic Shock

Nursing Diagnoses

Fatigue related to decreased mobility, stiffness

Risk for Impaired Oral Mucous Membrane related to effects of medications or Sjögren syndrome

(*continued*)

Disturbed Sleep Pattern related to pain or secondary to fibrositis (refer to Disturbed Sleep Pattern in Unit II)

(Specify) Self-Care Deficit related to limitations secondary to disease process

Ineffective Sexuality Patterns related to pain, fatigue, difficulty in assuming positions, and lack of adequate lubrication (female) secondary to disease process

Impaired Physical Mobility related to pain and limited joint motion

Chronic Pain related to inflammation of joints and juxta-articular structures

Risk for Ineffective Self-Health Management related to insufficient knowledge of condition, pharmacologic therapy, home care, stress management, and quackery

Interrupted Family Processes related to difficulty / inability of ill client to assume role responsibilities secondary to fatigue and limited motion (refer to Multiple Sclerosis)

Powerlessness related to physical and psychological changes imposed by the disease (refer to Chronic Obstructive Pulmonary Disease)

Related Care Plans

Corticosteroid Therapy

Raynaud Disease

Congestive Heart Failure

Diabetes Mellitus

**This medical condition was not included in the validation study.

Transition Criteria

Before transition the client or family will:

1. Identify components of a standard treatment program for inflammatory arthritis.
2. Relate proper use of medications and other treatment modalities.
3. Identify factors that restrict self-care and home maintenance.
4. Relate signs and symptoms that must be reported to a health care professional.

Transitional Risk Assessment Plan (TRAP)

Begin this plan on admission.

Implement the Transitional Risk Assessment Plan (TRAP):

- Refer to inside back cover.
- Add each validated risk diagnosis to client's problem list with the risk code in ( ).
- Refer to Unit II to the individual risk nursing diagnoses / collaborative problems for outcomes and interventions.

R: "Close coordination of care in the post-acute period, early transition follow-up care, enhanced client education and self-management training, proactive end-of-life counseling, and extending the resources and clinical expertise over time via multidisciplinary team management" can lower readmission rates and improve health outcomes (Boutwell & Hwu, 2009, p. 14).

Collaborative Problems

Risk for Complications of Septic Arthritis

Risk for Complications of Sjögren Syndrome

Risk for Complications of Neuropathy

Risk for Complications of Avascular Necrosis

Risk for Complications of Cardiopulmonary Effects (pericarditis, pericardial effusion, cardiomyopathy, pleurisy, pleural effusions, and congestive heart failure)

Risk for Complications of Septic Shock

Collaborative Outcomes

The client will be monitored for early signs and symptoms of (a) septic arthritis, (b) Sjögren syndrome, (c) neuropathy, (d) anemia, (e) avascular necrosis, (f) cardiopulmonary effects, and (g) septic shock, and will receive collaborative interventions if indicated to restore physiologic stability.

Indicators of Physiologic Stability

- Temperature 98° to 99.5° F (a, h)
- No change in usual level of pain (a)
- Moist mucous membranes (b)
- No c/o paresthesias and numbness (c)
- Hemoglobin (d)
  - Male: 14–18 g/dL
  - Female: 12–16 g/dL
  - WBC 4,300–10,800 cells/mm^3 (a, g)
- Joint pain with weight-bearing (e)
- Limited to no range of movement (e)
- Shortness of breath (f)
- Chest pain (sharp, or relieved by sitting up and forward and worsens by laying down) (f)
- Dry cough (f)
- Friction rub with respirations (f)
- Weight loss or gain (f)
- Dizziness (f)
- Refractory hypotension (g)
- Tachypnea (g)
- Decreased level of consciousness (f, g)

Interventions	*Rationales*

1. Monitor for signs and symptoms of septic arthritis:
  a. Chills, fever, temp >100.5° F
  b. Inability to move the limb with the infected joint
  c. New onset severe pain in the affected joint, especially with movement
  d. Swelling (increased fluid within the joint)
  e. Warmth (the joint is red and warm to touch because of increased blood flow)
	1. Septic arthritis which causes joint inflammation resulting from a viral, bacterial, or fungal organism invading the synovium and synovial fluid. Bacteria travels through the bloodstream from another site of active infection, resulting in hematogenous seeding of the joint. Inflammation of a joint cavity causes severe pain, erythema, and swelling. Because infection often spreads from a primary site elsewhere in the body, fever or shaking chills often accompany articular manifestations (Horowitz et al., 2012).

CLINICAL ALERT
- New onset or worsening of swelling, pain, fever and chills needs an urgent evaluation.
- "Prompt diagnosis and treatment of infectious arthritis can help prevent significant morbidity and mortality. The acute onset of monoarticular joint pain, erythema, heat, and immobility should raise suspicion of sepsis" (Horowitz et al., 2012).

(continued)

Documentation

Exercises (type, frequency)

Chronic Pain Related to Inflammation of Joints and Juxta-articular Structures

NOC

Comfort Level, Pain:
Disruptive Effects, Pain
Control, Depression
Level

Goal

The client will relate improvement of pain and, when possible, increase daily activities.

NIC

Pain Management,
Medication
Management, Exercise
Promotion, Mood
Management, Coping
Enhancement

Indicators

* Receive validation that pain exists.
* Practice selected noninvasive pain relief measures to manage pain.
* Relate improvement of pain and, when possible, increase daily activities.

Interventions	Rationales
1. Teach the client to differentiate between joint pain and stiffness.	1. When there is joint pain, techniques for joint protection are instituted. When flares are diminished, active ROM exercises are indicated (Arthritis Foundation, 2008).
2. If joints are inflamed, let the client rest and avoid activities that stress joints. Gentle ROM exercises may be tried.	2. ROM exercises can prevent contractures. Inflamed joints are at risk for injury.
3. Apply local heat or cold to affected joints for approximately 20–30 minutes three to four times a day. Check the temperature of warm soaks or covering a cold / ice pack with a towel.	3. Avoid temperatures likely to cause skin or tissue damage.
4. Encourage a warm bath or shower first thing in the morning to reduce morning stiffness.	4. Treatment of inflammatory joint pain focuses on the reduction of discomfort and inflammation by the use of local comfort measures, joint rest, and the use of anti-inflammatory or disease-modifying medications.
5. Encourage the use of adjunctive pain control measures: a. Progressive relaxation b. Transcutaneous electrical nerve stimulation (TENS) c. Biofeedback d. Imagery / music / acupuncture	5. Pain is a subjective, multifactorial experience that can be modified by the use of cognitive and physical techniques to reduce the intensity or perception of pain (Arthritis Foundation, 2008; Lewis et al., 2004; Maclean et al., 2000).

Documentation

Assessment of affected joints: pain, swelling, warmth, erythema
Response to pain relief measures

TRANSITION TO HOME / COMMUNITY CARE

If indicated, review the risk diagnoses identified for this individual on admission:

* Is the person still at risk?
* Can the family reduce the risks?
* Is the person at higher risk at home?
* Is a Home Health Nurse assessment needed?
* Refer to transition planner / case manager / social service
* When is this person scheduled for follow-up with primary provider? Specialists? Record dates of appointments.
* Complete a medication reconciliation prior to transition. Refer to index.

STAR   **Stop**

Think   Is this person at risk for injury, falls, medical complications, and / or inability to care for self (activities of daily living)?

        Is there a support person available?

        Is the person competent to manage self-administration of medications, treatment procedures? Are additional resources needed?

        Can the person explain how to monitor the condition (e.g., blood glucose, sign / symptoms of complications, dietary / mobility restrictions, and when to call his or her primary provider or specialist)?

Act   Contact or provide the appropriate resource (e.g., contacting a support person, home health assessment, additional teaching, printed materials).

Review   Has the problem been addressed? If not, use SBAR to communicate to the appropriate person.

Risk for Ineffective Self-Health Management Related to Insufficient Knowledge of Condition, Pharmacologic Therapy, Home Care, Stress Management, and Quackery

NOC

Compliance Behavior, Knowledge: Treatment Regimen, Participation in Health Care Decisions, Treatment Behavior: Illness or Injury

NIC

Anticipatory Guidance, Learning Facilitation, Risk Identification, Health Education, Teaching: Procedure / Treatment, Health System Guidance

Goals

The goals for this diagnosis represent those associated with transition planning. Refer to the transition criteria.

Interventions	*Rationales*

1. Explain inflammatory arthritis using teaching aids appropriate to the client's and family members' levels of understanding. Explain the following:
a. Inflammatory process
b. Joint function and structure
c. Effects of inflammation on joints and juxta-articular structures
d. Extra-articular manifestations of the disease process
e. Chronic nature of the disease
f. Disease course (remission / exacerbation)
g. Low incidence of significant or total disability
h. Components of the standard treatment program:
  • Medications (e.g., aspirin, nonsteroidal anti-inflammatory drugs, disease-modifying agents, cytotoxic agents, corticosteroids)
  • Local comfort measures
  • Exercise / rest
  • Joint protection / assistive devices
  • Consultation with other disciplines
	1. Inflammatory joint disease is a chronic illness. Education should emphasize a good understanding of the inflammatory process and actions the client can take to manage symptoms and minimize their impact on his or her life.

2. Allow significant others opportunities to share feelings and frustrations, including the need for: a. Adequate nutrition b. Regular follow-up care	2. Persons with RA may be difficult to live with, demanding or manipulative (Arthritis Foundation, 2008; Lewis et al., 2004).

(continued)

Interventions	Rationales

3. Teach the client and family to identify characteristics of quackery:
  a. "Secret" formulas or devices for curing arthritis
  b. Advertisements using "case histories" and "testimonials"
  c. Rejection of standard components of a treatment program
  d. Claims of persecution by the "medical establishment"
	3. An accurate and full understanding of inflammatory joint disease and its treatment lessens the client's susceptibility to quackery.

4. Explain that some medications will worsen the symptoms of Sjögren Syndrome (dry mouth, dry eyes) a. Antihistamines, decongestants, antidepressants, diuretics (water pills), tranquilizers, some blood pressure medications, some diarrhea medications, some antipsychotic medications	
5. Teach the client to take prescribed medications properly and to report symptoms of side effects promptly.	5. Adhering to the schedule may help to prevent fluctuating drug blood levels and can reduce side effects. Prompt reporting of side effects enables intervention to prevent serious problems.

6. Explain the proper use of other treatment modalities:
  a. Local heat or cold application
  b. Assistive devices
  c. Exercises
	6. Injury can further decrease mobility and motivation to continue therapies.

7. Explain the relationship of stress to inflammatory diseases. Discuss stress management techniques:
  a. Progressive relaxation
  b. Guided imagery
  c. Regular exercise
	7. Stressful events may be associated with an increase in disease activity. Effective use of stress management techniques can help to minimize the effects of stress on the disease process.

8. Reinforce the importance of routine follow-up care.	8. Follow-up care can identify complications early and help to reduce disabilities from disuse.
9. Refer to appropriate community resources such as the Arthritis Foundation, P.O. Box 7669, Atlanta, GA 30357-0669. Telephone: 800 283 7800 (Arthritis Foundation, 2008).	9. Such resources can provide specific additional information to enhance self-care.

Documentation

Client and family teaching
Status on transition
Referrals, if indicated

Infectious and Immunodeficient Disorders

Human Immunodeficiency Virus / Acquired Immunodeficiency Syndrome

An infection caused by the human immunodeficiency virus (HIV), acquired immunodeficiency syndrome (AIDS) was first reported in the United States in 1981. AIDS represents the end-stage of a continuum of HIV infection and its sequelae. Major modes of infection transmission include sexual activity with an infected person and exposure to infected needles or drug paraphernalia, blood, or blood products. A fetus can contract HIV infection from an infected mother perinatally. HIV infects primarily the T4-cell lymphocytes; this interferes with cell-mediated immunity. The clinical consequences of this progressive immune deficiency are opportunistic infections and malignancies. Beginning in the 1990s, the increased number of available medications has slowed the course of HIV dramatically. Individuals who are compliant with their antiviral therapy are living well to become senior citizens.

Time Frame
Initial diagnosis
Recurrent acute episodes

DIAGNOSTIC CLUSTER

Collaborative Problems

▲ Risk for Complications of Opportunistic Infections

△ Risk for Complications of Malignancies

▲ Risk for Complications of Sepsis (refer to Risk for Complications of Sepsis in Unit II)

* Risk for Complications of Myelosuppression

* Risk for Complications of Peripheral Neuropathy

* Risk for Complications of HIV-Related Nephropathy

Nursing Diagnoses

▲ Risk for Impaired Oral Mucous Membrane related to compromised immune system

▲ Risk for Infection Transmission related to the infectious nature of the client's blood and body fluids

* Risk for Imbalanced Nutrition: Less Than Body Requirements related to HIV infection, opportunistic infections / malignancies associated with AIDS (refer to Imbalanced Nutrition in Unit II)

* Risk for Ineffective Coping related to situational crisis (e.g., new HIV or AIDS diagnosis, first hospitalization)

△ Anxiety related to perceived effects of illness on lifestyle and unknown future (refer to Cancer: Initial Diagnosis)

△ Grieving related to loss of body function and its effects on lifestyle (refer to Cancer: Initial Diagnosis)

▲ Risk for Infection related to increased susceptibility secondary to compromised immune system

▲ Fatigue related to effects of disease, stress, chronic infections, and nutritional deficiency

▲ Risk for Ineffective Self-Health related to insufficient knowledge of HIV, its transmission, prevention, treatment, and community resources

* Risk for Caregiver Role Strain related to AIDS-associated shame / stigma, and uncertainty about course of illness and demands on caregiver

(continued)

Related Care Plan

Palliative Care Plan

▲ This diagnosis was reported to be monitored for or managed frequently (75% to 100%).

Δ This diagnosis was reported to be monitored for or managed often (50% to 74%).

* This diagnosis was not included in the validation study.

Transition Criteria

Before transition, the client or family will

1. Relate the implications of the diagnosis.
2. Describe the prescribed medication regimen.
3. Identify modes of HIV transmission.
4. Identify infection-control measures.
5. Describe signs and symptoms that must be reported to a health care professional.
6. Identify available community resources.

> ### Transitional Risk Assessment Plan (TRAP)
>
> Begin this plan on admission.
> Implement the Transitional Risk Assessment Plan (TRAP):
> • Refer to inside back cover.
> • Add each validated risk diagnosis to client's problem list with the risk code in ( ).
> • Refer to Unit II to the individual risk nursing diagnoses / collaborative problems for outcomes and interventions.
>
> *R: "Close coordination of care in the post-acute period, early transition follow-up care, enhanced client education and self-management training, proactive end-of-life counseling, and extending the resources and clinical expertise over time via multidisciplinary team management" can lower readmission rates and improve health outcomes (Boutwell & Hwu, 2009, p. 14).*

Collaborative Problems

Risk for Complications of Opportunistic Infections

Risk for Complications of Malignancies

Risk for Complications of Sepsis

Risk for Complications of Peripheral Neuropathy

Risk for Complications of HIV-Related Nephropathy

Collaborative Outcomes

The client will be monitored for early signs and symptoms of (a) opportunistic infections (pneumonia, encephalitis, enteritis, cytomegalovirus, herpes simplex, herpes zoster, stomatitis, esophagitis, meningitis), (b) malignancies, (c) sepsis, and (d) HIV-associated peripheral neuropathy, and will receive collaborative interventions if indicated to restore physiologic stability.

Indicators of Physiologic Stability

• Temperature 98°–99.5° F (a, c)
• Respirations 16–20 breaths/min (a, c)
• SaO_2 arterial oxygen saturation (pulse oximeter >95%) (c)
• $PaCO_2$ arterial carbon dioxide 35–45 mm Hg (c)
• Urine output >0.5 mL/kg/h (c)
• No proteinuria (c)
• Creatinine 0.2–0.8 ng/mL (c)

- Serum albumin 3.5–5 g/dL (c)
- Blood urea nitrogen 10–20 mg/dL (c)
- Alert, oriented (a)
- No seizures, no headaches (a)
- Regular, formed stools (a)
- No herpetic or zoster lesions (a)
- Swallows with no difficulty (a)
- No change in vision (a)
- No weight loss (b)
- No new lesions (b)
- No lymphadenopathy (b)
- No leg pain, burning, or paresthesia (d)

 Carp's Cues

Individuals with undiagnosed HIV infections can often present with opportunistic infections, which leads to the diagnosis of AIDS.

Interventions	Rationales

1. Monitor for opportunistic infections:
  a. Protozoal:
    • *Pneumocystis carinii* pneumonia (dry, nonproductive cough, fever, dyspnea)
    • *Toxoplasma gondii* encephalitis (headache, lethargy, seizures)
    • *Cryptosporidium enteritis* (watery diarrhea, malaise, nausea, abdominal cramps)
  b. Viral:
    • Genital herpes simplex (cluster of blister-like lesions, pain), labial herpes simplex (single blister-like lesion or cluster, pain), perirectal abscesses (severe pain, bleeding, rectal discharge)
    • Cytomegalovirus (CMV) retinitis, colitis, pneumonitis, encephalitis, or other organ disease
    • Progressive multifocal leukoencephalopathy (headache, decreased mentation)
    • *Varicella zoster*, disseminated (shingles), a tract (horizontal pattern of blister-like lesions, painful, reddened)
  c. Fungal:
    • *Candida albicans* oral, stomatitis, and esophagitis (exudate, complaints of unusual taste in mouth, discomfort with hot drinks)
    • *Cryptococcus neoformans* meningitis (fever, headache, blurred vision, stiff neck, confusion)
    • *Mycobacterium aviumintracellulare* disseminated
    • *Mycobacterium tuberculosis* extrapulmonary and pulmonary.
	1. Severe immune deficiencies with CD4 <200% cause opportunistic infections (OI) and malignancies. Antiretroviral therapy has dramatically reduced OIs.
	
	  • Herpes simplex is common and painful. The CMV infections are responsible for significant morbidity (e.g., blindness).
	
	  c. Fungal infections can be chronic, with relapses, and frequently affect the pulmonary system.

> **CLINICAL ALERT**
> - Emphasize the need to report symptoms early.
> - Advise that if the client is severely compromised, some symptoms will not be present (e.g., increased temperature).
> - Early treatment can often prevent serious complications (e.g., septicemia) and increases the chance of a favorable response to treatment.

(continued)

Interventions	*Rationales*
2. Administer medications for opportunistic infections, as prescribed. Consult a pharmacologic reference for specific nursing implications (Arcangelo & Peterson, 2011; CDC, 2009).	2. Some treatments for opportunistic infections are life-long to prevent reoccurrences.

3. Monitor for malignancies:
 	
  a. Kaposi sarcoma: Painless, palpable lesions (purplish, pinkish, or red) frequently on trunk, neck, arms, and head.
  b. Extracutaneous lesions in GI tract, lymph nodes, buccal mucosa, and lungs
  c. Pruritus, weight loss
  d. Lymphoma (non-Hodgkin, Burkitt):
    • Painless lymphadenopathy (an early site at neck, axilla, inguinal area)
	3. The malignancies that affect AIDS clients are related to immunosuppression.
	  a. Kaposi sarcoma is cancer of the lymphatic vessel (endothelial wall). It is not skin cancer.
	
	  • Non-Hodgkin lymphomas can progress into the bone marrow, liver, spleen, gastrointestinal, and nervous systems.

4. Monitor for signs and symptoms of sepsis:	4. Gram-positive and gram-negative organisms can invade open wounds, causing septicemia. An immunocompromised individual is at increased risk. Sepsis produces massive vasodilation, resulting in hypovolemia and subsequent tissue hypoxia. Hypoxia leads to decreased renal function and cardiac output, triggering a compensatory response of increased respirations and heart rate in an attempt to correct hypoxia and acidosis. Bacteria in urine or blood indicate infection.
5. Refer to Risk for Complications of Sepsis in Unit II.	

6. Monitor and support use of prescribed prophylactic medication for opportunistic infections (Sax, Cohen & Kuritzkes, 2012; CDC, 2009):
 	
  a. *P. carinii* pneumonia
    • If indicated, Bactrim DS 3× week (Monday, Wednesday, Friday) is prophylaxis for *P. carinii* pneumonia.
  b. Toxoplasmosis (*toxoplasma*-seropositive individuals who have a CD4+ count of <100 cells/μL should be administered prophylaxis against TE
    • If indicated, the double-strength tablet daily dose of TMP-SMX recommended as the preferred regimen for PCP prophylaxis also is effective against TE and is therefore recommended. TMP-SMX, one double-strength tablet, three times weekly is an alternative.
  c. Disseminated mycobacterium avium complex (MAC) disease (MAC seronegative individuals, with a CD4+ count < 50 cells/*u*L should be administered prophylaxis against MAC.
    • If indicated, 1200 mg Azithromycin po once weekly or 60 mg twice weekly for MAC is recommended prophylaxis.
	6. "Individuals with HIV disease are at risk for infectious complications not otherwise seen in immunocompetent individuals" (Sax, Cohen, Kuritzkes, 2012, p. 66). Prophylactic medications can prevent serious infections that increase morbidity and mortality.
	  a. HIV-infected adults and adolescents, including pregnant women and those on ART, should receive chemoprophylaxis against PCP if they have a CD4+ count of <200 cells/μL or oropharyngeal candidiasis. Persons who have a CD4+ cell percentage of < 14% or a history of an AIDS-defining illness, but do not otherwise qualify, should be considered for prophylaxis (CDC, 2009).

Interventions	Rationales

7. Monitor for HIV-related peripheral neuropathy:
  a. Extremely sensitive to touch
  b. Sharp pain / cramping
  c. Tingling, prickling, or burning sensation
  d. Muscle weakness
  e. Reports of loss of balance / coordination
	7. The cause of nerve or brain damage is unknown, possibly due to chronic immune system inflammation. Moderate to severe peripheral neuropathy in individuals with HIV is a usually side effect of certain medications, which can cause mitochondrial damage, nerve damage, and peripheral neuropathy (Evans et al., 2011).

CLINICAL ALERT

• The risk of peripheral neuropathy may be higher still if these medications are used in people with a history of neuropathy, diabetes, heavy alcohol consumption, poor nutrition, and / or older age.

Clinical Alert Report

Prior to providing care, advise ancillary staff / student to report the following to the professional nurse assigned to the client:

• New onset or worsening of headaches
• New lesions (skin, oral mucosa)
• Change in cognitive status
• Oral temperature >100.5° F
• Systolic BP <90 mm/Hg
• Resting pulse >100, <50
• Respiratory rate >28, <10 /min.
• Oxygen saturation <90%

Related Physician / NP Prescribed Interventions

Medications

Antibiotics, antiretrovirals, antiemetics, antifungals, chemotherapy, antipyretics, nucleoside reverse transcriptase inhibitors (NRTI), antiviral agents, protease inhibitors (PI), antidiarrheals, non-nucleoside reverse transcriptase inhibitors (NNRTI), fusion inhibitors

Laboratory Studies

Creatinine, hyperalimentation, blood urea nitrogen, Liver function tests, viral load, enzyme-linked immunosorbent assay (ELISA), complete blood count, cultures, T-lymphocyte cells, hepatitis panel, CD4 count, Western blot test, CD8 count, serum protein, genotype testing, phenotype testing.

Diagnostic Studies

Magnetic resonance imaging (MRI), endoscopy, biopsies, chest x-ray film

Therapies

Nasogastric feeding

Documentation

Lesions (number, size, locations)
Respiratory assessment
Neurologic assessment (mentation, orientation, affect)
Mouth assessment

Risk for Infection Transmission Related to the Infectious Nature of the Client's Blood and Body Fluids**

NOC

Infection Severity, Risk Control, Risk Detection

Goal

The client will take necessary steps to prevent infection transmission.

NIC

Teaching: Disease Process, Infection Protection

Indicators

- Describe the factors that contribute to HIV transmission
- Describe how to disinfect infected objects or surfaces

Interventions	Rationales
1. Adhere to universal precautions. Wash hands before and after contact with client in care situation. Wear gloves when contact with blood/body fluids may occur.	1. Universal precautions are to prevent the transmission of blood-borne pathogens from client to caregiver. They are taken with all clients regardless of diagnosis, age, or sexual orientation of the client. The particular precautions taken with each individual client are dependent on the potential of transmission related to the care to be rendered and not to the client's diagnosis. Hand-washing is one of the most important means of preventing the spread of infection.
2. Refer to Risk for Infection for generic interventions in Unit II.	

CLINICAL ALERT
- The CDC estimates > 600,000 significant occupational exposures to blood-borne pathogens occur yearly (Sax, Cohen, & Kuritzkes, 2102).
- The risks seroconversion (becoming infected with HIV) is 0.3% to 0.9% after percutaneous / mucus membrane exposure (e.g., needlesticks) and no reported seroconversion with exposure to intact skin (Sax, Cohen, & Kuritzkes, 2102).
- If exposure to blood-borne pathogens occurs, immediately follow agency protocols for post exposure prophylaxis (PEP).

3. Provide facts to dispel myths regarding transmission of HIV.	
4. Explain that HIV lives and reproduces in blood and other body fluids. It is known that the following fluids can contain high levels of HIV (CDC, 2012a): • Blood • Semen (cum) • Pre-seminal fluid (pre-cum) • Breast milk • Vaginal fluids • Rectal (anal) mucous	

** This diagnosis is not currently on the NANDA-I list but has been included for clarity or usefulness.

Interventions	Rationales

5. Advise of some myths:
  a. HIV is not transmitted by skin-to-skin contact, mosquito bites, swimming pools, clothes, eating utensils, telephones, or toilet seats.
  b. HIV cannot be contracted while giving blood.
	5. Other body fluids and waste products—like feces, nasal fluid, saliva, sweat, tears, urine, or vomit—don't contain enough HIV to infect a person, *unless* they have blood mixed in them and you have *significant* and *direct* contact with them (CDC, 2012a).

6. If indicated, instruct and provide written material on safer sex guidelines and other risks for transmission that include:
  a. Correct and consistent use of a latex condom with every act of vaginal, anal, and / or oral intercourse; avoid spermicides with nonoxynol 9.
  b. Provision for adequate lubrication during intercourse by the use of a water-based lubricant.
  c. Maintenance of a faithful monogamous sexual relationship with partner.
  d. Advise of avoidance of risk behavior as:
 	
    • Sex with multiple partners.
 	
    • Engaging in sexual activity when not sober and on street drugs
    • Rough sexual practices
 	
    • Needle or straw sharing during drug use, tattooing, body piercing, acupuncture, or other such activities
	
	  d. Certain behaviors are conducive to transmission of blood-borne or sexually transmitted diseases.
	    • This increases the risk of sexually transmitted infections, which injure tissue and allow infected fluids to enter bloodstream.
	    • When under the influence, safe sex practices are usually omitted.
	    • This can lead to breaks in the mucosal lining of the rectum, mouth, or vagina, providing entry of infected fluids.
	    • Any injury to mucous membranes will provide an entry for infected fluids.

CLINICAL ALERT • Correct and consistent use of a latex condom with every act of intercourse has been shown to significantly reduce the risk of transmission of sexually transmitted diseases, including HIV. • Oil-based lubricants (e.g., Vaseline) and nonoxynol 9 spermicides can degrade latex condoms. Any object contaminated with blood must be cleaned with a bleach solution (one part bleach to 10 parts water).	

7. Instruct the client and provide written material on transmission precautions for the home setting, including:
  a. No sharing of toothbrushes, razors, enema or douche equipment, or other sharp objects
  b. Prompt and adequate disposal of needles and other sharps into a puncture-proof, locked container
  c. Proper hand-washing after any contact with the clients' blood or infectious body fluids
  d. Use of gloves for provision of client care involving contact with his or her blood or body fluids
  e. Cleaning up blood and body fluid spills by using gloves and paper towel to get up the majority of the spill before disinfecting area with a 1:10 solution of bleach
	7. Fear of HIV transmission is a common concern of caregivers of persons with HIV. HIV is rapidly inactivated by exposure to disinfecting agents. Household bleach solution (dilute 1:10 with water) is an inexpensive choice.

8. Provide the client and caregiver with the National CDC INFO hotline number (1-800-232-4636).	8. The hotline provides rapid access to accurate information or go to AIDS.com for basic information on HIV/AIDS.

Risk for Ineffective Coping Related to Situational Crisis (i.e., New HIV or AIDS Diagnosis and / or First Hospitalization)

NOC

Coping, Self-Esteem, Social Interaction Skills

Goal

The client will make decisions and follow through with appropriate actions to change provocative situations in his or her personal environment.

NIC

Coping Enhancement, Counseling, Emotional Support, Active Listening, Assertiveness Training, Behavior Modification

Indicators

- Verbalize feelings related to emotional state.
- Focus on the present.
- Identify response patterns and the consequences of resulting behavior.
- Identify personal strengths and accept support through the nursing relationship.

Interventions	Rationales
1. Encourage the client's expression of anxiety, anger, and fear. Listen attentively and nonjudgmentally.	1. Listening is credited as a helpful strategy to assist clients coping with AIDS. Anger at AIDS-associated prejudice or lack of understanding of others occurs commonly among the HIV-infected.
2. Encourage the client to share her or his feelings regarding the multiple fears associated with AIDS (e.g., friends, community, family structure, and social networks).	2. Complex social issues of morality, sexuality, contagion, and shame are associated with AIDS-related losses and interfere with grieving and coping (Cotton et al., 2006; Mallison, 1999).
3. Encourage the individual to share his or her experiences with other individual with HIV/AIDS.	3. Disenfranchised grief occurs when social stigma is associated with a death or illness (e.g., suicide, AIDS); the person may be alone, emotionally isolated, or fearful of public expressions of grief (Bateman, 1999). Gay men who have experienced multiple AIDS-related losses (e.g., loss of friends and community, disintegrating family structures and social networks) may receive little understanding from heterosexuals (Cotton et al., 2006; Mallinson, 1999).
4. Determine the client's past coping strategies and assist him or her to develop coping strategies based on previously successful outcomes and personal strengths.	4. Interventions constructed using the client's personal style and character are likely to be of lasting use to her or him. Previous successes should be built on when possible.
5. Discourage coping mechanisms that are maladaptive or self-defeating (e.g., alcohol, drugs, denial, and compulsive behavior).	5. Substance abuse and destructive denial are behaviors often perceived to provide subjective relief. This relief, however, is usually temporary and ultimately self-defeating.
6. Assist the client with finding meaning in illness, and not assuming the victim role.	6. "Focus should be on living with AIDS, not dying of it. Nurses can rekindle the spark that is needed to discover the meaning and purpose in suffering and even death" (Carson & Green, 1992, p. 217).
7. Encourage and reinforce the client's hopes, as appropriate.	7. "All life is based on hope and when hope is low or absent, people see their lives as finished . . . when professional caretakers see hope in the terminally ill as unrealistic and label it as denial, they lower the quality of the years remaining to the person, or force him or her to turn elsewhere for help" (Hall, 1990, p. 183).

Interventions	Rationales
8. Assist the client to identify appropriate support systems (e.g., support group, community resources) and encourage their use.	8. Feelings of alienation and social isolation are common among the HIV-infected. Support groups potentially are able to educate, support, and assist the client to anticipate and deal with the crises inevitable to the client's illness (Mallinson, 1999).
9. Encourage and provide exercise, recreation, diversional activities, and independent activities-of-daily-living (ADLs) performance.	9. Diversional activities can provide opportunities of rest from mental and emotional distress. Maximal independence and participation in activities can increase self-confidence and self-esteem.
10. Instruct the client on stress-management techniques (e.g., distraction, relaxation imagery), as appropriate.	10. Stress reduction techniques can assist the client in dealing with personal fears and anxieties.

> **TRANSITION TO HOME / COMMUNITY CARE**
>
> If indicated, review the risk diagnoses identified for this individual on admission:
>
> * Is the person still at risk?
> * Can the family reduce the risks?
> * Is the person at higher risk at home?
> * Is a Home Health Nurse assessment needed?
> * Refer to transition planner / case manager / social service.
> * When is this person scheduled for follow-up with primary provider? Specialists? Record dates of appointments.
> * Complete a medication reconciliation prior to transition. Refer to index.

STAR

Stop

Think   Is this person at risk for injury, falls, medical complications, and / or inability to care for self (activities of daily living)?

Is there a support person available?

Is the person competent to manage self-administration of medications, treatment procedures? Are additional resources needed?

Can the person explain how to monitor the condition (e.g., blood glucose, signs / symptoms of complications, dietary / mobility restrictions, and when to call his or her primary provider or specialist)?

Act   Contact or provide the appropriate resource (e.g., contacting a support person, home health assessment, additional teaching, printed materials).

Review   Has the problem been addressed? If not, use SBAR to communicate to the appropriate person.

Risk for Ineffective Therapeutic Regimen Management Related to Insufficient Knowledge of HIV, Its Transmission, Prevention, Treatment, Health Promotion Activities, and Community Resources

NOC

Compliance Behavior, Knowledge: Treatment Regimen, Participation in Health Care Decisions, Treatment Behavior: Illness or Injury

Goals

The goals for this diagnosis represent those associated with transition planning. Refer to the Transitional criteria.

NIC

Anticipatory Guidance, Risk Identification, Health Education, Learning Facilitation

Interventions	Rationales
1. Teach the client and family the basic pathophysiology of HIV infection and concepts of the immune system.	1. The client's understanding of HIV and its effects on the body is the basis of all further learning.
2. Explain HIV infection treatment including those decisions related to the CD4 level and viral load. These include the initiation of antiretroviral therapy and prophylaxis against certain opportunistic infections (e.g., pneumocystis carinii pneumonia [PCP], mycobacterium avium complex [MAC]).	2. Besides the symptoms the client may experience as a result of the progress of HIV infection, his or her CD4 and viral load levels are essential to the initiation of antiretroviral therapy and prophylaxis against such opportunistic infections as PCP (Bartlett & Finkbeiner, 2001; Sax, Cohen, & Kuritzkes, 2012).
3. Teach HIV routes of transmission and preventive measures / risk reduction activities.	3. The importance of efforts to prevent HIV transmission to infected persons as well as prevention of reinfection by a resistant strain of HIV or with other STIs, if a person is already infected cannot be overstated.
4. Stress the importance of close adherence to combination antiretroviral therapy to prevent viral resistance to therapy.	4. Combination antiretroviral therapy, taken as directed, offers more effective long-term suppression of HIV infection and prevents the emergence of resistant HIV strains by maintenance of a constant effective level in the bloodstream (Sax, Cohen, & Kuritzkes, 2012).
5. Teach avoidance of food / water-borne illnesses: a. Avoid raw or undercooked eggs, meat, fish. b. Use pasteurized juices and dairy products.	
6. Instruct that individuals with AIDS (e.g., CD4+ count <200 cells/μL) should avoid untreated water sources (well water, lakes, streams, swimming polls).	6. Viable oocysts (cryptosporidium) in feces can be transmitted directly through contact with infected humans or animals, particularly those with diarrhea. Oocysts can contaminate recreational water sources (e.g., swimming pools, lakes) and public water supplies and might persist despite standard chlorination. Person-to-person transmission is common, especially among sexually active men who have sex with men (MSM). Young children with cryptosporidial diarrhea might infect adults during diapering and cleaning after defecation.
7. Follow travel food precautions (e.g., raw vegetables, fruits). a. Avoid exposure to TB, varicella, salmonella, campylobacter, cryptococcus, and other organisms. b. Avoid bat droppings and dust storms. c. Use caution in homeless shelters, prisons, and day care facilities. d. Avoid ill animals and cat excreta.	7. These infections can seriously compromise the health of a person with HIV/AIDS.
8. Explain the factors that impinge on the attainment of the client's health-related goals: a. Unsafe sexual practices b. Substance abuse c. Tobacco use d. Lack of adherence to therapy e. For individual with peripheral neuropathy: • Avoid ill-fitting shoes. • Keep feet and hands cool.	8a. Sexually transmitted infection further compromises the immune system. b. Heroin, cocaine, alcohol (ETOH), marijuana, and amphetamines are all possible factors in immune suppression. Substance abuse also interferes with adherence to medication regimen (Dolin et al., 2003). c. The detrimental effects of nicotine addiction are well-known (e.g., circulatory, respiratory). d. Strict adherence to combination antiretroviral therapy is necessary to prevent subtherapeutic levels of medication conducive to the emergence of viral resistance and consequent disease progression. • Too tight shoes will cause throbbing, cramps, and irritations. Too loose shoes will not provide sufficient support. • Individuals with peripheral neuropathy report pain is worse in the summer and under the covers at night.

Interventions	Rationales
9. Provide information and encourage appropriate utilization of community resources supportive of persons living with HIV.	9. There are numerous organizations available locally and nationally for a variety of services and support to clients living with HIV and their caregivers.
10. Include significant other / family participation in all phases of client education (only with the client's consent).	
11. Instruct the client on signs and symptoms to report to health care provider: a. Visual changes b. Anorexia / weight loss c. Difficult or painful swallowing d. Persistent or severe diarrhea e. Dyspnea or resistant cough f. Headache / stiff neck g. Fever / chills / night sweats h. Fatigue	11a. Blurred vision, "floaters," and other visual complaints can signify CMV retinitis of HIV retinopathy. CMV retinitis causes blindness if not treated. b. Anorexia or weight loss can be a sign of disease progression, opportunistic disease, or HIV wasting syndrome. c. Dysphagia or odynophagia are symptomatic of esophageal candidiasis or other GI tract infection or ulceration requiring treatment. d. Besides causing dehydration and electrolyte imbalances, diarrhea in the HIV-infected client can be symptomatic of anything from a food intolerance or medication side effect to an opportunistic pathogen. e. Cough or dyspnea in the HIV-infected client can be a sign of TB, PCP, or other bacterial or opportunistic infection. f. A headache with a stiff neck can be a sign of meningitis, bacterial or otherwise. Persistent headache can indicate a central nervous system malignancy or infection, or sinusitis. g. This combination of signs and symptoms can signify HIV progression or a local systemic infection. h. Fatigue can be the first sign of infection or generalized sepsis even in the absence of other signs and symptoms.

Documentation

Client teaching
Referrals, if indicated

For Advanced / End-Stage AIDS

Risk for Caregiver Role Strain Related to AIDS-Associated Shame / Stigma, and Uncertainty About the Course of Illness and Demands on the Caregiver

NOC
Caregiver Well-Being,
Role Performance,
Care-Giving Endurance
Potential, Family
Coping, Family Integrity

NIC
Caregiver Support,
Respite Care, Coping
Enhancement, Family
Mobilization, Mutual
Goal Setting, Support
System Enhancement,
Anticipatory Guidance

Goals

The caregiver will relate a plan on how to continue social activities despite care-giving responsibilities.

Indicators

- Identify activities that are important for self.
- Relate intent to enlist the help of at least two people.

Interventions	Rationales
1. Explore the meanings and beliefs that caregivers hold regarding the client's HIV infection.	1, 2. The caregiver's feelings of shame or guilt regarding the client's HIV infection or lifestyle may prohibit optimal care-giving. The caregiver may need help in expressing his or her feelings regarding these traditionally taboo topics (Brown & Powell-Cope, 1991; Powell-Cope & Brown, 1992).
2. Explore the caregivers' prior knowledge of, and current feelings about, the client's sexual behavior or drug use.	
3. Encourage the caregiver's consistent acknowledgment of, and support for, the care-giving role.	3. AIDS caregivers often receive little to no support for their care-giving role. Their fear of discrimination and hatred toward themselves or the client stops them from disclosing their situation. This leads to feelings of isolation (Brown & Powell-Cope, 1991; Powell-Cope & Brown, 1992).
4. Assist the caregiver with anticipating the uncertainty, role changes, and unpredictability of their care-giving role, and course of the HIV infection itself.	4. Uncertainty is a common concern in caregivers of persons with life-threatening illnesses. The ability to anticipate certain events or changes can allay some anxiety for caregivers (Brown & Powell-Cope, 1991).
5. Assist the caregiver with decision-making regarding whom to tell about his or her AIDS care-giving role.	5. Fear of rejection and isolation can make the decision of whom to tell anxiety-provoking and overpowering to AIDS caregivers (Powell-Cope & Brown, 1992).
6. Assist the caregiver with the "staging" method of disclosure of the AIDS care-giving role, if they desire.	6. Disclosure by "staging" of the information is less anxiety-provoking than full disclosure (e.g., Stage I: "My son is sick." Stage II: "My son is under a doctor's care and needs to stay with me until he is back on his feet." Stage III: "My son has AIDS and needs my help.") (Powell-Cope & Brown, 1992).
7. Reinforce the caregivers' knowledge of HIV transmission, infection-control precautions for the home, and so on. Provide written information on same and be available for questions.	7. Fear of HIV transmission to self and other members of their household is a major concern of AIDS caregivers (Brown & Powell-Cope, 1991).
8. Instruct the caregiver on the signs and symptoms of burnout, and on stress-reduction techniques.	8. AIDS caregivers are subject to burnout and need help to avoid it, if possible. If burnout is inevitable, caregivers need to be able to identify it at early onset, so as to be able to plan for respite care.
9. Identify and assist—with help of community resources supportive of AIDS caregivers, such as community case management services—AIDS caregivers' support groups, day care, respite care, and the like.	9. AIDS caregivers need support that recognizes their unique needs, and support should be used to reinforce their care-giving.

Systemic Lupus Erythematosus

Systemic lupus erythematosus (SLE) is an autoimmune disorder characterized by multisystem inflammation with the generation of autoantibodies. Although the specific cause of SLE is unknown, multiple factors are associated with the development of the disease, including genetic, epigenetic, ethnic, immuno-regulatory, hormonal, and environmental factors (Bartels, 2013).

SLE can affect any organ system; SLE can affect pleural and pericardial membranes, joints, skin, blood cells, and nervous and glomerular tissue. Symptoms vary from person to person. Almost everyone with SLE has joint pain and swelling. This chronic disease follows a relapsing and remitting course.

The frequency of SLE varies by race and ethnicity, with higher rates reported in blacks, Asians, and Hispanics. The female preponderance of lupus clients is 10:1, with males. Incidence is higher in first-degree relatives. The Lupus Foundation of American estimates prevalence to be up to 1.5 million cases (Lupus Foundation of America, 2013), which likely reflects inclusion of milder forms of this disease (Bartels, 2013).

 Time Frame
Initial diagnosis
Secondary diagnosis

■■■ DIAGNOSTIC CLUSTER**

Collaborative Problems

Risk for Complications of Sepsis

Risk for Complications of Septic Arthritis

Risk for Complications of Pericarditis

Risk for Complications of Hematological abnormalities

Risk for Complications of Pulmonary Dysfunction

Risk for Complications of Neuropsychiatric Disorders

Risk for Complications of Nephritis

Risk for Complications of Sjögren Syndrome (refer to Inflammatory Joint Disease)

Nursing Diagnoses

Fatigue related to decreased mobility joint pain and effects of chronic inflammation (refer to Inflammatory Joint Disease)

Risk for Disturbed Self-Concept related to inability to achieve developmental tasks secondary to disabling condition and changes in appearance

Risk for Injury related to increased dermal vulnerability secondary to disease process

Risk for Ineffective Therapeutic Regimen Management related to insufficient knowledge of condition, rest versus activity requirements, pharmacologic therapy, signs and symptoms of complications, risk factors, and community resources

Related Care Plan

Corticosteroid Therapy

**This medical condition was not included in the validation study.

Transition Criteria

Before transition, the client or family will:

1. Identify components of a standard treatment program.
2. Relate proper use of medications.
3. Describe actions to reduce the risk of exacerbations.
4. Identify signs and symptoms that must be reported to a health care professional.

> **Transitional Risk Assessment Plan (TRAP)**
>
> Begin this plan on admission.
> Implement the Transitional Risk Assessment Plan (TRAP):
> - Refer to inside back cover.
> - Add each validated risk diagnosis to client's problem list with the risk code in ( ).
> - Refer to Unit II to the individual risk nursing diagnoses / collaborative problems for outcomes and interventions.
>
> *R: "Close coordination of care in the post-acute period, early transition follow-up care, enhanced client education and self-management training, proactive end-of-life counseling, and extending the resources and clinical expertise over time via multidisciplinary team management" can lower readmission rates and improve health outcomes (Boutwell & Hwu, 2009, p. 14).*

Collaborative Problems

Risk for Complications of Sepsis

Risk for Complications of Septic Arthritis

Risk for Complications of Pericarditis

Risk for Complications of Hematological Abnormalities

Risk for Complications of Pulmonary Dysfunction

Risk for Complications of Neuropsychiatric Disorders

Risk for Complications of Nephritis

Risk for Complications of Sjögren Syndrome

Collaborative Outcomes

The client will be monitored for early signs and symptoms of (a) sepsis, (b) septic arthritis, (c) pericarditis, (d) hematologic abnormalities, (e) pulmonary dysfunction, (f) neuropsychiatric disorders, and (g) nephritis and will receive collaborative interventions if indicated to restore physiologic stability.

Indicators of Physiologic Stability

- Oriented, calm (a, f)
- No new complaints of pain (a, b)
- No c/o of headache (f)
- No c/o chest pain, dyspnea (c)
- Intact sensation and motor function (b, c, f)
- Blood pressure >90/60 mm Hg (a, c, f)
- Pulse 60–100 beats/min (a, c, e)
- Respirations 16–20 breaths/min (a, b, c, f)
- Breath sounds throughout (a, d, f)
- Temperature 98°–99.5° F (a, b)
- Capillary refill <3 seconds (a, c, e)
- Liver function tests
  - Alanine aminotransferase (ALT) (d)
  - Aspartate aminotransferase (AST) (d)

- Bilirubin total D.1–1.2 mg/dL (d)
- Prothrombin time 9.5–12 seconds (d)
- Partial prothrombin time 20–45 seconds (d)
- Bleeding time 1–9 minutes (d)
- Stool for occult blood: negative (d)
- Arterial blood gases
  - Oxygen saturation (SaO_2) 94% to 100% (a, b, c)
  - Carbon dioxide ($PaCO_2$) 35–45 mm Hg (a, c, g)
  - Serum pH 7.35–7.45 (c)
- Renal function(g)
  - Creatinine 0.7–1.4 mg/dL
  - Blood urea nitrogen 10–20 mg/dL
  - Prealbumin
  - Urine creatinine clearance
- Complete blood count (d)
  - Hemoglobin: Male 13–18 g/dL; Female 12–16 g/dL
  - Hematocrit: Male 42% to 50%; Female 40% to 48%
  - Red blood cells: Male 4.6–5.9 million/mm³; Female 4.2–5.4 million/mm³
  - White blood cells 5000–10,800/mm³ (a, b, d)
  - Platelets 100,000–400,000/mm³
- No seizures (f)

Carp's Cues

A defective elimination of self-reactive B cells results in increase production of antibodies. These autoantibodies directly damage tissue causing inflammation in any body system (e.g., kidney, respiratory, muscular-skeletal, skin, cardiac, and central nervous system) (Porth, 2011). Thus careful assessment of all body system functioning is critical.

Interventions	Rationales
1. Monitor for septic shock and systemic inflammatory response syndrome (SIRS) (Halloran, 2009): a. Urine output >0.5 mL/kg/h b. Body temperature greater than 38° C or less than 36° C c. Heart rate greater than 90/min (decreased blood flow to brain, heart, and kidneys triggers baroreceptors and release of catecholamines, increasing heart rate / cardiac output and further increasing vasoconstriction).	1. Damage to cell membranes can provide sites for gram-positive and gram-negative organisms. a. Urine output is decreased when sodium shifts into the cells, which pulls water into cells. Decreased circulation to kidneys reduce their ability to detoxify the toxins that result from anaerobic metabolism.
d. Hyperkalemia	d. Potassium moves into the cell with the sodium, impairing nervous, cardiovascular, and muscle cell function.
e. Decreasing blood pressure f. Respiratory rate greater than 20/min	e. Movement of water into the cell causes hypovolemia. f. Anaerobic metabolism decreases circulating oxygen. The body attempts to increase oxygenation by increasing respiratory rate.
g. Hyperglycemia	g. The liver and kidneys produce more glucose in response to the release of epinephrine, norepinephrine, cortisol, and glucagon. Anaerobic metabolism reduces the effects of insulin. Insulin resistance contributes to multiple organ failure, nosocomial infection, and renal injury (Ball et al., 2007).
h. White blood cell count greater than 12,000/µL or less than 4,000/µL or presence of 10% immature neutrophils.	h. Increased white cells indicate an infectious process.

CLINICAL ALERT
- Immediately report any changes in vital signs or urine output as outlined above.

(continued)

Interventions	Rationales
2. If sepsis occurs, refer to risk for complications of sepsis in Unit II for additional intervention.	
3. Monitor for signs and symptoms of pulmonary complications such as including pleurisy, pleural effusion, pneumonitis, pulmonary hypertension, and interstitial lung disease: a. Shortness of breath or dyspnea may be due to many causes. Pulmonary embolism, lupus pneumonitis, chronic lupus interstitial lung disease, pulmonary hypertension, complement-mediated pulmonary leuko-aggregation, alveolar hemorrhage, or infection may be related to lupus disease. b. Dyspnea c. Cough d. Hemoptysis (blood in sputum) e. Chest pain f. Tachycardia, tachypnea g. Decreased breath sounds	3. SLE may lead to multiple pulmonary complications, which may manifest acutely or slowly. Pleurisy with pleuritic chest pain with or without pleural effusions is the most common feature of acute pulmonary involvement in SLE (Bartels, 2013). Thirty percent of individuals with SLE have pulmonary involvement of lung inflammation (pneumonitis) and changes in membrane transfer capability, leading to fluid leakage into the interpleural space (Porth, 2011). **CLINICAL ALERT** • Hemoptysis may indicate diffuse alveolar hemorrhage, a rare, acute, life-threatening pulmonary complication of SLE (Bartels, 2013).
4. Monitor for pericarditis: a. Chest pain beneath left clavicle and in the neck and left scapular region; aggravated by movement or deep breaths, relieved by leaning forward b. Pericardial rub c. Temperature >101° F	4. Excessive autoantibodies combine with antigens to form immune complexes. These complexes are deposited in vascular and tissue surfaces, triggering an inflammatory response and eventually local tissue injury. Thus, SLE can affect any organ system (Porth, 2011).
5. Monitor for hematologic disorders: a. Hemolytic anemia b. Leukopenia c. Lymphopenia d. Thrombocytopenia	5. Antibodies against red blood cells result in hemolytic anemia. Antibodies against platelets result in thrombocytopenia. B-lymphocyte production is regulated by a balance of CD4+ and CD8+ lymphocytes (T cells). This balance is disrupted by SLE (Porth, 2011).
6. Teach the client to report purpura and ecchymosis.	6. These are manifestations of platelet deficiencies.
7. Monitor for lupus nephritis (Hahn et al., 2012): a. Increasing serum creatinine proteinuria of 1.0 g per 24 hours (either 24-hour urine specimens or spot protein / creatinine ratios are acceptable). b. Elevated B/P	7. Renal involvement occur in one-half to two-thirds of individuals with SLE (Porth, 2011).
8. Monitor for neurologic / psychiatric disorders (Bartels, 2013): a. Seizures b. Fluctuating altered consciousness c. Psychosis may manifest as paranoia or hallucinations. d. Delirium **CLINICAL ALERT** • New onset delirium requires urgent evaluation.	8. The pathologic cause of CNS symptoms is unclear. They are thought to result from acute vasculitis that impedes blood flow, causing clots, hemorrhage, or both. Seizures can be related to renal failure. a. Seizures related to SLE may be generalized or partial and may precipitate status epilepticus. d. Delirium may be caused by CNS vasculitis, encephalopathy, cerebritis, or the manifestations previously called organic brain syndrome or aseptic meningitis, myelopathy, optic neuropathy, or other demyelinating disorder.

Clinical Alert Report

Prior to providing care, advise ancillary staff / student to report the following to the professional nurse assigned to the client:

- Any changes in mental status such as orientation, agitation, lethargy, confusion
- Blood pressure, pulse, or respirations outside of prescribed limits. See "Indicators." Individual parameters may vary depending on client's medications
- Temperature (oral) 1°–2° F over baseline
- Difficulty breathing or new onset of shortness of breath
- New onset of pain (chest, joint, head)
- Changes in urine from baseline.
- Chills, fever, temp >100.5° F
- New onset inability to move the limb or joint
- Reports of increased pain in the affected joint, especially with movement
- Increased swelling (increased fluid within the joint)
- Red and warm joint
- Chest pain
- C/o shortness of breath

Related Physician / NP Prescribed Interventions (Bartels, 2013)

Medications

Biologic DMARD therapy (Belimumab), cyclophosphamide, nonsteroidal anti-inflammatory agents, cytotoxic agents, corticosteroids nonbiologic DMARDS (e.g., hydroxychloroquine, azathioprine, methotrexate mycophenolate mofetil)

Laboratory Studies

Complete blood count with differential, BUN, serum creatinine, urinalysis, 24-hour urine, creatinine clearance, autoantibody tests for SLE (antinuclear antibody titer [ANA]), antibody to double-stranded DNA antigen (anti-ds DNA), additional evaluation of antibodies to dsDNA, complement, and ANA subtypes such as Sm, SSA, SSB, and ribonucleoprotein (RNP) (often called the ENA panel), as well as screening anticardiolipin antibodies, lupus anticoagulant, and +/- beta-2 glycoprotein antibodies.

Therapies

Plasmapheresis, stem-cell transplantation, immunoablative therapy, joint replacement

Diagnostic Studies

EEG, chest x-ray, brain magnetic resonance imaging (MRI) / magnetic resonance angiography (MRA) (to evaluate for central nervous system [CNS] lupus), white-matter changes, vasculitis, or stroke, EKG, echocardiogram (to assess for pericardial effusion, pulmonary hypertension, or endocarditis), arthrocentesis (with joint effusions), chest x-rays, computed tomography (CT) (to assess for pneumonitis, pulmonary emboli, and alveolar hemorrhage), lumbar puncture (may be performed to exclude infection with fever or neurologic symptoms), renal biopsy (to confirm the presence of lupus nephritis), skin biopsy (to diagnose SLE or unusual rashes)

Documentation

Vital signs
Peripheral pulses
Complaints
Responses to treatment

Nursing Diagnoses

Risk for Injury Related to Increased Dermal Vulnerability Secondary to Disease Process

NOC
Risk Control

Goal

The client will identify causative factors that may increase disease activity (e.g., sun exposure).

NIC
Fall Prevention,
Environmental
Management: Safety,
Health Education,
Surveillance: Safety, Risk
Identification

Indicators

- Identify measures to reduce damage to skin by the sun.
- Identify strategies to manage skin damage should it occur.
- Identify signs and symptoms of cellulitis.

Interventions	Rationales
1. Explain to the client the relationship between sun exposure and disease activity. Identify strategies to limit sun exposure: a. Avoid sun exposure between 10 a.m. and 2 p.m. b. Use sunscreen (15 SPF); reapply after swimming or exercise. c. Select lightweight, long-sleeved clothing and wide-brimmed hats.	1. Through an unknown mechanism, exposure to ultraviolet light can precipitate an exacerbation of both skin and systemic diseases. The client's understanding of this relationship should encourage him or her to limit sun exposure.
2. Explain the need to avoid fluorescent lighting or a too-hot stove.	2. Like sunlight, fluorescent lighting produces ultraviolet rays.
3. Teach the client to keep skin ulcers clean and skin moist.	3. Skin changes associated with SLE increase the vulnerability to injury. Reducing bacteria on the skin reduces risk of infection. Dry skin is more susceptible to breakdown.
4. Teach the client to recognize signs and symptoms of vasculitis and to report them promptly to a health care professional such as tenderness, swelling, warmth, and redness.	4. Vascular inflammation of the smallest blood vessels, capillaries, and venules can cause occlusion.

Documentation

Skin assessment

TRANSITION TO HOME / COMMUNITY CARE

If indicated, review the risk diagnoses identified for this individual on admission:

- Is the person still at risk?
- Can the family reduce the risks?
- Is the person at higher risk at home?
- Is a Home Health Nurse assessment needed?
- Refer to transition planner / case manager / social service.
- When is this person scheduled for follow-up with primary provider? Specialists? Record dates of appointments.
- Complete a medication reconciliation prior to transition. Refer to index.

STAR   **Stop**

Think   Is this person at risk for injury, falls, medical complications, and / or inability to care for self (activities of daily living)?

Is there a support person available?

Is the person competent to manage self-administration of medications, treatment procedures? Are additional resources needed?

Can the person explain how to monitor the condition (e.g., blood glucose, signs / symptoms of complications, dietary / mobility restrictions, and when to call his or her primary provider or specialist)?

Act   Contact or provide the appropriate resource (e.g., contacting a support person, home health assessment, additional teaching, printed materials).

Review   Has the problem been addressed? If not, use SBAR to communicate to the appropriate person.

Risk for Ineffective Self-Health Management Related to Insufficient Knowledge of Condition, Rest Versus Activity Requirements, Pharmacologic Therapy, Signs and Symptoms of Complications, Risk Factors, and Community Resources

NOC

Compliance Behavior, Knowledge: Treatment Regimen, Participation in Health Care Decisions, Treatment Behavior: Illness or Injury

Goals

The goals for this diagnosis represent those associated with transition planning. See the transition criteria.

NIC

Anticipatory Guidance, Risk Identification, Learning Facilitation, Support Group

Interventions	Rationales
1. Instruct clients with SLE to seek medical care for evaluation of new symptoms, including fever. Advise clients regarding heightened risks for infection and cardiovascular disease. Educate clients with SLE regarding aggressive lipid and blood pressure goals to minimize the risk of coronary artery disease.	
2. Instruct clients with SLE to avoid exposure to sunlight and ultraviolet light. Also, encourage them to receive nonlive vaccines during stable periods of disease, to quit smoking, and to carefully plan pregnancies.	

3. Explain SLE in terms appropriate to client's and family's levels of understanding. Discuss the following:
  a. The inflammatory process
  b. Organ systems at risk of involvement (see Potential Complications in this care plan for more information)
  c. Chronic nature of disease (remission / exacerbation)
	3. Understanding may help to improve compliance and self-manage.

4. Teach the client to take medications properly and to report symptoms of side effects.	4. Knowledge of and proper adherence to the medication regimen can help to reduce complications and detect side effects early.
5. Advise to promptly report s/s of infections (e.g., fever, dyspnea).	5. The chronic steroids prescribed to clients also place them at increased risk for atypical infections.

(*continued*)

Interventions	*Rationales*
6. Teach the need to balance activity and rest (refer to the Inflammatory Joint Disease Care Plan for specific strategies).	6. The chronic fatigue associated with SLE necessitates strategies to prevent exhaustion and maintain the highest level of independent functioning (Albano & Wallace, 2001).
7. Teach the need for meticulous, gentle mouth care.	7. Vasculitis can increase the risk of mouth lesions and injury.
8. Teach warning signs of a flare and to contact their specialist or PCP: a. Increased fatigue b. Pain c. Rash d. Fever e. Abdominal discomfort f. Headache g. Dizziness	8. Early treatment of a flare can reduce the severity of the flare and damage to joints, etc.
9. Teach the client to report signs and symptoms of complications: a. Chest pain and dyspnea b. Fever c. Ecchymoses d. Edema e. Decreased urine output, concentrated urine. f. Nausea and vomiting	9. Early detection of complications enables prompt interventions to prevent serious tissue damage or dysfunction. a. Chest pain and dyspnea may indicate pericarditis or pleural effusion. b. Fever may indicate infection. c. Ecchymoses may indicate a clotting disorder. d. Edema may signal renal or hepatic insufficiency. e. These urine changes may indicate renal insufficiency. f. Nausea and vomiting may indicate GI dysfunction.

> **CLINICAL ALERT**
> - Instruct the individual and family to be alert to new signs and symptoms.
> - Advise the client that he or she knows his or her chronic disease and to seek immediate advice / care when condition changes.
> - If this is a new diagnosis, advise to consult with PCP with any new complaints.

Interventions	*Rationales*
10. Explain the relationship of stress and autoimmune disorders. Discuss stress management techniques: a. Progressive relaxation b. Guided imagery c. Regular exercise (e.g., walking, swimming) d. Refer the client to a counselor and psychiatrist, as appropriate	10. Stress may be associated with an increase in disease activity. Stress management techniques can reduce the stress and fatigue associated with unmanaged conflicts (Albano & Wallace, 2001).
11. Discuss complementary therapies that may help to reduce inflammation of joints and tissues (Shirato, 2005) such as massage, acupuncture.	11. Studies have shown benefits (Shirato, 2005).
12. Refer to appropriate community resources: a. Arthritis Foundation, http://www.arthritis.org b. Lupus Foundation of America, http://www.lupus.org/ c. National Institute of Arthritis and Musculoskeletal and Skin Diseases (NIAMS), http://www.niams.nih.gov/	12. Additional self-help information may be very useful for self-care. Provide excellent support and education for the client and family.

Documentation

Client teaching
Referrals, if indicated

Neoplastic Disorders

Cancer: Initial Diagnosis

Cancer involves a disturbance in normal cell growth in which abnormal cells arise from normal cells, reproduce rapidly, and infiltrate tissues, lymph, and blood vessels. The destruction caused by cancer depends on its site, whether or not it metastasizes, its obstructive effects, and its effects on the body's defense system (e.g., nutrition, hematopoiesis). Cancer is classified according to the cell of origin: malignant tumors from epithelial tissue are called *carcinomas* and those from connective tissue are known as *sarcomas*. Treatment varies depending on classification, cancer stage, and other factors.

Time Frame
Initial diagnosis

■■■ DIAGNOSTIC CLUSTER

Nursing Diagnoses

▲ Anxiety related to unfamiliar hospital environment, uncertainty about outcomes, feelings of helplessness and hopelessness, and insufficient knowledge about cancer and treatment

△ Risk for Disturbed Self-Concept related to changes in lifestyle, role responsibilities, and appearance

▲ Interrupted Family Processes related to fears associated with recent cancer diagnosis, disruptions associated with treatments, financial problems, and uncertain future

△ Decisional Conflict related to treatment modality choices

▲ Grieving related to potential loss of body function and the perceived effects of cancer on lifestyle

△ Risk for Spiritual Distress related to conflicts centering on the meaning of life, cancer, spiritual beliefs, and death (refer to Palliative Care Plan)

Related Care Plans

Chemotherapy

Radiation Therapy

▲ This diagnosis was reported to be monitored for or managed frequently (75% to 100%).
△ This diagnosis was reported to be monitored for or managed often (50% to 74%).

Transition Criteria

Before transition, the client or family will:
1. Relate the intent to share concerns with a trusted confidante.
2. Describe early signs of family dysfunction.
3. Identify signs and symptoms that must be reported to a health care professional.
4. Identify available community resources.

Collaborative Problems

The collaborative problems caused by cancer depend on its site, whether it metastasizes, its obstructive effects, and its effects on the body's defense system (e.g., white blood count, renal insufficiency). For example, cancer of the breast can metastasize to the brain, lung, liver, and bone. In this case, the collaborative problems Risk for Complications of Increased Intracranial Pressure, Risk for Complications of Hepatic Insufficiency, Risk for Complications of Respiratory Insufficiency, and Risk for Complications of Pathological Fractures would be appropriate. Refer to the collaborative problems in Unit II for specific collaborative problems.

Nursing Diagnoses

Anxiety Related to Unfamiliar Hospital Environment, Uncertainty about Outcomes, Feelings of Helplessness and Hopelessness, and Insufficient Knowledge about Cancer and Treatment

NOC
Anxiety Self-Control

Goal

The client will report increased psychological comfort.

NIC
Anxiety Reduction,
Anticipatory Guidance

Indicators

- Share concerns regarding the cancer diagnosis.
- Identify one strategy that reduces anxiety.

Interventions	Rationales
1. Provide opportunities for the client and family members to share feelings (anger, guilt, loss, and pain): 　a. Initiate frequent contacts and provide an atmosphere that promotes calm and relaxation. 　b. Convey a nonjudgmental attitude and listen attentively. 　c. Explore own feelings and behaviors.	1. Frequent contact by caregiver indicates acceptance and may facilitate trust. The client may be hesitant to approach the staff / student because of negative self-concept. The nurse should not make assumptions about a client's or family member's reaction; validating the client's particular fears and concerns helps to increase awareness. The nurse should be aware of how the client and family are reacting and how their reactions are influencing the nurse's feeling and behavior (Barsevick, Much, & Sweeney, 2000).
2. Encourage an open discussion of cancer, including experiences of others and potential for a cure or control of the disease.	2. The nurse who can talk openly about life after a cancer diagnosis offers encouragement and hope.
3. Explain hospital routines and reinforce the physician's / NP's explanations of scheduled tests and proposed treatment plan. Focus on what the client can expect.	3. Accurate descriptions of sensations and procedures help to ease anxiety and fear associated with the unknown (Christman & Kirchoff, 1992).
4. Identify those at risk for unsuccessful adjustment: 　a. Poor ego strength 　b. Ineffective problem-solving ability 　c. Poor motivation 　d. External focus of control 　e. Poor overall health 　f. Lack of positive support systems 　g. Unstable economic status 　h. Rejection of counseling (Shipes, 1987)	4. A client identified at risk may need referrals for counseling. Successful adjustment is influenced by factors such as previous coping success, achievement of developmental tasks, extent to which the disorder and treatment interfere with goal-directed activity, sense of self-determination and control, and realistic perception of the disorder.
5. Convey a sense of hope.	5. Clients who are reacting to a new cancer diagnosis must begin with hope. Hope is necessary to cope with the rigors of treatment (Barsevick, Much, & Sweeney, 2000).
6. Promote physical activity and exercise. Assist the client to determine the level of activity advisable.	6. Physical activity provides diversion and a sense of normalcy. Clients who exercise may improve their quality of life. Refer to Getting Started to Increase Activity on the Point at http://thePoint.lww.com/Carpenito6e.

Documentation

Present emotional status
Interventions utilized

Risk for Disturbed Self-Concept Related to Changes in Lifestyle, Role Responsibilities, and Appearance

NOC
Quality of Life, Depression Level, Coping, Self-Esteem

Goal

The client will relate the intent to continue previous lifestyle as much as possible.

NIC
Hope Instillation, Counseling, Coping Enhancement

Indicators

- Communicate feelings about possible changes.
- Participate in self-care.

Interventions	Rationales
1. Encourage the client to express feelings and thoughts about the following: a. Condition, Progress, Prognosis, Effects on lifestyle, Support system, Treatments	1. Encouraging the client to share feelings can provide a safe outlet for fears and frustration and can increase self-awareness.
2. Provide reliable information and clarify any misconceptions.	2. Misconceptions can needlessly increase anxiety and damage self-concept.
3. Encourage visitors.	3. Frequent visits by support persons can help the client feel that she or he is still a worthwhile, acceptable person; this should promote a positive self-concept.
4. Help the client to identify ways of integrating the cancer experience into her or his life, rather than allowing cancer to take it over.	4. The nurse can help the client learn how to balance relationships and preserve the family system. The experience of cancer is different for everyone. What is vitally important to one person may be inconsequential to another (Stevens, 1992).
5. Allow the client's family and support persons to share their feelings regarding the diagnosis and actual or anticipated effects (anger, rage, depression, or guilt).	5. Cancer can have a negative impact on the client's family financially, socially, and emotionally. All family members are affected by a cancer diagnosis, including children. This stressor on the children must be addressed; support groups are available (Su & Ryan-Wenger, 2007).
6. Assist with management of alopecia as necessary: a. Explain when the client should expect to begin to lose hair (usually within 2–3 weeks of initiation of therapy) and when hair would begin to regrow (usually 4–6 weeks after discontinuation of therapy). b. Suggest cutting long hair to minimize fallout. c. Suggest resources for wigs and hairpieces. d. Discuss measures to reduce hair loss in low-dose therapy (e.g., wash hair only twice a week, use a mild shampoo, or avoid brushing). e. Encourage good grooming, hygiene, and other measures to enhance appearance (e.g., makeup, manicures, and new clothes).	6. Embarrassment from alopecia can contribute to isolation and negative self-concept.
7. Refer an at-risk client for professional counseling.	7. Some clients may need follow-up therapy to aid with effective adjustment.

Documentation

Present emotional status

Interrupted Family Processes Related to Fears Associated with Recent Cancer Diagnosis, Disruptions Associated with Treatments, Financial Problems, and Uncertain Future

NOC

Family Coping, Family Normalization, Parenting Performance

Goal

The family will maintain a functional system of mutual support.

NIC

Family Involvement Promotion, Coping Enhancement, Family Integrity Promotion

Indicators

- Verbalize feelings regarding the diagnosis and prognosis.
- Identify signs of family dysfunction.
- Identify appropriate resources to seek, when needed.

Interventions	Rationales
1. Explore family members' perceptions of the situation. Explore their fears.	1. Verbalization can provide an opportunity for clarification and validation of feelings and concerns; this contributes to family unity. Spouses report increased anxiety prior to transition from hospital and anger at the client for ego-centricity during home-care period.
2. Determine if present coping mechanisms are effective.	2. If needed, refer families to community resources (e.g., counseling). This can help to maintain the existing family structure and its function as a supportive unit. Cancer challenges one's values and beliefs; this can result in changed cognitive, affective, and behavioral responses.
3. Encourage the family to call on its social network (e.g., friends, relatives, church members) for emotional and other support.	3. Outside assistance may help to reduce the perception that the family must "go it alone."
4. Identify dysfunctional coping mechanisms: a. Substance abuse b. Continued denial c. Exploitation of one or more family members d. Separation or avoidance. Refer for counseling, as necessary.	4. A family with a history of unsuccessful coping may need additional resources. A family with unresolved conflicts before diagnosis is at risk.
5. Direct to community agencies and other sources of assistance (e.g., financial, housekeeping, direct care, childcare), as needed.	

Documentation

Referrals if indicated

Decisional Conflict Related to Treatment Modality Choices

NOC

Decision-Making, Information Processing, Participation in Health Care Decisions

Goal

The client and family members will:

1. Relate the advantages and disadvantages of choices.
2. Share their fears and concerns regarding a decision.
3. Make an informed choice.

NIC

Decision-Making Support, Learning Facilitation, Health System Guidance, Client Rights Protection

Interventions	Rationales
1. Provide, reinforce, and clarify information about the diagnosis, treatment options, and alternative therapies.	1. The client and family need specific and accurate information to make an informed decision. Cancer gives a sense of being out of control. Exploration of all options may help the client to regain a sense of control (Thome, Dykes, Gunnars, & Hallberg, 2003).
2. Give the client and family members opportunities to share feelings and concerns regarding the decision.	2. Conflict is more intense when the decision has potentially negative impacts or when conflicting opinions exist. Anxiety and fear have a negative impact on decision-making ability. Providing opportunities to share feelings and concerns can help to reduce anxiety (Thome et al., 2003).
3. Ensure that the client and family clearly understand what is involved in each treatment alternative.	3. Informed decisions support a person's right to self-determination. Clients must be prepared for the emotional and physical problems they will face.
4. Assure the client that he or she does not have to abide by decisions that others make, but can choose for him- or herself, as appropriate. Discourage family members and others from undermining the client's confidence in his or her decision-making ability.	4. Each client has the right to make his or her own decisions and to expect respect from others (Thome et al., 2003).

STAR

Stop

Think Does individual understand treatment options? Benefits? Risks?

Act Contact the physician/NP.

> **Situation:** I am calling about Mr. Aidol. In discussing his treatment decisions, he has asked some questions about his choices.
>
> **Background:** With his new diagnosis of pancreatic cancer, he is questioning if surgery is the best option.
>
> **Assessment:** I think the problem is that Mr. Aidol does not understand the risks / benefits of surgery and other treatment options as chemotherapy, radiation, palliative care.
>
> **Recommendation:** I would recommend that you (his oncologist) meet with him and his family to discuss all the treatment options available.

Review Has the problem been addressed? If not, use SBAR to communicate to the manager, department head.

Documentation

Progress notes
Dialogues

Grieving Related to Potential Loss of Body Function and the Perceived Effects of Cancer on Lifestyle

NOC
Coping, Family
Coping, Psychosocial
Adjustment: Life
Change

NIC
Family Support, Grief
Work Facilitation,
Coping Enhancement,
Anticipatory Guidance,
Emotional Support

Goal

The client and family members will:

1. Express grief.
2. Describe the personal meaning of the loss.
3. Report an intent to discuss his or her feelings with significant others.

Interventions	Rationales
1. Provide opportunities for the client and family members to express feelings, discuss the loss openly, and explore the personal meaning of the loss. Explain that grief is a common and healthy reaction.	1. A cancer diagnosis typically gives rise to feelings of powerlessness, anger, profound sadness, and other grief responses. Open and honest discussions can help the client and family members accept and cope with the situation and their responses to it.
2. Encourage the use of positive coping strategies that have proved successful in the past.	2. Positive coping strategies aid in acceptance and problem-solving.
3. Encourage the client to express positive self-attributes.	3. Focusing on positive attributes increases self-acceptance and acceptance of the diagnosis.
4. Implement measures to support the family and promote cohesiveness: a. Help family members acknowledge their losses. b. Explain the grieving process. c. Encourage the client to verbalize her or his feelings. d. Allow participation in care to promote comfort. e. Encourage discussing the significance of family relationships.	4. Family cohesiveness is important in client support.

5. Promote grief work with each response:
a. Denial:
  • Encourage acceptance of the situation; do not reinforce denial by giving false reassurance.
  • Promote hope through assurances of care, comfort, and support.
  • Explain the use of denial by one family member to other members.
  • Do not push a client to move past denial until he or she is emotionally ready.
b. Isolation:
  • Convey acceptance by encouraging expressions of grief.
  • Promote open, honest communication to encourage sharing.
  • Reinforce the client's self-worth by providing privacy, when desired.
  • Encourage socialization, as feasible (e.g., support groups, church activities).
c. Depression:
  • Reinforce the client's self-esteem.
  • Employ empathetic sharing and acknowledge grief.
  • Identify the degree of depression and develop appropriate strategies.
	5. Grieving involves profound emotional responses; interventions depend on the particular response.

Interventions	Rationales

d. Anger:
  - Explain to other family members that anger represents an attempt to control the environment; it stems from frustration at the inability to control the disease.
  - Encourage verbalization of anger.

e. Guilt:
  - Acknowledge the client's expressed self-image.
  - Encourage identification of the relationship's positive aspects.
  - Avoid arguing and participating in the client's system of "I should have . . ." and "I shouldn't have . . ."

f. Fear:
  - Focus on the present and maintain a safe and secure environment.
  - Help the client explore reasons for and meanings of the fears.

g. Rejection:
  - Provide reassurance by explaining what is happening.
  - Explain this response to other family members.

h. Hysteria:
  - Reduce environmental stressors (e.g., limit personnel).
  - Provide a safe, private area in which to express grief.
  - Contact physician/NP.

6. Act as a guide to the client through the grief experience by understanding her or his needs and providing help where needed (Bushkin, 1993).

7. Validate and reflect impressions with the client.

6, 7. It is important to realize that clients with cancer often have their own realities that may differ from the nurse's view (Yates, 1993).

Documentation

Progress notes
Present emotional status
Interventions
Response to nursing interventions

TRANSITION TO HOME / COMMUNITY CARE

If indicated, review the risk diagnoses identified for this individual on admission:
- Is the person still at risk?
- Can the family reduce the risks?
- Is the person at higher risk at home?
- Is a Home Health Nurse assessment needed?
- Refer to transition planner / case manager / social service.
- When is this person scheduled for follow-up with primary provider? Specialists? Record dates of appointments.
- Complete a medication reconciliation prior to transition. Refer to index.

STAR   **Stop**

Think   Is this person at risk for injury, falls, medical complications, and / or inability to care for self (activities of daily living)?

Is there a support person available?

Is the person competent to manage self-administration of medications, treatment procedures? Are additional resources needed?

Can the person explain how to monitor the condition (e.g., blood glucose, signs / symptoms of complications, dietary / mobility restrictions, and when to call his or her primary provider or specialist)?

Act   Contact or provide the appropriate resource (e.g., contacting a support person, home health assessment, additional teaching, printed materials).

Review   Has the problem been addressed? If not, use SBAR to communicate to the appropriate person.

Risk for Ineffective Self-Health Management Related to Insufficient Knowledge of Follow-up Care, Diagnostic Test Scheduled and Community Resources

Refer to specific care plans such as Breast Surgery, Colostomy Surgery.

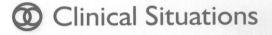

ⓓ Clinical Situations

Alcohol Dependency

More than 7 percent of the American population aged 18 and up have a drinking problem; this is nearly 13.8 million Americans, and 8.1 million of them are alcoholic (CDC, 2013). In addition, several million more partake in risky alcohol consumption that could potentially lead to abuse, and over three million American teenagers aged 14 to 17 have an alcohol problem (CDC, 2013).

It is estimated that one in every five hospitalized persons is an alcohol abuser (McKinley, 2005). Clinically, only one of every 10 alcoholics is diagnosed, and clinicians do not ask about alcohol use unless it is obvious. It is critical to identify people who abuse alcohol to prevent potentially fatal withdrawal symptoms. Surgical clients are at risk for alcohol withdrawal syndrome because of the preprocedural and postoperative fasting. Most signs and symptoms are caused by the rapid removal of the depressant effects of alcohol on the central nervous system. The focus of medical and nursing care is to prevent, not to observe for, the complications of alcohol withdrawal (Gordon, 2006). Prevention includes aggressive management of early withdrawal and close monitoring of the client's response.

 Time Frame
Secondary diagnosis

▪▪▪ DIAGNOSTIC CLUSTER**

Collaborative Problems

Risk for Complications of Delirium Tremens

Risk for Complications of Autonomic Hyperactivity

Risk for Complications of Seizures

Risk for Complications of Alcohol Hallucinosis

Risk for Complications of Hypovolemia (refer to Risk for Complications of Hypovolemia in Unit II)

Risk for Complications of Hypoglycemia (refer to Risk for Complications of Hypo / Hyperglycemia in Unit II)

Nursing Diagnoses

Risk for Violence related to (examples) impulsive behavior, disorientation, tremors, or impaired judgment

Ineffective Denial related to Acknowledgment of Alcohol Abuse or Dependency

Risk for Ineffective Self-Health Management related to insufficient knowledge of condition, treatments available, at risk situations, and community resources

**This clinical situation was not included in the validation study.

Transition Criteria

Before transition, the client or family will:

1. Recognize that alcoholism is a disease.
2. Acknowledge the negative effects of alcoholism in their lives.
3. Identify community resources available for treatment of alcoholism.

> **Transitional Risk Assessment Plan (TRAP)**
>
> Begin this plan on admission.
> Implement the Transitional Risk Assessment Plan (TRAP):
> * Refer to inside back cover.
> * Add each validated risk diagnosis to client's problem list with the risk code in ( ).
> * Refer to Unit II to the individual risk nursing diagnoses / collaborative problems for outcomes and interventions.
>
>   *R: "Close coordination of care in the post-acute period, early transition follow-up care, enhanced client education and self-management training, proactive end-of-life counseling, and extending the resources and clinical expertise over time via multidisciplinary team management" can lower readmission rates and improve health outcomes (Boutwell & Hwu, 2009, p. 14).*

Collaborative Problems

Risk for Complications of Delirium Tremens

Risk for Complications of Autonomic Hyperactivity

Risk for Complications of Seizures

Risk for Complications of Alcohol Hallucinosis

Risk for Complications of Hypovolemia

Risk for Complications of Hypoglycemia

Collaborative Outcomes

The client will be monitored for early signs and symptoms of (a) delirium tremens, (b) autonomic hyperactivity, (c) seizures, (d) alcohol hallucinosis, (e) hypovolemia, and (f) hypoglycemia, and will receive collaborative interventions if indicated to restore physiologic stability.

Indicators of Physiologic Stability

* No seizure activity (a, b, c)
* Calm, oriented (a, b, d)
* Temperature 98°–99.5° F (d)
* Pulse 60–100 beats/min (a, b, d)
* BP >90/60, <140/90 mm Hg (a, b, d)
* No reports of hallucinations (a, d)

Carp's Cues

It is estimated that one in five patients admitted to a hospital suffers from an alcohol use disorder (AUD) such as alcohol abuse or dependence (Doty et al., 2012). It is very common for individuals and their families to deny or underreport alcohol consumption. The nurse must routinely assess all individuals and their families for patterns of alcohol consumption. Five percent (5%) of individuals with alcohol withdrawal progress to delirium tremors; 5% of individuals with delirium tremors die.

Interventions	Rationales
1. Carefully attempt to determine if the client abuses alcohol on admission and during routine encounters. Consult with the family regarding perception of alcohol consumption. Explain why accurate information is necessary.	1. "In patients who are physically dependent on alcohol, the central nervous system adapts to the presence of alcohol and loses the ability to function normally in its absence. Signs and symptoms of AWS reflect declining blood alcohol levels. These usually appear within a few hours to a few days after cessation of alcohol consumption, although in some patients symptoms may develop up to 10 days after the last drink" (Doty et al., 2012, p. 2).
2. In a matter-of-fact manner, obtain history of drinking patterns from the client or significant others (Kappas-Larson & Lathrop, 1993): a. When did the client have his or her last drink? b. How much was consumed on that day? c. On how many days of the last 30 did the client consume alcohol? d. What was the average intake? e. What was the most consumed?	2. Alcoholics tend to underestimate alcohol consumed; therefore, multiply the amount a man tells you by two to three drinks and for a woman by four to five drinks (Smith-DiJulio, 2001).
3. Determine the client's attitude toward drinking by asking the CAGE questions: a. Have you ever thought you should cut down your drinking? b. Have you ever been annoyed by criticism of your drinking? c. Have you ever felt guilty about your drinking? d. Do you drink in the morning (i.e., "Eye-opener") (Ewing, 1984)?	3. These questions can be used to identify possible defensiveness and similar attitudes about drinking.
4. Obtain history of previous withdrawals, as applicable: a. Delirium tremens: Time of onset, manifestation b. Seizures: Time of onset, type **CLINICAL ALERT** • When surgery is anticipated, notify the surgeon / anesthesiologist / nurse anesthetist if alcohol abuse is confirmed or suspected. • Individuals with alcohol-related health problems (e.g., malnourished, hepatic disorders, immune deficiency, withdrawal) are at risk for perioperative and postoperative complications.	4. Withdrawal occurs between 6 and 96 hours after cessation of drinking. Withdrawal can occur in individuals who are considered "social drinkers" (6 ounces of alcohol daily for 3 to 4 weeks). Withdrawal patterns may resemble those of previous episodes. Seizure patterns, unlike previous episodes, may indicate another underlying pathology (Doty et al., 2012).

Interventions	Rationales

"Chronic alcohol use increases dose requirements for general anesthetic agents. These increased anesthetic requirements can exacerbate the risk of cardiovascular instability in patients who may be suffering from cardiomyopathy, heart failure, or dehydration. Chronic heavy alcohol use is associated with a 2–5-fold increase in postoperative complications. Depletion of coagulation factors and thrombocytopaenia increase the incidence of postoperative bleeding. Immune deficiency as a result of leucopoenia and altered cytokine production increase the risk of postoperative infection (especially, surgical wounds, respiratory system, or urinary tract). Electrolyte disturbances or periods of relative hypotension exacerbate the risk. Alcohol use is an independent risk factor for the development of acute confusion or delirium after operation."

Interventions	Rationales
5. Obtain complete history of prescription and nonprescription drugs taken.	5. Benzodiazepine or barbiturate withdrawal may mimic alcohol withdrawal and will complicate the picture. Substance abusers tend to cross-abuse substances (Doty et al., 2012).
6. Monitor all persons suspected of, or identified as, risk for alcohol withdrawal syndrome for early signs and symptoms (Clinical Institute Withdrawal Assessment of Alcohol Scale, McKinley, 2005): a. Do you feel sick to your stomach? b. Do you feel nervous? (Observe for restlessness, sweating.) c. Do you feel any pins-and-needles sensations? Any itching? d. Is the light too bright? Are sounds too loud? Are you afraid? e. Observe for tremors when the client's arms are extended and the fingers spread wide.	6. Identification of early signs and symptoms of central nervous system impairment can prompt early interventions and prevent mortality. Minor alcohol withdrawal symptoms often appear 6 to 12 hours after alcohol cessation, sometimes while clients still have a measurable blood alcohol level (Doty et al., 2012).
7. Consult with physician / NP regarding the client's risk and the initiation of benzodiazepine therapy, with dosage determined by assessment findings.	7. Benzodiazepine requirements in alcohol withdrawal are highly variable and client-specific. Fixed schedules may oversedate or undersedate (Doty et al., 2012).
8. Observe for desired effects of benzodiazepine therapy: a. Relief from withdrawal symptoms b. Client sleeping peacefully, but can be roused	8. Benzodiazepine is the drug of choice in controlling withdrawal symptoms. Neuroleptics cause hypotension and lower seizure threshold. Barbiturates may effectively control symptoms of withdrawal but have no advantages over benzodiazepines (Doty et al., 2012).
9. Monitor for alcohol hallucinosis: a. Visual, auditory, or tactile hallucinations	9a. "Between 12 and 24 hours after alcohol cessation, some patients may experience visual, auditory, or tactile hallucinations which usually end within 48 hours. Most patients are aware that the unusual sensations aren't real" (Doty et al., 2012).

(continued)

Interventions	Rationales

10. Monitor for withdrawal delirium or delirium tremens:
  a. Severe autonomic hyperactivity (hypertension, diaphoresis, fever tachycardia, tachypnea, tremors, seizures)
  b. Neuropsychiatric signs and symptoms (severe anxiety or agitation, hallucinations, confusion, disorientation, impaired attention)
	10. The most severe form of alcohol withdrawal is delirium tremens (DTs), characterized by altered mental status and severe autonomic hyperactivity that may lead to cardiovascular collapse (Doty et al., 2012). These signs and symptoms occur 48–96 hours after the last drink. If untreated, death can occur from respiratory and cardiovascular collapse (Doty et al., 2012).

11. Monitor for and intervene promptly in cases of status epilepticus. Follow the institution's emergency protocol.	11. Status epilepticus is life threatening if not controlled immediately with IV diazepam.
12. Monitor and restore fluid and electrolyte balances.	12. Fluid and electrolyte losses from vomiting, profuse perspiration, and decreased antidiuretic hormone (from alcohol ingestion) cause dehydration. Increased neuromuscular activity can deplete magnesium and IV glucose administration can cause intracellular shift of magnesium (Porth, 2011).
13. Monitor for hypoglycemia.	13. Alcohol depletes liver glycogen stores and impairs gluconeogenesis. Alcoholics are also malnourished (Porth, 2011).
14. Monitor vital signs every 30 minutes initially.	14. Clients in withdrawal will have elevated heart rate, respirations, and fever. Those experiencing delirium tremens can be expected to have a low-grade fever. A rectal temperature greater than 99.9° F; however, is a clue to possible infection. Hypotension may be associated with pneumonia and a clue to infection (Porth, 2011).
15. Monitor laboratory values: White blood cell count (WBC), liver function studies, serum glucose, occult blood, albumin, prealbumin, serum alcohol level, electrolytes	15. Laboratory values may indicate alcohol-related conditions. Alcohol abuse causes a range of immunopathologic events. In alcoholic liver disease, albumin is lowered because of decreased synthesis by liver and malnutrition (Porth, 2011).

16. Observe for side effects or overmedication of benzodiazepine therapy:
  a. Oversedation
  b. Slurred speech
  c. Ataxia
  d. Nystagmus
	16. All medications have a therapeutic window and are not without their side effects.

17. Maintain the client IV, running continuously.	17. Necessary for fluid replacement, dextrose, thiamin bolus, benzodiazepine, and magnesium sulfate administrations. Chlordiazepoxide and diazepam should not be given intramuscularly because of unpredictable absorption (Doty et al., 2012).

Related Physician / NP Prescribed Interventions

Medications
Benzodiazepines, dilantin, thiamin, multivitamins, folic acid, magnesium

Intravenous Therapy
Fluid replacement, dextrose 1 g/kg

Laboratory Studies
Complete blood cell count (CBC), serum prealbumin, liver function studies, serum potassium, serum glucose, serum sodium, serum alcohol level, serum magnesium, occult blood (stool), serum albumin, uric acid, carbohydrate deficient transferrin, mean corpuscular volume

Diagnostic Studies
Electroencephalogram, if first occurrence of seizure or pattern changes, EKG

Therapies
Well-balanced diet with multivitamin supplement

Documentation

Vital signs
Alcohol withdrawal symptoms

Nursing Diagnoses

Risk for Violence Related to (Examples) Impulsive Behavior, Disorientation, Tremors, or Impaired Judgment

NOC

Abuse Cessation, Abusive Behavior Self-Restraint, Aggression Self-Control, Impulse Self-Control

Goal

The client will have fewer violent responses.

NIC

Abuse Protection Support, Anger Control Assistance, Environmental Management: Violence Prevention, Impulse Control Training, Crisis Intervention, Seclusion, Physical Restraint

Indicators

- Demonstrate control of behavior with assistance from others.
- Relate causative factors.

Interventions	*Rationales*
1. Promote interactions that increase the client's sense of trust and value of self.	1. In agitated state, the client may not be able to verbally express feelings but may act out these feelings in an aggressive manner.
2. Establish an environment that decreases stimuli: a. Decrease noise level b. Soft lighting c. Personal possessions d. Single / semiprivate room e. Control number of people entering the client's room	2. The client is already in an agitated / mentally compromised state; environmental stimuli will unnecessarily aggravate this state and send the client "over the edge."
3. Assess situations that have contributed to past violent episodes and attempt to modify the circumstances to prevent similar occurrences.	3. There can be a pattern to violence. Detecting and changing the pattern can eliminate the violence.
4. If indicated, refer to Risk for Violence to Others in Unit II for specific interventions.	

Documentation

Observations (cognition, anxiety, tremors)
Aggressive incident
Actions taken
Evaluation / outcome

Ineffective Denial Related to Acknowledgment of Alcohol Abuse or Dependency

NOC

Anxiety Level, Coping, Social Support, Substance Addiction Consequences, Knowledge: Substance Abuse Control, Knowledge: Disease Process

Goal

The client will acknowledge an alcohol / drug abuse problem.

NIC

Coping Enhancement, Anxiety Reduction, Counseling, Mutual Goal Setting, Substance Abuse Treatment, Support System Enhancement, Support Group

Indicators

- Explain the psychological and physiologic effects of alcohol or drug use.
- Abstain from alcohol / drug use.

Interventions	Rationales
1. Approach client nonjudgmentally. Some causes of pancreatitis are not alcohol related. Be aware of your own feelings regarding alcoholism.	1. The client probably has been reprimanded by many and is distrustful. The nurse's personal experiences with alcohol may increase or decrease empathy for the client.
2. Help the client to understand that alcoholism is an illness, not a moral problem.	2. Historically alcoholics have been viewed as immoral and degenerate. Acknowledgment of alcoholism as a disease can increase the client's sense of trust.
3. Assist the client to examine how drinking has affected relationships, work, and so on. Ask how he or she feels when not drinking.	3. During alcohol-related health problems, the individual may be more likely to acknowledge his or her drinking problem.
4. Allow family members as individuals and a group to share pent-up feelings. a. Validate feelings as normal. b. Correct inaccurate beliefs.	4. Alcoholism disturbs family communication. Sharing feelings is uncommon because of a history of disappointment. Diminished sharing and silence can maintain disturbed families for long periods. Communication focuses mainly on family members trying to control the other client's drinking behavior (Grisham & Estes, 1982).
5. Emphasize that family members are not responsible for the client's drinking (Carlson, Smith, & Julio, 2006; Starling & Martin, 1990). a. Explain that emotional difficulties are relationship based rather than "psychiatric." b. Instruct that their feelings and experiences are associated frequently with family alcoholism.	5. "The potential value of reaching the alcoholic client by first assisting family members should not be underestimated" (Grisham & Estes, 1982, p. 257). The family and health care professional must accept that no certain outcome can be promised for the alcoholic, even when the family gets help.
6. Assist the family to gain insight into behavior. Discuss ineffective methods families use such as: a. Hiding alcohol or car keys b. Anger, silence, threats, crying c. Making excuses for work, family, or friends d. Bailing the client out of jail	
7. Explain how these behaviors do not stop drinking, increase family anger, remove the responsibility for drinking from the client, and prevent the client from suffering the consequences of his or her drinking behavior.	7. Interventions focus on assisting the family to change their ineffective communication and response patterns (Carson & Smith-DiJulio, 2006).

Interventions	Rationales
8. Emphasize that helping the alcoholic means first helping themselves. a. Focus on the effects of their response. b. Allow the client to be responsible for his or her drinking behavior. c. Describe activities that will improve their lives, as individuals and a family. d. Initiate one stress management technique (e.g., aerobic exercise, assertiveness course, meditation).	8. Family members use denial to avoid admitting the problem and dealing with their contribution to it, and in the hope that the problem will disappear if not disclosed (Collins et al., 1990).
9. Discuss with family that recovery will dramatically change usual family dynamics. a. The alcoholic is removed from the center of attention. b. All family roles will be challenged. c. Family members will have to focus on themselves instead of on the alcoholic client. d. Family members will have to assume responsibility for their behavior, rather than blaming others. e. Behavioral problems of children serve a purpose for the family.	9. Ending the drinking behavior threatens the family integrity because the family functioning is centered around the alcoholism (Halter & Carson, 2010).
10. Initiate health teaching regarding community resources and referrals as indicated. a. Al-Anon b. Alcoholics anonymous family therapy c. Individual therapy d. Self-help groups	10. The family is the unit of treatment when one member is an alcoholic. Referrals are needed for long-term therapy.

Documentation

Dialogues

TRANSITION TO HOME / COMMUNITY CARE

If indicated, review the risk diagnoses identified for this individual on admission:

- Is the person still at risk?
- Can the family reduce the risks?
- Is the person at higher risk at home?
- Is a Home Health Nurse assessment needed?
- Refer to transition planner / case manager / social service.
- When is this person scheduled for follow-up with primary provider? Specialists? Record dates of appointments.
- Complete a medication reconciliation prior to transition. Refer to inside back cover.

STAR

Stop

Think   Is this person at risk for injury, falls, medical complications, and / or inability to care for self (activities of daily living)?

Is there a support person available?

Is the person competent to manage self-administration of medications, treatment procedures? Are additional resources needed?

Can the person explain how to monitor the condition (e.g., blood glucose, signs / symptoms of complications, dietary / mobility restrictions, and when to call his or her primary provider or specialist)?

Act   Contact or provide the appropriate resource (e.g., contacting a support person, home health assessment, additional teaching, printed materials).

Review   Has the problem been addressed? If not, use SBAR to communicate to the appropriate person.

Risk for Ineffective Self-Health Management Related to Insufficient Knowledge of Condition, Treatments Available, Risk Situations, and Community Resources

NOC

Compliance Behavior, Knowledge: Treatment Regimen, Participation in Health Care Decisions, Treatment Behavior: Illness or Injury

NIC

Substance Use Prevention, Substance Use Treatment, Behavior Modification, Support System Enhancement, Health System Guidance

Goals

The goals for this diagnosis represent those associated with transition planning. Refer to the transition criteria.

Interventions	Rationales
1. Educate the client regarding the disease of alcoholism and its effects on self, family, job, and finances: loss of control, social problems, legal problems, family problems, employment difficulties.	1. Acknowledging alcoholism's effects on one's life can motivate a client to change behavior. It may be especially useful to do this after the person experiences the discomforts of withdrawal.
2. Teach the client to recognize and respond to the various alcohol-related medical conditions that are present.	2. Continued alcohol abuse will lead to varying alcohol-related medical conditions as described in the collaborative problems.
3. Refer the client to community skill-building activities: assertiveness training, stress management, anger management.	3. The disease of addiction prevents individuals from learning adaptive social and other coping skills.
4. Improve family functioning through referral to community programs (e.g., counseling, Al-Anon).	4. Family functioning and individuals have suffered from the disease of alcoholism.

Documentation

Referrals

Immobility or Unconsciousness

This care plan addresses the needs of clients who are immobile and either unconscious or conscious. All of these collaborative problems and nursing diagnoses can be found in other sections of this book. In addition to the following diagnostic cluster, refer to the specific coexisting medical disease or condition (e.g., renal failure and cancer).

■■■ DIAGNOSTIC CLUSTER

Collaborative Problems

▲ Risk for Complications of Pneumonia, Atelectasis (refer to Unit II)

▲ Risk for Complications of Fluid / Electrolyte Imbalance (refer to Unit II)

▲ Risk for Complications of Sepsis (refer to Unit II)

▲ Risk for Complications of Thrombophlebitis (refer to Unit II)

△ Risk for Complications of Renal Calculi (refer to Unit II)

△ Risk for Complications of Osteoporosis (refer to Corticosteroid Therapy Care Plan)

Nursing Diagnoses

△ Disuse Syndrome related to effects of immobility on body systems (refer to Unit II)

▲ (Specify) Self-Care Deficit related to immobility (refer to Unit II)

△ Powerlessness related to feelings of loss of control and the restrictions placed on lifestyle (refer to Unit II)

▲ Risk for Ineffective Airway Clearance related to stasis of secretions secondary to inadequate cough and decreased mobility (refer to COPD Care Plan)

▲ Total Incontinence related to unconscious state (refer to Neurogenic Bladder Care Plan)

△ Risk for Impaired Oral Mucous Membrane related to immobility to perform own mouth care and pooling of secretions (refer to Unit II)

▲ This diagnosis was reported to be monitored for or managed frequently (75% to 100%).
△ This diagnosis was reported to be monitored for or managed often (50% to 74%).

Palliative Care

Both hospice care and palliative care have the same principles of comfort and support (National Cancer Institute [NCI], 2010). Hospice care is provided to individuals with terminal illness with a likelihood of dying in 6 months or less. Palliative care is offered earlier in the disease process than hospice care for someone with a life-threatening disease at the time of diagnosis or anytime throughout the course of illness. Hospice care is usually defined as "When cure is no longer realistic, the aim is to achieve the best death and dying process possible in the circumstances" (Australian DHHS, 2007a, p. 2).

Palliative care is a multidisciplinary medical specialty dedicated to the care of clients with serious, life-threatening illnesses such as cancer, cardiac disease, chronic obstructive pulmonary disease (COPD), kidney failure, Alzheimer's, HIV/AIDS, and amyotrophic lateral sclerosis (ALS). The focus of palliative care is symptom management—relief from pain, shortness of breath, anxiety, fatigue, constipation, nausea, loss of appetite, and difficulty sleeping. The goal is to improve the quality of life for both the client and the family. It is appropriate at any age and can be provided along with curative treatment at any stage of an illness. The goal is accomplished through interventions that maintain physical, social, and spiritual well-being; improve communication and coordination of care, and ensure culturally appropriate care that is consistent with the values and preferences of the individual. A holistic approach is necessary in palliative care to encompass the wide range of human responses to serious illness (Jacqueline Finerson, personal communication, 2013).

The Support Study's findings are as follows (Support Study, 1995):

A 2-year prospective observational study "of 9,105 adults hospitalized with one or more of nine life-threatening diagnoses; and overall 6-month mortality rate of 47%, was designed to improve end-of-life decision making and reduce the frequency of a mechanically supported, painful, and prolonged process of dying."

"The phase I observation documented shortcomings in communication, frequency of aggressive treatment, and the characteristics of hospital death: only 47% of physicians knew when their patients preferred to avoid CPR; 46% of do-not-resuscitate (DNR) orders were written within 2 days of death; 38% of patients who died spent at least 10 days in an intensive care unit (ICU); and for 50% of conscious patients who died in hospital, family members reported moderate to severe pain at least half the time."

In phase II, "Physicians in the intervention group received estimates of the likelihood of 6-month survival for every day up to 6 months, outcomes of cardiopulmonary resuscitation (CPR), and functional disability at 2 months. A specially trained nurse had multiple contacts with the client, family, physician, and hospital staff / student to elicit preferences, improve understanding of outcomes, encourage attention to pain control, and facilitate advance care planning and client–physician communication."

"During the phase II intervention, patients experienced no improvement in client–physician communication (e.g., 37% of control patients and 40% of intervention patients discussed CPR preferences) or in the five targeted outcomes, i.e., incidence of timing of written DNR orders (adjusted ratio, 1.02; 95% confidence interval [CI], 0.90 to 1.15) physicians' knowledge of their patients' preferences not to be resuscitated (adjusted ratio, 1.22; 95% CI, 0.99 to 1.49), number of days spent in an ICU, receiving mechanical ventilation, or comatose before death (adjusted ratio, 0.97; 95% CI, 0.87 to 1.07), or level of reported pain (adjusted ratio, 1.15; 95% CI, 1.00 to 1.33). The intervention also did not reduce use of hospital resources (adjusted ratio, 1.05; 95% CI, 0.99 to 1.12)."

The researchers concluded "The phase I observation of SUPPORT confirmed substantial shortcomings in care for seriously ill hospitalized adults." The phase II intervention failed to improve care of client outcomes. Enhancing opportunities for more client–physician communication, although advocated as the major method for improving client outcomes, may be inadequate to change established practices. To improve the experience of seriously ill and dying patients, greater individual and societal commitment and more proactive and forceful measures may be needed.

Carp's Cues

Eighteen years later, how far have we come? A systematic analysis of the nursing literature (from 1996 to 2011) concerning the nurse's roles and strategies in end-of-life (EOL) decision making concluded with a promising trend (Adams et al., 2011). Nurses have three roles in EOL decision-making: information brokers, supporters, and advocates. Of most significant, "whereas earlier literature indicated that nurses were involved in a indirect manner, recent literature indicates that nurses are more actively engaged as advocates in EOL decision-making with both physicians and family members, challenging the status quo and helping all of the parties see the big picture" (Adams et al., 2011). The researchers reported that the "literature suggests that when nurses are actively engaged with family members by interpreting and explaining to them what is happening and explaining prognoses, family members are more satisfied and able to move forward in their acceptance and decision-making" (Adams et al., 2011) Through their roles as information brokers, supporters, and advocates, nurses were "a voice to speak up" (Baggs, 2007, p. 504) coaching, challenging, and arguing for individuals to have a "good death" (Adams et al., 2011).

In contrast, our physician colleagues have not progressed as well. Sixty percent of oncologists prefer to wait until there are no more treatments to give before they will discuss advanced medical directives, hospice care, or code status. Unfortunately, 50 percent of individuals with lung cancer, when referred to hospice, are within 2 months of their death (Huskamp et al., 2009). Physicians continue to hesitate to discuss poor prognostic outcomes and end-of-life issues with individuals and their families (Mack & Smith, 2012). Reasons given for their failure to disclose are that this information is depressing, takes away hope, unsure of prognosis, and that these discussions are difficult. The literature disputes all of these reasons except the last (Mack & Smith, 2012).

Physicians, especially specialists, have limited relationships with individuals and their families. Their time to disclose is limited and thus the encounter of disclosure, if it occurs, is often the individual / family listening, with little dialogue occurring.

Nurses have the privilege of having multiple opportunities to dialogue with clients and their families. They know them. They can explore what and how much information the individual desires. Their presence as the physician discloses the diagnosis and prognosis can be very beneficial for all involved. Nurse expertise can lend support to physician colleagues, who do not have the nurses' expertise nor the time. Specialists are particularly vulnerable because of their limited relationship with the individual / family. With subsequent encounters, nurses can explore with individuals and families the meaning of this information and their perceptions of its impact on their lives. More discussions, feelings, and questions will surface and that is the goal: meaningful dialogue.

DIAGNOSTIC CLUSTER

Collaborative Problems

Risk for Complications of Hypercalcemia

Risk for Complications of Delirium

Risk for Complications of Pleural Effusions

Risk for Complications of Opioid-Induced Side Effects Toxicity

Risk for Complications of Pathologic Fractures

Risk for Complications of Spinal Cord Compression

Risk for Complications of Superior Vena Cava Obstruction

Risk for Complications of Bowel Obstruction

Risk for Complications of End-Stage Medical Condition (e.g., CHF, COPD, AIDS, Renal Failure) (refer to the related care plan in index)

Risk for Complications of Chemotherapy (refer to Chemotherapy Care Plan)

Risk for Complications of Radiation Therapy (refer to Radiation Therapy Care Plan)

Nursing Diagnoses

Risk for Compromised Human Dignity related to multiple factors associated with end-of-life treatments and decision-making

Altered Comfort related to breathlessness (e.g., pleural effusion, severe anemia, agitation)

Death Anxiety related to (specify the unknown, uncertainty, fears, conflicts, suffering and the impact on others as perceived by the individual and significant others)

Anticipatory Grieving related to losses associated with illness, disabilities and impending death and their effects on loved ones

Acute / Chronic Pain related to disease process (refer to Unit II)

Constipation related to the effects of disease and / or opioids on intestinal function, inactivity, and / or low fiber intake (refer to Unit II)

Nausea / Vomiting related to the effects of medications and disease process (refer to Unit II)

Fatigue related to the effects of disease activity, complications, nausea, anemia, and the presence of comorbidities (refer to Unit II)

Risk for Disturbed Sleep Patterns related to multiple factors / discomforts (refer to Unit II)

Acute Confusion related to (e.g., fever, infection, electrolyte disturbances, dehydration) (refer to Unit II)

Risk for Caregiver Role Strain related to multiple care responsibilities (refer to Unit II)

Risk for Spiritual Distress related to challenge to spiritual beliefs secondary to terminal illness (refer to Unit II)

Risk for Ineffective Self-Health Management related insufficient knowledge of actions needed for exacerbated symptoms or sudden onset of new symptoms, home management, resources available

Interventions	Rationales

2. Explain palliative sedation to client and / or significant others (e.g., prevalent indications for sedation were dyspnea and / or delirium).

CLINICAL ALERT

Statement on Palliative Sedation (American Association of Hospice and Palliative Care Medicine, 2006):

- Palliative care seeks to relieve suffering associated with disease. Unfortunately, not all symptoms associated with advanced illness can be controlled with pharmacologic or other interventions. Patients need and deserve assurance that suffering will be effectively addressed, as both the fear of severe suffering and the suffering itself add to the burden of terminal illness.
  - Ordinary sedation: The ordinary use of sedative medications for the treatment of anxiety, agitated depression, insomnia, or related disorders, in which the goal of treatment is the relief of the symptom without reducing the patient's level of consciousness.
  - Palliative sedation (PS): The use of sedative medication at least in part to reduce client awareness of distressing symptoms that are insufficiently controlled by symptom-specific therapies. The level of sedation is proportionate to the patient's level of distress, and alertness is preserved as much as possible.
  - Palliative sedation (PS) to unconsciousness: The administration of sedatives to the point of unconsciousness, when less extreme sedation has not achieved sufficient relief of distressing symptoms. This practice is used only for the most severe, intractable suffering at the very end-of-life.

Carp's Cues

The fact that dying people require symptom relief does not mean that symptom relief causes death. Studies demonstrate that symptom relief near death does not hasten death (Maltoni et al., 2012; Mercadante et al., 2009). To the contrary, untreated symptoms such as pain, stress, and anxiety lead to worsening strain and exhaustion in clients and family members alike. Intractable pain itself, in fact, may hasten death.

Health care providers have a responsibility to do no harm and to relieve suffering. This is as true with palliative sedation as with any other aspect of medical treatment. In the United States, Supreme Court rulings (*Vacco v. Quill*, 1997, and *Washington v. Glucksberg*, 1997) supported the concept of sedation when used to relieve intractable suffering.

2. "Palliative sedation, when appropriately indicated and correctly used to relieve unbearable suffering, does not seem to have any detrimental effect on survival of patients with terminal cancer. In this setting, palliative sedation is a medical intervention that must be considered as part of a continuum of palliative care" (Maltoni et al., 2012, p. 1378). Controlled sedation is successful in dying clients with untreatable symptoms, did not hasten death, and yielded satisfactory results for relatives.

Interventions	*Rationales*
3. Monitor for calcium levels and for signs and symptoms of hypercalcemia:	3. Severe hypercalcemia is life threatening. Hypercalcemia is the most common life-threatening metabolic complication occurring in an estimated 20% to 30% of all adults with cancer, with an incidence of 40% to 50% with breast cancer and malignant myeloma (Horwitz, 2012). These symptoms accompany mild hypercalcemia. They are distressing to the individuals and carers. Treatment can improve remaining quality of life even when time is limited if desired (Australian DHHS, 2007b).
a. Corrected serum calcium level range 2.10–2.55	a. Serum calcium >2.6 is diagnostic. Mild hypercalcemia <3 mmol/L is usually asymptomatic.
b. Nausea c. Anorexia and vomiting d. Constipation e. Thirst, polyuria f. Altered mental status, confusion > coma g. Dysrhythmias (shortened QT interval and widened T wave) h. Numbness or tingling in fingers and toes i. Severe dehydration	
4. If the decision is made to treat hypercalcemia, rehydration with intravenous fluids will be initiated and possibly bisphosphonate infusion. **CLINICAL ALERT** • Following bisphosphonate infusions, the serum calcium will fluctuate up and down giving an unreliable reading until 48 hours after infusion (Australian DHHS, 2007b).	4. Bisphosphonate inhibits osteoclast resorption and thus reduces the amount of serum calcium (Porth, 2011).
5. Monitor for signs and symptoms of pleural effusion: a. Dyspnea b. Cough c. Chest pain d. Decreased breath sounds **CLINICAL ALERT** • Notify physician / NP for an evaluation of symptoms (e.g., chest x-ray, CT scan). If the decision is made to treat pleural effusion, e.g., thoracentesis will be initiated.	5. A pleural effusion may be caused by cancer of lung, breast, lymphoma, and leukemia, or by cancer treatments such as radiation and chemotherapy. Some individuals with cancer have other conditions that can cause pleural effusion such as congestive heart failure, pneumonia, pulmonary embolus, and malnutrition. **CLINICAL ALERT** • Removal of the fluid may help to relieve severe symptoms for a short time.
6. Monitor for signs and symptoms of pathologic fracture: a. Localized pain that becomes continuous and unrelenting b. Visible bone deformity c. Crepitation on movement d. Loss of movement or use e. Localized soft tissue edema f. Skin discoloration g. Tenderness to percussion over involved spine	6. Pathologic fractures can be caused by any type of bone tumor, but the majority of pathologic fractures in the elderly are secondary to metastatic carcinomas. Metastatic cancer deposits in the proximal femur may weaken the bone and cause a pathologic hip fracture. Bones most susceptible to tumor invasion are those with the greatest bone marrow activity and blood flow—the vertebrae, pelvis, ribs, skull, and sternum. The most common sites for long bone metastasis are the femur and humerus (Lindqvist, Widmarkt, & Rasmussen, 2006).
7. Maintain alignment and immobilize the site if fracture is suspected.	7. Immobilization helps reduce soft tissue damage from dislocations.

(continued)

Interventions	*Rationales*
8. Notify physician / NP for evaluation of possible fracture (e.g., x-ray and treatment).	8. The goal of treatment of impending or pathologic fracture is to provide pain relief and a functionally stable immobilization device.
9. Monitor for signs and symptoms of spinal cord compression: a. Back pain • Localized at first • Described as belt-like pain at the level of the compression • Worse when lying down, coughing, sneezing, or moving b. Neurologic symptoms: • C/o muscle weakness, heaviness or stiffness of limbs • Change in gait • Change in or loss of sensation (e.g., numbness and tingling) • Change in bowel or urinary habits (e.g., constipation or inability to urinate)	9. Spinal cord compression (SCC) occurs when a spinal cord tumor or metastatic tumor grows in the spine and destroys the bony vertebral body that surrounds the cord, or wraps around the spinal cord and its nerve roots. This can cause the vertebral body to collapse and compress the spinal cord. a. The most common area for spinal cord metastases is the thoracic spine (70%). Back pain is caused by irritation of the nerve roots by the tumor. b. If untreated, spinal cord compression may progress to cause serious neurologic problems such as paralysis. Fewer than 25% of people who are paralyzed at the time they are diagnosed with SCC will regain their ability to walk after treatment.
10. Notify physician / NP for an evaluation of possible spinal cord compression (e.g., imaging tests [x-rays, MRI, or myelogram]) and treatment (e.g., steroids, palliative chemotherapy, radiation).	10. Goals of treatment are to relieve compression, which will reduce or control pain, and to stabilize the spine. Individuals in final stage of terminal illness will likely have corticosteroid therapy.
11. Monitor for signs and symptoms of superior vena cava obstruction (SVCO) (Wilson, 2004): a. Early signs: • Facial, trunk, upper extremity edema • Pronounced venous pattern on trunk • Shortness of breath b. Late signs: • Hoarseness, stridor • Engorged conjunctiva, visual disturbances • Headache, dizziness • Decreased cardiac output • Flushed edematous face • Tachypnea, orthopnea c. Raise the head of the bed	11. The most common cause of superior vena cava syndrome is cancer. Primary or metastatic cancer in the upper lobe of the right lung can compress the superior vena cava. Lymphoma or other tumors located in the mediastinum can also cause compression of the superior vena cava. a. These symptoms are caused by the inability of the blood to return to the heart. b. SVCO occurs when the superior vena cava becomes occluded by a tumor or thrombus. Commonly associated with lung cancer, breast cancer, and lymphomas, SVCS causes impaired venous return from the head and upper extremities, resulting in upper body edema and prominent collateral circulation (Nickloes, 2012; Wilson, 2004). c. Individuals with clinical superior vena cava syndrome (SVCO) can have significant symptomatic improvement with elevation of the head of the bed and supplemental oxygen (Nickloes, 2012).
12. Notify physician / NP for an evaluation of possible SVCO (e.g., imaging tests [x-rays, MRI, or myelogram]) and treatment (e.g., steroids, palliative chemotherapy, radiation) (Nickloes, 2012).	12. Goals of treatment are to relieve compression, which will reduce or control pain, and to stabilize the spine. Individuals in final stage of terminal illness will likely have corticosteroid therapy.

Interventions	Rationales
13. Explain palliative chemotherapy (Weissman, 2009).	13. Palliative chemotherapy can shrink cancer tumors and improve or eliminate distressing symptoms for a period of time, such as dyspnea, pain.
14. Ensure that the individual / family understand the median duration of response. If not, access oncologist for this information (Bruera, 2012).	14. The median duration of response is how long the client's cancer can be expected to respond to chemotherapy. The number ranges from 3 to 12 months. Clients and family need this information to evaluate if the benefits outweigh the side effects of chemotherapy (Bruer, 2012).

Clinical Alert Report

Prior to providing care, advise ancillary staff / student to report the following to the professional nurse assigned to the client:
- Change in cognitive status
- Oral temperature >100.5° F
- Systolic BP <90 mm/Hg
- Resting Pulse >100, <50
- Respiratory rate >28, <10 /min
- C/o of new onset:
  - Back pain
  - Numbness
  - Edema
  - Shortness of breath
  - Localized bone pain
  - Inability to defecate, urinate

Nursing Diagnoses

Risk for Compromised Human Dignity Related to Potential Barriers to a Peaceful End-of-Life Transition

 Carp's Cues

Determine if the agency has a policy for prevention of compromised human dignity. This type of policy or standard may be titled differently. Agency policies can assist the nurse when problematic situations occur; however, the moral obligation to protect and defend the dignity of clients or groups does not depend on the existence of a policy.

NOC

Abuse Protection, Comfort Level, Knowledge: Illness Care, Self-Esteem, Dignified Dying, Spiritual Well-Being, Information Processing

Goal

The individual / significant others will report respectful and considerate care according to their end-of-life wishes.

NIC

Patient Rights Protection, Anticipatory Guidance, Counseling, Emotional Support, Preparatory Sensory Information, Family Support, Humor, Mutual Goal Setting, and Teaching: Procedure / Treatment, Touch

Indicators

- Respect for privacy
- Facilitate shared decision-making process
- Priority to individual's or designated surrogate decision-maker requests / decisions
- Clear, accurate, timely explanations with options
- Optimal control of distressful symptoms

Carp's Cues

The ANA's position statement on *Registered Nurses' Roles and Responsibilities in providing Expert Care and Counseling at the End of Life* (2010a) *states:*

"*Nurses* are leaders and vigilant advocates for the delivery of dignified and humane care. Nurses actively participate in assessing and assuring the responsible and appropriate use of interventions in order to minimize unwarranted or unwanted treatment and patient suffering" (ANA, 2010a, pp. 7–8). "Nursing interventions are intended to produce beneficial effects, contribute to quality outcomes, *and—above all—do no harm*. . . ." (ANA, 2010b, p. 15).

Do not participate in lying, do not ignore it for any reason, and if what you are witnessing is just wrong, speak up.

Interventions	Rationales
1. Determine and accept your own moral responsibility. Be "a voice to speak up" (Bach, Plooeg, & Black, p. 504). **CLINICAL ALERT** • If the nurse is a student or inexperienced in navigating the issues and potential conflicts in providing care to individuals / significant others, consultation with a nurse competent with end-of-life conflicts is imperative. • Attempts to go it alone can be responsible for interventions / interactions that are problematic and even worse than harmful to clients and significant others.	1. Nurses have reported feelings of powerlessness within the work environment because of not addressing unacceptable care conditions and their own moral distress (Hamric, 2000).
2. Provide care to each client and family as you would expect or demand for your family, partner, child, friend, or colleague.	2. Setting this personal standard can spur you to defend the client / group, especially when they do not belong to the same socioeconomic group as you.
3. Explore "how well the client and family understand the patient's relevant medical conditions and what their expectations, hopes, and concerns are."	3. "This listening phase can provide insight into the patient's values and goals and how much the patient and family want to engage in these discussions."
4. Allow the client an opportunity to share his or her feelings after a difficult situation and maintain privacy for the client's information and emotional responses.	4. Allowing the client to share his or her feelings can help him or her maintain or regain dignity. Recognition of the client as a living, thinking, and experiencing human being enhances dignity (Walsh & Kowanko, 2002).
5. Advocate for the client / family with their physician / NP before conflicts arise: a. Elicit the client's and / or family's perception of the situation b. Explore everyone's expectations. c. Explore if the client's and / or family's expectations are realistic. d. Offer your observations of the client / family understanding of the situation to involved health care professionals (e.g., manager, nurse colleagues, physicians, nurse practitioners).	5. Being less than truthful and / or unrealistic is a barrier to providing appropriate care and eventually a "good death" (Beckstrand & Callister, 2006).
6. Seek to accompany the physician / NP when he or she is going to disclose the diagnosis, prognosis, and / or treatment plan.	6. Knowing exactly what the individual / family has been told will help the nurse continue dialogue and to provide clarity when questions arise.

Interventions	Rationales

7. Explore with individual and family what their understanding of the situation is:
   a. What did your physician / NP tell you?
   b. Is there anything else that you want to know?
   c. Does the family want to restrict information to the individual?
   d. If needed, instruct client or family to write down specific questions for physician / NP.

> **CLINICAL ALERT**
> - Individuals will vary regarding how much information they desire.
> - Despite what the nurse believes an individual should know, all discussions regarding diagnosis and prognosis must be carefully approached.
> - Some individuals do not want to know their prognosis.
> - Some are overwhelmed with the information and cannot cope with the reality at the present time.

7. Individuals have the right to as much or as little information that they can manage at this time.

8. If the individual in the last stages of end-of-life, engage in a dialogue with the client and family separately regarding their assumptions of the individual's prognosis (Murray, Boyd, Sheikh, 2005).
   a. Consider how the individual and / or significant others would respond to the following theoretical questions:
   - If death is approaching, would they be surprised if the individual were to die in a few hours or days?
   - If death is not imminent but expected, would they be surprised if the individual were to die in 6 months, a year?
   b. If their actions / discussions indicate that they are unaware or unable to deal with the end-of-life reality, consult with an expert nurse and / or specialist in ethics for assistance.

8. Survival estimates are not viewed with an emphasis of when someone will die, but instead to provide information to allow all involved to be aware of the transition as needed as the individual deteriorates. The process of dying has many uncertainties and is unstable with the individual's condition oscillating from day to day with eventual deterioration.

9. Avoid giving a specific time for the expected time of death. "It is helpful to give a range of time, such as 'hours to days,' 'days to weeks' or 'weeks to months'" (Yarbro, Wujeck & Gobel, 2011, p. 1836).

9. Family members and friends will be able to better plan their time spent with their loved one with this information (Yarbro, Wujeck & Gobel, 2011).

10. Develop strategies to transition clients from acute care to palliative care.
   a. Explain the difference between acute care and palliative care. Address:
   - Change for a focus from curing to caring
   - The focus of care must be solely to relieve suffering. Painful treatments to prolong dying are inhumane and unethical.
   - "Appropriately negotiated treatment abatement and symptom relief does not constitute causing death" (Australian DHHS, 2007a, p. 2).
   - "By working in harmony of the reality of the situation, health care professionals can improve the journey considerably, but failure to recognize the dying process can make it worse, and prevent the timely deployment of appropriate palliative care" (Australian DHHS, 2007a, p. 2).
   - "The best possible pain and symptom relief in the clinical circumstances is both the patient's right and the clinician's duty" (Australian DHHS, 2010a, p. 2).

10. "Neither patients nor persons responsible can insist on treatment that is futile and therefore medically contraindicated in the circumstances, nor can they insist on actions that are illegal or contrary to professional ethics" (Australian, DHHS, 2007a, p. 3).

(continued)

Interventions	*Rationales*
11. Access physician / NP to discuss the options for treatment. Emphasize that the persons involved in the decision making (clients, significant others) can change their minds anytime.	11. The options for the treatment plan must be discussed with the benefits and hazards of each option. If the individual is capable of decision making, his or her wishes are priority. If not capable, the designated decision making should honor what the individual would choose if he or she could.
12. Ensure that all members of the health care team understand the individual / significant others decisions. Document clearly. Alert the next nurse at the handover.	12. In the moment of an emergency, panic can cause undesirable decisions that create only more pain and suffering.
13. Enlist the services of hospice when indicated.	13. Hospice organizations have the expertise and resources for palliative care.
14. Seek if possible to transfer individual out of the ICU. a. If feasible, plan to transition or transfer the client out of the hospital. b. Explore the Going Home Initiative at Baystate Medical Center, Springfield, Massachusetts (Lusardi et al., 2011).	14. ICU environments have many barriers to a palliative care environment (e.g., noise, frequent interruptions, close quarters, futile treatments).
15. When extreme measures that are futile are planned or are being provided for a client, initiate STAR: **STAR** **Stop** 　　**Think** Is this situation wrong? 　　**Act** Discuss situation with instructor / another nurse / manager / physician / NP using SBAR 　　　　**Situation:** Invasive treatments, increased pain, no improvement 　　　　**Background:** Terminal status, previous treatments 　　　　**Assessment:** Client's desire to stop present treatments. Family "wants to try everything" 　　　　**Recommendation:** Family conference with nurse, physician / NP, and / or ethics consultant to discuss the situation, (futility, pain) vs. palliative care 　　**Review**	15. "Extreme measures, when futile, are an infringement of the basic respect for the dignity innate in being a person" (Walsh & Kowanko, 2002, p. 146). "Practice expecting that honoring and protecting the dignity of individual / groups is not a value but a way of being" (Sodenberg et al., 1998).
16. Discuss with involved personnel an incident that was disrespectful to a client or family. Report any incident that may be a violation of a client's dignity to the appropriate person	16. Professionals have a responsibility to practice ethically and morally and to address situations and personnel that compromise human dignity.
17. Advocate for end-of-life decision dialogues with all clients and their families and your friends and relatives, especially when the situation is not critical. Direct them to create written documents of their decisions and to advise family of the document.	17. Exploring end-of-life decisions when there are no imminent threats to survival provide the most optimal setting for discussions. Decisions that are viewed as well-thought-out may assist the family with honoring their loved one's decision.

Clinical Alert Report

Advise ancillary staff / student to report any questions or concerns that the client / family ask in regard to condition, prognosis, treatments immediately.

Documentation

Significant discussions
Incident report, if indicated for unacceptable staff / student behavior.

Impaired Comfort Related to Episodes of Breathlessness, Agitation, and / or Pruritus

NOC

Symptom Control; Comfort Status

Goal

The client / significant others will report preservation of individual dignity, comfort, and safety and a reduction of stress and distress in individual / significant others.

NIC

Pruritus Management, Fever Treatment, Environmental Management: Comfort

Indicators

* Modification of agitation and aggressive behaviors
* Improvement in sleep quality
* Reduction in anxiety in individual / significant others

Interventions	Rationales

1. Assess for sources of discomfort:
  a. Pruritus > Refer to Cirrhosis Care Plan
  b. Breathlessness
  c. Delirium (hypoactive / hyperactive [agitation])	

2. For breathlessness, ensure that the individual's breathlessness has been fully evaluated, if indicated:
  a. Provide interventions to reduce breathlessness, acknowledge fears (Australian DHHS, 2007c).
    • Sit individual up, avoid abdominal or chest compressions, avoid restrictive clothing.
    • Provide cool airflow over face (e.g., fan).
    • Teach controlled diaphragmatic breathing.
    • Engage in distractions that are enjoyed (e.g., music, company, massage).
  b. Evaluate if supplemental oxygen is beneficial with a trial. Evaluate the risks versus benefits (Australian DHHS, 2007c)
    • Benefits: Individuals with oxygen saturation < 90% may have benefit.
    • Adverse effects
      • Dependency on equipment can increase anxiety if equipment problems occur.
      • Initially perceived benefits can be placebo and when this effect diminishes, anxiety can increase.
      • Causes nasal dryness, crusting, bleeding, trauma to nares
      • Irritates upper airways > cough
      • Increases risk for tripping / falls (tether line)
      • Noisy day and night
  c. Consult with physician / NP for pharmacologic management (e.g., opioids, anti-anxiety, dexamethasone).
	2. Some causes of breathlessness such as pain, anxiety, infection, pleural effusion, airway obstruction, and anemia may be corrected.
	
	b. Supplemental oxygen is often used to quickly solve episodes of breathlessness. It is thought to be benign, when in fact it comes with risks. Individuals with COPD will benefit: while individuals with cancer probably will not.
	
	c. Certain medications can reduce the perception of dyspnea.

(continued)

Interventions	*Rationales*
3. For delirium (hypoactive / hyperactive (agitation): "When deciding whether to investigate and treat underlying causes if present consider if this would be:" (Australian DHHS, 2007d, p. 4)	
a. Appropriate to the goals of care and stage of illness	
b. Realistic and reasonably likely to be achievable	
c. Likely to improve quality of life	
d. Overly burdensome	
e. Consistent with client's understanding and wishes / advances directives	
f. If indicated, ensure that hypoactive / hypoactive behavior has been fully evaluated.	f. Some causes of hypoactive / hypoactive behavior are treatable as sleep deprivation, nicotine withdrawal, multiple medications, hypercalcemia, infection, oversedation, pain, constipation, urinary retention, and drug / alcohol withdrawal.
g. Provide interventions to reduce agitation, acknowledge fears of significant others (Australian DHHS, 2007d). • Attempt to keep immediate environment familiar. • Encourage familiar objects (e.g., pictures). • Reduce unnecessary noise / stimulation (e.g., loud talking, disturbing TV shows). • Approach individual slowly in a quiet voice. Reorient individual with each encounter. • Use simple, brief sentences • Ensure frequent rest periods	g. Interventions should focus on calming the environment to reduce stressors.
h. Allow significant others to express their fears and concerns.	h. Witnessing confusion / agitation in a loved one is one of the most distressing situations.
i. Consult with physician / NP for pharmacologic management (e.g., opioids, anti-anxiety, dexamethasone).	i. Certain medications can reduce the perception of dyspnea.

Clinical Alert Report

Advise ancillary staff / student to report
- Any questions or concerns that the client / family ask in regard to condition, prognosis, treatments immediately.
- Increase / decrease in activity
- Change in cognition

Documentation

Exacerbation of symptoms
Interventions
Response

Death Anxiety Related to (Specify the Unknown, Uncertainty, Fears, Conflicts, Suffering and the Impact on Others as Perceived by the Individual and Significant Others)

NOC

Dignified Life Closure, Fear Self-Control, Client Satisfaction, Decision-Making, Family Coping

Goal

The client will report diminished anxiety or fear.

NIC
Limit Setting, Client
Rights Protection, Family
Support, Dying Care,
Coping Enhancement,
Active Listening,
Emotional Support,
Spiritual Support

Indicators

- Share feelings regarding dying.
- Identify specific requests that will increase psychological comfort.

Interventions	Rationales
1. For a client with a new or early diagnosis of a potentially terminal condition: a. Allow the client and family separate opportunities to discuss their understanding of the condition. Correct misinformation. b. Access valid information regarding condition, treatment options, and stage of condition from primary provider (physician, nurse practitioner). c. Ensure a discussion of the prognosis if known.	1. With a diagnosis of a potential terminal illness, clients and families should be given opportunities to talk about treatments, cures, and goals regarding quality of life (e.g., curative vs. symptomatic comfort care).
2. For the client experiencing a progression of a terminal illness: a. Explore with the client his or her understanding of the situation and feelings. b. Ensure that the primary physician or nurse practitioner initiate a discussion regarding the situation and options desired by the client. c. Discuss with family and client palliative care and strategies that can be used for dyspnea, pain, and other discomforts (Yabro, Wujcik & Gobel, 2011). d. Elicit from the client and client's family specific requests for end-of-life care	2a. It is important to determine the client's understanding of the situation and personal preferences or requests. b. These discussions provide insight into the client's understanding and directs treatment decisions. Research reports that only 31% of persons with terminal conditions reported end-of-life discussions with a physician (Wright, 2008b). c. During the final stage of life, anxiety for the client and family is highly correlated with the presence or fear of other symptoms such as dyspnea, pain, and fear of the unknown (Yabro, Wujcik, & Gobel, 2011). d. Persons with advanced cancer identified their priorities as protection of dignity, sense of control, pain control, inappropriate prolongation of dying, and strengthening relationships (Singer, 1999; Volker, 2004).
3. Provide opportunities for the person to discuss end-of-life decisions. Be direct and empathetic.	3. Clover et al. (2004) found that a person's readiness to participate in end-of-life decisions depends on the skills of the professional nurse to encourage the client to share his or her wishes.
4. Encourage the client to reconstruct his or her worldview: a. Allow the client to verbalize feelings about the meaning of death. b. Advise the client that there are no right or wrong feelings. c. Advise the client that responses are his or her choice. d. Acknowledge struggles. e. Encourage dialogue with a spiritual mentor or trusted friend.	4. When a client is facing death, reconstructing a world view involves balancing thoughts about the painful subject with avoiding painful thoughts.
5. Allow significant others opportunities to share their perceptions and concerns. Advise them that sadness is expected and normal.	5. Clarification is needed to determine if their concerns regarding end-of-life care is consistent with the client. "It is normal and healthy to feel sad at the end-of-life, to grieve the impending loss of everything a person holds dear" (Coombs-Lee, 2008, p. 12).

(continued)

Interventions	Rationales
6. Encourage difficult but truthful conversations (e.g., sorrow, mistakes, disagreements).	6. "Avoiding truthful conversations does not bring hope and comfort: it brings isolation and loneliness" (Coombs-Lee, 2008, p. 12).
7. To foster psycho-spiritual growth, open dialogue with the client specifically (Yokimo, 2009, p. 700): a. If your time is indeed shortened, what do you need to get done? b. Are there people whom you need to contact in order to resolve feelings or unfinished business? c. What do you want to do with the time you have left?	
8. If appropriate, offer to help the client contact others to resolve conflicts (old or new) verbally or in writing. Validate that forgiveness is not a seeking reconciliation, "but a letting go of a hurt" (Yakimo, 2006). a. The nurse through listening can help the client with personal growth.	8. "Asking for or providing forgiveness is a powerful healing tool" (Yakimo, 2006).
9. Explain preparatory depression and associated behaviors to significant others (Yakimo, 2006). a. Realization of impending death b. Reviewing what their life has meant c. Reflections on life review and sorrow of impeding losses	9. Preparatory depression is when the person realizes his or her approaching death and desires to be released from suffering (Yakimo, 2006).
10. Encourage significant others to allow for life review and sorrow and not to try and cheer him or her up. Encourage the client to: a. Tell life stories and reminisce. b. Discuss leaving a legacy: donation, personal articles, or taped messages.	10. Strategies that help the client find meaning in failures and successes can reduce anxiety and depression. Acceptance of the final separation in life is not reached until the dying client's life review and sorrow is listened to (Yakimo, 2006).
11. Respect the dying client's wishes (e.g., few or no visitors, modifications in care, no heroic measures, or food or liquid preferences). a. Encourage reflective activities such as personal prayer, meditation, and journal writing. b. Return to a previously pleasurable activity. Examples include painting, music, woodworking, and quilting. c. Return the gift of love to others by listening, praying for others, sharing personal wisdom gained from illness, and creating legacy gifts.	11. If the person is ready to release life and die, and others expect him or her to want to continue to live, that person's own depression, grief, and turmoil are increased (Yakimo, 2006). b. Promoting and restoring interests, imagination, and creativity enhance quality of life (Brant, 1998).
12. Aggressively manage unrelieved symptoms such as nausea, pruritus, pain, vomiting, and fatigue.	12. Serious unrelieved symptoms can cause a distressing death and needless added suffering for families (Nelson et al., 2000). Fatigue and pain consume excess energy and reduce energy needed for optimal dialogue (Matzo & Sherman, 2001).
13. Prepare significant others for changes in their loved one that may occur as death nears: a. Early: sleep more, eat / drink less, trouble swallowing, become more confused. have less pain, withdraw from others, trouble hearing b. Moaning sounds, moist breathing sounds, long periods without breathing followed by several quick, deep breaths, cool hands, arms, feet or legs, turning blue around nose, mouth, fingers, toes) (Hospice and Palliative Nurse's Association, 2012; Yarbro, Wujeck, & Gobel, 2011).	13. Clear, direct discussions can reduce the family's anxiety when these signs and symptoms occur and reduce attempts to reduce these signs and symptoms such as trying to force fluids (Yarbro, Wujeck, & Gobel, 2011).

Interventions	Rationales
14. Avoid giving a specific time for the expected time of death. "It is helpful to give a range of time, such as 'hours to days,' 'days to weeks' or 'weeks to months'" (Yarbro, Wujeck, & Gobel, 2011, p.1836).	14. Family members and friends will be able to better plan their time spent with their loved one with this information (Yarbro, Wujeck, & Gobel, 2011).

Documentation

Significant discussions

Anticipatory Grieving Related to Losses Associated with Illness, Disabilities and Impending Death and their Effects on Loved Ones

NOC
Coping, Family Coping, Grief Resolution, Psychosocial Adjustment: Life Change

Goal

Client / family will identify expected loss and grief reactions will be freely expressed.

NIC
Family Support, Grief Work Facilitation, Coping Enhancement, Anticipatory Guidance, Emotional Support

Indicators

- Participate in decision-making for the future.
- Share concerns with significant others.

Interventions	Rationales
1. Assess for causative and contributing factors of anticipated or potential loss (e.g., terminal illness, role changes, financial burden, loss of relationships, physical changes).	

2. Assess individual response:
  a. Denial
  b. Shock
  c. Rejection
  d. Anger
  e. Bargaining
  f. Depression
  g. Isolation
  h. Guilt
  i. Helplessness / hopelessness
  j. Fear
  k. Sadness
  l. Anxiety	

3. Encourage the client to share concerns:
  a. Use open-ended questions and reflection
  b. Acknowledge the value of the client and his or her grief by using touch, sitting with him or her, and verbalizing your concern.
  c. Recognize that some people may choose not to share their concerns, but convey that you are available if they desire to do so later.
	a. "What are your thoughts today?" "How do you feel?"
	b. "This must be very difficult." "What is most important to you now?"
	
	c. "What do you hope for?"

(continued)

Interventions	Rationales

4. Assist the client and family to identify strengths:
   a. "What do you do well?"
   b. "What are you willing to do to address this issue?"
   c. "Is religion / spirituality a source of strength for you?"
   d. "Do you have close friends?"
   e. "Whom do you turn to in times of need?"
   f. "What does this person do for you?"
   g. "What sources of strength have you called upon successfully in the past?"

5. Promote integrity of the client and family by acknowledging strengths:
   a. "Your brother looks forward to your visit."
   b. "Your family is so concerned for you."

6. Support the client and family with grief reactions:
   a. Prepare them for possible grief reactions.
   b. Explain possible grief reactions.
   c. Focus on the current situation until the client or family indicates the desire to discuss the future.

7. Promote family cohesiveness:
   a. Identify availability of a support system:
      • Meet consistently with family members.
      • Identify family member roles, strengths, and weaknesses.
   b. Identify communication patterns within the family unit:
      • Assess positive and negative feedback, verbal and nonverbal communication, and body language.
      • Listen and clarify messages being sent.
   c. Provide for the concept of hope:
      • Supply accurate information.
      • Resist the temptation to give false hope.
      • Discuss concerns willingly.
      • Help the family reframe hope (i.e., for a peaceful death).
   d. Promote group decision-making to enhance group autonomy:
      • Establish consistent times to meet with the client and family.
      • Encourage members to talk directly with and to listen to one another.

7. Mourners who were busy with the practical and necessary caregiving tasks of the dying client may not address the impending loss and, therefore, are at risk for delayed grieving response (Stuart & Sundeen, 2002).

8. Provide for expression of grief:
   a. Encourage emotional expressions of grieving.
   b. Caution the client about use of sedatives and tranquilizers, which may prevent or delay expressions.
   c. Encourage verbalization by clients of all age groups and families.
      • Support family cohesiveness.
      • Promote and verbalize strengths of the family group.
   d. Encourage the client and family to engage in life review:
      • Focus and support the social network relationships.
      • Reevaluate past life experiences and integrate them into a new meaning.
      • Convey empathic understanding.
      • Explore unfinished business.

Interventions	Rationales
9. Provide health teaching and referrals, as indicated:	9. The knowledge that no further treatment is warranted and that death is imminent may give rise to feelings of powerlessness, anger, profound sadness, and other grief responses. Open, honest discussions can help the client and family members accept and cope with the situation and their response to it (O'Mallon, 2009).
a. Refer the client with potential for dysfunctional grieving responses for counseling (psychiatrist, nurse therapist, counselor, psychologist).	a. Research validates that professional interventions and professionally supported voluntary and self-help services are capable of reducing the risk of psychiatric and psychoanalytic disorders resulting from bereavement (Bonnano & Lillenfied, 2008).

9. Provide health teaching and referrals, as indicated:

a. Refer the client with potential for dysfunctional grieving responses for counseling (psychiatrist, nurse therapist, counselor, psychologist).
b. Explain what to expect:
- Sadness
- Rejection
- Feelings of aloneness
- Anger
- Guilt
- Labile emotions
- Fear
- Feeling of "going crazy"
c. Teach the client and family signs of resolution:
- Grieving client no longer lives in the past but establishes new goals for life.
- Grieving client redefines relationship with the lost object / person.
- Grieving client begins to resocialize.
d. Teach signs of complicated responses and referrals needed:
- Defenses used in uncomplicated grief work that become exaggerated or maladaptive responses
- Persistent absence of any emotion
- Prolonged intense reactions of anxiety, anger, fear, guilt, and helplessness
e. Identify agencies that may enhance grief work:
- Self-help groups
- Widow-to-widow groups
- Parents of deceased children
- Single-parent groups
- Bereavement groups

Documentation

Significant discussions

TRANSITION TO HOME / COMMUNITY CARE

If indicated, review the risk diagnoses identified for this individual on admission:
- Is the person still at risk?
- Can the family reduce the risks?
- Is the person at higher risk at home?
- Is a Home Health Nurse assessment needed?
- Refer to transition planner / case manager / social service
- When is this person scheduled for follow-up with primary provider? Specialists? Record dates of appointments.
- Complete a medication reconciliation prior to transition. Refer to index.

STAR	**Stop**
Think	Is this person at risk for injury, falls, medical complications, and / or inability to care for self (activities of daily living)?
	Is there a support person available?
	Is the person competent to manage self-administration of medications, treatment procedures? Are additional resources needed?
•	Can the person explain how to monitor the condition (e.g., blood glucose, signs / symptoms of complications, dietary / mobility restrictions, and when to call his or her primary provider or specialist)?
Act	Contact or provide the appropriate resource (e.g., contacting a support person, home health assessment, additional teaching, printed materials).
Review	Has the problem been addressed? If not, use SBAR to communicate to the appropriate person.

Risk for Care Giver Role Strain Related to the Multiple Changes / Stressors Associated with Transition to Palliative Home Care

NOC

Caregiver Well-Being, Caregiver Lifestyle Disruption, Caregiver Emotional Health, Caregiver Role Endurance Potential, Family Coping, Family Integrity

Goals

The caregiver will:

- Relate what needs to be completed prior to transition to home care
- Identify the services to expect from palliative / hospice agencies
- Share frustrations regarding caregiving responsibilities
- Identify one source of support
- Identify two changes that, would improve daily life if implemented

The family will:

- Relate two strategies to increase weekly support or help
- Convey empathy to caregiver regarding daily responsibilities

NIC

Caregiver Support, Respite Care, Coping Enhancement, Family Mobilization, Mutual Goal Setting, Support System Enhancement, Anticipatory Guidance

Interventions	Rationales
1. Educate yourself regarding palliative / hospice services in the home.	1. To prepare individuals and their families for care at home, nurses need to clearly understand what they will experience during the time between care provided by the "sending" (hospital) and "receiving" (home hospice) providers (Does et al., 2011).
2. Ensure that family understand the services that will be provided at home (e.g., when, what, how often).	2. Failure to prepare individuals / family for transition to home care has proven to result in suboptimal outcomes, the development of new or worsening symptoms, unplanned rehospitalizations, medical errors, and other adverse events (Does et al., 2011).
3. Elicit from caregivers their concerns, fears.	3. Does et al. reported that many family members were not yet comfortable with their new roles as caregivers, were not sure what to expect, and identified feeling scared (2011, p. 400). Lack of clarity regarding hospice care entailed a tension between "hospice will take care of everything" and uncertainty over what exactly was meant by "everything" (Does et al., 2011, p. 400).
4. Elicit for the client his or her expectations, concerns, fears.	4. For many individuals at end of their life "going home" is the most important task remaining to achieve (Does et al., 2011).

Interventions	Rationales
5. Access palliative / hospice specialist to clarify the type and timing of services to be provided. Request that they instruct them on management of "emergencies."	5. Lack of clarity causes a tension during the transition from hospital to home hospice: "The period between leaving the hospital and the first home hospice visit is one in which the client and family are particularly vulnerable" (Does et al., 2011). Frank discussions are needed to differentiate on managing deterioration, impending death, and emergencies (e.g., when to call 911, when not to).
6. Allow the family to share their expectation of home care. Clarify their understanding of: a. Necessary supplies (e.g., dressings, hospital bed, commode) b. Current medication regimen available for doses needed (e.g., same day after transition at home) c. Knowledge of management of pain, other symptoms d. Ability to manage treatments (e.g., wounds, catheters) e. Who to call for advice f. Manage medication regimen	6. Managing care transitions require clear communication among providers to prevent complications in home care. In addition, hospital staff / student frequently overestimate client / family knowledge and capabilities or inadequately assess their abilities to provide care, and clinicians may not be as attuned to specialized end-of-life (EOL) care deemed critical by clients and their families.
7. If prescribed, initiate a discussion regarding acquiring a hospital bed and its placement prior to bringing the family member home. a. Ordering the bed for delivery prior to transition b. Criteria for selecting and preparing the space	7. Families have reported difficulty accessing equipment prior to transition. Optimal placement of the bed should permit interactions with visitors and ease of access to care (Does et al., 2011).
8. Explain the disruptions that will occur and that their home life will be different than before. "Going home on palliative / hospice services is different from just going home" (Does et al., 2011, p. 396).	8. This home will now become an "Open House," with numerous persons coming into the house (Does et al., 2011).

Documentation

Teaching
Referrals

Sexual Assault

There were 125,910 reported rapes in 2009. If about half of violent crimes are reported, this rate rises to over 250,000 in the U.S. (Bureau of Justice, 2010). Females knew their offenders in almost 70% of violent crimes committed against them; males knew their offenders in 45% of violent crimes committed against them (Bureau of Justice, 2010). Rape is a crime using sexual means to humiliate, dominate, and degrade the victim (Symes, 2000). Sexual assault is forced and violent oral, vaginal, or anal penetration of a person without his or her consent. This care plan focuses on nursing for a client who has been sexually assaulted and is hospitalized for injuries.

Carp's Cues

As a nurse practitioner, this author has interacted with numerous girls and women who have shared their sexual assaults with me; some for the first time in their lives. Two themes were woven into their stories: (1) Guilt that they contributed to the assault, and (2) profound disappointment with their mother's response. Many mothers blame their daughter for the event and sometimes refuse to believe their daughter if a relative or paramour is involved; or they suggest that their daughter provoked the event.

Perhaps that was the only reaction her mother could have at the time, for whatever reason. I discuss forgiveness with these girls / women. Forgiveness never means you accept what happened, only that you are going to release the pain from yourself. Stop carrying it around with you. Forgiveness is a gift you give yourself (Carpenito, 2013, p. 485).

Time Frame

Coexisting with (trauma requiring hospitalization)

▚▚▚▪▪ DIAGNOSTIC CLUSTER**

Collaborative Problems

Risk for Complications of Sexually Transmitted Infection (STI)

Risk for Complications of Unwanted Pregnancy

Collaborative Problems associated with physical injuries sometimes caused by sexual assault include fractures, head injuries, abdominal injuries, and burns (refer to the collaborative problem index for specific problems)

Nursing Diagnoses

Rape Trauma Syndrome

**This situation was not included in the validation study.

Transition Criteria

Before transition, the client or family will:

1. Share feelings.
2. Describe rationales and treatment procedures.
3. Identify what needs to be done now and take steps toward the goals.
4. Relate the intent to seek professional help after transition.
5. Identify members of support system available.

Transitional Risk Assessment Plan (TRAP)

Begin this plan on admission.
Implement the Transitional Risk Assessment Plan (TRAP):
- Refer to inside back cover.
- Add each validated risk diagnosis to client's problem list with the risk code in ( ).
- Refer to Unit II to the individual risk nursing diagnoses/collaborative problems for outcomes and interventions.

> *R:* *"Close coordination of care in the post-acute period, early transition follow-up care, enhanced client education and self-management training, proactive end-of-life counseling, and extending the resources and clinical expertise over time via multidisciplinary team management" can lower readmission rates and improve health outcomes (Boutwell & Hwu, 2009, p. 14).*

Collaborative Problems

Risk for Complications of Sexually Transmitted Infection

Risk for Complications of Unwanted Pregnancy

Collaborative Outcomes

The client will be advised of measures to prevent and / or treat (a) STIs and (b) unwanted pregnancy.

Indicators of Physiologic Stability

- Evidence of treatment for chlamydia
- Evidence of treatment for gonorrhea
- Prophylactic treatment for pregnancy
- Negative results for trichomonal infection or evidence of treatment
- Negative results on rapid plasma reagin test (RPR) or evidence of treatment
- Evidence of postexposure prophylaxis for HIV

Interventions	Rationales
1. Explain the risks of STIs and pregnancy.	1. The Centers for Disease Control and Prevention (CDC) and other expert groups recommend preventive treatment if the mouth, vagina, anus, or nonintact skin (e.g., a cut) was exposed to the assailant's blood or bodily fluids (CDC, 2010).
2. Discuss the implications of STI screening (cervical, urethral, rectal, oral) and blood specimens (syphilis, HIV). **CLINICAL ALERT** • If specimens were collected for STD testing and the individual does not want to be tested or has changed his or her mind, contact the physician / NP to discuss the situation (e.g., allowing the lab to dispose of the specimens).	2. "Testing for chlamydia, gonorrhea, trichomonas, hepatitis B, and HIV is recommended if the individual has signs or symptoms of one of these infections. However, testing for these infections in the days following the acute assault will only confirm prior infection, not an infection as a result of the assault. If one is tested for sexually transmitted infections during the evaluation, it is important to understand that the results will become part of the medical record and will be available to the assailant's attorney if the case goes to trial. Thus, the information could potentially be used to discredit the victim. For these reasons, some victims choose to avoid STI testing at this time and receive prophylactic treatment for STIs" (Bates, 2013, p. 4).
3. As prescribed, provide treatment prophylaxis for: a. Chlamydia: Zithromax 1 g b. Gonorrhea: Rocephin 250 mg IM (with 1% lidocaine as dilutant) c. Trichomonas: Flagyl 2 g in two divided doses over 24 h	
4. Explain risks of HIV transmission. The risks seroconversion (becoming infected with HIV) is 0.3% to 0.9% after percutaneous/mucus membrane exposure (e.g., needlesticks) and no reported seroconversion with exposure to intact skin (Sax, Cohen, & Kuritzkes, 2102).	
5. Explain postexposure prophylaxis for 2 weeks and the importance of starting as soon as possible (preferably within 48 h of assault but can be instituted 1–2 weeks after the assault) (Sax, Cohen, & Kuritzkes, 2102).	
6. Follow CDC protocols (CDC, 2011).	
7. Explain side effects of medications, need for adherence, and specific instruction regarding food and other drug interactions.	7. Taking every dose increases its effectiveness
8. Determine if the client is at risk for pregnancy: a. No contraceptive uses b. No surgical sterilization c. History of infertility d. Premenopausal or postmenopausal	
9. Explain how emergency contraceptive pills (ECPs) prevents implantation of fertilized egg.	9. ECP delays ovulation and interferes with tubal transport of egg or sperm (Arcangelo & Peterson, 2011).
10. If desired, and within 72 h of assault, provide ECP medication. Explain ECP can cause nausea and vomiting from high estrogen content.	

Related Physician/NP Prescribed Interventions

Medications

(Refer to collaborative problems for specific medications.) STD prophylaxis, ECP, HIV prophylaxis, antiemetics, analgesics, sedatives

Laboratory Studies
Vaginal, urine, urethra, rectal cultures; HIV testing; RPR test; serum/urine drug screens

Diagnostic Studies
Microscopic examination of vaginal fluid smear (wet mount)

Documentation

Present emotional status
Interventions
Responses in nursing interventions, police and counselor interviews, examination for evidence
Subjective, objective, and general reactions
Availability of significant others for support
Medications given and collection of specimens

Nursing Diagnoses

Rape Trauma Syndrome

NOC

Abuse Protection, Abuse Recovery Status, Coping

Goals

Refer to transition criteria.

Interventions	Rationales
1. Provide interventions to decrease anxiety. a. Limit people to whom the client—victim must describe assault. b. Do not leave individual alone. c. Maintain a nonjudgmental attitude. Show concern for the client. d. Gently explore with the individual her or his feelings regarding why she or he thinks the assault occurred. e. Some girls or women have reported that they: • Worn too sexy clothes • Drank too much. • Walked home after dark • Had engaged in kissing and hugging • Went with him alone to another place	1a. Repeatedly relating the incident increases shame and anxiety. b. Isolation can increase anxiety.

 Carp's Cues

I share with each girl / woman this scenario. "Instead of being sexually assaulted, imagine that you were hit over the head with a shovel. Would it matter what you were wearing, how much alcohol you drank or what you were saying or doing at the time? Sexual assault is not sex; it is a violent act, like hitting someone on the head with a shovel. I suggest that the next time they have self-blame, they think of the shovel" (Carpenito, 2013, p. 486).

Interventions	Rationales
f. Explore the available support systems. g. Create a plan to increase sense of safety. Be specific.	f. Support system provides some stability and safety. g. This will reduce fear and anxiety.
2. Assist the client to identify major concerns (psychological, medical, and legal) and his or her perception of needed help.	2. Sexual assault is always associated with coercion and threatened or actual violence. It is by this means the assailant takes control from the victim. Involving the victim in decision-making begins reestablishing a sense of control (Smith-DiJulio, 2001).
3. Whenever possible, provide crisis counseling within 1 hour of rape trauma event: a. Ask permission to contact the rape crisis counselor. Victim empowerment is the primary antidote to the trauma of sexual assault (Smith-DiJulio, 2001).	

Interventions	Rationales
4. Promote a trusting relationship by providing emotional support with unconditional positive regard and acceptance:	4. Providing immediate and ongoing empathy and support prepares victims for referral to more in-depth psychological counseling. Main issues in the acute stage are being in control, fearing being left alone, and having someone to listen (Smith-DiJulio, 2001).
a. Stay with the client during acute stage, or arrange for other support.	a.–i. Victims are vulnerable to any statement that can be construed as blaming. Their normal defenses are weakened. When asked too many questions, clients can feel "grilled." This interferes with the rapport between helper and client.
b. Brief the client on police and hospital procedures during acute stage.	
c. Assist during medical examination and explain all procedures in advance.	
d. Help the client to meet personal needs (bathing after examination and after evidence has been acquired).	
e. Listen attentively to the client's requests.	
f. Maintain unhurried attitude toward the client and her or his family.	
g. Avoid rescue feelings toward the client.	
h. Maintain nonjudgmental attitude.	
i. Support the client's beliefs and value system; avoid labeling.	
j. Reassure the individual that the symptoms are normal responses that will lessen and improve with time.	j. The victim needs to understand that a wide range of behavior and emotional responses is normal.
5. Explain the care and examination she or he will experience:	5. Because the victim's right to deny or consent has been violently violated, it is important to seek permission for subsequent care (Heinrich, 1987). It is important to tell the client as much as is practical or possible about what is happening and why. Even in life-threatening situations, any sense of control given to the individual is helpful.
a. Maintaining eye contact, conduct the examinations in an unhurried manner.	a. Unhurried and confident actions, eye contact, and affirming the victim is safe help to calm and assure that he or she is alive and worthy.
b. Explain every detail slowly before action.	b. Cognitive dysfunction impairs short-term memory.
c. Make every attempt to provide privacy, draping body parts, limit exposure.	c. The victim of rape needs to understand the common reactions to this experience. Any exposure or loss of privacy is especially distressing, because it can be reminiscent of the assault (Ledray, 2001).
6. Provide interventions to assist with regaining control (Smith-DiJulio, 2001):	
a. Listen, listen, listen.	6a. Probably the best response is simply for the nurse to listen without judgment and ask more than once what to do to support the client's recovery (Carosella, 1995).
b. "How can I help you?"	b. Many traumatized people repeat their stories over and over. This is part of the healing and diminishes with time.
7. Reassure that feelings and reactions are normal responses and accept where the client is in the recovery process.	7. Emotional care must aim to convey respect and understanding; communicate empathy, reassurance, and support; encourage ventilation of feelings; preserve dignity; empower the victim; provide anticipatory guidance; and ensure adequate follow-up.
8. Explore available support systems. Involve significant others:	
a. Share with family and friends the victim's immediate needs for love and support.	
b. Refer to counseling services.	8b. Postponing professional help lengthens the time reactions persist and lengthens recovery.

> ### *Clinical Alert Report*
>
> Prior to providing care, advise ancillary staff / student to report the following to the professional nurse assigned to the client:
> - Any change in levels of anxiety
> - Increase in distress
> - Distressful visitors

Documentation

Injuries
Emotional state
Documentation protocol for sexual assault

Section 2

Surgical Procedures

Generic Care Plan for the Surgical Client

This care plan presents nursing diagnoses and collaborative problems that commonly apply to clients (and their significant others) experiencing all types of surgery. Nursing diagnoses and collaborative problems specific to a surgical procedure (e.g., fortotal knee replacement, cholecystectomies are presented in the care plan for that procedure). Basic postoperative nursing care will not be repeated in the specific surgical procedure care plans.

Time Frame
Preoperative and postoperative periods

Carp's Cues
Prior to planned surgery, the majority of clients arrive the morning of surgery. It is the responsibility of the nursing staff / student in the presurgical unit and surgical suite to provide simple explanations prior to interventions and some teaching on what to expect after surgery. High levels of anxiety will impair the individual's level of comprehension.

■■■ DIAGNOSTIC CLUSTER

Preoperative

Nursing Diagnoses

Anxiety / Fear related to surgical experience, loss of control, unpredictable outcome, and insufficient knowledge of preoperative routines, postoperative exercises and activities, and postoperative changes and sensations

Postoperative

Collaborative Problems

Risk for Complications of Hemorrhage

Risk for Complications of Hypovolemia / Shock

Risk for Complications of Evisceration / Dehiscence

Risk for Complications of Paralytic Ileus

Risk for Complications of Infection (Peritonitis, Incision)

Risk for Complications of Urinary Retention

Risk for Complications of Thrombophlebitis

(continued)

Nursing Diagnoses

Risk for Ineffective Respiratory Function related to immobility secondary to postanesthesia state and pain

Risk for (Surgical Site) Infection related to access for organism invasion secondary to surgery

Acute Pain related to surgical interruption of body structures, flatus, and immobility

Risk for Imbalanced Nutrition: Less Than Body Requirements related to increased protein and vitamin requirements for wound healing and decreased intake secondary to pain, nausea, vomiting, and diet restrictions

Risk for Constipation related to decreased peristalsis secondary to immobility and the effects of anesthesia and narcotics

Activity Intolerance related to pain and weakness secondary to anesthesia, tissue hypoxia, and insufficient fluid and nutrient intake

Risk for Ineffective Self-Health Management related to insufficient knowledge of care of operative site, restrictions (diet, activity), medications, signs and symptoms of complications, and follow-up care

Transitional Criteria

Before transition, the client and / or family will:

1. Describe any at-home activity restrictions.
2. Describe at-home wound and pain management.
3. Discuss fluid and nutritional requirements for proper wound healing.
4. List the signs and symptoms that must be reported to a health care professional.
5. Describe necessary follow-up care.

Transitional Risk Assessment Plan (TRAP)

Begin this plan on admission.
Implement the Transitional Risk Assessment Plan (TRAP):
- Refer to inside back cover.
- Add each validated risk diagnosis to client's problem list with the risk code in ( ).
- Refer to Unit II to the individual risk nursing diagnoses / collaborative problems for outcomes and interventions.

  R: "Close coordination of care in the post-acute period, early transition follow-up care, enhanced client education and self-management training, proactive end-of-life counseling, and extending the resources and clinical expertise over time via multidisciplinary team management" can lower readmission rates and improve health outcomes (Boutwell & Hwu, 2009, p. 14).

Preoperative: Nursing Diagnosis

Anxiety / Fear Related to Surgical Experience, Loss of Control, Unpredictable Outcome, and Insufficient Knowledge of Preoperative Routines, Postoperative Exercises and Activities, and Postoperative Changes and Sensations

NOC
Anxiety Reduction, Coping, Impulse Control

Goal

The client will communicate feelings regarding the surgical experience, including the limitations and restrictions, and discuss any therapeutic medical devices (e.g., braces, crutches, plasters), that will apply postoperatively.

NIC
Anxiety Reduction, Impulse Control Training, Anticipatory Guidance

Indicators

- Verbalize, if asked, what to expect regarding routines, environment, and sensations.
- Demonstrate postoperative exercises, splinting, and respiratory regimen.

Carp's Cues

Please refer to the Generic Care Plan for the Surgical Client for detailed interventions for managing all surgical conditions. This care plan addresses specific additional interventions associated with any type of surgery performed.

Interventions	Rationales
1. Providing emotional support and encouraging the client to share her or his feelings / fears.	1. Preoperative teaching provides the client with information; this can help to reduce anxiety and fear associated with the unknown, and to enhance the client's sense of control over the situation.
2. Correct any misconceptions and inaccurate information.	2. Modifiable contributing factors to anxiety include incomplete and inaccurate information. Providing accurate information and correcting misconceptions may help to eliminate fears and reduce anxiety.
3. Allow and encourage family members and significant others to share their fears and concerns. Correct inaccurate information. a. Explain all interventions prior to providing them. b. Explain what to expect in operating room and recovery room.	3. Effective support from family members, other relatives, and friends can help the client to cope with surgery and recovery.
4. Notify the physician / NP if the client exhibits severe or panic anxiety.	4. Immediate notification enables prompt assessment and possible pharmacologic intervention.
5. Notify the physician / NP if the client needs any further explanations about the procedure.	5. The physician / NP is responsible for explaining the surgery to the client and family; the nurse, for determining their level of understanding and then notifying the physician / NP of the need to provide more information, if necessary.
6. Provide instruction on general information pertaining to preoperative routines and transport to OR. Elicit questions.	6. Preoperative teaching can help to reduce anxiety and fear associated with the unknown, and to enhance the client's sense of control over the situation.

Documentation

Vital signs
Medications administered

Postoperative: Collaborative Problems

Risk for Complications of Hemorrhage

Risk for Complications of Hypovolemia / Shock

Risk for Complications of Evisceration / Dehiscence

Risk for Complications of Paralytic Ileus

Risk for Complications of Infection (Peritonitis, Incision)

Risk for Complications of Urinary Retention

Risk for Complications of Thrombophlebitis

Collaborative Outcomes

The client will be monitored for early signs and symptoms of (a) hemorrhage, (b) hypovolemia / shock, (c) evisceration / dehiscence, (d) paralytic ileus, (e) infection, (f) urinary retention, and (g) thrombophlebitis, and will receive collaborative interventions if indicated to restore physiologic stability.

Indicators of Physiologic Stability

- Respirations 16–20 breaths/min, relaxed and rhythmic (a, b)
- Breath sound present all lobes (a, b)
- No rales or wheezing (a, b)
- Pulse 60–100 beats/min (a, b)
- BP > 90/60, <140/90 mm Hg (a, b)
- Capillary refill <3 seconds (a, b)
- Peripheral pulses full, equal (a, b)
- Temperature 98.5°–99° F (a, b, e)
- Urine output >0.5 mL/kg/h (a, b)
- No bladder distension (f)
- No difficulty voiding (f)
- Surgical wound intact (c, e)
- Minimal serosanguinous drainage (e)
- Bowel sounds present (b, d)
- No nausea and vomiting (b, d)
- No abdominal distention (b, d)
- No calf tenderness, warmth, or edema (g)
- White blood cells 4,000–10,000/mm^3 (e)
- Hemoglobin (a)
  - Male 14–18 g/dL
  - Female 12–16 g/dL
- Hematocrit (a)
  - Male 42% to 52%
  - Female 37% to 47%
- Oxygen saturation (SaO$_2$) >94% (a, b)

Interventions	Rationales
1. Monitor for signs and symptoms of hemorrhage / hypovolemia / shock (when fluid volume decreases, the body responds to compensate) (Porth, 2011).	1. The compensatory response to decreased circulatory volume aims to increase blood oxygen through increased heart and respiratory rates and decreased peripheral circulation (manifested by diminished peripheral pulses and cool skin).

a. Urine output <0.5 mL/kg/h (early sign)
  b. Thirst
  c. Increased pulse rate with normal or slightly decreased blood pressure
  d. Increased capillary refill >3 seconds
  e. Decreased oxygen saturation <94% (pulse oximetry)
  f. Increased respiratory rate
  g. Diminished peripheral pulses
  h. Cool, pale, or cyanotic skin
  i. Restlessness, agitation, decreased mentation (late sign)
	a. The kidney responds to decrease fluid volume by increasing the release of the antidiuretic hormone, which increases sodium retention and reduce urine production (Porth, 2011).
	
	  i. Decreased oxygen to the brain results in altered mentation.

2. Determine the risk status of the individual for postoperative hypovolemia (oliguria). a. Causes of oliguria are can be divided into three categories: prerenal (blood-flow related), renal (intrinsic kidney disorders), and postrenal (outlet obstruction).	2a. Prerenal causes can be fluid loss during surgery and as a result of NPO status can disrupt fluid balance in a high-risk client. Stress can cause sodium and water retention. Postoperative decreased urine output can be caused by hypovolemia (bleeding, fluid loss, NPO status, inadequate fluid replacement). Postrenal causes can be blocked urinary catheter or postoperative urinary retention.

Interventions	Rationales
3. Assess for additional risk factors.	3. Individuals at higher risk should have more frequent monitoring and may need a urinary catheter for frequent measurements.

CLINICAL ALERT
- Prerenal causes of hypovolemia are low cardiac output (myocardial infarction, heart failure, pulmonary embolism) and decreased systemic vascular resistance (sepsis).
- Specific renal (intrinsic) causes are due to acute tubular necrosis and are hypoperfusion (prolonged, e.g., over 4 hours), X-ray contrast dye, rhabdomyolysis, nephrotoxic drugs (e.g., aminoglycosides and other antibiotics, NSAIDs).
- Postrenal causes are mechanical urinary obstruction (blocked urinary catheter, prostatic hypertrophy, urinary calculi) or bladder / sphincter dysfunction (anticholinergic drug use, postoperative urinary retention, fecal impaction if severe).

4. Institute hourly urine output monitoring according to protocol and individual risks:
   a. Intake (parenteral and oral)
   b. Output and other losses (urine, drainage, and vomiting)

5. Palpate for bladder distention and evaluate patency of urinary catheter.	5. This will assess for outlet obstruction and blocked urinary catheter.

CLINICAL ALERT
- The kidneys respond to changes in blood volume and hypoxemia by reducing urine production.
- Decreased urine output is an earlier sign of hypovolemia than changes in pulse and blood pressure.
- Promptly report decreasing urine output.

6. Monitor the surgical site for bleeding, dehiscence.	6. Wound dehiscence is the partial or complete separation of the outer layers of the joined incision and evisceration. Evisceration is the protrusion of the intestines through the open incision.
7. Assess for risk factors: a. Advanced age (65 years or older) b. Chronic disease (diabetes, hypertension, renal urea, pulmonary or liver disease, immune deficiency, cancer) c. History of chemotherapy or radiation d. Malnutrition e. Hypoalbuminemia f. Increased intra-abdominal pressure or tension (ileus or distended bowel, coughing, straining, vomiting) g. Obesity h. Tobacco use i. Use of certain medications (anticoagulants, aspirin, colchicines, systemic corticosteroids, penicillamine, cyclosporine, metronidazole, cytotoxic chemotherapeutics)	7. Careful monitoring enables early detection of complications (Heller, Levin, & Butler, 2006).

(continued)

j. Wound complication (incisional infection, hematoma, inadequate incisional closure).

> **CLINICAL ALERT**
>
> If dehiscence or evisceration occurs, contact the surgeon or rapid response team immediately and do the following:
> - Rapid interventions can reduce severity of complications.
> - Either soak the dressings in a basin of NS or lay the dressings over the wound and irrigate them using the sterile syringe. (A wet sterile dressing helps to maintain tissue viability.)
> - Keep the client in bed in a low Fowler's position—about 15° to 45° C. Flex the knees. (This will reduce tension in the wound area.)
> - Change the client's intake status to NPO (In anticipation of surgery).
> - Instruct the client to lie still and quiet. Lying still and quiet also minimizes tissue protrusion.
> - Cover any protruding viscera with a wet sterile dressing. (Do not initiate fluids until bowel sounds are present; then, begin with small amounts. Monitor the client's response to resumption of fluids and foods and note the nature and amount of any emesis.)

j. The seepage of serosanguineous fluid through a closed abdominal wound is an early sign of abdominal wound dehiscence with possible evisceration. When this occurs, the surgeon should remove one or two sutures in the skin and explore the wound manually, using a sterile glove. If there is separation of the rectus fascia, the client may be taken to the operating room for primary closure. Wound dehiscence may or may not be associated with intestinal evisceration. When the latter complication is present, the mortality rate is dramatically increased and may reach 30%.

8. Monitor for signs of paralytic ileus:
   a. Absent bowel sounds
   b. Nausea, vomiting
   c. Abdominal distention

8. Intraoperative manipulation of abdominal organs and the depressive effects of narcotics and anesthetics on peristalsis can cause paralytic ileus, usually between the third and fifth postoperative day. Pain typically is localized, sharp, and intermittent.

9. Monitor for septic shock and systemic inflammatory response syndrome (SIRS) (Halloran, 2009):
   a. Urine output <0.5 mL/kg/h
   b. Body temperature greater than 38° C or less than 36° C

   c. Heart rate greater than 90/min

   d. Hyperkalemia

   e. Decreasing blood pressure
   f. Respiratory rate greater than 20/min

   g. Hyperglycemia

   h. White blood cell count greater than 12,000/µL or less than 4,000/µL or presence of 10% immature neutrophils

9a. Urine output is decreased when sodium shifts into the cells, which pulls water into cells. Decreased circulation to kidneys reduce their ability to detoxify the toxins that result from anaerobic metabolism.
   c. Decreased blood flow to brain, heart, and kidneys triggers baroreceptors and release of catecholamines, increasing heart rate / cardiac output and further increasing vasoconstriction.
   d. Potassium moves into the cell with the sodium, impairing nervous, cardiovascular, and muscle cell function.
   e. Movement of water into the cell causes hypovolemia.
   f. Anaerobic metabolism decreases circulating oxygen. The body attempts to increase oxygenation by increasing respiratory rate.
   g. The liver and kidneys produce more glucose in response to the release of epinephrine, norepinephrine, cortisol, and glucagon. Anaerobic metabolism reduces the effects of insulin. Insulin resistance contributes to multiple organ failure, nosocomial infection, and renal injury (Ball et al., 2007).
   h. Increased white cells indicate an infectious process

Interventions	Rationales
10. Ensure blood culture is done prior to the start of any antibiotic. Culture any suspected infection sites (urine, sputum, invasive lines). **CLINICAL ALERT** • Blood culture obtained after antibiotic therapy has been initiated can be inaccurate. • Research of individuals with septic shock demonstrated that the time to initiation of appropriate antimicrobial therapy was the strongest predictor of mortality (Schmidt & Mandel, 2012). • Microorganisms can be introduced into the body during surgery or through the incision. • Circulating pathogens trigger the body's defense mechanisms: WBCs are released to destroy some pathogens, and the hypothalamus raises the body temperature to kill others. Wound redness, tenderness, and edema result from lymphocyte migration to the area.	10. "Poor outcomes are associated with inadequate or inappropriate antimicrobial therapy (i.e., treatment with antibiotics to which the pathogen was later shown to be resistant in vitro. They are also associated with delays in initiating antimicrobial therapy, even short delays (e.g., an hour") (Schmidt & Mandel, 2012).
11. Monitor for signs of urinary retention: a. Bladder distention and unrelieved associated pain (Wagner, Johnson, & Kidd, 2006) b. Urine overflows (30–60 mL, or urine every 15–30 minutes)	11. Anesthesia relaxes the muscles, affecting the bladder. As muscle tone returns, spasms of the bladder sphincter prevent urine outflow, causing bladder distention. When urine retention increases the intravesical pressure, the sphincter releases urine and control of flow is regained. Pain medications interfere with the perception of bladder fullness and urge to void.
12. Instruct the client to report bladder discomfort or inability to void.	12. Bladder discomfort and failure to void may be early signs of urinary retention.
13. If the client does not void within 8–10 hours after surgery or complains of bladder discomfort, do the following: a. Warm the bedpan. b. Encourage the client to get out of bed to use the bathroom, if possible. c. Instruct a male client to stand when urinating, if possible. d. Run water in the sink as the client attempts to void. e. Pour warm water over the client's perineum.	13. These measures may help to promote relaxation of the urinary sphincter and facilitate voiding.
14. If the client still cannot void, follow the protocols for straight catheterization, as ordered.	14. Straight catheterization is preferable to indwelling catheterization, because it carries less risk of urinary tract infection from ascending pathogens.

(continued)

Interventions	Rationales
15. Monitor the status of venous thrombosis, noting:	15. Avoid performing Homans' sign (*dorsiflexion of the foot*). (Numerous studies have documented the unreliability of Homans' sign. Urbano [2001] reported "Estimates of the accuracy of Homans' sign range from it being positive in 8% to 56% of cases of proven DVT and positive in greater than 50% of symptomatic clients without DVT") (p. 23).
a. Diminished or absent peripheral pulses	a. Insufficient circulation causes pain and diminished peripheral pulses.
b. Unusual warmth and redness or coolness and cyanosis, increased leg swelling	b. Unusual warmth and redness point to inflammation; coolness and cyanosis indicate vascular obstruction.
c. Increasing leg pain	c. Leg pain results from tissue hypoxia.
16. Monitor for signs and symptoms of pulmonary embolism: a. Acute, sharp chest pain b. Acute dyspnea, restlessness, cyanosis, decreased mental status or anxiety c. Cool, moist and / or bluish-colored skin d. Tachycardia e. Tachypnea (Shaughnessy, 2007) f. Neck vein distention g. Crackles	16. Occlusion of pulmonary arteries impedes blood flow to the distal lung, producing a hypoxic state (Porth, 2011).

> **CLINICAL ALERT**
> • Call a code or rapid response team if sudden, severe chest pain, increased dyspnea, tachypnea occur.
> • Begin emergency care, as indicated (e.g., bag-mask, IV access).

Interventions	Rationales
17. Consult with physician / NP for intermittent pneumatic compression devices or graduated compression stockings.	17. These should be used for clients who are bleeding or at risk for it.
18. Evaluate hydration status based on urine specific gravity, intake / output, weights, and serum osmolality. Take steps to ensure adequate hydration.	18. Increased blood viscosity and coagulability and decreased cardiac output may contribute to thrombus formation.
19. Encourage client to perform isotonic leg exercises.	19. They promote venous return.
20. Ambulate as soon as possible with at least 5 minutes of walking each waking hour. Avoid prolonged chair sitting with legs dependent. Explain risk of DVT and PE. If client is resistant, evaluate the reason for pain.	20. Walking contracts leg muscles, stimulates the venous pump, and reduces stasis.
21. Elevate the affected extremity above the level of the heart unless contraindicated (e.g., CHF).	21. This positioning can help reduce interstitial swelling by promoting venous return.
22. Explain the effects of nicotine (cigarettes, cigars, smokeless) on circulation. Refer to Getting Started to Quit Smoking on thePoint at http://thePoint.lww.com/Carpenito6e.	22. Nicotine can cause vasoconstriction and hypercoagulable state which contributes to poor circulation and clot formation (Giardina, 1999).

Clinical Alert Report

Prior to providing care, advise ancillary staff / student to report the following to the professional nurse assigned to the client:

- Change in cognitive status
- Sudden restlessness, agitation, decreased mentation
- Oral temperature >100.5° F
- Systolic BP <90 mm/Hg
- Resting Pulse >100, <50
- Respiratory rate >28, <10/min.
- Oxygen saturation <90%
- A report of leg pain, soreness. Increased leg swelling
- Diminished peripheral pulses
- Unusual warmth and redness
- Cool, pale, moist, or cyanotic skin
- Increased immobility (e.g., refusal to ambulate)
- Urine output <0.5 mL/kg/h
- Increased drainage for wound
- Increased tenderness / c/o of pain

Related Physician / NP Prescribed Interventions

Medications
Preoperative: Sedatives, opioid analgesics, anticholinergics
Postoperative: Opioid analgesics, antiemetics

Intravenous Therapy
Fluid and electrolyte replacement

Laboratory Studies
Complete blood count, urinalysis, chemistry profile (especially magnesium, potassium, and calcium, coagulation studies)

Diagnostic Studies
Chest x-ray film, electrocardiography, computed tomography, ultrasound

Therapies
Indwelling catheterization, incentive spirometry, wound care, liquid diet (progressed to full diet) as tolerated, preoperative NPO status, and pulse oximetry

Documentation

Vital signs (pulses, respirations, blood pressure, and temperature)
Circulation (color, peripheral pulses)
Intake (oral, parenteral)
Output (urinary, tubes, specific gravity)
Bowel function (bowel sounds, defecation, distention)
Wound (color, drainage)
Unusual complaints or assessment findings

Postoperative: Nursing Diagnoses

Risk for Ineffective Respiratory Function Related to Immobility Secondary to Postanesthesia State and Pain

NOC
Aspiration Control,
Respiratory Status

NIC
Airway Management,
Cough Enhancement,
Respiratory Monitoring,
Positioning

Goal

The client will exhibit clear lung fields.

Indicators

- Breath sounds present in all lobes
- Clear breath sounds in all lobes (no wheezes or congestion)
- Relaxed rhythmic respirations

Interventions	Rationales
1. Monitor respiratory status: Vital signs, pulse oximetry.	
2. Auscultate lung fields for diminished and abnormal breath sounds.	2. Presence of rales indicates retained secretions. Diminished breath sounds may indicate atelectasis.
3. Take measures to prevent aspiration. Position the client on his or her side, with pillows supporting the back and knees slightly flexed.	3. In the postoperative period, decreased sensorium and hypoventilation contribute to increased risk of aspiration.
4. Reinforce preoperative client teaching about the importance of turning, coughing, deep breathing, and of leg exercises every 1–2 hours.	4. Postoperative pain may discourage compliance; reinforcing the importance of these measures may improve compliance.
5. Promote the following as soon as the client returns to the unit: a. Deep breaths b. Coughing (except if contraindicated) c. Frequent turning d. Early ambulation e. Incentive spirometry every hour (10 breaths each time, or as ordered) (Wagner, Johnson, & Kidd, 2006).	5. Exercises and movement promote lung expansion and mobilization of secretions. Incentive spirometry promotes deep breathing by providing a visual indicator of the effectiveness of the breathing effort. Coughing assists in dislodging mucus plugs. Coughing is contraindicated in clients who have had a head injury, intracranial surgery, eye surgery, or plastic surgery, because it increases intracranial and intraocular pressure and tension on delicate tissues (plastic surgery).
6. Encourage adequate oral fluid intake, as indicated.	6. Adequate hydration liquefies secretions, which enables easier expectoration and prevents stasis of secretions that provide a medium for microorganism growth. It also helps to decrease blood viscosity, which lowers the risk of clot formation.

Documentation

Temperature
Respiratory rate and rhythm
Breath sounds
Respiratory treatments and client responses

Risk for (Surgical Site) Infection Related to Access for Organism Invasion Secondary to Surgery

NOC
Infection Status, Wound
Healing: Primary
Infection, Immune
Status

Goal

The client will demonstrate healing of wound.

NIC

Infection Control,
Wound Care, Incision
Site Care, Health
Education

Indicators

- No abnormal drainage
- Intact, approximated wound edges

Interventions	Rationales

1. Identify individuals at risk for delayed wound healing:
  a. Malnourishment
  b. Tobacco use
  c. Obesity
  d. Anemia
  e. Diabetes
  f. Cancer
  g. Corticosteroid therapy
  h. Renal insufficiency
  i. Hypovolemia
  j. Hypoxia
  k. Surgery >3 hours
  l. Night or emergency surgery
  m. Zinc, copper, magnesium deficiency
  n. Immune system compromise
	1. Delayed wound healing can allow microorganisms to enter the wound.

2. Closely monitor the surgical sites in obese individuals.	2. Obese individuals have a higher rate of surgical site infection. Subcutaneous adipose tissue has decreased circulation, which slows healing and the absorption of antibiotics. The increased tension on the wound edges increases tissue pressure, reducing micro perfusion and the availability of oxygen to the wound needed for healing. This also contributes to wound dehiscence (Wilson & Clark, 2004).

3. Monitor normal wound healing by noting the following (Beattie, 2007; Mercandetti, 2013):
  a. Evidence of intact, approximated wound edges (primary intention). Within 48 hours after surgery, fibrin and epithelial cells, as well as strands of collagen fill in the gaps and seal the incision.
  b. Slight swelling, slight scabbing around sutures or staples and wound edges and some redness and warmth.
  c. Expected drainage (1–5 days after surgery: sanguineous (bloody) to serosanguineous / watery mixture of serum and blood to serous (yellowish, clear).
  d. By day 5, a "healing ridge" of granulation tissue can be palpated directly under the incision and extending approximately 1 cm on both sides of the wound.
	3. These observations are the normal inflammatory reaction triggered by the surgical procedure. Any deviations from this normal healing process—especially between post-op days 5 and 10—could spell trouble. Most dehiscence occurs 4–14 days after surgery (Mercandetti, 2013).

> **CLINICAL ALERT**
> - A surgical wound with edges approximated by sutures usually heals by primary intention.
> - Granulation tissue is not visible and scar formation is minimal.
> - In contrast, a surgical wound with a drain or an abscess heals by secondary intention or granulation and has more distinct scar formation.
> - A restructured wound heals by third intention and results in a wider and deeper scar.

(continued)

Interventions	Rationales
4. Maintain normothermia. Monitor temperature every 4 hours; notify physician / NP if temperature is greater than 100.8° F	4. Hypothermia also increases the risk of surgical wound infection hypothermia directly impairs immune function including T-cell-mediated antibody production. Thermoregulatory vasoconstriction decreases subcutaneous oxygen tension and increases the risk of wound infection (Sessler, 2006).
5. Monitor for inadequate tissue oxygen in risk clients (e.g., pulse oximetry): a. Advise smokers that the risk of wound infection is tripled in smokers (Sessler, 2006). b. Monitor for hyperglycemia in diabetic and nondiabetic clients. c. Consult with physician / NP for interventions to achieve rigorous postoperative glucose control. d. Aggressively manage postoperative pain using prevention vs. prn medication administration. e. Prevent hypovolemia.	5. Deceased tissue oxygen impairs tissue repair (Sessler, 2006). b. Surgical site infections have been found to double in both diabetic and nondiabetic clients postcardiac surgical clients when blood glucose exceeds 200 mg/dL in the first 48 hours (Sessler, 2006). c. Aggressive insulin infusion protocol has shown to reduce wound infections, multiple organ failure, sepsis, and mortality in critical care clients (Sessler, 2006). d. Postoperative pain provokes an autonomic response that produces arteriolar vasoconstriction and reduces circulation needed for wound healing (Sessler, 2006). e. Small-volume deficits can substantially reduce peripheral circulation (Sessler, 2006).
6. Assess wound site every 24 hours and apply dressing if indicated; report any abnormal findings (e.g., increased redness, change in drainage, failure for edges to seal).	6. Wound healing by primary intention requires a dressing to protect it from contamination until the edges seal (usually 24 hours). Wound healing by secondary intention requires a dressing to maintain adequate hydration; the dressing is not needed after wound edges seal.
7. Monitor for signs and symptoms of wound infection: a. Increased swelling and redness b. Wound separation c. Increased serosanguineous or purulent drainage d. Prolonged subnormal temperature or significantly elevated temperature	7. Tissue responds to pathogen infiltration with increased blood and lymph flow (manifested by edema, redness, and increased drainage) and reduced epithelialization (marked by wound separation). Circulating pathogens trigger the hypothalamus to elevate the body temperature; certain pathogens cannot survive at higher temperatures.
8. Explain when a dressing is indicated for a wound healing by primary intention, and for one healing by secondary intention.	8. A wound healing by primary intention requires a dressing to protect it from contamination until the edges seal (usually by 24 hours). A wound healing by secondary intention requires a dressing to maintain adequate hydration; the dressing is not needed after wound edges seal.
9. Teach and assist the client in the following: a. Supporting the surgical site when moving b. Splinting the area when coughing, sneezing, or vomiting	9. A wound typically requires 3 weeks for strong scar formation. Stress on the suture line before this occurs can cause disruption.
10. If indicated, consult with an enterostomal or clinical nurse specialist for specific skin care measures.	10. Management of a complex wound or impaired healing requires expert nursing consultation.

Documentation

Status of wound
Signs and symptoms of infection
Temperature

Acute Pain Related to Surgical Interruption of Body Structures, Flatus, and Immobility

NOC
Comfort Level, Pain Control

NIC
Pain Management, Medication Management, Emotional Support, Teaching: Individual, Hot / Cold Application, Simple Massage

Goal

A client will report progressive reduction of pain and an increase in activity.

Indicators

- Relate factors that increase pain.
- Report effective interventions.

Interventions	Rationales
1. Collaborate with the client to determine effective pain-relief interventions.	1. A client experiencing pain may feel a loss of control over his or her body and life. Collaboration can help minimize this feeling.
2. Teach the client to splint the surgical wound with a pillow when coughing, sneezing, or vomiting.	2. Splinting reduces stress on the suture line by equalizing pressure across the wound.
3. Listen attentively to the client's complaints, and convey that you are assessing the pain because you want to understand it better, not because you are trying to determine if it really exists.	3. A client who feels the need to convince health-care providers that she or he actually is experiencing pain is likely to have increased anxiety that can lead to greater pain.
4. Provide optimal pain relief with prescribed analgesics: a. Determine the preferred administration route—by mouth, intramuscular, intravenous, or rectal. Consult with the physician or advanced practice nurse. b. Assess vital signs—especially respiratory rate—before and after administering any narcotic agent. c. Take a preventive approach to pain medication; that is, administer medication before an activity (e.g., ambulation) to enhance participation (but be sure to evaluate the hazards of sedation); instruct the client to request pain medication as needed before pain becomes severe. d. After administering the pain medication, return in ½ hour to evaluate its effectiveness.	4a. The proper administration route optimizes the efficacy of pain medications. The oral route is preferred in most cases; for some drugs, the liquid dosage form may be given to a client who has difficulty swallowing. If frequent injections are necessary, the intravenous (IV) route is preferred to minimize pain and maximize absorption; however, IV administration may produce more profound side effects than other routes. b. Narcotics can depress the respiratory center of the brain. c. The preventive approach may reduce the total 24-hour dose as compared with the PRN approach; it also provides a more constant blood drug level, reduces the client's craving for the drug, and eliminates the anxiety associated with having to ask for and wait for PRN relief. d. Each client responds differently to pain medication; careful monitoring is needed to assess individual response (Lehne, 2004; Lewis et al., 2011).
5. Explain and assist with noninvasive and nonpharmacologic pain relief measures (e.g., splinting the incision site, proper positioning, heat or cold application). Refer to Unit II *Acute Pain* for additional interventions.	5. These measures can help to reduce pain by substituting another stimulus to prevent painful stimuli from reaching higher brain centers. In addition, relaxation reduces muscle tension and may help enhance the client's sense of control over pain.
6. Teach the client to expel flatus by the following measures: a. Walking as soon as possible after surgery b. Changing positions regularly, as possible (e.g., lying prone, assuming the knee–chest position)	6. Postoperatively, sluggish peristalsis results in accumulation of nonabsorbable gas. Pain occurs when unaffected bowel segments contract in an attempt to expel this accumulated gas. Activity speeds the return of peristalsis and the expulsion of flatus; proper positioning helps cause the gas to rise and be expelled.

Documentation

Type, route, and dosage schedule of all prescribed medications
Unsatisfactory relief from pain-relief measures

Risk for Imbalanced Nutrition: Less Than Body Requirements Related to Increased Protein and Vitamin Requirements for Wound Healing and Decreased Intake Secondary to Pain, Nausea, Vomiting, and Diet Restrictions

NOC
Nutritional Status,
Teaching: Nutrition

Goal

The client will resume ingestion of the daily nutritional requirements.

NIC
Nutrition Management,
Nutritional Monitoring

Indicators

- Selections from the four basic food groups, taking into account cultural preferences and allergies (Lewis et al., 2004).
- 2000–3000 mL of fluids.
- Adequate fiber, vitamins, and minerals.

Interventions	Rationales
1. Start clear liquids when signs of bowel function returns.	1. Clear liquid diets supply fluid and electrolytes in a form that requires minimal digestion and little stimulation of the GI tract.
2. Explain that a well-balanced diet is needed to meet your body's needs for surgical wound healing.	2. To support proper wound healing your body needs adequate intake of calories, protein, iron, vitamin A, vitamin C, zinc, and adequate hydration for vascular transport of oxygen and wastes.
a. Iron	a. Iron-rich foods include beef, poultry, pork, baked potato with skin, chickpeas, kidney beans, peas, apricots, egg, whole grain bread, tamarind, iron-fortified cereals.
b. Vitamin A: Cellular differentiation, proliferation, epithelialization, collagen synthesis, counteract catabolic effect of steroids with renal failure due to greater potential for toxicity.	b. Vitamin A-rich foods include sweet potatoes, grape fruit, cantaloupe, carrots, mango, peaches, papaya, collard greens, kale, spinach, fish, dairy products.
c. Vitamin C: Collagen synthesis. Not for individuals with renal failure due to risk for renal oxalate stone formation.	c. Vitamin C-rich foods include oranges, cantaloupe, honeydew melon, strawberries, papaya, broccoli, bell peppers, baked potato, tomato, cauliflower.
d. Zinc: Protein synthesis, cellular replication, collagen formation; large wounds, chest tubes, and wound drains contribute to further zinc loses.	d. Zinc-rich foods include meat, pork, seafood, dark poultry, dairy products, beans.
3. Restrict fluids before meals and large amounts of fluids at any time; instead, encourage the client to ingest small amounts of ice chips or sip cool, clear liquids (e.g., dilute tea, Jell-O water, flat ginger ale, or cola) frequently, unless vomiting persists.	3. Gastric distention from fluid ingestion can trigger the vagal visceral afferent pathways that stimulate the medulla oblongata (vomiting center) (Wagner, Johnson, & Kidd, 2012).
4. Teach the client to move slowly.	4. Rapid movements stimulate the vomiting center by triggering vestibulocerebellar afferents.
5. Reduce or eliminate unpleasant sights and odors.	5. Noxious odors and sights can stimulate the vomiting center.
6. Provide good mouth care after the client vomits.	6. Good oral care reduces the noxious taste.

Interventions	Rationales
7. Instruct the client to avoid lying down flat for at least 2 hours after eating. A client who must rest should sit or recline with her or his head at least 4 inches higher than the feet.	7. Pressure on the stomach can trigger vagal visceral afferent stimulation of the vomiting center in the brain.
8. Teach the client to practice relaxation exercises during episodes of nausea. Refer also to Unit II *Nausea*.	8. Concentrating on relaxation activities may help to block stimulation of the vomiting center.
9. Maintain good oral hygiene at all times.	9. A clean, refreshed mouth can stimulate the appetite.
10. Administer an antiemetic agent before meals, if indicated.	10. Antiemetics prevent nausea and vomiting.

> **CLINICAL ALERT**
> * If individual is unable or unwilling to drink, notify physician / NP for antiemetics or parenteral fluids.

Documentation

Intake and output (amount, type, time)
Vomiting (amount, description)
Multidisciplinary client education record

Risk for Constipation Related to Decreased Peristalsis Secondary to Immobility and the Effects of Anesthesia and Narcotics

NOC
Bowel Elimination, Hydration, Symptom Control

Goal

The client will resume effective preoperative bowel function.

NIC
Bowel Management, Fluid Management, Constipation / Impaction Management

Indicators

* No bowel distention
* Bowel sounds in all quadrants

Interventions	Rationales
1. Monitor for bowel sounds, abdominal distention, and bowel movements. After surgery, opioid pain medications, anticholinergic, anesthesia, decreased oral intake, and immobility can cause constipation. a. Explain that a bowel movement should occur 2–3 days after surgery. Drink 6–8 glasses of water daily. b. Assess bowel sounds to determine when to introduce liquids. Advance diet as tolerated.	1. Manipulation of the bowel during surgery can decrease peristalsis. Decreased oral intake and decreased activity the first few days after the surgery will decrease bowel motility. b. Bowel sounds indicate the return of peristalsis.
2. Explain the effects of daily activity on elimination. Assist with ambulation when possible.	2. Activity influences bowel elimination and expelling of gas by improving abdominal muscle tone and stimulating appetite and peristalsis.

(*continued*)

Interventions	Rationales
3. Promote factors that contribute to optimal elimination. 　a. Balanced diet: Review a list of foods high in bulk (e.g., fresh fruits with skins, bran, nuts and seeds, whole grain breads and cereals, cooked fruits and vegetables, and fruit juices). 　b. Encourage intake of fluids at least 8–10 glasses (about 2,000 mL) daily, unless contraindicated.	3a. A well-balanced diet high in fiber content stimulates peristalsis. 　b. Sufficient fluid intake is necessary to maintain bowel patterns and promote proper stool consistency.

> **CLINICAL ALERT**
> - Notify the physician / NP if bowel sounds do not return within 6–10 hours, or if elimination does not return within 2–3 days postoperatively.
> - Absence of bowel sounds may indicate paralytic ileus; absence of bowel movements may indicate obstruction.

Documentation

Bowel movements
Bowel sounds

Activity Intolerance Related to Pain and Weakness Secondary to Anesthesia, Tissue Hypoxia, and Insufficient Fluid and Nutrient Intake

NOC
Activity Tolerance

Goal

The client will increase tolerance to activities of daily living (ADLs).

NIC
Activity Tolerance, Energy Management, Exercise Promotion, Sleep Enhancement, Mutual Goal Setting

Indicators

- Progressive ambulation
- Ability to perform ADLs

Interventions	Rationales
1. Encourage progress in the client's activity level during each shift, as indicated: 　a. Allow the client's legs to dangle first; support the client from the side. 　b. Place the bed in high position and raise the head of the bed. 　c. Encourage the client to increase activity when pain is at a minimum or after pain relief measures take effect.	1. A gradual increase in activity allows the client's cardio-pulmonary system to return to its preoperative state without excessive strain. 　a. Dangling the legs first helps to minimize orthostatic hypotension. 　b. Raising the head of the bed helps to reduce stress on suture lines.
2. Assess for abnormal responses to increased activity: 　a. Decreased pulse rate 　b. Decreased or unchanged systolic blood pressure 　c. Excessively increased or decreased respiratory rate 　d. Confusion or vertigo	2. Activity tolerance depends on the client's ability to adapt to the physiologic requirements of increased activity. The expected immediate physiologic responses to activity are increased blood pressure and increased respiratory rate and depth. After 3 minutes, the pulse rate should decrease to within 10 beats/minute of the client's usual resting rate. Abnormal findings represent the body's inability to meet the increased oxygen demands imposed by activity.

Documentation

Ambulation (time, amount)

Abnormal or unexpected response to increased activity

> ### TRANSITION TO HOME / COMMUNITY CARE
> If indicated, review the risk diagnoses identified for this individual on admission:
> * Is the person still at risk?
> * Can the family reduce the risks?
> * Is the person at higher risk at home?
> * Is a Home Health Nurse assessment needed?
> * Refer to transition planner / case manager / social service.
> * When is this person scheduled for follow-up with primary provider? Specialists? Record dates of appointments.
> * Complete a medication reconciliation prior to transition. Refer to index.

STAR

Stop

Think   Is this person at risk for injury, falls, medical complications, and / or inability to care for self (activities of daily living)?

Is there a support person available?

Is the person competent to manage self-administration of medications, treatment procedures? Are additional resources needed?

Can the person explain how to monitor the condition (e.g., blood glucose, signs / symptoms of complications, dietary / mobility restrictions, and when to call his or her primary provider or specialist)?

Act   Contact or provide the appropriate resource (e.g., contacting a support person, home health assessment, additional teaching, printed materials).

Review   Has the problem been addressed? If not, use SBAR to communicate to the appropriate person.

Risk for Ineffective Self-Health Management Related to Insufficient Knowledge of Care of Operative Site, Restrictions (Diet, Activity), Medications, Signs and Symptoms of Complications, and Follow-up Care

NOC

Compliance Behavior, Knowledge: Treatment Regimen, Participation: Health-Care Decisions, Treatment Behavior: Illness or Injury

NIC

Anticipatory Guidance, Learning Facilitation, Risk Management, Health Education, Teaching: Procedures / Treatments, Health System Guidance

Goals

The goals for this diagnosis represent those associated with transition planning. Refer to the transitional criteria.

Interventions	Rationales
1. Explain the process of normal wound healing by noting the following (Beattie, 2007): a. Within 48 hours the wound edges are together. b. Slight swelling, slight scabbing around sutures or staples and wound edges with some redness and warmth is normal. c. Some drainage (1–5 days after surgery, bloody to watery rose colored to pink to yellowish / clear) d. By day 5, a "healing ridge" of scar tissue can be palpated directly under the incision and extending on both sides of the wound. e. Advise to report to surgeon / primary care provider if the condition of the wound or drainage changes.	1. Teaching what is expected will prepare the person to identify abnormal signs and the need to report. These observations are the normal inflammatory reaction triggered by the surgical procedure. Any deviations from this normal healing process—especially between post-op days 5 and 10—can indicate infection or dehiscence. Most dehiscence occurs 4–14 days after surgery.
2. As appropriate, explain and demonstrate care of an uncomplicated surgical wound: a. Washing with soap and water b. Dressing changes using clean technique	2. Uncomplicated wounds have sealed edges after 24 hours and therefore do not require aseptic technique or a dressing; however, a dressing may be applied if the wound is at risk for injury.
3. As appropriate, explain and demonstrate care of a complicated surgical wound.	3. Aseptic technique is necessary to prevent wound contamination during dressing changes. Hand-washing helps to prevent contamination of the wound and the spread of infection. Proper handling and disposal of contaminated dressings helps to prevent infection transmission. Daily assessment is necessary to evaluate healing and detect complications.
4. If a home health nurse is needed for wound care, initiate a referral.	
5. Teach the client about factors that can delay wound healing: a. Keep wound covered until the wound is sealed to prevent dehydrated wound tissue, b. Wound infection c. Inadequate nutrition and hydration d. Compromised blood supply e. Increased stress or excessive activity	5a. Epithelial migration is impeded under dry crust; movement is three times faster over moist tissue (Porth, 2011). b. The exudates in infected wounds impairs epithelialization and wound closure. c. To repair tissue, the body needs increased protein and carbohydrate intake and adequate hydration for vascular transport of oxygen and wastes. d. Blood supply to injured tissue must be adequate to transport leukocytes and remove wastes. e. Increased stress and activity result in higher levels of chalone, a mitotic inhibitor that depresses epidermal regeneration.
6. Reinforce activity restrictions, as indicated (e.g., bending, lifting). Advise to ask surgeon at post-op office visit regarding activity restrictions.	6. Avoiding certain activities decreases the risk of wound dehiscence before scar formation (usually after 3 weeks).
7. Explain that a bowel movement should occur 2–3 days after surgery. Advise to: a. Drink 6–8 glasses of water daily. b. Eat light meals.	

Interventions	Rationales
8. Explain that a well-balanced diet is needed to meet the body's needs for surgical wound healing.	8. To support proper wound healing, your body needs adequate intake of calories, protein, iron, vitamin A, vitamin C, zinc, and adequate hydration for vascular transport of oxygen and wastes.
a. Iron: The practice of avoiding transfusions due to risks and shorter postoperative stays results in clients leaving hospital after surgery with lower hemoglobin (Hb) than previously. Iron is needed to replenish red blood cells decreased with the blood loss during surgery.	a. Iron-rich foods include meat, shellfish, baked potato with skin, legumes, chickpeas, kidney beans, peas, apricots, egg, whole grain bread, tamarind, iron-fortified cereals.
b. Vitamin A: Cellular differentiation, proliferation, epithelialization, collagen synthesis (scar tissue) counter-act catabolic effect of steroids with renal failure due to greater potential for toxicity.	b. Vitamin A-rich foods include fish,* dairy products,* grape fruit, cantaloupe, mango, peaches, papaya, collard greens,* sweet potatoes, carrots, kale,* spinach.*
c. Vitamin C: Collagen synthesis (scar tissue). Not for individuals with renal failure due to risk for renal oxalate stone formation.	c. Vitamin C-rich foods include oranges, melons strawberries, papaya, broccoli, bell peppers, baked potato, tomato, cauliflower.
d. Zinc: Protein synthesis, cellular replication, collagen formation; large wounds, chest tubes, and wound drains contribute to further zinc losses.	d. Zinc rich foods include meat, pork, seafood, dark poultry, dairy products, beans
9. Teach the client and family to watch for and report signs and symptoms of possible complications: a. Persistent temperature elevation b. Difficulty breathing, chest pain c. Change in sputum characteristics d. Increasing weakness, fatigue, pain, or abdominal distention e. Wound changes (e.g., separation, unusual or increased drainage, increased redness or swelling) f. Voiding difficulties, burning on urination, urinary frequency, or cloudy, foul-smelling urine g. Pain, swelling, and warmth in calf	9. Early detection and reporting danger signs and symptoms enables prompt intervention to minimize the severity of complications.

CLINICAL ALERT
- Instruct to promptly report any of the above signs / symptoms to surgeon for an evaluation of complications as infections, deep vein thrombosis, urinary retention or go to the ER.

*also rich in iron

Documentation

Transition instructions
Follow-up instructions arranging appointment with surgeons / physicians, as ordered, prior to the client leaving the hospital
Status at transition (pain, activity, wound healing)

Abdominal Aortic Aneurysm Repair

"The prognosis is guarded in individuals who suffer rupture of an AAA prehospital. More than 50% do not survive to the emergency department; of those who do, survival rate drops by about 1% per minute. However, the survival rate is good in the subset of clients who are not in severe shock and who receive timely, expert surgical intervention" (Pearce, 2011).

"Mortality in elective AAA repair is drastically lower than that associated with rupture. Consequently, the emphasis must be on early detection and repair free from complications" (Pearce, 2011).

The major risk factors or accelerators for AAA include older age, male gender, positive family history of aneurysm, cardiovascular disease, a history of ever smoking, and hypertension.

"Clients with an incidentally discovered AAA that is less than 3 cm require no further follow-up. If the AAA is 3-4 cm, annual ultrasound imaging should be used to monitor for further dilatation. AAAs 4–4.5 cm should be evaluated by ultrasound every 6 months, and clients with AAAs greater than 4.5 cm in diameter should be referred to a vascular surgeon" (Pearce, 2011).

The two primary methods of AAA repair are open and endovascular. Open AAA repair requires direct access to the aorta through an abdominal or retroperitoneal approach. Open thoracic and abdominal aneurysm repair has a mortality rate of around 8% (Pearce, 2011).

More frequently utilized is endovascular repair of an AAA, which involves gaining access to the lumen of the abdominal aorta, usually via small incisions over the femoral vessels. The graft serves to contain aortic flow and decrease the pressure on the aortic wall, leading to a reduction in AAA size over time and a decrease in the risk of aortic rupture. While endovascular repair has less operative morbidity, it has significant long-term morbidity and is much more expensive (Beese-Bjurstrom, 2004; Dillion, 2007; Mukherjee, 2003; Pearce, 2013).

 Time Frame
Preoperative
Postoperative periods

▪▪▪▪▪ DIAGNOSTIC CLUSTER

Postoperative Period

Collaborative Problems

Risk for Complications of Endoleaks

Risk for Complications of Distal Vessel Thrombosis or Emboli

Risk for Complications of Renal Failure

Risk for Complications of Mesenteric Ischemia / Thrombosis

Risk for Complications of Spinal Cord Ischemia

Nursing Diagnoses

▲ Risk for Infection related to location of surgical incision (refer to Arterial Bypass Graft)

▲ Risk for Ineffective Self-Health Management related to insufficient knowledge of home care, activity restrictions, signs and symptoms of complications, and follow-up care

Related Care Plan

General Surgery Generic Care Plan

▲ This diagnosis was reported to be monitored for or managed frequently (75% to 100%).
Δ This diagnosis was reported to be monitored for or managed often (50% to 74%).

Transitional Criteria

Before transition, the client or family will:

1. State wound care measures to perform at home.
2. Verbalize precautions regarding activities.
3. State signs and symptoms that must be reported to a health care professional.

Transitional Risk Assessment Plan (TRAP)

Begin this plan on admission.

Implement the Transitional Risk Assessment Plan (TRAP):

• Refer to inside back cover.
• Add each validated risk diagnosis to client's problem list with the risk code in ( ).
• Refer to Unit II to the individual risk nursing diagnoses / collaborative problems for outcomes and interventions.

R: "Close coordination of care in the post-acute period, early transition follow-up care, enhanced client education and self-management training, proactive end-of-life counseling, and extending the resources and clinical expertise over time via multidisciplinary team management" can lower readmission rates and improve health outcomes (Boutwell & Hwu, 2009, p. 14).

Collaborative Outcomes

The client will be monitored for early signs and symptoms of (a) rupture of aneurysm(preoperative), (b) distal vessel thrombosis / emboli, (c) renal failure, (d) mesenteric ischemia / thrombosis, and (e) spinal cord ischemia, and will receive collaborative interventions if indicated to restore physiologic stability.

Indicators of Physiologic Stability

• Calm, oriented (a, d)
• All pulses palpable and strong (a, b, e)
• No abdominal pelvic chest pain (a, b)
• Nontender abdomen (a, b, d)
• Capillary refill <3 seconds (b)
• No numbness of extremities (b, e)
• Urine output >0.5 mL/kg/h (c, e)
• Blood urea nitrogen 5–25 mg/dL (c)
• Serum creatinine
    • Male 0.6–1.5 g/dL
    • Female 0.6–1.1 g/dL
• Sensory / motor intact (e)
• Bowel sounds present 5–30 times/min (d)
• Flatus present (d)
• Soft-formed bowel movements (d)

Carp's Cues

Please refer to the Generic Care Plan for the Surgical Client for detailed interventions for managing all surgical conditions. This care plan addresses specific additional interventions associated with the type of surgery performed.

Interventions	Rationales
1. Monitor all pulses (carotid, brachial, radial, ulnar, femoral, popliteal, dorsalis pedis, and posterior tibial) and blood pressure.	1. A carotid bruit must be evaluated preoperatively to rule out risk of stroke during the operation. Assessing upper extremity pulses establishes a baseline for follow-up after arterial lines are in place and arterial punctures are made for blood gas analysis. Assessing lower extremity pulses establishes a baseline for postoperative assessment. A potential complication of aneurysm repair is thrombosis or embolus of distal vessels. Also, clients with abdominal aneurysm have a higher incidence of popliteal aneurysm than the general population.
2. If prior to surgery, monitor for signs and symptoms of aneurysm rupture:	2. The larger the aneurysm, the greater the risk of rupture. Risk of rupture increases significantly when aneurysm size >5 cm (Anderson, 2010).
CLINICAL ALERT • If there is a sudden change in the client's hemodynamic status, c/o of acute abdominal pain with intense back, chest, or pelvic pain; pain sometimes described as "tearing," call Rapid Response Team. • Pain results from massive tissue hypoxia and profuse bleeding into the abdominal cavity (Beese-Bjurstrom, 2004).	
a. Tender, pulsating abdomen	a. Abdominal pulsations and tenderness result from rhythmic pulsations of the artery and tissue hypoxia, respectively.
b. Restlessness	b. Restlessness is a response to tissue hypoxia.
c. Shock	c. Shock may result from massive blood loss and tissue hypoxia.

Postoperative: Collaborative Problems

Risk for Complications of Distal Vessel Thrombosis or Emboli

Risk for Complications of Renal Failure

Risk for Complications of Mesenteric Ischemia / Thrombosis

Risk for Complications of Spinal Cord Ischemia

Risk for Complications of Aortoenteric Fistula

Risk for Complications of Endoleak

Carp's Cues

The most common cause of secondary surgical intervention is endoleak in the new generation of devices, and migration was the prime indication in half of all secondary interventions with older generation devices (Walker et al., 2010). All endoleaks do not require surgical repair. Type II endoleaks are seen in 20% to 30% of clients, with half of early leaks sealing spontaneously. Some leaks persist in 11% to 15% of individuals. Radiographic evidence of expansion of the AA sac with a type II endoleak requires surgery. (Walker et al., 2010)

Interventions	Rationales
1. Monitor for complications of Anticoagulant therapy. Refer to Risk for Complications of Anticoagulant Therapy.	1. Heparin is utilized intraoperatively to prevent thrombosis formation.
2. Monitor for signs of ischemic complications (Walker et al., 2010).	2. Ischemic complications are the result of thrombosis, embolization, endoleaks, or malpositioning of graft (Walker et al., 2010).
3. Monitor for DVT: a. Diminished distal pulses, increased capillary refill time (>3 seconds) b. Pallor or darkened patches of skin c. Refer to Unit II to Risk for Complications of DVT for specific complications.	
4. Monitor for colinic ischemia: a. Decreased bowel sounds. b. Constipation or diarrhea (may be bloody) (Beese-Bjurstrom, 2004). c. Increasing abdominal pain or girth (Beese-Bjurstrom, 2004). d. New onset nausea / vomiting.	4. The mesenteric artery, like the renal artery, is at risk for thrombosis. b. A liquid bowel movement before the third postoperative day may point to bowel ischemia; may be bloody. c. Postoperative pain normally decreases each day.
5. Monitor for spinal cord ischemia: a. Urinary retention or incontinence b. C/o of numbness of legs, feet c. Change in sensation or ability to move toes	5. Inadequate perfusion above the second lumbar vertebra (L2) can result in bladder dysfunction.
6. Monitor for renal ischemia: a. Urinary retention or incontinence b. Decreased urine output	6. Thrombosis can cause renal artery compromise
7. Monitor for limb occlusion (kinking of graft or poor outflow supplying the leg results in a cool, pale, numb, tingling, or painful): a. Lower extremity pulses b. C/o of pain in legs with ambulation **CLINICAL ALERT** • Any change in clinical assessment data indicating possible thrombosis or impaired circulation, requires immediate notification of surgeon.	
8. If the client complains of pain, assess its location and characteristics.	8. It is important to differentiate pain of surgical manipulation from ischemic pain. Microembolization from the aneurysm to the distal skin causes skin infarctions manifested by point discomfort at the infarct and a dark pink-purple discoloration.

(continued)

Interventions	Rationales
9. Post AAA surgery, monitor for signs of renal failure (may be due to cross-clamping, hypotension, emboli, or contrast medium) (Anderson, 2001).	9. During abdominal aorta surgery, the renal arteries are at risk for thrombosis if they are involved in the aneurysm, are clamped for the operation, or are hypoperfused any time during periods of hypotension. Impaired renal function can result. The endovascular technique reduces risks for subclinical renal damage and colonic ischemia (Solomon, Yee, & Soulen, 2000).
10. Carefully monitor intake, output, and hydration and renal status (e.g., central venous pressure / hemodynamic monitoring every hour for the first 24 hours postoperatively) (Anderson, 2001).	10. Hypovolemia can cause thrombosis of graft and decrease renal perfusion. Cross-clamping during surgery will disrupt blood flow to the renal arteries.
11. Monitor blood pressure and report elevations from baseline.	11. Hypertension can result from vasoconstrictor and can potentiate graft rupture.
12. Monitor for retroperitoneal bleeding (Anderson, 2001): a. Decreased hematocrit b. Hypotension c. Tachycardia d. Back pain e. Grey Turner sign (ecchyomotic [bluish] discoloration in flank area	12. Retroperitoneal bleeding can occur after endovascular surgery.
13. Monitor for intra-abdominal bleeding: a. Increased abdominal girth b. Decreased hematocrit c. Hypotension d. Tachycardia	13. Intra-abdominal bleeding can occur during the first 24 hours postoperatively.
14. Palpate or Doppler peripheral pulses every hour for the first 24 hours.	14. Early detection of graft failure can prevent limb loss.
15. Monitor for ileus: a. Absence of bowel sounds b. Absence of flatus c. Abdominal distention	15. Manual manipulation and displacement of the bowel during surgery will cause bruising and resultant decreased peristalsis.
16. Monitor for signs of infection. Refer to Risk for Infection in Unit II.	16. Wound and endovascular graft infections can occur.

Clinical Alert Report

Prior to providing care, advise ancillary staff / student to report the following to the professional nurse assigned to the client:

* Change in cognitive status
* New onset abdominal / back pain
* Oral temperature >100.5° F
* Systolic BP <90 mm/Hg
* Resting Pulse >100, <50
* Respiratory rate >28, <10/min
* Oxygen saturation <90%
* Decreased / absent bowel sounds
* Urine output < 0.5 mg/kg/h

Related Physician / NP Prescribed Interventions

Medications

Dependent on underlying etiology, antihypertensive (e.g., nitroprusside), beta blockers. Antiplatelet therapy.

Intravenous Therapy

Fluid and electrolyte replacement.

Laboratory Studies

Refer to the General Surgery care plan, Appendix II.

Diagnostic Studies

Plain radiograph, Computed tomography scanning, Angiography, MRI, Ultrasonography.

Therapies

Oxygen, endovascular stent-graft.

Documentation

Vital signs
Circulation (distal, pulses, color)
Bowel sounds, presence of occult blood
Lower extremities (sensation, motor function)
Urine (output, occult blood)
Characteristics of pain
Unrelieved pain
Interventions, response to interventions

Postoperative: Nursing Diagnoses

> **TRANSITION TO HOME / COMMUNITY CARE**
> If indicated, review the risk diagnoses identified for this individual on admission:
> - Is the person still at risk?
> - Can the family reduce the risks?
> - Is the person at higher risk at home?
> - Is a Home Health Nurse assessment needed?
> - Refer to transition planner / case manager / social service.
> - When is this person scheduled for follow-up with primary provider? Specialists? Record dates of appointments.
> - Complete a medication reconciliation prior to transition. Refer to index.

STAR

Stop

Think   Is this person at risk for injury, falls, medical complications, and / or inability to care for self (activities of daily living)?

Is there a support person available?

Is the person competent to manage self-administration of medications, treatment procedures? Are additional resources needed?

Can the person explain how to monitor the condition (e.g., blood glucose, signs / symptoms of complications, dietary / mobility restrictions, and when to call his or her primary provider or specialist)?

Act   Contact or provide the appropriate resource (e.g., contacting a support person, home health assessment, additional teaching, printed materials).

Review   Has the problem been addressed? If not, use SBAR to communicate to the appropriate person.

Risk for Ineffective Self-Health Management Related to Insufficient Knowledge of Home Care, Activity Restrictions, Signs and Symptoms of Complications, and Follow-up Care

NOC

Compliance Behavior, Knowledge: Treatment Regimen, Participation: Health Care Decisions, Treatment Behavior: Illness or Injury

NIC

Anticipatory Guidance, Risk Identification, Health Education, Learning Facilitation

Goal

The goals for this diagnosis represent those associated with transition planning. Refer to the transitional criteria.

Interventions	Rationales
1. For wound care measures and rationale, refer to the General Surgery Care Plan.	
2. If an aorto-bifemoral graft was performed, reinforce the need for a slouched position when sitting.	2. A slouched position helps to prevent graft kinking and possible occlusion.
3. Reinforce activity restrictions (e.g., car riding, stair climbing, lifting). Specifically ask surgeon how long to continue restrictions at post-op office visit.	3. About 5–6 weeks after abdominal surgery for a client in good nutritional status, the collagen matrix of the wound becomes strong enough to withstand stress from activity. The surgeon may prefer to limit activity for a longer period, because certain activities place tension on the surgical site (Walker et al., 2010). The period of activity restriction is significantly less with endovascular repair, as incisions are smaller.
4. Explain lifelong imaging surveillance following the EVAR procedure and at 1, 6, and 12 months and yearly thereafter (Walker et al., 2010).	4. "Surveillance after EVAR is critical for the detection and, if possible, the characterization of endoleaks and evidence of expansion or shrinkage of the residual AAA sac, detection of mechanical changes in the stent-graft, such as migration, kinking, or fracture; and evaluation of the long-term performance of the endoprosthesis" (Walker et al., 2010, pp. 1645–1646).
5. If prescribed, explain the need to continue antiplatelet therapy, especially in clients with PAD (e.g., aspirin, statins, clopidogrel).	5. Antiplatelet therapy is needed to prevent complications such as graft-limb thrombosis and peripheral arterial disease.
6. If the client smokes, reinforce the health benefits of quitting and refer the client to a smoking cessation program, if available. Refer to Getting Started to Quit Smoking on thePoint at http://thePoint.lww.com/Carpenito6e.	6. Tobacco acts as a potent vasoconstrictor that increases stress on the graft.
7. Stress the importance of managing hypertension, if indicated.	7. Hypertension can cause false aneurysms at the anastomosis site.
8. Instruct to immediately call the surgeon if: a. Any changes in color, temperature, or sensation in the legs. b. Blood in stools of darkening of stools. c. New onset diarrhea / constipation	8a. These signs and symptoms may indicate thrombosis or embolism that requires immediate evaluation. b. Duodenal bleeding may be a sign of erosion of the aortic graft into the duodenum.

Interventions	*Rationales*

9. Seek emergency treatment if (call 911 if needed):
  a. C/o of sudden abdominal / back pain
  b. Change in cognitive status
  c. Sudden increasing pulse rate, respirations
  d. New onset cool, pale, numb, tingling, or painful lower limb(s)
  e. New onset urinary retention / incontinence	

Documentation

Teaching / instructions given
Referrals, if indication

Amputation

"In the United States, 30,000–40,000 amputations are performed annually. There were an estimated 1.6 million individuals living with the loss of a limb in 2005; these estimates are expected to more than double to 3.6 million such individuals by the year 2050 (Ertl, 2012).

Most amputations are performed for ischemic disease of the lower extremity. Of dysvascular amputations, 15% to 28% of clients undergo contralateral limb amputations within 3 years. Of elderly persons who undergo amputations, 50% survive the first 3 years (Ertl, 2012).

Amputation is the surgical severing and removal of a limb. Amputations are caused by accidents (23%), disease (74%), and congenital disorders (3%). The most common reason for amputation is peripheral vascular disease, especially for those over 50 years old (Society for Vascular Surgery, 2007). Lower extremity amputation is about 15–20 times greater in people with diabetes (Calvert, Penner, Younger, & Wing, 2007). Lower-limb constitutes 80 to 85% of all amputations, with nearly two-thirds related to diabetes (Philbin, DeLuccia, Nitsch, & Maurus, 2007). "Of dysvascular amputations, 15% to 28% of clients undergo contralateral limb amputations within 3 years.

"The following factors will affect the outcome of amputation: the client's nutritional status, age, tissue perfusion, smoking habits, infection and the presence of coexisting diseases such as diabetes, anemia, and renal failure. This paper describes a number of problems associated with amputation wound healing, including infection, tissue necrosis, pain, difficulties associated with the surrounding skin, bone erosion, hematoma, edema, and dehiscence / wound breakdown" (Harker, 2006, p. 2).

Time Frame
Preoperative and postoperative periods

DIAGNOSTIC CLUSTER

Preoperative Period

Nursing Diagnoses

▲ Anxiety related to insufficient knowledge of postoperative routines, postoperative sensations, and crutch-walking techniques

Related Care Plan

▲ General Surgery Generic Care Plan

(continued)

Postoperative Period

Collaborative Problems

▲ Risk for Complications of Edema of Stump

▲ Risk for Complications of Wound Hematoma

▲ Risk for Complications of Hemorrhage

* Risk for Complications of Delayed Wound Healing

Nursing Diagnoses

Δ Risk for Disturbed Body Image related to perceived negative effects of amputation and response of others to appearance

▲ Risk for Impaired Physical Mobility related to limited movement secondary to pain

▲ Grieving related to loss of limb and its effects on lifestyle

▲ Acute / Chronic Pain related to phantom limb sensations secondary to peripheral nerve stimulation and abnormal impulses to central nervous system

▲ Risk for Falls related to altered gait and hazards of assistive devices (refer to Unit II Risk for Falls)

Δ Risk for Ineffective Self-Health Management related to insufficient knowledge of activity of daily living (ADL) adaptations, stump care, signs/symptoms of complications gait training, and follow-up care

▲ This diagnosis was reported to be monitored for or managed frequently (75% to 100%).
Δ This diagnosis was reported to be monitored for or managed often (50% to 74%).

Transition Criteria

Before transition, the client and family will:

1. Share their fear and concerns regarding the effects of amputation.
2. Describe daily stump care.
3. Explain phantom sensations and interventions to reduce them.
4. Describe measures to protect the stump from injury.
5. Identify what to report to surgeon after transition.
6. Demonstrate self-care activities correctly and safely for physical therapists.

Transitional Risk Assessment Plan (TRAP)

Begin this plan on admission.
Implement the Transitional Risk Assessment Plan (TRAP):

• Refer to inside back cover.
• Add each validated risk diagnosis to client's problem list with the risk code in ( ).
• Refer to Unit II to the individual risk nursing diagnoses / collaborative problems for outcomes and interventions.

R: *"Close coordination of care in the post-acute period, early transition follow-up care, enhanced client education and self-management training, proactive end-of-life counseling, and extending the resources and clinical expertise over time via multidisciplinary team management"* can lower readmission rates and improve health outcomes (Boutwell & Hwu, 2009, p. 14).

Preoperative: Nursing Diagnosis

Anxiety Related to Insufficient Knowledge of Postoperative Routines, Postoperative Sensations, and Crutch-walking Techniques

NOC
Anxiety Control, Coping, Impulse Control

Goal

The client will identify his or her expectations of the postoperative period.

NIC
Anxiety Reduction, Impulse Control Training, Anticipatory Guidance

Indicators

- Ask questions.
- Express concerns.

 Carp's Cues

Please refer to the Generic Care Plan for the Surgical Client for detailed interventions for managing all surgical conditions. This care plan addresses specific additional interventions associated with the type of surgery performed.

Interventions	Rationales

1. Explore the client's feelings about the impending surgery.
  a. Allow the client to direct discussion.
  b. Do not assume or project how the client feels.
	1. Some clients may perceive amputation as a devastating event, while others will view the surgery as an opportunity to eliminate pain and improve quality of life.

2. Help to establish realistic expectations.	2. Successful prosthetic rehabilitation requires cooperation, coordination, tremendous physical energy and fitness, and a well-fitting, comfortable prosthesis (Chin, Sawamura, & Shiba, 2006; Piasecki, 2000; Yetzer, 1996).
3. Consult with other team members (e.g., physical therapy) to see the client preoperatively.	3. Preoperative instructions on postoperative activity help the client to focus on rehabilitation instead of on the surgery; this may help to reduce anxiety.

4. Discuss postoperative expectations, including the following:
  a. Appearance of the stump
  b. Positioning
 	
  c. Phantom pain
	4. These explanations help to reduce fears associated with unknown situations and to decrease anxiety.
	
	  b. The stump will be elevated for 24 hours after surgery to prevent edema. The client will be assisted into the prone position three to four times a day to prevent hip contractures (Piasecki, 2000).
	  c. Research suggests that 85% of amputees have phantom limb pain ranging from daily to weekly to yearly (Richardson, Glenn, & Horgan, 2006).

5. Explain that immediately following surgery, the client will perceive the amputated limb as if it were still intact and of the same shape and size as before surgery.	5. Immediately after surgery, most amputees feel the phantom limb as it was before surgery.

Documentation

Assessment of learning readiness and ability
Client teaching
Response to teaching

Postoperative: Collaborative Problems

Risk for Complications of Edema of Stump

Risk for Complications of Wound Hematoma

Risk for Complications of Tissue Necrosis

Risk for Complications of Infection

Risk for Complications of Delayed Wound Healing

Collaborative Outcomes

The client will be monitored for early signs and symptoms of (a) edema of stump, (b) wound hematoma, (c) tissue necrosis, and (d) infection, and will receive collaborative interventions if indicated to restore physiologic stability.

Indicators of Physiologic Stability

- Diminishing edema (a)
- No evidence of boggy tissue, discoloration, skin changes (c)
- Approximated suture line (a, b, d)
- No point tenderness (b, c)
- Temperature 98°–99.5° F (d)
- White blood cells 4,300–10,800 mm³ (d)

Interventions	Rationales
1. Elevate the stump with calf tilted 15 degrees as prescribed, usually for the first 24 hours only.	1. Elevation for the first 24 hours will reduce edema and promote venous and lymphatic return. Elevation of the limb over 15 degrees can cause flexion contractions (Williamson, 1998).
2. Aggressively, monitor the incision for the following: a. Edema along suture lines b. Ruddy color changes c. Oozing dark blood d. Point tenderness on palpation	2. Peripheral vascular disorders are the major cause for lower limb amputations. After amputation, peripheral vascular disorders continue and thus increase the risk for infection and tissue necrosis. Individuals with diabetes are 5 times more at risk for postsurgical infections (Harker, 2006).
3. Monitor for surgical site infection.	
4. Monitor for tissue necrosis: a. Dusky skin changes b. Mottled / purple discoloration c. Dry or wet gangrene d. Sloughy tissue (necrotic tissue separating from healthy tissue) e. Cool tissue, very painful **CLINICAL ALERT** • Any sign of necrosis must be reported immediately.	4. Poor tissue perfusion prior to surgery increases the risk of tissue necrosis postoperatively.
5. Monitor for edema along suture line and signs of delayed healing (Calvert, Penner, Younger, & Wing, 2007).	5. Traumatized tissue responds with lymphedema. Excessive edema must be detected to prevent tension on the suture line that can cause bleeding. Tissue compression from edema can compromise circulation (Williamson, 1998). Delayed wound healing is the most common complication, especially among diabetics (Calvert, Penner, Younger, & Wing, 2007).

Interventions	Rationales

6. Monitor for signs of hematoma:
  a. Unapproximated suture line
  b. Ruddy color changes of skin along suture line
  c. Oozing dark blood from suture line
  d. Point tenderness on palpation
	6. Amputation flaps may be pulled over large areas of "space," creating pockets that may contain old blood. Hematoma may compromise flap healing and delay rehabilitation (Ray, 2000).

7. Maintain the same wound dressing postoperatively, unless changed by surgeon.	7. Proper bandaging provides wound protection, controls tissue edema, molds the limb for prosthetic fitting, and remains secure with movement (Williamson, 1998).

Clinical Alert Report

Prior to providing care, advise ancillary staff / student to report the following to the professional nurse assigned to the client:
- Oral temperature >100.5° F
- Appearance of wound. The nurse supervising the student and / or ancillary staff should ask to be notified when the dressing is removed, to perform a detailed assessment.

Related Physician / NP Prescribed Interventions

Medications

Analgesics, antibiotics, and antidepressants

Laboratory Studies

CBC, C-reactive protein, serum albumin

Diagnostic Studies

CT scanning Bone scanning, Transcutaneous oxygen, laser Doppler flowmetry

Therapies

Physical therapy, occupational therapy, prosthesis fittings

Documentation

Appearance of suture line
Appearance of skin around suture line
Drainage
Abnormal findings

Postoperative: Nursing Diagnoses

Risk for Disturbed Body Image Related to Perceived Negative Effects of Amputation and Response of Others to Appearance

NOC

Body Image, Child Development: (specify age), Grief Resolution, Psychosocial Adjustment: Life Change, Self-Esteem

Goal

The client will communicate feelings about his or her changed appearance.

NIC

Self-Esteem
Enhancement,
Counseling, Presence,
Active Listening, Body
Image Enhancement,
Grief Work Facilitation,
Support Group, Referral

Indicators

- Express an interest in dress and grooming.
- Discuss feelings with family.

>> **Carp's Cues**

"We all get older. Unfortunately, many of us have to deal with amputation at the same time. Though we don't have much control over aging, we do have some power over the way we see ourselves" (Saberi & Pouresmail, 2007). This quote is from a three-page article from the National Limb Loss Information Center: Coping With Aging and Amputation: *How Changing the Way You Think Could Change Your Health* (http://www.amputee-coalition.org/senior_step/coping_aging.html).

I would recommend that the nurse / student read this prior to giving care to an individual who has had or is approaching a limb amputation. This would be also very appropriate to give the individual and family. Don't be surprised if you find it meaningful for your life and practice, even though you have both your legs.

Interventions	*Rationales*
1. Contact the client frequently to inquire about condition or requests.	1. Frequent contact by the caregiver indicates acceptance and may facilitate trust. The client may be hesitant to approach staff / student because of negative self-concept; the nurse must reach out (Dudas, 1997).
2. Encourage the client to verbalize feelings about appearance and perceptions of lifestyle impacts. What are you most concerned about? Validate the client's perceptions and assure him or her that they are normal and appropriate.	2. Expressing feelings and perceptions increases the client's self-awareness and helps the nurse to plan effective interventions to address the client's needs. Validating the client's perceptions provides reassurance and can decrease anxiety (Dudas, 1997).
3. Assist the client in identifying personal attributes and strengths.	3. These can help the client to focus on the positive characteristics that contribute to the whole concept of self, rather than only on the change in body image. The nurse should reinforce these positive aspects and encourage the client to reincorporate them into his or her new self-concept (Dudas, 1997). Body image is strongly related to depression, perception of poor quality of life, low self-esteem, increased general anxiety, lowers levels of satisfaction with prosthetic, participation in activity, and social isolation (Gallagher, Horgan, Franchignoni, Giordano, & MacLachlan, 2007; Yazicioglu et al., 2007).
4. Encourage optimal hygiene, grooming, and other self-care activities.	4. Participation in self-care and planning promotes positive coping with the change.
5. Encourage the client to perform as many activities as possible unassisted.	5. Nonparticipation in self-care and overprotection by caregivers tends to promote feelings of helplessness and dependence.
6. When appropriate, discuss the anticipated changes in lifestyle.	6. Open, honest discussions—expressing that changes will occur but that they are manageable—promote feelings of control.
7. Prepare the client's family and significant others for physical and emotional changes.	7. Support can be given more freely and more realistically if others are prepared (Dudas, 1997).
8. Discuss with the client's support system the importance of communicating honestly.	8. This will enhance trust, confidence and promote adjustment.
9. Refer a client to counseling, as appropriate.	9. Professional counseling is indicated for a client post amputation.

Documentation

Present emotional status
Dialogues

Risk for Impaired Physical Mobility Related to Limited Movement Secondary to Pain

NOC

Ambulation: Walking,
Joint Movement: Active,
Mobility Level

Goal

The client will report increased use of affected limb.

NIC

Exercise Therapy:
Joint Mobility, Exercise
Promotion: Strength
Training, Exercise
Therapy: Ambulation,
Positioning, Teaching:
Prescribed Activity /
Exercise, Teaching:
Assistive Device,
Teaching: Strategy

Indicators

* Demonstrate safe use of adaptive devices.
* Use safety measures to prevent injury.

Interventions	Rationales
1. Explain the importance of exercises and participation in activities of daily living in spite of discomforts.	1. Successful adaption to prosthesis use is dependent on the client's belief that one's behavior will improve one's situation (Bandura, 1982).
2. Elevate the limb for the first 24 hours only.	2. Elevation will reduce edema. Continued elevation after 24 hours can cause flexion contractures (Williamson, 1992).
3. Initiate transfer to chair and ambulation as soon as prescribed.	3. These activities are usually initiated 12–24 hours after surgery (Williamson, 1992).
4. Consult with a physical therapist regarding bedside exercises and activity recommendations.	4. Exercises are indicated for muscle strengthening and to prevent abduction and flexion contractures (Williamson, 1992).
5. Assist the client into a prone position three to four times a day for at least 15 minutes. Encourage the client to sleep in this position.	5. Abdominal lying places the pelvic joints in an extended position that extends the extensor muscles and prevents contractures (Williamson, 1992).
6. Reinforce the need to perform active ROM exercises on unaffected limbs at least four times a day. (Note: Perform passive ROM only if the client cannot do active ROM.)	6. Active ROM increases muscle mass, tone, and strength, and improves cardiac and respiratory functioning
7. Avoid prolonged sitting.	7. Prolonged sitting can cause hip flexion contractures.
8. Explain the increased energy requirements needed to use a prosthesis.	8. Walking with a prosthesis requires more effort because of its weight and the loss of the usual muscle coordination. Clients who are successful see more advantages than disadvantages with prosthetic use (Williamson, 1992).
9. Emphasize the client's progress with all activities, no matter how small. Convey that the client can successfully manage adaptation to the prosthesis.	9. Other people's belief that they can successfully cope increases one's own confidence (Bandura, 1982).

Documentation

Exercises
Range of motion

Nursing Diagnosis

Grieving Related to Loss of a Limb and Its Effects on Lifestyle

NOC

Coping, Family Coping, Grief Resolution, Psychosocial Adjustment: Life Change

Goal

The client will describe the meaning of the loss.

NIC

Anticipatory Guidance, Risk Management, Health Education, Learning Facilitation

Indicators

• Express grief.
• Report an intent to discuss feelings with family members or significant others.

Interventions	*Rationales*
1. Provide opportunities for the client and family members to ventilate feelings, discuss the loss openly, and explore the personal meaning of the loss. Explain that grief is a common and healthy reaction.	1. Amputation may give rise to feelings of powerlessness, anger, profound sadness, and other grief responses. Open, honest discussions can help the client and family members to accept and cope with the situation and their responses to it (Butler, Turkal, & Seidl, 1992; Williamson, 1998).
2. Assess the family's or significant others' responses to the situation.	2. Successful adjustment depends on the client's and their support system's realistic perceptions of the situation (Piasecki, 2000).
3. Encourage family members and significant others to maintain usual roles and behaviors.	
4. Discuss the reality of everyday emotions such as anger, guilt, and jealousy; relate the hazards of denying these feelings.	4. A positive response by client's family or significant others is one of the most important factors in the client's own acceptance of the loss (Butler, Turkal, & Seidl, 1992).
5. Refer the client to amputee support group. Determine if a trained amputee visitor can see the client, if indicated.	5. This allows the client and his or her family the opportunity to ventilate and ask questions.
6. Refer to Grieving in Unit II.	

Documentation

Present emotional status
Interventions
Response to interventions

Acute / Chronic Pain Related to Phantom Limb Sensations Secondary to Peripheral Nerve Stimulation and Abnormal Impulses to Central Nervous System

NOC
Comfort Level, Pain:
Disruptive Effects, Pain
Control, Symptom
Control

Goal

The client will differentiate between surgical pain and phantom pain and will report decreased phantom pain.

NIC
Pain Management,
Medication
Management, Emotional
Support, Symptom
Control

Indicators

- Describe the difference of surgical pain and phantom pain
- State the reasons for phantom sensation.
- Demonstrate techniques for managing phantom sensation.

Carp's Cues

The incidence of post-op phantom limb pain / sensation has been reported to be 72% to 84%; at 6 months is 67% to 90%. The incidence of pre amputation pain increases the incidence of phantom pain.

Interventions	Rationales

1. Explain the two types of pain that may be present post amputation:
  a. The pain of surgery is dull, throbbing, or aching.
  b. The pain resulting from severed nerves is sharp, shooting, tingling, or burning (phantom pain).
 	
CLINICAL ALERT
• The differentiation of surgical pain from phantom pain is important since the treatment for each is different.	

2. Explain that the phantom limb pain sensations are normal and encourage the client to report them. Sensations are physiologic, not psychological in origin. Clients prefer personal education regarding phantom sensations rather than reading about it.	2. The client may be hesitant to discuss phantom sensations for fear of appearing abnormal. Nearly 100% of clients with amputations report phantom pain sensation of varying degree during their first six months. Education reduces anxiety and opens lines of communication.

3. Explain that phantom sensations and / or pain are common phenomena.
  a. Phantom sensations are non painful sensations that may manifest as sensations of position of the amputated limb (proprioception or kinesthetic); of movement (kinetic); of feelings within the missing limb (exteroceptive) such as paresthesia, tickling, itching, warmth or cold, something touching the phantom limb, or numbness; or sensations as if an object, such as a ring, watch, or shoe, is still on the limb (superadded).
  b. Phantom pain is any sensation so intense it manifests as pain (Bosmans et al., 2007; Richardson, Glenn, & Hogan, 2006). Phantom sensations occur in 29% to 78% of clients with amputations; phantom pain occurs in 49% to 83% (Bosmans et al., 2007).
	3. Phantom sensations are caused by stimulation of the nerve proximal to the amputation that previously extended to the limb. The client perceives the stimulation as originating from the absent limb. There is no agreement on the exact cause of phantom limb pain. Stimulus of peripheral nerves proximal to the amputation is thought to be a cause. Another explanation is that severed nerves may send impulses that are perceived by the brain as abnormal (Davis, 1993; Katz, 1996).

Interventions	Rationales
4. Explain that stress, anxiety, fatigue, depression, excitement, and weather changes may intensify phantom limb pain (Wilkens, McGrath, Finley, & Katz, 2004).	4. Psychological stressors do not cause phantom limb pain, but can trigger or increase it (Katz, 1996).

5. Describe some techniques used to reduce or alleviate phantom pain after the surgical site has healed. Consult with physical therapist:
  a. Wrapping the residual limb in a warm, soft towel, heating pad
  b. Wrapping the residual limb in a cold pack or applying a cooling cream or gel
  c. Soaking in a warm bath or using the shower to massage the residual limb.
  d. Massaging the residual limb with both hands
  e. Transcutaneous electrical nerve stimulation (TENS)
  f. Mentally exercising the missing limb in the area where the pain occurs
  g. Mentally relaxing the missing limb and the residual limb
  h. Tightening the muscles in the residual limb and slowly releasing them
  i. For people with a prosthesis, putting it on and taking a short walk
  j. Increase the time walking on prosthesis.
  k. Changing position, moving around, or standing up
	5. Stimulation causing a second sensation may serve to override the phantom sensation (Williamson, 1992).

6. For management of pain related to surgical wound, refer to Generic Care Plan for the Surgical Client.	

Documentation

Reports of pain
Interventions
Response to interventions

TRANSITION TO HOME / COMMUNITY CARE

If indicated, review the risk diagnoses identified for this individual on admission:

- Is the person still at risk?
- Can the family reduce the risks?
- Is the person at higher risk at home?
- Is a Home Health Nurse assessment needed?
- Refer to transition planner / case manager / social service.
- When is this person scheduled for follow-up with primary provider? Specialists? Record dates of appointments.
- Complete a medication reconciliation prior to transition. Refer to index.

STAR   **Stop**

> **Think**   Is this person at risk for injury, falls, medical complications, and / or inability to care for self (activities of daily living)?
>
> > Is there a support person available?
> >
> > Is the person competent to manage self-administration of medications, treatment procedures? Are additional resources needed?
> >
> > Can the person explain how to monitor the condition (e.g., blood glucose, signs / symptoms of complications, dietary / mobility restrictions, and when to call his or her primary provider or specialist)?
>
> **Act**   Contact or provide the appropriate resource (e.g., contacting a support person, home health assessment, additional teaching, printed materials).
>
> **Review**   Has the problem been addressed? If not, use SBAR to communicate to the appropriate person.

Risk for Ineffective Self-Health Management Related to Insufficient Knowledge of Activity of Daily Living (ADL) Adaptations, Stump Care, Signs / Symptoms of Complications Gait Training, and Follow-up Care

NOC

Compliance Behavior, Knowledge: Treatment Regimen, Participation: Health Care Decisions, Treatment Behavior: Illness or Injury

NIC

Anticipatory Guidance, Risk Identification, Health Education, Learning Facilitation, Amputation Care

Transition Goal

The goals for this diagnosis represent those associated with transition planning. Refer to the transition criteria.

Interventions	*Rationales*
1. Reinforce the importance of preventing injury to the remaining foot with: a. Daily inspection for corns, calluses, blisters, and signs of infection b. Wearing sturdy slippers or shoes c. Prompt reporting of early signs of infection (e.g., a minor cut that does not heal in 1–2 days)	1. Daily care is necessary to deflect or prevent injury, especially if a circulatory disorder was a contributing factor to amputation.
2. Instruct the client to place a chair or other large object next to the bed at home to prevent him or her from getting out of bed at night and attempting to stand on the stump when not fully awake.	2. Phantom sensations include a kinesthetic awareness of the absent limb. A half-asleep client arising during the night may fall and damage the healing stump (Davis, 1993).
3. Instruct the client to avoid tobacco; refer to a smoking cessation program, if necessary. Refer to Getting Started to Quit Smoking on thePoint at http://thePoint.lww.com/Carpenito6e (printable to give to client)	3. Nicotine in tobacco constricts arterial vessels, which decreases blood flow to the healing stump. If amputation was related to atherosclerosis, tobacco use may threaten the stump's survival (CDC 2011).
4. Ensure the individual / family can properly clean, examine and bandage the stump.	4. It is necessary to regularly examine the stump for expected changes (e.g., muscle and scar atrophy) and unexpected changes (e.g., skin breakdown, redness, tenderness, increased warmth or coolness, numbness or tingling).

(continued)

Interventions	*Rationales*

5. Follow directions for stump care to prepare for prosthesis and when instructed to initiate per physical therapist:
  a. Walk short distances three to four times a day. Slowly increase how far you walk each time.
  b. When you are resting, keep your leg raised above the level of your heart to prevent leg swelling:
    • Lie down and place a pillow under the lower part of your leg.
    • Do not sit for more than 1 hour at a time when you first come home. If you can, raise your feet and legs when you are sitting. Rest them on another chair or a stool.
  c. You will have more leg swelling after walking or sitting. If you have a lot of swelling, you may be doing too much walking or sitting, or eating too much salt in your diet.
  d. When you climb stairs, use your good leg first when you go up. Use your leg that had surgery first when you go down. Rest after taking several steps.
  e. Your doctor will tell you when you can drive. You may take short trips as a passenger, but try to sit in the backseat with your leg that had surgery raised up on the seat.
	5. Elastic compression reduces edema in the stump. Edema interferes with wound healing and prolongs the rehabilitation time. Wrapping using figure-of-eight turns also helps to shape the stump for better fit into the prosthesis. Ace bandages wrapped horizontally can impede circulation.

6. Reinforce the need to continue exercises at home. (For more information, see the nursing diagnosis Risk for Impaired Physical Mobility in this care plan.)	6. Active ROM exercises increase muscle mass, tone, strength and joint mobility; and improve cardiac and respiratory function.
7. Recommend an online publication Lower Extremity Amputations http://svnnet.org/uploads/File/PatientEd/AmputationBk.pdf from the *Education Committee of the Society for Vascular Nursing,* which addresses living with an amputation.	

8. Explain the risks for infection and the need to report immediately to surgeon:
  a. Fever (oral temperature of 100.5° F or greater)
  b. Increased pain
  c. Increased swelling, boggy tissue
  d. Dusky skin changes
  e. Mottled / purple discoloration
  f. Increase wound drainage
  g. Cool tissue
 	
CLINICAL ALERT
• The factors that contributed to the individual's infection and amputation continue after surgery.
• The nurse must emphasize that any changes that can indicate an infection in the amputated limb and the non amputated limb need aggressive management to prevent further surgery on the stump and / or on the non amputated limb
	8. Hematomas of the wound contribute to infection. Coexisting diabetes mellitus reduces resistance to bacteria and causes diminished circulation. Tissue necrosis also can result from decreased circulation, chronic swelling, and infection.

9. Explain the transition to a rehabilitative facility.	9. The sooner the client engages in rehabilitation, the more successful the prosthetic ambulation.

Documentation

Client and family teaching
Response to teaching
Referrals, if indicated

Arterial Bypass Grafting in the Lower Extremity

"Peripheral artery disease (PAD) results from the build-up of plaque (atherosclerosis) in the arteries of the legs. For most people with PAD, symptoms may be mild or absent, and no treatment of the artery blockages is required. However as these blockages become more extensive, clients may experience pain and disability that limits their walking, and in the most advanced cases individuals may be at risk for loss of the limb unless circulation is improved. For these clients with severe PAD, attempts to improve blood flow in the leg are usually indicated. The goals of improving blood flow to the limb are to reduce pain, improve functional ability and quality of life, and to prevent amputation" (Conti, 2009).

Surgical treatments for PAD can be minimally invasive as angioplasty or stenting or arterial bypass surgery, depending on the severity and location of the arterial blockage (Conti, 2009).

There are three types of arterial bypass surgeries (Creager & Libby, 2007):

* Aortobifemoral bypass on the major abdominal artery (aorta) and the large arteries that branch off of it.
* Femoropopliteal (fem-pop) bypass on the arteries above and below the knee.
* Femoral-tibial bypass on the arteries in the lower leg or foot.

Endarterectomy is less common surgery and is done to remove fatty build-up (plaque) and to increase blood flow to the leg. This surgery may be done by itself, or it may be done at the same time as bypass surgery or angioplasty.

Time Frame
Postoperative periods

■■■ DIAGNOSTIC CLUSTER

Collaborative Problems

*   Risk for Complications of Deep Vein Thrombosis / Pulmonary Embolism (refer to Unit II Risk for Complications of DVT / PE)

Δ   Risk for Complications of Thrombosis of Graft

Δ   Risk for Complications of Compartment Syndrome

Δ   Risk for Complications of Lymphocele

▲   Risk for Complications of Disruption of Anastomosis or Puncture Site

▲   Risk for Complications of Renal Failure (refer to Unit II Risk for Complications of Renal Insufficiency)

Nursing Diagnoses

▲   Acute Pain related to increased tissue perfusion to previous ischemic tissue

Δ   Risk for Ineffective Self-Health Management related to insufficient knowledge of wound care, signs and symptoms of complications, activity restrictions, and follow-up care

Related Care Plans

▲ General Surgery Generic Care Plan

▲ Abdominal Aortic Aneurysm Resection

▲ This diagnosis was reported to be monitored for or managed frequently (75% to 100%).
Δ This diagnosis was reported to be monitored for or managed often (50% to 74%).

Transition Criteria

Before transition, the client and / or family will:

1. Demonstrate proper wound care.
2. Demonstrate correct pulse palpation technique.
3. State the signs and symptoms that must be reported to a health care professional.

> ### Transitional Risk Assessment Plan (TRAP)
>
> Begin this plan on admission.
> Implement the Transitional Risk Assessment Plan (TRAP):
> * Refer to inside back cover.
> * Add each validated risk diagnosis to client's problem list with the risk code in ( ).
> * Refer to Unit II to the individual risk nursing diagnoses / collaborative problems for outcomes and interventions.
>
> *R: "Close coordination of care in the post-acute period, early transition follow-up care, enhanced client education and self-management training, proactive end-of-life counseling, and extending the resources and clinical expertise over time via multidisciplinary team management" can lower readmission rates and improve health outcomes (Boutwell & Hwu, 2009, p. 14).*

Collaborative Problems

Risk for Complications of Thrombosis of Graft

Risk for Complications of Compartment Syndrome

Risk for Complications of Lymphocele

Risk for Complications of Disruption of Anastomosis or Puncture Site

Collaborative Outcomes

The client will be monitored for early signs and symptoms of (a) thrombosis of graft, (b) compartment syndrome, (c) lymphocele, and (d) disruption of anastomosis, and will receive collaborative interventions if indicated to restore physiologic stability.

Indicators of Physiologic Stability

* Capillary refill <3 seconds (a, b, d)
* Peripheral pulses: full, present (a)
* Warm, not mottled limbs (a, b)
* Intact sensation (a, b)
* Minimal limb edema (b)
* No pain with passive stretching (a, b)
* Intact muscle tension (a, b)
* Increasing wound drainage (c)
* Increasing local swelling (b, c)
* No bounding pulsation over graft (d)
* Can move toes (b)

Carp's Cues

Please refer to the Generic Care Plan for the Surgical Client for detailed interventions for managing all surgical conditions. This care plan addresses specific additional interventions associated with this type of surgery performed.

Interventions	Rationales
1. Monitor graft patency, palpate a graft patency, palpate a graft near the skin surface, and assess distal pulses for changes from the baseline (e.g., Doppler pressure).	1. Graft patency is essential to arterial circulation.
2. Monitor peripheral circulation hourly initially per protocol, compare extremities (pulses, sensation, capillary refill, skin color, temperature). **CLINICAL ALERT** • Report any changes, which may indicate thrombolic occlusion of the graft, immediately. • Sudden decrease in arterial flow, indicating thrombosed graft, is an emergency requiring immediate surgical exploration of the graft (Edwards, Abullarade, & Turnbull, 1996).	2. A sudden change in temperature, drop in pressure, or absence of pulses indicates graft thrombosis. Changes in sensation or motor function can indicate arterial thrombosis or compartment syndrome. (Edwards, Abullarade, & Turnbull, 1996)
3. Maintain bed rest as prescribed usually 1–2 days.	3. Bed rest helps to prevent graft trauma from injury.
4. Keep the limb warm but do not use electric heating pads or hot water bottles.	4. Peripheral nerve ischemia causes diminished sensation. High temperatures of heating devices may damage tissue without the client feeling discomfort.
5. Instruct the client to sit in a "slouched" position and not to cross legs. If leg elevation is ordered, elevate the entire leg and pelvis to heart level unless contraindicated.	5. Sharp flexion and pressure on the graft must be avoided to prevent graft damage (Edwards, Abullarade, & Turnbull, 1996).
6. Monitor for signs and symptoms of compartment syndrome: a. Edema of revascularized limb b. Complaints of pain with passive stretching of the muscle c. Decreased sensation, motor function, or paresthesias of the distal limb d. Increased tension and firmness of muscle **CLINICAL ALERT** • Postoperative edema is expected in the new revascularized limb. • Careful assessment alerts the nurse to edema severe enough to cause compartment syndrome. • Access surgeon for an evaluation when excess edema is suspected (Edwards, Abullarade, & Turnbull, 1996).	6. After a period of ischemia comes a period of increased capillary wall permeability. Restoration of arterial flow causes plasma and extracellular fluid to flow into the tissues, producing massive swelling in the calf muscles. The edema compresses the blood vessels and nerves within the nonexpanding fascia (Sieggreen, 2007). The nerves become anoxic, causing paresthesias and motor deficits. Urgent fasciotomy is required to relieve pressure and preserve the limb (Sieggreen, 2007).
7. Monitor for signs and symptoms of lymphocele: a. Discomfort accompanied by local swelling b. Large amounts of clear or pink-tinged drainage **CLINICAL ALERT** • Contact the surgeon. • Although compression may possibly halt the flow of lymph long enough for the lymphatic vessel to seal, this usually is not the case; surgical intervention may be required to repair the draining lymphatic chain. • Compression should be used only on the physician's / NP's order; overly vigorous compression may damage the new graft.	7. A major lymphatic channel courses through the inner thigh area. If the lymphatic chain is lacerated during the operation, drainage may occur. The large amount of accumulated fluid seeks the path of least resistance and usually drains through the incision.
8. Monitor for disruption of anastomosis: a. Decrease in perfusion of distal extremity b. Bounding aneurysmal pulsation over the anastomosis site. If bleeding occurs, apply firm, constant pressure over the site and notify the physician / NP.	8. Hemorrhage from anastomotic disruption is an emergency requiring immediate surgical intervention.

Clinical Alert Report

Prior to providing care, advise ancillary staff / student to report the following to the professional nurse assigned to the client:

- Capillary refill >3 seconds
- Decreased peripheral pulses
- Cool, mottled limbs
- Decreased sensation
- Increasing limb edema
- New c/o of pain, difficulty in moving toes
- Increasing wound drainage

Related Physician / NP Prescribed Interventions

Medications

Vasodilators, anticoagulant therapy, mannitol, analgesics antiplatelet therapy, cholesterol-reducing medications, antihypertensive

Intravenous Therapy

Fluid / electrolyte replacement

Laboratory Studies

Prothrombin time, platelet count, serum creatinine phosphokinase, urine creatinine clearance, triglycerides, complete blood cell count, partial prothrombin time

Diagnostic Studies

Doppler ultrasonography, angiography, ankle-brachial index, magnetic resonance angiography (MRA), computed tomographic angiography

Therapies

Hyperbaric oxygen therapy; also refer to the General Surgery Care Plan

Documentation

Vital signs
Distal pulses
Circulatory status
Presence and description of pain
Unusual events, actions, responses
Wound drainage and appearance

Nursing Diagnoses

Acute Pain Related to Increased Tissue Perfusion to Previous Ischemic Tissue

NOC
Comfort Level, Pain Control

Goal

The client will report pain relief after interventions.

NIC
Pain Management, Medication Management, Emotional Support, Teaching: Individual, Heat / Cold Application, Simple Massage

Indicators

- State the reason for the pain.
- Relate signs and symptoms of ischemia.

Interventions	Rationales
1. Monitor the "Six P's" of acute ischemia related to arterial occlusion: pain, coolness, pulselessness, pallor, paresthesia, and paralysis (begins with generic motor deficits) (Sieggreen, 2007).	1. Acute ischemia related to arterial occlusion needs early identification to prevent permanent damage.
2. Explain the source of pain and reassure the client that the sensation is temporary and will decrease each day.	2. Pain results from the reperfusion of previously ischemic sensory nerve endings. Pain lessens as reperfusion progresses.
3. Assess carefully to differentiate between the pain of reperfusion and the pain of ischemia (reperfused tissue is warm and edematous; ischemic tissue is cool). Notify the surgeon immediately if ischemia is suspected.	3. Ischemic pain may indicate graft failure and warrants immediate evaluation.
4. Refer to the nursing diagnosis Acute Pain in the General Surgery Care Plan for additional interventions.	

Documentation

Unrelieved pain
Interventions
Response to interventions

TRANSITION TO HOME/COMMUNITY CARE

If indicated, review the risk diagnoses identified for this individual on admission:

- Is the person still at risk?
- Can the family reduce the risks?
- Is the person at higher risk at home?
- Is a Home Health Nurse assessment needed?
- Refer to transition planner / case manager / social service.
- When is this person scheduled for follow-up with primary provider? Specialists? Record dates of appointments.
- Complete a medication reconciliation prior to transition. Refer to index.

STAR   **Stop**

Think   Is this person at risk for injury, falls, medical complications, and / or inability to care for self (activities of daily living)?
Is there a support person available?
Is the person competent to manage self-administration of medications, treatment procedures?
Are additional resources needed?
Can the person explain how to monitor the condition (e.g., blood glucose, signs / symptoms of complications, dietary / mobility restrictions, and when to call his or her primary provider or specialist)?

Act   Contact or provide the appropriate resource (e.g., contacting a support person, home health assessment, additional teaching, printed materials).

Review   Has the problem been addressed? If not, use SBAR to communicate to the appropriate person.

Risk for Ineffective Self-Health Management Related to Insufficient Knowledge of Wound Care, Signs and Symptoms of Complications, Activity Restrictions, and Follow-up Care

NOC

Compliance Behavior, Knowledge: Treatment Regimen, Participation: Health Care Decisions, Treatment Behavior: Illness or Injury

NIC

Anticipatory Guidance, Risk Management, Health Education, Learning Facilitation

Goals

The goals for this diagnosis represent those associated with transitional planning. Refer to the transition criteria.

Interventions	Rationales
1. Teach the client and family the proper wound care techniques. (Refer to the nursing diagnosis Risk for Ineffective Therapeutic Regimen Management in the General Surgery Care Plan, Appendix II, for specific measures.)	1. Proper wound care can prevent infection that delays healing (Edwards, Abullarade, & Turnbull, 1996).
2. Reinforce teaching regarding activity restrictions and mobility (Edwards, Abullarade, & Turnbull, 1996). a. Increase activity as prescribed. b. Avoid long periods (>20 minutes) of standing or sitting with legs bent at the groin and knee. c. Ambulate as advised; plan a walking or exercise program (Sieggreen, 2006).	2. The client's understanding may encourage compliance with the therapeutic regimen. a. Activity should be increased gradually to promote circulation and reduce loss of strength. b. Dependent positioning of the legs increases postoperative swelling. Positions of hip–knee flexion impede venous return. c. Early ambulation is recommended to restore muscle activity and enhance venous blood return.
3. Teach the client and family or support persons how to assess graft patency. a. Assess pulses and capillary refill. b. Palpate the graft for pulsations, if near the surface.	3. Monitoring circulatory status must be continued at home.
4. Teach the client and family or significant others to recognize signs and symptoms of problems and report them immediately. a. Sudden onset of shortness of breath (call 911) b. Absence of pulses c. Change in temperature of the leg or foot d. Paresthesias and other changes in sensation e. Increased pain f. Increased swelling g. Wound or sore in the affected leg h. Changes in the incision site (e.g., redness, drainage) i. Fever (>100.5° F)	4. Reporting these signs of compromised circulation, infection, or possible graft failure promptly enables intervention to prevent serious complications. Diminished circulation impedes healing; infection can cause graft failure (Edwards, Abullarade & Turnbull, 1996; Hirsch et al., 2006).
5. Reinforce teaching regarding foot care and prevention of injury to the leg. Refer to Peripheral Arterial Care Plan for specific teaching.	5. Continued care and precautions are necessary at home.

Interventions	Rationales
6. Teach the client and family about the vascular disease process and prevention of further arterial occlusions (Sieggreen, 2007): a. The development of atherosclerosis and PAD is influenced by heredity and also by lifestyle factors, such as dietary habits and levels of exercise. The risk factors for atherosclerosis that can be modified or eliminated are: • Elevated blood cholesterol and triglycerides. • Hypertension • Tobacco use or exposure to tobacco smoke • Diabetes, types 1 and 2 • Obesity • Inactivity, lack of exercise	6. Addressing risk factors and encouraging regular follow-up with the physician / NP may prevent the client from experiencing a similar event (Bick, 2003; Hirsch et al., 2006; Sieggreen, 2007).

 Carp's Cues

Refer to Getting Started to Quit Smoking, Getting Started to Increase Activity, and Getting Started to Healthy Eating on thePoint at http://thePoint.lww.com/Carpenito6e for printable handouts to give to client.

Documentation

Client and family teaching
Response to teaching

Breast Surgery (Lumpectomy, Mastectomy)

The primary treatment for breast cancer is removal of the cancerous tissue. The type of surgery is based on the type of tumor, size of tumor, grade of tumor, estrogen and progesterone receptors, and client preference. With either a lumpectomy or mastectomy one or several axillary lymph nodes may be examined and / or removed. *Lumpectomy*, also known as breast-conserving surgery or partial mastectomy, is the removal of the cancerous tissue and a small amount of adjacent tissue with overlying skin left in place. Axillary nodes may be dissected through a separate incision. Lumpectomy is not usually recommended for tumors larger than 5 cm. However, women with a strong desire to save their breast may opt for chemotherapy or hormone therapy given prior to surgery to shrink the tumor. Lumpectomy followed by radiation therapy is currently the standard of care and research has shown equally as effective as a mastectomy for early stage breast cancer (Giuliano & Hurvitz, 2012).

Mastectomy is the removal of the whole breast performed in several ways, including the following: *simple, skin sparing or nipple / areolar sparing* based on surgeon expertise training and individual assessment; a *total or complete mastectomy*, removal of the entire breast tissue, is routinely performed for tumors larger than 5 cm with known cancer spreading to the lymph nodes; *modified radical mastectomy* is the removal of the entire breast and some of the axillary lymph nodes; *radical mastectomy* is the removal of the entire breast, skin, pectoral muscles, and all axillary lymph nodes. This procedure is rarely done and only for extensive tumors that have invaded the chest wall. Post mastectomy clients can choose breast reconstruction with implant, reconstruction with their own tissue, or choose to wear prostheses. Axillary lymph node removal is important in staging, preventing axillary recurrence, and in treatment planning. More common sentinel node biopsy is done intraoperative, if negative for spread of disease, axillary dissection may be omitted. Surgery may be followed by radiation, chemotherapy, hormonal therapy, or combinations of these.

Time Frame

Each breast cancer case is individualized based on a number of factors, including treatment decisions and tumor characteristics. With each case careful consideration includes the kind of surgery, the desire for reconstruction of the breast, genetic profile of likelihood of recurrence, targeted therapy, and hormonal therapy. Balance must be placed on the characteristic and staging of the cancer inclusive of the client's wishes, and impact on quality of life. Hospital stay is routinely not needed for a lumpectomy, and a 1–2 day hospital stay for mastectomy.

Preoperative and Postoperative Periods

Clients should be offered a consultation with a reconstructive plastic surgeon to discuss options and ensure *preoperatively* they understand and have made informed decisions on treatment and reconstruction.

Breast conserving surgery followed by radiation therapy should be considered as primary treatment whenever possible. For most women, a lumpectomy can leave the breast structurally, preserving the appearance and sensation of the breast with good cosmetic results. It can, however, in some cases leave the breast smaller and distorted. Postoperatively the tumor is assessed for margins, to ensure that the area around the tumor is free of cancer cells. Final pathology can take up to a week to review, and if margins are found positive, clients will need to endure another surgery. Postoperatively clients are likely to have 5–7 weeks of radiation therapy. Radiation may affect the timing of reconstruction and limit reconstruction options due to changes in the skin. The most common reasons for hospitalization following breast surgery is postoperative pain, nausea, vomiting, and anxiety.

▪▪▪▪▪▪ DIAGNOSTIC CLUSTER

Nursing Diagnoses

Preoperative Period

▲ Anxiety / Fear related to perceived effects of surgery (immediate: pain, nausea, vomiting; post transition: relationships, edema, work) and prognosis

▲ Psychological distress related to diagnosis of cancer and subsequent alterations in body image.

Postoperative Period

Collaborative Problems

Risk for Complications of Neurovascular Compromise

Nursing Diagnoses

Risk for Impaired Physical Mobility (arm, shoulder) related to lymphedema, nerve / muscle damage, and pain

Risk for Injury related to compromised lymph drainage, motor, and sensory function in affected arm

Risk for Disturbed Self-Concept related to perceived negative effects of loss on functioning (refer to Unit II)

Grieving related to loss of breast and change in appearance (refer to Unit II)

Risk for Ineffective Self-Health Therapeutic Regimen Management related to insufficient knowledge of wound care, exercises, breast prosthesis, signs and symptoms of complications, hand / arm precautions, community resources, and follow-up care

Related Care Plan

General Surgery Generic Care Plan

Transitional Criteria

Before transition, the client and family will:

1. Demonstrate hand and arm exercises.
2. Verbalize understanding of ways to reduce the risk of lymphedema (i.e., wear loose clothes or jewelry on the surgical side, elevate surgical arm to a point higher than the heart when resting, do not let arm hang down, do not apply heat to limb).
3. Demonstrate breast self-examination.
4. State care measures to perform at home.
5. Discuss strategies for performing ADLs.
6. State necessary precautions.
7. State the signs and symptoms that must be reported to a health care professional.
8. Verbalize an intent to share feelings and concerns with significant others.
9. Identify available community resources and self-help groups.

> ### Transitional Risk Assessment Plan (TRAP)
>
> Begin this plan on admission.
> Implement the Transitional Risk Assessment Plan (TRAP):
> - Refer to inside back cover.
> - Add each validated risk diagnosis to client's problem list with the risk code in ( ).
> - Refer to Unit II to the individual risk nursing diagnoses / collaborative problems for outcomes and interventions.
>
>   *R: "Close coordination of care in the post-acute period, early transition follow-up care, enhanced client education and self-management training, proactive end-of-life counseling, and extending the resources and clinical expertise over time via multidisciplinary team management" can lower readmission rates and improve health outcomes (Boutwell & Hwu, 2009, p. 14).*

Collaborative Problems

Risk for Complications of Neurovascular Compromise

Collaborative Outcomes

The client will be monitored for early signs and symptoms of neurovascular compromise and will receive collaborative interventions if indicated to restore physiologic stability.

NIC
Fall Prevention,
Environmental
Management: Safety,
Health Education,
Surveillance: Safety,
Risk Identification

Indicators of Physiologic Stability

- Radial pulses full, bounding
- No numbness or tingling of hand
- Capillary refill <3 seconds
- Warm, not mottled extremity
- Intact finger flexion and extension

Carp's Cues

Please refer to the Generic Care Plan for the Surgical Client for detailed interventions for managing all surgical conditions. This care plan addresses specific additional interventions associated with the type of surgery performed.

Interventions	Rationales

1. Monitor for signs and symptoms of neurovascular compromise by comparing findings between limbs:
  a. Diminished or absent radial pulse
  b. Numbness or tingling in hand
  c. Capillary refill time >3 seconds
  d. Pallor, blanching, or cyanosis, and coolness of extremity
  e. Inability to flex or extend fingers
	1. Significant edema of the arm occurs in 10% to 30% of clients after axillary dissection (Yarbro, Wujcik, & Gobel, 2011).

Related Physician / NP Prescribed Interventions

Medications

Refer to the Cancer: Initial Diagnosis and General Surgery care plans.

Diagnostic Studies

Mammogram; thermography; ultrasound; computed tomography (CT) scan; xeroradiography; breast node biopsies (fine-needle core, wire localization); positron emission tomography (PET); scintimammography, magnetic resonance imaging (MRI), and galactography (Nettina, 2006)

Therapies

Back brace, physical therapy, temporary soft prosthesis, radiation, breast reconstruction, prosthesis, implants

Documentation

Radial pulse assessment
Affected arm: color, sensation, capillary refill time, movement

> **CLINICAL ALERT**
> Notify surgeon for:
> • C/O numbness or tingling of hand
> • Capillary refill >3 seconds
> • Cool, mottled extremity
> • Diminished finger flexion and extension

Nursing Diagnosis

Anxiety / Fear Related to Perceived Effects of Surgery (Immediate: Pain, Edema; Post Transition: Relationships, Work) and Prognosis

Goal

The client will share concerns regarding the surgery and its outcome. A clear explanation of expectations during the hospital should be explained during preoperative counseling.

Indicators

• Describe actions that can help to reduce postoperative edema and immobility.
• State the intent to share feelings with family, significant other, or friends.

CLINICAL ALERT
- Research has shown levels of preoperative stress and worries about outcomes directly relate to the incidence of post surgical nausea, fatigue, pain, and discomfort (Montgomery & Bowbjerg, 2004).

Interventions	*Rationales*
1. Encourage the client to verbalize her concerns and fears. Stay with the client and family as much as possible and convey empathy and concern.	1. A significant number of women face survivorship issues once diagnosed with breast cancer. Psychological struggles, upper extremity lymphedema, weight management, and the fear of uncertainty.
2. Explore with individual sources of his or her distress. **CLINICAL ALERT** - Clients are at an increased risk of distress with fear and worry about the future. - Clients may express anger, fear, and feeling out of control. - Physical symptoms may include poor sleep, appetite, concentration, preoccupation with thoughts of illness and dealt, and concerns of role changes (NCCN, 2013).	2. Distress is a multifactorial unpleasant emotional experience of psychological (cognitive, behavioral, emotional), social, and / or spiritual nature that may interfere with the ability to cope effectively with cancer, its physical symptoms and its treatment. Distress extends along a continuum, ranging from common normal feelings of vulnerability, sadness, and fears to problems that can become disabling, such as depression, anxiety, panic, social isolation, and existential and spiritual crisis (NCCN, 2013).
3. Ensure that the individual / families understanding of diagnosis, treatment, and possible side effects: a. Access physician / NP for clarification of misinformation or inadequate information b. Assess client readiness to learn; provide appropriate client education materials acknowledge fear, build trust, maintain continuity of care.	3. Clients / family who are empowered with knowledge, resources, and a sense of control, will ultimately manage their care to reduce risk of side effects, to make informed treatment decisions, and to receive the follow-up care needed.
4. Explain expected events simply, such as the following: a. Postoperative routines b. Possible development of lymphedema and sensory changes after surgery c. Positioning and exercises d. Presence of drainage tubes	4. Previous research has confirmed uncertainty in illness (UIL) is common to individuals with breast cancer, also confirming the negative emotions that are associated with UIL impact client's ability to seek information about the disease but also prevent them from having treatment (Wu, Li, & Jin, 2008).
5. Explain that a temporary soft prosthesis can be worn immediately, inside a bra. Permanent breast prosthesis can be fitted after the individual has healed.	5. A temporary prosthesis enhances the appearance and reduces the sense of imbalance that can result from breast removal. Understanding that prosthesis can be worn immediately after recovery can help to allay anxiety associated with appearance.
6. Allow the client's partner to share his or her concerns in private. Assure partner that his or her concerns and fears are normal and expected.	6. Research has shown that satisfaction with marital support and support from other adults positively affects the woman's adjustment (Hoskins et al., 2000). Partners may feel unsure of how to show support and affection (Susan B. Komen for the Cure, 2007d).
7. Providing access to psycho-social interventions is needed for oncology clients and their family members to achieve quality of life outcomes (Fitch, 2006).	7. Validation can help to reduce fear associated with such feelings as rejection, repulsion, abandonment, and loss of attractiveness. Open communication between partners is very important (Susan B. Komen for the Cure, 2007d).

Documentation

Dialogues
Interventions

Risk for Impaired Physical Mobility (Arm, Shoulder) Related to Lymphedema, Nerve / Muscle Damage, and Pain

NOC
Ambulation: Walking, Joint Movement: Active, Mobility Level

Goal

The client will demonstrate progressive mobility to the extent possible within limitations imposed by the surgery.

NIC
Ambulation, Positioning, Teaching: Prescribed Activity / Exercise, Teaching: Procedure / Treatment

Interventions	Rationales
1. Explain not to exercise postoperative arm exercise plan until recommended by surgeon / NP.	1. The current American College of Sports Medicine (ACSM, 2010) recommendations specific to mastectomy and lumpectomy indicate to wait up to 8 weeks before exercise to ensure sufficient time for healing.
2. When exercise is permitted, explain the need to increase mobility to the maximum extent tolerated, and specify the hazards of immobility.	2. Explanations can help to elicit cooperation despite discomfort or fear of falling. Early mobilization and arm exercise after surgery is important for enhancing recovery.
3. Explain the reasons for poor balance; accompany client while she walks.	3. A large compression bandage and impaired arm movement can interfere with balance and increase the risk of falling.
4. Instruct client to elevate the affected arm on a pillow when sitting or reclining.	4. Elevation facilitates lymphatic drainage and prevents pooling.

Documentation

Level of function
Exercises (type, frequency)

Risk for Injury Related to Compromised Lymph Drainage, Motor, and Sensory Function in Affected Arm

NOC
Risk Control, Safety Status: Falls Occurrence

Goal

The client will report no injuries to the affected arm.

NIC
Fall Prevention, Environmental Management: Safety, Health Education, Surveillance: Safety, Risk Identification

Indicators

• Relate the factors that contribute to lymphedema.
• Describe activities that are hazardous to the affected arm.

Interventions	Rationales

CLINICAL ALERT
- Unfortunately there is no accepted definition of clinically significant lymphedema, and as a result it is difficult to advise the woman of the amount of lymphedema post breast cancer surgery (Koul et al., 2007).

1. Monitor for signs and symptoms of sensorimotor impairment:
   a. Impaired joint movement
   b. Muscle weakness
   c. Numbness or tingling

1. These signs can indicate entrapment of nerves at the cervical outlet or wrist from lymphedema or damage to the thoracodorsal nerve.

2. Monitor regular measurements of arm circumference for changes.

2. Regular measurements can detect increasing lymphedema.

CLINICAL ALERT
- Rarely, edema may be severe enough to interfere with the use of the limb.
- Consult with provider if edema persists or worsens.
- Mild diuretic, compressor pump, manual compression, or use of a lymphedema sleeve may be indicated.

3. Monitor for increase in lymphedema, as more aggressive therapy may be indicated.

3. Late or secondary edema can develop years after treatment; client should be evaluated by provider to rule out infection or recurrence of disease.

4. Teach the client to avoid the following:
   a. Vaccines, blood samples, injections, and blood pressure measurements on affected arm
   b. Constrictive jewelry and clothing
   c. Carrying a shoulder bag or heavy object with the affected arm
   d. Brassieres with thin shoulder straps (use wide-strap or no-strap brassieres instead)
   e. Lifting objects weighing more than 5–10 pounds; leaning on arm

4a, b. Constriction of the arm can exacerbate lymphedema.

   c. Shoulder bags and heavy objects increase pressure at the shoulder joint and increase blood flow to the affected arm.
   d. Thin straps also produce constriction on the shoulder.
   e. Anything that increases blood flow to the affected area contributes to lymphedema (Yarbro, Wujcik, & Gobel, 2011).

5. Teach the client precautions to prevent trauma to the affected arm and hand:
   a. Using long-gloved potholders
   b. Avoiding cuts, scratches, and bruises (e.g., using a thimble when sewing)
   c. Avoiding injections and venipunctures of any kind
   d. Avoiding strong detergents or other chemical agents
   e. Wearing heavy gardening gloves and avoiding gardening in thorny plants
   f. Using electric razor under arms
   g. Protecting from sunburn and avoiding excessive heat (e.g., saunas, hot tubs, or tanning beds)
   h. Keeping skin clean and well moisturized
   i. Not cutting cuticles
   j. Promptly treating infections of hand and arm (National Cancer Institute, 2007; Susan B. Komen for the Cure, 2007c)

5. Skin care is a priority with lymphedema. The body has a difficult time clearing bacteria in tissue affected with lymphedema, resulting in a higher risk of infection to the area (Cheville & Gergich, 2004).

(continued)

Interventions	Rationales
6. Teach the client to cleanse arm or hand wounds promptly, and to observe carefully for early signs of infection (e.g., redness, increased warmth). Stress the need to report any signs promptly.	6. Compromised lymph drainage weakens the body's defense against infection; this necessitates increased emphasis on infection prevention. Studies show that prophylactic antibiotics significantly reduce the incidence of surgical site infection, lowering potential morbidity (Cunningham, Bunn, & Handscomb, 2006).
7. Teach the client to keep the wrist higher than the elbow and the elbow higher than the heart whenever possible.	7. This will reduce edema.
8. Follow exercise program directed by physician / NP to teach methods of reducing lymphedema.	8. Complete decongestive physiotherapy exercise (e.g., opening and closing the hand), manual lymphatic drainage (a specific type of massage), and physical therapy have been shown to reduce swelling and lymphedema-related infection (Susan B. Komen for the Cure, 2007c).

Documentation

Client teaching

> **TRANSITION TO HOME / COMMUNITY CARE**
> If indicated, review the risk diagnoses identified for this individual on admission:
> * Is the person still at risk?
> * Can the family reduce the risks?
> * Is the person at higher risk at home?
> * Is a Home Health Nurse assessment needed?
> * Refer to transition planner / case manager / social service.
> * When is this person scheduled for follow-up with primary provider? Specialists? Record dates of appointments.
> * Complete a medication reconciliation prior to transition. Refer to index.

STAR

Stop

Think Is this person at risk for injury, falls, medical complications, and / or inability to care for self (activities of daily living)?
Is there a support person available?
Is the person competent to manage self-administration of medications, treatment procedures?
Are additional resources needed?
Can the person explain how to monitor the condition (e.g., blood glucose, signs / symptoms of complications, dietary / mobility restrictions, and when to call his or her primary provider or specialist)?

Act Contact or provide the appropriate resource (e.g., contacting a support person, home health assessment, additional teaching, printed materials).

Review Has the problem been addressed? If not, use SBAR to communicate to the appropriate person.

Risk for Ineffective Self-Health Management Related to Insufficient Knowledge of Wound Care, Exercises, Breast Prosthesis, Signs and Symptoms of Complications, Hand / Arm Precautions, Community Resources, and Follow-up Care

NOC

Compliance Behavior, Knowledge: Treatment Regimen, Participation: Health Care Decisions, Treatment Behavior: Illness or Injury

NIC

Anticipatory Guidance, Risk Identification, Health Education, Learning Facilitation

Goals

The goals for this diagnosis represent those associated with transition planning. Refer to the transition criteria.

Interventions	Rationales
1. Teach the client breast self-examination techniques; instruct her to examine both breasts periodically.	1. Periodic, careful breast self-examination can detect problems early; this improves the likelihood of successful treatment (Nettina, 2006).
2. Teach the client wound care measures (refer to Generic Care Plan for the Surgical Client for details) and to avoid using strong deodorants and shaving of axilla for two weeks after surgery (Yarbro, Wujcik, & Gobel , 2011).	2. Proper wound care is essential to reduce risk of infection. Irritation of the axilla should be avoided to decrease risk of infection (Yarbro, Wujcik, & Gobel, 2011).
3. Provide information about breast prostheses. Emphasize the importance of a properly fitted prosthesis.	3. A prosthesis of optimal contour, size, and weight provides normal appearance, promotes good posture, and helps to prevent back and shoulder strain.
4. Explain the benefits of strengthening and aerobic exercises.	4. Strengthening exercises increase lymph flow with muscle-pumping action. Aerobic activity elevates the heart and respiratory rates; this stimulates the lymphatic transport (Yarbro, Wujcik, & Gobel, 2011).
5. Encourage the client to maintain ideal body weight.	5. Adipose tissue compresses and reduces lymphatic transport (Yarbro, Wujcik, & Gobel, 2011).
6. Refer to a specialist in lymphedema, if needed.	6. Early interventions at the first sign of lymphedema can reduce long-term complications.
7. Explain the use of a compression sleeve, if ordered.	7. Compression increases lymphatic return and reduces edema.
8. Explain to expect fatigue in the months after surgery (Badger, Braden, & Michel, 2001).	8. Fatigue has been found to be the most frequently reported side effect (Badger, Braden, & Michel, 2001).
9. Encourage the client to seek professional counseling for assistance with coping and depression.	9. Depression is common and affects the client's quality of life significantly (Badger, Braden, & Michel, 2001).
10. Provide written instructions for exercises to perform at home and reemphasize their importance.	10. Research has shown that, after breast surgery, women experience significant attention deficits, regardless of the extent of surgery (Cimprich, 1992).

(continued)

Interventions	Rationales
11. Instruct the client to inspect her arm and hand daily, and to report promptly any signs and symptoms of complications, including these: a. Increasing edema or weakness b. Numbness or tingling c. Impaired hand or arm movement d. Warmth, redness, or rashes e. Pain	11. These signs and symptoms point to increasing lymphedema, which can lead to impaired sensorimotor function or infection.
12. Discuss available community resources (e.g., Reach for Recovery, ENCORE). Encourage contact and initiate referrals, if appropriate. Home health care may be helpful due to short length of hospitalization after surgery (Nettina, 2006).	12. Personal sources of information have been found to be more important than written materials.
13. As appropriate, explore the client's feelings concerning radiation therapy or chemotherapy, if planned.	13. Both radiation and chemotherapy have side effects that necessitate client teaching to enhance self-care and coping.

Documentation

Client and family teaching
Referrals, if indicated

Carotid Endarterectomy

A Multidisciplinary Consensus Statement from the American Heart Association concluded that carotid endarterectomy, performed in medical centers with documented combined perioperative morbidity and mortality for asymptomatic endarterectomy of less than 3%, in conjunction with aggressive modifiable risk factor management is beneficial for clients who have an asymptomatic stenosis exceeding 60% diameter reduction confirmed by angiography (Jauch et al., 2013).

Symptomatic occlusion indicates the occurrence of a transient ischemic attack (TIA) or cerebral vascular accident (Greelish, Mohler, & Fairman, 2006b). The procedure may be performed under general or local anesthesia; local anesthesia significantly reduces morbidity and mortality.

Time Frame
Postoperative periods

■■■■■ DIAGNOSTIC CLUSTER

Postoperative Period

Collaborative Problems

Circulatory

▲ Risk for Complications of Thrombosis

▲ Risk for Complications of Hypotension

▲ Risk for Complications of Hypertension

▲ Risk for Complications of Hemorrhage

▲ Risk for Complications of Cerebral Infarction

Neurologic

▲ Risk for Complications of Cerebral Infarction

▲ Risk for Complications of Cranial Nerve Impairment

▲ Risk for Complications of Respiratory / Airway Obstruction

Nursing Diagnoses

▲ Risk for Injury Falls related to syncope secondary to vascular insufficiency (refer to Unit II Risk for Falls)

Δ Risk for Ineffective Self-Health Management related to insufficient knowledge of home care, signs and symptoms of complications, risk factors, activity restrictions, and follow-up care

Related Care Plan

General Surgery Generic Care plan

▲ This diagnosis was reported to be monitored for or managed frequently (75% to 100%).
Δ This diagnosis was reported to be monitored for or managed often (50% to 74%).

Transition Criteria

Before transition, the client and family will:

1. Describe wound care techniques.
2. State activity restrictions for home care.
3. Demonstrate range-of-motion (ROM) exercises.
4. State the signs and symptoms that must be reported to a health care professional.
5. Identify risk factors and describe their relationship to arterial disease.

> ### Transitional Risk Assessment Plan (TRAP)
>
> Begin this plan on admission.
> Implement the Transitional Risk Assessment Plan (TRAP):
> • Refer to inside back cover.
> • Add each validated risk diagnosis to client's problem list with the risk code in ( ).
> • Refer to Unit II to the individual risk nursing diagnoses / collaborative problems for outcomes and interventions.
>
> *R: "Close coordination of care in the post-acute period, early transition follow-up care, enhanced client education and self-management training, proactive end-of-life counseling, and extending the resources and clinical expertise over time via multidisciplinary team management" can lower readmission rates and improve health outcomes (Boutwell & Hwu, 2009, p. 14).*

Collaborative Problems

Risk for Complications of Circulatory Problems, Thrombosis, Hypotension, Hypertension, Hemorrhage, Cerebral Infarction

Risk for Complications of Neurologic Problems, Cerebral Infarction, Cranial Nerve Impairment, Local Nerve Impairment

Risk for Complications of Respiratory / Airway Obstruction

Collaborative Outcomes

The client will be monitored for early signs and symptoms of (a) vascular problems, (b) neurologic deficits, and (c) respiratory obstruction, and will receive collaborative interventions if indicated to restore physiologic stability.

Indicators of Physiologic Stability

- Respirations—quiet, regular, unlabored (a, b, c)
- Respirations 16–20 breaths/min (a, b, c)
- BP >90/60, <140/90 mm Hg (a, b)
- Pulse 60–100 beats/min (a, b, c)
- Temperature 98°–99.5° F (a)
- Alert, oriented (b)
- Pupils, equal, reactive to light (b)
- Intact motor function (b)
- Clear speech (b)
- Swallowing reflex intact (b)
- Facial symmetry (b)
- Full ROM upper / lower limbs (b)
- Urine output >0.5 mL/kg/h (a, b, c)
- Oxygen saturation (SaO_2) 94–100 mm Hg (a, b, c)
- Carbon dioxide ($PaCo_2$) 35–45 mm Hg (a, b, c)
- pH 7.35–7.45 (a, b, c)
- Hemoglobin
  - Male 13–15 g/dL (a, b, c)
  - Female 12–10 g/dL (a, b, c)
- Hematocrit
  - Male 42% to 50% (a, b, c)
  - Female 40% to 48% (a, b, c)
- Mean arterial pressure 60–160 mm Hg (a, b, c)
- White blood count 4,000–10,800 mm^3 (a, b, c)

Carp's Cues

Please refer to the Generic Care Plan for the Surgical Client for detailed interventions for managing all surgical conditions. This care plan addresses specific additional interventions associated this is type of surgery performed.

Interventions	Rationales
1. Monitor for the following: 　a. Respiratory obstruction (check trachea for deviation from midline; listen for respiratory stridor) 　b. Peri-incisional swelling or bleeding	1. Edema or hematoma at the surgical site can cause mechanical obstruction.
2. Monitor for changes in neurologic function (Greelish et al., 2006b): 　a. Level of consciousness 　b. Pupillary response 　c. Motor / sensory function of all four extremities (check hand grasps and ability to move legs)	2. Stroke is a possible, and most common, complication of carotid endarterectomy. Manifestations of cerebral infarction include neuromuscular impairment of the contralateral body side (Greelish et al., 2006b).
3. Monitor for cranial nerve dysfunction (Greelish et al., 2006c): 　a. Difficulty with speech 　b. Dysphagia 　c. Upper airway obstruction 　d. Upward protrusion of lower lip 　e. Sagging shoulder 　f. Difficulty raising arm or shoulder 　g. Loss of gag reflex 　h. Hoarseness 　i. Asymmetrical movements of vocal cords 　j. Numbness / weakness of face on the surgical side.	3. The surgical procedure can temporarily or permanently disrupt cranial nerve functions (Greelish et al., 2006c; National Library of Medicine, 2006). Most cranial nerve injuries resolve over a few months; permanent injuries are rare (Greelish et al., 2006c). Nerve damage affects around 8% of people but is usually temporary and disappears within a month. 　a. The hypoglossal nerve controls intrinsic and extrinsic muscles for tongue movement. 　d. The facial nerve controls facial motor function and taste. 　e. The accessory nerve controls the trapezius and sterno-cleidomastoid muscles. 　g. The vagus nerve regulates movements of swallowing and sensation to the pharynx and larynx. Laryngeal nerve (branches of vagus nerve) damage may cause unilateral vocal cord paralysis (Greelish et al., 2006c). Stimulation of the glossopharyngeal nerve may cause hypotension and bradycardia. Dissection of trigeminal nerve may lead to sensory loss in affected area.
4. Monitor for hypertension.	4. Hypertension can be anticipated in certain clients exhibiting predisposing factors, such as preoperative hypertension or postoperative hypoxia and excessive fluid replacement.
5. As necessary, consult with the physician / NP for IV pharmacologic management to prevent hypertensive episodes.	5. Hypertension can increase the risk of hemorrhage or disruption of arterial reconstruction.
6. Monitor for hypotension and bradycardia.	6. The removal of atherosclerotic plaque may cause increased pressure waves on the carotid sinus, leading to hypotension. Bradycardia may result from pressure on the carotid sinus during the operation or from postoperative edema. Postoperative cardiac complications are the leading cause of morbidity following carotid endarterectomy (Greelish et al., 2006c; Hickey, 1996).

Clinical Alert Report

Prior to providing care, advise ancillary staff / student to report the following to the professional nurse assigned to the client:

- Change in cognitive status
- Change in voice
- Difficulty swallowing
- Oral temperature >100.5° F
- Systolic BP <90 mm/Hg
- Resting Pulse >100, <50
- Respiratory rate >28, <10/min
- Oxygen saturation <90%

Related Physician / NP Prescribed Interventions

Medications
Antiplatelet therapy, statins

Diagnostic Studies
Ultrasound, carotid angiography, arteriography, magnetic resonance angiography, computed tomography angiography

Intravenous Therapies
Refer to Generic Care Plan for the Surgical Client

Documentation

Vital signs
Patency of the temporal artery on the operative side
Level of consciousness
Pupillary response
Motor function (hand grasp, leg movement)
Cranial nerve function
Wound assessment

Nursing Diagnoses

TRANSITION TO HOME / COMMUNITY CARE

If indicated, review the risk diagnoses identified for this individual on admission:

- Is the person still at risk?
- Can the family reduce the risks?
- Is the person at higher risk at home?
- Is a Home Health Nurse assessment needed?
- Refer to transition planner / case manager / social service.
- When is this person scheduled for follow-up with primary provider? Specialists? Record dates of appointments.
- Complete a medication reconciliation prior to transition. Refer to index.

STAR

Stop

Think Is this person at risk for injury, falls, medical complications, and / or inability to care for self (activities of daily living)?

Is there a support person available?

Is the person competent to manage self-administration of medications, treatment procedures? Are additional resources needed?

Can the person explain how to monitor the condition (e.g., blood glucose, signs / symptoms of complications, dietary / mobility restrictions, and when to call his or her primary provider or specialist)?

Act Contact or provide the appropriate resource (e.g., contacting a support person, home health assessment, additional teaching, printed materials).

Review Has the problem been addressed? If not, use SBAR to communicate to the appropriate person.

Risk for Ineffective Self-Health Management Related to Insufficient Knowledge of Home Care, Signs and Symptoms of Complications, Risk Factors, Activity Restrictions, and Follow-up Care

NOC

Compliance Behavior, Knowledge: Treatment Regimen, Participation: Health Care Decisions, Treatment Behavior: Illness or Injury

NIC

Anticipatory Guidance, Risk Management, Health Education, Learning Facilitation

Goals

The goals for this diagnosis represent those associated with transition planning. Refer to the transition criteria.

Interventions	Rationales
1. Advise the individual will have neck pain and difficulty swallowing for a few days. Advise to eat soft foods.	
2. Advise to seek emergency care if: a. Numbness or weakness of the face, arms, or legs, especially on one side of the body b. Confusion and trouble speaking or understanding speech c. Trouble seeing in one or both eyes d. Dizziness, trouble walking, loss of balance or coordination, and unexplained falls e. Severe headache with no clear cause f. Increased swelling in neck	2. These signs / symptoms may be indicative a stroke or a transient ischemic attack. Individuals with both a prior stroke and contralateral total occlusion had a 7.5% perioperative stroke rate. Clients with both a prior stroke and hypertension had a 6.1% perioperative stroke rate (Rockman, 1997).
3. Teach the client and family to watch for and report the following to their surgeon: a. Swelling of, or drainage from, the incision b. Temperature >100.5° F.	3. These signs are indicative of infection.
4. Teach the client and family about the vascular disease process and prevention of further arterial occlusions (Sieggreen, 2007).	4. The development of atherosclerosis is influenced by heredity and also by lifestyle factors, such as dietary habits and levels of exercise.
5. Teach the client and family about the risk factors for atherosclerosis that can be modified or eliminated are: a. Elevated blood cholesterol and triglycerides b. Hypertension c. Tobacco use or exposure to tobacco smoke d. Diabetes, types 1 and 2 e. Obesity f. Inactivity, lack of exercise	5. Addressing risk factors and encouraging regular follow-up with the physician / NP may prevent the client from experiencing a similar event (Bick, 2003; Hirsch et al., 2006; Sieggreen, 2007).

Carp's Cues

Refer to Getting Started to Quit Smoking, Getting Started to Increase Activity, and Getting Started to Healthy Eating on thePoint at http://thePoint.lww.com/Carpenito6e.

Documentation

Client teaching
Referrals, if indicated

Colostomy

A colostomy is an opening between the colon and the abdominal wall. The proximal end of the colon is sutured to the skin. Indications for colostomy include diverticulitis, trauma, and cancer (tumors) of the mid-transverse colon. This procedure bypasses the rectum by diverting feces into an external appliance (Minkes, 2013).

There are different names for colostomies, which are dependent on where the stoma is created. There is the *ascending colostomy*, which has an opening created from the ascending colon, and is found on the right abdomen. Because the stoma is created from the first section of the colon, stool is more liquid and contains digestive enzymes that irritate the skin. This type of colostomy is the least common.

The *transverse colostomy* may have one or two openings in the upper abdomen, middle, or right side, which are created from the transverse colon. If there are two openings in the stoma, (called a double-barrel colostomy) one is used to pass stool and the other, mucus. The stool has passed through the ascending colon, so it tends to be liquid to semi-formed. This method is mostly used for temporary colostomies.

In a *descending or sigmoid colostomy*, the descending or sigmoid colon is used to create the stoma, typically on the left lower abdomen. This is the most common type of colostomy surgery and generally produces stool that is semi-formed to well-formed because it has passed through the ascending and transverse colon (Lewis et al., 2004).

Carp's Cues

Prior to surgery to create a colonoscopy, the site for the stoma should be marked. Preoperative site marking reduces the incidence of postoperative ostomy complications and related pouching problems (Park et al., 1999). Stoma site marking is jointly recommended by the American Society of Colorectal Surgeons and the Wound, Ostomy, Continence Nurses Society. "Stoma site marking should be performed by an Enterostomal Nurse (ETN) or a health care professional who has been trained in the principles of stoma site marking and is aware of the implications of ostomy care and poor stoma site marking," Canada.

Ensure the stoma site marking is done prior to transport to or whenever possible. Consult with the ETN or wound specialist nurse. The stoma site should be selected to avoid fat folds, scars, and bony prominences. The individual should be marked in both the sitting and supine positions to ensure that the stoma appliance fits securely. This could make the difference between an ostomy pouch leaking or not for the person's lifetime. Types of skin damage included erosion, maceration, erythema and irritant dermatitis. Collectively, these accounted for 77% of all complications (Canada).

Time Frame
Preoperative and postoperative periods

■■■■■ DIAGNOSTIC CLUSTER

Collaborative Problems

▲ Risk for Complications of Peristomal Tissue

▲ Risk for Complications of Stoma

* Risk for Complications of Intra-abdominal sepsis

* Risk for Complications of Large Bowel Obstruction

* Risk for Complications of Perforation of Genitourinary Tract

Nursing Diagnoses

▲ Risk for Disturbed Self-Concept related to effects of ostomy on body image and lifestyle

Δ Risk for Loneliness related to Anxiety related to possible odor and leakage from appliance in public.

△ Grieving related to implications of cancer diagnosis Refer to: Cancer: Initial Diagnosis.

▲ Risk for Ineffective Self-Health Regimen Management related to insufficient knowledge of stoma pouching procedure, colostomy irrigation, peristomal skin care, perineal wound care, and incorporation of ostomy care into activities of daily living (ADLs)

Related Care Plan

General Surgery Generic Care Plan

▲ This diagnosis was reported to be monitored for or managed frequently (75% to 100%).
△ This diagnosis was reported to be monitored for or managed often (50% to 74%).
* This diagnosis was not included in the validation study.

Transitional Criteria

Before transition, the client and family will:

1. Elicit concerns or problems with ostomy care at home, including stoma, pouching, irrigation, and skin care.
2. State signs and symptoms that must be reported to a health care professional.
3. Verbalize intent to share with significant others' feelings and concerns related to ostomy.
4. Identify available community resources and self-help groups:
   a. Home health nurse
   b. United Ostomy Association
   c. American Cancer Foundation

Transitional Risk Assessment Plan (TRAP)

Begin this plan on admission.
Implement the Transitional Risk Assessment Plan (TRAP):
• Refer to inside back cover.
• Add each validated risk diagnosis to client's problem list with the risk code in ( ).
• Refer to Unit II to the individual risk nursing diagnoses / collaborative problems for outcomes and interventions.

R: "Close coordination of care in the post-acute period, early transition follow-up care, enhanced client education and self-management training, proactive end-of-life counseling, and extending the resources and clinical expertise over time via multidisciplinary team management" can lower readmission rates and improve health outcomes (Boutwell & Hwu, 2009, p. 14).

Collaborative Problems

Risk for Complications of Peristomal Tissue

Risk for Complications of Stoma

Risk for Complications of Intra-abdominal Sepsis

Risk for Complications of Large Bowel Obstruction

Risk for Complications of Perforation of Genitourinary Tract

Collaborative Outcomes

The client will be monitored for early signs and symptoms of (a) peristomal complications (b) stomal complications, (c) intra-abdominal sepsis, (d) large bowel obstruction, and (e) perforation of genitourinary tract, and will receive collaborative interventions if indicated to restore physiologic stability.

Indicators of Physiologic Stability

- Intact bowel sounds in all quadrants (d)
- Intact peristomal muscle tone (a, b)
- Free-flowing ostomy fluid (a, b)
- No evidence of bleeding (a, b)
- No evidence of infection (c)
- No complaints of nausea / vomiting / hiccups (c, d)
- Nondistended abdomen (d)
- Perineal wound intact (if sutured) (c)
- Temperature 98°–99.5° F; no chills (c)
- BP >90/60, <140/90 mm Hg (c)
- Pulse 60–100 beats/min (c)
- Respirations 16–20 breaths/min
- Urine output >0.5 mL/kg/h (e, j)

>> **Carp's Cues**

Please refer to the Generic Care Plan for the Surgical Client for detailed interventions for managing all surgical conditions. This care plan addresses specific additional interventions associated with this type of surgery performed.

Interventions	Rationales
1. Monitor for stomal complications: a. Parastomal hernia defect in the abdominal fascia allowing the gut to bulge into the parastomal area b. Prolapsed (telescoping of the bowel through the stoma) c. Necrosis (death of stomal tissue with impaired local blood flow) d. Mucocutaneous separation, retraction, (disappearance of normal stomal protrusion in line with or below skin level) e. Stenosis, fistula, trauma	1. The most common complications were stomal retraction, peristomal hernia, prolapse, necrosis, and peristomal skin problems.
2. Monitor for peristomal complications: a. Varices b. Candidiasis, folliculitis, necrosis c. Irritant contact dermatitis d. Trauma	2. Complications affect the skin immediately surrounding the stoma (Colwell & Beitz, 2007).

CLINICAL ALERT

- Stomal and peristomal complications can occur postoperatively, or months later (Registered Nurses' Association of Ontario, 2009).
- Incidence of stomal and peristomal complications at 3 and 12 months, respectively:
  - Retraction 3% to 7% 10% to 24%
  - Peristomal hernia 0.8% 12% to 40%
  - Prolapse 0% to 3% 4% to 10%
  - Necrosis 0% to 3% 7%
  - Peristomal skin problems 14.7% 15% to 43%
- Obesity (defined as a body mass index .25kg/m^2) has been associated with stomal (retraction, prolapse, and necrosis) and peristomal skin problems in multiple studies (Canada).

Interventions	Rationales
3. Monitor the peristomal area for the following: a. Decreased peristomal muscle tone b. Bulging beyond the normal skin surface and musculature c. Persistent ulceration	3. Early detection of ulcerations and herniation can prevent serious tissue damage (Colwell & Beitz, 2007).
4. Monitor the following: a. Color, size, and shape of the stoma; and mucocutaneous separation b. Color, amount, and consistency of ostomy effluent c. Complaints of cramping abdominal pain, nausea and vomiting, and abdominal distention d. Fit of ostomy appliance and appliance belt	4a. These changes can indicate inflammation, retraction, prolapse, or edema. b. These changes can indicate bleeding or infection. Decreased output can indicate obstruction. c. These complaints may indicate obstruction. d. An improperly fitting appliance or belt can cause mechanical trauma to the stoma (Colwell & Beitz, 2007).
5. If mucocutaneous separation occurs, notify wound / ostomy nurse specialist or surgeon.	5. Special techniques are needed to prevent fecal contamination.
6. Monitor perineal wound for signs and symptoms of infection, bleeding. drainage	
7. Monitor for intra-abdominal sepsis: a. Complaints of nausea, hiccups b. Spiking fevers, chills c. Tachycardia d. Elevated WBC	

> **CLINICAL ALERT**
> - Immediately notify surgeon.
> - Leakage of GI fluid into the peritoneal cavity (e.g., a leak at the anastomotic site) can cause serious infections (e.g., staphylococcal).

Interventions	Rationales
8. Monitor for intestinal obstruction (Minkes, 2013): a. Increasing pain b. Decreased / absent bowel sounds or hyperperistalsis c. Clinical evidence of hypovolemia	8. "Intestinal obstruction is also common. Stoma strictures can occur at the skin level, fascial level, or both. Partial obstruction can result in hyperperistalsis and hypersecretion; massive fluid losses through the stoma may result in dehydration. Other causes of obstruction include luminal plugging caused by ingested food, adhesive intestinal obstruction, internal hernia, and volvulus" (Minkes, 2013).
9. Monitor for large bowel obstruction; notify the physician / NP, if detected: a. Decreased bowel sounds b. Nausea, vomiting c. Abdominal distension	9. Intraoperative manipulation of the abdominal organs and the depressive effects of anesthesia and narcotics can cause decreased peristalsis.
10. Monitor for perforation of bladder: a. Acute pelvic pain b. Nausea, vomiting, malaise c. Abdominal distension d. Costovertebral angle tenderness, ileus, fever, flank pain	10. Intraoperatively, the bladder can be punctured during the colon resection. Urine leakage into perineum will cause infection.
11. Notify surgeon for radiographic evaluation.	

Clinical Alert Report

Prior to providing care, advise ancillary staff / student to report the following to the professional nurse assigned to the client:

- Change in cognitive status
- Oral temperature >100.5° F
- Systolic BP <90 mm/Hg
- Resting Pulse >100, <50
- Respiratory rate >28, <10/min
- Oxygen saturation <90%
- New onset pelvic pain
- Nausea / vomiting
- Change in stoma appearance
- Urine output <0.5 mL/kg/h

Related Physician / NP Prescribed Interventions

Refer also to the General Surgery care plan.

Medications

Antibiotics (e.g., kanamycin, erythromycin, neomycin); chemotherapy; immunotherapy; laxatives (preoperative)

Laboratory Studies

Carcinoembryonic antigen (CEA)

Diagnostic Studies

Flat plate of abdomen, computed tomography (CT) scan of abdomen

Therapies

Radiation therapy (preoperative, intraoperative, postoperative)

Documentation

Intake and output
Bowel sounds
Wound status
Stoma condition

Postoperative: Nursing Diagnoses

Risk for Disturbed Self-Concept Related to Effects of Ostomy on Body Image and Lifestyle

NOC

Anxiety Reduction, Coping, Impulse Control

Goal

The client will communicate feelings about the ostomy, addressing the changes in his or her body and function, and acknowledge the reason for the surgery (Haugen, Bliss, & Savik, 2006).

NIC

Hope Instillation, Mood Management, Values Clarification, Counseling, Referral, Support Group, Coping Enhancement

Indicators

- Acknowledge changes in body structure and function.
- Participate in stoma care.

Carp's Cues

"The average period of time needed to resolve the psychological distress produced by ostomy surgery and restore optimal quality of life is not known, but existing evidence suggests that this process requires 12 months or longer" (Registered Nurses' Association of Ontario, 2009). Long-term recovery is characterized initially by taking control of ostomy care, followed by seeking to recover a sense of normalcy and reestablishing work-related and social activities (Registered Nurses' Association of Ontario, 2009).

Interventions	*Rationales*
1. Contact the client frequently and treat him or her with warm, positive regard.	1. Frequent contact by caregiver indicates acceptance and may facilitate trust. The client may be hesitant to approach staff / student because of a negative self-concept (Colwell & Beitz, 2007).
2. Incorporate emotional support into technical ostomy self-care sessions. Encourage the individual to perform as much self-care as possible.	2. Nursing interventions that enable clients to increase self-efficacy in ostomy management act as enablers as they struggle to reestablish a sense of normalcy following ostomy surgery. Impaired body image is associated with symptoms of weakness, fragility, unattractiveness and feelings of stigma (Registered Nurses' Association of Ontario, 2009).
3. Assess if individual looks at and touches the stoma.	3. Persson and Helstrom (2002) reported that individuals postostomy, emphasized the initial shock and emotional distress they experienced when the stoma was first visualized. The nurse should not make assumptions about a client's reactions to ostomy surgery. The client may require help in accepting the reality of the altered body appearance and function, or in dealing with an overwhelming situation (Richbourg, Thorpe, & Rapp, 2007).
4. Encourage the client to verbalize feelings (both positive and negative) about the stoma and perceptions of its anticipated effects on his or her lifestyle. Direct the client to the appropriate professional to help overcome negative feelings and perceptions (Junkin & Beitz, 2005; Registered Nurses' Association of Ontario, 2009; Richbourg, Thorpe, & Rapp, 2007).	4. Multiple studies reveals that psychological distress is prevalent following creation of an ostomy, resulting in impaired body image and self-esteem, and diminished quality of life (Registered Nurses' Association of Ontario, 2009). Impaired body image is associated with symptoms of weakness, fragility, unattractiveness, and feelings of stigma. Sharing gives the nurse an opportunity to identify and dispel misconceptions and allay anxiety and self-doubt (Registered Nurses' Association of Ontario, 2009).
5. Validate the client's perceptions and reassure that such responses are normal and appropriate.	5. Validating the client's perceptions promotes self-awareness and provides reassurance.
6. Ensure that support persons have been included in learning ostomy care principles. Assess the client's interactions with support persons.	6. Other people's response to the ostomy is one of the most important factors influencing a client's acceptance of it.
7. Initiate the topic of sexuality and sexual function and the individual's and partner's concerns	7. "Ostomy surgery can significantly affect sexual function, thereby impacting intimacy and sexual relationships, not only for the client but for their partner as well. The opportunity to listen, support and encourage open dialogue with clients and their partner is critical" (Registered Nurses' Association of Ontario, 2009).

(continued)

Interventions	Rationales
8. Encourage the individual / partner to initiate future discussions with primary care provider and / or ostomy nurse specialist.	8. Future discussions will be needed; however, when the nurse postoperatively initiates the discussion, it gives the concerned individuals permission for future dialogue.

> **CLINICAL ALERT**
> • Undergoing ostomy surgery, whether the ostomy is temporary or permanent, can have a profound impact on intimacy and sexuality.
> • Although sexual function may be altered, sexuality cannot be destroyed (Junkin & Beitz, 2005).
> • Altered sexual function in men can result from damage of the prostatic nerve plexus and the autonomic nerves that are close to the rectum during colorectal or bladder cancer surgery, resulting in sensory loss and erectile failure.
> • In women, there may be nerve, vascular, and tissue damage resulting in dyspareunia, damage to the vagina, altered vaginal lubrication, problems with engorgement, reduced vaginal space, and possible prolapse of the vaginal wall or bladder (Black, 2004).

Documentation

Present emotional status
Interventions
Response to interventions

Anxiety related to Possible Odor and Leakage from Appliance in Public

NOC
Loneliness, Social Involvement

Goal

The client will state the intent to reestablish preoperative socialization pattern.

NIC
Socialization Enhancement, Spiritual Support, Behavior Modification: Social Skills, Presence, Anticipatory Guidance

Indicators

• Discuss methods to control odor and appliance leakage.
• Participate in self-help groups with similar experiences.

Interventions	Rationales
1. Elicit from individual his or her concerns regarding resuming preoperative activities,	1. Fear of accidents and odor can reduce previously pleasurable activities.
2. Discuss methods for reducing odor learned from wound care / ostomy specialist: a. Avoid odor-producing foods, such as onions, fish, eggs, cheese, and asparagus (Hyland, 2002). b. Use internal chlorophyll tablets or a liquid appliance deodorant (Hyland, 2002). c. Empty or change the ostomy pouch regularly, when the pouch is one-third to one-half full (Hyland, 2002).	2. Minimizing odor improves self-confidence and can permit more effective socialization. Bacterial proliferation in retained effluent increases odor with time. A full pouch also puts excessive pressure on seals, which increases risk of leakage.
3. Encourage the client to reestablish his or her preoperative socialization pattern. Help the client through such measures as progressively increasing his or her socializing time in the hospital, role-playing possible situations that the client feels may cause anxiety, and encouraging him or her to visualize and anticipate solutions to "worst-case scenarios" for social situations.	3. Encouraging and facilitating socialization help to prevent isolation. Role playing can help the client to identify and learn to cope with potential anxiety-causing situations in a nonthreatening environment.
4. Suggest that the client meet with a person from the United Ostomy Associations (UOA) who can share similar experiences.	4. Others in a similar situation can provide a realistic appraisal and may provide information to answer the client's unasked questions.

Documentation

Dialogues

> **TRANSITION TO HOME / COMMUNITY CARE**
>
> If indicated, review the risk diagnoses identified for this individual on admission:
>
> - Is the person still at risk?
> - Can the family reduce the risks?
> - Is the person at higher risk at home?
> - Is a Home Health Nurse assessment needed?
> - Refer to transition planner / case manager / social service.
> - When is this person scheduled for follow-up with primary provider? Specialists? Record dates of appointments.
> - Complete a medication reconciliation prior to transition. Refer to index.

S T A R

Stop

Think   Is this person at risk for injury, falls, medical complications, and / or inability to care for self (activities of daily living)?

Is there a support person available?

Is the person competent to manage self-administration of medications, treatment procedures? Are additional resources needed?

Can the person explain how to monitor the condition (e.g., blood glucose, signs / symptoms of complications, dietary / mobility restrictions, and when to call his or her primary provider or specialist)?

Act   Contact or provide the appropriate resource (e.g., contacting a support person, home health assessment, additional teaching, printed materials).

Review   Has the problem been addressed? If not, use SBAR to communicate to the appropriate person.

Risk for Ineffective Self-Health Management Related to Insufficient Knowledge of Stoma Poaching Procedure, Colostomy Irrigation, Peristomal Skin Care, Perineal Wound Care, and Incorporation of Ostomy Care into Activities of Daily Living (ADLs)

NOC

Compliance Behavior, Knowledge: Treatment Regimen, Participation: Health Care Decisions, Treatment Behavior: Illness or Injury

NIC

Anticipatory Guidance, Ostomy Care, Learning Facilitation, Risk Management, Health Education

Goals

The goals for this diagnosis represent those associated with transition planning. Refer to the transition criteria.

Interventions	Rationales
1. Continuously, assess the individual's ability to manage colostomy care. Consult / refer to ostomy nurse specialist as indicated.	1. The details of ostomy management are taught by the nurse specialist. The unit nurse is responsible for evaluating the individual's competency.
2. Observe the condition of the stoma and peristomal skin during pouch changes.	2. Regular observation enables early detection of skin problems.
3. Watch for and report signs and symptoms of infection or abscess (e.g., pain or purulent drainage).	

> **CLINICAL ALERT**
> - Removal of the rectum results in a large perineal wound that may be left open to heal by secondary intention.
> - Some clients with a colostomy do not have the rectum and anus removed but have a rectal stump sutured across the top.
> - This becomes a nonfunctioning internal pouch (Hartmann pouch).
> - In this situation, the client continues to expel mucus through the anus, produced by the remaining rectal mucosa.

4. Ensure that a consult with nutritionist has occurred.	4. The colonoscopy affects absorption and use of nutrients

Interventions	Rationales

5. Explain that stoma monitoring is important for months at home (WOCN, 2011). For example:
 	
  a. Mucosal transplantation (moist tissue along suture line, resulting from seeding of viable intestinal mucosa).
 	
  b. Pseudo-verrucous lesions (wart-like lesions [hyperplasia]) that are caused by years of improper fitting appliance.
 	
  c. Pyoderma gangrenosum (rare skin condition that causes painful open sores [ulcers]).
 	
  d. Suture granulomas (granualar tissue in area of retained or reactive suture material [e.g., allergic response]).
	5. Some stoma complications take months and years to occur. Once they occur they interfere with successful pouching.

6. Discuss:
 	
  a. Exercise:
    • Normal activities (even strenuous sports, in most cases) can be resumed after recovery from surgery.
    • Be aware that increased incidence of peristomal herniation is associated with heavy lifting.
    • Also keep in mind that increased perspiration from strenuous exercise may require more frequent ostomy appliance changes due to increased melting of the appliance skin barrier.
 	
  b. Travel:
    • Take all ostomy supplies along when traveling; if by air, put them in a carry-on bag (Collett, 2002).
    • Do not leave ostomy appliances in automobiles parked in the sun, because the heat will melt the skin barrier.
    • When flying, always keep appliances in carry-on luggage to avoid loss.	

7. Discuss community resources / self-help groups, including:
 	
  a. Home health nurse
  b. United Ostomy Associations, www.uoaa.org
  c. National Foundation for Ileitis and Colitis (800-343-3637)
  d. American Cancer Foundation
  e. Community suppliers of ostomy equipment
  f. Financial reimbursement for ostomy equipment
	7. Personal sources of information have been found to be more important than written materials (Richbourg, Thorpe, & Rapp, 2007).

Documentation

Client and family teaching

Response to teaching as well as achieved outcomes or the status of each goal

Coronary Artery Bypass Grafting

Indicated for clients with coronary artery disease, coronary artery bypass grafting (CABG) increases blood flow to the heart by either anastomosis of an autograft vessel (e.g., saphenous vein or inferior epigastric artery) to an area proximal and distal to the coronary artery occlusion, or by use of an autograft vessel (i.e., internal mammary or gastroepiploic artery) grafted distal to the coronary artery occlusion. Internal mammary grafts have a 90% patency rate at 10 years compared to 40% to 60% for saphenous veins.

Surgery most often involves a median sternotomy incision with cardiopulmonary bypass, or extracorporeal circulation, to circulate and oxygenate the blood while diverting it from the heart and lungs to provide a bloodless operative field for the surgeon. A more recent trend in cardiac surgery is a minimally invasive procedure known as "off-pump coronary artery bypass," in which the heart is not stopped for suturing of the bypass graft(s). Cardiopulmonary bypass is not used; the incision is smaller and may have a thoracotomy approach; complications are reduced and recovery is faster (American Heart Association, 2007a; Martin & Turkelson, 2006; Shatzer, George, & Wei, 2007).

Over the last few years, advancements have allowed the robot-assisted endoscopic CABG approach to expand with substantially less complications and more rapid recovery (Pike & Gundry, 2003).

Time Frame
Preoperative and postoperative periods (not intensive care period)

DIAGNOSTIC CLUSTER

Preoperative Period

Nursing Diagnosis

▲ Fear (individual / family) related to the client's health status, need for coronary artery bypass graft surgery, and unpredictable outcome

Postoperative Period

Collaborative Problems

▲ Risk for Complications of Cardiovascular Insufficiency

▲ Risk for Complications of Respiratory Insufficiency

▲ Risk for Complications of Renal Insufficiency

* Risk for Complications of Hyperthermia

* Risk for Complications of Postcardiotomy Delirium

Nursing Diagnoses

Δ Fear related to transfer from intensive environment of the critical care unit and potential for complications

Δ Interrupted Family Processes related to disruption of family life, fear of outcome (death, disability), and stressful environment (ICU)

Δ Risk for Disturbed Self-Concept related to the symbolic meaning of the heart and changes in lifestyle

Δ Risk for Ineffective Therapeutic Regimen Management related to insufficient knowledge of incisional care, pain management (angina, incisions), signs and symptoms of complications, condition, pharmacologic care, risk factors, restrictions, stress management techniques, and follow-up care

▲ Impaired Comfort related to surgical incisions, chest tubes, and immobility secondary to lengthy surgery (refer to General Surgery)

Related Care Plans

General Surgery Generic Care Plan

Thoracic Surgery

▲ This diagnosis was reported to be monitored for or managed frequently (75% to 100%).

Δ This diagnosis was reported to be monitored for or managed often (50% to 74%).

* This diagnosis was not included in the validation study.

Transition Criteria

Before transition, the client and family will:

1. Demonstrate insertion site care.
2. Relate at-home restrictions and follow-up care.
3. State signs and symptoms that must be reported to a health-care professional.
4. Relate a plan to reduce risk factors, as necessary.

Transitional Risk Assessment Plan (TRAP)

Begin this plan on admission.

Implement the Transitional Risk Assessment Plan (TRAP):

- Refer to inside back cover.
- Add each validated risk diagnosis to client's problem list with the risk code in ( ).
- Refer to Unit II to the individual risk nursing diagnoses / collaborative problems for outcomes and interventions.

R: "Close coordination of care in the post-acute period, early transition follow-up care, enhanced client education and self-management training, proactive end-of-life counseling, and extending the resources and clinical expertise over time via multidisciplinary team management" can lower readmission rates and improve health outcomes (Boutwell & Hwu, 2009, p. 14).

Preoperative: Nursing Diagnosis

Fear (Individual / Family) Related to the Client's Health Status, Need for Coronary Artery Bypass Graft Surgery, and Unpredictable Outcome

NOC
Anxiety Control, Fear Control

NIC
Anxiety Reduction, Coping Enhancement, Presence, Counseling

Goals

The client or family will verbalize concerns regarding surgery.

Indicators

- Verbalize, if asked, what to expect before surgery (e.g., routines and tests).
- Verbalize, if asked, an understanding of the CABG procedure.
- Verbalize, if asked, what to expect post-CABG (e.g., monitoring and care).
- Demonstrate postoperative exercises, turning, splinting, and respiratory regimen.

Carp's Cues

Please refer to the Generic Care Plan for the Surgical Client for detailed interventions for managing all surgical conditions. This care plan addresses specific additional interventions associated with the type of surgery performed.

Interventions	Rationales
1. Reinforce previous teaching about coronary artery disease, as necessary.	1–6. Preoperative teaching provides information to help reduce the client's and family's fears of the unknown, and enhance their sense of control over the situation (Kirkeby-Garstad et al., 2006).
2. Reinforce, as necessary, the physician's / NP's explanation of CABG surgery and why it is needed. Notify the physician / NP if additional explanation is indicated.	
3. Explain necessary preoperative tests and procedures, such as the following: a. 12-lead electrocardiogram (ECG) b. Chest x-ray film c. Cardiac catheterization d. Urinalysis e. Blood work: electrolytes, coagulation studies, complete blood count, type, and cross-match f. Nuclear studies, if indicated	
4. Provide instruction about preoperative routines beyond those of general surgery, such as the following: a. Chlorhexidine gluconate (Hibiclens or Betadine) shower the night before and the morning of surgery b. Sending belongings home with family members c. Measures in operating room holding area: skin preparation, IV and other invasive line insertions, and indwelling (Foley) catheter insertion	
5. Discuss postoperative measures, routines, and expectations, including the following (Kirkeby-Garstad et al., 2006): a. Endotracheal intubation and mechanical ventilation b. Chest tubes c. Multiple IV lines d. Sedative the evening before e. Pulmonary artery catheter f. Arterial line g. Epidural cardiac pacing h. Cardiac monitoring i. Indwelling urinary catheter j. Autotransfusion / blood replacement k. Weight increase l. Nasogastric tube m. Pain n. Frequent assessment of vital signs, dressing, heart and lung sounds, peripheral pulses, skin, and capillary refill time o. TEDs stockings	
6. Discuss expectations for intensive care (Kirkeby-Garstad et al., 2006): a. Environment, noises b. Length of stay c. Care measures d. Visiting policies e. Early ambulation (Kirkeby-Garstad et al., 2006) f. Cough and deep breathing exercises / incentive spirometry (Kirkeby-Garstad et al., 2006)	

Interventions	*Rationales*
7. Explain specific pain-relief measures that will be used and the comfort level goals (e.g., splinting) (Kirkeby-Garstad et al., 2006).	7. Knowledge of the pain expected and the ability to control pain can reduce fear and increase pain tolerance (Kirkeby-Garstad et al., 2006).
8. Discuss possible emotional and mental reactions post-CABG surgery.	8. The heart is a symbol of life; cardiac dysfunction and surgery typically invoke a profound emotional reaction. Anesthesia, fluid loss from surgery, and pain medications can temporarily cloud thinking.
9. Present information or reinforce learning using written materials (e.g., booklets, posters, or instruction sheets) and audiovisual aids (e.g., slides, videotapes, models, or diagrams).	9. Using various teaching materials and approaches provides multisensory stimulation that can enhance effectiveness of teaching and learning and improve retention.
10. Offer a tour of intensive care unit.	10. Individuals who have a preoperative tour of ICU report a benefit from the experience (Lynn-McHale Wiegand, 2010).

Documentation

Present emotional status
Interventions
Response to interventions
Client and family teaching
Response to teaching
Outcome achievement or status

Postoperative: Collaborative Problems

Risk for Complications of Cardiovascular Insufficiency

Risk for Complications of Respiratory Insufficiency

Risk for Complications of Renal Insufficiency

Risk for Complications of Hyperthermia

Risk for Complications of Postcardiotomy Delirium

Goal

The nurse will detect early signs and symptoms of (a) cardiovascular insufficiency, (b) respiratory insufficiency, (c) renal insufficiency, (d) hyperthermia, and (e) postcardiotomy delirium, and will collaboratively intervene to stabilize the client.

Indicators of Physiologic Stability

- Oriented, calm (a, b, c, d, e)
- No change in vision (a)
- Normal sinus rhythm (EKG) (a, b)
- Heart rate 60–100 beats/min (a, b)
- BP >90/60, <140/90 mm Hg (a, b)
- No complaints of syncope, palpitations (a, b)
- Mean arterial pressure 70/90 mm Hg (a, b)
- Pulmonary artery wedge pressure 4–12 mm Hg (a, b)

- Cardiac output / index >2.4 (a, b)
- Pulmonary artery systolic pressure 20–30 mm Hg (a, b)
- Pulmonary artery diastolic pressure 10–15 mm Hg (a, b)
- Temperature 98°–99.5° F (d)
- Minimal change in pulse pressure (a, b)
- Respirations 16–20 breaths/min (a, b)
- Urine output >0.5 mL/kg/h (a, b, c)
- Capillary refill <3 seconds (a, b)
- Skin warm, no pallor, cyanosis, or grayness (a, b)
- No complaints of palpitations, syncope, chest pain (a, b)
- No neck vein distension (a, b)
- Cardiac enzymes (a)
  - Myoglobin up to 85 mg/mL
  - Creatine phosphokinase (CK)
    - Male 50–325 mU/mL
    - Female 50–250 mU/mL
  - Troponin complex (C, I, T)
  - Hemoglobin (a)
    - Males 13–18 g/dL
    - Females 12–16 g/dL
  - Hematocrit (a)
    - Males 42% to 50%
    - Females 40% to 48%
- Partial thromboplastin time (PTT) 20–45 seconds (a)
- International Normalized Ratio (INR) 1.0 (a)
- Platelets 100,000–400,000/mm^3 (a)
- Prothrombin time (PT) >20 seconds (a)
- Urine specific gravity 1.005–1.025 (a, b, c)
- Blood urea nitrogen 8–20 mg/dL (a, b, c)
- Creatinine 0.6–1.2 mg/dL (c)
- Potassium 3.5–5.0 mEq/L (c)
- Magnesium 1.84–3.0 mEq/L (c)
- Sodium 135–145 mEq/L (c)
- Calcium 8.5–10.5 mg/dL (c)
- Oxygen saturation (SaO$_2$) 4–100 mm Hg (a, b)
- Carbon dioxide (PaCO$_2$) 35–45 mm Hg (a, b)
- pH 7.35–7.45 (a, b)
- Relaxed, regular, deep, rhythmic respirations (a, b)
- No rales, crackles, wheezing (b)
- Wound approximated, minimal drainage (d)
- Chest tube drainage <200 mL/h (d)
- Full, easy to palpate pulses (a, b)
- No evidence of petechiae (pinpoint round, reddish lesions) or ecchymoses (bruises) (a)
- No seizure activity (a, d, e)

Interventions	Rationales
1. Monitor for the following as per unit standard (Martin & Turkelson, 2006): a. Dysrhythmias, abnormal rate, or conduction b. ECG changes: ST segment depression or elevation; T-wave changes; PR, QRS, or QT interval changes c. Peripheral pulses (pedal, tibial, popliteal, femoral, radial, brachial)	1. Myocardial ischemia results from reduction of oxygen to myocardial tissue. Ischemic muscle is electrically unstable, leading to dysrhythmias. Dysrhythmias also may result from surgical manipulation, hypothermia, and acidosis. Atrial dysrhythmias may also be due to mechanical remodeling or injury or conductive delays (Porth, 2005).

Interventions	Rationales
d. Blood pressure (arterial, left atrial, pulmonary artery) e. Pulmonary artery diastolic pressure (PAD) f. Pulmonary artery wedge pressure (PAWP) g. Cardiac output / index h. Cardiac enzymes daily (e.g., creatine phosphokinase, troponin complex) i. Urine output j. Skin color, temperature k. Capillary refill l. Palpitations m. Syncope n. Cardiac emergencies (e.g., arrest or ventricular fibrillation)	
2. Monitor select electrolytes (Porth, 2011): a. Potassium b. Magnesium c. Sodium d. Calcium	2. Specific levels of electrolytes are necessary for both extracellular and intracellular body fluids. a. Inadequate intake, diuretics, vomiting, nasogastric drainage, and stress can decrease potassium. Renal insufficiency, increased intake, tissue necrosis, and adrenal cortical insufficiency can increase potassium levels. b. Decreased intake, alcoholism, excess intake of calcium, and increased excretion after surgery; diabetic ketoacidosis; primary aldosteronism; and primary hyperparathyroidism cause decreased magnesium levels. Renal failure and excess intake of medications with magnesium (antacids, cathartics) increase magnesium levels. c. Increased water intake causes decreased sodium levels. d. Alkalosis and multiple transfusions of citrated blood products cause low calcium levels. Prolonged immobility causes increased calcium levels.
3. Monitor for signs and symptoms of hypotension and low cardiac output syndrome (Martin & Turkelson, 2006): a. Cardiac index <2.4 b. Increased pulmonary arteriole wedge pressure (PAWP) c. Increased central venous pressure (CVP) d. SvO2 <60% e. Development of S3 or S4 f. Neck vein distention g. Decreased systolic BP (90 mm Hg or 30 mm Hg below baseline) h. Irregular pulse i. Cool, moist skin j. Decreased urine output (<0.5 mL/kg/h) k. Increased pulse and respirations l. Increased restlessness m. Lethargy or confusion n. Increased rales / crackles o. Weak peripheral pulses	3. These effects can result from severe pain or greatly reduced cardiac output secondary to severe tissue hypoxia; inadequate preload and inadequate myocardial contractility; dysrhythmias; and ventricular failure. Decreased circulating volume and cardiac output can lead to kidney hypoperfusion and overall decreased tissue perfusion, triggering a compensatory response of decreased circulation to the extremities, and increased heart and respiratory rates. Cerebral hypoperfusion also may result.
4. Monitor for signs and symptoms of cardiac tamponade: a. Decreased systolic BP (90 mm Hg or 30 mm Hg below baseline) b. Muffled heart sounds c. Pericardial friction rub	4. Cardiac tamponade is a condition in which excess fluid collects within the pericardial space and impairs cardiac filling. It occurs because of graft leakage, inadequate hemostasis, or inadequate chest tube drainage (Porth, 2005).

(continued)

Interventions	Rationales
d. Pulsus paradoxus e. Kussmaul respirations f. Neck vein distention g. Narrowing pulse pressure h. Anginal pain i. Restlessness or stupor j. Equalizing CVP and pulmonary arterial wedge pressure (PAWP) k. Significant increase in or cessation of chest tube drainage l. Decreased electrocardiograph (ECG) voltage	
5. Monitor for signs and symptoms of respiratory failure: a. Increased respiratory rate b. Dyspnea c. Use of accessory muscles of respiration d. Cyanosis e. Increasing crackles or wheezing f. Increased pCO_2, decreased O_2 saturation, decreased pH g. Decreased SvO_2 h. Restlessness i. Decreased capillary refill time >3 seconds	5. In the immediate postoperative period, hypoventilation may result from central nervous system depression caused by narcotics and anesthesia, impaired respiratory effort resulting from pain, fatigue, and immobility, or incomplete reinflation of lungs collapsed during surgery. Pulmonary dysfunction occurs in 30% to 60% of postoperative CABG clients (Martin & Turkelson, 2006).
6. Monitor for signs and symptoms of hypertension or hypervolemia (Martin & Turkelson, 2006): a. Systolic blood pressure >140 mm Hg b. Diastolic blood pressure >90 mm Hg c. Mean arterial pressure >90 mm Hg d. Increased systemic vascular resistance	6. Hypervolemia and hypertension can result from a response to circulating catecholamines and renin secretion following cardiopulmonary bypass, which causes sodium and water retention. Hypertension can lead to bleeding at anastomosis sites (Martin & Turkelson, 2006).
7. Monitor for signs and symptoms of hemorrhage or hypovolemia: a. Incisional bleeding b. Chest tube drainage >200 mL/h c. Increased heart rate, decreased blood pressure, increased respirations d. Weak or absent peripheral pulses e. Cool, moist skin f. Dizziness g. Petechiae h. Ecchymoses i. Bleeding gums j. Decreased hemoglobin and hematocrit k. Increased prothrombin time (PT), partial thromboplastin time (PTT), international normalized ratio (INR), and decreased platelet count	7. Hemorrhage can be caused by inadequate surgical hemostasis, inadequate heparin reversal, or hypertension.
8. Monitor for signs and symptoms of myocardial infarction: a. Chest pain or pressure b. Increased heart rate c. Hypotension d. Tachypnea e. Abnormal heart sounds f. Restlessness, lethargy, or confusion g. Elevated CVP and PAWP h. Nausea and vomiting	8. Cardiac pain results from cardiac tissue hypoxia secondary to narrowing or blockage of the coronary arteries, increased myocardial oxygen consumption, or collapse of the newly grafted bypass.

Interventions	Rationales
i. ECG changes: ST segment elevation, abnormal Q waves j. Increased cardiac enzymes k. Decreased SvO2 l. Neck vein distention m. Weak peripheral pulses n. Moist, cool skin o. Decreased urine output (<0.5 mL/kg/h)	

9. Monitor for signs and symptoms of renal failure (Martin & Turkelson, 2006):
  a. Elevated BUN, creatinine, and potassium
  b. Decreased urine output (<0.5 mL/kg/h)
  c. Elevated urine specific gravity (>1.030)
  d. Weight gain
  e. Elevated CVP and PAP
	9. Cardiopulmonary bypass causes destruction of some red blood cells (RBCs), producing free hemoglobin that may occlude renal arteries. Hypovolemia or poor myocardial contractility may decrease circulation to the kidneys, resulting in hypoperfusion and eventual renal failure.

10. Monitor for signs and symptoms of cerebrovascular accident (stroke):
  a. Unequal pupil size and reaction
  b. Paralysis or paresthesias in extremities
  c. Decreased level of consciousness
  d. Dizziness
  e. Blurred vision
  f. Seizure activity
  g. Slurred speech
  h. Confusion
  i. Altered motor and sensory function (Martin & Turkelson, 2006)
	10. CVA may result from embolization or hypoperfusion that obstructs or interrupts blood flow to the central nervous system.

11. Monitor for signs and symptoms of postcardiotomy delirium:
  a. Disorientation
  b. Confusion
  c. Hallucinations or delusions
	11. This disorder may result from surgery-related microemboli, sensory overload or deprivation, altered sleep pattern, hypoxia, medications, metabolic disorders, or hypotension.

12. Monitor for hyperthermia:
  a. Increased temperature
  b. Increased heart rate
  c. Hypotension
	12. Hyperthermia can indicate infection or postpericardiotomy syndrome (pericarditis) (Porth, 2005).

13. Assess readiness for early extubation (Martin & Turkelson, 2006).	13. Early extubation promotes reduced pulmonary complications (Martin & Turkelson, 2006).

14. Monitor for gastrointestinal (GI) complications (Martin & Turkelson, 2006):
  a. GI bleeding
  b. Decreased Hct & Hgb
  c. Reduced or absent bowel sounds
  d. Nausea & vomiting
  e. Abdominal distention
  f. Nasogastric tube output
	14. GI complications occur in 0.12% to 2% of clients and include: peptic ulcer disease, perforated ulcer, pancreatitis, bowel ischemia, diverticulitis, acute cholecystitis, and liver failure (Martin & Turkelson, 2006).

15. Monitor for sleep disturbance (Martin & Turkelson, 2006).	15. Sleep disturbances can result from poor pain control. Sleep deprivation can lead to negative outcomes (Martin & Turkelson, 2006).

Related Physician / NP Prescribed Interventions

Medications

Antibiotics, anticoagulants, analgesics, stool softeners, diuretics, beta-blockers, aspirin (postoperatively), antidysrhythmics, calcium-channel blockers, H_2 blockers, vasoactive medications

Intravenous Therapy

Fluid / electrolyte replacement

Laboratory Studies

Complete blood count, arterial blood gas analysis, glucose, creatinine, cardiac enzymes, amylase, electrolytes, BUN, blood chemistry profile, coagulation levels

Diagnostic Studies

Ear / pulse oximetry, chest x-ray film, ECG, cardiac echocardiogram, cardiac catheterization

Nuclear Studies

Egthallium-221

Therapies

Supplemental oxygen, pulse oximetry, hemodynamic monitoring and others, dependent on symptomatology

Documentation

Vital signs
Cardiac rhythm
Peripheral pulses
Skin color, temperature, moisture
Neck vein distention
Respiratory assessment
Neurologic assessment
Intake (oral, IVs, blood products)
Incisions (color, drainage, swelling)
Output (chest tubes, nasogastric tube)
Bowel function (bowel sounds, distention)
Sputum (amount, tenaciousness, color)
Change in physiologic status
Interventions
Response to interventions

Postoperative: Nursing Diagnoses

Fear Related to Transfer From Intensive Environment of the Critical Care Unit and Potential for Complications

NOC
Anxiety Control, Fear Control

Goal

The client will report a decreased level of anxiety or fear.

NIC
Anxiety Reduction, Coping Enhancement, Presence, Counseling

Indicators

- Verbalize any concerns regarding the completed surgery, possible complications, and the critical care environment.
- Verbalize the intent to share fears with one person after transition.

Interventions	Rationales

1. Take steps to reduce the client's levels of anxiety and fear:
  a. Reassure the client that you or other nurses are always close by and will respond promptly to requests.
  b. Convey a sense of empathy and understanding.
  c. Minimize external stimuli (e.g., close the room door, dim the lights, speak in a quiet voice, decrease the volume level of equipment alarms, and position equipment so that alarms are diverted away from the client).
  d. Plan care measures to provide adequate periods of uninterrupted rest and sleep.
  e. Promote relaxation; encourage regular rest periods throughout the day.
  f. Explain each procedure before performing it.
	1. Reducing anxiety, fear, and stress can decrease demands made on an already compromised heart.

2. Encourage the client to verbalize concerns and fears. Clarify any misconceptions and provide positive feedback regarding progress.	2. This sharing allows the nurse to correct any erroneous information the client may believe and to assure the client that concerns and fears are normal; this may help to reduce anxiety.
3. Encourage the client to identify and call on reliable support persons and to recall coping mechanisms that have worked well in the past.	3. Support persons and coping mechanisms are important factors in anxiety reduction.
4. Consult with the physician / NP for medications, as necessary.	4. Pharmacologic assistance may be necessary if anxiety is at an unmanageable level; severe pain may also be interfering with the client's ability to cope.
5. Prepare the client for progression through the intensive care unit (ICU) and for stepdown to the general care unit.	5. Explanations can prevent serious complications related to unexpected relocations or transfers.

Documentation

Present emotional status
Interventions
Response to interventions

Interrupted Family Processes Related to Disruption of Family Life, Fear of Outcome (Death, Disability), and Stressful Environment (ICU)

NOC

Family Coping, Family Environment: Internal, Family Normalization, Parenting

Goal

The family members or significant others will report continued adequate family functioning during the client's hospitalization.

NIC

Family Involvement Promotion, Coping Enhancement, Family Integrity Promotion, Family Therapy, Counseling, Referral

Indicators

- Verbalize concerns regarding CABG outcome and client prognosis.
- Verbalize concerns regarding the transition.

Interventions	Rationales
1. Spend time with family members or significant others and convey a sense of empathetic understanding.	1. Frequent contact and communicating a sense of caring and concern can help to reduce stress and promote learning.
2. Allow family members or significant others to express their feelings, fears, and concerns.	2. Sharing allows the nurse to identify fears and concerns, then plan interventions to address them.
3. Explain the ICU environment and equipment. 4. Explain expected postoperative care measures and progress, and provide specific information on the client's progress, as appropriate.	3, 4. This information can help to reduce anxiety associated with the unknown.
5. Teach family members or significant others ways in which they can be more supportive (e.g., show them how they can touch the client; encourage them to talk with and touch the client and to maintain a sense of h umor, as appropriate).	5. This information can ease fears associated with doing or saying the wrong thing and can promote normal interaction with the client.
6. Encourage frequent visits and participation in care measures.	6. Frequent visits and participation in care can promote continued family interaction and support.
7. Consult with, or provide referrals to, community and other resources (e.g., social service agency) as necessary.	7. Families with problems such as financial needs, unsuccessful coping, or unresolved conflicts may need additional resources to help maintain family functioning.

Documentation

Present family functioning
Interventions
Response to interventions
Referrals, if indicated

Risk for Disturbed Self-Concept Related to the Symbolic Meaning of the Heart and Changes in Lifestyle

NOC
Quality of Life, Depression Level, Self-Esteem, Coping

Goal

The client will demonstrate healthy coping skills.

NIC
Hope Instillation, Mood Management, Values Clarification, Counseling, Referral, Support Group, Coping Enhancement

Indicators

- Report realistic changes in lifestyle.
- Appraise situation realistically.

Interventions	Rationales
1. Encourage the client to express feelings and concerns about necessary lifestyle changes and changes in level of functioning.	1. Sharing gives nurse the opportunity to correct misconceptions, provide realistic feedback, and reassure the client that his or her concerns are normal.
2. Stress the client's role in preventing recurrence of atherosclerosis. Emphasize steps the client can take and encourage progress.	2. The client's knowledge of control over the situation can enhance ego strength. Stressing the positive promotes hope and reduces frustration.
3. Allow the client to make choices regarding daily activities.	3. A decrease in power in one area can be counterbalanced by providing opportunities for choices and control in other areas.
4. Encourage the client to participate actively in the care regimen.	4. Participation in self-care mobilizes the client and promotes decision making, which enhances self-concept.

5. Identify a client at risk for poor ego adjustment (Shipes, 1987).
  a. Poor ego strength
  b. Ineffective problem-solving ability
  c. Difficulty learning new information or skills
  d. Lack of motivation
  e. External locus of control
  f. Poor health
  g. Unsatisfactory preoperative sex life
  h. Lack of positive support systems
  i. Unstable economic status
  j. Rejection of counseling
	5. Successful adjustment to CABG surgery is influenced by factors such as the following:
	  a. Previous coping success
	  b. Achievement of development tasks before surgery
	  c. The extent to which resulting lifestyle changes interfere with goal-directed activity
	  d. Sense of control over the situation
	  e. Realistic perceptions by the client and support persons

6. Refer an at-risk client for counseling.	6. Follow-up therapy is indicated to assist with effective adjustment.

TRANSITION TO HOME / COMMUNITY CARE

If indicated, review the risk diagnoses identified for this individual on admission:

- Is the person still at risk?
- Can the family reduce the risks?
- Is the person at higher risk at home?
- Is a Home Health Nurse assessment needed?
- Refer to transition planner / case manager / social service.
- When is this person scheduled for follow-up with primary provider? Specialists? Record dates of appointments.
- Complete a medication reconciliation prior to transition. Refer to index.

STAR

Stop

Think Is this person at risk for injury, falls, medical complications, and / or inability to care for self (activities of daily living)?

Is there a support person available?

Is the person competent to manage self-administration of medications, treatment procedures? Are additional resources needed?

Can the person explain how to monitor the condition (e.g., blood glucose, signs / symptoms of complications, dietary / mobility restrictions, and when to call his or her primary provider or specialist)?

Act Contact or provide the appropriate resource (e.g., contacting a support person, home health assessment, additional teaching, printed materials).

Review Has the problem been addressed? If not, use SBAR to communicate to the appropriate person.

Risk for Ineffective Self-Health Management Related to Insufficient Knowledge of Incisional Care, Pain Management (Angina, Incisions), Signs and Symptoms of Complications, Condition, Pharmacologic Care, Risk Factors, Restrictions, Stress Management Techniques, and Follow-up Care

NOC

Compliance Behavior,
Knowledge: Treatment
Regimen, Participation:
Health-Care Decisions,
Treatment Behavior:
Illness or Injury

NIC

Anticipatory Guidance,
Risk Identification,
Health Education,
Learning Facilitation

Goal

The goals for this diagnosis represent those associated with transition planning. Refer to the transition criteria.

Interventions	Rationales
1. Explain and demonstrate care of uncomplicated surgical incisions: a. Wash with soap and water (bath and shower, as permitted; use lukewarm water). b. Wear loose clothing until incision areas are no longer tender.	1. Correct technique is needed to reduce the risk of infection.
2. Provide instruction for pain management: a. For incision pain (sore, sharp, stabbing): • Take pain medication as prescribed and before activities that cause discomfort. • Continue to use the splinting technique, as needed. b. For angina (tightness, squeezing, pressure, pain, or mild ache in chest; indigestion; choking sensation; pain in jaw, neck, and between shoulder blades; numbness, tingling, and aching in either arm or hand): • Stop whatever you are doing and sit down. • Take nitroglycerin, as prescribed (e.g., one tablet every 5 minutes sublingually until pain subsides or a maximum of three tablets have been taken). • If pain is unrelieved by three nitroglycerin tablets, call for immediate transportation to the emergency room.	2a. Adequate instruction in pain management can reduce the fear of pain by providing a sense of control. Combining analgesics and nonsteroidal anti-inflammatory agents may increase the effectiveness of pain management (Martin & Turkelson, 2006). b. Angina is a symptom of cardiac tissue hypoxia. Immediate rest reduces the tissues' oxygen requirements. Nitroglycerin causes coronary vasodilation, which increases coronary blood flow in an attempt to increase myocardial oxygen supply.
3. Provide instruction regarding the client's condition and reduction of risk factors: a. Reinforce the purpose and outcome of CABG surgery. b. Explain the risk factors that need to be eliminated or reduced (e.g., obesity, smoking, high cholesterol, sedentary lifestyle, regular heavy alcohol intake, excessive stress, hypertension, or uncontrolled diabetes mellitus).	3. Surgery does not replace the need to reduce risk factors. a. Preoperative anxiety may have interfered with retention of preoperative teaching. b. Emphasizing those risk factors that can be reduced may decrease the client's sense of powerlessness regarding those factors that cannot be reduced, such as heredity.
4. Teach the client about safe and effective weight loss methods, if indicated. Consult a dietitian, and refer the client to appropriate community resources.	4. Weight reduction reduces peripheral resistance and cardiac output.

Interventions	*Rationales*
5. Provide instruction about smoking cessation, if indicated; refer to a community program.	5. Smoking's immediate effects include vasoconstriction and decreased blood oxygenation, elevated blood pressure, increased heart rate, and possible dysrhythmias, and increased cardiac workload. Long-term effects include an increased risk of coronary artery disease and myocardial infarction. Smoking also contributes to hypertension, peripheral vascular disease (e.g., leg ulcers), and chronically abnormal arterial blood gases (low oxygen, or PO_2, and high carbon dioxide, or PCO_2).
6. Teach about a low-fat, high-fiber, low-cholesterol diet; consult with a dietitian.	6. A low-fat, high-fiber, and low-cholesterol diet can reduce or prevent arteriosclerosis in some clients.
7. Provide instruction in a progressive activity program: a. Increase activity gradually. b. Consult with a physical therapist and cardiac rehabilitation specialist. c. Schedule frequent rest periods throughout the day for the first 6–8 weeks. Balance periods of activity with periods of rest. d. Consult with the physician before resuming work, driving, strenuous recreational activities (e.g., jogging, golfing, and other sports), and travel (airplane or automobile). e. Try to get 8–10 hours of sleep each night. f. Avoid isometric exercises (e.g., lifting anything over 10 lb). Avoid pushing anything weighing more than 10 lb (e.g., vacuum cleaner, grocery cart) for 6–8 weeks. g. Limit stair climbing to once or twice a day.	7a. Progressive regular exercise increases cardiac stroke volume, thus increasing the heart's efficiency without greatly altering rate. b. These professionals can provide specific guidelines. c. Rest periods reduce myocardial oxygen demands. d. Caution is needed to reduce risk of myocardial hypoxia from overexertion. e. Sleep allows the body restorative time. f. Isometric exercises and straining increase cardiac workload and peripheral resistance. They also place stress on the healing sternum. g. Stair climbing increases cardiac workload.
8. Provide instructions for stress management strategies (Cheng et al., 2005): a. Identify stressors. b. Avoid stressors, if possible. c. Use techniques to reduce stress response (e.g., deep breathing, progressive relaxation, guided imagery, or exercise within postoperative constraints).	8. Although the relationship of stress and atherosclerotic changes is not clear, stress may increase cardiac workload.
9. Provide instructions for sexual activity: a. Consult with the physician about when sexual activity can be resumed. b. Rest before and after engaging in sexual activity. c. Stop sexual activity if angina occurs. d. Try different positions to decrease exertion (e.g., both partners side-lying or the client on bottom). e. If prescribed, take nitroglycerin before sexual activity. f. Avoid sexual activity in very hot or cold temperatures, within 2 hours of eating or drinking, when tired, after alcohol intake, with an unfamiliar partner, and in an unfamiliar environment.	9. Although resumption of sexual activity is encouraged, the client needs specific instructions focusing on reducing cardiac workload and avoiding certain situations that increase anxiety or vasoconstriction.
10. Provide instructions regarding prescribed medications (i.e., purpose, dosage and administration techniques, and possible side effects).	10. Understanding can help to improve compliance and reduce the risk of overdose and morbidity.

(continued)

Interventions	Rationales

11. Teach the client and family to report these signs and symptoms of complications to the physician:
  a. Redness, drainage, warmth, or increasing pain at incision site
  b. Increasing weakness, fatigue
  c. Elevated temperature
  d. Anginal pain
  e. Difficulty breathing
  f. Weight gain exceeding 3 lb in one day or 5 lb in one week
  g. Calf swelling, tenderness, warmth, or pain
  h. Dehiscence (Cheng et al., 2005)
	11. Early reporting of complications enables prompt interventions to minimize their severity.
	  a–c. These signs and symptoms may indicate infection. Wounds from graft donation sites may be more painful than the sternotomy site; endovascular harvesting reduces these risks (Cheng et al., 2005).
	  d. Anginal pain indicates myocardial hypoxia.
	  e, f. Difficulty breathing and abnormal weight gain may point to fluid retention.
	
	  g. These signs and symptoms may indicate thrombophlebitis.

12. Provide information regarding community services (e.g., American Heart Association, "Mended Hearts Club").	12. Community resources after discharge can assist with adaptation and self-help strategies (Cheng et al., 2005), including home health and telehealth interventions (Barnason, Zimmerman, Nieveen, & Hertzog, 2006).

Documentation

Client and family teaching
Response to teaching
Referrals, if indicated

Fractured Hip and Femur

The CDC (2010A) reports that in 2007, there were 281,000 hospital admissions for hip fractures among people age 65 and older. Falls cause over 90% of hip fractures (CDC, 2010A). One out of five individuals who fracture a hip will die within a year of their injury (CDC, 2010A).

Elderly clients are more vulnerable to hip fractures because of osteoporosis, mobility. and deconditioning problems. "Up to one in four adults who lived independently before their hip fracture remains in a nursing home for at least a year after their injury" (CDC, 2010A).

The type of surgery for hip fractures depends on the location of the break and bone fragments and the age of the individual. Surgery may include internal fixation (screws, rods, or plates) to stabilize broken bones or hip replacement (partial or total) (American Academy of Orthopaedic Surgeons and American Academy of Pediatrics, 2010).

Carp's Cues

Please refer to the Generic Surgical Care Plan for detailed interventions for managing all surgical conditions. This care plan addresses specific additional interventions associated with the type of surgery performed.

Time Frame
Postoperative periods

■■■■ DIAGNOSTIC CLUSTER

Postoperative Period

Collaborative Problems

▲ Risk for Complications of Fat Emboli

▲ Risk for Complications of Displacement of Hip Joint

▲ Risk for Complications of Compartment Syndrome (refer to Unit II)

▲ Risk for Complications of Peroneal Nerve Palsy

△ Risk for Complications of Venous Stasis / Thrombosis (refer to Unit II)

△ Risk for Complications of Avascular Necrosis of Femoral Head (refer to Inflammatory Joint Disease)

△ Risk for Complications of Sepsis (refer to Unit II)

Risk for Complications of Hemorrhage / Shock (refer to Generic Care Plan for the Surgical Client)

Risk for Complications of Pulmonary Embolism (refer to Generic Care Plan for the Surgical Client)

Nursing Diagnoses

▲ Acute Pain related to trauma and muscle spasms

▲ Risk for Constipation related to immobility (refer to Unit II)

▲ Risk for Impaired Skin Integrity related to immobility and urinary incontinence secondary to inability to reach toilet quickly enough between urge to void and need to void (refer to Unit II)

▲ Risk for Ineffective Self-Health Management related to insufficient knowledge of activity restrictions, assistive devices, home care, follow-up care, and supportive services

Related Care Plan

General Surgery Generic Care Plan

▲ This diagnosis was reported to be monitored for or managed frequently (75% to 100%).
△ This diagnosis was reported to be monitored for or managed often (50% to 74%).

Transition Criteria

Before transition, the client and family will:

1. Demonstrate care of the surgical site and use of assistive devices.
2. Relate at-home restrictions and follow-up care.
3. State the signs and symptoms that must be reported to a health-care professional.
4. Demonstrate a clear understanding of medications.

Transitional Risk Assessment Plan (TRAP)

Begin this plan on admission.
Implement the Transitional Risk Assessment Plan (TRAP):
• Refer to inside back cover.
• Add each validated risk diagnosis to client's problem list with the risk code in ( ).
• Refer to Unit II to the individual risk nursing diagnoses / collaborative problems for outcomes and interventions.

R: "Close coordination of care in the post-acute period, early transition follow-up care, enhanced client education and self-management training, proactive end-of-life counseling, and extending the resources and clinical expertise over time via multidisciplinary team management" can lower readmission rates and improve health outcomes (Boutwell & Hwu, 2009, p. 14).

Postoperative: Collaborative Problems

Risk for Complications of Fat Emboli

Risk for Complications of Peroneal Nerve Palsy

Risk for Complications of Hip Joint Displacement

Collaborative Outcomes

The client will be monitored for early signs and symptoms of (a) fat emboli, (b) compartment syndrome, (c) peroneal nerve palsy, (d) hip joint displacement, (e) venous stasis / thrombosis, (f) avascular necrosis of femoral head, and (g) sepsis, and will receive collaborative interventions if indicated to restore physiologic stability.

Indicators of Physiologic Stability

- Alert, calm, oriented (g)
- Temperature 98.5°–99° F (a, f, g)
- Heart rate 60–100 beats/min (a, g)
- Respirations 16–20 breaths/min (a, g)
- BP >90/60, <140/90 mm Hg (a, g)
- Peripheral pulses: full, equal, strong (b)
- Sensation intact (b)
- No pain with passive dorsiflexion (calf, toes) (b)
- Pain relieved by analgesics (b)
- No tingling in legs (b, c)
- Can move legs (b, c, d)
- No calf or thigh redness, warmth (e)
- Affected extremity aligned (d)
- No petechiae (upper trunk, axilla) (a)
- Urine output >0.5 mL/kg/h (a, g)
- White blood cells 4,000–10,800 (g)
- Oxygen saturation 94% to 100% (a, g)
- Capillary refill <3 seconds (b)

 Carp's Cues

Please refer to the Generic Care Plan for the Surgical Client for detailed interventions for managing all surgical conditions. This care plan addresses specific additional interventions associated with the type of surgery performed.

Interventions	Rationales
1. Monitor for signs and symptoms of fat embolism (de Feiter et al., 2007; Nucifora et al., 2007): a. Respiratory hypoxia (tachypnea, dyspnea, and cyanosis)	1. Fat emboli, unlike other emboli, is gradual, with respiratory and neurological sign / symptoms of hypoxemia, fever, and a petechial rash occurring 12–36 hours following injury. Fat droplets act as emboli, becoming impacted in the pulmonary microvasculature and other microvascular beds such as in the brain. Embolism begins rather slowly and attains a maximum in about 48 hours.
b. Cerebral changes (nonspecific, ranging from acute confusion to drowsiness, rigidity, convulsions, or coma)	b. Cerebral changes are seen in 86% of clients with FES.
c. Petechial rash	c. It occurs in up to 60% of cases and is due to embolization of small dermal capillaries leading to extravasation of erythrocytes. This produces a petechial rash in the conjunctiva, oral mucous membrane, and skin folds of the upper body, especially in the neck and axilla.

Interventions	Rationales

CLINICAL ALERT
- The risk factors for the development of FES are young age, closed fractures, multiple fractures, and conservative therapy for long-bone fractures.
- Factors which increase the risk of FES after intramedullary nailing are over-zealous nailing of the medullary cavity, reaming of the medullary cavity, increased velocity of reaming, and increase in the gap between nail and cortical bone.
- The literature reports "to give prophylactic steroid therapy only to those clients at risk for fat embolism syndrome, for example, those with long bone or pelvic fractures, especially closed fractures.
- "Methylprednisolone i.v. can be administered every 8 h for six doses" (Gupta & Reilly, 2007, p. 5).

Interventions	Rationales
2. Monitor for hypoxemia with pulse oximetry.	2. Pulmonary dysfunction is the earliest sign of fat embolism to manifest and is seen in 75% of clients; it progress to respiratory failure in 10% of the cases. Hypoxemia may be detected hours before the onset of respiratory complaints.
3. Monitor for signs and symptoms of peroneal nerve palsy: a. Decreased sensation to light touch (numbness and tingling at the top of the foot) (Baird, Keen, & Swearingen, 2005) b. Inability to distinguish between sharp and dull sensations c. Paralysis d. Foot drop (Baird, Keen, & Swearingen, 2005) e. Walking abnormalities (Baird, Keen, & Swearingen, 2005) f. Slapping gait (Baird, Keen, & Swearingen, 2005) g. Toes drag while walking (Baird, Keen, & Swearingen, 2005)	3. Pressure of the strap from skeletal traction (Buck traction) over the fibular head can compress the perineal nerve, resulting in paresthesias and ultimately paralysis due to nerve ischemia (Buck traction is not commonly used in acute care settings) (Wagner, Johnson, & Kidd, 2006).
4. Prevent dislocation during turning by placing a pillow between the client's legs.	4. The pillow will maintain abduction and alignment.
5. Monitor for signs and symptoms of hip joint displacement: a. External rotation of affected extremity b. Affected extremity shorter than unaffected extremity c. Increased pain	5. Damaged tissue and muscles may not provide adequate support for the hip joint, resulting in displacement.

TRANSITION TO HOME/COMMUNITY CARE

If indicated, review the risk diagnoses identified for this individual on admission:

• Is the person still at risk?
• Can the family reduce the risks?
• Is the person at higher risk at home?
• Is a Home Health Nurse assessment needed?
• Refer to transition planner / case manager / social service.
• When is this person scheduled for follow-up with primary provider? Specialists? Record dates of appointments.
• Complete a medication reconciliation prior to transition. Refer to index.

S T A R   **Stop**

Think   Is this person at risk for injury, falls, medical complications, and / or inability to care for self (activities of daily living)?

Is there a support person available?

Is the person competent to manage self-administration of medications, treatment procedures? Are additional resources needed?

Can the person explain how to monitor the condition (e.g., blood glucose, signs / symptoms of complications, dietary / mobility restrictions, and when to call his or her primary provider or specialist)?

Act   Contact or provide the appropriate resource (e.g., contacting a support person, home health assessment, additional teaching, printed materials).

Review   Has the problem been addressed? If not, use SBAR to communicate to the appropriate person.

Risk for Ineffective Self-Health Management Related to Insufficient Knowledge of Activity Restrictions, Assistive Devices, Home Care, Follow-up Care, and Supportive Services

NOC

Compliance Behavior, Knowledge: Treatment Regimen, Participation: Health-Care Decisions, Treatment Behavior: Illness or Injury

NIC

Anticipatory Guidance, Risk Management, Learning Facilitation, Health Education, Teaching: Procedure / Treatment, Health System Guidance

Goals

The goals for this diagnosis represent those associated with transition planning. Refer to the transition criteria.

Interventions	Rationales
1. Ensure that the client's ability to ambulate and perform ADLs. has been evaluated	1. The client's self-care abilities before transition need to be assessed to determine the need for referrals.
2. Evaluate mental status and presence of depression and / or confusion.	2. Individuals with confusion and depressive symptomatology have very risk for prolonged disability and death (Lewis et al., 2004).

Interventions	Rationales
3. Consult with a specialist for management of depression, as necessary.	3. Early detection and treatment of depression can reduce hospital stay and long-term disabilities.
4. Ensure written instructions are provided for exercises and activity restrictions	4. These measures may help to reduce risk of injury.
5. Advise to report any changes in gait and an increase in pain	5. This may indicate a dislocation.
6. Explain the importance of progressive care (i.e., from early non–weight-bearing ambulation to self-care within the client's abilities).	6. The risk of complications increases with each day of immobility, particularly in an elderly client (Baird, Keen, & Swearingen, 2005; Lewis et al., 2004; Wagner, Johnson, & Kidd, 2006).
7. Teach the client and family to watch for and report subtle signs of infection: a. Increased temperature chills. b. Malaise c. Pain unrelieved with analgesia (Lewis et al., 2004).	7. Hip fracture typically affects elderly clients who have a decreased ability to compensate for physiologic and immunologic system changes that may mask pronounced signs and symptoms of infection.
8. Teach the client and family to watch for and report subtle signs of DVT and to seek medical evaluation. a. Change in sensation in leg (aching, warmer, pain)	8. The risk for DVT continues after surgery for 3 months.
9. Teach the importance of avoiding immobility and exercises such as ankle pumping.	
10. Explain the possibility of delirium and contributing factors (electrolyte imbalances, metabolic abnormalities, infection, hypoxia, pain, medications, unfamiliar environment (Brauer et al., 2000).	
11. Refer to Unit II Acute Confusion if indicated.	

Documentation

Client and family teaching and return demonstration of understanding of education
Outcome achievement or status
Referrals, if indicated

Hysterectomy

A hysterectomy is a surgery to remove a woman's uterus for a variety of reasons such as (Gor, 2012):

- Uterine fibroids that cause pain, bleeding, or other problems
- Uterine prolapse, which is a sliding of the uterus from its normal position into the vaginal canal
- Cancer of the uterus, cervix, or ovaries
- Endometriosis
- Abnormal vaginal bleeding
- Chronic pelvic pain
- Adenomyosis, or a thickening of the uterus

There are various types of hysterectomies performed today, depending on the client diagnosis. The *supracervical* hysterectomy (subtotal hysterectomy) involves removal of the uterus while leaving the cervix intact. *Total hysterectomy* removes both the uterus and the cervix. *Radical hysterectomy* or *modified radical hysterectomy* is indicated if cancer is diagnosed. This method removes the uterus and cervix, may remove part of the vagina (if cancer is involved), ovaries (oophorectomy), fallopian tubes (salpingectomy), and lymph nodes (in order to stage the cancer and to determine how far the cancer is spread, if involved) (Gor, 2012; Harmanli et al., 2004; Paparella et al., 2004).

There are several approaches to performing a hysterectomy and again it is dependent on client diagnosis. The *open approach* (*abdominal hysterectomy*) is where the uterus, fallopian tubes and such are removed from a 6 to 12-inch incision in the lower abdomen. The *vaginal approach* is where the uterus is removed through the vagina. *Laparoscopic hysterectomy* removes the uterus either vaginally or through a small incision made in the abdomen. This method offers the surgeon better visualization of affected structures than either *vaginal* or *abdominal* alone, as a 2D video monitor is used (Gor, 2012).

A new method, called the *da Vinci hysterectomy*, is said to be one of the most effective and least invasive treatments. It is performed by using the da Vinci Surgical System, which enables the surgeons to perform with unmatched precision and control—using only a few small incisions. The benefits of this surgery include a considerable decrease in postoperative pain, blood loss, fever complications, scarring, length of hospitalization, and faster return to normal daily living.

 Time Frame
Postoperative periods

▪▪▪▪▪▪ DIAGNOSTIC CLUSTER

Postoperative Period

Collaborative Problems

▲ Risk for Complications of Ureter, Bladder, Bowel Trauma

▲ Risk for Complications of Vaginal Bleeding

▲ Risk for Complications of Deep Vein Thrombosis

▲ Risk for Complications of Neurological Deficits Secondary to Epidural Therapy

Nursing Diagnoses

△ Risk for Disturbed Self-Concept related to perceived effects on sexuality and feminine role

△ Risk for Ineffective Self-Health Management related to insufficient knowledge of perineal / incisional care, signs of complications, activity restrictions, loss of menses, hormone therapy, and follow-up care

▲ This diagnosis was reported to be monitored for or managed frequently (75% to 100%).
△ This diagnosis was reported to be monitored for or managed often (50% to 74%).

Transition Criteria

Before transition, the client and family will:

1. State wound care procedures to follow at home, especially ensuring that the client can monitor for wound infection and separation, if the abdominal approach is used.
2. Verbalize precautions to take regarding activities, especially the lifting restrictions of no more that 5 lb until cleared by doctor (usually after 6 weeks).
3. State the signs and symptoms that must be reported to a health-care professional, such as fever, drainage, redness, swelling, unresolved pain, and transition associated with itching and bad-smelling odors.
4. Verbalize an intent to share feelings and concerns with significant others.

> **Transitional Risk Assessment Plan (TRAP)**
>
> Begin this plan on admission.
> Implement the Transitional Risk Assessment Plan (TRAP):
> * Refer to inside back cover.
> * Add each validated risk diagnosis to client's problem list with the risk code in ( ).
> * Refer to Unit II to the individual risk nursing diagnoses / collaborative problems for outcomes and interventions.
>
> > *R:* "*Close coordination of care in the post-acute period, early transition follow-up care, enhanced client education and self-management training, proactive end-of-life counseling, and extending the resources and clinical expertise over time via multidisciplinary team management*" *can lower readmission rates and improve health outcomes (Boutwell & Hwu, 2009, p. 14).*

Postoperative: Collaborative Problems

Risk for Complications of Ureter, Bladder, Bowel Trauma

Risk for Complications of Vaginal Bleeding

Risk for Complications of Deep Vein Thrombosis

Risk for Complications of Neurological Deficits Associated with Epidural Injection

Collaborative Outcomes

The client will be monitored for early signs and symptoms of (a) ureter, bladder, and bowel trauma, (b) vaginal bleeding, (c) deep vein thrombosis, (d) infection, (e) hemodynamic instability, and (f) neurologic and neuromuscular deficits and will receive collaborative interventions if indicated to restore physiologic stability.

Indicators of Physiologic Stability

* Urine output >0.5 mL/kg/h (a)
* Clear urine (a)
* Intact bowel sounds all quadrants (a)
* Flatus present (a)
* No leg pain (c)
* No leg edema (c)
* Light-colored vaginal drainage (b)
* No headache (particularly, spinal headache due to epidural therapy) (e, f) (Lehne, 2004)
* Monitor signs of hypotension (due to epidural therapy) (e, f) (Lehne, 2004)
* No fever (d)
* No cardiac arrhythmias (e, f)
* No decreased level of consciousness (e, f)

Carp's Cues

Please refer to the Generic Care Plan for the Surgical Client for detailed interventions for managing all surgical conditions. This care plan addresses specific additional interventions associated with the type of surgery performed.

Interventions	Rationales
1. Monitor for signs and symptoms of ureter, bladder, or rectal trauma: a. Urinary retention b. Prolonged diminished bowel sounds c. Bloody, cloudy urine d. Absence of flatus	1. Proximity of these structures to the surgical site may predispose them to atony because of edema or nerve trauma.

(continued)

Interventions	Rationales
2. Monitor for signs and symptoms of deep-vein thrombosis (DVT). a. Refer to Unit II for intervention for Risk for Complications of DVT.	2. Gynecologic surgery increases the risk of DVT because of operative time and surgical positioning.

3. Monitor for adverse reactions to epidural therapy, if in place (Lehne, 2004):
   a. Hemodynamic stability
   b. Decreased level of consciousness
   c. Decreased respiratory rate and effort
   d. Allergic reactions
	3. An opioid or a combination of opioid and local anesthetic is infused into the space just before the dura mater. The opioid diffuses across the dura mater and binds to the opioid receptors. This route requires lower doses of analgesia and, as a result, minimizes the potential side effects. Providing analgesia outside of the central nervous system (CNS), on the other hand, affects drowsiness and respiratory depression. The rationale for hourly assessment is to recognize early signs and symptoms of systemic toxicity before signs of bradycardia, heart blocks, cardiac arrest, CNS excitation (possible convulsion), followed by CNS depressions and coma, occur. This is achieved by monitoring blood pressure, heart rate and rhythm, respiratory rate and regulation, and level of consciousness (Lehne, 2004; Wagner, Johnson, & Kidd, 2006).

4. Perform leg exercises every hour while client is in bed. Ambulate the client early, unless she is on epidural anesthesia, then mobilize as ordered (Baird, Keen, & Swearingen, 2005; Wagner et al., 2006).	4. Leg exercises and ambulation contract leg muscles, stimulate the venous pump, and reduce stasis. Movement reduces stasis and vascular pooling in legs; pressure under knees can interfere with peripheral circulation (Harmanli et al., 2004; Paparella, Sizzi, De Benedictine et al., 2004).

5. If the surgical route is vaginal, monitor vaginal bleeding every 2–4 hours:
   a. Monitor vaginal drainage. Record amount and color.
   b. If packing is used, notify the physician / NP if packing is saturated or clots are passed.
   c. Notify the physician / NP if perineal pad is saturated.
	5a. Drainage is expected. Frank vaginal bleeding, if it occurs, should be light (Porth, 2005).
	
	b, c. Packing is used if hemostasis is a problem during surgery. Excess bleeding or clots can indicate abnormal bleeding.

6. If the route is abdominal, monitor for incisional and vaginal bleeding every 2 hours.	6. The female pelvis has an abundant supply of blood vessels, creating a risk for bleeding (Porth, 2011).

Clinical Alert Report

Prior to providing care, advise ancillary staff / student to report the following to the professional nurse assigned to the client:

- Change in cognition / consciousness
- Oral temperature >100.5° F
- Systolic BP <90 mm/Hg
- Resting pulse >100, <50
- Respiratory rate >28, <10/min
- Oxygen saturation <90%
- Bright red bleeding

Related Physician / NP Prescribed Interventions

Medications
Estrogen therapy (selected cases)

Intravenous Therapy
Refer to the Generic Care Plan for the Surgical Client

Laboratory Studies
STD screening

Diagnostic Studies
Ultrasound or computed tomography (CT) scan, Papanicolaou test, endometrial sampling

Therapies
Urinary or suprapubic catheter, pelvic ultrasound, hysterosalpingography

Documentation

Vital signs (including adverse reactions to epidural therapy)
Perineal drainage
Intake and output
Turning, ambulation

Postoperative: Nursing Diagnoses

Risk for Disturbed Self-Concept Related to Significance of Loss

NOC
Quality of Life, Depression Level, Self-Esteem, Coping

NIC
Hope Instillation, Mood Management, Values Clarification, Counseling, Referral, Support Group, Coping Enhancement

Goal

The client will acknowledge change in body structure and function.

Indicators

- Communicate feelings about the hysterectomy.
- Participate in self-care within the restricted guidelines set by surgeon.

Interventions	Rationales
1. Contact the client frequently and treat her with warm, positive regard.	1. Frequent contact by the caregiver indicates acceptance and may facilitate trust. The client may be hesitant to approach staff because of a negative self-concept.
2. Incorporate emotional support into the technical care teaching sessions (e.g., wound care and bathing) (Katz, 2005; Zalon, 2004).	2. This encourages resolution of emotional issues while teaching technical skills (Katz, 2005; Zalon, 2004).
3. Encourage the client to verbalize her feelings about the surgery and its consequent impact on her lifestyle. Validate her perceptions and reassure her that the responses are normal and appropriate.	3. Sharing concerns and ventilating feelings provides an opportunity for the nurse to correct any misinformation. Validating the client's perceptions increases self-awareness (Katz, 2005; Zalon, 2004).
4. Replace myths with facts (e.g., hysterectomy usually does not affect physiologic sexual response) (Katz, 2005; Zalon, 2004).	4. Misinformation may contribute to unfounded anxiety and fear. Providing accurate information can help to reduce these emotional stressors.

(continued)

Interventions	Rationales
5. Discuss the surgery and its effects on functioning with family members or significant others; correct any misconceptions. Encourage client to share her feelings and perceptions with family and significant others (Katz, 2005; Zalon, 2004).	5. The support of family members or significant others is often critical to client's acceptance of changes and positive self-concept (Katz, 2005; Zalon, 2004).
6. Refer the client at high risk for unsuccessful adjustment for professional counseling.	6. Follow-up therapy to assist with effective adjustment may be indicated.

Documentation

Present emotional status
Response to interventions

> ### TRANSITION TO HOME / COMMUNITY CARE
> If indicated, review the risk diagnoses identified for this individual on admission:
> * Is the person still at risk?
> * Can the family reduce the risks?
> * Is the person at higher risk at home?
> * Is a Home Health Nurse assessment needed?
> * Refer to transition planner / case manager / social service.
> * When is this person scheduled for follow-up with primary provider? Specialists? Record dates of appointments.
> * Complete a medication reconciliation prior to transition. Refer to index.

STAR   **Stop**

Think Is this person at risk for injury, falls, medical complications, and / or inability to care for self (activities of daily living)?

Is there a support person available?

Is the person competent to manage self-administration of medications, treatment procedures? Are additional resources needed?

Can the person explain how to monitor the condition (e.g., blood glucose, signs / symptoms of complications, dietary / mobility restrictions, and when to call his or her primary provider or specialist)?

Act Contact or provide the appropriate resource (e.g., contacting a support person, home health assessment, additional teaching, printed materials).

Review Has the problem been addressed? If not, use SBAR to communicate to the appropriate person.

Risk for Ineffective Self-Health Management Related to Insufficient Knowledge of Perineal / Incisional Care, Signs of Complications, Activity Restrictions, Loss of Menses, Hormone Therapy, and Follow-up Care

NOC
Compliance Behavior, Knowledge: Treatment Regimen, Participation: Health-Care Decisions, Treatment Behavior: Illness or Injury

NIC
Anticipatory Guidance, Health Education, Risk Management, Support Group, Learning Facilitation

Goals

The goals for this diagnosis represent those associated with transition planning. Refer to the transition criteria.

Interventions	Rationales
1. Encourage the client to verbalize her feelings about the surgery and its consequent impact on her lifestyle. Validate her perceptions and reassure her that the responses are normal and appropriate.	1. Sharing concerns and ventilating feelings provides an opportunity for the nurse to correct any misinformation. Validating the client's perceptions increases self-awareness. (Katz, 2005; Zalon, 2004).
2. Replace myths with facts (e.g., hysterectomy usually does not affect physiologic sexual response) (Katz, 2005; Zalon, 2004).	2. Misinformation may contribute to unfounded anxiety and fear. Providing accurate information can help to reduce these emotional stressors.
3. Discuss expectations for recovery based on type and extent of surgery. Explain that vaginal hysterectomy generally affords more rapid recovery and causes less postoperative discomfort but has several disadvantages, including the following: a. Greater risk of postoperative infection. b. Reduced ability (as compared with abdominal hysterectomy) to deal with unexpected difficulties of surgery or complications (Katz, 2005; Zalon, 2004). Explain that abdominal hysterectomy allows better visualization during surgery and has fewer contraindications, but it involves longer recovery periods, increased use of anesthesia, and greater postoperative pain.	3. Understanding expectations for recovery can help the client and family to plan strategies for complying with the postoperative care regimen.
4. Explain care of an uncomplicated wound (abdominal hysterectomy).	4. Proper wound care helps to reduce microorganisms at the incision site and prevent infection.
5. Explain perineal care (vaginal hysterectomy); teach the client to do the following: a. Wash thoroughly with soap and water. b. Change the peripad frequently. c. After elimination, wipe from the front to back using a clean tissue for each front-to-back pass.	5. Proper perineal care reduces microorganisms around the perineum and minimizes their entry into the vagina.
6. Explain the need to increase activity, as tolerated, while maintaining restrictions such as no lifting greater than 5 lb for 6 weeks after the surgery (Zalon, 2004).	6. Physical activity, especially early and frequent ambulation, can help to prevent or minimize abdominal cramps, a common complaint during recovery from abdominal hysterectomy
7. Explain it is usual to return to normal sexual activities after 6 weeks of surgery.	7. After the surgery, it takes 4-6 weeks to recover. Recovery is earlier in cases of vaginal hysterectomy and laparoscopically assisted vaginal hysterectomy.
8. Teach the client and family to watch for and report the following: a. Temperature greater than 100° F (37.7° C) b. Vaginal bleeding that is greater than a typical menstrual period or is bright red c. Urinary incontinence, urgency, burning, or frequency d. Severe pain	8. Because of the abundance of blood vessels in the female pelvis, hysterectomy carries a higher risk of postoperative bleeding than most other surgeries. Bleeding most often occurs within 24 hours after surgery, but risk also occurs on the fourth, ninth, and 21st postoperative days, when the sutures dissolve. A small amount of pink, yellow, or brown serous drainage or even minor frank vaginal bleeding (no heavier than normal menstrual flow) is normal and expected.

(*continued*)

Interventions	Rationales
9. If ovaries are removed, explain the effects of surgery on cessation of menses menstruation and ovulation a symptoms to expect: a. Hot flashes b. Headache c. Nervousness d. Palpitations e. Fatigue f. Depression, feelings of uselessness, and other emotional reactions	9. Removal of the uterus but keeping the ovaries theoretically should not produce menopausal symptoms; however, the client may experience them temporarily, apparently because of increased estrogen levels resulting from surgical manipulation of the ovaries. Removal of both ovaries artificially induces menopause; this causes more severe symptoms than typically experienced in a normal climacteric. To help reduce these symptoms, a portion of the ovary often is left in place unless contraindicated. Estrogen therapy relieves symptoms and may be indicated except in cases of malignancy (Zalon, 2004; Thakar et al., 2002).
10. Explore the client's concerns regarding the impact of surgery on sexual feelings and function. Explain that she should be able to resume intercourse anywhere from 3 weeks (with a vaginal hysterectomy) to 16 weeks after surgery; confirm a specific time frame with the physician / NP.	10. In most cases, hysterectomy should not affect sexual response or functioning. For 3–4 months after surgery, intercourse may be painful due to abdominal soreness and temporary shrinking of the vagina. Deep penetration intercourse should be avoided initially. Intercourse helps to stretch the vaginal walls and eventually relieves the discomfort (Katz, 2005).
11. Discuss follow-up care and that a postoperative check is scheduled for 4–6 weeks after transition. Reinforce the importance of keeping scheduled appointments (Zalon, 2004).	11. Regular follow-up care is necessary to evaluate the results of surgery and estrogen therapy, if indicated, and to detect any complications.

Documentation

Client and family teaching
Outcome achievement or status

Ileostomy

Ileostomy is the surgical creation of an opening between the ileum and the abdominal wall for the purpose of fecal diversion. An ileostomy is typically indicated for clients with pathologic small bowel conditions, such as ulcerative colitis, cancer complications, Crohn's disease, and familial polyposis (Hyland, 2002; Lewis et al., 2004). An ileostomy may be temporary or permanent, and may be constructed as an end stoma, a loop stoma, or a double-barrel stoma.

Loop ileostomies are usually temporary and are formed to (Adkins, 2011):

- Protect a distal anastomosis;
- Protect the anastomosis of an ileal-anal pouch or a colo-anal pouch during the healing process;
- Aid healing in Crohn's disease, which affects the colon and the anus;
- Aid healing of fistula tracts (the result of underlying pathology; e.g. abscess, malignancy, Crohn's disease, trauma, sepsis).

Time Frame
Postoperative periods

■■ DIAGNOSTIC CLUSTER

Postoperative Period

Collaborative Problems

▲ Risk for Complications of Peristomal Ulceration / Herniation

▲ Risk for Complications of Stomal Necrosis, Retraction Prolapse, Stenosis, Obstruction

▲ Risk for Complications of Fluid and Electrolyte Imbalances

△ Risk for Complications of Ileal Reservoir Pouchitis (Kock Pouch)

△ Risk for Complications of Failed Nipple Valve (Kock Pouch)

△ Risk for Complications of Ileoanal Kock Pouchitis

△ Risk for Complications of Cholelithiasis

△ Risk for Complications of Urinary Calculi

Nursing Diagnoses

▲ Risk for Disturbed Self-Concept related to effects of ostomy on body image and lifestyle

△ Anxiety related to lack of knowledge of ileostomy care and perceived negative effects on lifestyle (refer to Colostomy Care Plan)

△ Risk for Ineffective Self-Health Management related to insufficient knowledge of stoma pouching procedure, peristomal skin care, perineal wound care, and incorporation of ostomy care into activities of daily living (ADLs)

Related Care Plan

Generic Care Plan for the Surgical Client

▲ This diagnosis was reported to be monitored for or managed frequently (75% to 100%).
△ This diagnosis was reported to be monitored for or managed often (50% to 74%).

Transitional Criteria

Before transition, the client and family will:

1. Discuss and give return demonstration in relation to ostomy care at home, including stoma, pouching, irrigation, skin care.
2. Discuss strategies for incorporating ostomy management into ADLs.
3. Verbalize precautions for medication use and food intake.
4. State signs and symptoms that must be reported to a health-care professional.
5. Verbalize an intent to share feelings and concerns related to ostomy with significant others.
6. Identify available community resources and self-help groups.

Transitional Risk Assessment Plan (TRAP)

Begin this plan on admission.
Implement the Transitional Risk Assessment Plan (TRAP):
• Refer to inside back cover.
• Add each validated risk diagnosis to client's problem list with the risk code in ( ).
• Refer to Unit II to the individual risk nursing diagnoses / collaborative problems for outcomes and interventions.

R: "Close coordination of care in the post-acute period, early transition follow-up care, enhanced client education and self-management training, proactive end-of-life counseling, and extending the resources and clinical expertise over time via multidisciplinary team management" can lower readmission rates and improve health outcomes (Boutwell & Hwu, 2009, p. 14).

Preoperative Period

Carp's Cues

"The presence of a stoma is associated with significant psychological morbidity, including fears of bad hygiene, limitation in social or athletic activities, and elimination of intimate relationships."

Individuals and their significant others should have had at least one session with an ostomy / wound specialist to prepare for the surgery. Individual and their significant others are "provided with real-life experiences and encouraged to engage in frank discussions regarding odor, leakage, diet, clothing and sexuality"; teaching and reinforcement will continue post-operatively.

> **CLINICAL ALERT**
> Prior to surgery, even in an emergency, the nurse should make every attempt to have soma site selection done. A joint statement from the American Society of Colon & Rectal Surgeons and the Wound Ostomy Continence Nurses Society states that "all clients undergoing intestinal ostomy surgery should have preoperative stoma site marking by an experienced, educated, competent clinician" (Butler, 2009, p. 514). These position statements caution that poor stoma placement can lead to unavoidable postoperative morbidity, including pain, leakage from the pouching system, peristomal skin irritation, fitting challenges, and impaired psychological health (ASCRS & WOCN, 2007).

For elective procedures, stoma site marking should be preformed prior to surgery with the person supine, sitting, standing, and bending forward." The site must be visible to the individual and, to improve adherence skin creases, bony prominences, scars, and drain sites should be avoided.

Postoperative: Collaborative Problems

Risk for Complications of Intra-abdominal Hypertension (refer to Unit II)

Risk for Complications of Peristomal Ulceration / Herniation

Risk for Complications of Stomal (Necrosis, Retraction, Prolapse, Stenosis, Obstruction)

Risk for Complications of Fluid and Electrolyte Imbalances

Risk for Complications of Pouchitis

Risk for Complications of Failed Nipple Valve

Risk for Complications of Cholelithiasis

Risk for Complications of Urinary Calculi

Collaborative Outcomes

The client will be monitored for early signs and symptoms of peristomal complications as (a) peristomal ulceration / herniation; (b) stomal necrosis, retraction; (c) prolapse, stenosis, obstruction; (e) pouchitis; (f) fluid and electrolyte imbalances; (g) cholelithiasis; (h) urinary calculi; and will receive collaborative interventions if indicated to restore physiologic stability.

Indicators of Physiologic Stability

- Intact peristomal muscle tone (a)
- No stomal ulceration (a)
- No complaints of abdominal cramping or pain (b, e,)
- No abdominal or flank pain (g, h)
- No nausea or vomiting (b, g, e,)
- No abdominal distention (b, h, f)
- Urine output >0.5 mL/h (g, e, h)

- Minimal or no weight loss (e, f)
- Clear, pale urine (e, f, h)
- Urine specific gravity 1.005–1.030 (e, f)
- No change in stool color (e, f)
- No epigastric fullness (g)
- No jaundice (g)
- Temperature 98.5°–99° F (e, f)

 Carp's Cues

Please refer to the Generic Care Plan for the Surgical Client for detailed interventions for managing all surgical conditions. This care plan addresses specific additional interventions associated with the type of surgery performed.

Interventions	Rationales
CLINICAL ALERT • Complications after stoma creation surgery can occur shortly after surgery, in 10 days, 3–6 months and 1–2 years with a rate of 0% to 22%.	
1. Monitor for signs of peristomal ulceration or herniation: a. Decreased peristomal muscle tone b. Bulging beyond normal skin surface and musculature c. Persistent ulceration	1. The acid content in the small bowel intestinal effluent is high. Early detection of ulcerations and herniation can prevent serious tissue damage (Colwell & Beitz, 2007).
2. Monitor for stomal necrosis, prolapse, retraction, stenosis, and obstruction. Assess the following: a. Color, size, and shape of stoma b. Color, amount, and consistency of ostomy effluent c. Complaints of cramping, abdominal pain, nausea and vomiting, and abdominal distension d. Ostomy appliance and appliance belt fit	2. Daily assessment is necessary to detect early changes in stoma condition: a. These changes can indicate inflammation, retraction, prolapse, or edema. b. These changes can indicate bleeding or infection. Decreased output can indicate obstruction. c. These complaints may indicate obstruction. d. Contributing factors are excessive tension, necrosis, retraction, or mucocutaneous. Improperly fitting appliance or belt can cause mechanical trauma to the stoma (Colwell & Beitz, 2007).
3. Monitor for bulging around the stoma.	3. This finding may indicate herniation, which is caused by loops of intestine protruding through the abdominal wall.
4. Monitor for obstruction: a. Crampy abdominal pain and may feel bloated b. Pain very severe and constant c. Loss of appetite, and nausea and / or vomiting d. Very liquid output , no solids, explosive force (partial obstruction) e. No liquid, solid, or gas output (complete obstruction) **CLINICAL ALERT** • Notify surgeon immediately	4. A partial obstruction will allow fluid but no solids to pass leading to complete obstruction.
5. Monitor for ischemia: a. Stoma narrows or contracts at the skin or fascia b. Decrease effluent from stoma	5. Factors that contribute to ischemia are excessive tension, necrosis, retraction, mucocutaneous separation.

(continued)

Interventions	Rationales
6. Monitor for signs and symptoms of ileal reservoir or ileoanal pouchitis: a. Acute increase in effluent flow b. Evidence of dehydration c. Abdominal pain and bloating, nausea and vomiting d. Fever	6. Pouchitis or ileitis involves inflammation of the internal pouch. The cause is unknown, but bacterial growth in the pouch is a suspected causative factor. Insufficiently frequent pouch emptying increases the risk of infection.
7. Connect an indwelling catheter to continuous straight drainage.	7. This measure promotes continuous urine drainage of the Kock pouch.
8. Monitor output closely. Consult with surgeon or wound / ostomy specialist for treatment.	8. Insertion of an indwelling catheter may be indicated to permit continuous straight drainage.
9. Monitor for signs of fluid and electrolyte imbalance: a. High volume of watery ostomy output (more than five $^1/_3$- to $^1/_2$-filled pouches or >1,000 mL daily) b. Decreased serum sodium, potassium, magnesium levels (Lewis et al., 2004; Wagner, Johnson, & Kidd, 2006). c. Weight loss d. Nausea and vomiting, anorexia, abdominal distention	9. Fluid and electrolyte imbalances most commonly result from diarrhea. Major causes of acute diarrhea include infection, diuretic therapy, obstruction, and hot weather. Chronic diarrhea can result from ileal resection or "short gut syndrome," radiation therapy, or chemotherapy (Lewis et al., 2004; Richbourg, Thorpe, & Rapp, 2007; Wagner, Johnson, & Kidd, 2006).
10. Administer fluid and electrolyte replacement therapy, as ordered. Monitor fluid status cautiously.	10. Replacement therapy may be needed to prevent serious electrolyte imbalance or fluid deficiency, and cardiac arrhythmias (ventricular ectopic, ventricular tachycardia and Torsades de pointes) (Lewis et al., 2004; Wagner, Johnson, & Kidd, 2006). "In contrast aggressive postoperative fluid resuscitation may distort the ostomy, resulting in retraction and necrosis if the stoma is under tension" (Butler, 2009).
11. Monitor for cholelithiasis (gallstones): a. Epigastric fullness b. Abdominal distention c. Vague pain d. Very dark urine e. Grayish or clay colored stools f. Jaundice g. Elevated cholesterol	11. Changes in absorption of bile acids postoperatively increase cholesterol levels and can cause gallstones (Colwell & Beitz, 2007; Wagner, Johnson, & Kidd, 2006).
12. If symptoms occur, collaborate with the surgeon, wound / ostomy nurse specialist / NP to prepare for a diagnostic evaluation (e.g., ultrasound, cholecystography).	12. Diagnostic studies will be indicated to confirm gallstones and to determine severity.
13. Monitor for urinary calculi (stones): a. Lower abdominal pain b. Flank pain c. Hematuria d. Decreased urine output e. Increased urine specific gravity	13. Large volumes of fluid lost through the ileostomy can cause urinary stones as a result of dehydration.

Clinical Alert Report

Prior to providing care, advise ancillary staff / student to report the following to the professional nurse assigned to the client:

- Change in cognitive status
- Oral temperature >100.5° F
- Systolic BP <90 mm/Hg
- Resting Pulse >100, <50
- Respiratory rate >28, <10/min.
- Oxygen saturation <90%
- Change in effluent, amount, presence of blood
- No effluent
- C/o of nausea, abdominal pain

Related Physician / NP Prescribed Interventions

Depending on the underlying problem (e.g., cancer, inflammatory bowel disease), refer to the care plan of the condition.

Documentation

Intake and output
Bowel sounds
Wound status
Stoma condition
Changes in physiologic status

Postoperative: Nursing Diagnoses

Risk for Disturbed Self-Concept Related to Effects of Ostomy on Body Image

NOC
Quality of Life, Coping, Depression, Self-Esteem

Goal

The client will acknowledge change in body structure and function.

NIC
Hope Instillation, Mood Management, Values Clarification, Counseling, Referral, Support Group, Coping Enhancement

Indicators

- Communicate feelings about the ostomy.
- Participate in stoma care.

Carp's Cues

Anderson et al. compared Health Related Quality of Life index in 105 individuals with ulcerative colitis (and 5 clients with familial adenomatous polyposis), all with an intact pouch, with that of 4,152 individuals from the general population. Individuals 2–22 years post surgery reported slightly lower but significant scores in 4 of the 6 health domains (2011). "Frequency of defecation was a median of 7 (3–12) bowel movements during the day and 2 (0–6) at night. The majority had some degree of fecal incontinence, median (range) Wexner score of 8 (0–17), and 40% reported urgency of defecation necessitating alterations in lifestyle" (Anderson et al., 2011).

Interventions	*Rationales*
1. Connect with the individual frequently. Ask, what are you most concerned about? **CLINICAL ALERT** • Nurses are often fearful of asking a question to which they may not know how to respond to the client's response. • This fear creates dialogue that is superficial and meaningless. • Your response could acknowledge the situation: "I am sorry you are in this situation" or "Tell me more about this." • Then just listen. Listening to someone pour out his or her soul to you never means you take away the fears, BUT you can listen to them. • If there are some answers to the client's concerns that someone else, such as an ostomy nurse specialist, is better qualified to address, consult that specialist. • Nurses must learn to be comfortable sitting in a dark cave with individuals without talking about the light.	1. Frequent contact by the caregiver indicates acceptance and may facilitate trust. This question will help the nurse focus on the concern of the individual, not what "we think the concerns are."

2. Incorporate emotional support into technical ostomy self-care sessions. Richbourg, Thorpe, and Rapp (2007) have identified four stages of psychological adjustment that ostomy clients may experience:
  a. Narration. The client recounts his or her illness experience and reveals understanding of how and why he or she finds self in this situation.
  b. Visualization and verbalization. The client looks at and expresses feelings about his or her stoma.
  c. Participation. The client progresses from observer to assistant, then to independent performer of the mechanical aspects of ostomy care.
  d. Exploration. The client begins to explore methods of incorporating the ostomy into her or his lifestyle.
	2. This allows resolution of emotional issues during acquisition of technical skills.

3. Involve support persons in learning ostomy care principles. Assess the client's interactions with support persons.	3. Other people's response to the ostomy is one of the most important factors influencing the client's acceptance of it.
4. Encourage the client to discuss plans for incorporating ostomy care into his or her lifestyle. Is the client concerned about a specific situation (e.g., travel, eating out)? Share the client's concerns with the nurse specialist	4. Evidence that the client will pursue his or her goals and resume lifestyle reflects positive adjustment (Junkin & Beitz, 2005).
5. Suggest that the client meet with a person from the United Ostomy Associations (UOA) who can share similar experiences.	5. In addition to the professional nurse's clinical expertise, the ostomy client may choose to take advantage of a UOA visitor's actual experience with an ostomy (Junkin & Beitz, 2005).

Documentation

Present emotional status
Discussions

TRANSITION TO HOME / COMMUNITY CARE

If indicated, review the risk diagnoses identified for this individual on admission:

* Is the person still at risk?
* Can the family reduce the risks?
* Is the person at higher risk at home?
* Is a Home Health Nurse assessment needed?
* Refer to transition planner / case manager / social service.
* When is this person scheduled for follow-up with primary provider? Specialists? Record dates of appointments.
* Complete a medication reconciliation prior to transition. Refer to index.

STAR

Stop

Think   Is this person at risk for injury, falls, medical complications, and / or inability to care for self (activities of daily living)?

Is there a support person available?

Is the person competent to manage self-administration of medications, treatment procedures? Are additional resources needed?

Can the person explain how to monitor the condition (e.g., blood glucose, signs / symptoms of complications, dietary / mobility restrictions, and when to call his or her primary provider or specialist)?

Act   Contact or provide the appropriate resource (e.g., contacting a support person, home health assessment, additional teaching, printed materials).

Review   Has the problem been addressed? If not, use SBAR to communicate to the appropriate person.

Risk for Ineffective Self-Health Management Related to Insufficient Knowledge of Stoma Pouching Procedure, Peristomal Skin Care, Perineal Wound Care, and Incorporation of Ostomy Care into Activities of Daily Living (ADLs)

NOC

Compliance Behavior, Knowledge: Treatment Regimen, Participation: Health-Care Decisions, Treatment Behavior: Illness or Injury

Goals

The goals for this diagnosis represent those associated with transition planning. Refer to the transition criteria.

NIC

Ostomy Care, Anticipatory Guidance, Risk Identification, Learning Facilitation, Health Education

---

Interventions   *Rationales*

CLINICAL ALERT

* Most clinical nurses are not responsible for the specific teaching of ostomy care and its implications on lifestyle and function.
* The wound care / ostomy specialist will provide an organized teaching plan.
* However, since nurses are responsible for care 24/7, each nurse needs to be confident in basic ostomy care.
* A good method to learn this care is to watch the nurse specialist provide / teach ostomy care

(continued)

Interventions	Rationales
1. When providing care, explore fears and concerns. Identify and dispel any misinformation or misconceptions the client / significant others has regarding ileostomy (Richbourg, Thorpe, & Rapp, 2007).	1. Replacing misinformation with facts can reduce anxiety.
2. Emphasize the importance of adequate fluid and salt intake; explain also risk situations for dehydration such as: a. Hot weather b. Exercising in hot weather c. Episodes of diarrhea d. When intake is reduced (e.g., illness)	2. Loss of the reabsorptive surface of the large bowel increases the amount of water and sodium loss in the stool. If the ileostomy is high (more proximal in the ileum), additional potassium losses may also occur.
3. Advise to: a. Drink enough fluid to have at least 1 quart of ostomy output daily and pale urine. b. Drink more fluids and consume extra salt in hot weather c. Eat foods high in potassium (e.g., bananas, oranges)	
4. Discuss signs and symptoms of fluid and electrolyte imbalances: a. Extreme thirst b. Dry skin and oral mucous membrane c. Dark yellow urine output d. Weakness, fatigue e. Muscle cramps f. Orthostatic hypotension (feeling faint when suddenly changing positions)	
5. Ensure that a consult with nutritionist / wound / ostomy nurse specialist has occurred.	5. The nutritionist or wound / ostomy nurse specialist will review foods to avoid controlling odor and preventing food blockage.
6. Teach s/s of food blockage (Canadian Association of Endostomal Therapy, 2005): a. Abdominal cramping b. Swelling of the stoma c. Absence of ileostomy output for over 4 to 6 hours	
7. Advise to (Canadian Association of Endostomal Therapy, 2005): a. Not eat solid food b. Not take a laxative c. Remove pouching system and increase the size of the pouch opening to accommodate the swollen stoma. d. Drink as much fluid as possible if tolerated (e.g., there is no vomiting and if the stoma is still active). e. If there is NO stoma output, DO NOT DRINK FLUIDS	

Interventions	Rationales

8. Advise to call surgeon / wound / ostomy specialist, if self-care measures taught to relieve blockage are not effective .

> **CLINICAL ALERT**
> • A client with a stoma is at increased risk for peristomal skin breakdown.
> • Factors that influence skin integrity include composition, quantity, and consistency of the ostomy effluent; allergies; mechanical trauma; the underlying disease and its treatment (including medications); surgical construction and location of the stoma; the quality of ostomy and periostomal skin care; availability of proper supplies; nutritional status; overall health status; hygiene; and activity level.

9. Teach to check the stoma and peristomal skin with each pouch change. Report changes to skin to physician / ostomy nurse specialist:
 	
  a. Allergic or contact dermatitis
 	
  b. Purulent ulcerated areas surrounding the stoma
 	
  c. A red, scaly, itchy rash, or white-coated area
	9. Ongoing assessment is important for optimal health and function of the stoma and surrounding skin. Stripping of tape or excessively frequent pouch removal may cause mechanical trauma to peristomal skin.
	  a. A rash may result from contact with fecal drainage or indicate sensitivity to pouch, paste, tape, or sealant.
	  b. Disruption of the protective barrier of the skin allows bacterial entry.
	  c. This is a manifestation of *Candida albicans*, a yeast infection.

10. Instruct to report abnormal appearance of the stoma or surrounding skin to the surgeon, primary care provider or wound / ostomy nurse specialist:
  a. Narrowing of the stoma lumen
 	
  b. Lacerations or cuts in the stoma
 	
  c. Separation of the stoma from the abdominal surface
	10a. This indicates stenosis and may interfere with fecal elimination.
	  b. The stoma contains no nerves, so trauma may occur without pain.
	  c. This potential complication may require surgical repair.

11. Explain the possibility of stoma retraction and the importance of not gaining weight. > **CLINICAL ALERT** > • A retracted stoma will have a poor adherence of the pouches with leakage and skin irritation.	11. Ileostomy stomas can retract early due to a too-short exteriorized segment, which may require a surgical revision. Weight gain can also cause the stoma to retract with less or no protrusion.

(continued)

Interventions	*Rationales*

12. Discuss community resources / self-help groups:
   a. Printed Self-Help Guidelines
      • A Guide to Living with an Ileostomy access, Canadian Association of Endostomal Therapy at http://www.caet.ca/caet-english/documents/caet-guide-to-living-with-an-ileostomy.pdf
      • Ileostomy Care. American Cancer Society, at http://www.cancer.org/acs/groups/cid/documents/webcontent/002870-pdf.pdf
   b. Organizations
      • Visiting nurse
      • United Ostomy Associations of America, Inc. (UOAA),
        1-800-826-0826, www.uoaa.org.
        For local support group information; the interactive website includes discussion boards.
      • International Ostomy Association (IOA), www.ostomyinternational.org.
        Advocates for and outlines the rights of ostomates.
      • Wound, Ostomy and Continence Nurses Society (WOCN),
        1-888-224-9626, www.wocn.org
      • Community suppliers of ostomy equipment
      • Financial reimbursement for ostomy equipment

Clinical Alert Report

Prior to providing care, advise ancillary staff / student to report the following to the professional nurse assigned to the client:
• Any questions regarding home care, self-care

Documentation

Client and family teaching
Outcome achievement or status

Lumbar Laminectomy

Surgery of the spine is performed for several reasons, such as trauma, removal of tumors / lesions, spinal stenosis, and for disk disease when diagnostic tests reveal a herniation that is not responding to conservative treatment. A lumbar laminectomy may also be indicated when significant pain, neural impingement, or persistent neurologic deficits are affecting daily life. Several different approaches may be used; however, this is dependent on the disease / injury process which surgical intervention is indicated for (Lewis et al., 2004). The surgical excision can be done with one of the following techniques:

• *Discectomy* is the removal of a herniated or fragmented intervertebral disk. This can include an anterior or posterior approach, with or without fusion involved. Anterior cervical discectomy with fusion (ACDF) is used to treat various pathologic conditions such as spondylosis and forminal stenosis. A discectomy with fusion is a small discectomy with a bone graft (donor or from client) to fuse the spinous process to stabilize the spine. Anterior cervical discectomy without fusion (ACD) is not advocated by modern neurosurgeons and is considered antiquated (Bader & Littlejohns, 2004).

   Anterior corpectomy with fusion is indicated when a large anterior decompression of the spinal canal is required; often multiple spinal segments are involved, such as in severe spondylosis and / or stenosis with associated reversal of normal lordosis. This method is more often used in trauma, tumors, or osteomyelitis. Interbody fusion options for anterior corpectomy are the same as for ACDF: allograft, autologous graft, or titanium cage. Anterior plating is desirable to promote osseous fusion (Bader & Littlejohns, 2004).

- *Laminectomy* is the surgical procedure that removes a part of the posterior arch of a vertebra (lamina) to provide access to the spinal canal and to remove pathology and relieve compression (Bader & Littlejohns, 2004; Lewis et al., 2004).
- *Hemi-laminectomy* is the surgical removal of part of a lamina and part of the posterior arch (usually one side of a vertebral lamina) (Bhardwaj, Mirski, & Ulatowski, 2004).
- *Foraminotomy* is the surgical removal of the intervertebral foramen to increase space for a spinal nerve and to reduce compression.
- *Laminoplasty* is performed to decompress the cord when multiple vertebral segments are compressing (e.g., central cord syndrome from cervical stenosis). It requires normal lordotic curvature of the cervical spine (Bader & Littlejohns, 2004; Bhardwaj, Mirski, & Ulatowski, 2004).
- *Laminotomy*, bilateral or unilateral, is performed when a client has decreased functional ability, especially ambulation, associated with pain. A laminotomy preserves the central ligamentous structure and allows for adequate central foraminal decompression (Bader & Littlejohns, 2004; Bhardwaj, Mirski, & Ulatowski, 2004).

    Microsurgical techniques make removal of tissue more precise with less damage to normal tissue.

 Time Frame
Preoperative and postoperative periods
Healthcare settings:
Neuro Specialty Unit
Inpatient Surgical Unit
Orthopedic Unit

■■ DIAGNOSTIC CLUSTER

Preoperative Period

Nursing Diagnoses

▲ Risk for Injury related to lack of knowledge of postoperative position restrictions and log-rolling technique

Postoperative Period

Collaborative Problems

▲ Risk for Complications of Paralytic Ileus

▲ Risk for Complications of Neurological Sensory and Motor Impairments

▲ Risk for Complications of Urinary Retention

▲ Risk for Complications of Cerebrospinal Fistula

Nursing Diagnoses

▲ Acute Pain related to muscle spasms (back, thigh) secondary to nerve irritation during surgery, edema, skeletal malalignment, or bladder distention

▲ Risk for Falls related to altered mobility secondary to gait unsteadiness and lumbar instability

▲ Risk for Ineffective Self-Health Management related to insufficient knowledge of home care, activity restrictions, and exercise program

Related Care Plan

General Surgery Generic care plan

▲ This diagnosis was reported to be monitored for or managed frequently (75% to 100%).

Transition Criteria

Before transition, the client or family will:

1. Describe proper wound care at home and verify knowledge gained related to maintaining wound cleanliness, understanding the importance of not applying any type of lotions, creams, or ointments to wound site.
2. Verbalize necessary activity precautions, including those regarding time frames for sitting, standing, lifting, and twisting, and the correct procedure in applying a brace, if ordered by the surgeon.
3. State signs and symptoms that must be reported to a health-care professional, no matter how insignificant they may appear, especially neurologic deficits, wound leakage, and bulging at the incision site.
4. Describe proper personal hygiene techniques, including the use of no pools, bathtubs, or whirlpools.
5. State the need to make a postoperative visit for follow-up, usually around 10–14 days after surgery.
6. Describe possible treatments for incision pain, including the use of prescribed analgesics and / or narcotics, ice / heat therapy to incision site, and diversion techniques as needed.
7. Verbalize the importance of not driving, especially while taking prescribed analgesics, until further instructions are given by the MD.

> **Transitional Risk Assessment Plan (TRAP)**
>
> Begin this plan on admission.
> Implement the Transitional Risk Assessment Plan (TRAP):
> • Refer to inside back cover.
> • Add each validated risk diagnosis to client's problem list with the risk code in ( ).
> • Refer to Unit II to the individual risk nursing diagnoses / collaborative problems for outcomes and interventions.
>
> *R: "Close coordination of care in the post-acute period, early transition follow-up care, enhanced client education and self-management training, proactive end-of-life counseling, and extending the resources and clinical expertise over time via multidisciplinary team management" can lower readmission rates and improve health outcomes (Boutwell & Hwu, 2009, p. 14).*

Preoperative: Nursing Diagnosis

Risk for Injury Related to Lack of Knowledge of Postoperative Position Restrictions and Log-rolling Technique

NOC
Risk Control, Safety Status: Falls Occurrence

Goal

The client will demonstrate correct positioning and log-rolling technique.

NIC
Fall Prevention, Environmental Management: Safety, Health Education, Surveillance: Safety, Risk Identification

Indicators

• State why precautions are needed.
• State necessary restrictions.

Carp's Cues

Please refer to the Generic Care Plan for the Surgical Client for detailed interventions for managing all surgical conditions. This care plan addresses specific additional interventions associated with the type of surgery performed.

Interventions	*Rationale*

1. Teach the client the correct body alignment to maintain while lying in bed, sitting, and standing. Teach the correct log-rolling technique to use to get in and out of bed; show the client how to do the following:
  a. Roll to the edge of the bed, keeping the lower back flat and the spine straight.
  b. Raise the head and simultaneously swing both legs (bent at the knees) over the side of the bed.
  c. Use the upper hand to support the stomach muscles and the lower arm to push away from the mattress (Bhardwaj, Mirski, & Ulatowski, 2004; Wagner, Johnson, & Kidd, 2006).
	1. Maintaining proper positioning, good posture, and using proper procedure for getting in and out of bed will minimize back strain, muscle spasms, and discomfort.

Documentation

Client teaching
Client / Family Education
Outcome achievement or status

Postoperative: Collaborative Problems

Risk for Complications of Neurological Sensory and / or Motor Impairment

Risk for Complications of Urinary Retention

Risk for Complications of Paralytic Ileus

Risk for Complications of Cerebrospinal Fistula

Collaborative Outcomes

The client will be monitored for early signs and symptoms of (a) sensory and / or motor impairment, (b) urinary retention, (c) paralytic ileus, and (d) cerebrospinal fistula, and collaboratively intervene to stabilize the client.

Indicators of Physiologic Stability

- Motor function equal and intact (a)
- Sensory function equal and intact (a)
- Strength equal and intact (a)
- Urinary output >0.5 mL/kg/h (a, b)
- Can verbalize bladder fullness (a, b)
- No complaints of lower abdominal pain (a, b)
- Bowel sounds present and all quadrants (c)
- Reports flatus (c)
- Bowel movement by third day (c)
- Minimal or no drainage (d)
- Negative glucose test of drainage (d)
- No complaints of headache (d)

Interventions	Rationales
1. Monitor symmetry of sensory and motor function in extremities: 　a. To touch, pin scratch 　b. Strength (have the client push your hands away with his or her soles, then pull his or her feet up against resistance). 　Compare findings from right side to left side and preoperative baseline.	1. Cord or nerve root edema, pressure on a nerve root from herniated disk fragments, or hematoma at the operative site can cause or exacerbate deficits in motor and sensory functions postoperatively. Surgical manipulation can result in nerve damage causing paresthesias, paralysis, and possibly respiratory insufficiency.
2. Monitor bladder function: 　a. Ability to void sufficient quantities, and to empty the bladder completely. If urinary retention is suspected, use the bladder ultrasound as needed to assess amount of residual urine. The use of bladder scanners provides a safe alternative in comparison to urinary catheterization and is fast becoming the safest and most reliable option for urinary retention (Davis, Chrisman, & Walden, 2012). 　b. Ability to sense bladder fullnes	2. Cord edema or disruption of autonomic pathways during surgery can cause a temporary loss of bladder tone (Bader & Littlejohns, 2004; Bhardwaj, Mirski, & Ulatowski, 2004; Hickey, 2009).
3. If possible, stand a male client 8–12 hours after surgery to void (mobilize as soon as possible either by nursing staff or physical therapy) (Bader & Littlejohns, 2004).	3. Urinary retention, especially when client lies flat, may be due to difficulty voiding in a horizontal position, the depressant effects of perioperative drugs, or sympathetic fiber stimulation during surgery (Hickey, 2009).
4. Monitor bowel function: 　a. Bowel sounds in all quadrants returning within 24 hours of surgery 　b. Flatus and defecation resuming by the second or third postoperative day	4. Surgery on the lumbosacral spine decreases innervation of the bowels, reducing peristalsis and possibly leading to transient paralytic ileus.
5. Monitor for signs and symptoms of cerebrospinal fistula: 　a. Clear or pink ring around bloody drainage 　b. Positive glucose test of drainage 　c. Severe headache, which becomes worse when sitting up and gets better while lying down, light sensitivity, nausea, and complaints of neck stiffness	5. Incomplete closure of the dura causes CSF drainage. Glucose is present in CSF, but not in normal wound drainage. Changes in CSF volume cause headache.
6. Monitor and report incisional dressing for drainage. Note color, consistency, odor, and amount and notate if erythema or edema is present. If incision appears to be unapproximated, suspect wound dehiscence. Report immediately.	6. Drainage should be minimal and if drainage does occur, suspect cerebrospinal fluid leakage.
7. If the client smokes, advise him or her of increased risks. Discuss the possibility of quitting or cutting back.	7. Smokers are at risk for postoperative cardiopulmonary complications and risk of developing pseudoarthrosis or delayed healing.
8. Monitor output from drains. Expect minimal to approximately 200 mL/12 hours and notify surgeon if output exceeds 200 mL/12 hours.	8. Hypovolemia can cause decreased cardiac output.
9. Monitor for and report the following: 　a. Restlessness, confusion, apprehension, tachypnea 　b. Progressive weakness of lower extremities 　c. Increased numbness and tingling in limbs (Bhardwaj, Mirski, & Ulatowski, 2004) 　d. Decreased sensitivity, inability to perform neurologic exam or deviation from last neurologic exam	9a. Symptoms of fat embolism can occur during surgery or 72 hours postoperatively. 　b. Surgical trauma, hematoma formation, or vascular injury can cause cauda equina syndrome.

Related Physician / NP Prescribed Interventions

Medications

Analgesics, corticosteroids, muscle relaxants, narcotics

Intravenous Therapy

Refer to the General Surgery Care Plan

Laboratory Studies

Refer to the General Surgery Care Plan

Diagnostic Studies

CT scan, spinal x-ray film, myelography, MRI of lumbar spine, electromyelography

Therapies

Physical therapy, brace, refer to the General Surgery Care Plan

Documentation

Vital signs (hemodynamics, neurologic, and neurovascular)
Intake and output (strict)
Circulation (color, peripheral pulses)
Neurologic sensory and motor status (reflexes, sensory, and motor function)
Bowel function (bowel sounds, defecation)
Wound condition (color, drainage, swelling, amount of drainage, if any)
Changes in status
Worsening pain

Postoperative: Nursing Diagnoses

Acute Pain Related to Muscle Spasms (Back or Thigh) Secondary to Nerve Irritation During Surgery, Edema, Skeletal Misalignment, or Bladder Distention

NOC

Comfort Level, Pain Control

Goal

The client will report progressive pain reduction and / or alleviation after pain-relief interventions.

NIC

Pain Management, Medication Management, Emotional Support, Teaching: Individual, Heat / Cold Application, Simple Massage

Indicators

- Describe and / or demonstrate pharmacologic and nonpharmacologic techniques to reduce pain
- Report movements to avoid, ensuring that the client and family understand the limitations and expectations required postsurgery.

Interventions	Rationales
1. Explain to client that muscle spasms and paresthesias commonly occur after surgery.	1. Surgical trauma and edema cause pain and muscle spasms. Spasms may begin on the third or fourth postoperative day. Postoperative paresthesias in the affected leg and back may result from impaired neural function due to edema. As edema subsides, normal sensation should return.
2. Teach the importance of complying with the brace regimen.	2. Wearing a brace can prevent future hardware failure and pseudoarthrosis.
3. Evaluate if brace fits properly and is correctly aligned,	3. Mobilizing devices can cause sustained pressure on tissues leading to ischemia and tissue necrosis.

(continued)

Interventions	Rationales
4. Teach the client the importance of evaluating skin for pressure areas.	4. Low pressure for long periods can cause damage and may not be noticed by the client.
5. Teach the client to use arms and legs to transfer weight properly when getting out of bed.	5. Using the stronger muscles of the arms and legs can reduce strain on the back.
6. Encourage walking, standing, and sitting for short periods from the first postoperative day or as soon as possible after surgery, ensuring that client understands that the nurse or physiotherapist will ambulate him or her the first time and continue to do so until he or she is deemed at low risk for falls (Bader & Littlejohns, 2004; Bhardwaj, Mirski, & Ulatowski, 2004). Assess carefully in the first few days after surgery to ensure proper use of body mechanics and to detect any gait or posture problems.	6. Activity goals depend on the client's pain level and functional ability. Gait or posture problems can contribute to pain on walking, standing, or sitting. Ensure that client is wearing brace, if prescribed.
7. Teach the client the following precautions to maintain proper body alignment: a. Use the log-rolling technique to turn and reposition in bed. (Refer to the nursing diagnosis Risk for Injury in this care plan for details.) b. Avoid stress or strain on the operative site. c. Use the side-lying position in bed with the legs bent up evenly and the abdomen and back supported by pillows. d. Teach the client to keep her or his spine straight and when on side to place a pillow between the legs. Place pillow to support upper arm as well and to prevent the shoulder from sagging. e. Sit with knees higher than hips. f. When standing, regularly shift weight bearing from one foot to the other.	7. Proper body alignment avoids tension on the operative site and reduces spasms. Techniques are taught to keep the lower spine as flat as possible and prevent twisting, flexing, or hyperextending.
8. Ask the client to rate pain from 0 to 10 before and after medication administration. Consult with the physician / NP or advanced practice nurse if relief is unsatisfactory. Also, be sure to observe for visual cues and facial expressions showing that the client appears to be in pain.	8. An objective rating scale can help to evaluate the subjective experience of pain.
9. Refer to the General Surgery Care Plan for general pain-relief techniques.	

Documentation

Type, dose, route, frequency of all medications
Pain scale reassessment (30 minutes after narcotics have been administered, reassess pain level and 1 hour for all others)
Activity level
Client's response to pain medication

Risk for Falls related to neurocognition, decreased sensory in lower extremities, and the use of narcotics, opiates, psychotropics, or diuretics

NOC

Balance, Body Mechanics Performance, Fall Prevention Behavior, Knowledge: Fall Prevention, Knowledge: Medication, Knowledge: Personal Safety, Medication Response, Sensory Function Status

Goals

The client will practice all safety interventions during his or her stay.
The client will remain free from falls.

NIC

Analgesic Administration, Environmental Management: Safety, Fall Prevention, Health Education

Indicators

- State why safety precautions are still needed.
- State all necessary restrictions.
- State possible side effects of medication regimen.

Interventions	Rationales
1. The nurse will educate the client on all safety precautions, including use of the call bell for assistance out of bed and the use of yellow fall-risk bracelets and yellow nonskid socks.	1. The combined use of a yellow fall-risk bracelet and yellow nonskid socks increases safety of the client by allowing for a visual identifier for at-risk clients.
2. Orient client to environment and ensure all proper safety interventions are in place (call bell in working order and at client's bedside, bed in the lowest position and the brakes locked, side rails × 2 up).	2. Client orientation to room, unit, and surroundings alleviates perceived fear and anxiety. Education regarding safety techniques helps to ensure that client is aware of safety hazards and is properly instructed on safety interventions, such as the call bell.
3. The nurse will educate client on potential side effects from medication regimen and focus on the possible risks for falls associated with the medication use.	3. The use of certain medications, such as narcotics, opiates, psychotropics, and diuretics have the ability to contribute to possible weakness, balance problems, confusion, and gait disturbances.

Documentation

Fall Risk Score
Medication Administration Record:
    The use of narcotics, opiates, psychotropics, or diuretics
Safety Interventions
Hourly Rounding

> **TRANSITION TO HOME/COMMUNITY CARE**
> If indicated, review the risk diagnoses identified for this individual on admission:
> - Is the person still at risk?
> - Can the family reduce the risks?
> - Is the person at higher risk at home?
> - Is a Home Health Nurse assessment needed?
> - Refer to transition planner / case manager / social service.
> - When is this person scheduled for follow-up with primary provider? Specialists? Record dates of appointments.
> - Complete a medication reconciliation prior to transition. Refer to index.

STAR

Stop

Think Is this person at risk for injury, falls, medical complications, and / or inability to care for self (activities of daily living)?

Is there a support person available?

Is the person competent to manage self-administration of medications, treatment procedures? Are additional resources needed?

Can the person explain how to monitor the condition (e.g., blood glucose, signs / symptoms of complications, dietary / mobility restrictions, and when to call his or her primary provider or specialist)?

Act Contact or provide the appropriate resource (e.g., contacting a support person, home health assessment, additional teaching, printed materials).

Review Has the problem been addressed? If not, use SBAR to communicate to the appropriate person.

Risk for Ineffective Self-Health Management Related to Insufficient Knowledge of Home Care, Activity Restrictions, and Exercise Program

NIC

Anticipatory Guidance, Learning Facilitation, Risk Management, Health Education, Teaching: Procedure / Treatment, Health System Guidance

Goals

The goals for this diagnosis represent those associated with transition planning. Refer to the transition criteria.

Interventions	Rationales
1. Explain the rationale for activity restrictions and for gradual activity progression as tolerance increases.	1. Activity restrictions allow the spinal supporting structures time to heal. Complete healing of ligaments and muscles takes approximately 6 weeks.
2. Teach the client to avoid the following: a. Prolonged sitting b. Twisting the spine c. Bending at the waist d. Climbing stairs e. Long automobile trips	2. These activities increase spinal flexion and create tension at the surgical site.
3. Teach the client the proper use of a back brace, if indicated.	3. A brace may be indicated to stabilize the spine and reduce pain; instruction in proper use is necessary.
4. Explain the importance of following a regular exercise program after recovery.	4. Regular, safe exercise increases spinal muscle strength and flexibility, helping protect against future injury.

Interventions	Rationales
5. Encourage the use of heat on the operative area, as indicated.	5. Heat increases circulation to the operative site; this promotes healing and removal of wound exudate.
6. Teach the client postlaminectomy recovery precautions, such as the following: a. Sleeping on a firm mattress b. Maintaining proper body mechanics c. Wearing only moderately high-heeled shoes d. Avoiding lifting objects over 10 lb e. Sitting in a straight-backed chair with feet on a stool and knees flexed slightly higher than the hips f. For at least 3 weeks postsurgery, limit sitting time to 15–20 minutes	6. Techniques that reduce stress and strain on the lumbosacral spine can decrease spasms and help to prevent other disk herniation.
7. As appropriate, explain the connection between obesity and lower back problems; encourage weight loss.	7. Excess weight, particularly in the abdomen, strains and stretches muscles that support the spine, predisposing the client to spinal injury. Explaining these effects may encourage the client to lose weight.
8. Explain that normal neurologic status may not return immediately.	8. Irritation of the nerve root during surgery may increase deficits temporarily (Hickey, 2002; Bhardwaj, Mirski, & Ulatowski, 2004).
9. Teach the client and family to report the following: a. Change in mobility, sensation, color, or pain in extremities b. Increased pain at the operative site c. Persistent headaches d. Elevated temperature e. Change in bowel or bladder function f. Drainage at incision site	9. Early detection and reporting enable prompt intervention to prevent or minimize serious complications such as infection (marked by headache, fever, and increased pain) and cord compression (indicated by changes in bowel and bladder functions, movement, and sensation).

Clinical Alert Report

Prior to providing care, advise ancillary staff / student to report the following to the professional nurse assigned to the client:
- Vital signs (heart rate, temperature, respirations, and blood pressure)
- Intake and output
- Drain output
- Change in level of consciousness, decreased sensation in lower extremities, or any neurologic changes
- Complaints of pain or discomfort

Documentation

Client and family teaching, including the understanding of the teaching from both client and family (Lewis et al., 2004).

Nephrectomy

Nephrectomy is the surgical procedure of removing a kidney or a section of a kidney. A nephrectomy is performed on clients with cancer of the kidney (renal cell carcinoma); a disease in which cysts (sac-like structures) displace healthy kidney tissue (polycystic kidney disease); massive trauma to the kidney, serious kidney infections, and renal failure. It is also used to remove a healthy kidney from a donor for the purposes of kidney transplantation (National Kidney Foundation, 2007; Parekattil et al., 2005).

The removal of the kidney can be classified in various ways: a *simple nephrectomy* is the removal of the kidney while a *radical nephrectomy* is removal of the kidney and possibly the surrounding perinephritic fat, Gerota's fascia, and lymph nodes. Laparoscopic techniques are also utilized for *partial nephrectomies*, which are referred to as a nephron-sparing nephrectomy (Mattar & Finelli, 2007; Parekattil et al., 2005).

 Time Frame
Preoperative and postoperative periods

▪▪▪▪▪ DIAGNOSTIC CLUSTER

Preoperative Period

Collaborative Problems

▲ Risk for Complications of Hemorrhage / Shock

▲ Risk for Complications of Paralytic Ileus

▲ Risk for Complications of Renal Insufficiency

△ Risk for Complications of Pyelonephritis

△ Risk for Complications of Pneumothorax Secondary to Thoracic Approach Thoracic Surgery

Nursing Diagnoses

▲ Risk for Ineffective Self-Health Management related to insufficient knowledge of hydration requirements, nephrostomy care, and signs and symptoms of complications

△ Acute Pain related to distention of renal capsule and incision (refer to General Surgery)

▲ Risk for Ineffective Respiratory Function related to pain on breathing and coughing secondary to location of incision (refer to General Surgery)

Related Care Plans

General Surgery Generic Care Plan

Cancer (Initial Diagnosis)

▲ This diagnosis was reported to be monitored for or managed frequently (75% to 100%).
△ This diagnosis was reported to be monitored for or managed often (50% to 74%).

Transitional Criteria

Before discharge, the client and family will:

1. Demonstrate nephrostomy tube care.
2. State measures for at-home wound care.
3. Share feelings regarding loss of kidney.
4. State signs and symptoms that must be reported to a health-care professional.
5. Explain the difference between incisional pain and the pain of infection.

> ### Transitional Risk Assessment Plan (TRAP)
>
> Begin this plan on admission.
>
> Implement the Transitional Risk Assessment Plan (TRAP):
>
> - Refer to inside back cover.
> - Add each validated risk diagnosis to client's problem list with the risk code in ( ).
> - Refer to Unit II to the individual risk nursing diagnoses / collaborative problems for outcomes and interventions.
>
>   *R:* *"Close coordination of care in the post-acute period, early transition follow-up care, enhanced client education and self-management training, proactive end-of-life counseling, and extending the resources and clinical expertise over time via multidisciplinary team management" can lower readmission rates and improve health outcomes (Boutwell & Hwu, 2009, p. 14).*

Postoperative: Collaborative Problems

Risk for Complications of Hemorrhage / Shock

Risk for Complications of Paralytic Ileus

Risk for Complications of Renal Insufficiency

Risk for Complications of Pyelonephritis

Collaborative Outcomes

The client will be monitored for early signs and symptoms of (a) hemorrhage / shock, (b) paralytic ileus, (c) renal insufficiency (partial nephrectomy), and (d) pyelonephritis (partial nephrectomy), and will receive collaborative interventions if indicated to restore physiologic stability.

Indicators of Physiologic Stability

- Calm, oriented, alert (a)
- Pulse 60–100 beats/min (a)
- Respirations 16–20 breaths/min (a)
- BP >90/60, <120–129/80–84 mm Hg (a) (JNC, 2007)
- No chills (d)
- Temperature 98.5°–99° F (d)
- Urine specific gravity 1.005–1.030 (c, d)
- Urine output >0.5 mL/h (a, c, d)
- Full peripheral pulses (a)
- Capillary refill <3 seconds (a)
- Dry, warm skin (a)
- Hemoglobin (a)
    - Male 13–18 g/dL
    - Female 12–16 g/dL
- Hematocrit (a)
    - Male 42% to 50%
    - Female 40% to 48%
- Bowel sounds present all quadrants (b)
- No abdominal distention (b)
- White blood cells 5,000–10,000/mm³ (d)
- Urine sodium 130–200 mEq/24 h (c)
- Blood urea nitrogen 10–20 mg/dL (c)
- Potassium 3.8–5 mEq/L (c)
- Serum sodium 135–145 mEq/L (c)
- Phosphorus 2.5–4.5 mg/dL (c)
- Creatinine clearance 100–150 mL of blood cleared per mm (c)

- No costovertebral angle (CVA) tenderness (d)
- Urine negative bacteria (d)
- No complaints of dysuria or frequency (d)
- No bladder distention (d)

 Carp's Cues

Please refer to the Generic Care Plan for the Surgical Client for detailed interventions for managing all surgical conditions. This care plan addresses specific additional interventions associated with the type of surgery performed.

Interventions	*Rationales*
1. Monitor for signs and symptoms of hemorrhage / shock every hour for the first 24 hours, then every 4 hours: a. Increasing pulse rate with normal or slightly decreased blood pressure b. Decreased oxygen saturation (pulse oximetry) <94% c. Urine output <0.5 mL/kg/h (normal value for urine output is 0.5 to 1.0 mL/kg/h) (Wagner, Johnson, & Kidd, 2006, p. 228) d. Restlessness, agitation, change in mentation e. Increasing respiratory rate f. Diminished peripheral pulses g. Cool, pale, or cyanotic skin h. Thirst	1. Because the renal capsule is very vascular, massive blood loss can occur. The compensatory response to decreased circulatory volume is to increase blood oxygen by increasing the heart and respiratory rates and decreasing circulation to extremities (manifested by decreased pulses and cool skin). Diminished cerebral oxygenation can cause changes in mentation. Decreased oxygen to kidneys results in decreased urine output.
2. Monitor fluid status hourly: Accurate daily assessment of body weight is more reliable in measuring fluid loss than intake-vs-output, because it accounts for water loss during fever, diaphoresis, and respiration: 1 L (1,000 mL) of water weighs 1 kg or 2.2 lb (Wagner, Johnson, & Kidd, 2006). a. Intake (parenteral, oral) b. Output and loss (urinary, drainage, vomiting) c. Weigh daily at same time in same clothes, if needed.	2. Fluid loss due to surgery and nothing-by-mouth (NPO) status can disrupt fluid balance in some clients. Stress can produce sodium and water retention.
3. Monitor surgical site for bleeding, dehiscence, and evisceration.	3. Frequent monitoring enables early detection of complications. Hypotension and vasospasm during surgery can cause temporary hemostasis and can result in delayed bleeding.
4. Teach the client to splint the incision site with a pillow when coughing and deep breathing (to decrease / prevent occurrences of postoperative pneumonia secondary to the inability to breathe deeply due to pain).	4. Splinting reduces stress on suture lines by equalizing the pressure across the incision site.
5. Monitor for signs and symptoms of paralytic ileus: a. Decreased or absent bowel sounds b. Abdominal distention c. Abdominal discomfort 6. Do not initiate fluids until bowel sounds are present. Begin with small amounts. Note the client's response and the type and amount of emesis, if any.	5, 6. Reflex paralysis of intestinal peristalsis and manipulation of the colon to gain access place the client at risk for ileus. The depressive effects of narcotics, and anesthetics on peristalsis, as well as the handling of the bowel during surgery, can also cause paralytic ileus. Ileus can occur between the third and fifth postoperative day. Pain can be localized, sharp, and intermittent (Wagner, Johnson, & Kidd, 2006, pp. 722–723).

Interventions	Rationales
7. Monitor for early signs and symptoms of renal insufficiency:	7. Renal insufficiency can result from edema caused by surgical manipulation (partial nephrectomy) or by a nonpatent nephrostomy tube.
a. Sustained elevated urine specific gravity b. Elevated urine sodium level	a, b. Ability of renal tubules to reabsorb electrolytes results in increased urine sodium levels and urine specific gravity.
c. Sustained insufficient urine output (<30 mL/h) d. Elevated blood pressure	c, d. Decreased glomerular filtration rate eventually leads to insufficient urine output and increased renin production, resulting in elevated blood pressure in the body's attempt to increase renal blood flow.
e. Elevated BUN and serum creatinine, potassium, phosphorus, and ammonia; decreased creatinine clearance	e. These changes result from decreased excretion of urea and creatinine in urine.

> **CLINICAL ALERT**
> • Report signs of renal insufficiency.

8. Monitor the client for signs and symptoms of infection:	8. Microorganisms can be introduced into the body during surgery or through the incision. Urinary tract infections can be caused by urinary stasis (e.g., from a nonpatent nephrostomy tube) or by irritation of tissue by calculi.
a. Chills and fever	a. Endogenous pyrogens are released and they reset the hypothalamic setpoint to febrile levels. The body temperature is sensed as "too cool"; shivering and vasoconstriction result, to generate and consume heat. The core temperature rises to the new setpoint level, resulting in fever. The leukocytes (WBCs) are the circulating cells of the immune system; although their quantities are limited, they are an extremely quick and powerful defense system and respond immediately to foreign invaders by going to the site of involvement (Kee, 2004, p. 352; Wagner, Johnson, & Kidd, 2006, p. 524). Wound redness, tenderness, and edema result from lymphocyte migration to the area (Wagner, Johnson, & Kidd, 2006, p. 802).
b. Change in the type of pain	b. The literature states that a client may experience considerable discomfort in the area around the incision and may need to be taught the difference between incisional pain and infection pain. Incisional pain will decrease each day while infection pain will increase and is usually accompanied by fever (Kok, Alwayn, Tran, Hop, Weimar, & Ijzermans, 2006).
c. Costovertebral angle (CVA) pain (a dull, constant backache below the 12th rib)	c. CVA pain results from distention of the renal capsule.
d. Leukocytosis	d. Leukocytosis reflects an increase in WBCs to fight infection through phagocytosis.
e. Bacteria and pus in urine	e. Bacteria and pus in urine indicate a urinary tract infection.
f. Dysuria and frequency	f. Bacteria irritate bladder tissue, causing spasms, and frequency.

9. Monitor for signs of urinary retention: a. Bladder distention b. Urine overflow (30–60 mL of urine every 15–30 minutes)	9. Trauma to the detrusor muscle and injury to the pelvic nerves during surgery can inhibit bladder function. Anxiety and pain can cause spasms of the reflex sphincters. Bladder neck edema can also cause retention. Sedatives and narcotics can affect the central nervous system and the effectiveness of the smooth muscles (Gillenwater et al., 1996).

(continued)

Interventions	Rationales
10. Instruct the client to report bladder discomfort or inability to void.	10. Overdistention of the bladder can aggravate a client's ability to empty the bladder (Gillenwater et al., 1996).

Clinical Alert Report

Prior to providing care, advise ancillary staff / student to report the following to the professional nurse assigned to the client:

- Please add data that need to be reported for the collaborative problems. Most often this is applicable to physiologic problems such as significant change in vital signs, change in cognition, skin, new onset of pain, etc.

Related Physician / NP Prescribed Interventions

Refer to the Surgical Client Care Plan.

Documentation

Vital signs
Circulatory status
Intake (oral, parenteral)
Output (urinary drainage color, clarity, sediment, drainage tubes)
Bowel function (bowel sounds, defecation pattern, abdominal distention)
Wound status (color, drainage, pain around incision, tenderness)

TRANSITION TO HOME/COMMUNITY CARE

If indicated, review the risk diagnoses identified for this individual on admission:

- Is the person still at risk?
- Can the family reduce the risks?
- Is the person at higher risk at home?
- Is a Home Health Nurse assessment needed?
- Refer to transition planner / case manager / social service.
- When is this person scheduled for follow-up with primary provider? Specialists? Record dates of appointments.
- Complete a medication reconciliation prior to transition. Refer to index.

STAR

Stop

Think   Is this person at risk for injury, falls, medical complications, and / or inability to care for self (activities of daily living)?

Is there a support person available?

Is the person competent to manage self-administration of medications, treatment procedures? Are additional resources needed?

Can the person explain how to monitor the condition (e.g., blood glucose, signs / symptoms of complications, dietary / mobility restrictions, and when to call his or her primary provider or specialist)?

Act   Contact or provide the appropriate resource (e.g., contacting a support person, home health assessment, additional teaching, printed materials).

Review   Has the problem been addressed? If not, use SBAR to communicate to the appropriate person.

Postoperative: Nursing Diagnosis

Risk for Ineffective Therapeutic Regimen Self-Health Management Related to Insufficient Knowledge of Hydration Requirements, Nephrostomy Care, and Signs and Symptoms of Complications

NIC
Anticipatory Guidance,
Risk Identification,
Health Education,
Learning Facilitation

Goals

The goals for this diagnosis represent those associated with discharge planning. Refer to the discharge criteria.

Interventions	Rationales
1. Explain the need to maintain optimal hydration.	1. Optimal hydration reduces urinary stasis, decreasing the risk of infection and calculi formation.
2. Teach and have the client perform a return demonstration of nephrostomy care measures, including: a. Aseptic technique b. Skin care c. Tube stabilization	2. Proper techniques can reduce the risk of infection. Movement of the tube can cause dislodgement or tissue trauma.
3. Teach the client to use pillows to support the back when lying on side.	3. Certain positions will decrease tension on the incisional area.
4. Explain why the pain is severe, as well as other discomforts. Teach the client to avoid lifting any weight more than 10 lb for 6 weeks.	4. The client's position and the incision's size cause severe pain. The client's position on the operating room table will cause muscular aches and pains.
5. Teach the client to report the following: a. Decreased urine output b. Fever or malaise c. Purulent, cloudy drainage from or around the tube	5. Early detection enables prompt intervention to prevent serious complications such as renal insufficiency and infection.
6. Refer the client and family to a home health-care agency for follow-up care.	6. A home care nurse evaluates the client's ability for home care and provides periodic assessment of renal function and development of infection.

Documentation

Discharge summary record
Client and family teaching, and clarification of understanding towards education
Outcome achievement or status
Referrals

Radical Prostatectomy

Radical prostatectomy is the surgical removal of the prostate gland, ejaculatory ducts, seminal vesicles, some pelvic fasciae, and sometimes the pelvic lymph nodes due to cancer of the prostate (James, 2007). The procedure takes about 3 to 4 hours. There are three generations of radical prostate surgery: open, laparoscopic, and robot assisted. The open approach can be performed via a perineal, suprapubic, or retropubic incision. Laparoscopic surgery involves smaller incisions and the use of a scope, but the equipment is difficult to manipulate accurately. Robot-assisted laparoscopic approaches provide improved dexterity for surgeons (Rigdon, 2006). Forty percent of laparoscopic approaches are now robot assisted, also known as the da Vinci Surgical System, allowing nerve-sparing outcomes and reducing complications, blood loss, and surgical time (Challacombe & Dasgupta, 2007; Starnes & Sims, 2006; Tewari, Peabody, Sarle, Balakrishnan, Hemal, Shrivastava, et al., 2002; Vattikuti Urology Institute, 2007).

 Time Frame
Postoperative periods

▪▪▪▪▪▪ DIAGNOSTIC CLUSTER

Collaborative Problems

▲ Risk for Complications of Hemorrhage

▲ Risk for Complications of Clot Formation

△ Risk for Complications of Thrombophlebitis

Nursing Diagnoses

▲ Acute Pain related to bladder spasms; clot retention; and back, leg, and incisional pain

△ Risk for Ineffective Sexuality Patterns related to fear of impotence resulting from surgical intervention

▲ Risk for Ineffective Therapeutic Regimen Management related to insufficient knowledge of fluid restrictions, catheter care, activity restrictions, urinary control, and signs and symptoms of complications

Related Care Plan

General Surgery Generic Care Plan

▲This diagnosis was reported to be monitored for or managed frequently (75% to 100%).
△ This diagnosis was reported to be monitored for or managed often (50% to 74%).

Transitional Criteria

Before transition, the client and family will:

1. Identify the need for increased oral fluid intake.
2. Demonstrate care of the indwelling (Foley) catheter.
3. Demonstrate wound care for home care
4. Verbalize necessary precautions for activity and urination.
5. State the signs and symptoms that must be reported to a health-care professional.
6. Verbalize an intent to share feelings and concerns related to sexual function with significant others.

Transitional Risk Assessment Plan (TRAP)

Begin this plan on admission.
Implement the Transitional Risk Assessment Plan (TRAP):
- Refer to inside back cover.
- Add each validated risk diagnosis to client's problem list with the risk code in ( ).
- Refer to Unit II to the individual risk nursing diagnoses / collaborative problems for outcomes and interventions.

R: "Close coordination of care in the post-acute period, early transition follow-up care, enhanced client education and self-management training, proactive end-of-life counseling, and extending the resources and clinical expertise over time via multidisciplinary team management" can lower readmission rates and improve health outcomes (Boutwell & Hwu, 2009, p. 14).

Postoperative: Collaborative Problems

Risk for Complications of Hemorrhage

Risk for Complications of Clot Formation

Risk for Complications of Urinary Leak from Anastomosis Site

Risk for Complications of Thrombophlebitis (refer to Generic Surgical Care Plan)

Collaborative Outcomes

The client will be monitored for early signs and symptoms of (a) hemorrhage, (b) clot formation, (c) urinary retention, and (d) urinary leak at anastomosis site, and will receive collaborative interventions if indicated to restore physiologic stability.

Indicators of Physiologic Stability

- Calm, oriented, alert (a)
- Pulse 60–100 beats/min (a)
- Respirations 16–20 breaths/min (a)
- BP >90/60, <140–90 mm Hg (a)
- Temperature 98°–99.5° F
- Urine output >0.5 mL/h (a,)
- Pink or clear red urine in the first 24 h (a)
- Amber pink urine after 24 h (a)
- Warm, dry skin (a)
- Hemoglobin (a) Male 13–18 g/dL, Female 12–16 g/dL
- Hematocrit (a) Male 42% to 50%, Female 40% to 48%
- Continuous flowing bladder irrigation (b, c)
- No bladder distention (c)
- No increase in drainage from JP drain (d)

Carp's Cues

Please refer to the Generic Care Plan for the Surgical Client for detailed interventions for managing all surgical conditions. This care plan addresses specific additional interventions associated with the type of surgery performed.

Interventions	Rationales

1. Monitor for signs and symptoms of hemorrhage:
  a. Abnormal urine characteristics (e.g., highly viscous, clots, bright red, or burgundy color)
  b. Increased pulse rate
  c. Urine output <30 mL/h
  d. Restlessness, agitation
  e. Cool, pale, or cyanotic skin
  f. Hemoglobin and hematocrit values
	1. The prostate gland is highly vascular, receiving its blood supply from the internal iliac artery. Elderly clients and those who have had prolonged urinary retention are vulnerable to rapid changes in bladder contents and fluid volume. During the first 24 hours after surgery, urine should be pink or clear red, gradually becoming amber to pink-tinged by the fourth day. Bright red urine with clots indicates arterial bleeding. Burgundy-colored urine indicates venous bleeding, which usually resolves spontaneously. Clots are expected; their absence may point to blood dyscrasias. Hemoglobin and hematocrit values decline if significant postoperative bleeding occurs (Kantaff, Carroll, D'Amico, Isaacs, Ross, & Scherett, 2001; Porth, 2011).

(continued)

Interventions	*Rationales*

2. Monitor dressings, catheters, and drains that vary depending on the type of surgery performed:
  a. Suprapubic approach:
    • Urethral catheter
    • Suprapubic tube
    • Abdominal drain
  b. Retropubic approach:
    • Urethral catheter
    • Abdominal drain
  c. Perineal approach:
    • Urethral catheter
    • Perineal drain
	2. Heavy venous bleeding is expected the first 24 hours for all approaches except the perineal approach. Blood loss can occur from the catheter or incision (Kantaff et al., 2001).

3. Instruct the client to do the following:
  a. Avoid straining for bowel elimination.
  b. Do not sit in a firm, upright chair.
  c. Recline slightly while on the toilet.
	3. Increased pressure on the rectum can trigger bleeding and perforated rectal tissue.

4. Provide bladder irrigation as prescribed; maintain aseptic technique:
  a. Continuous (closed)
  b. Manual: Using a bulb syringe, irrigate the catheter with 30–60 mL normal saline solution every 3–4 hours, as needed.
	4. Continuous bladder irrigation with normal saline dilutes blood in the urine to prevent clot formation. Manual irrigation provides the negative pressure needed to remove obstructive clots or tissue particles.

5. Ensure adequate fluid intake (oral, parenteral).	5. Optimal hydration dilutes urine and prevents clot formation.
6. Monitor for urine leak from anastomosis site (Starnes & Sims, 2006): a. High-volume Jackson-Pratt (JP) drain output **CLINICAL ALERT** • Consult with an experienced nurse to define expected drainage amounts.	6a. A JP drain is placed at the anastomosis site between the bladder neck and urethra. If hemostasis is disrupted , urine can leak into the site and drain. Increased wound drainage may suggest a urine leak, lymph leak, or pelvic bleeding (Rigdon, 2006).
7. Notify surgeon of possible urine leak for assessment (e.g., testing the drainage fluid for the presence of creatinine, cystogram) and treatment (e.g., urinary catheter is placed on traction).	7. Traction will allow the leak site to heal. If drainage fluid is positive for creatinine, a leak is confirmed. Cystogram can confirm the location and extent of leak (Starnes & Sims, 2006).

Clinical Alert Report

Prior to providing care, advise ancillary staff / student to report the following to the professional nurse assigned to the client:
- Change in cognitive status
- Oral temperature >100.5° F
- Systolic BP <90 mm/Hg
- Resting pulse >100, <50
- Respiratory rate >28, <10 /min.
- Oxygen saturation <90%
- Increase in drainage
- Decreased urine output
- New onset bloody urine
- New c/o of leg pain

Related Physician / NP Prescribed Interventions

Medications

Antispasmodics (oral: oxybutynin, belladonna; suppository: belladonna & opium [B&O]); analgesics; antibiotics (Rigdon, 2006)

Intravenous Therapy

Refer to the General Surgery Care Plan, prostatic fluid, cytology, urine cytology

Laboratory Studies

CBC, PTT, BC, magnesium, electrolytes, prostate-specific antigen (PSA), urine culture, serum prostatic acid phosphatase level

Diagnostic Studies

Cystourethroscopy, bone scans, prostatic biopsy, transrectal ultrasound, CT, flow cytometry, MRI (abdomen, pelvis), voiding cystourethrogram

Therapies

Indwelling catheterization, wound drains, catheter traction, bladder irrigation (manual or continuous), radiotherapy, sitz baths, endocrine manipulation, sequential compression stocking device, chemotherapy, nasogastric tube

Documentation

Vital signs
Intake and output
Urine (color, viscosity, presence of clots)
Drains
Continuous irrigations / manual irrigations (times, amounts)

Postoperative Nursing Diagnoses

Acute Pain Related to Bladder Spasms; Clot Retention; and Back, Leg, and Incisional Pain

NOC

Comfort Level, Pain Control

Goal

The client will report decreased pain after pain relief interventions.

NIC

Pain Management, Medication Management, Emotional Support, Teaching: Individual, Heat / Cold Application, Simple Massage

Indicators

- Can do leg exercises.
- Increase activity progressively.

Interventions	Rationales
1. Monitor for intermittent suprapubic pain: bladder spasms, burning sensation at the tip of the penis.	1. Irritation from an indwelling catheter can cause bladder spasms and pain in the penis.
2. Monitor for persistent suprapubic pain: bladder distention with sensations of fullness and tightness, inability to void.	2. Catheter obstruction can cause urinary retention, leading to increased bladder spasms and increased risk of infection.
3. Monitor for lower back and leg pain. Provide gentle massage to the back, and heat to the legs, if necessary.	3. During surgery, the client lies in the lithotomy position that can stretch and aggravate muscles that normally may be underused.

(continued)

Interventions	Rationales
4. Anchor the catheter to the leg with a catheter leg strap.	4. Pressure from a dangling catheter can damage the urinary sphincter, resulting in urinary incontinence after catheter removal. Catheter movement also increases the likelihood of bladder spasms.
5. Monitor for testicular pain.	5. Clipping the vas deferens causes congestion of seminal fluid and blood. This congestion takes several weeks to resolve.
6. Administer medication, as ordered, for pain and spasms.	6. Antispasmodic medications (e.g., opioid and belladonna suppositories) prevent bladder spasms. Analgesic medications diminishes the incisional pain.
7. Encourage adequate oral fluid intake (at least 2,000 mL/day, unless contraindicated).	7. Adequate hydration dilutes urine that helps to flush out clots.
8. Manually irrigate the indwelling catheter only when prescribed.	8. Each time the closed system is opened for manual irrigation, risk of bacterial contamination increases.
9. Monitor output of wound drains (Rigdon, 2006).	
10. Refer to Generic Surgical Care Plan for pain management strategies	

Documentation

Type, dose, route of all medications
Complaints of pain (type, site, duration)
Unsatisfactory pain relief

Risk for Ineffective Sexuality Patterns Related to Fear of Impotence Resulting From Surgical Intervention

NOC
Body Image, Self-Esteem, Role Performance, Sexual Identity: Acceptance

Goals

The client will discuss his feelings and concerns regarding the effects of surgery on sexuality and sexual functioning.

NIC
Behavior Management: Sexual, Sexual Counseling, Emotional Support, Active Listening, Teaching: Sexuality

Indicators

* Engages in discussions on fears and concern regarding sexual activity after discharge from hospital.
* Explains effects of surgery on sexual function and expected course of resolution.

Interventions	Rationales

CLINICAL ALERT
- Initially, incontinence will be the side effect that poses the most concern.
- As incontinence decreases; interest in resuming sexual activity increases.

1. Explain the effects of surgery on sexual function (orgasms, erections, fertility, ejaculations).	1. If one or both nerve bundles responsible for erections are spared during surgery, erections will return. Orgasms will occur without ejaculations. It may take more than a year after wound healing and all edema from surgery subsides for full function to return. Men older than 70 years probably will not regain erections; ejaculate will be reduced but will still contain sperm. Robot-assisted laparoscopic approaches report 90% return to good sexual function after surgery (Vattikuti Urology Institute, 2007).
2. Explore previous sexual function prior to surgery. Use familiar terms, when possible, and explain unfamiliar terms.	2. Previous patterns of functioning need to be considered as they do influence postsurgical functioning. Unfamiliar medical terminology may cause confusion and misunderstanding.
3. Explain that the surgeon's permission to resume sexual activity is needed. Clearly state that cancer of the prostate is not transmitted sexually.	3. Complete healing is needed to prevent bleeding and to resolve edema, which usually takes 6 weeks to 3 months.
4. Provide opportunities for the partner to share concerns and questions.	4. Partners are crucial to the recovery process. They manage their own anxiety and also assist their partner in managing his (Maliski, Heilemann, & McCorkle, 2001). Cultural and religious beliefs may affect the spouse's participation and queries (Sublett, 2007).
5. Encourage the client to continue to discuss concerns with significant others and professionals post discharge.	5. At some point post discharge, PDE5 inhibitors (e.g., sildenafil, tadalafil) may be prescribed to stimulate erections if not medically contraindicated.

Documentation

Expressed concerns
Client teaching

TRANSITION TO HOME/COMMUNITY CARE

If indicated, review the risk diagnoses identified for this individual on admission:
- Is the person still at risk?
- Can the family reduce the risks?
- Is the person at higher risk at home?
- Is a Home Health Nurse assessment needed?
- Refer to transition planner / case manager / social service.
- When is this person scheduled for follow-up with primary provider? Specialists? Record dates of appointments.
- Complete a medication reconciliation prior to transition. Refer to index.

STAR   **Stop**

Think   Is this person at risk for injury, falls, medical complications, and / or inability to care for self (activities of daily living)?

Is there a support person available?

Is the person competent to manage self-administration of medications, treatment procedures? Are additional resources needed?

Can the person explain how to monitor the condition (e.g., blood glucose, signs / symptoms of complications, dietary / mobility restrictions, and when to call his or her primary provider or specialist)?

Act	Contact or provide the appropriate resource (e.g., contacting a support person, home health assessment, additional teaching, printed materials).
Review	Has the problem been addressed? If not, use SBAR to communicate to the appropriate person.

Risk for Ineffective Self-Health Management Related to Insufficient Knowledge of Fluid Restrictions, Catheter Care, Activity Restrictions, Urinary Control, and Signs and Symptoms of Complications

NOC

Compliance Behavior, Knowledge: Treatment Regimen, Participation: Health-Care Decisions, Treatment Behavior: Illness or Injury

NIC

Anticipatory Guidance, Risk Identification, Health Education, Learning Facilitation

Goals

The goals for this diagnosis represent those associated with transition planning. Refer to the transition criteria.

Interventions	Rationales
1. Reinforce the need for adequate oral fluid intake (at least 2,000 mL/day, unless contraindicated).	1. Optimal hydration helps to reestablish bladder tone after catheter removal by stimulating voiding, diluting urine, and decreasing susceptibility to urinary tract infections and clot formation.
2. Explain that scrotal / penile swelling and bruising are normal and strategies to reduce symptoms (Starnes & Sims, 2006). a. Elevate scrotum with a small towel or washcloth when sitting or lying down. b. Wear supportive briefs or an athletic support.	2. Scrotal / penile swelling, resulting from trauma during surgery will resolve in 7–10 days.
3. Teach indwelling catheter care: a. Explain that the duration for needing the urinary catheter will be 7–10 days. b. Gently, wash the urinary meatus with soap and water twice a day. If it becomes irritated, apply antibiotic cream to the irritated area twice a day. c. Increase the frequency of cleansing if drainage is evident around the catheter insertion site. d. Instruct individual / family member on use of: • Leg collection bag: • Observe individual applying, removing, and connecting equipment. • Instruct to reposition every 4–6 hours • Urinary drainage bag: • Observe individual applying, changing, and connecting equipment. • Advise to use when frequent emptying of leg bag is not possible, care trip, nighttime. e. Always keep any type of collection bag below the level of the bladder.	3. The indwelling catheter provides a route for bacteria that are normally found on the urinary meatus to enter the urinary tract. These measures help to reduce risk of urinary tract infection. • Repositioning to other leg or lower or higher on the leg will prevent prolonged pressure to skin / tissues.

Interventions	Rationales
4. Instruct on care of pelvic drain at home, if needed.	4. This drain is usually removed the first day postoperatively; however, sometimes it is left in a week or more (University of Michigan Health System, 2007).
5. Reinforce activity restrictions that may include the following: a. Avoid straining with bowel movements; increase intake of dietary fiber or take stool softeners, if indicated. b. Do not use suppositories or enemas. c. Avoid sitting with legs dependent. d. Avoid heavy lifting and strenuous activity or sport for 4 weeks. e. Avoid sexual intercourse until the physician / NP advises otherwise.	5. These restrictions are necessary to reduce the risk of internal bleeding.
6. Advise that the client may do the following: a. Take long walks. b. Use stairs as tolerated. c. Drive 3 weeks after surgery if power steering is used.	6. These activities can stress the surgical site and impede healing of surgical site.
7. Explain that urinary continence will return in phases after the catheter is removed (University of Michigan Health System, 2007): Phase 1—You are dry when you are lying down at night. Phase 2—You have periods of good urinary control in the early morning. Phase 3—Urinary control lasts for longer intervals and later into the afternoon and evening. a. Dribbling, frequency, and urgency may occur initially, but will gradually subside over weeks.	7. Continence will return gradually in phases from anywhere to a few weeks to several months. Continence returns sooner after robotic surgery. Long-term incontinence occurs at a 1% to 3% rate (Starnes & Sims, 2006; Walsh et al., 2000). a. Difficulty resuming normal voiding patterns may be related to bladder neck trauma, urinary tract infection, or catheter irritation. While the indwelling catheter is in place, constant urine drainage decreases muscle control and increases flaccidity.
8. Teach exercises to strengthen perineal muscles: explain that when you tighten your pelvic muscles to stop the flow of urine or prevent the passing of gas, you are performing a Kegel exercise. a. Tighten and tense buttocks, hold for 10 seconds, then relax for 10 seconds; repeat 10 times. b. Tighten only the pelvic muscles; keep your abdominal, thigh, and buttock muscles relaxed. c. Do exercises frequently (6–12 times a day; 10 at a time). d. Advise that Kegel exercises can be performed while sitting or standing, anywhere and anytime.	8. Regular contracture of the sphincter muscles will strengthen the pelvic floor muscles and decrease incontinence in 4–6 weeks. Use of biofeedback or anal electrical stimulation may help prevent continued incontinence (Hunter, Moore, & Glazener, 2007).
9. Advise to: a. Avoid drinking fluids near bedtime b. Avoiding caffeine and alcohol can help to prevent problems. c. Wear a pants liner or diaper initially, if needed.	9b. Caffeine acts as a mild diuretic and makes it more difficult to control urine. Alcohol may increase the burning sensations on urination.

(continued)

Interventions	Rationales

10. Instruct to call 911 or to go to the nearest emergency room if (University of Michigan Health System [2007]:
    a. Any signs of pulmonary embolus (blood clot from pelvis that has gotten into the blood circulation of the lung)
    b. Sudden onset chest pain
    c. New onset of difficulty breathing or worsening of usual breathlessness
    d. Sensation of heart racing

> **CLINICAL ALERT**
> • The above symptoms require immediate attention to prevent serious complication and death.

11. Instruct on the signs and symptoms to report to surgeon without delay (University of Michigan Health System, 2007):
    a. Signs of a blood clot in the legs or pelvis (deep vein thrombosis)
       • Pain in the back of the thigh, calf, or groin
       • Swelling of the leg
       • Red streaking color or warmth of the leg
    b. Problems with the surgical incision
       • Redness and / or warmth around incision
       • Pus draining from the incision
       • Separation of the skin at the incision line
    c. Problems with the urethral catheter
       • Urine not draining
       • Red blood that does not clear soon after resting and increasing fluid intake
       • Urethral catheter inadvertently pulled out from the bladder or penis
    d. Other
       • Fever with temperature by mouth greater than 101° F
       • Nausea, vomiting, or severe abdominal bloating
       • Pain not relieved by prescribed medications
       • Inability to urinate after catheter removal
       • Decreased force of stream and sensation of incomplete emptying after catheter removal

12. Refer to community services (e.g., home care, counseling) and sources of information (e.g., www.cancer-prostate.com).

Documentation

Client teaching
Referrals, if indicated

Thoracic Surgery

A term encompassing various procedures involving a surgical opening into the chest cavity, thoracic surgery may be a pneumonectomy (removal of entire lung), lobectomy (removal of a lobe), segmentectomy (removal of a segment), wedge resection (small localized section of lung removed), sleeve resection with bronchoplastic reconstruction (partial removal of bronchus), or exploratory thoracotomy (internal view of the lung). Thoracic surgery usually is indicated for lung cancer but also may be indicated to repair a traumatized lung, treat pleural, and interstitial lung diseases, and to isolate tuberculosis, abscesses, bronchiectasis, blebs, and bulla caused by emphysema (Khraim, 2007).

Thoracic surgery may be open or endoscopic, also known as video-assisted, or minimally invasive. Both require general anesthesia and possibly single lung ventilation, using a double-lumen endotracheal tube (Khraim, 2007; Stanbridge, Hon, Bateman, & Roberts, 2007). However, video-assisted thoracic surgery (VATS) can also be performed under local anesthesia with less postoperative pain, decreased morbidity, shorter hospitalization, reduced postoperative shoulder dysfunction, and quicker return to preoperative activities / functions (Khraim, 2007; Stanbridge et al., 2007). VATS provides real-time, two-dimensional video images of the thoracic cavity (Khraim, 2007).

 Time Frame
Postoperative periods

■■■ DIAGNOSTIC CLUSTER

Collaborative Problems

▲ Risk for Complications of Mediastinal Shift

▲ Risk for Complications of Subcutaneous Emphysema

▲ Risk for Complications of Acute Pulmonary Edema

▲ Risk for Complications of Dysrhythmias

* Risk for Complications of Acute Lung Injury

* Risk for Complications of Bronchopleural Fistula

▲ Risk for Complications of Respiratory Insufficiency (refer to Unit II)

▲ Risk for Complications of Pulmonary Embolism (refer to Unit II)

△ Risk for Complications of Thrombophlebitis (refer to Unit II)

Nursing Diagnoses

▲ Ineffective Airway Clearance related to increased secretions and diminished cough secondary to pain and fatigue (refer to Unit II)

▲ Impaired Physical Mobility related to restricted arm and shoulder movement secondary to pain and muscle dissection and imposed position restrictions (refer to Unit II)

▲ Acute Pain related to surgical incision, chest tube sites, and immobility secondary to lengthy surgery (refer to Generic Surgical Care Plan)

Risk for Ineffective Self-Health Management Related to Insufficient Knowledge of Activity Restrictions

Related Care Plans

Generic Surgery Care Plan

Cancer: Initial Diagnosis

Transitional Criteria

Before transition, the client or family will:

1. Describe at-home wound care.
2. Relate the need to continue exercises at home.
3. Verbalize precautions for activities.
4. State signs and symptoms that must be reported to a health-care professional.
5. Identify appropriate community resources and self-help groups.
6. Describe at-home pain management.

Transitional Risk Assessment Plan (TRAP)

Begin this plan on admission.

Implement the Transitional Risk Assessment Plan (TRAP):

• Refer to inside back cover.
• Add each validated risk diagnosis to client's problem list with the risk code in ( ).
• Refer to Unit II to the individual risk nursing diagnoses / collaborative problems for outcomes and interventions.

R: "Close coordination of care in the post-acute period, early transition follow-up care, enhanced client education and self-management training, proactive end-of-life counseling, and extending the resources and clinical expertise over time via multidisciplinary team management" can lower readmission rates and improve health outcomes (Boutwell & Hwu, 2009, p. 14).

Collaborative Problems

Risk for Complications of Acute Pulmonary Edema

Risk for Complications of Mediastinal Shift

Risk for Complications of Subcutaneous Emphysema

Risk for Complications of Dysrhythmias

Risk for Complications of Acute Lung Injury (ALI)

Risk for Complications of Bronchopleural Fistula

Collaborative Outcomes

The client will be monitored for early signs and symptoms of (a) increased pneumothorax, (b) pulmonary edema, (c) mediastinal shift, (d) subcutaneous emphysema, and (e) dysrhythmias, and will receive collaborative interventions if indicated to restore physiologic stability.

Indicators of Physiologic Stability

• Respirations 16–20 breaths/min (a, b, c)
• Symmetrical, easy, rhythmic respirations (a, b, c)
• Breath sounds all lobes (a, b, c)
• No crackles or wheezing (a, b, c)
• Capillary refill <3 seconds (a, b, c)
• Oxygen saturation (PaO_2) >94% (a, b, c)
• pH 7.35–7.45 (a, b, c)
• Carbon dioxide ($PaCO_2$) 35–45 mm Hg (a, b, c)
• Pulse 60–100 beats/min (a, b, c)
• BP >90/60, <140/90 mm Hg (a, b, c)
• Peripheral pulses equal full (a, b, c)
• Normal EKG (e)

- Larynx / trachea midline (c)
- No neck vein distention (c)
- Minimal subcutaneous air (d)

 ## Carp's Cues

Please refer to the Generic Care Plan for the Surgical Client for detailed interventions for managing all surgical conditions. This care plan addresses specific additional interventions associated with the type of surgery performed.

Interventions	Rationales
1. Follow institution procedures for chest drainage systems. **CLINICAL ALERT** • Students and nurses who are inexperienced with management of chest drainage system must work with an experienced nurse.	

2. Monitor for malfunction of system:
  a. No fluctuation in water seal chamber
  b. Respiratory distress (excessive bubbling in water seal chamber)
  c. Subcutaneous air under skin (e.g., neck, chest, face)
 	
CLINICAL ALERT
• Report signs and symptoms system malfunction immediately.
	2. Malfunction of the chest drainage system causes air accumulation in the pleural space, compromising respirations, and forcing air into the subcutaneous tissue (subcutaneous emphysema).

3. If a tube disconnects, reattach or place end under water as the client exhales. Do not clamp the tube. Notify the surgeon and plan for a stat chest x-ray (Coughlin & Parchinsky, 2006).	3. Exhalation prior to reconnection will force excess air from pleural space. Clamping the tube can cause a tension pneumothorax.

4. Assess chest tube insertion site every 2 hours:
  a. Evidence of bleeding
  b. Intact occlusive dressing
 	
  c. Correct position of chest tubes
  d. Evidence of subcutaneous emphysema (Coughlin & Parchinsky, 2006)
	4a. Recent bleeding can be detected early
	  b. An occlusive dressing is needed to prevent air from entering pleural space.
	  c. Improper positioning of tubes can increase air and drainage in pleural space.

5. Document amount, consistency, and color of chest tube drainage every hour according to protocol. Notify the surgeon if drainage increases. Color and consistency of drainage in the chamber may be mixed and not appear accurately; assess drainage in the tubing for changes (Coughlin & Parchinsky, 2006).	5. Increased drainage can indicate bleeding; no drainage can indicate a nonpatent tube that can cause an increase in intrapleural pressure.
6. Prior to removal of chest tubes (3–4 days postop), assess for absence of chest tube drainage, no tidaling with respirations, and breath sounds in affected area (Coughlin & Parchinsky, 2006).	6. These clinical findings indicate lung reexpansion.
7. Provide pain medication ½ to 1 hour prior to removal.	7. This reduces the pain during chest tube removal.
8. Apply an occlusive dressing.	8. An occlusive dressing is needed to prevent air leaks and infection.

(continued)

Interventions	Rationales
9. After tube removal, evaluate respiratory status: no distress, breath sounds present in all lobes, even chest movement, calm, and no dysrhythmias	9. Complications after tube removal can be pneumothorax, hemothorax, or mediastinal shift. Early detection in respiratory or cardiac function can prevent serious complications.
CLINICAL ALERT • Modifiable risk factors that increase the risk for pneumonia or atelectasis post chest surgery are >75 years, have BMI > or = 30 kg/m, smoking history and COPD (Agostini et al., 2010).	
10. Instruct the client to use a spirometer at least 10 breaths an hour: a. Sit up as much as possible. b. Breathe in slowly and as deeply as possible. c. Breathe normally for a few breaths.	
11. After using the spirometer, instruct how to cough. Hold pillow to incision, apply gentle pressure, and cough.	11. Frequent use of a spirometer increases lung volumes and prevents pneumonia.
12. Monitor vital signs, pulse oximetry, respiratory function (rate, rhythm, capillary refill, breath sounds, skin color) according to protocol.	12. Frequent respiratory assessments are needed to evaluate early signs and symptoms of atelectasis, pneumothorax, and hemothorax.
13. Provide oxygen as prescribed and position the client in semi-Fowler's or full-Fowler's.	13. The semi-Fowler's position aids in lung expansion. Oxygen may be needed until lungs are fully expanded.
14. Monitor for signs of acute pulmonary edema (severe dyspnea, tachycardia, adventitious breath sounds, persistent cough).	14. Circulatory overload can result from the reduced size of the pulmonary vascular bed caused by removal of pulmonary tissue and the yet-unexpanded lung postoperatively. Hypoxia produces increased capillary permeability, causing fluid to enter pulmonary tissue and triggering signs and symptoms.
15. Cautiously administer IV fluids as prescribed.	15. Caution is needed to prevent circulatory overload.
16. Monitor for signs of mediastinal shift: increased weak, irregular pulse rate, severe dyspnea, cyanosis, hypoxia, increased restlessness and agitation, deviation of larynx or trachea from midline, shift in the point of apical impulse, asymmetric chest excursion. **CLINICAL ALERT** • Activate Rapid Response Team	16. Mediastinal shift is caused by increased intrapleural pressure on the operative side from fluid and air accumulations or excessive negative pressure on the operative side from inadequate fluid accumulation. These changes in pressure provide a space for the contents of the mediastinum (heart, trachea, esophagus, pulmonary vessels) to shift. Constriction of vessels (aorta, vena cava) creates hypoxia and its resultant signs and symptoms.
17. If signs and symptoms of a mediastinal shift occur, do the following: a. Position the client in a semi-Fowler's position. b. Maintain oxygen therapy.	17a. Sitting upright reduces mediastinal shifting. b. Oxygen therapy reduces hypoxia.
18. Monitor for signs of pneumothorax (Khraim, 2007; Roman et al., 2003): a. Reduced or absent breath sounds in affected area b. Subcutaneous emphysema (also known as crepitus) c. Dyspnea	18. Pneumothorax can cause acute respiratory failure (Roman et al., 2003).

Interventions	Rationales
d. Chest pain (pleuritic), usually increasing with respiratory effort e. Clinical signs of respiratory failure: cyanosis, tachycardia, tachypnea f. Reduced chest wall movement on affected side g. Clinical signs of mediastinal shift **CLINICAL ALERT** • Activate Rapid Response Team.	
19. Monitor status of subcutaneous emphysema: a. Mark periphery of the emphysematous tissue with a skin-marking pencil; reevaluate frequently. b. Monitor for neck involvement.	19. Subcutaneous emphysema can occur after thoracic surgery as air leaks out of incised pulmonary tissue: a. Serial markings help the nurse to evaluate the rate of progression. b. Severe subcutaneous emphysema can indicate air leakage through the bronchial stump and can compress the trachea.
20. If subcutaneous emphysema worsens, check patency of the chest drainage system and notify the surgeon.	20. Some subcutaneous emphysema may be present. Severe manifestations need to be corrected.
21. Monitor for cardiac dysrhythmias. Report any changes immediately and initiate protocol.	21. Decreased oxygen to the myocardium causes cardiac dysrhythmias.

Clinical Alert Report

Prior to providing care, advise ancillary staff / student to report the following to the professional nurse assigned to the client:
- Change in cognitive status
- New onset chest pain or shortness of breath
- Oral temperature >100.5° F
- Systolic BP <90 mm/Hg
- Resting pulse >100, <50
- Respiratory rate >28, <10 /min
- Oxygen saturation <90%

Related Physician / NP Prescribed Interventions

Medications
Bronchodilators, opioids, expectorants, local anesthetics, narcotic, nonsteroidal anti-inflammatory

Intravenous Therapy
Refer to the General Surgery Care Plan

Laboratory Studies
Arterial blood gas analysis; also refer to the General Surgery Care Plan

Diagnostic Studies
Chest x-ray film, pulmonary function studies, fiberoptic bronchoscopy, computed tomography (CT) scan, continuous pulse oximetry, sputum cytology, fine-needle aspiration, gallium scan, MRI, pulse oximetry, pulmonary artery pressure monitoring, central venous pressure monitoring.

Therapies

Intermittent positive-pressure breathing (IPPB) treatments, chest drainage system, client-controlled analgesia, chest physiotherapy, epidural analgesia, antiembolism devices, chemotherapy, radiation, and pleurodesis (Roman, Weinstein, & Macaluso, 2003)

Documentation

Vital signs
Intake and output records
Chest tube drainage (description, amount)

Nursing Diagnoses

Impaired Physical Mobility Related to Restricted Arm and Shoulder Movement Secondary to Pain and Muscle Dissection and Imposed Position Restrictions

NOC
Ambulation: Walking, Joint Movement: Active, Mobility Level

Goal

The client will return or progress to preoperative arm and shoulder function.

NIC
Exercise Therapy: Joint Mobility, Exercise Promotion: Strength Training, Exercise Therapy: Ambulation, Positioning, Teaching: Prescribed Activity / Exercise

Indicators

- Demonstrate knowledge of the need to maintain certain positions.
- Demonstrate ROM exercises.

Interventions	Rationales
1. Position conscious client in semi-Fowler position (30–45 degrees).	1. Supine position until consciousness is regained, then semi-Fowler's position. This position allows the diaphragm to resume its normal position, which reduces the effort of respiration.
2. Explain the need for frequent turning. Gently turn the client from side to side every 1–2 hours, unless contraindicated.	2. Turning mobilizes drainage of secretions, promotes circulation, inhibits thrombus formation, and aerates all parts of the remaining lung tissue. Lying on the operative side can be contraindicated following a wedge resection and pneumonectomy.
3. Avoid extreme lateral turning following a pneumonectomy.	3. This can cause a mediastinal shift (refer to Risk for Complications of Mediastinal Shift in this care plan).
4. Avoid traction on chest tubes during movement; check for kinks after repositioning.	4. Traction can cause dislodgment; kinks can inhibit drainage or negative pressure.
5. Explain the need for frequent exercises of arms, shoulders, and trunk, even in the presence of some pain and discomfort.	5. The muscle groups transcended by a thoracotomy form the shoulder girdle and maintain the trunk's posture. Failure to perform exercises can result in muscle adhesions, contractures, and postural deformities.
6. Initiate passive ROM exercises on the operative arm and shoulder within 4 hours per protocol after recovery from anesthesia. Begin with two times every 4 hours for the first 24 hours; progress to 10–20 times every 2 hours.	6. Passive ROM exercises help to prevent ankylosis of the shoulder and contractures of the arm.

Interventions	Rationales
7. Consult with a physical therapist for active ROM exercises for the client to perform, starting 1–2 days after surgery.	7. Active ROM exercises help to prevent adhesions of two incised muscle layers.
8. Encourage use of the affected arm in ADLs and stress the need to continue exercises at home.	8. Regular use increases ROM and decreases contractures and shift (refer to Risk for Complications of Mediastinal Shift in this entry for more information).

Documentation

Limitations on performing activities
Therapeutic exercises performed
Turning, positioning
Client teaching

TRANSITION TO HOME/COMMUNITY CARE

If indicated, review the risk diagnoses identified for this individual on admission:

* Is the person still at risk?
* Can the family reduce the risks?
* Is the person at higher risk at home?
* Is a Home Health Nurse assessment needed?
* Refer to transition planner / case manager / social service.
* When is this person scheduled for follow-up with primary provider? Specialists? Record dates of appointments.
* Complete a medication reconciliation prior to transition. Refer to index.

S T A R   **Stop**

Think   Is this person at risk for injury, falls, medical complications, and / or inability to care for self (activities of daily living)?

Is there a support person available?

Is the person competent to manage self-administration of medications, treatment procedures? Are additional resources needed?

Can the person explain how to monitor the condition (e.g., blood glucose, signs / symptoms of complications, dietary / mobility restrictions, and when to call his or her primary provider or specialist)?

Act   Contact or provide the appropriate resource (e.g., contacting a support person, home health assessment, additional teaching, printed materials).

Review   Has the problem been addressed? If not, use SBAR to communicate to the appropriate person.

Risk for Ineffective Self-Health Therapeutic Regimen Management Related to Insufficient Knowledge of Activity Restrictions, Wound Care, Shoulder Exercises, Signs and Symptoms of Complications, and Follow-up Care

NOC

Compliance Behavior, Knowledge: Treatment Regimen, Participation: Health-Care Decisions, Treatment Behavior: Illness or Injury

NIC

Anticipatory Guidance, Risk Identification, Health Education, Learning Facilitation

Goals

The goals for this diagnosis represent those associated with the discharge planning. Refer to the discharge criteria.

Interventions	Rationales

1. Explain restrictions:
  a. Avoid heavy lifting or moving heavy objects for 3–6 months.
  b. Avoid excessive fatigue.
  c. Avoid crowds and bronchial irritants (smoke, fumes, aerosol sprays).
	1a. Heavy lifting can increase tension on the incision, which can prolong healing.
	  b. Fatigue can prolong the healing process.
	  c. Attempts should be made to prevent infection and irritations.

2. Practice breathing exercises and shoulder exercises (refer to Impaired Physical Mobility and Ineffective Airway Clearance for specifics). Provide written exercise instructions.	2. These will prevent complications of contractures, pneumonia, and atelectasis.
3. Apply local heat to the intracostal region. Use analgesics, as needed.	3. All attempts to relieve pain are needed to promote mobility and exercises.

4. Instruct to call the surgeon if any of the following occur:
  a. New onset or increasing chest pain
  b. Increasing shortness of breath
  c. Increasing fatigue
  d. Oral temperature >100.5° F, chills
  e. New drainage from wound
  f. Increasing incisional pain
	4. These signs and symptoms can indicate infection, bleeding, and / or respiratory insufficiency.

5. Provide information on community resources (e.g., American Cancer Society, smoking cessation programs, support groups, home health agencies, Meals-On-Wheels), and follow-up plan.	5. The client and / or family may need assistance after discharge.

Documentation

Client teaching
Referrals (e.g., PT)
Exercises taught

Total Joint Replacement (Hip, Knee, Shoulder)

Joint replacement (arthroplasty) is the surgical replacement of all or part of a joint. This surgery is indicated for irreversibly damaged joints caused by osteoarthritis or rheumatoid arthritis, fractures of hip or femoral neck with avascular necrosis, trauma, and congenital deformity. Osteoarthritis remains the most common cause of arthroplasty (Branson & Goldstein, 2001).

For hip replacements, a ball and socket prosthesis is implanted, either with cement or uncemented. Uncemented prostheses have porous surfaces that allow the client's bone to grow into and stabilize the prosthesis.

For knee joint replacements, the prosthesis is tricompartmental, with femoral, tibial, and patellar components. As with hip prostheses, the knee prosthesis can be cemented or uncemented. Cemented fixation reduces blood loss because the cement seals open bone edges; it is therefore the most common fixation technique (Branson & Goldstein, 2001).

Knee and hip arthroplasty can now be done with minimally invasive and small-incision techniques. These techniques reduce postoperative pain, length of hospital stay, rehabilitation requirements, and complications. Clients are able to return to usual activities faster with fewer complications (McGrory et al., 2005).

 Time Frame
Postoperative periods

▬▬ DIAGNOSTIC CLUSTER

Postoperative Period

Collaborative Problems

▲ Risk for Complications of Hemorrhage / Hematoma Formation

▲ Risk for Complications of Dislocation / Subluxation of Joint

▲ Risk for Complications of Neurovascular Compromise (refer to Unit II)

▲ Risk for Complications of Fat Emboli (refer to Unit II)

▲ Risk for Complications of Sepsis (refer to Unit II)

▲ Risk for Complications of Thromboemboli (refer to Unit II)

Nursing Diagnoses

▲ Impaired Physical Mobility related to pain, stiffness, fatigue, restrictive equipment, and prescribed activity restrictions (refer to Unit II)

▲ Risk for Impaired Skin Integrity related to pressure and decreased mobility secondary to pain and temporary restrictions (refer to Unit II)

▲ Risk for Injury related to altered gait and use of assistive devices (refer to Unit II)

△ Risk for Ineffective Therapeutic Regimen Management related to insufficient knowledge of activity restrictions, use of assistive devices, signs of complications, and follow-up care (refer to Unit II)

Related Care Plans

General Surgery Generic Care Plan

Anticoagulant Therapy

Amputation

Discharge Criteria

Before discharge, the client and family will:

1. Describe activity restrictions.
2. Describe a plan for resuming ADLs.
3. Regain mobility while adhering to weight-bearing restrictions.
4. State signs and symptoms that must be reported to a health-care professional.

> ### Transitional Risk Assessment Plan (TRAP)
>
> Begin this plan on admission.
> Implement the Transitional Risk Assessment Plan (TRAP):
> * Refer to inside back cover.
> * Add each validated risk diagnosis to client's problem list with the risk code in ( ).
> * Refer to Unit II to the individual risk nursing diagnoses / collaborative problems for outcomes and interventions.
>
> *R: "Close coordination of care in the post-acute period, early transition follow-up care, enhanced client education and self-management training, proactive end-of-life counseling, and extending the resources and clinical expertise over time via multidisciplinary team management" can lower readmission rates and improve health outcomes (Boutwell & Hwu, 2009, p. 14).*

Collaborative Problems

Risk for Complications of Hemorrhage / Hematoma

Risk for Complications of Dislocation of Joint (Hip, Knee)

Risk for Complications of Neurovascular Compromise

Collaborative Outcomes

The client will be monitored for early signs and symptoms of (a) hemorrhage / hematoma, (b) dislocation (hip, knee), and (c) neurovascular compromise, and will receive collaborative interventions if indicated to restore physiologic stability.

Indicators of Physiologic Stability

- Pulse 60–100 beats/min (a)
- Respirations 16–20 breaths/min (a)
- BP >90/60, <140/90 mm Hg (a)
- Capillary refill <3 seconds (a, c)
- Peripheral pulses full, bilateral (a, c)
- Warm, dry skin, no blanching (a, c)
- Urine output >0.5 mL/kg/h (a)
- Hip in abduction or neutral rotation (b)
- Leg length even (b)
- Knee in neutral position (b)
- No complaints of tingling, numbness (c)
- Ability to move toes (c)
- Hemoglobin (a)
  - Male 13–18 g/dL
  - Female 12–16 g/dL
- Hematocrit (a)
  - Male 42% to 50%
  - Female 40% to 48%

If on anticoagulant therapy:
- Partial thromboplastin time 1.5 × control (a)
- Prothrombin time 1.5–2 × normal (a)
- International Normalized Ratio (INR) 2–3 (a)

Carp's Cues

Please refer to the Generic Care Plan for the Surgical Client for detailed interventions for managing all surgical conditions. This care plan addresses specific additional interventions associated with the type of surgery performed.

Interventions	Rationales
1. Identify individuals at risk for compromised wound healing: a. History of cardiac problems b. Poor nutritional status c. Obesity d. Diabetes mellitus e. History of deep vein thrombosis (DVT) or pulmonary embolism (PE) f. Blood dyscrasias g. Deconditioned state h. Older adults	1. Wound healing is compromised by diabetes mellitus, inadequate nutrition, obesity, and impaired oxygen transport. Older adults, with associated comorbidities, are most vulnerable to postoperative complications and mortality. Preoperative identification of potential complications permits development of preventative strategies (Graul, 2002; Lopez-Bushnell et al., 2004).

Interventions	Rationales
2. Ensure appropriate prophylaxis's has been initiated to prevent DVTs. For-risk individuals (e.g., CHF, those who have a history of prior DVT, are on estrogen therapy, and / or have a recent history of cancer) are often started on anticoagulants such as warfarin, Coumadin, or heparin, the night before surgery, with an initial dose of 5–10 mg depending on age, weight, and medical. Low-risk individuals are placed on aspirin (Ennis, 2012). At the time of discharge, individuals, who are at a risk for deep vein thrombosis (DVT) will remain on anticoagulation therapy for 4–6 weeks, and then transition to aspirin for an additional 6 weeks.	2. The incidence of pulmonary embolism is 7% of individuals undergoing surgery for fractured hips. The American College of Chest Physicians (ACCP) recommends early prophylaxis in surgical clients with low-molecular-weight-heparin (LMWH) to prevent venous thrombosis. Studies have shown that initiation of therapy within 8 hours of surgery has the greatest effect (Hull, 2001).
3. Monitor drainage from suction device every hour.	3. The hip is a very vascular area and the use of anticoagulants creates a risk for bleeding. Expect 200–500 mL in the first 24 hours reducing to approximately 50 mL in 48 hours. Some drainage systems permit salvage and autologous transfusion (Graul, 2002).
4. Maintain pressure dressing and ice to surgical area as ordered.	4. Pressure can reduce bleeding at site, reducing hematoma formation.
5. Monitor for early signs and symptoms of bleeding and hypoxia: increased pulse rate, increased respirations, urinary output >0.5 mL/kg/h). **CLINICAL ALERT** • Promptly report change in clinical status.	5. Early signs and symptoms of bleeding and hypoxia can prompt rapid interventions to prevent hemorrhage.
6. Monitor for hematoma: increased pain at site (e.g., tense swelling in buttock and thigh [post THR], knee [post TKR]).	6. Bleeding into the surgical area can cause hematoma formation.
7. Maintain correct positioning: a. Hip: Maintain hip in abduction, neutral rotation, or slight external rotation. b. Hip: Avoid hip flexion over 60 degrees. c. Knee: Keep knees apart at all times and slightly elevated from hip; avoid gatching bed under knee or placing pillows under knee (to prevent flexion contractures); pillows should be placed under calf.	7. These positions prevent dislocation.
8. Assess for signs of joint (hip, knee) dislocation: a. Hip: • Acute groin pain in operative hip • Shortening of leg and in external rotation b. Hip, knee: • "Popping" sound heard by client • Inability to move • Bulge at surgical site **CLINICAL ALERT** • Promptly call surgeon.	8. Until the surrounding muscles and joint capsule heal, joint dislocation may occur if positioning exceeds the limits of the prosthesis, such as when flexing or hyperextending the knee or abducting the hip more than 45 degrees.
9. Keep affected joint in a neutral position with rolls, pillows, or specified devices.	9. This maintains alignment and prevents dislocation.

(continued)

Interventions	Rationales
1. Monitor drainage amount and color every hour for the first 24 hours from: a. Incision b. Cecostomy catheter c. Urethral stents and bile catheters d. Stomal catheter e. Urethral catheter	1. A sudden decrease in urine flow may indicate obstruction (edema, mucus) or dehydration.
2. Irrigate cecostomy tube, as prescribed. **Clinical Alert** • Report a sudden change (increased or decreased) in drainage or bleeding from the stoma. • A change in drainage can indicate bleeding or infection (increased) or blockage (decreased).	2. Irrigation removes mucus to prevent blockage.
3. Monitor every hour for the first 24 hours: a. Vital signs b. Capillary refill <3 seconds c. Oxygen saturation (pulse oximetry) d. Urine output e. Bowel sounds	3. Changes in vital signs (increased pulse, decreased BP, decreased urine output, decreased oxygen saturation, and increased capillary fill time) can indicate dehydration, bleeding, and / or hypoxia.
4. Monitor for signs of internal urine leakage: a. Abdominal distention with decrease bowl motility b. Fever c. Elevated serum creatinine level d. Decreased urine output despite adequate hydration	4. Urine leakage either from the ureteroileal anastomosis or from the base of the conduit, occurs in as many as 8% of clients with a urostomy. Leakage is confirmed through fluoroscopy. Small leaks may seal themselves with continuous drainage of the conduit via a stomal catheter.
5. Explain the reason for cloudy urine.	5. Because the intestine produces mucus, mucus in the diversion will cause urine to appear cloudy (Clark, 2006; Early & Poquette, 2000).
6. Monitor for signs and symptoms of urinary tract infection (Ewing, 1989): a. Fever b. Flank pain c. Malodorous, cloudy urine d. Alkaline urine pH	6. Between 10% and 20% of clients with a urinary diversion develop pyelonephritis. The major cause is poor urine flow through the conduit, leading to urinary stasis and bacterial contamination through the stoma.
7. Consult with the physician / NP / Ostomy Nurse Specialist for a urine culture from a double-lumen catheter specimen.	7. Cultures enable identification of the causative organism and guide pharmacologic therapy.
8. Monitor for signs of peristomal ulceration or herniation: a. Decreased peristomal muscle tone b. Bulging beyond normal skin surface and musculature c. Persistent ulceration d. Redness, skin breakdown or irritation, itching, warmth or pain in the peristomal area (Colwell & Beitz, 2007). Teach proper assessment of the peristomal area.	8. Early detection of ulcerations and herniation enables prompt intervention to prevent serious tissue damage.
9. Consult with Ostomy Nurse Specialist therapist regarding persistent ulceration.	9. Expert assistance may be needed for prevention and treatment of persistent skin problems.

Interventions	Rationales
10. Monitor for stomal necrosis, prolapse, retraction, stenosis, and obstruction. Assess the following:	10. Daily assessment is necessary to detect early changes in stoma condition.
a. Color, size, and shape of stoma	a. Changes can indicate inflammation, retraction, prolapse, edema.
b. Color and amount of urine from the urostomy or from each stent	b. Changes can indicate bleeding or infection. Decreased output can indicate obstruction.
c. Complaints of cramping abdominal pain, nausea and vomiting, abdominal distention	c. These complaints may indicate obstruction.

Clinical Alert Report

Prior to providing care, advise ancillary staff / student to report the following to the professional nurse assigned to the client:
- Change in cognitive status
- Oral temperature >100.5° F
- Systolic BP <90 mm/Hg
- Resting pulse >100, <50
- Respiratory rate >28, <10 /min.
- Decreased urine output despite adequate hydration
- Oxygen saturation <90%
- Changes in peristomal tissue
- C/o cramping abdominal pain, nausea and vomiting, abdominal distention
- Abdominal distention with decrease bowel motility

Related Physician / NP Prescribed Interventions

Medications
Refer to the General Surgery Care Plan.

Intravenous Therapy
Refer to the General Surgery Care Plan.

Laboratory Studies
Refer to the General Surgery Care Plan.

Diagnostic Studies
Intravenous pyelography, CT scan, cystoscopy, conduitogram, bone scan, endoscopy, flow cytometry, pouchogram

Therapies
Sitz baths, urinary diversion collection appliances

Documentation

Vital signs
Intake and output
Abdomen (girth, bowel sounds)
Condition of peristomal area

Postoperative: Nursing Diagnoses

> **TRANSITION TO HOME/COMMUNITY CARE**
>
> If indicated, review the risk diagnoses identified for this individual on admission:
> * Is the person still at risk?
> * Can the family reduce the risks?
> * Is the person at higher risk at home?
> * Is a Home Health Nurse assessment needed?
> * Refer to transition planner / case manager / social service.
> * When is this person scheduled for follow-up with primary provider? Specialists? Record dates of appointments.
> * Complete a medication reconciliation prior to transition. Refer to index.

STAR

Stop

Think   Is this person at risk for injury, falls, medical complications, and / or inability to care for self (activities of daily living)?

Is there a support person available?

Is the person competent to manage self-administration of medications, treatment procedures? Are additional resources needed?

Can the person explain how to monitor the condition (e.g., blood glucose, signs / symptoms of complications, dietary / mobility restrictions, and when to call his or her primary provider or specialist)?

Act   Contact or provide the appropriate resource (e.g., contacting a support person, home health assessment, additional teaching, printed materials).

Review   Has the problem been addressed? If not, use SBAR to communicate to the appropriate person.

Risk for Ineffective Self-Health Management Related to Insufficient Knowledge of Stoma Pouching Procedure, Peristomal Skin Care, Perineal Wound Care, and Incorporation of Ostomy Care Into Activities of Daily Living (ADLs)

NOC

Compliance Behavior, Knowledge: Treatment Regimen, Participation: Health-Care Decisions, Treatment Behavior: Illness or Injury

NIC

Anticipatory Guidance, Risk Identification, Health Education, Learning Facilitation

Goals

The goals for this diagnosis represent those associated with discharge planning. Refer to the discharge criteria.

Interventions	Rationales

> **CLINICAL ALERT**
> - Most clinical nurses are not responsible for the specific teaching of ostomy care and its implications on lifestyle and function.
> - The wound care / ostomy specialist will provide an organized teaching plan.
> - However, since nurses are responsible for care 24/7, each nurse needs to be confident in basic ostomy care.
> - A good method to learn this care is to watch the nurse specialist provide / teach ostomy care.

Interventions	Rationales
1. When providing care, explore fears and concerns. Identify and dispel any misinformation or misconceptions the client / significant others has regarding ileostomy (Richbourg, Thorpe, & Rapp, 2007).	1. Replacing misinformation with facts can reduce anxiety.
2. Emphasize the importance of adequate fluid intake; Explain also risk situations for dehydration such as: a. Hot weather b. Exercising in hot weather c. With episodes of diarrhea d. When intake is reduced (e.g., illness)	2. Concentrated urine is more prone to bacterial growth.
3. Explain why urine should be kept in an acid state and how: a. Drink cranberry juice. b. Take vitamin C supplements daily. c. Avoid orange juice or other citrus juices. d. Prevent urostomy oxalate crystal formation (Collett, 2002).	3. Acid urine reduces bacterial growth and prevents infections c. Citrus juices make the urine more alkaline.
4. Explain how to prevent urinary crystals forming on the stoma or skin (Collett, 2002): a. Soak a wash cloth in a mixture of equal parts of water and white vinegar. b. Hold the moist cloth on the stoma before applying a new drainage bag.	4. The crystals look like white, gritty particles and may cause stoma irritation or bleeding. They are caused by alkaline urine.
5. Discuss signs and symptoms of fluid and electrolyte imbalances: a. Extreme thirst b. Dry skin and oral mucous membrane c. Dark yellow urine output d. Weakness, fatigue e. Muscle cramps f. Orthostatic hypotension (feeling faint when suddenly changing positions)	
6. Teach sign and symptoms of infection include: a. Dark urine or urine containing excess mucus b. Strong-smelling urine c. Pain in the back d. Poor appetite e. Nausea f. Vomiting	

(continued)

Interventions	Rationales
7. Stress importance of connecting the appliance to a straight drainage when the client is sleeping in bed.	7. Bacteria multiply rapidly as urine collects in the pouch. Bacterial contamination of the urinary tract can result from backflow of urine from a full pouch. Nighttime drainage systems hold large amounts of urine and drain urine away from the stoma.
8. Explain to report any of these changes in the client's stoma or skin around it to surgeon, PCP, or ostomy nurse specialist: a. Is purple, gray, or black b. Has a bad odor c. Is dry d. Pulls away from the skin e. Opening gets big enough for your intestines to come through it f. Is at skin level or deeper g. Pushes farther out from the skin and gets longer h. Skin opening becomes narrower	8. These changes can indicate infection, ulceration, prolapse, and retraction.
9. Call your surgeon, PCP, or ostomy nurse specialist, if your stoma: a. Has a pale color b. Is dark red or purple c. Has moderate to severe swelling d. Has moderate to heavy bleeding	9. The stoma is normally pink to red; changes can indicate necrosis, ischemia, infection.
10. Teach measures to help prevent urinary calculi: a. Ensure optimal hydration. b. Avoid sulfa drugs and vitamin C supplements. c. Engage in regular physical activity.	10. Inadequate hydration promotes urinary stasis and calculi formation. Certain drugs and inactivity can predispose to calculi formation (Goshorn, 2000).

11. Discuss community resources / self-help groups:
a. Printed Self-Help Guideline, such as American Cancer Society (2011) "Urostomy: A Guide," accessed 6/29/2013 at http://www.cancer.org/acs/groups/cid/documents/webcontent/002931-pdf.pdf
b. Organizations
  • Visiting nurse
  • United Ostomy Associations of America, Inc. (UOAA),
   1-800-826-0826, www.uoaa.org.
   For local support group information; the interactive website includes discussion boards.
  • International Ostomy Association (IOA), www.ostomyinternational.org. Advocates for and outlines the rights of ostomates
  • Wound, Ostomy and Continence Nurses Society (WOCN),
   1-888-224-9626, www.wocn.org
  • Community suppliers of urostomy equipment
  • Financial reimbursement for ostomy equipment	

Documentation

Client and family teaching
Outcome achievement or status

Section 3

Diagnostic and Therapeutic Procedures

Anticoagulant Therapy

Anticoagulant therapy is treatment for a coagulation disorder (e.g., deep vein thrombosis, pulmonary embolism, atrial fibrillation, ischemic stroke) or prophylaxis for coagulation for people undergoing orthopedic surgery or receiving prosthetic cardiac valves.

Anticoagulants for therapy or prophylaxis include warfarin (Coumadin), heparin, low-molecular-weight heparin (Lovenox, Fragmin, Orgaran, Normiflo), all of which prevent clot extension and formation; antiplatelet agents (aspirin, Plavix, Ticlid) that interfere with platelet activity; and thrombolytic agents that dissolve existing thrombi. This care plan addresses the use of heparin and warfarin (Coumadin).

Time Frame
Intratherapy

Refer to Unit II Risk for Complications of Anticoagulant Therapy Adverse Effects.

Casts

Casts are used to immobilize a fractured bone or dislocated joint, support injured tissues during the healing process, correct deformities, prevent movement of joints during healing, and provide traction force. Casting materials can be dehydrated gypsum that recrystallizes when reconstituted with water, fiberglass, and casting tape. The material used depends on the severity of the fracture's displacement. Plaster casts take 24–72 hours to dry; fiberglass casts usually dry in 5–30 minutes. After the fiberglass cast is dry, keep it dry, or it will get soft or crack.

Time Frame
Intratherapy

■■■ DIAGNOSTIC CLUSTER

Collaborative Problems

▲ Risk for Complications of Compartment Syndrome

▲ Risk for Complications of Infection / Sepsis

Nursing Diagnoses

▲ Risk for Impaired Skin Integrity related to pressure of cast on skin surface

▲ Risk for Ineffective Self-Health Management related to insufficient knowledge of cast care, signs and symptoms of complications, use of assistive devices, and hazards

▲ This diagnosis was reported to be monitored for or managed frequently (75% to 100%).

Transition Criteria

Before transition, the client or family will:

1. Describe precautions to take with the cast.
2. Identify how to monitor for signs and symptoms of complications.
3. Identify barriers in the home environment and relate strategies for overcoming these barriers.
4. Identify a plan to meet role responsibilities.

Collaborative Problems

Risk for Complications of Compartment Syndrome

Risk for Complications of Infection/Sepsis

Collaborative Outcomes

The client will be monitored for early signs and symptoms of (a) compartment syndrome and (b) infection / sepsis, and will receive collaborative interventions if indicated to restore physiologic stability.

Indicators of Physiologic Stability

- Alert, calm, oriented (b)
- Temperature 98.5°–99° F (b)
- Heart rate 60–100 beats/min (b)
- Respirations 16–20 breaths/min (b)
- Blood pressure >90/60, 140/90 mm Hg (b)
- Peripheral pulses full, equal, strong (a)
- Sensation intact (a)
- No pain with passive dorsiflexion (calf and toes) (a)
- Mild edema (a)
- Pain relieved by analgesics (a)
- No tingling in legs (a)
- Can move arms / legs (a)
- White blood cells 4,800–10,000/mm^3 (b)
- Oxygen saturation 94% to 100% (b)
- Capillary refill <3 seconds (a)
- Blood urea nitrogen (BUN) 10–20 mg/dL (a)
- Creatinine 0.7–1.4 mg/dL (b)

Interventions	Rationales
1. Instruct client to report any changes however slight. Determine if these changes are new and different.	1. Nerve deficit is one of the earliest signs of compartment syndrome. Close monitoring and early detection can help save an extremity or prevent permanent deformity (Altizer, 2004).
2. Monitor for signs and symptoms of compartment syndrome: a. Deep, throbbing pain at fracture site b. Increasing pain with passive movement c. Decreased sensation to light touch d. Inability to distinguish between sharp and dull sensation in first web space of toes, sole, and dorsum and lateral aspect of foot e. Diminished or absent pedal pulses f. Increased edema and induration in extremity g. Increased capillary refill (toes or fingers) >3 seconds	2. These signs and symptoms are indicative of venous or arterial obstruction and nerve compression. Edema at the fracture site can compromise muscular vascular perfusion. Stretching damaged muscle causes pain. Sensory deficit is an early sign of nerve ischemia. Utilize the five "Ps" of assessment on both the affected and unaffected limb to determine a baseline; assess for pain, pallor, paresthesia, paralysis, and pulselessness (Altizer, 2004).

Interventions	Rationales

> **CLINICAL ALERT**
> - Immediately, advise physician / NP of the need for immediate evaluation of the neurovascular changes assessed or reported by the client.
> - Immediate medical assessment will determine what specific interventions are needed (e.g., emergency surgery [fasciotomy], removal of cast, splints).

Interventions	Rationales
3. Warn client not to mask pain with analgesics until the exact cause has been identified.	3. Identifying the location and nature of pain assists in differential diagnosis.
4. Investigate any complaints of pain, burning, or an offensive odor from inside the cast. Smell the cast to check for odors.	4. These signs and symptoms may indicate that a pressure sore is forming or has become infected. Pathologic tissue necrosis emits a musty, offensive odor that can easily be detected.
5. Feel cast surface to identify areas that are appreciably warmer than other areas ("hot spots"). Particularly evaluate areas over pressure points.	5. Areas of tissue necrosis or infection often cause the overlying area of the cast to feel warmer.
6. If drainage is noted on cast, draw a mark around drainage area and record date and time on cast. Notify surgeon if drainage increases.	6. Marking the initial drainage will provide a baseline for comparison.
7. When moving client or body part, support plaster cast during hardening with palms of hands. Avoid pressure or sharp edges on cast.	7. Maximum hardness of plaster cast takes 24–72 hours depending on thickness. Careful hardening will prevent dents that can cause pressure on underlying tissue.

Clinical Alert Report

Advise ancillary staff / student to report the following to the professional nurse assigned to the client:
- Unrelieved or increasing pain
- Pain with passive stretch movement or flexion of toes or fingers
- Skin changes mottled or cyanotic skin, rash
- C/o numbness (paresthesia)
- Inability to move toes or fingers
- Change in cognitive status
- Oral temperature >100.5° F
- Systolic BP <90 mm/Hg
- Resting pulse >100, <50
- Respiratory rate >28, <10/min
- Oxygen saturation <90%
- Oral temperature >100.5° F

Related Physician / NP Prescribed Interventions

Diagnostic Studies

X-ray films (preapplication and postapplication)

Therapies

Assistive devices, physical therapy, casts (plaster, nonplaster)

Documentation

Skin color (distal to injury)

Pulses (distal to injury)

Sensations (pain, paresthesias, paralysis)

Odor (under cast)

Temperature of cast surface

Temperature of distal digits

Mobility of distal digits

Elevation of casted limb, if applicable

Progress notes

Unusual complaints

Any drainage noted

Client's acceptance of cast

Nursing Diagnoses

Risk for Ineffective Self-Health Management Related to Insufficient Knowledge of Cast Care, Signs and Symptoms of Complications, Use of Assistive Devices, and Hazards

NOC

Compliance Behavior, Knowledge: Treatment Regimen, Participation: Health-Care Decisions, Treatment Behavior: Illness or Injury

NIC

Anticipatory Guidance, Learning Facilitation, Health Education, Cast Care: Maintenance

Goal

The goals for this diagnosis represent those associated with transition planning. Refer to the transition criteria.

Interventions	Rationales
1. Teach client and family to watch for and report the following symptoms: a. Severe pain b. Numbness or tingling c. Swelling d. Skin discoloration e. Paralysis or reduced movement f. Cool, white toes, or fingertips g. Foul odor, warm spots, soft areas, or cracks in the cast	1. Early detection of possible problems enables prompt intervention to prevent serious complications such as infection or impaired circulation.
2. Instruct client never to insert objects down inside edges of cast.	2. Sharp objects used for scratching may cause breaks in skin continuity that provide an entry point for infectious microorganisms.

Interventions	Rationales
3. Teach client and family to handle a drying plaster cast with palms of hands only; using fingertips may cause indentations.	3. Cast indentations may lead to pressure sores.
4. Instruct client to keep cast uncovered until it is completely dry.	4. A damp, soiled cast can weaken and may cause skin irritation or promote bacteria growth.
5. Instruct client to avoid weight bearing or other stress on cast for at least 24 hours after application.	5. Covers restrict escape of heat, especially in a large cast, and prolong the drying process.
6. Instruct client to avoid getting plaster cast wet; teach how to protect cast from moisture.	6. Ultimate cast strength is obtained after cast is dry—within 48–72 hours, depending on factors such as environmental temperature and humidity.

Documentation

Client and family teaching

Chemotherapy / Targeted Therapy

Over the last decade significant advancements have been made in personalized medicine. For years, chemotherapy was the gold standard to treat many cancers, based on the site of the cancer. It was given systemically according to protocols researched; infused like a recipe with no consideration of an individual's genes, proteins, and personal response to treatment. Chemotherapy works best on fast growing cells, and cannot differentiate between normal and cancer cells. Monoclonal antibodies, anti-angiogenesis, and other therapies are types of targeted therapies. Targeted therapy is the result of over 100 years of research dedicated to understanding the differences between cancer cells and normal cells and how the body responds to treatment. As research continues to boom around personalized medicine, chemotherapy / targeted therapy will be an ever moving target. Consider a missile with a global positioning unit on it, with a direct path of destruction specific to the biologics of each cell, or receptors on the cell "targeted" to destroy, block, or disrupt the specific molecules needed for tumor growth or progression. This type of treatment is now considered "personalized medicine" unique to each cancer diagnosis, down to the genetic level of the client. While this chapter will not touch the surface of the hundreds of agents currently being used in treatment, it will offer you a broad understanding.

Indications for chemotherapy treatment is for cure, palliative to reduce tumor burden, to increase the sensitivity of radiation, or given presurgery to shrink the tumor for optimal surgical treatment (Lowitz & Casciato, 2009).

Drug reactions, side-effects, and toxicities must be anticipated, and rigorously monitored for during administration or follow-up assessments (Cornett & Dea, 2012). The extent of side effects will vary based on dose, type of treatment, and frequency of treatment. Side-effect management is very individualized to the treatment given, and how it is disrupting the cell pathway. Systemic cancer treatment modality aims to safely eradicate or control the growth of cancerous cells by producing maximum cancer cell death with minimum toxicity. Chemotherapy or targeted therapy may be the sole treatment provided, or it may be used in combination with surgery and / or radiation. Administration of these agents is also very specific to the disease being treated, administered either continuously or intermittently using various routes, techniques, and special equipment. Detailed guidelines for the treatments recommended for all diagnoses can be found at www.nccn.org.

Time Frame
Pretherapy and intratherapy

▪▪▪▪▪ DIAGNOSTIC CLUSTER

Collaborative Problems

▲ Risk for Complications of Anaphylactic Reaction

△ Risk for Complications of Cardiotoxicity

▲ Risk for Complications of Electrolyte Imbalance

▲ Risk for Complications of Extravasation of Vesicant Drugs

△ Risk for Complications of Hemorrhagic Cystitis

▲ Risk for Complications of Bone Marrow Depression

  Risk for Complications of Renal Insufficiency (refer to Unit II)

△ Risk for Complications of Pulmonary Toxicity

△ Risk for Complications of Neurotoxicity

  Risk for Complications of Renal Calculi

△ Risk for Complications of Infection (refer to Unit II)

Nursing Diagnoses

▲ Anxiety related to prescribed chemotherapy, insufficient knowledge of chemotherapy, and self-care measures

▲ Nausea related to gastrointestinal cell damage, stimulation of vomiting center, fear, and anxiety

▲ Imbalanced Nutrition: Less Than Body Requirements related to anorexia, taste changes, persistent nausea / vomiting, and increased metabolic rate (refer to Unit II)

▲ Impaired Oral Mucous Membrane related to dryness and epithelial cell damage secondary to chemotherapy (refer to Unit II)

▲ Fatigue related to effects of anemia, malnutrition, persistent vomiting, and sleep pattern disturbance (refer to Unit II)

△ Risk for Constipation related to autonomic nerve dysfunction secondary to Vinca alkaloid administration and inactivity (refer to Unit II)

▲ Diarrhea related to intestinal cell damage, inflammation, and increased intestinal mobility (refer to Unit II)

▲ Risk for Impaired Skin Integrity related to persistent diarrhea, malnutrition, prolonged sedation, and fatigue (refer to Unit II)

△ Disturbed Self-Concept related to change in lifestyle, role, alopecia, and weight loss or gain (refer to Cancer [Initial Diagnosis])

▲ This diagnosis was reported to be monitored for or managed frequently (75% to 100%).
△ This diagnosis was reported to be monitored for or managed often (50% to 74%).

Transitional Criteria

Before transition, the client and family will:

1. Verbalize understanding of treatment plan.
2. Describe signs and symptoms that must be reported to a health-care professional.
3. Relate an intent to share feelings and concerns with significant others and health-care professionals.
4. Identify available community resources.

Collaborative Problems

Risk for Complications of Anaphylactic Reaction

Risk for Complications of Cardiotoxicity

Risk for Complications of Electrolyte Imbalance

Risk for Complications of Extravasation of Vesicant Drugs

Risk for Complications of Hemorrhagic Cystitis

Risk for Complications of Bone Marrow Depression

Risk for Complications of Renal Insufficiency

Risk for Complications of Pulmonary Toxicity

Risk for Complications of Neurotoxicity

Risk for Complications of Renal Calculi

Collaborative Outcomes

The client will be monitored for early signs and symptoms of (a) anaphylactic reaction, (b) cardiotoxicity, (c) electrolyte imbalance, (d) extravasation of vesicant drugs, (e) hemorrhagic cystitis, (f) bone marrow depression, (g) renal insufficiency, (h) pulmonary toxicity, (i) neurotoxicity, and (j) renal calculi, and will receive collaborative interventions if indicated to restore physiologic stability.

Indicators of Physiologic Stability

- Calm, alert, oriented (a, i)
- No complaints of urticaria or pruritus (a)
- No complaints of tightness in throat (a)
- No complaints of shortness of breath or wheezing (a, h)
- Temperature 98.5°–99° F (h)
- Pulse 60–100 beats/min (b, h)
- BP >90/160, <140/90 mm Hg (b, g)
- Normal sinus rhythm (b)
- Flat neck veins (b)
- Serum sodium 135–145 mEq/L (c, g)
- Serum potassium 3.8–5 mEq/L (c, g)
- Serum magnesium 1.3–2.4 mEq/L (c, g)
- Serum phosphorous 2.5–4.5 mEq/L (c, g)
- Serum calcium 8.5–10.5 mEq/L (c, g)
- Urine output >0.5 mL/kg/h (c, g, j)
- Intact strength (c, i)
- Intact sensation (c, i)
- Stable gait (c, i)
- No seizures (c, i)
- No complaints of headache (c)
- No muscle cramps or twitching (c)
- No nausea or vomiting (c, j)
- Stools soft and formed (c, i)
- No swelling at IV site (d)
- No erythema or pain at IV site (d)
- No dysuria, frequency or urgency (e, j)
- White blood cells 4,800–10,000/mm^3 (f)
- Red blood cells (f)
    - Male 4,600,000–6,200,000
    - Female 4,200,000–5,400,000/mm^3
- Platelet 100,000–400,000/mm^3 (f)

- Monocytes 2% to 6% (f)
- Blood urea nitrogen 10–20 mg/dL (g)
- Serum creatinine 0.7–1.4 mg/dL (g)
- Serum pH 7.35–7.45 (h)
- Oxygen saturation (SaO_2) 94% (h)
- Carbon dioxide ($PaCO_2$) 34–45 mm/Hg (h)
- Normal chest x-ray (h)
- Normal pulmonary function tests (h)
- No complaints of flank or abdominal pain (j)

Interventions	Rationales
1. Perform a thorough assessment of past reactions to other medications, food, contrast dye, and bee stings **CLINICAL ALERT** • Hypersensitivy reaction (HSR) is defined as "as exaggerated immune response to an antigen or foreign substance" (Gobel, 2005). • Previous research supports that clients with a history of environmental or medication allergies may be at an increased risk of having a hypersensitivity reaction.	1. If a medication has a high probability of a reaction, premedication protocols are indicated (Kuntzsch & Voge, 2009). Premedications include antihistamine (H_1 receptor antagonist), H_2 antagonist, and steroids. The H_1 receptor blockade results in decreased vascular permeability, reduction of pruritus, and relaxation of smooth muscle in the respiratory and gastrointestinal tracts. Routinely given by intravenous route; however, studies have shown safe protection against hypersensitivity reactions when given orally (Zidan et al., 2008). Decadron is often given as a premedication to stabilize mast cell membranes and prevent mast cell degranulation.
2. Record baseline vital signs and mental status before administering chemotherapy.	2. Antibodies are released in response to an allergen (chemotherapy or targeted therapy is the antigen), so if the body is not feeling under attack or senses an allergic reaction, little IgE would be found in the body (Timoney et al., 2003).
3. Ensure skin tests or test dose given when administering a drug known to have increased incidence of hypersensitivity. Stay with your client for the first 15 minutes, monitoring vital signs.	3. Reactions can occur on first exposure and repeat doses. "Anaphylaxis is caused by the interaction of a foreign antigen with specific immunoglobulin E (IgE) antibodies found on the tissue of mast cells and peripheral blood basophils. The subsequent release of bioactive mediators from these cellular components results in smooth muscle spasm, mucosal edema and inflammation, and increased capillary permeability" (Timoney et al., 2003).
4. Monitor for symptoms of anaphylactic reaction: a. Urticaria, pruritus b. Sensation of lump in throat c. Shortness of breath / wheezing d. Flushing of skin, drop in BP e. Edema	4. Remember, histamine promotes inflammation causing vasodilation and increased capillary permeability. A hypersensitivity reaction will most likely occur within minutes of administration or shortly after an increased rate. Missing one step in premedication, length of time between premedications, and titration of paclitaxel can be detrimental to the individual. a. Stimulation of nerve endings, causing itching and pain to skin c. Constricted bronchial airways, wheezing and difficulty breathing, stimulation of mucous secretion causing congestion d. Dilatation of blood vessels, flushing to skin, drop in blood pressure, will progress to shock e. Increased capillary permeability causing swelling of tissues (edema), if severe untreated reaction, decreased blood volume, shock

Interventions	*Rationales*
5. If symptoms of anaphylaxis develop, discontinue chemotherapy and apply a tourniquet proximal to the injection site. Call Rapid Response Team. Administer emergency drugs per protocol (epinephrine, diphenhydramine, hydrocortisone). Emergency drugs reduce histamine release, relieve edema and spasm, and prevent shock. Remain calm, assess all symptoms and (1) stop the infusion, infuse normal saline, and continue to monitor the individual or (2) slow the infusion and monitor for symptoms to alleviate.	5. Increased vascular permeability, a characteristic feature of anaphylaxis, allows transfer of as much as 50% of the intravascular fluid into the extravascular space within 10 minutes. As a result, hemodynamic collapse might occur rapidly with little or no cutaneous or respiratory manifestations. This means individuals may not complain of any shortness of breath, itching, or any forewarning prior to reacting (Lieberman et al., 2005).

CLINICAL ALERT
- Reactions are very frightening for you, the individual and his or her family.
- The more rapidly anaphylaxis occurs during an infusion the more likely it is to be severe and potentially life threatening.
- Most reactions will occur within minutes, but some individual may have a delayed reaction such as 30 minutes into the infusion. Some individual may have a delayed reaction called "late phase" or "biphasic reactions," which may occur 8–12 hours after the individual is home.
- Once an individual is reacting despite the best interventions and aggressive treatment, individuals may experience protracted and severe anaphylaxis up to 32 hours.

6. Monitor vital signs every 15 minutes until client is stable.	6. Careful monitoring can detect early signs of hypotension and shock.
7. Monitor for signs and symptoms of cardiotoxicity, which can occur within 24 hours, subacute at 4 to 5 weeks, or chronic occurring weeks or months following therapy. Report promptly: a. Gradual increase in heart rate b. Increased shortness of breath c. Diminished breath sound, rales d. Decreased systolic blood pressure e. Presence of or increase in S_3 or S_4 gallop f. Peripheral edema g. Distended neck veins h. Arrhythmia i. Asymptomatic ECG changes	7, 8, 9. Cardiotoxicity can be (1) acute, occurring soon after administration of chemotherapy; (2) subacute, associated with pericarditis and myocardial dysfunction that occur 4–5 weeks after treatment; and (3) "Cardiotoxicity can be . . . cardiomyopathic," which occurs within months of treatment. Anthracyclines, such as doxorubicin and daunorubicin, are known for their potential to cause cardiotoxicity. In high doses, anthracyclines damage heart cells, causing loss of pumping ability and increased oxygen need. A QRS voltage change in an ECG may signal a life-threatening condition.

CLINICAL ALERT
- Stop infusion. Call Rapid Response Team, if indicated

8. Recline the individual, elevating legs to slow progression of hemodynamic compromise, prevent hypotension, and encourage blood flow to the head, heart, and kidneys.

9. Maintain airway, monitor pulse oximetry, administer oxygen to individual. Follow protocols.

(continued)

Interventions	Rationales
10. Ensure that individuals receiving potentially cardio-toxic drugs have baseline cardiac workup prior to administration.	10. Factors putting clients at increased risk of cardiotoxicity include cumulative dose of anthracycline, over the age of 70, previous chest radiation, preexisting cardiac disease, and concurrent treatment with targeted therapy (Cornett & Dea, 2012).
11. Monitor for electrolyte imbalances:	11. Chemotherapeutic agents, as well as cancers themselves, often precipitate electrolyte imbalance (Astle, 2005).
a. Hyponatremia or hypernatremia	a. Hyponatremia is caused by secretion of antidiuretic hormone secondary to vincristine or cyclophosphamide therapy, excessive hydration, or decrease in peripheral blast count secondary to daunorubicin or cytosine therapy. Hypernatremia may result from renal failure secondary to drug nephrotoxicity.
b. Hypokalemia or hyperkalemia	b. Hypokalemia may be due to intercellular shift, excessive diarrhea, or renal tubular injury. Hyperkalemia is caused by cell lysis and renal damage.
c. Hypomagnesemia	c. Hypomagnesemia can result from vomiting, diarrhea, or cisplatin therapy, which causes excretion of divalent ions.
d. Hypophosphatemia	d. Hypophosphatemia is associated with hypercalcemia, hypokalemia, and hypomagnesemia.
e. Hypocalcemia or hypercalcemia (refer to the Collaborative Problems section of the Chronic Renal Failure Care Plan for specific signs and symptoms of each electrolyte imbalance).	e. Hypercalcemia is secondary to hypophosphatemia, renal failure, or mithramycin therapy; hypocalcemia is secondary to hyperphosphatemia or renal failure.
12. Monitor and teach client and family to monitor for and report the following: a. Excessive fluid loss or gain b. Change in orientation or level of consciousness c. Weakness or ataxia d. Paresthesias e. Persistent headache f. Muscle cramps, twitching, or tetany g. Nausea and vomiting h. Diarrhea	12. Electrolyte imbalances affect neurotransmission, muscle activity, and fluid balance.

> **CLINICAL ALERT**
> • Take steps to reduce extravasation of vesicant medications—agents that cause severe necrosis, tissue destruction, ulcers, or blisters (Chmielowski, Casciato, & Wagner, 2009) if they leak from blood vessels into tissue.
> • Signs and symptoms of extravasation include edema and changes of the appearance of the skin.
> • The individual may complain of pain, numbness, or tightness at the site.
> • The American Society of Clinical Oncology (ASCO) and the Oncology Nursing Society (ONS) have partnered on a collaborative effort to develop evidence-based standards for safe administration of chemotherapy.
> • Current ASCO / ONS standards address safety of all routes of chemotherapy administration to adult clients in the outpatient setting and inpatient setting.
> • Refer to http://www.ons.org/CNECentral/Chemo/Standards to review the 2013 standards.

A central line significantly reduces the risk of a drug extravasation. Extravasation may occur secondary to improper placement, damaged vein, or obstructed venous drainage secondary to superior vena cava syndrome, edema, or tumor. The back of the hand or near joints should be avoided as functional damage can occur with extravasations (Chmielowski et al., 2009).

Interventions	Rationales

- Preventive measures are as follows:
  - Avoid infusing vesicants over joints, bony prominences, tendons, neurovascular bundles, or the antecubital fossa.
  - Avoid multiple punctures, or probing to find a site of the same vein within 24 hours.
  - Recommendation to administer drug through a central line.
  - Do not administer drug if edema is present or blood return is absent.
  - If peripheral IV site is used, evaluate its status and if it is less than 24 hours old.
  - Observe peripheral infusion continuously.
  - Provide infusion through a central line and check every 1–2 hours.

13. Advise individual / family of the possibility of extravasation.

13. Clients must have informed consent of the potential of an extravasation (local infiltration of the chemotherapy / targeted therapy).

14. Ensure that a document is posted clearly in the infusion area outlining vesicants and irritants, recommended antidotes, and hot or cold compress indication.

14. This will ensure a rapid and correct response.

15. Monitor during drug infusion. Assess patency of intravenous (IV) infusion line by gently withdrawing blood and infusing normal saline. Instruct individual to report any changes in sensation immediately:
    a. Observe tissue at the IV site every 30 minutes for the following:
       - Swelling (most common)
       - Leakage
       - Burning / pain (not always present)
       - Inflammation
       - Erythema (not seen initially)
       - Hyperpigmentation

15. Prior to initiation of the vesicant, the nurse and client should be aware of any potential complications. Extravasation usually causes immediate pain (however, it can be painless—detected late with a potential for increased tissue damage) with increased signs / symptoms over a few days, in some clients (Chmielowski et al., 2009).

16. If extravasation occurs, take the following steps with gloves on:
    a. Stop administration of drug.
    b. Leave needle in place.
    c. Gently aspirate residual drug and blood in tubing or needle.
    d. Avoid applying direct pressure on site.
    e. Give antidote as ordered by physician / NP or institutional policy.
    f. If plant alkaloid or etoposide extravasation, apply warm compresses 15–20 minutes QID for 24 hours.
    g. If anthracycline extravasation, apply ice for 15–20 minutes every 3–4 hours for 24–48 hours.
    h. Outline area of extravasation with pen.
    i. Never flush the line.

17. If extravasation occurs, monitor site: Elevate limb above heart for 48 hours. After 48 hours, encourage client to use limb normally. Follow your hospital policy on extravasations.

17. Detecting signs of extravasation early enables prompt intervention to prevent serious complications, including tissue necrosis.

(continued)

Interventions	Rationales
18. Monitor for erythema, pain, and indication every hour for 4 hours and then every 4–8 hours according to protocol. 　a. For periferal intravenous sites, avoid sites that infuse vesicants over joints, bony prominences, tendons, neurovascular bundles, and antecubital fossa. 　b. Avoid multiple punctures in the same vein within 24 hours.	18. Extravasation can cause underlying tissue damage resulting in permanent damage. 　a. These sites, if extravasated, into can cause permanent damage or deformity (Chmielowski et al., 2009). 　b. Multiple punctures make the vessel more vulnerable to infiltration.
19. When administering cyclophosphamide, monitor for signs and symptoms of hemorrhagic cystitis: 　a. Dysuria 　b. Frequency 　c. Urgency 　d. Hematuria	19. Cyclophosphamide administration is associated with the development of hemorrhagic cystitis.
20. Administer cyclophosphamide early in the day.	20. Administration early in the day reduces the high drug concentration that can occur during the night secondary to reduced intake.
21. Teach client to do the following: 　a. Void every 2 hours. 　b. Increase fluid intake to 2,500–3,000 mL/day unless contraindicated.	21. Frequent voiding and optimal hydration reduce drug concentration in the bladder.
22. Monitor for signs of bone marrow depression: 　a. Decreased WBC and RBC counts 　b. Decreased platelet count 　c. Decreased granulocyte count	22. Bone marrow toxicity is dependent on the treatment used. Most chemotherapeutic agents can cause suppression of the bone marrow.

> **CLINICAL ALERT**
> * The earlier the symptoms are realized, the faster they can be treated (Forsythe & Faulkner, 2004).
> * Chemotherapy interferes with cell division of bone marrow stem cells that form blood cells.
> * Granulocytes are mainly neutrophils that are the first line of defense against infection.
> * The American Society of Clinical Oncology and NCCN guidelines provide recommendations for clients at risk for complications of myelosupression.

Interventions	Rationales
23. Explain risks of bleeding and infection. (Refer to the Corticosteroid Therapy Care Plan for strategies to reduce these risks.)	23. Chemotherapy may cause a depression in bone marrow production, especially when the bone marrow of skeletal sites is irradiated. Leukocytes, thrombocytes, and RBCs are decreased, predisposing the client to infection, bleeding, and anemia, in that order (Twite, 2005).
24. Monitor for signs of renal insufficiency: 　a. Sustained elevated urine specific gravity 　b. Elevated urine sodium levels 　c. Sustained insufficient urine output (<30 mL/h) 　d. Elevated blood pressure 　e. Hypomagnesemia or hypocalcemia 　f. Increasing BUN and serum creatinine, potassium, phosphorus, ammonia, and decreased creatinine clearance	24. Chemotherapy-induced renal toxicity can occur (1) directly, as with cisplatin, methotrexate, and mitomycin, which can produce toxic effects on renal glomeruli and tubules and (2) indirectly because of rapid tumor cell lysis, causing hyperuricemia and nephropathy (Camp-Sorrell, 2007).

Interventions	Rationales
25. Monitor for pulmonary toxicity (pneumonitis or fibrosis) when administering bleomycin and nitrosoureas; signs and symptoms include the following: a. Cough b. Fever c. Tachycardia d. Dyspnea e. Rales f. Weakness g. Cyanosis h. Abnormal arterial blood gas analysis i. Abnormal chest x-ray film j. Abnormal pulmonary function tests	25. Lung inflammation and fibrosis are associated with administration of bleomycin and nitrosoureas (e.g., carmustine and busulfan). The extent of fibrosis determines the severity of respiratory dysfunction.
26. Instruct client to cough and do deep breathing every 2 hours.	26. These activities help to reduce retention of secretions and dilate alveoli.
27. Monitor for signs and symptoms of neurotoxicity: a. Paresthesias b. Gait disturbance c. Altered fine motor activity d. Lethargy e. Muscle weakness f. Foot or wrist drop g. Somnolence h. Disorientation i. Confusion j. Hearing loss	27. Chemotherapy may cause peripheral or central neurotoxicity. Peripheral neurotoxicity is usually noted as a peripheral neuropathy, with mixed sensory motor deficits and may be associated with painful parenthesias. Monitor for cumulative doses of Cisplatin. Neurotoxicity can progress to total hearing loss (Cornett & Dea, 2012).
28. Monitor for signs and symptoms of renal calculi: a. Flank pain b. Nausea and vomiting c. Abdominal pain	28. Renal calculi may result from chemotherapy because rapid cell lysis of tumor cells produces hyperuricemia. Pain is caused by pressure of calculi on the renal tubules. Afferent stimuli in renal capsule may cause pylorospasm of the smooth muscle of the enteric tract and adjacent structures.
29. Refer to the Urolithiasis Care Plan for specific interventions to reduce risk of renal calculi.	

Clinical Alert Report
Prior to providing care, advise ancillary staff / student to report the following to the professional nurse assigned to the client:
- Change in cognitive status
- Increased sombulence
- Complaints of itching,
- Complaints of pain, burning, or redness at infusion site
- Oral temperature >100.5° F
- Systolic BP <90 mm/Hg
- Resting pulse >100, <50
- Respiratory rate >28, <10/min
- Oxygen saturation <90%
- Complaints of headache (c)
- Complaints of muscle cramps or twitching
- Complaints of nausea or vomiting

Related Physician / NP Prescribed Interventions

Medications

Antiemetics, antianxiety, dexamethasone, chemotherapeutic agents, targeted therapy

Laboratory Studies

Complete blood count, urinalysis, electrolytes, BUN, serum albumin, pulmonary function test

Diagnostic Studies

Chest x-ray, pulse oximetry

Documentation

Vital signs
Abnormal laboratory values (electrolytes, complete blood count [CBC], platelets, and BUN)
Condition of injection sites
Intake and output
Urine specific gravity
Client teaching
New complaints and interventions provided

Nursing Diagnoses

Anxiety Related to Prescribed Chemotherapy, Insufficient Knowledge of Chemotherapy, and Self-Care Measures

NOC

Anxiety Level, Coping, Impulse Control

NIC

Anxiety Reduction, Impulse Control Training, Anticipatory Guidance

Goal

The client will share feelings regarding scheduled chemotherapy / targeted therapy.

Indicators

- Describe the anticipated effects of chemotherapy.
- Relate signs and symptoms of toxicity.
- Identify important self-care measures.

Interventions	Rationales
1. Encourage client to share feelings and beliefs regarding chemotherapy. Delay teaching if high levels of anxiety are present.	1. Verbalization can identify sources of client anxiety and allow the nurse to correct misinformation. High anxiety impairs learning. Despite dramatic advances in understanding cancer biology and subsequent progression in the development of treatment options, cancer continues to cause devastating emotional and physical suffering in clients who are dealing with the diagnosis of cancer each year in the United States. Pain, anxiety, depression, and fatigue are prominent contributors to the impact of psychosocial distress (McQuellon et al., 1998). Depression has been identified as the only psychological diagnosis more prevalent in clients with cancer than in the general population (Satin, Linden, & Phillips, 2009).
2. Reinforce physician / NP's explanations of the chemotherapeutic regimen—the drugs, dosage schedules, and management of side effects.	
3. Explain the therapeutic effects of cytotoxic drugs; provide written information. (Note: Client education booklets are available from the National Cancer Institute and the American Cancer Society.)	

Interventions	Rationales

4. Explain the common side effects and toxicities of chemotherapy:
  a. Decreased WBC count
  b. Decreased platelet count
  c. Infection
  d. GI alterations
  e. Hair loss
  f. Fatigue
  g. Emotional responses
  h. Neuropathies
	4. Specific explanations provide information to help reduce anxiety associated with fear of the unknown and loss of control.

5. Discuss self-care measures to reduce risk of toxicities:
  a. Nutrition
  b. Hygiene
  c. Rest
  d. Activity
  e. Managing bowel elimination problems
  f. Managing hair loss
  g. Monitoring for infection
  h. Prioritizing activities
	5. Providing clients with the appropriate amount of information tends to increase their sense of control, and ability to adapt to the situation, facilitate participation in their treatment plan, decrease anxiety, and increase ability to cope (McQuellon et al., 1998).

6. Refer also to the Cancer (Initial Diagnosis) Care Plan for additional information.	

Documentation

Client teaching
Outcome achievement or status
Dialogues

Nausea Related to Gastrointestinal Cell Damage, Stimulation of Vomiting Center, Fear, and Anxiety

NOC
Comfort Level,
Nutritional Status,
Hydration

Goal

The client will report decreased nausea.

NIC
Medication
Management, Nausea
Management, Fluid /
Electrolyte Management,
Nutrition Management

Indicators

- Name foods or beverages that do not increase nausea
- Describe factors that increase nausea

Client adhering to antiemetic schedule

Interventions	Rationales
1. Promote a positive attitude about chemotherapy; reinforce its cancer cell-killing effects.	1. Frank discussions can increase motivation to reduce and tolerate nausea.
2. Explain possible reasons for nausea and vomiting.	2. Chemotherapy-induced nausea and vomiting is thought to be due to a stimulation of the chemoreceptor trigger zone located in the medulla. This area of the brain reacts according to the level of circulating chemicals found in the blood (Porth, 2011). Cytotoxic drugs damage GI cells, which can produce a vagal response. They also can stimulate the vomiting center in the brain. Anxiety and fear contribute to the problem. Chemotherapy effects can lead to marked disruption in self-care, requiring more family support.

(continued)

Interventions	Rationales

> **CLINICAL ALERT**
> * The importance of assessing, managing, and treating chemotherapy-induced nausea and vomiting (CINV) cannot be over stressed.
> * Ensure that individuals are able to verbalize understanding of their antiemetic schedule (Cornett & Dea, 2012).

Interventions	Rationales
3. Explain the rationale for antiemetic agents; administer them before initiating chemotherapy and during the time chemotherapy drugs are most likely to cause nausea and vomiting.	3. Antiemetics are given before chemotherapy to reduce nausea.
4. Infuse cytotoxic drugs slowly.	4. Slow infusion can decrease stimulation of the vomiting center.
5. Eat only lightly before therapy.	5. This will avoid gastric overstimulation.
6. Administer emetic and cytotoxic drugs at night (during sleep if possible) or have client lie quietly for 2 hours after administration.	6. Activity stimulates the GI tract, which can increase nausea and vomiting.
7. If delayed nausea develops 3–4 days after treatment, consult with physician / NP.	7. Delayed nausea is usually unresponsive to standard antiemetics. Antianxiety agents (e.g., lorazepam), are often as effective as dexamethasone.
8. If taste alterations occur, suggest that the client suck on hard candy during chemotherapy.	8. Hard candy can reduce the metallic or bitter taste that client may experience from chemotherapy.
9. Encourage client to eat small, frequent meals and to eat slowly. Cool, bland foods and liquids are usually well tolerated. Vary diet.	9. Intake of small amounts prevents gastric distention from stimulating vomiting.
10. Eliminate unpleasant sights and odors from the eating area.	10. Eliminating noxious stimuli can decrease stimulation of the vomiting center.
11. Instruct client to avoid the following: a. Hot or cold liquids b. Foods containing fat and fiber c. Spicy foods, caffeine	11. Certain foods increase peristalsis and provoke nausea and vomiting: a. Cold liquids can induce cramping; hot liquids can stimulate peristalsis. b. High-fat and high-fiber food and drinks increase peristalsis. c. These substances can stimulate intestinal motility.
12. Encourage client to rest in semi-Fowler's position after eating and to change position slowly.	12. Muscle relaxation can reduce peristalsis.
13. Teach stress reduction techniques such as these: a. Relaxation exercises b. Visual imagery c. Massage d. Music therapy	13. These techniques reduce muscle tension and decrease client's focus on nausea.
14. Additional resources can be accessed at: http://www.cancer.org/treatment/treatmentsandsideeffects/treatmenttypes/ http://www.cancer.gov/cancertopics/factsheet/Therapy/targeted http://www.chemocare.com/chemotherapy/drug-info/default.aspx http://www.ons.org/Research/PEP	

Documentation

Intake and output
Tolerance of intake

Corticosteroid Therapy

Corticosteroid is the generic name for commercial adrenocortical hormones and synthetic analogues. Corticosteroids are indicated as replacement therapy for adrenal insufficiency, inflammation suppression, allergic reaction control, and reducing the risk of graft rejection in transplantation. A client on long-term corticosteroid therapy has suppressed pituitary and adrenal functions. Some indications for corticosteroid therapy are severe autoimmune diseases, rheumatoid arthritis, severe asthma, cancer, multiple sclerosis, and psoriasis.

"Short-term corticosteroid use is associated with generally mild side effects, including cutaneous effects, electrolyte abnormalities, hypertension, hyperglycemia, pancreatitis, hematologic, immunologic, and neuropsychologic effects, although occasionally, clinically significant side effects may occur. Long-term corticosteroid use may be associated with more serious sequel, including osteoporosis, aseptic joint necrosis, adrenal insufficiency, gastrointestinal, hepatic, and ophthalmologic effects, hyperlipidemia, growth suppression, and possible congenital malformations" (Buchman, 2001, p. 289).

Time Frame
Intratherapy

Refer to Unit II Risk for Complications of Adrenocorticosteroid Therapy Adverse Effects.

Enteral Nutrition

Enteral nutrition is the administration of an elemental liquid diet (calories, minerals, and vitamins) to the GI tract through a nasogastric, nasojejunostomy, gastric, or jejunostomy tube. Enteral nutrition can include both oral supplements and tube-feeding techniques. The client with a functioning intestine but who is unable to eat sufficient calories is a candidate.

Evaluation by a multidisciplinary team is indicated prior to insertion of a long-term feeding device to establish whether (Enteral Nutrition Practice Recommendations Task Force, 2009, p. 143):

- benefit outweighs the risk of access placement;
- insertion of feeding tubes near end of life is warranted; or
- insertion of feeding tubes is indicated in the situation where clients are close to achieving oral feeding.

Carp's Cues
"The decision concerning placement of long-term access is dependent on the estimated length of therapy, the client's disposition, and the special needs of the client and caregivers" (Enteral Nutrition Practice Recommendations Task Force, 2009, p. 143).

Researchers have reported adult clients with persistent dysphagia due to neurological diseases had better outcomes with percutaneous endoscopic gastrostomy (PEG) feedings than those randomized to NG feedings (Norton et al., 1996; Park et al., 1992). Individuals with PEG access had greater weight gain and fewer missed feedings (Norton et al., 1996; Park et al., 1992). Clients with persistent dysphasia should have a long-term enteral access device placed (Enteral Nutrition Practice Recommendations Task Force, 2009).

Time Frame
Preprocedure and postprocedure

■■■■■ DIAGNOSTIC CLUSTER

Collaborative Problems

▲ Risk for Complications of Hypoglycemia / Hyperglycemia

▲ Risk for Complications of Hypervolemia

△ Risk for Complications of Hypertonic Dehydration

▲ Risk for Complications of Electrolyte Imbalances

△ Risk for Complications of Mucosal Erosion

Nursing Diagnoses

▲ Impaired Comfort: Cramping, Distention, Diarrhea, Nausea, Vomiting related to type of formula, administration rate, route, or formula temperature

▲ Risk for Aspiration related to position of tube and client

△ Risk for Ineffective Self-Health Management related to lack of knowledge of nutritional indications / requirements, home care, and signs and symptoms of complications

▲ This diagnosis was reported to be monitored for or managed frequently (75% to 100%).
△ This diagnosis was reported to be monitored for or managed often (50% to 74%).

Transition Criteria

Before transition, the client or family will

1. Identify therapeutic indications and nutritional requirements.
2. Demonstrate tube feeding administration and management.
3. Discuss strategies for incorporating enteral management into ADLs.
4. State signs and symptoms that must be reported to a health-care professional.

Collaborative Problems

Risk for Complications of Hypoglycemia or Hyperglycemia

Risk for Complications of Hypervolemia

Risk for Complications of Hypertonic Dehydration

Risk for Complications of Electrolyte and Trace Mineral Imbalance

Risk for Complications of Mucosal Erosion

Collaborative Outcomes

The client will be monitored for early signs and symptoms of of (a) hypoglycemia / hyperglycemia, (b) hypervolemia, (c) hypertonic dehydration, (d) electrolyte imbalances, and mucosal erosion, and will receive collaborative interventions if indicated to restore physiologic stability.

Indicators of Physiologic Stability

• Alert, oriented, calm (a)
• Pulse 60–100 beats/min (a, b)
• Respirations easy, rhythmic 16–20 breaths/min (b)
• Respiratory, no rales or wheezing (b)
• BP >90/60, <140/90 mm Hg (b)
• No complaints of dizziness (a)
• Urine output 0.5 mL/kg/h (a)
• Urine specific gravity 1.005–1.030 (c)
• Blood glucose 60–140 mg/dL
• Serum potassium 3.8–5 mEq/L (c, d)

- Serum sodium 135–145 mEq/L (c, d)
- Serum osmolality 280–300 mOsm/kg H_2O (c, d)
- No peripheral edema (b)
- Moist mucous membranes (oral) (c)
- Intact mucosa at tube exit site (d)
- No complaints of fatigue (a)
- No complaints of nausea (a)

Interventions	Rationales

CLINICAL ALERT

- If inappropriate use of enteral therapy is suspected (e.g., NG feedings, PEG tube feedings or any type of tube feeding due to end-of-life situation), proceed with STAR.

Situation 1

STAR

Stop

Think Is this individual inappropriate for enteral nutrition (e.g., not in end-of-life stage)?

Act If this treatment is inappropriate and causing unnecessary suffering, consult an experienced nurse.

Review Has the problem been addressed? If not, use SBAR to communicate to the appropriate person (e.g., manager, physician / NP). Initiate a family conference with nurse, physician / NP, ethics consultant to discuss the situation (futility, pain) vs. palliative care.

Situation 2

STAR

Stop

Think If enteral nutrition is indicated, is the method appropriated? "Long-term feeding devices should be considered when the need for enteral feeding is at least 4 weeks in adults, children, and infants after term age" (Enteral Nutrition Practice Recommendations Task Force, 2009, p. 146).

Act If PEG tube indicated, consult an experienced nurse for assistance or contact the physician / NP.

Review Has the problem been addressed? If not, use SBAR to communicate to the appropriate person (e.g., manager, physician / NP).

1. Cleanse incision and tube insertion site regularly following standard protocol.	1. Cleaning removes microorganisms and reduces risk of infection.

(continued)

Interventions	*Rationales*
2. Protect skin around the external feeding tube with a protective barrier film. Apply a loose dressing cover and change it when moist. For excessive drainage, protect skin with an adhesive barrier square and ostomy pouch to capture drainage; change the barrier when nonadherent or soiled.	2. The catheter can irritate skin and mucosa. Gastric juices can cause severe skin breakdown.
3. For a temporary gastrostomy or jejunostomy tube, anchor tube to an external surface to minimize tube migration and retraction.	3. Movement can cause tissue trauma and create entry points for opportunistic microorganisms.
4. Monitor for symptoms of hypoglycemia after completion of tube feeding: a. Tachycardia b. Diaphoresis c. Confusion d. Dizziness e. Generalized weakness	4. Sudden cessation of enteral feedings in a physiologically stressed client may trigger a hypoglycemic reaction.
5. Monitor for symptoms of hyperglycemia during formula administration: a. Thirst b. Increased urination c. Fatigue d. Generalized weakness e. Increased respirations f. Increased pulse g. Nausea	5. Hyperglycemia most commonly occurs in clients with inadequate insulin reserves. Enteral formulas with a higher fat percentage are less likely to contribute to hyperglycemic reaction.
6. Monitor for signs and symptoms of overhydration during formula administration: a. Tachycardia b. Elevated blood pressure c. Pulmonary edema d. Shortness of breath e. Peripheral edema	6. Hypervolemia usually is associated with the high water and sodium contents of the enteral formula. This complication most often occurs as feeding is initiated or reintroduced in a client with compromised cardiac, renal, or hepatic function.
7. Monitor for signs and symptoms of hypertonic dehydration during formula administration: a. Dry mucous membranes b. Thirst c. Decreased serum sodium d. Circulatory overload (increased BP, increased respirations) e. Decreasing urine output f. Concentrated urine	7. Hypertonic dehydration most often results when a formula of high osmolarity and protein content is administered to a client unable to recognize or respond to thirst. It causes circulatory overload and cellular dehydration.
8. Monitor tube exit and entrance sites for: a. Mucosal erosion b. Pain and tenderness c. Bleeding d. Ulceration	8, 9. External pressure or tension on delicate structures can produce mucosal erosion. Prolonged use of large-bore polyvinyl chloride (PVC) catheters has been linked to the development of rhinitis, pharyngitis, nasal cartilage destruction, and esophageal erosion (Best, 2007). After 10 days PVC tubes begin to break down and lose their flexibility, increasing the risk of complications. Graded tubes improve the accuracy of measurement during insertion, and at subsequent client assessments.

Interventions	*Rationales*

9. Take steps to reduce tube irritation:
   a. Tape tubes securely without causing pressure or tension.
   b. Prepare skin prior to taping with a skin protective agent.
   c. Use a PVC tube only if the feeding is needed for 10 days or less. Fine-bore polyurethane tubes are preferable for longer term nasogastric enteral therapy (Best, 2007).
   d. All tubes should be clearly marked in centimeters or line markers (Best, 2007).

Clinical Alert Report

Prior to providing care, advise ancillary staff / student to report the following to the professional nurse assigned to the client:
- Change in cognitive status
- Blood glucose >200 mg/dL
- Oral temperature > 100.5° F
- Systolic BP <90 mm/Hg
- Resting pulse >100, <50
- Respiratory rate >28, <10 /min
- Oxygen saturation <90%
- Drainage (characteristics, amount)
- Site condition

Related Physician / NP Prescribed Interventions

Medications
Formula (frequency and dilution) and flush or free water amount

Intravenous Therapy
Not applicable

Laboratory Studies
Serum prealbumin, electrolytes, serum glucose, serum transferrin

Diagnostic Studies
Radiogram (verification)

Therapies
Dependent on the type of tube used, weights

Documentation

Vital signs
Intake and output
Urine specific gravity
Serum glucose
Tube site condition
Drainage (characteristics, amount)
Site condition

Nursing Diagnoses

Risk for Aspiration Related to Position of Tube and Client

NOC
Aspiration Control

Goal

The client will not experience aspiration.

NIC
Aspiration Precautions,
Airway Management,
Positioning, Airway
Suctioning

Indicators

Relate measures to prevent aspiration

Interventions

1. "Obtain radiographic confirmation that any blindly placed tube (small-bore or large-bore) is properly positioned in the GI tract prior to its initial use for administering feedings and medications" (Enteral Nutrition Practice Recommendations Task Force, 2009, p. 145):
   a. Once radiographic confirmation is complete, mark the tube at the nares with permanent marker.

   b. "After feedings have been started, it is necessary to assure that the tube has remained in the desired location (either the stomach or small bowel)" (Enteral Nutrition Practice Recommendations Task Force, 2009, p. 144).

   > **CLINICAL ALERT**
   > • Do not assume because previous feeding have been reported as satisfactory that aspiration is not occurring.

   c. Testing the pH of feeding tube aspirates is most likely to be helpful when intermittent feedings are used (Enteral Nutrition Practice Recommendations Task Force, 2009, p. 144). If using pH aspirate, administer a scheduled intermittent tube feeding only if gastric pH is 4.0 or less (intrinsically higher in neonates), or postpyloric pH is greater than 6.

   > **CLINICAL ALERT**
   > • In adult clients, do not rely on the auscultatory method to differentiate between gastric and respiratory placement. The auscultatory method cannot distinguish between gastric and small bowel placement, nor can it detect when a tube's tip is in the esophagus (Enteral Nutrition Practice Recommendations Task Force, 2009, p. 144).

Rationales

1. Radiographic confirmation is the only valid confirmation that the tube is in the proper position. Proper tube position must be verified before feeding to prevent introducing formula into the respiratory tract.

   a. Mark the exit site of a feeding tube at the time of the initial radiograph; observe for a change in the external tube length during feedings. If a significant increase in the external length is observed, use other bedside tests to help determine if the tube has become dislocated. If in doubt, obtain a radiograph to determine tube location" (Enteral Nutrition Practice Recommendations Task Force, 2009, p. 145).
   b. "Unfortunately, a small bowel tube may dislocate upward into the stomach or a gastric tube may migrate downward into the small bowel; a worse scenario is when a tube's tip dislocates upward into the esophagus" (Enteral Nutrition Practice Recommendations Task Force, 2009, p. 144).

Interventions	Rationales

d. Elevate the backrest to a minimum of 30 degrees, and preferably to 45 degrees, for all individuals receiving EN unless medically contraindicated. An alternative is to use the reverse Trendelenberg position to elevate the HOB, unless contraindicated, when the client cannot tolerate a backrest elevated position (Enteral Nutrition Practice Recommendations Task Force, 2009).

d. Upper body elevation can prevent reflux through use of gravity.

e. "If necessary to lower the HOB for a procedure or a medical contraindication, return the client to an HOB elevated position as soon as feasible. There is no benefit from stopping the feedings during short periods of HOB lowering" (Enteral Nutrition Practice Recommendations Task Force, 2009, p. 154).

e. McClave et al. (2002) reported that 30% crucially ill individuals in the study received inadequate calories due to suspended feedings during the delivery of nursing care.

CLINICAL ALERT
• Continuous feedings and pH altering medications (e.g., proton-pump will affect accuracy of pH testing) (Huffman, 2004). When aspirating for residual contents, administer a scheduled intermittent tube feeding only if residual contents are less than residual limit set by physician/NP or policy. When a high residual is identified, return it to the stomach. Delay feeding if it is intermittent; stop it for 1 hour if it is continuous. Recheck the residual in 1 hour; if it is still high, notify physician/NP. A different rate, method, route, or formula change may be indicated.

Although there is no one volume of gastric residual determined to be a cutoff point, administering feedings in the presence of excessive residual contents increases risks of reflux and aspiration.

2. Regulate intermittent gastric feedings to allow gastric emptying between feedings and to allow periods of rest so client can ambulate unencumbered by feeding apparatus.

2. Such regulation is necessary to prevent overfeeding and increased risk of reflux and aspiration. Gastric feedings should be administered intermittently when the potential for aspiration is high. When clients are predisposed to aspiration, jejunal tube placement for continual feeding is preferred.

3. Flush feeding tube with 30 mL water every 4 hours during continuous feedings, before and after intermittent feedings and after residual volume measurement.

3. Flushing is necessary to remove formula that can provide a medium for microorganism growth.

CLINICAL ALERT
• Use sterile water for tube flushing in immuno-compromised or critically ill individuals to prevent contaminated water causing a water-borne infection (Enteral Nutrition Practice Recommendations Task Force, 2009).

4. Monitor for GI intolerance (Enteral Nutrition Practice Recommendations Task Force, 2009):
   a. Emesis
   b. Distention
   c. Constipation
   d. Signs of regurgitation
   e. Gastric residual volume GRV of 200–500 mL

CLINICAL ALERT
• Stop enteral feeding if overt regurgitation or aspiration is suspected.
• Notify physician / NP.

(continued)

Interventions	*Rationales*

5. When administering medications directly into the enteral feeding tube (Enteral Nutrition Practice Recommendations Task Force, 2009):
  a. Follow protocols for administering medication into enteral tube.
  b. Do not add medications to the feeding formula.
  c. Dilute medications but do not mix medications together.
  d. Do not use (crush) extended release tablets.
  e. Flush with 15 mL of water before med. administration, between each medication and before reconnecting to feeding formula.
	5. Adhering to the standards of medication administration can reduce risks for physical and chemical incompatibilities, tube obstruction, and altered therapeutic (Enteral Nutrition Practice Recommendations Task Force, 2009).

CLINICAL ALERT
- Consult with pharmacist for direction and clarification if needed.

6. Ensure that a misconnection of the enteral tubing to nonenteral system such as an intravascular catheter, peritoneal dialysis catheter, tracheostomy, medical gas tubing, etc. does not occur:
   a. At hand-off or at transfers, check all connections and trace tubes to their origin.
   b. Label all enteral bags with "For enteral use only."
   c. Prior to reconnecting, nurses should routinely trace each line back to their site of origin and ensure that they are secure. "Route tubes and catheters that have different purposes in unique and standardized directions (e.g., IV lines should be routed toward the client's head, and enteric lines should be routed toward the feet)" (Enteral Nutrition Practice Recommendations Task Force, 2009, p. 157).

CLINICAL ALERT
- The Joint Commission that reports of misconnections may be greatly underestimated (2006). This type of error commonly results in the death of the client by embolus or sepsis. (IBID)

Clinical Alert Report

Prior to providing care, advise ancillary staff / student to report the following to the professional nurse assigned to the client:
- C/o feeling full, distended
- Coughing
- Nausea, vomiting
- Decreased bowel sounds

Documentation

Tube type, tip location, and external markings
pH readings prior to feedings
Breath sounds
Intake and output
Unusual complaints

Impaired Comfort: Cramping, Distention, Nausea, Vomiting Related to Type of Formula, Administration Rate, Route, or Formula Temperature

NOC

Symptom Control,
Comfort Level,
Nutrition Status,
Hydration

Goal

The client will tolerate enteral feedings.

NIC

Environmental
Management:
Comfort, Medication
Management, Nausea
Management,
Fluid/Electrolyte
Management, Nutrition
Management

Indicators

Will report no episodes of cramping, distention, nausea, or vomiting.

Interventions	Rationales
1. Review enteral product information for formula characteristics (i.e., lactose, osmolarity, calories, fiber). Consult with nutritional expert.	1. Many current enteral products have a significantly lower osmolarity and are now lactose free. Specialty formulas (i.e., specific for renal or liver conditions) tend to have higher osmolarities because of their increased calorie-to-milliliter ratio.
2. Initiate feedings slowly; gradually increase rate based on tolerance. Begin with an isotonic, lactose-free formula or alternately dilute other types of feedings with water to decrease osmolality.	
3. Prevent diarrhea by: a. Initiate feedings slowly; progress gradually as tolerated. Begin with an isotonic, lactose-free, fiber-enriched supplement.	3a. The feeding regimen itself may cause problems. For example, a bolus feeding of high osmolality at cold temperature can provoke gastric and digestive problems. Uncontrolled feedings by jejunal route are particularly prone to these complications because the feeding is not processed in the stomach before it reaches the intestines.
b. Instill formula at room temperature directly from the can when possible.	b. Administering cold formula can cause cramping and possibly lead to elimination problems.
c. Discard unused portions or store in a tightly sealed container.	c. These precautions can minimize growth of microorganisms.

(continued)

Interventions	Rationales
d. For continuous feeding, fill container with enough formula for a 4-hour feeding. Do not overfill or allow formula to stand for a longer period.	d. Each type of formula has an individual shelf-life after opening. Follow the institution's policy for safe preparation and administration. Formula should be protected from environmental contaminants to prevent bacterial growth and possible resultant diarrhea. Jejunal intestinal feedings are particularly sensitive to diarrhea because they lack hydrochloric acid. For example, sterile, decanted formula should have an 8-hour hang time or less (Enteral Nutrition Practice Recommendations Task Force, 2009).
4. For intermittent feeding, instill formula gradually over a 15- to 45-minute period. Do not administer as a bolus or at a rapid rate.	4. Intermittent feedings simulate a normal feeding regimen and allow for stomach digestion and emptying. Intermittent stomach feedings also allow for unencumbered physical care between feedings.
5. Consult with physician / NP for antidiarrheal medications as necessary.	5. Medications may be needed to control severe diarrhea.
6. Instill formula at room temperature directly from the can whenever possible.	
7. Discard unused portions or store in a tightly sealed container.	7, 8. Extended exposure of a feeding to room temperature promotes microorganism growth.
8. For continuous feeding, fill container with enough formula for a 4-hour feeding. Do not overfill or allow formula to stand for a longer period.	
9. For intermittent feeding, instill formula gradually over a 15- to 45-minute period. Do not administer as a bolus or at a rapid rate.	9. Slow administration can reduce cramping, nausea, and vomiting.
10. Chew gum, if indicated.	10. Gum can help to keep the mouth moist.
11. Brush teeth and use mouthwash three to four times a day.	11. Frequent mouth care can maintain moist mucous membranes and remove microorganisms.

Documentation

Intake and output
Unusual events or problems

Risk for Ineffective Self-Health Management Related to Lack of Knowledge of Nutritional Indications / Requirements, Home Care, and Signs and Symptoms of Complications

NOC

Compliance Behavior, Knowledge: Treatment Regimen, Participation: Health-Care Decisions, Treatment Behavior: Illness or Injury

Goal

The goals for this diagnosis represent those associated with transition planning. Refer to the transition criteria.

NIC

Anticipatory Guidance, Learning Facilitation, Risk Identification, Health Education, Teaching: Procedure / Treatment, Health System Guidance

Interventions	Rationales
1. For individuals who receive enteral at home, refer to home health nursing agency for home care assessment on the day of transition.	1. A home health-care agency can provide ongoing assistance and support.
2. Have client or support person perform return demonstration of selected care measures.	2. Return demonstration lets nurse evaluate client's and family's abilities to perform feedings safely.
3. Explain measures to prevent aspiration. (Refer to the nursing diagnosis Potential for Aspiration in this entry for more information.)	3. Aspiration is a potential complication of all types of oral / pharyngeal tube feedings.
4. Refer to the care plan for the specific condition that necessitated enteral feeding.	

> **CLINICAL ALERT**
>
> • If there are concerns over the ability of the caregivers at home to safely administer enteral feeding:
>
> | STAR | Stop | |
> |---|---|---|
> | | Think | If enteral nutrition is indicated, is the method appropriated? "Are there barriers for the caregivers to provide safe enteral feedings?" (e.g., motivation, manual skills, anxiety, practice, knowledge) |
> | | Review | Can the barriers be removed for successful transition? Is it safe for transition to proceed? Can a home health nurse be at the home the day of transition? If not use SBAR, to communicate to the appropriate person (e.g., manager, physician / NP). |

Documentation

Client and family teaching
Demonstrated ability of home caregiver to provide treatments safely
Outcome achievement or status
Referrals, if indicated

Hemodialysis

Hemodialysis is the removal of metabolic wastes and excess electrolytes and fluids from the blood to treat acute or chronic kidney disease. The procedure uses the principles of diffusion, osmosis, and filtration. Blood is pumped into an artificial kidney through a semipermeable, cellophane-like membrane surrounded by a flow of dialysate, which is a solution composed of water, glucose, sodium, chloride, potassium, calcium, and acetate or bicarbonate. The amounts of these constituents vary depending on the amount of water, waste products, or electrolytes to be removed. Hemodialysis does not correct renal dysfunction; it only corrects metabolic waste, fluid, electrolyte, and acid–base imbalances (King, 2008).

Time Frame
Predialysis, intradialysis, postdialysis

▪▪▪▪▪▪ DIAGNOSTIC CLUSTER

Collaborative Problems

▲ Risk for Complications of Electrolyte Imbalance (Potassium, Sodium, and Magnesium)

* Risk for Complications of Hemolysis

△ Risk for Complications of Dialysis Disequilibrium Syndrome

▲ Risk for Complications of Clotting

▲ Risk for Complications of Air Embolism

▲ Risk for Complications of Pyrogen Reaction

▲ Risk for Complications of Fluid Imbalances Refer to Peritoneal Dialysis Care Plan

* Risk for Complications of Anaphylaxis / Allergies

Nursing Diagnoses

▲ Risk for Infection Transmission related to frequent contacts with blood and risk of hepatitis B and C

Related Care Plans

Chronic Kidney Disease or Acute Kidney Injury

External Arteriovenous Shunting

▲ This diagnosis was reported to be monitored for or managed frequently (75% to 100%).
△ _ This diagnosis was reported to be monitored for or managed often (50% to 74%).
* This diagnosis was not included in the validation study.

Transitional Criteria

The client and / or family will:

1. Describe the purpose of hemodialysis.
2. Discuss feelings and concerns regarding the effects of long-term therapy on self and family.
3. State signs and symptoms that must be reported to a health-care professional.

Transitional Risk Assessment Plan (TRAP)

Begin this plan on admission and involve the client, family, and support persons.
Risk for Infection Transmission: client / family need education regarding good handwashing, avoidance of ill individuals, using appropriate bactericidal agent to clean up any blood spills, no sharing of personal items such as toothbrushes.
If appropriate client / family should consider hepatitis B vaccine, annual influenza vaccine, and pneumonia vaccine.

Collaborative Problems

Risk for Complications of: Electrolyte Imbalance (Potassium, Sodium, Magnesium)

Risk for Complications of Hemolysis

Risk for Complications of Dialysis Disequilibrium Syndrome

Risk for Complications of Clotting

Risk for Complications of Air Embolism

Risk for Complications of Anaphylaxis or Allergies

Collaborative Outcomes

The client will be monitored to detect early signs and symptoms of (a) electrolyte imbalance, (b) hemolysis, (c) dialysis disequilibrium syndrome, (d) clotting, (e) air embolism, (f) fluid imbalances, (g) sepsis, and (h) anaphylaxis / allergies, and will receive collaborative interventions if indicated to restore physiologic stability.

Indicators of Physiologic Stability

- No itching / hives (e, h, i)
- No or minimal edema (f)
- BP >90/60, <140/90 mm Hg (c, e, h, i)
- Pulse 60–100 beats/min with regular rate and rhythm (c, e, h, i)
- Respirations 16–20 breaths/min, relaxed, rhythmic, with no rales, or wheezing (e, h, i)
- Weight change of no more than 1–2 kg between dialysis treatment (f)
- No headache (c)
- No chest pain (e, i)
- No complaints of nausea / vomiting (c)
- Serum potassium 3.5–5 mEq/L (a)
- Serum sodium 135–148 mm/dL (a)
- Serum creatinine 0.6–1.2 mg/dL (a)
- Blood urea nitrogen 7–18 mg/dL (a)

Interventions	Rationales
1. Assess the following:	1. Predialysis assessment and documentation of client's status are mandatory before initiation of the hemodialysis procedure to establish a baseline and to identify problems (Salai, 2008).
a. Skin (color, turgor, temperature, moisture, and edema)	a. Skin assessment can provide data to evaluate circulation, level of hydration, fluid retention, and uremia.
b. Blood pressure (lying, sitting and standing, as appropriate for client)	b. Low blood pressure may indicate intolerance to transmembrane pressure, hypovolemia, or the effects of antihypertensive medication given predialysis. High blood pressure may indicate overhydration, increased renin production, or dietary and fluid indiscretion.
c. Apical pulse (rhythm and rate and abnormalities)	c. Cardiac assessment evaluates the heart's ability to compensate for changes in fluid volume. Pericardial rub indicates uremia, gallops occur with fluid overload, arrhythmias can indicate volume changes, uremia, changes in cardiac function.
d. Respirations (rate, effort, and abnormal sounds)	d. Respiratory assessment evaluates compensatory ability of the system and presence of fluid or infection.
e. Weight (gain or loss)	e. Predialysis weight indicating gain or loss may necessitate a need to reevaluate dry weight.
f. Vascular access (site and patency and infection)	f. The vascular access site is assessed for signs of infection (warmth, redness, tenderness) or abnormal drainage. Patency is evaluated by assessment of bruits (swishing sound heard with a stethoscope) and thrills (vibration felt with light palpation) in fistulas and grafts. Notify the physician or advanced practice nurse before using a potentially compromised access (Dinwiddie, 2008).
g. Pretreatment BUN, serum creatinine, sodium, and potassium levels	g. Pretreatment serum levels are used as a baseline for evaluation of the effectiveness of the dialysis.

(continued)

Interventions	*Rationales*
2. Assess the client's pretreatment condition (chest pain, shortness of breath, cramps, headache, dizziness, blurred vision, nausea and vomiting, change in mentation, or speech	2. These assessment data help to determine if there has been a change in the client's condition since last treatment or if a change in treatment is indicated. When a client presents with problems predialysis, underlying etiology needs to be determined before initiation of treatment.
3. Intradialysis—monitor for signs and symptoms of potassium and sodium imbalance. (Refer to the Peritoneal Dialysis Care Plan for more information.)	3. Dialysate fluid composition and rates of inflow and outflow determine electrolyte imbalances.
4. Monitor for manifestations of hemolysis: bright red and / or translucent blood in venous line, burning at the circulatory return site, pink- to red-tinged dialysate, abdominal or back pain, dyspnea	4. Rupture of red blood cells can result from the hypotonic dialysate, high dialysate temperature, mechanical problems (e.g., pressure on RBCs from narrowed or occluded lines, or chloramines, nitrates, copper, zinc, or formaldehyde in the dialysate) (Hlebovy & King, 2008).

CLINICAL ALERT
- Hemolysis is a rare but ever-present potential complication of hemodialysis.
- Symptoms may be subtle and similar to hypotension or may not manifest until after treatment.
- Hemoglobin levels can drop dramatically so immediate care and investigation is necessary (Dutka, 2008; Harman & Dutka, 2007).

Interventions	*Rationales*
5. Monitor for signs and symptoms of dialysis disequilibrium syndrome (DDS): headache, nausea, vomiting, restlessness, hypertension, increased pulse pressures, altered sensorium, arrhythmias, and blurred vision	5. As a result of hemodialysis, the concentration of BUN is reduced more rapidly than the urea nitrogen level in cerebrospinal fluid and brain tissue, because of the slow transport of urea across the blood–brain barrier. Urea acts as an osmotic agent, drawing water from the plasma and extracellular fluid into the cerebral cells and producing cerebral edema. Other factors, such as rapid pH changes and electrolyte shifts, also can cause cerebral edema. DDS more likely in acute dialysis with high pretreatment BUNs (Bogle et al., 2008).

CLINICAL ALERT
- DDS symptoms may be delayed for up to 24 hours after dialysis.
- In addition to acute clients with high BUNs, more susceptible populations are the elderly and pediatric, and chronic clients who have missed several treatments (Hlebovy & King, 2008, p. 710).

Interventions	*Rationales*
6. Monitor for clotting: a. Observe for clot formation in the dialyzer and drip chambers. b. Monitor pressure readings every 15 minutes. c. Observe for clots when aspirating fistula needles, arteriovenous access, or intravenous dialysis catheter. d. Provide anticoagulation therapy as ordered.	6. Blood contacting the nonvascular surface of the extracorporeal circuit activates the normal clotting mechanism. During dialysis, fibrin formation and a gradual increase in the circuit's venous pressure (resulting from clotting in the venous drip chamber or needle) may indicate inadequate heparinization. Clot formation elevates blood pressure readings (Salai, 2008). d. increased clotting may indicate need for adjustments in anticoagulation therapy.
7. Monitor for signs and symptoms of air embolism: sudden onset of cyanosis, shortness of breath, chest pain, anxiety, persistent cough although symptoms may vary depending on position of client at time of event (Hlebovy & King, 2008).	7. As little as 10 mL of air introduced into the venous circulation is clinically significant. Large air bubbles are changed to foam as they enter the heart. Foam can decrease the volume of blood entering the lungs, decreasing left heart blood flow and cardiac output. Entry of air into the respiratory circulatory system causes a profound negative response.

Interventions	Rationales
8. If signs and symptoms of air embolism occur, take these steps (Hlebovy & King, 2008): 　a. Clamp the venous line and stop the blood pump. 　b. Position client on his or her left side with feet elevated for 30 minutes. 　c. Give 100% oxygen by mask.	8a. Clamping the line and stopping the pump can halt infusion of air. 　b. This prevents air from going to the head and traps air in the right atrium and in the right ventricle away from the pulmonic valve. 　c. Oxygen will aid in the reabsorption of the embolized air.
9. Monitor for signs and symptoms of anaphylaxis, which can include itching, hives, feeling of warmth, restlessness, feeling of impending doom, chest / back pain, shortness of breath, cough, cardiac arrest and death (Hlebovy & King, 2008). 　a. Stop dialysis and do not return blood. 　b. Administer oxygen 　c. Per protocol and / or physician / nurse practitioner order administer intravenous antihistamines, steroids, and / or epinephrine.	9. This is due to an allergic response to the ingredients in the dialysate or dialysis membrane, which involves the interaction between immunoglobin E (IgE) and mast cells. Anaphylaxis is a severe hypersensitivity response caused by a massive release of chemical mediators and other substances. The cardiovascular, respiratory, cutaneous, and gastrointestinal systems are generally involved in anaphylaxis. The IgE antibodies interact with mast cells, triggering the release of histamine, which, because of its potent vasodilator effect, causes widespread edema and vascular congestion (Hlebovy & King, 2008). 　a. This will prevent further contact with the offending agent. 　b. Oxygen will ease symptoms and provide additional oxygen for cardiac function. 　c. Medications will block allergic reaction.

Clinical Alert Report

Advise ancillary staff / student to report the following to the professional nurse assigned to the client:

- Any new change or deterioration in behavior, cognition, or level of consciousness
- Change in systolic BP > 200 mm/Hg or < 90 mm/Hg; diastolic BP > 90 mm/Hg or outside of specifically prescribed parameters
- Resting pulse > 120 or < 55 bpm or outside of specifically prescribed parameters
- Onset or changes in cardiac rhythm or heart sounds
- Change in respiratory rate > 28 or < 10 / minute
- Onset of new lung sounds (e.g., wheezes, rales, or increased respiratory effort)
- Changes in urinary output from usual baseline if applicable
- Temperature > 100° F oral
- Bleeding from dialysis access
- Decrease in thrill or bruit of dialysis access
- New coolness, pain, or cyanosis in hand or foot below the dialysis access

Related Physician / NP Prescribed Interventions

Medications
Refer to the Chronic Kidney Disease Care Plan

Laboratory Studies
Refer to the Chronic Kidney Disease Care Plan

Diagnostic Studies
Refer to the Chronic Kidney Disease Care Plan

Therapies
Dialysate solution

Documentation

Vital signs
Weight
Vascular access site
Dialysis (time, solution)
Predialysis complaints
Intradialysis complaints

Nursing Diagnoses

Risk for Infection Transmission Related to Frequent Contacts with Blood and People at Risk for Hepatitis B and C

NOC

Infection Status, Risk Control, Risk Detection

Goal

The client will relate the risks of hepatitis B virus (HBV) transmission.

NIC

Teaching: Disease Process, Infection Protection (Wiseman et al., 2008).

Indicators

- Have antibodies to HBV.
- Take precautions to prevent transmission of HBV.

Interventions	Rationales

1. Follow universal precautions for all dialysis treatments:
  a. Wear personal protective equipment: face shield, impervious gown, and gloves for all client or machine contact.
  b. All blood or dialysis effluent spills must be cleaned up immediately with antimicrobial soap and water.
  c. Do not permit staff and other personnel or visitors to eat or drink anything within the dialysis treatment area.
  d. Use individual supplies (e.g., thermometers, dressing change supplies, and individual medication vials for each client).	

2. Observe strict isolation procedure for clients who do not have the serologic marker for hepatitis B surface antibody:
  a. Wear an isolation gown and mask during dialysis treatment.
  b. Dialysis should be performed in client's private room or a dialysis unit isolation area.
  c. All blood or dialysis effluent spills must be cleaned up immediately with antimicrobial soap and water.
  d. Observe isolation disposal procedure for all needles, syringes, and effluent.
  e. Do not permit staff and other personnel or visitors to eat or drink anything within the dialysis treatment area.
  f. Ensure that all specimens for laboratory analysis are labeled "Isolation" and placed in bags also labeled "Isolation."
	2. Clients who are hepatitis C positive dialyze with the general population using universal precautions. HBV / HCV is found in the blood, saliva, semen, and vaginal secretions. Transmission is usually through blood (percutaneous or permucosal). Hepatitis B virus is stable on and viable on environmental surfaces for 7 days. Regularly practicing certain precautions provides protection (Wiseman et al., 2008).

Interventions	Rationales
g. Use special disposable thermometers to assess temperature. h. Avoid contact with other dialysis clients, if staffing level permits. If contact is necessary, change isolation gowns and wash hands carefully. i. Avoid any skin contact with the client's blood. j. Follow isolation procedure for waste and linen disposal per institutional protocol. k. Follow the recommended sterilization procedure for the hemodialysis machine after use.	
3. Administer hepatitis B immunizations, as appropriate, following facility policies.	3. High-risk clients and others should be immunized.
4. Explain that there is no prophylaxis for hepatitis C virus (HCV) and that it can go unnoticed for years.	4. Only 10% of people report an acute illness.
5. Minimize use of anticoagulants in clients with liver disease. 6. Collaborate with physician and / or advanced practice nurse to adjust medications with potential hepatotoxicity, including immunosuppressants. 7. Reinforce to client and family the serious nature of HBV / HCV, precautions, and risks.	5–7. Reiterating the seriousness of HBV / HCV and its possible sequelae may encourage compliance with instructions and precautions.

TRANSITION TO HOME/COMMUNITY CARE

Review risk diagnoses identified on admission.

- Does the client / family know how to follow-up the transition plan?
- If dialysis is to continue, ascertain that outpatient dialysis has been arranged, all necessary results have been obtained and transferred (labs, including hepatitis status, chest XRay, EKG, history and physical, medications, and dialysis prescription), time and location of next treatment have been confirmed.
- Discuss dietary changes and client / family understanding.
- Medication reconciliation has been done and written list and instructions are provided.
- Does client have contact information for questions and concerns?
- Use STAR (Stop, Think, Act, Review) to determine if transition plan is complete.
- Use SBAR (Situation, Background, Assessment, Recommendation) to relay necessary information to appropriate professional.

SBAR   *Situation:* Client is being transition and next dialysis treatment is scheduled at outpatient facility 10 miles from client's home.

Background: Client does not drive and family member will be at work during dialysis treatment.

Action: Discuss with case manager / transition planner / social worker. (This potential problem may have already been addressed and resolved during hospitalization.)

Recommendation: Client may be eligible for public assistance, car pool, or be considered for a different dialysis shift.

Risk for Ineffective Self-Health Management Related to Insufficient Knowledge of Condition, Dietary Restrictions, Daily Recording, Pharmacological Therapy, Signs / Symptoms of Complications, Follow-up Visits, and Community Resources

NOC

Compliance Behavior, Knowledge: Treatment Regimen, Participation in Health-Care Decisions, Treatment Behavior: Illness

NIC

Anticipatory Guidance, Learning Facilitation, Risk Identification, Health Education, Teaching: Procedure / Treatment, Health System Guidance

Goals

The goals for this diagnosis represent those associated with transition planning. Refer to the transition criteria.

Interventions	Rationales
1. Review care of the dialysis access. a. Signs and symptoms of problems and who to contact for questions. b. No blood draws or blood pressure measurements on access arm. **CLINICAL ALERT** • A dialysis access should NEVER be used as an intravenous access or for phlebotomy, unless specified by the vascular access physician or nephrologist.	1. An infected or poorly functioning access will not provide safe or adequate dialysis. Many problems can be dealt with quickly and without hospitalization. Drawing blood or taking blood pressures in the access arm increases the risk of thrombosis and infection (Dinwiddie, 2008).
2. Review each medication, including dosing, purpose, and specific instructions (e.g., take the phosphate binders with the meal rather than between meals).	2. Kidney disease requires a large number of medications. Clients will have more success with medication management if they understand why and how to take them (e.g., the antihypertensive regime may be different on dialysis vs. nondialysis days).
3. Discuss client's choice of therapy.	3. The type of renal replacement therapy may change as the client's health status or interests change. Ideally, all choices have been discussed but due to circumstances this may not have been possible during the hospitalization. Clients can be directed to educational material as well as professionals for further information.
4. Reinforce importance of adhering to the prescribed dietary plan.	4. All clients on dialysis have access to the professional dietitian who will review labs and adjust diet as needed. Clients are encouraged to write down questions and participate in their diet plan.

Interventions	Rationales
5. Provide opportunities for client to voice concerns and questions regarding kidney disease and treatment.	5. Kidney disease and dialysis is a life-altering experience that depends on clients being able to participate in their care. Additional support systems may be needed. Dialysis social workers can assist clients with local or regional support groups. Accurate information and support are also available on the Internet through organization such as the American Association of Kidney Patients (AAKP) at www.aakp.org and the National Kidney Foundation (NKF) at www.kidney.org.

Documentation

Client and family teaching
Monthly HBV screening results

Long-Term Venous Access Devices

Long-term venous access devices (VADs) are used for clients who have a need for frequent venous access to deliver chemotherapy, intravenous fluids, and blood products. They also provide access for blood samples.

The procedures outlined below pertain to the access and maintenance of long-term central venous catheters (e.g., vascular access devices). These include peripherally inserted central catheters (PICCs), tunneled catheters (e.g., Broviac®, Hickman®, and Groshong® catheters), including tunneled apheresis catheters, and implanted ports. These devices can last weeks, months, or years. Percutaneous central catheters have the shortest duration.

The risks and possible complications differ according to the choice of VAD and the vessel in which it is placed. Both the catheter choice and placement site should be tailored to the needs of the client.

Carp's Cues

The Centers for Disease Control (CDC) recommends the following (2011, pp. 8–9):

1. Educate health care personnel regarding the indications for intravascular catheter use, proper procedures for the insertion and maintenance of intravascular catheters, and appropriate infection control measures to prevent intravascular catheter-related infections. Category IA**
2. Periodically assess knowledge of and adherence to guidelines for all personnel involved in the insertion and maintenance of intravascular catheters. Category IA**
3. Designate only trained personnel who demonstrate competence for the insertion and maintenance of peripheral and central intravascular catheters. Category IA**
4. Ensure appropriate nursing staff levels in ICUs. Observational studies suggest that a higher proportion of "pool nurses" or an elevated client-to-nurse ratio is associated with catheter-related bloodsteam infection (CRBSI) in ICUs where nurses are managing clients with CVCs. Category IB**

Time Frame
Preprocedure and postprocedure

** Category IA. Strongly recommended for implementation and strongly supported by well-designed experimental, clinical, or epidemiologic studies. Category IB. Strongly recommended for implementation and supported by some experimental, clinical, or epidemiologic studies and a strong theoretical rationale; or an accepted practice. Refer to http://www.cdc.gov/hicpac/pdf/guidelines/bsi-guidelines-2011.pdf for the complete CDC Guidelines for the Prevention of Intravascular Catheter-Related Infections, 2011

DIAGNOSTIC CLUSTER

Collaborative Problems

▲ Risk for Complications of Hemorrhage

▲ Risk for Complications of Air Embolism (refer to Parenteral Nutrition Care Plan)

Δ Risk for Complications of Embolism / Thrombosis

† Risk for Complications of Infection / Sepsis

  Risk for Complications of Phlebitis (site)

  Risk for Complications of Extravasation (site)

Nursing Diagnoses

▲ Risk for Infection related to catheter's direct access to bloodstream (refer to Unit II)

Δ Risk for Ineffective Self Care Management related to insufficient knowledge of home care, signs and symptoms of complications, and community resources

Related Care Plans

  Cancer: Initial Diagnosis

  Chemotherapy

▲ This diagnosis was reported to be monitored for or managed frequently (75% to 100%).
Δ This diagnosis was reported to be monitored for or managed often (50% to 74%).

Transition Criteria

Before transition, the client and / or family will:

1. Demonstrate procedure and discuss conditions of catheter care and administration at home.
2. Discuss strategies for incorporating catheter management in activities of daily living (ADLs).
3. Verbalize necessary precautions.
4. State signs and symptoms that must be reported to a health care professional.
5. Identify available community resources.

Collaborative Problems

Risk for Complications of Hemorrhage

Risk for Complications of Embolism / Thrombosis

Risk for Complications of Infection / Sepsis

Risk for Complications of Phlebitis (site)

Risk for Complications of Extravasation (site)

Collaborative Outcomes

The client will be monitored for early signs and symptoms of (a) hemorrhage, (b) embolism / thrombosis, (c) infection / sepsis, (d) phlebitis (site), and (e) extravasation (site), and will receive collaborative interventions if indicated to restore physiologic stability.

Indicators of Physiologic Stability

* Calm, alert, oriented (b, c)
* BP >90/60, <140/90 mm Hg (a, b, c)
* Pulse 60–100 beats/min (a, b, c)
* Respirations 16–20 breaths/min (a, b, c)
* Respirations easy, rhythmic (a, b, c)

- Temperature 98.5°–99° F (c, d)
- Urine output >0.5 mL/kg/h (a, c)
- Urine negative for bacteria, WBC (c)
- Negative blood culture (c)
- Intact insertion site (d, e)
- Client catheter with blood return (d, e)
- No swelling, tenderness, drainage at site (d, e)
- No complaints of stinging, pain, or burning at insertion site (d, e)

Carp's Cues

The U.S. Centers for Medicare and Medicaid Services (CMS) Inpatient Prospective Payment System (IPPS) (Centers of Medicare and Medicaid Services, 2012) identified vascular catheter-associated infections as one of the targeted conditions. Under those reforms, vascular catheter-associated infections may not qualify for higher payment rates. Infections related to Hickman catheters, peripherally inserted central catheters (PICC), portacaths (port-a-cath) triple lumen catheter, or umbilical venous catheter are addressed. Infections associated with peripheral lines or urinary catheters are not included.

Interventions	Rationales
1. Follow agency protocols for insertion, maintenance, and management of local complications. If chemotherapeutic agents are administered, refer to Chemotherapy Care Plan. **CLINICAL ALERT** • Nurses inexperienced with long-term venous access devices must shadow an experienced nurse. • Deviations from the protocol must be reported. • Use SBAR format to communicate your concerns about providing safe care.	1. Institutional policies will specifically outline monitoring and interventions for catheter care and local complications (e.g., phlebitis, extravasation [leakage of chemotherapeutic or other caustic agents into surrounding tissues]).
2. Monitor for signs and symptoms of pneumothorax: a. Acute chest pain b. Dyspnea **CLINICAL ALERT** • Call rapid response team	2. Pneumothorax is the most common acute complication with central venous access, with reported rates of up to 4%. For this reason, an upright chest radiograph (or lateral decubitus image if the individual cannot sit upright) should be obtained after central venous access is attempted. The physician / NP should personally view the image after the procedure and obtain radiologic interpretation if necessary.
3. Monitor for catheter displacement, damage, infiltration, and extravasation: a. Superior vena cava syndrome (facial edema, distention of thoracic, and neck veins) b. Swelling, redness, tenderness, or drainage from insertion site (extravasation) c. Leakage of fluid from catheter d. Inaccurate infusion rate e. Inability to infuse or draw blood f. Bulging of catheter during infusion g. Chest or infraclavicular pain, paresthesia of the arm, dysrhythmias, palpitations, or an extra heart sound (Schummer, Schummer, & Schelenz, 2003) h. Report abnormal signs and symptoms to physician / NP for immediate evaluation	3. Catheters can malfunction, obstruct, or displace from misuse or defects.
4. Monitor for signs and symptoms of hemorrhage: a. Hypotension b. Tachycardia c. Evidence of bleeding d. Hematoma around insertion site (Hamilton, 2006) e. Cool, clammy skin (Hamilton, 2006)	4. Hemorrhage is a serious surgical complication of long-term venous access catheter placement. It can occur within several hours of insertion after blood pressure returns to preinsertion levels and puts increased pressure on a newly formed clot. It also can develop later, secondary to vascular erosion due to infection.

(continued)

Interventions	Rationales
5. Adhere to protocols for preventing CVC occlusions. **CLINICAL ALERT** • Causes of occlusions can be mechanical (positioning) or thrombosis.	5. CVC occlusions occur at a rate 14% to 36% within 1–2 years of catheter placement (Baskin et al., 2009). An occlusion can be partial that allows infusion but not aspiration or complete when neither are possible (IBID).
6. Check for mechanical obstruction (Baskin et al., 2009): a. Kink in catheter b. Suture too tight c. Clamp left closed in error d. Catheter tip blocked by blood vessel e. Malpositioned subcutaneous port	6. The initial assessment of catheter occlusion should be to rule out a mechanical cause.
7. Perform repositioning maneuvers as: (Baskin et al., 2009): a. Raise the arm on the side of the catheter insertion site. b. Have individual sit or stand up if possible. c. Roll onto one side. **CLINICAL ALERT** • If positioning can affect the catheter flow, occlusion can reoccur.	7. These maneuvers can reposition the catheter and relieve the pressure on the catheter.
8. If mechanical obstruction is ruled out, consult with clinical pharmacist / physician / NP to determine if medication or parenteral nutrition is causing occlusion. **CLINICAL ALERT** • If the above analyses are not diagnostic, a contrast study of the catheter may be ordered.	8. High pH medications can precipitate in an acidic environment, calcium phosphate crystals can occur in basic solutions, and lipid can precipitate from parenteral nutrition (Baskin et al., 2009).
9. Monitor for signs and symptoms of thrombosis: a. Pain and swelling of the ipsilateral arm or supraclavicular fossa b. Dilatation of the subcutaneous veins	9. "Thrombosis can occur at the point of vein entry or where a catheter tip irritates the vein intima. It can surround the catheter, occlude the tip or the entire vessel, and lead to pulmonary embolus. There is no definite evidence that rates differ between insertion sites, but incorrect tip position and infection are thought to increase the risk" (Hudman & Bodenham, 2013).
10. Report findings immediately to physician / NP for evaluation (e.g., ultrasound, venogram).	10. A thrombosis obstructs the catheter and can dislodge as a pulmonary embolism.
11. If thrombosis is confirmed, an antithrombolytic agent (e.g., alteplase, reteplase, urokinase, tenecteplase) will be injected into the access device. **CLINICAL ALERT** • Thrombosis and infection must be promptly diagnosed and vigorously treated. Both complications may require removal of the catheter.	11. The mechanism of action of antithrombolytic agents is as a tissue plasminogen activator. Tissue plasminogen activator catalyzes the conversion of plasminogen to plasmin, which then cleaves fibrin into fibrin degradation products to dissolve the thrombus (Baskin et al., 2009). "Alteplase, one of the current therapies, clears 52% of obstructed catheters within 30 min with 86% overall clearance (after 2 doses, when necessary)." (Baskin et al., 2009, p. 4e).

Interventions	Rationales

12. Monitor for signs and symptoms of air embolism. Report changes to physician and advanced nurse practitioner:
  a. Anxiety, restlessness
  b. Altered level of consciousness
  c. Shortness of breath (SOB), cyanosis
  d. Tachycardia
  e. Shoulder or back pain (Hamilton, 2006)
	12. A client with a long-term VAD is at increased risk for air embolism. Accidental leakage of air from catheter can occlude a major pulmonary artery; obstruction of blood flow to the alveoli decreases alveolar perfusion, shunts air to patent alveoli, and leads to bronchial constriction and possible collapse of pulmonary tissue. There is an increased risk of air embolism in those individuals with compromised circulation from hemorrhage or dehydration, and in dyspneic clients due to fluctuations in chest pressures (Hamilton, 2006).

13. Monitor for signs and symptoms of hematoma:
  a. Tenderness and swelling at insertion site
  b. Discoloration at insertion site
	13. Long-term VAD placement can cause soft tissue injury resulting in rupture of small vessels. As blood collects at insertion site, hematoma forms.

14. Monitor for signs and symptoms of infection:
  a. Tenderness and erythema along the track of the catheter
  b. Fever
  c. Bacteremia
	14. "Catheter-related bloodstream infections (CRBSIs) and catheter microbial colonization are thought to occur in three ways; by 'tracking' from the skin exit site (most common in short-term catheters), by intraluminal / hub contamination (most common in catheters *in situ* >30 days), and by seeding from hematogenous spread (in immunocompromised patients)" (Hudman & Bodenham, 2013, section 4e).

15. Monitor for septic shock and systemic inflammatory response ryndrome (SIRS) (Halloran, 2009):
 	
  a. Urine output 0.5 mL/kg/h
 	
  b. Body temperature greater than 38° C or less than 36° C
  c. Heart rate greater than 90/min
 	
  d. Hyperkalemia
 	
  e. Decreasing blood pressure
  f. Respiratory rate greater than 20/min
 	
  g. Hyperglycemia
 	
  h. White blood cell count greater than 12,000/µL or less than 4,000/µL or presence of 10% immature neutrophils
	15. The invasive nature of a VAD puts client at risk for opportunistic infection and septicemia. If the VAD is used to instill chemotherapy, the possibility of chemotherapy-induced leukopenia further increases risk. Sepsis causes massive vasodilatation and resultant hypovolemia, leading to tissue hypoxia and decreased renal and cardiac function. The body's compensatory response increases respiratory and heart rates in an attempt to correct hypoxia and acidosis.
	  a. Urine output is decreased when sodium shifts into the cells which pulls water into cells. Decreased circulation to kidneys reduces their ability to detoxify the toxins that result from anarobic metabolism.
	
	  c. Decreased blood flow to brain, heart, and kidneys triggers baroreceptors and release of catecholamines, increases heart rate / cardiac output, and further increases vasoconstriction
	  d. Potassium moves into the cell with the sodium, impairing nervous, cardiovascular, and muscle cell function
	  e. Movement of water into the cell causes hypovolemia.
	  f. Anaerobic metabolism decreases circulating oxygen. The body attempts to increase oxygenation by increasing respiratory rate.
	  g. The liver and kidneys produce more glucose in response to the release of epinephrine, norepinephrine, cortisol, and glucagon. Anaerobic metabolism reduces the effects of insulin. Insulin resistance contributes to multiple organ failure, nosocomial infection, and renal injury (Ball et al., 2007).
	  h. Increased white cells indicate an infectious process

(*continued*)

Interventions	Rationales
16. Ensure that blood culture is done prior to the start of any antibiotic. Culture any suspected infection sites (urine, sputum, invasive lines).	16. "Poor outcomes are associated with inadequate or inappropriate antimicrobial therapy (i.e., treatment with antibiotics to which the pathogen was later shown to be resistant in vitro). They are also associated with delays in initiating antimicrobial therapy, even short delays (e.g., an hour)" (Schmidt & Mandel, 2012).

CLINICAL ALERT
- Blood culture obtained after antibiotic therapy has been initiated can be inaccurate.
- Research of clients with septic shock demonstrated that the time to initiation of appropriate antimicrobial therapy was the strongest predictor of mortality (Schmidt & Mandel, 2012).

Interventions	Rationales
17. Refer to Unit II Risk for Complications of sepsis for additional interventions.	
18. Monitor for phlebitis:	18. Phlebitis is inflammation of a vein, usually from chemical or mechanical infiltration. An infective phlebitis is the inflammation of the intima from a bacterial infection. The incidence of phlebitis increases with the length of time the IV line is in place.
a. Evaluate the catheter insertion site daily by palpation through the dressing to discern tenderness and by inspection if a transparent dressing is in use.	
b. If there is local tenderness or other signs of possible CRBSI, an opaque dressing should be removed and the site inspected for redness or streak of red at insertion site or purulent drainage.	b. Gauze and opaque dressings should not be removed if there are no clinical signs of infection (Centers for Disease Control, 2011).
c. Evaluate for elevated temperature and elevated WBC.	
d. Report to physician / NP if the site develops signs of phlebitis (warmth, tenderness, and erythema).	

Clinical Alert Report

Prior to providing care, advise ancillary staff / student to report the following to the professional nurse assigned to the client:
- Change in cognitive status
- New c/o dyspnea, chest pain, pain at insertion site, shoulder / back pain
- Oral temperature >100.5° F
- Systolic BP <90 mm/Hg
- Resting pulse >100, <50
- Respiratory rate >28, <10/min.
- Oxygen saturation <90%
- Swelling, redness at insertion site
- Urine output <0.5 mL/kg/h

Related Physician / NP Prescribed Interventions

Refer to the care plan for the underlying condition necessitating VAD use (e.g., Cancer: Initial Diagnosis)
Medications
thrombolytic agents

Diagnostic studies
Ultrasound, venogram, chest xray

Laboratory
CBC, blood cultures

Documentation

Vital signs
Respiratory assessment
Catheter site / patency assessment

Nursing Diagnoses

Risk for Ineffective Self-Health Management Related to Insufficient Knowledge of Home Care, Signs and Symptoms of Complications, and Community Resources

NOC

Compliance Behavior, Knowledge: Treatment Regimen, Participation: Health Care Decisions, Treatment Behavior: Illness or Injury

Goal

The goals for this diagnosis represent those associated with transition planning. Refer to the transition criteria.

NIC

Anticipatory Guidance, Learning Facilitation, Risk Identification, Health Education, Teaching: Procedure / Treatment

Interventions	Rationales
1. For individuals who will have a venous access device at home, refer to home health nursing agency for home care assessment on the day of transition to home.	1. A home health care agency can provide ongoing assistance and support and will be needed to assess caregiver's knowledge and skills at home in as timely a manner as possible.
2. Have client or support person perform return demonstration of selected care measures.	2. Return demonstration lets nurse evaluate client's and family's abilities to manage the device safely.
3. Refer to the care plan for the specific condition that necessitated long-term venous access device.	

CLINICAL ALERT
- If there are concerns over the ability of the caregivers at home to safely manage venous access device initiate STAR.

(continued)

Interventions	Rationales

STAR   Stop

Think   Are there barriers for the caregivers to provide safe management of venous access device (e.g., motivation, manual skills, anxiety, practice, knowledge)?

Review   Can the barriers be removed for successful transition? Is it safe for transition to proceed? Can a home health nurse be at the home the day of transition? If not use SBAR, to communicate to the appropriate person (e.g., manager, physician / NP).

---

4. Explain signs and symptoms of VAD complications:

> **CLINICAL ALERT**
> • Ensure that the caregiver comprehends the seriousness of any of these possible complications and the need for immediate evaluation (e.g., emergency room).

a. Fever
b. Tenderness, swelling, and drainage at site

c. VAD occlusion
d. Inability to infuse

e. Facial edema and distended neck veins

4. Understanding signs and symptoms of complications enables early detection and reporting to a health care professional for timely intervention:

b. Fever and changes at the insertion site may indicate infection, phlebitis.

d. Inaccurate infusion rate or inability to infuse points to obstruction or catheter damage.

e. Facial edema and neck vein distention may indicate superior vena caval syndrome.

Documentation

Client and family teaching
Demonstrated ability of home caregiver to provide treatments safely
Outcome achievement or status
Referrals, if indicated
Evaluation of ability to perform treatments safely.

Peritoneal Dialysis

Peritoneal dialysis (PD)—the repetitive instillation and drainage of dialysis solution into and from the peritoneal cavity—uses the processes of osmosis, ultrafiltration, and diffusion to remove wastes, toxins, and fluid from the blood. PD uses the client's own peritoneal lining to serve as the semipermeable membrane through which diffusion, osmosis, and filtration occur (Ponferrada & Prowant, 2008). The procedure is indicated for acute or chronic kidney disease and severe fluid or electrolyte imbalances unresponsive to other treatments.

Numerous techniques for instillation and drainage of dialysis fluid have been developed. These methods are both manual and automated. Therapy can be continuous or automated.

Continuous therapies include continuous ambulatory peritoneal dialysis (CAPD), carried out manually by the client or caregiver, and automated peritoneal dialysis (APD) carried out by a PD machine. The variations of APD include continuous cycling peritoneal dialysis (CCPD), nocturnal peritoneal dialysis (NPD), intermittent peritoneal dialysis (IPD), and tidal peritoneal dialysis (TPD). Other terms may be occasionally encountered (Ponferrada & Prowant, 2008). CAPD is most commonly used and provides dialysate inflow with a disposable bag and tubing, which is sterilely connected then covered with a sterile cap during dwell time. Exchanges are done four times per day with 2.0–2.5 L. CCPD uses an automated cycler to perform exchanges during sleep and the abdomen is left full during the day. IPD consists of treatment periods with dwell time and alternates with periods of peritoneal cavity draining. Intermittent techniques use multiple short dwell exchanges three or four times a week. Automated intermittent exchanges may occur with repeated small TPD or at night (NPD). Manual IPD also may be done in hospitals for a prescribed number of cycles and length of time based on client requirements. Manual peritoneal dialysis requires careful control of dialysate instillation (2 L), dwell time, and outflow.

 Time Frame
Pretherapy and intratherapy

███ DIAGNOSTIC CLUSTER

Collaborative Problems

▲ Risk for Complications of Fluid Imbalances

▲ Risk for Complications of Electrolyte Imbalances

▲ Risk for Complications of Uremia

△ Risk for Complications of Hemorrhage

△ Risk for Complications of Hyperglycemia

△ Risk for Complications of Bladder / Bowel Perforation

▲ Risk for Complications of Inflow / Outflow Problems

* Risk for Complications of Sepsis

Nursing Diagnoses

▲ Risk for Infection related to access to peritoneal cavity

△ Risk for Ineffective Breathing Pattern related to immobility, pressure, and pain

△ Altered Comfort related to catheter insertion, instillation of dialysis solution, outflow, suction, and chemical irritation of peritoneum

△ Risk for Ineffective Self-Health Management related to insufficient knowledge of rationale of treatment, medications, home dialysis procedure, signs and symptoms of complications, community resources, and follow-up care

△ Imbalanced Nutrition: Less Than Body Requirements related to anorexia and loss of protein in peritoneal dialysis fluid (refer to Chronic Kidney Disease)

△ Interrupted Family Processes related to the effects of interruptions of the treatment schedule on role responsibilities (refer to Chronic Kidney Disease)

△ Powerlessness related to chronic illness and the need for continuous treatment (refer to Chronic Kidney Disease)

▲ This diagnosis was reported to be monitored for or managed frequently (75% to 100%).
△ This diagnosis was reported to be monitored for or managed often (50% to 74%).
* This diagnosis was not included in the validation study.

Transitional Criteria

Before transition, the client or family will:

1. Be able to demonstrate home peritoneal dialysis procedures, if appropriate.
2. State signs and symptoms of infection.
3. Discuss the expected effects of long-term dialysis on the client and family.
4. State signs and symptoms that must be reported to a health care professional.

Transitional Risk Assessment Plan (TRAP)

Begin this plan on admission.

If peritoneal dialysis is to be the ongoing treatment of choice, the client / caregiver will be ultimately responsible for all aspects of the treatment procedure. Training may begin during the hospitalization and continue in a formal outpatient clinic setting. Arrangements need to be completed prior to transition.

* Risk for infection: in addition to general infection control education (handwashing, avoidance of sick individuals, maintenance of routine vaccinations) client / family need instruction in peritoneal dialysis catheter care, avoidance of contamination during PD procedure, possible home risks (e.g., pets, swimming pool or pond / Jacuzzi, or lack of private space for procedure).
* Imbalance nutrition: nutritional requirements may change dramatically from predialysis diet. Current dietary habits, pain, abdominal distension from PD fluid, or anorexia may all impact nutritional intake. Dietary consult with reinforcement from nursing may be helpful.

Collaborative Problems

Risk for Complications of Fluid Imbalances

Risk for Complications of Electrolyte Imbalances

Risk for Complications of Uremia

Risk for Complications of Hemorrhage

Risk for Complications of Hyperglycemia

Risk for Complications of Bladder or Bowel Perforation

Risk for Complications of Inflow or Outflow Problems

Risk for Complications of Sepsis

Collaborative Outcomes

The nurse will detect early signs and symptoms of (a) fluid imbalances, (b) electrolyte imbalances, (c) uremia, (d) hemorrhage, (e) hyperglycemia, (f) bladder or bowel perforation, (g) inflow or outflow problems, and (h) sepsis, and will intervene collaboratively to stabilize the client.

Indicators of Physiologic Stability

* Alert, oriented, calm (a, b, c, g)
* Skin warm, dry, usual color, no lesions (a, c, d, e, g)
* No or minimal edema (a)
* BP >90/60, <140/90 mm Hg (a, b, d, g)
* Pulse pressure (40 mm Hg difference in systolic or diastolic) (a, b, d, g)
* Pulse 60–100 beats/min (a, b, d, g)
* Respirations 16–20 breaths/min; relaxed, rhythmic; no rales or wheezing (a, g)
* No weight change (a)
* Flat neck veins (a)
* No headache (b, g)
* Bowel sounds present (b)
* No chest pain (c)
* No abdominal pain (b, e, g)

- Intact reflexes (b)
- No change in vision (c)
- No complaints of nausea / vomiting (c, g)
- Intact muscle strength (b, c)
- No seizures (b)
- Serum potassium 3.5–5 mEq/L (b, c)
- Fasting blood glucose 70–110 mg/dL (e)
- Hemoglobin (d)
  - Male 13.5–17.5 g/dL
  - Female 13–16 g/dL
- Hematocrit (d)
  - Male 40% to 54%
  - Female 37% to 47%
- Serum sodium 135–148 mm/dL (c)
- Patent inflow and outflow (g)
- Intact connections, no kinks (g)
- No urinary urgency (f)
- No glucose in urine (e, f)
- No bowel urgency (f)
- No diarrhea (c, f)
- No fecal material in dialysate (f)
- White blood cell count >4,000 cells/mms or <12,000 with bands <10% (g)
- Temperature >96.8° F or <100.4° F (g)

Interventions	Rationales
1. Monitor for signs and symptoms of hypervolemia: a. Edema b. Dyspnea or tachypnea c. Rales or frothy secretions d. Rapid, bounding pulse e. Hypertension f. Jugular vein distention g. S_3 heart sounds	1. Hypervolemia may occur if dialysate does not drain freely or if excess IV or oral fluids have been infused or injected (Satalowich & Prowant, 2008). Excess fluid greater than 5% of body weight is needed to produce edema. Fluid in lungs produces signs and symptoms of hypoxia. Increasing flow rate will increase fluid removal with little change in clearance of solutes.
2. Monitor for signs and symptoms of hypovolemia: a. Dry skin and mucous membranes b. Poor skin turgor c. Thirst d. Tachycardia e. Tachypnea f. Hypotension with orthostatic changes g. Narrowed pulse pressure h. Altered level of consciousness	2. Hypovolemia may occur from excessive or too-rapid removal of dialysate fluid, inadequate salt and fluid intake, increased insensible loss, or overuse of hypertonic solution. Decreasing dextrose concentration to 1.5% may remove solutes without fluid (Ponferrada & Prowant, 2008).
3. Monitor intake and output.	3. Urine output varies depending on renal status.
4. Enforce fluid restrictions, as ordered.	4. Physician / NP may restrict fluid intake to insensible losses or the previous day's urine output.
5. Weigh daily or before and after each dialysis treatment.	5. Daily weights help to evaluate fluid balance.
6. Add medications to dialysate, as ordered.	6. Heparin commonly is added to decrease fibrin clots in the catheter. Potassium is added to prevent hypokalemia.

(continued)

Interventions	Rationales
7. Monitor peritoneal dialysis inflow, dwell time, and outflow.	7. *Inflow* (usually taking less than 15 minutes) is the infusion of dialysis solution by gravity into the peritoneal cavity. *Dwell time* is the length of time that the dialysis solution remains in the peritoneal cavity, which determines the amount of diffusion and osmosis that occurs. The time depends on the type of PD and can range from 0 minutes to hours. *Drain* (usually less than 20 minutes) is the emptying of the peritoneal cavity by gravity.
8. Monitor for signs and symptoms of hypernatremia with fluid overload: a. Thirst b. Agitation c. Convulsions	8. Dialysate solution >4.25% or rapid outflow or no long swell can cause hypernatremia (Ponferrada & Prowant, 2008; Satalowich & Prowant, 2008).
9. Monitor for signs and symptoms of hyponatremia: a. Lethargy or coma b. Weakness c. Abdominal pain d. Muscle twitching or convulsions	9. Hyponatremia results from the dilutional effects of hypervolemia. Extracellular volume decrease lowers blood pressure and leads to hypoxia.
10. Monitor for signs and symptoms of hyperkalemia: a. Weakness or paralysis b. Muscle irritability c. Paresthesias d. Nausea, vomiting, abdominal cramping, or diarrhea e. Irregular pulse	10. Prolonged dwell time can increase potassium fluctuations that can affect neuromuscular transmission, reduce action of GI smooth muscles, and impair electrical conduction of the heart. Strategies to lower serum potassium include using dialysate without potassium, performing extra dialysis exchanges, and decreasing dietary potassium. Severe hyperkalemia may require emergency medical management (Satalowich & Prowant, 2008).
11. Monitor for signs and symptoms of hypokalemia: a. Weakness or paralysis b. Leg cramps c. Decreased or absent tendon reflexes d. Hypoventilation e. Polyuria f. Hypotension g. Constipation or paralytic ileus	11. Hypokalemia impairs neuromuscular transmission and reduces action of respiratory muscles and GI smooth muscles. Potassium can be repleted through diet, oral supplements, or as addition to dialysate (Satalowich & Prowant, 2008).
12. Monitor for signs and symptoms of uremia: a. Skin and mucous membrane lesions b. Pericardial friction rub c. Pleural friction rub d. GI disturbances e. Peripheral neuropathy f. Vision changes g. Central nervous system impairment h. Tachypnea i. Musculoskeletal changes	12. A multisystem syndrome, uremia is a manifestation of end-stage renal disease resulting from waste products of protein metabolism, including urea, creatinine, and uric acid. To increase removal of wastes, the number of exchanges can be increased.
13. Monitor for blood in dialysate drainage: a. Trauma to bowel or blood vessel during catheter insertion b. Menstruation / ovulation c. Disease / illness (e.g., cyst, infection, neoplasm)	13. Perforation of a blood vessel during catheter insertion can cause bloody dialysate, urine, or stool, or bleeding at insertion site. The fallopian tubes and ovaries open into the peritoneum so blood effluent is common during ovulation and menses (Satalowich & Prowant, 2008).

Interventions	Rationales

14. If bleeding persists, apply a pressure dressing and carefully monitor vital signs.

> **CLINICAL ALERT**
> - In addition to pressure and vital sign monitoring, rapid PD exchanges, ice packs, fluid / blood replacement, and surgery may be required (Prowant, 2008).

15. Monitor for signs and symptoms of hyperglycemia:
    a. Elevated or depressed blood glucose level
    b. Polyuria
    c. Polyphagia
    d. Polydipsia
    e. Abdominal pain
    f. Diaphoresis

15. The amount of dextrose absorbed from the dialysate varies with dextrose concentration and number of cycles. In two cycles of 1.5% solution, 41 kcal are absorbed. After dialysis is complete, hypoglycemia may occur because of increased insulin production during instillation of high dextrose concentrations.

16. Monitor for signs and symptoms of bladder or bowel perforation:
    a. Fecal material in dialysate
    b. Complaints of urgency
    c. Increased urine output with high glucose concentrations
    d. Complaints of pressure in the sensation to defecate
    e. Watery diarrhea

16. Catheter insertion may perforate bowel or bladder, allowing dialysate to infuse into bowel or bladder (Prowant, 2008).

> **CLINICAL ALERT**
> - Notify physician / NP immediately.

17. Have client empty bladder and bowel before insertion of peritoneal dialysis catheter.

17. Emptying bladder and bowel decreases risk of perforation during catheter insertion (Prowant, 2008).

18. Monitor drug levels during dialysis to maintain therapeutic treatment (Ponferrada & Prowant, 2008).

18. Drugs may be added to the dialysate.

19. If inflow or outflow problems occur, do the following:

    a. Increase height of the dialysate bag and lower the bed.

    b. Reposition client and instruct him or her to cough.

    c. Check for kinks and closed clamps.
    d. Remove a nontransparent dressing to check for catheter obstruction.
    e. Check dressing for wetness. Dialysate leaking from exit site presents as a clear fluid testing strongly for glucose.
    f. Assess abdominal or shoulder pain on outflow.

    g. Assess amount of dialysate return.

19. These measures can enhance the effectiveness of dialysis and prevent complications (Satalowich & Prowant, 2008):
    a. Raising the bag and lowering the bed can help to maximize gravity drainage.
    b. Repositioning and coughing may help to clear a blocked or kinked catheter.

    d. Dressing can obscure an external obstruction or kink.

    e. Leakage at site may be from poor insertion technique or delayed healing and infection.

    f. Abdominal pain may result from excessive suction on abdominal viscera or incorrect catheter position. Shoulder pain may indicate air in the abdomen.
    g. If catheter does not drain, omentum may be obstructing or fibrin may have formed in the catheter.

Interventions	*Rationales*
CLINICAL ALERT • Notify Physician / NP if 50% of inflow is retained.	
h. Ascertain if heparin has been added to dialysate. i. If ordered, irrigate with heparinized saline. j. If ordered, irrigate with fibrinolytic agents. k. Assess for constipation.	h, i. Heparin can help to prevent catheter blockage from fibrin or blood clots. j. Fibrinolytic agents may be effective in removing blockage. k. Constipation may lead to shifting of catheter position, drainage failure, and catheter loss.
20. Calculate inflow and outflow volume at the end of each dialysis cycle. Report discrepancies in accordance with hospital protocol.	20. Accurate inflow and outflow records determine fluid loss or retention by client (Ponferrada & Prowant, 2008).

Clinical Alert Report

Advise ancillary staff / student to report the following to the professional nurse assigned to the client:
- Any changes in mental status such as agitation, lethargy, confusion
- Blood pressure, pulse, or respirations outside of prescribed limits. See Indicators. Individual parameters may vary depending on client's medications
- Temperature (oral) 1–2° F over baseline. Uremia suppresses temperature so lower readings may still indicate fever
- Difficulty breathing or new onset of shortness of breath
- New onset of pain
- Inability of peritoneal dialysis fluid to drain
- Cloudy or blood tinged peritoneal dialysis fluid drainage
- Any redness, warmth, drainage, or tenderness at peritoneal catheter site
- Genital edema

Related Physician / NP Prescribed Interventions

Medications
Heparinized saline, fibrinolytic agents

Laboratory Studies
Refer to either the Acute Kidney Failure or Chronic Kidney Disease Care Plan.

Therapies
Dialysate solution, dwell time, number of cycles

Documentation

Vital signs
Intake and output
Weight and medications
Dialysate color
Abdominal girth
Serum glucose
Urine specific gravity
Other laboratory values
Changes in status
Inflow or outflow problems
Interventions

Nursing Diagnoses

Risk for Infection Related to Access to Peritoneal Cavity

NOC
Infection Status, Wound Healing: Primary Intention, Immune Status

Goal

The client will be infection free at catheter site and will not develop peritonitis or a systemic infection.

NIC
Infection Control, Wound Care, Incision Site Care, Health Education

Indicators (Ponferrada & Prowant, 2008; Prowant, 2008; Satalowich & Prowant, 2008)

- Temperature >96.8° F or <100.4° F
- No edema or drainage at site

Interventions	Rationales
1. Ensure use of sterile technique when setting up equipment.	1–5. Aseptic technique reduces microorganisms and helps prevent their introduction into the system (Prowant, 2008).
2. Ensure complete skin preparation before catheter insertion.	
3. Use sterile technique when assisting with catheter insertion or removal and when performing dialysis. Wear gloves to examine exit site.	
4. Apply masks to all staff / student and the client during catheter insertion, removal, and dressing changes.	
5. Minimize catheter movement at exit site (not to be used until site healed postinsertion, preferably 10–14 days).	
6. Warm dialysate solution in a dedicated peritoneal dialysis microwave oven for the institution's recommended time frame. Agitate bag before infusing. Other heating methods include heating pad, laying bag in sunshine, or near other heat source. Avoid heating in water bath.	6. Because microwave ovens vary in rate, consistency, and method of heating, each institution needs to establish its own time frame and protocol. Heating in water may lead to possible contamination. High heat over a prolonged time can change the composition and clarity of the dialysate (Ponferrada & Prowant, 2008).
7. Determine that dialysate is between 36.5° C and 37.5° C (97.7° F and 99.5°F) before infusing.	7. External temperature may be measured by folding the bag over an electronic thermometer. Bag should be tepid to touch (Ponferrada & Prowant, 2008).
8. When performing manual peritoneal dialysis, prevent contamination of spikes when changing dialysate bags.	8. Peritoneal dialysate may be done manually with a manifold setup or by an automatic cycler. Use of bags allows the peritoneal dialysis system to remain closed except when connecting (Ponferrada & Prowant, 2008).
9. Monitor dialysate return for color and clarity. Obtain culture of any drainage.	9–13. Turbidity may indicate infection, noninfectious eosinophilia, or menstruation (Satalowich & Prowant, 2008).
10. Perform routine exit site care using aseptic technique.	
11. Increase frequency of exit site care, as needed.	
12. Change cleansing agent for exit site care, as indicated.	
13. Teach alternative methods of exit site care.	

Documentation

Signs and symptoms of infection

Dressing changes

Risk for Ineffective Breathing Pattern Related to Immobility, Pressure, and Pain

NOC

Respiratory Status: Gas Exchange, Vital Sign Status, Anxiety Control

NIC

Respiratory Monitoring, Progressive Muscle Relaxation, Teaching, Anxiety Reduction

Goal

The client will demonstrate optimal respiratory function.

Indicators

- Bilateral breath sounds, clear lung fields globally with no rales or crepitus
- Arterial blood gases

Interventions	Rationales
1. Encourage regular coughing and deep-breathing exercises.	1. Hypoventilation may result from increased pressure on the diaphragm as a result of dialysate instillation and position during cycle. Pulmonary edema, pleuritis, infection, or uremic lung also may contribute to respiratory distress (Satalowich & Prowant, 2008).
2. Evaluate effect of smaller dialysate solution volumes on adequacy and initiate if appropriate. Evaluate potential for PD modality change to cycling therapy.	2. Stopping flow reduces pressure on the diaphragm, possibly relieving distress (Satalowich & Prowant, 2008).

CLINICAL ALERT
- If client experiences respiratory distress, immediately stop inflow or begin outflow.
- Respiratory distress can indicate an acute hydrothorax from a leak in the diaphragm.
- The negative pressure in the thoracic cavity and the positive pressure in the intra-abdominal cavity moves the peritoneal fluid from the peritoneal to the pleural cavity (Satalowich & Prowant, 2008).

Documentation

Abnormal respiratory status

Impaired Comfort Related to Catheter Insertion, Instillation of Dialysis Solution, Outflow Suction, and Chemical Irritation of Peritoneum

NOC

Comfort Level, Pain Control

NIC

Respiratory Monitoring, Progressive Muscle Relaxation, Pain Management, Anxiety Reduction

Goal

The client will be as comfortable as possible during peritoneal dialysis.

Indicators

Explain reason for discomforts

- No pressure or pain during the procedure
- Report measures used that reduced pain

Interventions	Rationales
1. Instruct client to report excessive pain on catheter insertion or dialysate instillation. Have client describe pain's severity on a scale of 0–10 (0 = no pain; 10 = most severe pain).	

> **CLINICAL ALERT**
> • Pain on catheter insertion calls for catheter repositioning; pain during dialysate instillation may result from various factors including too-rapid inflow rate, dialysate temperature too cool or too warm, and complications of treatment. (Satalowich & Prowant, 2008).

Interventions	Rationales
2. Position client to minimize pain while maintaining good air exchange and free-flowing dialysate.	2. Certain positions can reduce abdominal discomfort during instillation.
3. Drain effluent to assess for cloudy or bloody fluid. Initiate protocol for peritonitis, if indicated.	3. Lidocaine may be used as an intraperitoneal analgesic.
4. As necessary, use nonpharmacologic pain relief techniques such as distraction, massage, guided imagery, and relaxation exercises.	4. Nonpharmacologic pain relief techniques can offer effective, safe alternatives to medication in some clients.
5. Check temperature of dialysate before and during instillation.	5. A too-cool dialysate temperature can cause abdominal cramps; too warm a temperature can cause tissue damage. A slower instillation rate reduces intra-abdominal pressure and may decrease pain. A decrease in volume reduces degree of abdominal distention, especially on initiation of dialysis.

> **CLINICAL ALERT**
> • If client reports extreme pain during dialysis, decrease inflow rate and consult with physician / NP to decrease temporarily the amount of dialysate instilled.

Interventions	Rationales
6. Investigate carefully any client reports of pain in the shoulder blades.	6. Referred pain to the shoulders may be from diaphragmatic irritation or from air infused on insertion.

Documentation

Pain
Relief measures instituted
Client's response

> **TRANSITION TO HOME / COMMUNITY CARE**
> • Review the risk diagnoses identified at admission.
> • Review medications including purpose, dose and schedule with client. Provide written list including instructions.
> • Ascertain that the follow-up plan for dialysis is in place and that the client / family knows the schedule, time, and place of follow-up. Provide contact information for dialysis services.
> • Discuss dietary changes. If client is still uncertain, contact dietitian or refer to outpatient dietitian.
> • Use STAR (Stop, Think, Act, Review) to determine if transition plan is complete.
> • Use SBAR (Situation, Background, Assessment, Recommendation) to relay necessary information to appropriate professional.

■■■■■■■ SBAR   **Situation:** client is being transitioned on chronic dialysis but has not yet learned how to do own treatment. PD catheter was inserted one week ago.

Background: client is scheduled to start training in one week. Client has been receiving hemodialysis with a temporary catheter.

Assessment: verify with health team (a) is dialysis continuing? and (b) where will client be receiving dialysis? (This potential problem may have already been addressed and resolved during hospitalization but client and outpatient facility need clear plan.)

Recommendation: client may be eligible for public assistance, car pool, or be considered for a different dialysis shift.

Risk for Ineffective Self-Heath Management Related to Insufficient Knowledge of Rationale of Treatment, Medications, Home Dialysis Procedure, Signs and Symptoms of Complications, Community Resources, and Follow-up Care

NOC

Compliance Behavior, Knowledge: Treatment Regimen, Participation: Health Care Decisions, Treatment Behavior: Illness or Injury

NIC

Anticipatory Guidance, Learning Facilitation, Risk Identification, Health Education, Teaching: Procedure / Treatment, Health System Guidance

Goals

The goals for this diagnosis represent those associated with transition planning. Refer to the transition criteria.

Interventions	Rationales
1. Reinforce physician's / NP's explanations of renal disease and of peritoneal dialysis procedure and its effects. 2. Discuss all prescribed medications, covering purpose, dosage, and side effects.	1, 2. Client's understanding can help to increase compliance and tolerance of treatment.
3. As appropriate, teach client the following and ask client to perform return demonstrations so nurse can evaluate client's ability to do procedures safely and effectively: a. Aseptic technique b. Catheter care c. Dialysate preparation d. Positioning during treatment e. Instilling additives to dialysate f. Inflow and outflow procedure g. Obtain fluid sample for infection or peritoneal membrane characteristic study.	3. Many clients can perform home peritoneal dialysis without assistance. Proper technique can help to prevent infection and inflow and outflow problems (Ponferrada & Prowant, 2008).
4. Discuss how to manage inflow pain by ensuring proper temperature and flow rate of dialysate.	4. Cold dialysate, too-rapid inflow, acid dialysate, and stretching of diaphragm can cause inflow pain.
5. Teach client to maintain adequate protein and calorie intake.	5. Protein malnutrition is a major concern. Large protein losses occur with peritoneal dialysis. Low serum albumin levels are known to be associated with an increased risk of death. Because glucose is absorbed from the dialysate and weight gain may be a problem, high glucose solutions should be used sparingly and dietary intake of simple carbohydrates avoided (Ponferrada & Prowant, 2008).

Interventions	Rationales
6. Teach client to prevent constipation through adequate diet, fluid intake, and physical activity.	6. Constipation or bowel distention impedes dialysate outflow (Satalowich & Prowant, 2008).

7. Teach client to watch for and promptly report:
 	
  a. Unresolved pain from inflow
  b. Outflow failure
 	
  c. Low-grade fever, cloudy outflow, malaise, and catheter site changes (redness, inflammation, drainage, tenderness, warmth, and leaks).
	7. Early detection of complications enables prompt intervention to minimize their seriousness (Satalowich & Prowant, 2008):
	  a. This finding can indicate intraperitoneal infection.
	  b. This finding may result from catheter obstruction, peritonitis, dislodged catheter, or a full colon.
	  c. These signs can point to infection.

CLINICAL ALERT
- Advise to notify physician / NP immediately.

Interventions	Rationales

d. Signs of fluid / electrolyte imbalance (see Risk for Complications of Fluid Imbalance, Risk for Complications of Electrolyte Imbalances for specific signs and symptoms of various imbalances)
  e. Abdominal pain, stool changes, constipation
	d. Dialysis alters fluid and electrolyte levels, possibly resulting in imbalance.
	
	  e. Bowel distention impedes outflow.

CLINICAL ALERT
- Advise to call physician / NP with symptoms.

Interventions	Rationales
8. Ensure that client knows how to order / obtain necessary supplies.	8. Knowledge of sources of supplies can prevent incorrect substitutions.

9. Teach client to record the following:
  a. Vital signs and weight before and after dialysis
  b. Percent of dialysate and amount of inflow
  c. Amount of outflow
  d. Number of exchanges required
  e. Medications taken
  f. Problems
  g. Urine output and number and character of stools
	9. Accurate records aid in evaluating effectiveness of treatment.

10. Initiate referral to a home health care agency if indicated.	10. Home health referral may be needed for services such as medication management, physical and occupational therapy. Services managed by home dialysis are generally covered by that program.
11. Provide information on available community resources and self-help groups (e.g., National Kidney Foundation at www.kidney.org, American Association of Kidney Patients [AAKP] at www.aakp.org).	11. Access to resources and self-help groups may ease difficulties of home dialysis and help to minimize its effects on home life.

Documentation

Client and family teaching
Outcome achievement or status
Referrals, if indicated

Radiation Therapy

As a key modality in the management of cancer; radiation therapy (RT) is neither chemical nor invasive. RT is used as palliative or curative treatment in multiple cancer diagnoses. RT works by damaging the DNA molecules within the cancer cell using high-energy ionizing radiation (x-rays or proton beams) to destroy or damage cancer cells. Radiation oncologists are physicians specializing in use of radiologic imaging working in collaboration with surgical and medical oncologists. Palliative treatment is used to relieve pain, prevent fracture, or mobilize a client following cord compression. When used in cancer treatment, radiation therapy aims to kill maximum cancer cells while causing minimal damage to normal tissue; ultimately designed to preserve quality of life and functionality while eradicating disease (Pollock, 2010).

RT uses ionizing radiation can be delivered in two ways. In *external beam radiation (teletherapy)*, a radioactive source or electromagnetic energy from a linear accelerator placed at some distance from the target site delivers the treatment. The distance is advantageous because the dose is relatively uniform across a given volume and allows for dose-shaping or modifying devices (wedges, blocks, etc.) to be interposed between the accelerator and patient to direct the RT, sparing normal tissue while targeting tumors. Proton-beam radiation is the latest development in RT. Protons are atomic particles that are easier to manage than traditional x-ray beams, concentrating treatment on oddly shaped tumors or specific direct areas such as the brain. These newer techniques enable doctors to allow RT as a targeted dose directly on the precise site of the tumor, limiting damage to healthy cells.

In *internal therapy*, the radioactive sources are placed directly into the tumor or tumor bed, swallowed, or injected. In brachytherapy, seeds are planted as temporary or may stay in place permanently. This treatment is most common in prostate, gynecologic, head and neck, lung, and breast cancers. A high dose is near the sources in the tumor bed and a much lower dose in the normal tissues. Radiopharmaceuticals are given systemically, delivering a radioactive component to destroy cancer cells. This type of treatment is most common in bone, lymphomas, and thyroid cancer. Combination teletherapy and brachytherapy is used in the treatment of many neoplasms. *Radiation sensitizers* are compounds that enhance the damaging effects of ionizing radiation. *Radioprotector* compounds protect cells and tissues from the damaging effects of radiation. A *radiolabeled antibody* is an antibody with a radioactive substance attached to its molecular structure that binds the antibody and radioisotope.

When radiation oncologists are determining the best course of RT to be delivered, four fundamental principles are considered: cellular repair, repopulation, redistribution, and reoxygenation. Normal cells maintain the ability to repair RT damage, while cancerous cells are vulnerable to permanent damage. Guidelines have been published to guide the total doses, frequency, and volume based on the areas receiving radiation. **Cellular repopulation** is the foundation to complete RT as soon as possible without treatment breaks to combat the regrowth of cells not killed by RT in each cycle. **Cellular redistribution** refers to the portion of the cell cycle at which tumors are dividing. RT is most effective in the G2-M phase. Dividing RT over many weeks allows the potential to destroy the cell at that phase of the cell cycle. Tissues with a rapid rate of cellular division are more sensitive to the effects of radiation therapy. Some examples of radiosensitive tissues include bone marrow, epithelial cells lining the GI and genitourinary (GU) tracts, gonads, and hair follicles. Radioresistant tissues with a slow generation time, such as muscles, tendons, and nerves, have a less dramatic response. **Cellular reoxygenation** is the process of RT entering the tissue, inducing free radicals. The free radicals affect the tumor's DNA, promoting a lethal injury. Oxygen in the tissue is directly related to the electrons circulating. Research has shown low oxygen or low hemoglobin levels directly (negatively) affect the benefits of RT (Pollock, 2010). The response of tissues to radiation is divided into three specific time periods: *acute, subacute,* and *chronic.* Acute response period is the first 6 months after exposure to radiation. Subacute response period occurs 6 months to 1 year after exposure, and late or chronic response occurs 1–5 years longer after exposure to radiation.

Continuous improvements have been made to prevent, and address skin reactions. Greater than 90% of patients experience some degree of skin reactions; severity is based on treatment-related and patient-related factors (Chmielowski, Casciato, & Wagner, 2009). Skin reactions caused by RT are usually minor and monitored closely. Short-term side effects usually resolve within 2 months of treatment. General short-term side effects specific to the area of the body receiving RT include skin sensitivity (redness, dryness, peeling, itching) fatigue, anemia, anorexia, hair loss in the area of the body being treated, nausea / vomiting, mouth sores, or headaches. Long-term side effects can include fatigue, dry mouth, loss of changes in taste (if head and neck treated). Late effects again are site specific and can occur months after treatment ends. These can include pneumonitis, pulmonary fibrosis, memory problems (for brain radiation), loss of motion in joints (area of body specific), infertility (if pelvis radiated), cavities and tooth decay (jaw radiation), and lymphedema. Because radiation is often given in addition to other modalities of treatment, the nurse must be thorough in the systematic assessment and management of potential adverse effects.

To proactively decrease the risk of skin damage, patients should be instructed to wash the irradiated areas with lukewarm water and mild soap to decrease the risk of bacterial infections. Patients should be directed to avoid rubbing the skin, refrain from skin irritants or metallic based topical agents, encourage loose cotton clothing, and avoid direct exposure to sun or extreme temperatures.

Individuals experiencing erythema and dry desquamation will benefit from the use of nonscented, lanolin-free hydropholic or moisturizing creams; do not apply to skin breakdowns. Medications like low-dose steroids decrease the severity of inflammation and pruritis.

Site Specific Side Effects (Strobl, 2009)

- Brain: alopecia, late cognitive changes—avoid irritants to scalp, ongoing neurocognitive function assessments
- Head and neck: xerostomia, mucositis, cavities, dysphagia—encourage soft, bland foods, saliva replacement products, analgesics / numbing products, preventive dental care
- Chest: cough, pneumonitis, late fibrosis—expectorants, corticosteroids
- Abdomen / pelvis: nausea, vomiting, diarrhea, cystitis, infertility—encourage fluids, antiemetics, bland diet, antidiarrheals, promote fertility counseling prior to initiation of radiation
- Skin: erythema, dry and moist desquamation—avoid direct trauma to skin, adherence to skin care directions, using creams and lotions as prescribed

Time Frame
Pretherapy and intratherapy

▓▓ DIAGNOSTIC CLUSTER

Collaborative Problems

▲ Risk for Complications of Myelosuppression (Infection, Bleeding)

▲ Risk for Complications of Malabsorption

▲ Risk for Complications of Pleural Effusion

▲ Risk for Complications of Cerebral Edema

△ Risk for Complications of Mucositis, Esophagitis, Pneumonitis

△ Risk for Complications of Cystitis, Urethritis, and Tenesmus

△ Risk for Complications of Myelitis and Parotitis

△ Risk for Complications of Fluid and Electrolyte Imbalance (refer to Renal Failure)

Nursing Diagnoses

▲ Anxiety related to prescribed radiation therapy and insufficient knowledge of treatments and self-care measures

△ Risk for Impaired Oral Mucous Membrane related to dry mouth or inadequate oral hygiene

▲ Impaired Skin Integrity related to effects of radiation on epithelial and basal cells and effects of diarrhea on perineal area

△ Impaired Comfort related to stimulation of the vomiting center and damage to the gastrointestinal mucosa cells secondary to radiation (refer to Gastroenteritis)

(continued)

▲ Fatigue related to systemic effects of radiation therapy

▲ Impaired Comfort related to damage to sebaceous and sweat glands secondary to radiation (refer to Inflammatory Joint Disease Cirrhosis)

▲ Imbalanced Nutrition: Less Than Body Requirements related to decreased oral intake, reduced salivation, mouth discomfort, dysphasia, nausea / vomiting, increased metabolic rate, and diarrhea (refer to Unit II)

△ Disturbed Self-Concept related to alopecia, skin changes, weight loss, sterility, and changes in role, relationships and life styles (refer to Cancer: Initial Diagnosis)

△ Grieving related to changes in lifestyle, role, finances, functional capacity, body image, and health losses (refer to Cancer: Initial Diagnosis)

△ Interrupted Family Processes related to imposed changes in family roles, relationships, and responsibilities (refer to Cancer: Initial Diagnosis)

▲ This diagnosis was reported to be monitored for or managed frequently (75% to 100%).

△ This diagnosis was reported to be monitored for or managed often (50% to 74%).

Transitional Criteria

The client or family will:

1. Relate skin care, oral care, and rest requirements.
2. Verbalize importance of expressing concerns to support system and providers.
3. Identify signs and symptoms that must be reported to a health care professional.

Collaborative Problems (site specific to area receiving treatment)

Risk for Complications of Potential Complication: Myelosuppression (Infection, Bleeding)

Risk for Complications of Malabsorption

Risk for Complications of Pleural Effusion

Risk for Complications of Cerebral Edema

Risk for Complications of Mucositis, Esophagitis, Pneumonitis

Risk for Complications of Cystitis, Urethritis, and Tenesmus

Risk for Complications of Potential Complication: Myelitis and Parotitis

Collaborative Outcomes

The client will be monitored for early signs and symptoms of myelosuppression (infection, bleeding), malabsorption, pleural effusion, cerebral edema, mucositis, esophagitis, pneumonitis, cystitis, urethritis, and tenesmus, myelitis and parotitis, and will receive collaborative interventions if indicated to restore physiologic stability.

Indicators of Physiologic Stability

- Calm, alert oriented
- Temperature 98.5°–99° F
- Pulse 60–100 beats/min
- Stable pulse pressure (approximately 40 mm Hg difference between diastolic and systolic pressures)
- BP >90/60, <140/90 mm Hg
- Respirations 16–20 breaths/min
- No rales or wheezing
- Respirations relaxed, rhythmic
- Breath sound in all lobes
- Clear sputum
- No rectal, abnormal vaginal, or nasal bleeding

- No prolonged bleeding after invasive procedures
- No evidence of petechiae or ecchymoses
- No abdominal pain
- No chest pain
- Urine output >0.5 mL/kg/h
- Sensation intact, strength intact
- No change in vision
- Pupils equal and reactive to light
- Pinkish or brownish oral mucous membranes
- Oral mucous membranes intact
- No change in bowel function
- Normal chest x-ray

Interventions	Rationales
CLINICAL ALERT • Side effects of RT are dependent on the site treated. • As RT has progressed over the years to be more directed, the surrounding areas are spared of unwanted side effects. • The nurse will monitor to detect early signs and symptoms specific to the organs of the body receiving radiation.	

1. Monitor for signs of myelosuppression:
  a. Decreased WBC and RBC counts
  b. Decreased platelet count
	1. Myelosuppression (bone marrow depression) occurs when large volumes of active bone marrow are irradiated (e.g., pelvis, brain, chest, long bones). The results are destruction of the blood elements. RBCs are less affected because of their longer life span.

2. Monitor for signs and symptoms of spontaneous or excessive bleeding:
  a. Petechiae, ecchymoses, or hematomas
  b. Bleeding from nose or gums
  c. Prolonged bleeding from invasive procedures
  d. Hemoptysis
  e. Hematuria
  f. Vaginal bleeding
  g. Rectal bleeding
  h. Change in vital signs
  i. Change in neurologic status
  j. Change in respiratory status
	2. Radiation therapy alone usually does not cause thrombocytopenia, unless a significant amount of radiation is directed at the pelvis, the patient is receiving chemotherapy at the same time, or the cancer spreads to the bone. Failure of the bone marrow is the primary cause of death within the first few months following exposure of RT.

3. Instruct client to:
  a. Use soft toothbrushes.
  b. Use electric razors.
  c. Avoid injections.
  d. Avoid alcohol.
  e. Avoid medications that interfere with hemostasis / platelet function.
  f. Avoid venipuncture. If necessary, avoid prolonged tourniquet use. Apply direct pressure 3–5 minutes after.
  g. Avoid forceful coughing, sneezing, nose blowing.
  h. Avoid straining during defecation.
  i. Blow nose gently using soft tissue.
  j. Avoid contact sports or other activities that may cause injury.
	3. Clients with diminished clotting ability and at risk for infection are taught methods to prevent trauma, which can initiate bleeding or be a site for infection (Gobel, 2005).

(continued)

Interventions	*Rationales*

4. Monitor for signs and symptoms of infection:
  a. Fever
  b. Redness / swelling at site
  c. Pus formation
  d. Pain / discomfort
	4. Lymphocytes provide long-term protection against various microorganisms. They produce antibodies that neutralize foreign proteins and facilitate phagocytosis (Ellerhorst-Ryan, 2000; Shelton, 2005).

5. Explain risks of bleeding and infection. (Refer to the Corticosteroid Therapy Care Plan for strategies to reduce the risk of infection.)	

6. Monitor for signs and symptoms of malabsorption:
  a. Diarrhea
  b. Steatorrhea
  c. Abdominal pain
  d. Iron deficiency anemia
  e. Easy bleeding or bruising
  f. Paresthesias
  g. Skin and vision changes
  h. Weight loss
  i. Abnormal laboratory study results: vitamin B12, folic acid, hemoglobin, hematocrit, electrolytes, and prothrombin time and international normalized ratio (INR)
	6. Injury to the intestines can affect both the large and small intestine, is often progressive, and may lead to a variety of side effects. Presenting 6 or more months after radiation therapy. "Chronic radiation enteritis is due to an obliterative arteritis that leads to intestinal ischemia, which can result in stricture, ulceration, fibrosis, and occasionally fistula formation. The physiologic consequences can include altered intestinal transit, reduced bile acid absorption, increased intestinal permeability, bacterial overgrowth, and lactose malabsorption. Clinical manifestations may include nausea, vomiting, lactose intolerance, obstructive symptoms, diarrhea, weight loss, malnutrition, and bleeding" (Uptodate, 2012).

7. Monitor for signs and symptoms of radiation pleural effusion:
  a. Dyspnea
  b. Dry, nonproductive cough
  c. Chest pain—may be achy, heavy, or pleuritic
  d. Tachycardia
  e. Tachypnea
  f. Bulging of intercostal spaces
  g. Decreased breath sounds
  h. Abnormal chest x-ray film
  i. May be asymptomatic
  j. Anxiety, fear of suffocation
  k. Desire to lie on affected side
	7. Treatment of the primary tumor in the chest or mediastinum increases the risk of a malignant pleural effusion. Monitor 6 weeks to 6 months post RT as pleuritis can lead to pleural effusion. Late effects can present years post treatment including fibrosis, constrictive pericarditis, and vena cava obstruction (Story, 2006).

8. Monitor for signs and symptoms to the central nervous system. The CNS is highly susceptible to adverse effects from radiation. The severity of neural dysfunction is directly related to the total radiation dose, fraction, and volume of radiation given to the brain or spinal cord, and time duration between treatments (DeAngelis, 2009):
  a. Restlessness, irritability, memory loss
  b. Somnolence
  c. Headache
  d. Vomiting
  e. Seizure activity
  f. Increased systolic blood pressure with widening pulse pressure
  g. Bradycardia
  h. Depressed respirations
  i. Weakness
  j. Hemiparesis
  k. Vision changes
  l. Abnormal pupillary response to light
	8. RT adverse effects to the CNS can be acute, early, delayed, or late delayed and believed to be caused by a breakdown to the blood–brain barrier resulting in increased intracranial pressure (DeAngelis, 2009).

Interventions	Rationales

9. Monitor for signs and symptoms of mucositis. Mucositis can occur anywhere along the GI track presenting complications from the mouth to the anus. Occurring in up to 50% of patients receiving combination chemo-radiation:
  a. White patches on oral mucosa
  b. Reddened, swollen mucous membranes
  c. Ulcerated, bleeding lesions
  d. Weight loss due to eating difficulty
	9. Individuals with head and neck cancers, receiving concurrent chemotherapy are at a risk of developing severe mucositis (Cornett & Dea, 2012). RT can cause a decrease in salivation, therefore upsetting the natural balance of bacteria in the mouth leading to infections, mouth sores, and tooth decay.

10. Instruct client to do the following:
  a. Schedule a preventative visit to dentist for examination to assess for integrity / health of gums and assess dentures for fitting.
  b. Perform good oral hygiene, soft bristle tooth brush, brushing teeth 2–3 times daily, rinse and spit after eating.
  c. Avoid alcohol, smoking, and spicy or acidic foods.
  d. Avoid very hot or cold liquids and foods.
  e. Report any signs of mucositis early.
  f. Quit smoking.
  g. Suck on ice, chew gum, suck on sour candy such as lemon drops.
	10g. It is critically important to maintain moisture in the oral cavity, as saliva protects the mouth and gums from infection. Avoid any mouthwashes containing alcohol as it can burn the mouth.

11. Monitor for signs and symptoms of pneumonitis:
  a. Shortness of breath
  b. Hemoptysis
  c. Dry cough
	11. Acute radiation pneumonitis can develop 3 to 10 weeks post RT and is more common in higher radiation doses. Pneumonitis can progress into interstitial fibrosis (Prommer, 2009).

12. Monitor for signs and symptoms of esophagitis:
  a. Difficulty swallowing
  b. Sore throat
  c. Nausea and vomiting	

13. Monitor for signs and symptoms of cystitis or urethritis:
  a. Urinary urgency and frequency
  b. Hematuria
  c. Dysuria
  d. Negative urine cultures
	13. Bladder damage to the urinary tract may increase bacterial infection (radiation-induced cystitis). Serious damage to the bladder may require surgery. Nephritis and kidney dysfunction can present in immediate or delayed effects, is dose dependant.

14. Monitor for gastro-intestinal injury:
  a. Tenesmus (diarrhea and rectal urgency)
  b. Persistent sensation of need to void or defecate
  c. Diarrhea
	14. Radiation injury to the lower intestine may be encountered following treatment of cancers of the rectum, cervix, uterus, prostate, urinary bladder, and testes. Bowel damage secondary to RT may be complicated by previous bowel surgery. High doses of radiation exposure inhibit gastric secretion and cause inflammation and ulceration of the bowels.

15. Monitor for signs and symptoms of myelitis:
  a. Paresthesias in back or extremities
  b. Shocklike sensation on neck flexion
 	
16. Monitor for signs and symptoms of parotitis:
  a. Painful, swollen parotid glands
	15, 16. Radiation therapy to head and neck can cause myelitis or parotitis. These problems usually are transient, not serious, and resolve spontaneously (Hilderley, 2000; Maher, 2005).

(continued)

Interventions	Rationales

17. Monitor for Systemic Reaction of Acute Radiation Syndrome. Advise individual / family of its symptoms / signs to report:
  a. Anorexia
  b. Nausea and vomiting
  c. Weakness
  d. Exhaustion
  e. Lassitude
  f. Prostration
  g. Dehydration
  h. Anemia
  i. Infection
	17. While rare, symptoms can present within hours to days post treatment. The Centers for Disease Control and Prevention offers a comprehensive web-based education regarding this systemic reaction: http://emergency.cdc.gov/radiation/arsphysicianfactsheet.asp.

CLINICAL ALERT

- As RT is a complex, individualized, and a site-based modality, the above adverse effects are not all-inclusive.
- Refer to these websites for specific side effects and adverse effects depending on site of radiation:
  - American Cancer Society: www.cancer.org, Symptoms and Side Effects
  - American Society of Clinical Oncology: www.cancer.net, Managing Side Effects
  - National Cancer Institute: www.cancer.gov/cancertopics/coping, Coping with cancer
  - CancerSymptoms.org

Related Physician / NP Prescribed Interventions

Depend on cancer site, stage, and extent

Documentation

Flow records
Intake and output
Abnormal laboratory values
Assessments—full physical (skin, oral, respiratory, neurologic)
Distress assessment as needed
Stool for occult blood
Daily weights

Nursing Diagnoses

Anxiety Related to Prescribed Radiation Therapy and Insufficient Knowledge of Treatment and Self-Care Measures

NOC
Anxiety Level, Coping, Impulse Control

Goals

The client will report less anxiety after teaching.

NIC
Energy Management, Exercise Promotion, Sleep Enhancement, Mutual Goal Setting

Indicators

- Verbalize rationale for radiation treatment and treatment plan.
- Identify expected side effects and their management.
- Describe self-care measures to reduce fatigue, promote nutrition, manage skin problems, and prevent infection and bleeding.

See Neoplastic Disorders Care Plan for additional interventions.

Interventions	Rationales
1. Encourage client to share fears and beliefs regarding radiation therapy. Delay teaching if client is experiencing severe anxiety.	1. Sharing enables nurse to identify sources of client anxiety and to correct misinformation. Severe anxiety prevents retention of learning.
2. Review general principles of radiation therapy, as necessary. Provide written materials such as a client education booklet from the National Cancer Institute.	2. A client undergoing radiation therapy is likely to have many questions about the treatment and its effects. Reinforcing information provided by the physician / NP and radiologist and answering questions can help to reduce client's anxiety related to lack of knowledge (Hilderley, 2000; Maher, 2005).
3. Reinforce physician / NP's explanation of the treatment plan; cover the following items: a. Area to be irradiated b. Treatment schedule c. Dose to be administered d. Simulation to compute dose and delivery of radiation e. Markings and tattoos f. Shielding of vital organs	3. This information can help to reduce client's anxiety associated with fear of the unknown and the unexpected.
4. Help client understand that fatigue is common and to be expected during radiation therapy. Refer to Fatigue in Unit II for additional interventions.	4. Treatment-related fatigue is related to the body's need to conserve energy to repair the health cells damaged during treatment. Physical and mental fatigue may also be a direct result from medications taken in addition to radiation to treat the disease or side effects.
5. Explain skin reactions and precautions. Refer to Impaired Skin Integrity in this care plan.	

6. Explain site-specific radiation side effects:
a. Neck:
  • Mucositis
  • Dry mouth
  • Altered taste
  • Dental problems
  • Hoarseness
  • Dysphagia
b. Head
  • Headache
  • Alopecia
  • Nausea and vomiting
c. Chest and back
  • Pneumonitis
  • Esophagitis
d. Abdomen and pelvis:
  • Nausea and vomiting
  • Anorexia
  • Cystitis
  • Tenesmus
  • Diarrhea
  • Dehydration
  • Weakness
  • Abdominal cramps
	6. Understanding what to expect can decrease anxiety related to fear of the unknown and the unexpected and can help client to recognize and report adverse effects.
	
	c. Potential damage to heart and coronary arteries: Delayed effects such as obliterative endarteritis, constrictive pericarditis occurring months to years later:

Documentation

Anxiety level
Client teaching
Outcome achievement or status

Risk for Impaired Oral Mucous Membrane Related to Dry Mouth or Inadequate Oral Hygiene

NOC
Oral Hygiene

NIC
Oral Health Restoration, Chemotherapy Management, Oral Health Maintenance

Goals

The client will maintain intact oral mucosa.

Indicators

- Describe the possible effects of radiation on the oral cavity.
- Explain proper techniques for oral care.

Interventions	Rationales
1. Explain signs and symptoms of mucositis and stomatitis.	1. Client's understanding can help to ensure early detection and prompt intervention to minimize problems.
2. Stress the need to have dental visit prior to initiation of RT caries filled and bad or loose teeth extracted before initiation of radiation therapy to the head and neck.	2. Preexisting dental problems increase risk of radiation-induced infection.

3. Emphasize the need for regular oral hygiene during and after therapy. Instruct client to do the following:
  a. Brush with fluoridated toothpaste after meals.
  b. Use a soft-bristle toothbrush.
  c. Rinse mouth with topical fluoride solution after each brushing.
  d. Use a molded dental carrier and fluoride gel daily.
	3. Proper oral hygiene eliminates microorganisms and reduces risk of infection.

4. If gingival tissue becomes inflamed, suggest an oral rinse.	4. Rinsing removes debris and microorganisms without causing trauma to mucosal tissue.

5. Teach client to avoid the following:
  a. Commercial mouthwashes
  b. Very hot foods / drinks
  c. Alcoholic beverages
  d. Tobacco
  e. Highly seasoned foods
  f. Acidic foods (grapefruit, tomatoes, and oranges)
	5. These substances are irritating to oral mucosa and can increase inflammation.

6. Explain the need for dental examinations during and after course of treatment.	6. Increased risk of dental caries and gum disease persists for months to years after completion of radiation therapy. Long-term follow-up dental care decreases the risk.

Documentation

Mouth assessment
Oral care
Client teaching
Outcome achievement or status

Impaired Skin Integrity Related to Effects of Radiation on Epithelial and Basal Cells and Effects of Diarrhea on Perineal Area

NOC
Tissue Integrity: Skin and Mucous Membranes

NIC
Pressure Management, Pressure Ulcer Care, Skin Surveillance, Positioning

Goals

The client will demonstrate healing of tissue.

Indicators

- Relate strategies to reduce skin damage.
- Relate importance of good nutrition.

Interventions	Rationales
1. Explain the effects of radiation on skin (e.g., redness, tanning, peeling, itching, hair loss, decreased perspiration), and monitor skin in the irradiated area(s).	1. Radiation damages epithelial, sebaceous, and hair follicle cells, causing localized skin reactions. Understanding the reason for these effects can promote compliance with protective and preventive measures (Yarbro, Wujcik, & Gobel, 2011).
2. Explain the need for optimal nutritional intake; provide instruction.	2. During radiation treatments, the body must build and repair tissue and protect itself from infection. This process requires increased intake of protein, carbohydrates, vitamins, and minerals (Yarbro, Wujcik, & Gobel, 2011).
3. Teach client the precautions to protect skin integrity, avoid trauma: a. Do not wash treated area until therapist allows. b. If tattoos are used for skin markings, wash irradiated skin with a mild soap and tepid water; do not remove markings. c. Avoid harsh soap, ointments, creams, cosmetics, and deodorants on treated skin unless approved by health care professionals. d. Avoid exposure of radiated skin to sun, chlorinated pools, wind, and shaving. e. Wear loose-fitting cotton clothing over treated skin. f. Apply a thin layer of vitamin A and D ointment for dry skin if needed. g. Apply cool air to the affected area; avoid heat lamps and warmth. h. Use an electric razor only—no blades—to shave irradiated area. i. If moist desquamation is present, shower or irrigate the area frequently; use a moist wound healing dressing.	3. These measures can help to maintain skin integrity: a. Moisture enhances skin reactions. b. To reduce irritation, harsh soaps and hot water should be avoided. The tattoo must remain to guide evaluation and subsequent therapy, if necessary. c. Harsh substances may increase skin's vulnerability to damage. d. This exposure can cause additional damage. e. Loose-fitting cotton clothing can minimize irritation and injury to the epithelial surface. f. Vitamin A and D ointment can prevent or treat dry skin. g. Coldness reduces irritating sensory stimulation (e.g., pruritus) and prevents moist desquamation. h. An electric razor can protect sensitive skin from razor cuts. i. Showering or irrigation and moist wound dressings can help to debride the area and aid healing.
4. Instruct client to report any skin changes promptly.	4. Early detection of moist desquamation with shedding of surface epithelium enables prompt intervention to prevent severe skin damage and subsequent fibrosis.
5. Teach client to keep rectal and perineal areas clean and to apply protective ointment after each cleaning.	5. Good hygiene and application of nonwater-soluble ointments reduce erosion of acidic excreta on perineal area.
6. After skin is completely healed, teach client sun precautions: a. Use sun screen as directed by provider. b. Increase exposure time very slowly. c. Discontinue sun exposure if redness occurs. d. Protect treated skin with hats and long sleeves.	6. Skin reactions with erythema progressing to desquamation may occur, and is in direct relation to dose and amount of radiation received (Strobl, 2009; Yarbro, Wujcik, & Gobel, 2011).

Documentation

Skin assessments
Client teaching
Outcome achievement or status

Total Parenteral Nutrition

Total parenteral nutrition (TPN) involves intravenous (IV) administration of an elemental diet (dextrose, amino acids, and lipids) in a hypertonic solution to a client who cannot ingest or assimilate sufficient calories or who has increased metabolic needs that oral ingestion cannot meet. Total nutritional admixture (TNA) system combines IV lipids with the base TPN solution. This admixture is often referred to as three-in-one solution because it contains dextrose, amino acids, and lipids. TPN solutions that contain more than 10% dextrose may be infused only in a central line. Indications for TPN include cancer, chronic nausea, and vomiting of any etiology, prolonged bowel rest, anorexia nervosa, massive burns, and GI disorders such as inflammatory bowel disease, bowel obstruction, or fistula.

 Time Frame
Intratherapy

▄▄▄▄▄ DIAGNOSTIC CLUSTER

Collaborative Problems

△ Risk for Complications of Pneumothorax, Hemothorax, or Hydrothorax (refer to Long-Term Venous Access Devices Care Plan)

△ Risk for Complications of Air Embolism

▲ Risk for Complications of Infection / Sepsis (refer to Long-Term Venous Access Devices Care Plan)

▲ Risk for Complications of Hyperglycemia

▲ Risk for Complications of Metabolic Complications

Nursing Diagnoses

▲ Risk for Infection related to catheter's direct access to bloodstream (refer to Long-Term Venous Access Device)

△ Risk for Ineffective Self-Health Management related to insufficient knowledge of home care, signs and symptoms of complications, catheter care, and follow-up care (laboratory studies)

▲ This diagnosis was reported to be monitored for or managed frequently (75% to 100%).
△ This diagnosis was reported to be monitored for or managed often (50% to 74%).
* This diagnosis was not included in the validation study.

Transition Criteria

Before transition, the client or family will:

1. Demonstrate proper catheter care and TPN administration at home.
2. Discuss strategies for incorporating TPN management into ADLs.
3. Verbalize precautions for medication use.
4. Relate causes, prevention, and treatment of hypoglycemia and hyperglycemia.
5. State signs and symptoms that must be reported to a health care professional.

Collaborative Problems

Risk for Complications of Potential Complication: Pneumothorax, Hemothorax, or Hydrothorax

Risk for Complications of Air Embolism

Risk for Complications of Infection / Sepsis

Risk for Complications of Hyperglycemia

Risk for Complications of Metabolic Complications

Collaborative Outcomes

The client will be monitored for early signs and symptoms of (a) pneumothorax, hemothorax, or hydrothorax, (b) air embolism, (c) sepsis, (d) hyperglycemia, and (e) metabolic complications, and will receive collaborative interventions if indicated to restore physiological stability.

Indicators of Physiologic Stability

- Alert, calm, oriented (a, b, c, d, e)
- Respirations 16–20 breaths/min (a, b, e)
- Respirations relaxed, rhythmic (a, b, e)
- Pulse 60–100 beats/min (a, b, e)
- BP >90/60, <140/90 mm Hg (a, b, e)
- Temperature 98.5°–99° F (c)
- Flat neck veins (b)
- Skin usual color, dry, warm (a, b, e)
- No complaints of chest pain (a, b)
- Urine output >0.5 mL/kg/h (d, e)
- Specific gravity 1.005–1.030 (d, e)
- Urine negative for glucose (d, e)
- Negative blood cultures (c)
- Intact insertion site (c)
- No drainage at insertion site (c)
- No or minimal weight loss (d)
- Phosphorous 3.0–4.5 mg/dL (e)
- Calcium 8.5–10.5 mg/dL (e)
- Aspartate transaminase (AST) 7–21 u/L (e)
- Alanine transaminase (ALT) 5–35 u/L (e)
- Sodium 135–145 mEq/L (e)
- Magnesium 1.5–2.5 mEq/L (e)
- Potassium 3.5–5.0 mEq/L (e)
- Total cholesterol <200 mg/dL (e)
- Triglycerides (e)
    - Male 40–160 mg/dL
    - Female 35–135 mg/dL
- Blood glucose <140 mg/dL (e)
- Prealbumin 3–7 (e)
- Serum ammonia 20–120 µg/dL (e)
- Blood urea nitrogen 5–25 mg/dL (e)
- Creatinine 0.7–1.4 mg/dL (e)
- Oxygen saturation (SaO_2) >94% (e)
- Carbon dioxide ($PaCO_2$) 35–45 mm/Hg (e)
- Arterial pH 7.35–7.45 (e)
- White blood cell count 4,800–10,000/mm^3 (c)

Interventions	Rationales
1. Monitor for signs and symptoms of air embolism during dressing and IV tubing changes and on accidental separation of IV connections:	1. Intravascular air embolism occurs when two conditions are met: (1) there is direct connection between a source of air and the vascular system and (2) the pressure gradient favors the entry of this air into the bloodstream. They can occur with IV tubing changes, with accidental tubing separations, and during catheter insertion and disconnection. Often the person is asymptomatic. For example, client can aspirate as much as 200 mL of air from a deep breath during subclavian line disconnection. Entry of air into the circulatory system can block blood flow and cause cardiac arrest.

(continued)

Interventions	Rationales

CLINICAL ALERT

- Small volumes of air travel to the right side of the heart and into pulmonary vasculature, where the air is dissipated.
- Larger volumes with rapid infusion of air, cause pulmonary artery pressures to rise, putting strain on the right side of the heart. This can create an air lock in one or more of the pulmonary arteries, obstructing pulmonary circulation and causing circulatory collapse.
- The closer to the heart the air embolism enters into the venous system, the smaller the volume of air is required to be symptomatic.
- Even small air embolisms can cause tissue ischemia or inflammatory changes within blood vessels, leading to a host of potentially lethal complications (e.g., systemic inflammatory response syndrome, pulmonary edema, myocardial, and cerebral ischemia) (O'Dowd & Kelley, 2000; Pennsylvania Patient Safety Advisory, 2012).

a. Dyspnea
b. Light-headedness
c. Pallor
d. Tachypnea
e. Decreased oxygen saturation
f. Sense of impending doom, anxiety, agitation
g. Change in mental status
h. Chest pain, tachycardia, or bradycardia
i. Hypotension

CLINICAL ALERT

- Call rapid response team if air embolism is suspected.

Interventions	Rationales

2. Perform emergency interventions:
  a. Place the individual in a left side-lying position in Trendelenburg.
  b. Administer 100% oxygen.
	2. This position helps the air embolus to move toward the apex of the right ventricle, away from the pulmonary artery and right ventricular outflow tract. The administration of oxygen supports the individual with cardiovascular instability through its effects on the partial pressures of oxygen and nitrogen within the blood causes nitrogen to move from the embolus into the bloodstream, thus decreasing the size of the embolus (O'Dowd & Kelley, 2000; Pennsylvania Patient Safety Advisory, 2012).

3. Secure proximal catheter connection with a Luer-locking IV set and tape all connections.	3. These precautions can help prevent accidental disconnection.
4. Instruct client to perform Valsalva maneuver during IV tubing disconnections or removal. Instruct the individual to hold his or her breath, and perform a Valsalva maneuver as the last portion of the catheter is removed; if unable to do so, time the removal while the individual expires air.	4. Valsalva maneuver with breath-holding minimizes air aspiration and reduces risk of embolism.

Interventions	Rationales
5. Explain potential problems with tubing separation and instruct client to crimp tubing near entry site if it occurs.	5. Immediate action can prevent air embolism.
6. Monitor for signs and symptoms of sepsis or catheter-related infection: a. Refer to Long-term Venous Access Device Care Plan for interventions to prevent infection and sepsis.	6. The high glucose concentration of the TPN solution and frequent catheter manipulation put the client at risk for infection.

7. Monitor for signs and symptoms of hyperglycemia:
  a. Kussmaul respirations
  b. Polyuria
  c. Low urine specific gravity
  d. Glycosuria
  e. Mental status changes (e.g., lethargy or disorientation)
  f. Elevated serum glucose
  g. Weight change
	7. Osmotic diuresis can result from inability to compensate for rapid instillation of high-glucose solution. The subsequent rise in serum glucose causes fluid shifts to the vascular compartment in an attempt to dilute the hyperosmolar glucose concentration. Increased fluid volume along with the exogenous source is lost rapidly in urine. If unrecognized and untreated, this condition can progress rapidly to nonketotic hyperglycemic coma.

8. If possible, determine if hyperglycemia was present prior to initiation of TPN or occurred within 24 hours of initiation.	8. Pasquel et al. (2010) reported that "blood glucose values before and within 24 h of initiation of TPN are better predictors of hospital mortality and complications than blood glucose during the entire duration of TPN" (p. 740). The increased risk of complications during TPN therapy can be related, among other factors, to the development of hyperglycemia, which occurs in 10% to 88% of hospitalized patients receiving TPN therapy (Pasquel et al., 2010). Observational studies have reported a 33% mortality rate in TPN patients who developed hyperglycemias as well as an increased risk of cardiac complications, infections, systemic sepsis, and acute renal failure (Pasquel et al., 2010).
9. Monitor blood glucose level every 2 hours during and after discontinuation of TPN.	9. Fluctuations in blood glucose level need to be detected early.

10. Monitor for metabolic complications related to carbohydrate (CHO) content of TPN:
  a. Hyperglycemia (increased blood sugar, glycosuria)
 	
  b. Hypoglycemia
 	
  c. Hyperglycemic hyperosmolar, nonketotic dehydration (HHNKD):
    • Increased blood glucose
    • Increased urine output
    • Increased serum sodium
    • Changes in mental status
    • Report changes and early signs and symptoms of HHNKD.
	10a. The high CHO content of TPN makes hyperglycemia the most common metabolic complication.
	  b. Abrupt discontinuation of TPN can cause hypoglycemia.
	  c. HHNKD is a risk with rapid infusion to those with mild diabetes, renal insufficiency, or congestive heart failure.

11. Monitor for metabolic complications related to protein content of TPN:
  a. Increased BUN
  b. Increased creatinine
  c. Increased serum ammonia
  d. Increased AST
  e. Increased ALT
  f. Change in mental status
	11. The protein content in TPN can cause amino acid imbalance and azotemia (increased BUN and creatinine). The amount of protein produces increased urea that a compromised kidney (e.g., older adult, preexisting renal insufficiency) cannot excrete. People with hepatic insufficiency cannot metabolize certain amino acids: this causes increased ammonia levels and hepatic encephalopathy.

(continued)

Interventions	Rationales
12. Monitor for metabolic complications related to lipid content, especially triglyceride level.	12. Clients who cannot metabolize more lipids experience hypertriglyceridemia. Rapid infusion can precipitate this condition.
13. Monitor for gallbladder dysfunction commonly shown by dyspepsia.	13. Decreased bile flow is caused by the loss of enteric stimulation (NPO status), which then produces decreased gallbladder contractions. This causes gallbladder sludge and / or gallstones (Onizuka et al., 2001; Marinell, 2008).

14. Monitor for metabolic acidosis:
  a. Hyperkalemia
  b. Decreased thiamin levels
  c. Decreased biotin levels
  d. Decreased pH
  e. Decreased or normal $PaCO_2$
  f. Headache, confusion
  g. Decreased BP
  h. Cold, clammy skin
  i. Increased respiratory rate and depth
	14. Metabolic acidosis is produced by loss of bicarbonate or excess acid in extracellular fluid caused by excessive GI or renal losses, inadequate acetate in solution, impaired renal function, and inadequate thiamin and biotin intake.

Clinical Alert Report

Prior to providing care, advise ancillary staff / student to report the following to the professional nurse assigned to the client:

- Change in cognitive status
- Oral temperature >100.5° F
- Systolic BP <90 mm/Hg
- Resting pulse >100, <50
- Respiratory rate >28, <10/min
- Oxygen saturation <90%
- Blood glucose >200 mg/dL

Related Physician / NP Prescribed Interventions

Intravenous Therapy
Nutritional solution; additives (e.g., insulin)

Laboratory Studies
Serum albumin; prealbumin; thyroxine-binding prealbumin; CBC; electrolytes; liver enzymes; serum transferrin; amino acid profile; glucose, BUN, and PT; 24-hour creatinine excretion; arterial blood gases

Diagnostic Studies
Chest x-ray film

Therapies
Daily weights; anthropometric measurements; catheter site care

Documentation

Vital signs
Intake and output
Weight
Serum glucose
Urine specific gravity
Catheter site
Unusual complaints with related interventions

Nursing Diagnoses

Risk for Ineffective Self-Health Management Related to Insufficient Knowledge of Home Care, Signs and Symptoms of Complications, Catheter Care, and Follow-up Care (Laboratory Studies)

NOC

Compliance Behavior, Knowledge: Treatment Regimen, Participation: Health Care Decisions, Treatment Behavior: Illness or Injury

NIC

Anticipatory Guidance, Learning Facilitation, Risk Identification, Health Education, Teaching: Procedure / Treatment

Goals

The goals for this diagnosis represent those associated with transition planning. Refer to the transition criteria.

Interventions	Rationales
1. For individuals who will have a venous access device and TPN at home, refer to home health nursing agency for home care assessment on the day of transition to home.	1. The initial home care visit evaluates suitability for home TPN / TNA by considering client's ability, environment, financial needs, and support system. Subsequent visits are needed to assess client's nutritional status, blood glucose levels, laboratory results, insertion site, and catheter patency.
2. Have client or support person perform return demonstration of selected care measures.	2. Return demonstration lets nurse evaluate client's and family's abilities to manage the device safely.
3. Refer to the care plan for the specific condition that necessitated long-term venous access device with TPN.	

> **CLINICAL ALERT**
> • If there are concerns over the ability of the caregivers at home to safely manage venous access device initiate STAR.

STAR

Stop

Think Are there barriers for the caregivers to provide safe management of venous access device (e.g., motivation, manual skills, anxiety, practice, knowledge)?

Review Can the barriers be removed for successful transition? Is it safe for transition to proceed? Can a home health nurse be at the home the day of transition? If not, use SBAR to communicate to the appropriate person (e.g., manager, physician / NP).

4. Encourage client and family to ask questions and express concerns about TPN / TNA therapy.	4. Sharing concerns and questions identifies learning needs and misconceptions; this allows nurse to address problem areas.

(continued)

Interventions	Rationales

5. Teach about hyperglycemia:
  a. Signs and symptoms: nausea, weakness, thirst, headaches, elevated blood glucose level
  b. Prevention: maintain prescribed rate; avoid increasing rate to "catch up"
  c. Treatment: consult with physician / NP for possible insulin supplement
	5. Because TPN / TNA solution contains high glucose concentrations, sudden changes in rate can increase blood glucose levels.

6. Teach about hyperglycemia:
  a. Signs and symptoms: nausea, weakness, thirst, headaches, elevated blood glucose level
  b. Prevention: maintain prescribed rate; avoid increasing rate to "catch up"
  c. Treatment: consult with physician / NP for possible insulin supplement
	6. Because TPN / TNA solution contains high glucose concentrations, sudden changes in rate can increase blood glucose levels.

7. Teach about hypoglycemia and treatment (e.g., glass of orange juice, teaspoon of honey):
  a. Signs and symptoms: sweating, pallor, palpitations, nausea, headache, shaking feeling, hunger, blurred vision
  b. Prevention: avoid stopping TPN / TNA too abruptly; slow TPN / TNA rate gradually
	7. During TPN / TNA infusion, the body produces insulin in response to high glucose concentrations. Too much insulin in TPN / TNA or too-rapid discontinuation of TPN / TNA can produce hypoglycemia.

8. Explain signs and symptoms of VAD / TPN complications:	8. Understanding signs and symptoms of complications enables early detection and reporting to a health care professional for timely intervention

CLINICAL ALERT

• Ensure that the caregiver comprehends the seriousness of any of these possible complications and the need for immediate evaluation (e.g., emergency room).

a. Fever	a, b. Fever and changes at the insertion site may indicate infection, phebitis.
b. Tenderness, swelling, and drainage at site	
c. VAD occlusion	
d. Inability to infuse	d. Inaccurate infusion rate or inability to infuse points to obstruction or catheter damage.
e. Facial edema and distended neck veins	e. Facial edema and neck vein distention may indicate superior vena caval syndrome.
f. Mental status changes (e.g., lethargy, disorientation)	f, g. These symptoms may indicate air embolism, metabolic imbalances
g. Sudden onset anxiety, breathlessness, chest pain	

Documentation

Client and family teaching
Demonstrated ability of home caregiver to provide treatments safely
Outcome achievement or status

Section 4

Specialty Diagnostic Clusters

Section 4 outlines four specialty generic care plans for newborns, children, and adolescents; the family in the postpartum period; and individuals with mental health disorders. Diagnostic clusters of nursing diagnoses and collaborative problems are presented for each specialty plan. The reader can access the complete plan on thePoint at http://thePoint.lww.com/Carpenito6e, the website for additional supplements to this book.

Once the care plan is accessed on thePoint, it can be printed. Using the steps to create a care plan as outlined in Chapter 5, the nurse can also use nursing diagnoses and collaborative problems from Unit II. For example, for a child with diabetes mellitus, the nurse can access *Risk for Complications of Hypo / Hyperglycemia* (in Unit II) and add it to the specialty generic plan. For an adolescent on a postsurgical unit, voicing suicide threats, the nurse can access *Risk for Suicide* in Unit II and add it to the plan.

Normal Newborn Generic Care Plan

Newborn Transition from Intrauterine to Extrauterine Life: Birth to 4 Hours of Life

■■ DIAGNOSTIC CLUSTER

Collaborative Problems: Newborn Transition from Intrauterine to Extrauterine Life: Birth to 4 Hours of Life

Risk for Complications of Respiratory Dysfunction: Hypoxemia

Risk for Complications of Hypothermia

Risk for Complications of Hypoglycemia

Newborn Transition from Intrauterine to 4 Hours to 4 Days of Life

■■■■■ DIAGNOSTIC CLUSTER

Collaborative Problems: Normal Newborn Care: 4 Hours to 4 Days of Life

Risk for Complications of Hypothermia

Risk for Complications of Hypoglycemia

Risk for Complications of Infection

Risk for Complications of Hyperbilirubinemia

Risk for Complications of Bleeding (Circumcision)

Nursing Diagnoses: Normal Newborn Care: 4 Hours to 4 Days of Life

Risk for Aspiration

 related to decreased muscle tone of the inferior esophageal sphincter

 related to secretions of the oropharynx

Ineffective Thermoregulation

 related to newborn transition to extrauterine life

 related to immature temperature regulating mechanisms

 related to heat loss from exposure to cool temperature of birthing room, mother's room

Risk for Complications of Hypothermia

Risk for Infection

 related to vulnerability of newborn secondary to immature immune system

 related to lack of normal flora

 related to exposure of eyes to vaginal secretions

 related to open wound (umbilical cord, spiral electrode lesion, circumcision)

 related to colonization by / transmission of perinatal infection acquired in utero

 related to environmental hazards

Risk for Ineffective Breastfeeding

 related to incorrect positioning of newborn at the breast

 related to unsuccessful latch

 related to absence of regular and sustained suckling / swallowing at the breast

 related to maternal fatigue or anxiety due to inexperience with breastfeeding

Risk for Imbalanced Nutrition: Less than body requirements

 related to limited caloric intake during the first few days of life

 related to ineffective infant latch and sucking

 related to maternal nipple soreness

Risk for Impaired Skin Integrity

 related to diaper dermatitis, circumcision

Risk for Acute Pain / Impaired Comfort

related to injections, heel sticks, circumcision

Risk for Impaired Parent Attachment

related to unwanted pregnancy

related to prolonged or difficult labor and delivery

related to postpartum pain or fatigue

related to lack of positive support system

related to lack of positive role model

related to inability to prepare emotionally

Risk for Impaired Parenting

related to lack of access to resources

related to postpartum depression

related to adolescent parents

related to substance abuse

related to domestic violence

related to poor home environment

related to preterm birth

related to ineffective adaptation to stressors associated with parenting a new infant

related to impaired support system

Risk for Injury

related to parental lack of awareness of environmental hazards

Infants, Children, and Adolescents Generic Care Plans

This care plan presents nursing diagnoses and collaborative problems that commonly apply to infants, children, adolescents (and their significant others) undergoing hospitalization for any medical disorder. It represents a basic standard of care. For beginning students, it can represent the care that they are prepared to provide. As the student progresses in the curriculum, the care plans for specific medical conditions such as pneumonia, diabetes mellitus, fractures, and those focusing on the care of individuals undergoing surgery or therapies such as chemotherapy will be their focus of care.

 Carp's Cues

This plan is designed to focus on the expected care that is needed when infant, child, or adolescent is hospitalized for a medical condition. It addresses the care that is needed regardless of the specific medical condition that necessitated admission. (We assessed what the bedside nurse needs to be aware of upon admission and during daily assessment of his or her client regardless of the client's diagnosis.) If the child has diabetes mellitus, one can refer to Unit II Risk for Complications of Hypo / Hyperglycemia for specific interventions.

▪▪▪ DIAGNOSTIC CLUSTER

Collaborative Problems

Risk for Complications of Cardiovascular Dysfunction

Risk for Complications of Respiratory Dysfunction

Risk for Complications of Neurological Dysfunction

Risk for Complications of Dehydration / Hypovolemia

Risk for Complications of Sepsis

Nursing Diagnoses

Anxiety (child, caregivers) related to unfamiliar environment, routines, diagnostic tests, treatments, and loss of control

Risk for Injury related to unfamiliar environment, developmental considerations, and physical and mental limitations secondary to condition, medications, therapies, and diagnostic tests

Risk for Infection related to increased microorganisms in environment, risk of person-to-person transmission, and invasive tests and therapies

Acute Pain related to (specify)

Chronic Pain related to (specify)

(Specify) Self-Care Deficit related to sensory, cognitive, mobility, endurance, or motivation problems

Risk for Imbalanced Nutrition: Less Than Body Requirements related to developmental feeding issues, congenital or disease entities, altered route of nutrition (NG, ND, GT, Central Line / TPN) decreased appetite secondary to treatments, fatigue, environment, and changes in usual diet, and to increased protein and vitamin requirements for healing

Risk for Deficient Fluid Volume

related to insufficient intake secondary to fatigue, malaise, dyspnea, pain

related to fluid loss secondary to fever, diarrhea

related to difficult or painful swallowing

Risk for Constipation related to change in fluid and food intake, routine, and activity level; effects of medications; and emotional stress

Risk for Impaired Skin Integrity

related to adhesive tape, dressings, monitoring devices, IV infiltrates,

related to changes in stooling patterns, urinary / fecal incontinence

related to effects of certain medications (chemotherapy, antibiotics, Stevens Johnson Syndrome)

related to prolonged pressure on tissues associated with decreased mobility

related to increased fragility of the skin associated with dependent edema

related to decreased tissue perfusion, malnutrition

Disturbed Sleep Pattern related to unfamiliar, noisy environment, change in bedtime ritual, emotional stress, and change in circadian rhythm

Interrupted Family Processes related to disruption of routines, change in role responsibilities, and fatigue associated with increased

Risk for Impaired Parenting related to lack of control, anxiety, fear, multiple stressors associated hospitalizations, cultural barriers, and unfamiliar environment.

Risk for Compromised Human Dignity related to multiple factors (intrusions, unfamiliar procedures and personnel, loss of privacy) associated with hospitalization

Risk for Ineffective Child Health Management related to complexity and cost of therapeutic regimen, complexity of health care system, insurance / financial issues, coordination of care, shortened length of stay, insufficient knowledge of treatment, and barriers to comprehension secondary to language barriers, cognitive deficits, hearing and / or visual impairment, anxiety and lack of motivation

Generic Care Plan for Individuals With Mental Health Disorders

Individuals with mental disorders, who require hospitalization do so because they are not functioning well or appropriately. Their compromised coping disrupts their ability to self-care, relate to others effectively, and problem solve appropriately. They may in addition be at risk for harming themselves or others. This care plan focuses on functional health patterns that are disrupted with an attempt to stabilize and comfort the individual and significant others.

Most individuals hospitalized for a mental disorder also have comorbidities such as hypertension, diabetes mellitus, COPD, and asthma. If indicated, refer to Unit II Section 2 collaborative problems and select those that need monitoring such as *Risk for Complications of Hypertension*, *Risk for Complications of Asthmatic Exacerbation*, *Risk for Complications of Hypo / Hyperglycemia.*

In addition to nursing diagnoses associated with a mental disorder (in the diagnostic cluster below), the generic nursing diagnoses that relate to any individual in the hospital are applicable and can be found in the text under Generic Medical Care Plan:

- Anxiety related to unfamiliar environment, routines, diagnostic tests, treatments, and loss of control
- Risk for Injury related to unfamiliar environment and physical and mental limitations secondary to condition, medications, therapies, and diagnostic tests
- Risk for Infection related to increased microorganisms in environment, risk of person-to-person transmission, and invasive tests and therapies
- (Specify) Self-Care Deficit related to sensory, cognitive, mobility, endurance, or motivation problems
- Risk for Imbalanced Nutrition: Less Than Body Requirements related to decreased appetite secondary to treatments, fatigue, environment, and changes in usual diet, and to increased protein and vitamin requirements for healing
- Risk for Constipation related to change in fluid and food intake, routine, and activity level; effects of medications; and emotional stress
- Risk for Impaired Skin Integrity related to prolonged pressure on tissues associated with decreased mobility, increased fragility of the skin associated with dependent edema, decreased tissue perfusion, malnutrition, and urinary / fecal incontinence
- Disturbed Sleep Pattern related to unfamiliar, noisy environment, change in bedtime ritual, emotional stress, and change in circadian rhythm
- Interrupted Family Processes related to disruption of routines, change in role responsibilities, and fatigue associated with increased workload and visiting hour requirements
- Risk for Compromised Human Dignity related to multiple factors (intrusions, unfamiliar procedures and personnel, loss of privacy) associated with hospitalization
- Risk for Ineffective Self-Health Management related to complexity and cost of therapeutic regimen, complexity of health care system, shortened length of stay, insufficient knowledge of treatment, and barriers to comprehension secondary to language barriers, cognitive deficits, hearing and / or visual impairment, anxiety and lack of motivation

Carp's Cues

The following are examples of nursing diagnoses that represent dysfunction and ineffective coping in individuals with mental disorders. The nurse must focus on those problems that are most disruptive to the person's ability to function safely and effectively in society. Students should seek the advice of their instructor or experienced nurse for selection of this client's priority problems. It is not very helpful to focus on the psychiatric diagnosis because it will not help to determine nursing interventions. Instead focus on what functional health patterns are disrupted that prevent him or her from functioning well in the community.

▪▪▪▪▪▪ DIAGNOSTIC CLUSTER

Nursing Diagnoses

Risk for Disabled Family Coping

    related to chronicity of illness

    related to marital discord and role conflicts secondary to effects of chronic depression

Disturbed Self-Concept related to feelings of worthlessness and lack of ego boundaries

Chronic Low Self-Esteem related to feelings of worthlessness and failure secondary to (specify)

Ineffective Coping

    related to internal conflicts (guilt, low self-esteem) or feelings of rejection

    related to biochemical changes with faulty thinking secondary (specify mental disorder)

    related to biochemical changes with poor impulse control and low frustration level

Defensive Coping related to unrealistic expectations secondary to exaggerated sense of self-importance and abilities

Impaired Social Interaction

    related to alienation from others secondary to overt hostility, overconfidence, or manipulation of others

    related to effects of behavior and actions on forming and maintaining relationships

    related to feelings of mistrust and suspicion of others

Risk for Self-Harm related to feelings of hopelessness and loneliness

Risk for Other-Directed Violence

    related to responding to delusional thoughts or hallucinations

    related to impaired reality testing, impaired judgment, or compromised ability to control behavior

Disturbed Thought Processes

    related to negative cognitive set (overgeneralizing, polarized thinking, selected abstraction, arbitrary inference)

    related to unknown etiology (e.g., repressed fears, drug use, abuse)

    related to biochemical disturbances

Noncompliance related to feelings of no longer requiring medication, impaired judgments, and thought disturbances

Ineffective Denial related to substance abuse

Impaired Social Interaction

    related to unrealistic expectations of relationships and impaired ability to maintain enduring attachments

    related to biochemical disturbances with preoccupation with egocentric and illogical ideas and extreme suspiciousness

Deficient Dimensional Activity

    related to a loss of interest or pleasure in usual activities and low energy levels

    related to apathy, inability to initiate goal-directed activities, and loss of skills

Risk for Ineffective Self-Health Management related to insufficient knowledge of condition, behavior modification, therapy options (pharmacologic, electroshock), and community resources

Impaired Home Maintenance related to impaired judgment, inability to self-initiate activity, and loss of skills over long course of illness

Generic Care Plan for Women in the Postpartum Period

This care plan focuses on the care of the mother postdelivery and preparation of the family unit to transition to home. If the mother also has a medical condition such as diabetes mellitus, asthma, or hypertension, refer to Unit II for the specific collaborative problem such *as Risk for Complications of hypertension, Risk for Complications of asthma exacerbation*, or *Risk for Complications of hypo / hyperglycemia*, and add it to the problem list.

■■ DIAGNOSTIC CLUSTER

Collaborative Problems

Risk for Complications of Hemorrhage

Risk for Complications of Uterine Atony

Risk for Complications of Retained Placental Fragments

Risk for Complications of Lacerations

Risk for Complications of Hematomas

Risk for Complications of Urinary retention

Risk for Complications of Deep Vein Thrombosis

Nursing Diagnoses

Risk for Infection related to bacterial invasion secondary to trauma during labor, delivery, episiotomy or cesarean surgical site, urinary catheterization, breasts (refer to Unit II)

Risk for Ineffective Breastfeeding related to inexperience or pain secondary to engorged breasts, sore nipples (refer to Unit II)

Acute Pain related to trauma to perineum during labor and delivery, hemorrhoids, engorged breasts, and involution of uterus

Risk for Constipation related to decreased intestinal peristalsis (postdelivery), decreased activity, and fear of pain with defecation due to perineal discomfort (refer to Unit II)

Risk for Impaired Parent–Infant Attachment related to (examples) inexperience, feelings of incompetence, powerlessness, unwanted child, disappointment with child, lack of role models, high risk newborn

Stress Incontinence related to tissue trauma during delivery (refer to Unit II)

Risk for Injury: Falls related to orthostatic hypotension, blood loss, effect of epidural analgesia, fatigue (refer to Unit II)

Risk for Ineffective Infant Care Management Deficient Knowledge, Infant Care related insufficient knowledge and / or to primiparous status, inexperience with infant care (refer to Normal Newborn Care Plan)

Risk for Ineffective Coping related to history of anxiety or mood disorder, unmarried or not cohabiting with partner poor social support, low socioeconomic status, birth complications, smoking, multiparity, BMI >30, stressful life event during pregnancy and / or postpartum

Risk for Ineffective Self-Health Management related to insufficient knowledge of postpartum routines, hygiene (breast, perineum), exercises, sexual counseling (contraception), nutritional requirements (infant, maternal), infant care, stresses of parenthood, adaptation of father, sibling, parent–infant bonding, postpartum emotional responses, sleep / rest requirements, household management, community resources, management of discomforts (breast, perineum), adolescent parents, and signs and symptoms of complications.

References

Adams, C., Bailey, D., Anderson, R., & Docherty, S. (2011). Nursing roles and strategies in end-of-life decisions: A systematic review of the literature. *Nursing Practice and Research*. Retrieved from http://www.hindawi.com/journals/nrp/2011/527834/

Addams, S., & Clough, J. A. (1998). Modalities for mobilization. In A. B. Mahler, S. Salmond, & T. Pellino (Eds.), *Orthopedic nursing*. Philadelphia, PA: W. B. Saunders.

Adkins, E. S. (2011). *Surgical treatment of ulcerative colitis*. Retrieved from http://emedicine.medscape.com/article/937427-overview

Adler, N. E., Page, A., & Institute of Medicine (U.S.). (2008). *Cancer care for the whole patient: Meeting psychosocial health needs*. Washington, DC: National Academies Press.

Agency for Health Care Policy and Research. (1992). *Pressure ulcers in adults: Prediction and prevention: Clinical practice guideline 3*. Washington, DC: AHCPR, Public Health Service, U.S. Department of Health and Human Services.

Agency for Health Care Policy and Research. (1994). *Evaluation and management of early HIV infection. Clinical practice guideline 7*. Washington, DC: AHCPR, Public Health Service, U.S. Department of Health and Human Services.

Agency for Healthcare Research and Quality. (2012). Guidelines for prevention and treatment of opportunistic infections in HIV-infected adults and adolescents. Recommendations from CDC, the National Institutes of Health, and the HIV Medicine Association of the Infectious Diseases Society. Retrieved from http://guideline.gov/content.aspx?id=14320Idathic

Agostini, P., Cieslik, H., Rathinam, S., Bishay, E., Kalkat, M.S., Rajesh, P. B., . . . Naidu, B. (2010). Postoperative pulmonary complications following thoracic surgery are there any modifiable risk factors? *Thorax*, *65*(9), 815–818.

Akbari, C. M., Saouaf, R., Barnhill, D. F., Newman, P. A., LoGerfo, F. W., & Veves, A. (1998). Endothelium-dependent vasodilatation is impaired in both microcirculation and macrocirculation during acute hyperglycemia. *Journal of Vascular Surgery*, *28*(4), 687–694.

Albano, S. A., & Wallace, D. J. (2001). Managing fatigue in patients with SLE. *Journal of Musculoskelatal Medicine*, *18*, 149–152.

Alcee, D. (2000). The experience of a community hospital in quantifying and reducing patient falls. *Journal of Nursing Care Quality*, *14*(3), 43–53.

Alcoholics Anonymous. (2008). *A brief guide to Alcoholics Anonymous. Welcome to Alcoholics Anonymous*. Retrieved from www.aa.org

Allen-Burge, R., Stevens, A., & Burgio, L. (1999). Effective behavioural interventions for decreasing dementia-related challenging behaviour in nursing homes. *International Journal of Geriatric Psychiatry*, *14*, 213–228.

ALLHAT officers and coordinators for the ALLHAT collaborative research group. (2002). Major outcomes in high-risk hypertensive patients randomized to angiotensin-converting enzyme inhibitor or calcium channel blocker vs diuretic: The antihypertensive and lipid-lowering treatment to prevent heart attack trial (ALLHAT). *Journal of the American Medical Association*, *288*, 2981–2997.

Altizer, L. (2004). Compartment syndrome. *Orthopedic Nursing*, *23*(6), 391–396.

American Academy of Orthopaedic Surgeons and American Academy of Pediatrics. (2010). Fracture of the proximal femur. In L. Y. Griffin (Ed.), *Essentials of musculoskeletal care* (4th ed., pp. 563–567). Rosemont, IL: American Academy of Orthopaedic Surgeons.

American Association of Hospice and Palliative Care Medicine. (2006). *Statement on palliative sedation*. Retrieved from http://www.aahpm.org/positions/default/sedation.html

American Cancer Society. (2007). *Breast reconstruction after mastectomy*. Retrieved from http://www.cancer.org/docroot/CRI/content/CRI_2_6X)Breast_Reconstruction_After_Mastectomy_5.asp

American Cancer Society. (2011a). *Ileostomy care*. Retrieved from http://www.cancer.org/acs/groups/cid/documents/webcontent/002870-pdf.pdf

American Cancer Society. (2011b). *Urostomy: A guide*. Retrieved from http://www.cancer.org/acs/groups/cid/documents/webcontent/002931-pdf.pdf

American College of Chest Physicians (2012). Preventing DVT and PE in nonsurgical patients. *ACCP Guidelines* (9th ed.). Northbrook, IL: Author.

American College of Sports Medicine. (2010). Exercise and type 2 diabetes: American College of Sports Medicine and the American Diabetes Association: Joint Position Statement. *Medicine and Science in Sports and Exercise, 42*(12), 2282–2303.

American Diabetes Association. (2012a). Diagnosis and classification of diabetes mellitus. *Diabetes Care, 35*(Suppl. 1), S64–S71.

American Diabetes Association. (2012b). Executive summary: Standards of medical care in diabetes—2012. *Diabetes Care, 35*(Suppl. 1), S4–S10.

American Heart Association. (2003). *Let's talk about stroke and aphasia*. Retrieved from http://www.americanheart.org/downloadable/stroke/1079557856294500073%20ASA%20Strokeaphasia.pdf

American Heart Association. (2004a). *Overview of stroke systems plans*. Retrieved from http://www.strokeassociation.org/presenter.jhtml?identifier=3028498

American Heart Association. (2004b). *What is carotid endarectomy?* Retrieved from http://www.americanheart.org/downloadable/heart/110065676921546%20WhatIsCarotidEdarterect.pdf

American Heart Association. (2005). *Heart disease and stroke statistics: 2005 update*. Dallas, TX: Author.

American Heart Association. (2007a). *Bypass surgery, coronary artery*. Retrieved from http://www.americanheart.org/presenter.jhtml?indentifier=4484

American Heart Association. (2007b). *Let's talk about complications after stroke*. Retrieved from http://www.american-heart.org/downloadable/stroke/1181161981749500068%20ASA%20ComplicationsStrk_ 4-07.pdf

American Heart Association. (2012). About high blood pressure. Retrieved from www.http.heart.org/HEARTORG/Conditions/HighBloodPressure/AboutHighBloodPressure/Understanding-Blood-Pressure-Readings_UCM_301764_Article.jsp

American Heart Association. (2012). Prevention and treatment of heart failure. Retrieved from http://www.heart.org/HEARTORG/Conditions/HeartFailure/PreventionTreatmentofHeartFailure/Heart-Failure-Medications_UCM_306342_Article.jsp

American Lung Association. (2013). Measuring your peak flow rate. Retrieved from http://www.lung.org/lung-disease/asthma/living-with-asthma/take-control-of-your-asthma/measuring-your-peak-flow-rate.html

American Nurses Association. (2001). Code of ethics. Retrieved from http://www.nursingworld.org/

American Nurses Association. (2010a). ANA's position statement on *Registered Nurses' roles and responsibilities in providing expert care and counseling at the end of life*. Retrieved from http://nursingworld.org/MainMenuCategories/Ethics-Standards/Ethics-Position-Statements/etpain14426.pdf

American Nurses Association. (2010b). Social policy statement. Retrieved from http://www.nursingworld.org/MainMenuCategories/Policy-Advocacy/Positions-and-Resolutions/ANAPositionStatements/Position-Statements-Alphabetically/Nursess-Role-in-Ethics-and-Human-Rights.pdf

American Pain Society. (2005). *Guideline for the management of cancer pain in adults and children*. Glenview, IL: Author. Guideline for the Management of Cancer Pain in Adults and Children.

American Speech-Language-Hearing Association. (2007). *Laryngeal cancer*. Retrieved from http://www.asha.org/public/speech/disorderslaryngealCancer.htm

American Stroke Association. (2007). *What is stroke?* Retrieved from http://www.stroke association.org/presenter.jhtml?identifier=3030066

Anand, B. S. (2012). *Peptic ulcer disease*. Retrieved from http://emedicine.medscape.com/article/181753-overview

Anderson, F., & Audet, A. (1998). *Best practices: Preventing deep vein thrombosis and pulmonary embolism*. Worcester, MA: Massachusetts Medical School/Center for Outcomes Research. Retrieved from http://www.outcomes-umassmed.org/dvt/best_practice/

Anderson, L. A. (2001). Abdominal aortic aneurysm. *Journal of Cardiovascular Nursing, 15*(4), 1–14.

Andersson, T., Lunde, O. C., Johnson, E., Moum, T., & Nesbakken, A. (2011). Long-term functional outcome and quality of life after restorative proctocolectomy with ileo-anal anastomosis for colitis. *Colorectal Disease, 13*(4), 431–437.

Annon, J. S. (1976). The PLISS T model: A proposed conceptual scheme for the behavioral treatment of sexual problems. *Journal of Sexual Education and Therapy, 2*, 211–215.

Annweiler, C., Montero-Odasso, M., Schott, A., Berrat, G., Fautino, B., & Beauchet, O. (2010). Fall prevention and vitamin D in the elderly: An overview of the key role of the non-bone effects. *Journal of Neuroengineering and Rehabilitation, 7*, 50.

Apfel, C. C., Läärä, E., Koivuranta, M., Greim, C. A., & Roewer, N. (1999). A simplified risk score for predicting postoperative nausea and vomiting: Conclusions from cross-validations between two centers. *Anesthesiology, 91*(3), 693–700.

Araki, Y., Kumakura, H., Kanai, H., Kasama, S., Sumino, H., Ichikawa, A., . . . Kurabayashi, M. (2012, June 4). Prevalence and risk factors for cerebral infarction and carotid artery stenosis in peripheral arterial disease. *Atherosclerosis, 223*(2), 473–477.

Arcangelo, V., & Peterson, A. (2010). *Pharmacotherapeutics for advanced practice* (3rd ed.). Philadelphia, PA: Lippincott Williams & Wilkins.

Arcangelo, V., & Peterson, A. (2011). *Pharmacotherapeutics for advanced practice* (3rd ed.). Philadelphia, PA: Lippincott Williams & Wilkins.

Armstrong, J. A., & McCaffrey, R. (2006). The effects of mucositis on quality of life. *Clinical Journal of Oncology Nursing, 10*(1), 53–56. Retrieved from http://ensco.waldenu.edu/ehost/pdf?vid=68&hid=104&sid=781c7c0c-696c-44ec-9c5d-f6382763aca4%40sessionmgr106

Aronow, W. S. (2005). Management of peripheral arterial disease. *Cardiology in Review, 13*(2), 61–68.

Arsalaini-Zadeh, R., ELFadl, D., Yassin, N., & MacFie, J. (2011). Evidence-based review of enhancing postoperative recovery after breast surgery. *British Journal of Surgery, 98*, 181–196.

Arthritis Foundation. (2008). *Take control; We can help*. Retrieved from http://www.arthritis.org/index.php

Arthritis Foundation. (2012). Tips for improving your sleep. *Arthritis Today*. Retrieved from www.arthritis.org/sleep-tips.php

Askin, D., & Wilson, D. (2007). The high risk newborn and family. In M. J. Hockenberry & D. Wilson (Eds.), *Wong's nursing care of infants and children* (8th ed., pp. 314–389). St. Louis, MO: Mosby Elsevier.

Association of Community Cancer Centers. (n.d.). *Cancer Program Guidelines* (Chapter 4). Retrieved from http://accc-cancer.org/publications/CancerProgramGuidelines-4.asp#section 6

Astle, S. M. (2005). Restoring electrolyte balance. *RN, 68*(5), 34–39.

Aubyn Crump, V. S. (n.d.). Auckland Allergy Clinic – Idiopathic anaphylaxis: An update. Auckland Allergy Clinic – Diagnosis and treatment of allergy. Retrieved from http://www.allergyclinic.co.nz/guides/56.html

Austin, J. K. (2003). Childhood epilepsy: Child adaptation and family resources. *Journal of Child and Adolescent Psychiatric Nursing, 1*(1), 8–24.

Australian Department of Health & Human Services. (2007a). *Clinical decision-making at end of life in palliative care > Care management guidelines*. Retrieved from http://www.tas.gov.au/stds/codi.htm

Australian Department of Health & Human Services. (2007b). *Hypercalcemia in palliative care > Care management guidelines*. Retrieved from http://www.tas.gov.au/stds/codi.htm

Australian Department of Health & Human Services. (2007c). *Breathlessness in palliative care > Care management guidelines*. Retrieved from http://www.tas.gov.au/stds/codi.htm

Australian Department of Health & Human Services. (2007d). *Delirium in palliative care > Care management guidelines*. Retrieved from http://www.tas.gov.au/stds/codi.htm

Awaad, S., & Raid, M. (2011, July 27). *Ophthalmologic manifestations of myasthenia gravis*. Retrieved from http://emedicine.medscape.com/article/1216417-overview

Azer, S. A. (2011). *Intestinal perforation*. Retrieved from http://emedicine.medscape.com/article/195537-overview#a0102

Bach, V., Ploeg, J., & Black, M. (2009). Nursing roles in end-of-life decision making in critical care settings. *Western Journal of Nursing Research, 31*(4), 496–512.

Bader, M. K. (Speaker). (2009, May). Different strokes for different folks: Assessment, interventions and outcomes. Presentation of NTI 2009, New Orleans, LA. Podcast retrieved from http://www.aacn.org

Bader, M. K., & Lillejohns, L. R. (2004). *American Association of Neuroscience Nurses: Core curriculum for neuroscience nursing* (4th ed.). St. Louis, MO: Saunders.

Badger, T., Braden, C. J., & Michel, M. (2001). Depression burden, self-help. Interventions and side effects experience in women receiving treatment for breast cancer. *Oncology Nursing Forum, 28*(3), 567–574.

Baggs, J. (2007). Nurse-physician collaboration in intensive care units. *Critical Care Medicine, 35*(2), 641–642.

Bailey, P. P. (2008). Asthma. In T. M. Buttaro, J. Trybulski, P. P. Bailey, & J. Sandberg-Cook (Eds.), *Primary care: A collaborative practice* (3rd ed., pp. 398–422). St. Louis, MO: Mosby.

Baird, M. S., Keen, J. H., & Swearingen, P. L. (2005). *Manual of critical care nursing: Nursing interventions and collaborative management* (5th ed.). St Louis, MO: Elsevier Mosby.

Balach, T., & Peabody, T. (2011). Management of skeletal metastases. In W. M. Stadler (Ed.), *Renal cancer*. New York, NY: Demos Medical.

Ball, C., deBeer, K., Gomm, A., Hickman, B., & Collins, P. (2007). Achieving tight glycaemic control. *Intensive and Critical Care Nurisng, 23*(3), 137–144.

Ballas, S., & Delengowski, A. (1993). Pain measurement in hospitalized adults with sickle cell painful episodes. *Annals of Clinical and Laboratory Science, 23*(5), 358–361.

Bandura, A. (1982). Self efficacy mechanism in human agency. *American Psychologist, 37*(2), 122–147.

Barbar, S., Noventa, F., Rossetto, V., Ferrari, A., Brandolin, B., Perlati, M., . . . Prandoni, P. (2010). A risk assessment model for the identification of hospitalized medical patients at risk for venous thromboembolism: The Padua Prediction Score. *Journal of Thrombosis and Haemostasis, 8*, 2450–2457.

Bard, M. R., Goettler, C. E., Toschlog, E. A., Sagraves, S. G., Schenarts, P. J., Newell, M. A., . . . Rotondo, M. F. (2006). Alcohol withdrawal syndrome: Turning minor injuries into a major problem. *Journal of Trauma Injury, Infection and Critical Care, 61*(6), 1441–1446.

Barker, L. R., Burton, J., & Aieve, P. D. (Eds.). (2006). *Principles of ambulatory medicine* (6th ed.). Philadelphia, PA: Lippincott Williams & Wilkins.

Barnason, S., Zimmerman, L., Nieveen, J., & Hertzog, M. (2006). Impact of a telehealth intervention to augment home health care on functional and recovery outcomes of elderly patients undergoing coronary artery bypass grafting. *Heart & Lung: Journal of Acute & Critical Care, 35*(4), 225–233.

Barsevick, A. M., Much, J., & Sweeney, C. (2000). Psychosocial responses of cancer. In S. L. Groenwald, M. H. Frogge, M. Goodman, & C. Yarbro (Eds.), *Cancer nursing: Principles and practice* (5th ed.). Boston, MA: Jones & Bartlett.

Bartels, C. (2013). *Systemic lupus erythematosus (SLE) clinical presentation Medscape*. Retrieved from http://emedicine.medscape.com/article/332244-clinical

Bartick, M. (2009). Small changes promote better sleep. *Today's Hospitalist*. Retrieved from www.TodaysHospitalist.com/index.php?b=articles_read&cnt=899

Bartlett, J. G., & Finkbeiner, A. K. (2001). *The guide to living with HIV infection* (6th ed.). Baltimore, MD: The Johns Hopkins University Press.

Baskin, J. L., Ching-Hon Pui, C. H., Reiss, U., Wilimas, J. A., Metzger, M. L., Ribeiro, R. C., & Howard, S. C. (2009). Management of occlusion and thrombosis associated with long-term indwelling central venous catheters. *Lancet, 374*(9684), 159. Retrieved from http://www.ncbi.nlm.nih.gov/pmc/articles/PMC2814365/

Baskin, J. L., Reiss, U., Wilimas, J. A., Metzger, M. L., Ribeiro, R. C., Pui, C. H., & Howard, S. C. (2012). Thrombolytic therapy for central venous catheter occlusion. *Haematologica, 97*(5), 641–650.

Bateman, A. L. (1999). Understanding the process of grieving and loss: A critical social thinking perspective. *Journal of American Psychiatric Nurses Association, 5*(5), 139–149.

Bates, C. K. (2013). *Patient information: Care after sexual assault (beyond the basics) update*. Retrieved from http://www.uptodate.com/contents/care-after-sexual-assault-beyond-the-basics

Bauldoff, G., Hoffman, L., Sciurba, F., & Zullo, T. (1996). Home based upper arm exercises training for patients with chronic obstructive pulmonary disease. *Heart and Lung, 25*(4), 288–294.

Bautista, L., Cesar, J., & Sumpaico, M. (2007). Stevens-Johnson from hemodialysis-associated hypersensitivity reaction in a 61-year-old male. *World Allergy Organization Journal, 1*(6), 198–207.

Beattie, S. (2007). *Bedside emergency: Wound dehiscence modern medicine*. Retrieved from http://www.modernmedicine.com/modern-medicine/news/bedside-emergency-wound-dehiscence

Beckstrand, R. L., Callsiter, L. C., & Kirchhoff, K. T. (2006). Providing a "Good Death": Critical care nurse's suggestions for improving end-of-life care. *American Journal of Critical Care, 15*(1), 38–45.

Bednarski, D., Cahill, M. L., Castner, D., Counts, C. S., Groenhoff, C. L., Hall, L. M., . . . Witten, B. (2008). The individual with kidney disease. In C. S. Counts (Ed.), *Core curriculum for nephrology nursing* (5th ed.). Pitman, NJ: American Nephrology Nurses' Association.

Beese-Bjurstrom, S. (2004). Hidden danger: Aortic aneurysms & dissections. *Nursing, 34*(2), 36–41.

Beling, J., & Roller, M. (2009). Multifactorial intervention with balance training as a core component among fall-prone older adults. *Journal of Geriatric Physical Therapy, 32*(3),125–133.

Ben-Zacharia, A. B. (2001). Palliative care in patients with multiple sclerosis. *Neurol Epilepsia, 51*(4), 676–685. doi: 10.1111/j.1528-1167.2010.02522.x. Epub 2010 Feb 26.

Bennett, R. (2000). Acute gastroenteritis and associated conditions. In L. R. Barker, J. Burton, & P. Zieve (Eds.), *Principles of ambulatory medicine*. Baltimore, MD: Williams & Wilkins.

Bennett, S. J., Cordes, D., Westmoreland, G., Castro, R., & Donnelly, E. (2000). Self-care strategies for symptom management in patients with chronic heart failure. *Nursing Research, 49*(3), 139–145.

Benowitz, N. L. (2010). Nicotine addiction. *New England Journal of Medicine, 362*(24), 2295-2303. Retrieved from http://www.ncbi.nlm.nih.gov/pmc/articles/PMC2928221/

Berg, A. T., Berkovic, S. F., Brodie, M. J., Buchhalter, J., Cross, J. H., van Emde Boas, W., …Scheffer, I. E. (2010). Revised terminology and concepts for organization of seizures and epilepsies: Report of the ILAE Commission on Classification and Terminology, 2005-2009. *Epilepsia, 19*(4), 801–827.

Berkowitz, D., Lukes, C., Prker, V., Logan, C., Ayello, E., & Zulkowski, K. (2007a). *Preventing pressure ulcers in hospitals AHRQ*. Retrieved from http://www.ahrq.gov/professionals/systems/long-term-care/resources/pressure-ulcers/pressureulcertoolkit/putoolkit.pdf

Berlowitz, D., & Brienza, D. (2007b). Are all pressure ulcers the result of deep tissue injury? A review of the literature. *Ostomy Wound Management, 53*, 34–38.

Bernheisel, C. R., Schlauderecker, J. D., & Leopold, K. (2011). Subacute management of ischemic stroke. *American Family Physician, 84*(12), 1383–1388.

Berry, A. M., Davidson, P. M., & Masters, J. (2007). Systemic literature review of oral hygiene practices for intensive care patients receiving mechanical ventilation. *American Journal of Critical Care, 16*(4), 552–562.

Best, C., & Wilson, N. (2007). Administration of medication via a enteral tubing. *Nursing Times, 107*(41), 18–20.

Bhardwaj, A., Mirski, M. A., & Ulatowski, J. A. (2004). *Handbook of neurocritical care*. Totowa, NJ: Humana Press.

Bhatt, D., Lee, L., Casterella, P., Pulsipher, M., Rogers, M., Cohen, M., . . . Lincoff, A. M. (2003). Coronary revascularization using integrilin and single bolus enoxaparin study. *Journal of the American College of Cardiology, 41*(1), 20–25.

Bickley, B. (2003). *A guide to physical examination and history taking* (8th ed.). Philadelphia, PA: Lippincott Williams & Wilkins.

Black, P. K. (2004). Psychological, sexual and cultural issues for patients with a stoma. *British Journal of Nursing, 13*(12), 692–697.

Bliss, D. Z., Jung, H. J., Savik, K., Lowry, A., LeMoine, M., Jensen, L.,…Schaffer, K. (2001). Supplementation with dietary fiber improves fecal incontinence. *Journal of Nursing Research, 50*(4), 203–213.

Block, A. (2007). Chronic pain coping techniques. *Pain Management.* Retrieved from http://www.spine-health.com/conditions/chronic-pain/chronic-pain-coping-techniques-pain-management

Bluestein, D., & Javaheri, A. (2008). Pressure ulcers: Prevention, evaluation, and management. *American Family Physician, 78*(10), 1186–1194.

Boardman, M. B. (2008). Chronic obstructive pulmonary disease. In T. M. Buttaro, J. Trybulski, P. P. Bailey, & J. Sandberg-Cook (Eds.), *Primary care: A collaborative practice* (3rd ed., pp. 433–443). St. Louis, MO: Mosby.

Bodenheimer, T., MacGregor, K., & Sharifi, C. (2005). Helping patients manage their chronic conditions. Retrieved from www.chef.org/publications

Bogle, J. L., Craig, M., Williams, H. F., Garrigan, P. L., Davey-Tresemer, J., & Dalton, T. L. (2008). Hemodialysis in the acute care setting. In C. S. Counts (Ed.), *Core curriculum for nephrology nursing* (5th ed.). Pitman, NJ: American Nephrology Nurses' Association.

Bonanno G. A., & Lilienfeld S. O. (2008). Let's be realistic: When grief counseling is effective and when it's not. *Professional Psychology: Research and Practice, 39*(3), 377–378.

Bone, R., Balk, R. C., Cerra, F. B., Dellinger, R. P., Fein, A. M., Knaus, W. A., . . . Sibbald, W. J. (1992). Definitions for sepsis and organ failure and guidelines for the use of innovative therapies in sepsis. *Chest, 101*(6) 1644–1655.

Bonham, P. A. (2006). Get the LEAD out: Noninvasive assessment for lower extremity arterial disease using ankle brachial index and toe brachial index measurements. *Journal of Wound Ostomy Continence Nursing, 33*, 30–41.

Boonpongmanee, S., Fleischer, D. E., Pezzullo, J. C., Collier, K., Mayoral, W., Al-Kawas, F., . . . Benjamin, S. B. (2004). The frequency of peptic ulcer as a cause of upper-GI bleeding is exaggerated. *Gastrointestinal Endoscopy, 59*(7), 788–794. Retrieved from http://emedicine.medscape.com/article/187857-overview#aw2aab6b2b3aa

Bosmans, J. C., Suurmeijer, T. P. B. M., Hulsink, M., van der Schans, C. P., Geertzen, J. H. B., & Dijkstra, P. U. (2007). Amputation, phantom pain and subjective well-being: A qualitative study. *International Journal of Rehabilitation Research, 30*, 1–8.

Boulware, L. E., Daumit, G. L., & Frick, K. D. (2001). An evidence-based review of patient-centered behavioral interventions for hypertension. *American Journal of Preventive Medicine, 21*, 221–232.

Boutwell, A., & Hwu, S. (2009). *Effective interventions to reduce rehospitalization: A survey of published evidence.* Cambridge, MA: Institute for Healthcare Improvement.

Boyd, M. A. (2005). *Psychiatric nursing: Contemporary practice* (3rd ed.). Philadelphia, PA: Lippincott Williams & Wilkins.

Branson, J., & Goldstein, W. (2001). Sequential bilateral total knee arthroplasty. *AORN Journal, 73*(3), 608, 610, 613.

Brant, J. M. (1998). The art of palliative care: Living with hope, dying with dignity. *Oncology Nursing Forum, 25*(6), 995–1004.

Brauer, C., Morrison, R. S., & Silberzweig, S. B. (2000). The cause of delirium in patients with hip fracture. *Archives of Internal Medicine, 160*(12), 1856–1860.

BreastCancer.org. (2007). *The role of surgery in breast cancer treatment.* Retrieved from http://www.breastcancer.org/treatment/surgery/index.jsp

Brienza, D., Kelsey, S., Karg, P., Allegretti, A., Olson, M., Schmeler, M., . . . Holm, M. (2010). A randomized clinical trial on preventing pressure ulcers with wheelchair seat cushions. *Journal of American Geriatrics Society, 58*(12), 2308–2314.

Brown, M. A., & Powell-Cope, G. (1991). AIDS family caregiving transitions through uncertainty. *Nursing Research, 40*, 338–345.

Bruera, E. (2012). Palliative sedation: When and how? *Journal of Clinical Oncology, 30*, 1258–1259.

Bryant, R. A. (2000). *Acute and chronic wounds. Nursing management* (2nd ed.). Missouri, MO: Mosby.

Bryson, K. A. (2004). Spirituality, meaning, and transcendence. *Palliative and Supportive Care, 2*(3), 321–328.

Buchanan, R. J., Wang, S., & Ju, H. (2002). Analyses of the minimum data set: Comparisons of nursing home residents with multiple sclerosis to other nursing home residents. *Multiple Sclerosis, 8*(6), 512–522.

Buchman, A. L. (2001). Side effects of corticosteroid therapy. *Journal of Clinical Gastroenterology, 33*(4), 289–294.

Bulechek, G. M., Butcher, G. M., & Dochterman, J. M. (Eds.). (2013). *Nursing interventions: Treatments for nursing diagnoses* (5th ed.). Philadelphia, PA: W. B. Saunders.

Bullock, B., & Henze, R. (2000). *Focus on pathophysiology.* Philadelphia, PA: Lippincott Williams & Wilkins.

Burch, K., Todd, K., Crosby, F., Ventura, M., Lohr, G., & Grace, M. L. (1991). PVD: *Nurse patient interventions. Journal of Vascular Nursing, 9*(4), 13–16.

Bureau of Justice. (2010). *Female victims of sexual violence, 1994–2010.* Retrieved from http://www.bjs.gov/content/pub/pdf/fvsv9410.pdf

Burkhart, L., & Solari-Twadell, A. (2001). Spirituality and religiousness: Differentiating the diagnoses through review of the literature. *International Journal of Nursing Terminologies and Classification, 12*(2), 45–54.

Bushkin, E. (1993). Signposts of survivorship. *Oncology Nursing Forum, 20*(6), 869–875.

Butler, D. (2009). Early postoperative complications following ostomy surgery: A review. *Journal of Wound, Ostomy and Continence Nursing, 36*(5), 513–519.

Cagir, B. (Ed.). *Lower gastrointestinal bleeding.* Retrieved from http://emedicine.medscape.com/article/188478-overview

Calvert, E., Penner, M., Younger, A., & Wing, K. (2007). Transmetatarsal amputations. *Techniques in foot and ankle surgery, 6*(3), 140–146.

Camp-Sorrell, D. (2007). Chemotherapy: Toxicity management. In C. Yarbro, M. H. Frogge, M. Goodman, & S. Groenwald (Eds.), *Cancer nursing: Principles and practice.* Boston, MA: Jones and Barlett.

Campbell, K. E. (2009). A new model to identify shared risk factors for pressure ulcers and frailty in older adults. *Rehabilitation Nursing, 34*(6), 242–247.

Canadian Association of Endostomal Therapy. (2005). A guide to living with an ileostomy access therapy. Retrieved from http://www.caet.ca/caet-english/documents/caet-guide-to-living-with-an-ileostomy.pdf

Carek, P. J., Dickerson, L. M., & Sack, J. L. (2001). Diagnosis and management of osteomyelitis. *American Family Physician, 63*(12), 2413–2420.

Carlson, D. S., & Pfadt, E. (2012). Preventing deep vein thrombosis in perioperative patients. *OR Nursing 2013, 6*(5), 14–20.

Carosella, C. (1995). *Who's afraid of the dark?* New York, NY: HarperCollins.

Carpenito, L. J. (2013). *Nursing diagnoses: Application to clinical practice* (14th ed.). Philadelphia, PA: Lippincott Williams & Wilkins.

Carr, E. (2005). Head and neck malignancies. In C. H. Yarbo, M. H. Frogge, & M. Goodman (Eds.), *Cancer nursing: Principles and practice* (6th ed.). Boston, MA: Jones & Bartlett.

Carson, V. B. (1999). *Mental health nursing: The nurse-patient journey* (2nd ed.). Philadelphia, PA: W. B. Saunders.

Carson, V. B., & Alvarez, C. (2006). Anger and aggression. In E. M. Varcarolis, V. B. Carson, & N. C. Shoemaker (Eds.), *Foundations of psychiatric-mental health nursing* (5th ed.). Philadelphia, PA: W. B. Saunders.

Carson, V. B., & Green, H. (1992). Spiritual well-being: A predictor of hardiness in patients with acquired immunodeficiency syndrome. *Journal of Professional Nursing, 8,* 209–220.

Carson, V. M., & Smith-DiJulio, K. (2006). Family violence. In E. M. Varcarolis, V. M. Carson, & N. C. Shoemaker (Eds.), *Foundations of psychiatric mental health nursing* (5th ed.). Philadelphia, PA: W. B. Saunders.

Casey, K. (1997). Malnutrition associated with HIV/AIDS. Part two: Assessment and interventions. *Journal of the Association of Nurses in AIDS Care, 8*(5), 39–48.

Cassells, J. M., & Redman, B. K. (1989). Preparing students to be moral agents in clinical nursing practice. *Nursing Clinics of North America, 24,* 463–473.

Casswell, D., & Cryer H. G. (1995) When the nurse and the doctor don't agree. *Journal of Cardiovascular Nursing, 9,* 30–42.

Castillo-Bueno, M., Moreno-Pina, J. P., Martínez-Puente, M. V., Artiles-Suárez, M. M., Company-Sancho, M. C., García-Andrés, M. C.,…Hernández-Pérez, R. (2010). Effectiveness of nursing intervention for adult patients experiencing chronic pain: A systematic review. *JBI Library of Systematic Reviews, 28*(8), 1112–1168.

Centers for Disease Control and Prevention. (2002). *Guideline for hand hygiene in health-care settings.* Retrieved from https://www.premierinc.com/safety/topics/guidelines/downloads/03_cdchandhygfinal02.pdf

Centers for Disease Control and Prevention. (2007). *Infection control measures for preventing and controlling influenza transmission in long-term care facilities.* Retrieved from www.cdc.gov/flu/professionals/infectioncontrol/resphygiene.htm

Centers for Disease Control and Prevention. (2009). *Hepatitis B FAQs for the public.* Retrieved from http://www.cdc.gov/hepatitis/B/bFAQ.htm#transmission

Centers for Disease Control and Prevention. (2010). *Asthma's impact on the nation:* Data from the CDC National Asthma Control Program. Retrieved from http://www.cdc.gov/asthma/impacts_nation/AsthmaFactSheet.pdf

Centers for Disease Control and Prevention. (2010a). *Hip fractures among older adults.* Retrieved from http://www.cdc.gov/homeandrecreationalsafety/falls/adulthipfx.html

Centers for Disease Control and Prevention. (2010b). 2010 *Surgeon General's Report—How tobacco smoke causes disease: The biology and behavioral basis for smoking-tattributable disease.* Retrieved from www.cdc.gov/tobacco/data_statistics/sgr/2010/index.htm

Centers for Disease Control and Prevention. (2011a). *Leading causes of death in US.* Retrieved from http://www.cdc.gov/nchs/fastats/lcod.htm

Centers for Disease Control and Prevention. (2011b). *Tobacco-related mortality.* Retrieved from www.cdc.gov/tobacco/data/fact_sheets/health_effects

Centers for Disease Control and Prevention. (2012a). *Respiratory hygiene/cough etiquette in healthcare settings.* Retrieved from www.cdc.gov/flu/professionals/infectioncontrol/resphygiene.htm

Centers for Disease Control and Prevention. (2012b). Division of blood disorders. National Center on Birth Defects and Developmental Disabilities, Centers for Disease Control and Prevention. Retrieved from www.http.cdc.gov/ncbddd/dvt/facts.html

Centers for Disease Control and Prevention. (2012c). *Chronic obstructive pulmonary disease: Fact sheet.* Retrieved from http://www.who.int/mediacentre/factsheets/fs315/en/index.html

Centers for Disease Control and Prevention. (2012d). *Pneumonia can be prevented: Vaccines can help.* Retrieved from http://www.cdc.gov/features/pneumonia/

Centers for Disease Control and Prevention. (2013). *CDC state data shows high costs due to excessive alcohol use.* Retrieved from http://www.cdc.gov/media/releases/2013/p0813-excessive-alcohol-use.html

Centers for Medicare & Medicaid Services. (2005). *Health insurance reform.* Retrieved from http://www.cms.gov/Regulations-and-Guidance/Guidance/Transmittals/downloads/r8som.pdf

Centers of Medicare and Medicaid Services. (2012). Acute inpatient PPS. Retrieved from http://www.cms.gov/Medicare/Medicare-Fee-for-Service-Payment/AcuteInpatientPPS/index.html?redirect=/acuteinpatientpps/

Cesario, K. R., Choure, A., & Carey, W. D. (2010). *Complications of cirrhosis: Ascites, hepatic encephalopathy, and variceal hemorrhage.* Retrieved from http://www.clevelandclinicmeded.com/medicalpubs/diseasemanagement/hepatology/complications-of-cirrhosis-ascites/References

Chait, M. (2007). Lower GI bleeding in the elderly. *Annals of Long-Term Care: Clinical Care and Aging, 15*(4), 40–46.

Challacombe, B., & Dasgupta, P. (2007). Reconstitution of the lower urinary tract by laparoscopic robotic surgery. *Current Opinion in Urology, 17,* 390–395.

Chang, J. Y., & Tsai, P. F. (2004). Assessment of pain in elders with dementia. *MEDSURG Nursing, 13*(6), 364–369, 390.

Chapman, D., & Moore, S. (2005). Breast cancer. In C. Yarbo, M. H. Frogge, & M. Goodman (Eds.), *Cancer nursing: Principles and practice* (6th ed.). Boston, MA: Jones & Bartlett.

Cheadle, W. G. (2006). Risk factors for surgical site infection. *Surgical Infections, 7*(s1), S7–S11.

Cheng, D. M. D., Allen, K. M. D., Cohn W. M. D., Connolly, M. M. D., Edgerton, J. M. D., Falk, V. M. D., ... Vitali, R. (2005). Endoscopic vascular harvest in coronary artery bypass grafting surgery: A meta-analysis of randomized trials and controlled trials. *Innovations: Technology 7 Techniques in Cardiothoracic & Vascular Surgery, 1*(2), 61–74.

Cheng, S. (2011). Mineral and bone disorders. In J. T. Daugirdas (Ed.), *Handbook of chronic kidney disease management.* Philadelphia, PA: Lippincott Williams & Wilkins.

Cherny, N., Ripamonti, N., Pereira, J., Davis, C., Fallon, M.,... Vittorio Ventafridda for the Expert Working Group of the European Association of Palliative Care Network. (2001). Strategies to manage the adverse effects of oral morphine: An evidence-based report. *Journal of Clinical Oncology, 19*(9), 2542–2554.

Cheskin, L., & Lacy, B. (2003). Selected gastrointestinal problems: Bleeding, diarrhea, abdominal pain. In L. R. Barker, J. Burton, & P. D. Zieve (Eds.), *Principles of ambulatory medicine* (6th ed.). Philadelphia, PA: Lippincott Williams & Wilkins.

Chester, M., Wasko, M., Hubert, H., Lingala, V., Elliot, J., Luggen, M., . . . Ward, M. M. (2007). Hydroxychloroquine and risk of diabetes in patients with rheumatoid arthritis. *Journal of the American Medical Association, 298*(2), 187–193.

Cheville, A., & Gergich, N. (2004). Lymphedema: Implications for wound care. In P. J. Sheffield, A. P. S. Smith, & C. Fife (Eds.), *Wound care practice* (pp. 285–303). Flagstaff, AZ: Best.

Chin, T., Sawamura, S., & Shiba, R. (2006). Effect of physical fitness on prosthetic ambulation in elderly amputees. *American Journal of Physical Medicine & Rehabilitation, 85*(12), 992–996.

Chmielowski, B., Casciato, D. A., & Wagner, R. F. (2009). Cutaneous complications. In D. A. Casciato & M. C. Territo (Eds.), *Manual of clinical oncology* (pp. 585–605). Philadelphia, PA: Lippincott Williams & Wilkins.

Christman, N., & Kirchhoff, K. (1992). Preparatory sensory information. In G. Bulechek & J. McCloskey (Eds.), *Nursing interventions.* Philadelphia, PA: W. B. Saunders.

Chronic pain: What psychosocial interventions work? (2011). *Critical Science.* Retrieved from http://criticalscience.com/chronic-pain-psychosocial-interventions.html

Chu, Y-F., Jiang, Y., Meng, M., Jiang, J-J., Zhang, J-C., Ren, H-S., & Wang, C-T. (2010). Incidence and risk factors of gastrointestinal bleeding in mechanically ventilated patients. *World Journal of Emergency Medicine, 1*(1), 32–36. Retrieved from http://www.wjem.org/upload/admin/201103/48c45290d1d6f045db5aac2806d8f3ff.pdf

Cicirelli, V., & MacLean, A. P. (2000). Hastening death: A comparison of two end-of-life decisions. *Death Studies, 24*(3), 401–419.

Cimprich, B. (1992). Attentional fatigue following breast cancer surgery. *Research in Nursing and Health, 15,* 199–207.

Clanet, M., & Brassat D. (2000). The management of multiple sclerosis patients. *Current Opinion in Neurology, 13*(3), 263–270.

Clark, J. (2006). *Ileostomy guide.* Retrieved from http://www.cancer.org/docroot/CRI/content/CRI_2_6x_Ileostomy.asp.

Clark, J., & Dubois, H. (2004). *Urostomy guide.* United Ostomy Associations of America (UOAA). Retrieved from http://www.uoaa.org/ostomy_info/pubs/uoa_urostomy_

Clover, K., Carter, G. L., & Whyte, I. M. (2004). Posttraumatic stress disorder among deliberate self-poisoning patients. *Journal of Traumatic Stress, 17*(6), 509–517.

Cohen-Mansfield, J. (2000) Use of patient characteristics to determine non-pharmacologic interventions for behavioural and psychological symptoms of dementia. *International Psychogeriatrics, 12*(Suppl. 1), 373–380.

Cole, C., & Richards, K. (2007). Sleep disruption in older adults. *American Journal of Nursing.* Retrieved from www.nursingcenter.com/pordev/ce_article.asp?tid=714432

Collett, K. (2002). Practical aspects of stoma management. *Nursing Standard, 17*(8), 45–52.

Collier, J. D., Ninkovic, M. J., & Compston, E. (2002). Guidelines on the management of osteoporosis associated with chronic liver disease. *Gut, 50,* i1–i9.

Collins, R. L., Leonard, K., & Searles, J. (1990). *Alcohol and the family: Research and clinical perspectives.* New York, NY: Guilford.

Colten, H. R., & Altevogt, B. M. (Eds.). (2006). *Sleep disorders and sleep deprivation/An unmet public health problem*. Washington, DC: National Academies Press. Retrieved from www.ncbi.nlm.nih.gov/books/MBK199601/

Colwell, J. C., & Beitz, J. (2007). Survey of wound, ostomy and continence (WOC) nurse clinicians on stomal and peristomal complications. *Journal of Wound, Ostomy and Continence Nursing, 34*(1), 57–69.

Colwell, J. C., Goldberg, M. T., & Carmel, J. E. (2004). *Fecal and urinary diversions: Management principles*. St. Louis, MO: Mosby.

Conn, V. S., Hafdahl, A. R., Porock, D. C., McDaniel, R., & Nielsen, P. J. (2006). A meta-analysis of exercise interventions among people treated for cancer. *Support Care Cancer, 14*(7), 699–712.

Connors, A. F., Dawson, N. V., Desbiens, N. A., Fulkerson, W. J., Goldman, L., Knaus, W. A., . . . Oye, R. K. (1995). The SUPPORT study: A controlled trial to improve care for seriously ill hospitalized patients: The study to understand prognoses and preferences for outcomes and risks of treatments (SUPPORT). *Journal of the American Medical Association, 274*(20), 1591–1598.

Conte, M. S. (2009). *Lower extremity bypass surgery*. Retrieved from http://vascular.surgery.ucsf.edu/conditions—procedures/lower-extremity-bypass-surgery.aspx#SurgicalConsiderations

Conti, R. C. (2009). Myocardial revascularization: PCI/stent or coronary artery bypass graft—What is best for our patients? *Clinical Cardiology, 32*(11), 606–607.

Cook, D. J., Fuller, H. D., Guyatt, G. H., Marshall, J. C., Leasa, D., Hall, R., . . . Roy, P. (1994). Risk factors for gastrointestinal bleeding in critically ill patients. Canadian Critical Care Trials Group. *New England Journal of Medicine, 330*(6), 377–381.

Cook, S., & Lloyd, A. (2010). *Guidelines for the diagnosis, management and prevention of delirium (acute confusion) in adults age 18 years and older*. Retrieved from bolton.nhs.uk/Library/policies/SPOVO8.pdf

Coombs-Lee, B. (2004). A model that integrates assisted dying with excellent end of life care. In T. E. Quill, & M. P. Battin (Eds.), *Physician-assisted dying. The case for palliative care and patient choice* (pp. 190–201). Baltimore/London: The John Hopkins University Press.

Corley, M., Minick, P., Elswick, R., & Jacobs, M. (2005). Nurse moral distress and ethical work environments. *Nursing Ethics, 12*(4), 381–389.

Cornett, P. A., & Dea, T. O. (2012). Cancer. In S. J. McPhee & M. A. Papadakis (Eds.), *Current medical diagnosis and treatment*. New York, NY: McGraw-Hill Lange.

Correia de Sa, J. C. (2011). Symptomatic therapy in multiple sclerosis: A review for a multimodal approach in clinical practice. *Therapeutic Advances in Neurological Disorders, 4*(3), 139–168.

Cotton, A. B. (2008). Kidney disease and kidney replacement therapies in nutrition in kidney disease, dialysis, and transplantation. In C. S. Counts (Ed.), *Core curriculum for nephrology nursing* (5th ed.). Pitman, NJ: American Nephrology Nurses' Association.

Cotton, S., Puchalski, C. M., Sherman, S. N., Mrus, J. M., Peterman, A. H., Feinberg, J., . . . Tsevat, J. (2006). Spirituality and religion in patients with HIV/AIDS. *Journal of General Internal Medicine, 21*(Suppl. 5), S5–S13.

Coughlin, A. M., & Parchinsky, C. (2006). Go with the flow of chest tube therapy. *Nursing, 36*(3), 36–42.

Coughlin, A., & Parchinsky, C. (2006). Go with the flow of chest tube therapy. *Nursing, 36*(3), 36–41.

Counts, C. S., Benavente, G., McCarley, P. B., Pelfrey, N. J., Petroff, S., & Stackiewicz, L. (2008a). Chronic kidney disease: Deterring chronic kidney disease. In C. S. Counts (Ed.), *Core curriculum for nephrology nursing* (5th ed.). Pitman, NJ: American Nephrology Nurses' Association.

Counts, C. S., Benavente, G., McCarley, P. B., Pelfrey, N. J., Petroff, S., & Stackiewicz, L. (2008b). Chronic kidney disease: Empowering strategies and the introduction to kidney replacement therapies. In C. S. Counts (Ed.), *Core curriculum for nephrology nursing* (5th ed.). Pitman, NJ: American Nephrology Nurses' Association.

Coyne, D. W. (2007). Use of epoetin in chronic renal failure. *Journal of the American Medical Association, 297*(15), 1713–1716.

Creager, M. A., & Libby, P. (2007). Peripheral arterial disease. In P. Libby, R. O. Bonow, D. L. Mann, & D. P. Zipes (Eds.), *Braunwald's heart disease: A textbook of cardiovascular medicine* (8th ed., Chapter 57). Philadelphia, PA: Saunders.

Cukierman, T., Gatt, M. E., Hiller, N., & Chajek-Shaul, T. (2005, August 4). Fracture diagnosis. *New England Journal of Medicine, 353*, 509–514.

Cunningham, M., Bunn, F., & Handscomb, K. (2006). Prophylactic antibiotics to prevent surgical site infection after breast cancer surgery. *Cochrane Database of Systematic Reviews*. Retrieved from http://uhra.herts.ac.uk/bitstream/handle/2299/5242/AntibioticsCD005360.pdf?sequence=5

Cunningham, R. S., & Huhmann, M. B. (2011). Nutritional disturbances. In C. H. Yarbro, D. Wujcik, & B. H. Gobel (Eds.), *Cancer nursing: Principles and practice* (7th ed.). Boston, MA: Jones and Bartlett.

Currie, S. R., & Wang, J. (2005). More data on major depression as an antecedent risk factor for first onset of chronic back pain. *Psychological Medicine, 35*, 1275–1282.

Cutilli, C. C. (2005). Health literacy: What you need to know. *Orthopedic Nursing, 24*(3), 227–231.

Cutler, C. J., & Davis, N. (2005). Improving oral care in patients receiving mechanical ventilation. *American Journal of Care, 14*(5), 389–394.

Da Vinci Hysterectomy. (2007). *Da Vinci hysterectomy*. Retrieved from http://www.davinci hysterectomy.com/davincihysterectomy/index.aspx

Dadd, M. (1983). Self care for side effects. *Cancer Nursing, 6*, 63–66.

Dahlin, C. (2013). *Clinical practice guidelines for quality palliative care* (3rd ed.). Pittsburgh, PA: National Consensus Project for Quality Palliative Care.

Davies, E.T., Moxham, T., Rees, K. S., Singh, S., Coats, A., Ebrahim, S.,…. Taylor, R. (2010). Exercise training for systolic heart failure: Cochrane systematic review and meta-analysis. *European Journal of Heart, 12*(7), 706–715.

Davis, A. J. (1989). Clinical nurses' ethical decision making in situations of informed consent. *Advanced Nursing Science, 11*(3), 63–69.

Davis, C. (1998). *ABCs of palliative care. Breathlessness, cough, and other respiratory problems.* Retrieved from http://www.ncbi.nlm.nih.gov/pmc/articles/PMC2127624/pdf/9361545.pdf

Davis, C. P. (n.d.). Hepatitis A. Retrieved from http://www.emedicinehealth.com/hepatitis_a-health/article_em.htm

Davis, C., Chrisman, J., & Walden, P. (2012). To scan or not to scan? Detecting urinary retention. *Nursing made incredibly easy! 10*(4), 53–54. doi:10.1097/01.NME.0000415016.88696.9d

Davis, J. (2003). One-side neglect: Improving awareness to speedy recovery; Life after stroke. Retrieved from http://www.strokeassociation.org/STROKEORG/LifeAfterStroke/RegainingIndependence/EmotionalBehavioral-Challenges/One-side-Neglect-Improving-Awareness-to-Speed-Recovery_UCM_309735_Article.jsp

Davis, R. (1993). Phantom sensation, phantom pain, and stump pain. *Archives of Physical Medicine and Rehabilitation, 74*(1), 79–91.

de Feiter, P., van Hooft, M. A. A., Beets-Tan, R. G., & Brink, P. R. G. (2007). Fat embolism syndrome: Yes or no? *The Journal of TRAUMA Injury, Infection, and Critical Care, 63*(2), 429–431.

De Ridder, D. J., Everaert, K., Fernández, L. G., Valero, J. V., Durán, A. B., Abrisqueta, M. L., & Ventura, M. G. (2005). Intermittent catheterisation with hydrophilic-coated catheters (SpeediCath) reduces the risk of clinical urinary tract infection in spinal cord injured patients: A prospective randomised parallel comparative trial. *European Urology, 48*(6), 991–995.

Deandrea, S., Montanari, M., Moja, L., & Apolone, G. (2008). Prevalence of undertreatment in cancer pain. A review of published literature. *Annals of Oncology, 19*(12), 1985–1991.

DeAngelis, L. M. (2009). Cutaneous complications. In D. A. Casciato & M. C. Territo (Eds.), *Manual of clinical oncology* (pp. 639–640). Philadelphia, PA: Lippincott Williams & Wilkins.

Deegens, J. K., & Wetzels, J. F. M. (2011). Nephrotic range proteinuria. In J. T. Daugirdas (Ed.), *Handbook of Chronic Kidney Disease Management*. Philadelphia, PA: Lippincott Williams & Wilkins.

Defloor, T., & Grypdonck, M. F. (2005). Pressure ulcers: Validation of two risk assessment scales. *Journal of Nursing, 14*(3), 373–382.

Defloor, T., & Schoonhoven, L. (2004). Inter-rater reliability of the EPUAP pressure ulcer classification system using photographs. *Journal of Clinical Nursing, 13*, 952–959.

DeJong, N. W., Patiwael, J. A., de Groot, H., Burdorf, A., & Gerth van Wijk, R. (2011). Natural rubber latex allergy among healthcare workers: Significant reduction of sensitization and clinical relevant latex allergy after introduction of powder-free latex gloves. *Journal of Allergy and Clinical Immunology, 127*(2), AB70.

Denys, P., Schurch, B., & Fraczek,. S. (2005). Poster 59: Management of neurologic bladder with focal administration of botulinum toxin A: Minimizing risks associated with increased detrusor pressure. *Journal of Pelvic Medicine & Surgery, 11*(Suppl. 1), S52–S53.

Dewey, R., Delley, R., & Shulman, L. (2002). A better life for patients with Parkinson's disease. *Patient Care, 36*(7), 8–14.

Dillingham, T. (2007). Musculoskeletal rehabilitation: Current understandings and future directions. *American Journal of Physical Medicine and Rehabilitation, 86*, S19–S28.

Dillion, P. M. (2007). Assessing the respiratory system. In P. M. Dillion (Ed.), *Nursing health assessment: A critical thinking case studies approach* (2nd ed., pp. 393–436). Philadelphia, PA: F. A. Davis.

Dinwiddie, L. C. (2008). Vascular access for hemodialysis. In C. S. Counts (Ed.), *Core curriculum for nephrology nursing* (5th ed.). Pitman, NJ: American Nephrology Nurses' Association.

Dinwiddie, L., Burrows-Hudson, S., & Peacock, E. (2006). Stage 4 chronic kidney disease: Preserving kidney function and preparing patients for stage 5 kidney disease. *American Journal of Nursing, 106*(9), 40–51.

Dodd, M. J., Dibble, S. L., & Miaskowski, C. (2000). Randomized clinical trial of the effectiveness of 3 commonly used mouthwashes to treat chemotherapy-induced mucositis. *Oral Surgery, Oral Medicine, Oral Pathology, Oral Radiology, and Endodontics, 90*(1), 39–47.

Dodd, M., Miaskowski , C., Dibble, S., Paul, S., MacPhail, L., Greenspan, D., & Shiba, G. (2008). Factors influencing oral mucositis in patients receiving chemotherapy. *Cancer Practice, 8*(6), 291–297.

Does, A., Rhudy, L., Holland, D. E., & Olson, M. E. (2011). The experience of transition from hospital to home hospice. *Journal of Hospice and Palliative Nursing, 13*(6), 394–402.

Doley, J. (2010). Nutrition management of pressure ulcers. *Nutrition in Clinical Practice, 25*, 50–60.

Dolin, R., Masur, H., & Saag, M. (2003). *AIDS therapy* (2nd ed.). Philadelphia, PA: Churchill Livingston.

Doran, M. (2007). Rheumatoid arthritis and diabetes mellitus: Evidence for an association? *Journal of Rheumatology, 34*, 469–473.

Dorner, B., Posthauer, M. E., & Thomas, D. (2009). The role of nutrition in pressure ulcer prevention and treatment: National Pressure Ulcer Advisory Panel white paper. *Advances Skin and Wound Care, 22*(5), 212–221.

Dorsher, P. T., & McIntosh, P. M. (2010). Neurogenic bladder. *Advances in Urology, 2012*, Article ID 816274. Retrieved from http://www.hindawi.com/journals/au/2012/816274/ref/

Doty Y. Elliott, Geyer, C., Lionetti, T., & Doty, L. (2013). Managing alcohol withdrawal in hospitalized patients. *Nursing, 42*(4), 22–23.

Dougherty, M. (1998). Current status of research on pelvic muscles strengthening techniques. *Journal of Wound, Ostomy, and Continence, 25*(3), 75–83.

Douglas, S., & James, S. C. B. (2004). Non-pharmacological interventions in dementia *Advances in Psychiatric Treatment, 10*, 171–177.

Drews, R. E. (2007). *Superior vena cava syndrome.* Retrieved from www.Uptodate.com

Dudas, S. (1997). Altered body image and sexuality. In S. L. Groenwald, M. H. Frogge, M. Goodman, & C. Yarbro (Eds.), *Cancer nursing: Principles and practice* (4th ed.). Boston, MA: Jones and Bartlett.

Dudek, S. (2010). *Nutrition handbook for nursing practice* (6th ed.). Philadelphia, PA: Lippincott Williams & Wilkins.

Dutka, P. (2008). Journal club discussion: Guarding against hidden hemolysis during dialysis: An overview. *Nephrology Nursing Journal, 35*(1), 45–50.

Eachempati, S., Wang, J., Hydo, L., Shou, J., & Barie, P. (2007). Acute renal failure in critically ill surgical patients: Persistent lethality despite new modes of renal replacement therapy. *Journal of Trauma: Injury, Infection Critical Care, 63*(50), 987–993.

Early, L. M., & Poquette, R. (2000). Bladder and kidney cancer. In S. L. Groenwald, M. H. Frogge, M. Goodman, & C. H. Yarbro (Eds.), *Cancer nursing: Principles and practice* (5th ed.). Boston, MA: Jones & Bartlett.

Edelman, C., & Mandle, C. (2010). *Health promotion throughout the lifespan.* St. Louis, MO: Mosby.

Edelman, S., & Henry, R. (2011). *Diagnosis and management of type 2 diabetes* (4th ed.). New York, NY: Professional Communications.

Eisenberg, P. (1990). Monitoring gastric pH to prevent stress ulcer. *Focus on Critical Care, 17*(4), 316–322.

El-Salhy, M., Lillebø, E., Reinemo, A., Salmelid, L., & Hausken, T. (2010). Effects of a health program comprising reassurance, diet management, probiotics administration and regular exercise on symptoms and quality of life in patients with irritable bowel syndrome. *Gastroenterology Insights, 2*(1), 21–26.

Ellerhorst-Ryan, J. M. (2000). Infection. In S. Groenwald, M. Frogge, M. Goodman, & C. Yarbro (Eds.), *Cancer nursing: Principles and practice* (5th ed.). Boston, MA: Jones & Bartlett.

Elliot, D. (2002). The treatment of peptic ulcers. *Nursing Standards, 16*(23), 37–42.

Ellstrom, K. (2006). The pulmonary system. In J. Grif-Alspach (Ed.), *Core curriculum for critical care nursing* (6th ed., pp. 45–183). St. Louis, MO: Saunders-Elsevier.

Elpern, E., Covert, B., & Kleinpell, R. (2005). Moral distress of staff nurses in a medical intensive care unit. *American Journal Critical Care, 14*(6), 523–530.

Ennis, R. (2012). *Deep venous thrombosis prophylaxis in orthopedic surgery Medscape.* Retrieved from http://emedicine.medscape.com/article/1268573-overview

Enns, R. S. (n.d.). *Deep venous thrombosis prophylaxis in orthopedic surgery.* Retrieved from http://emedicine.medscape.com/article/1268573-overview#a1

Epilepsy Foundation. (2007). *What is epilepsy? Frequently asked questions.* Retrieved from http://epilepsyfoundation.org/about/faq/index.cfm

Errsser, S. J., Getliffe, K., Voegeli, D., & Regan, S. (2005). A critical review of the inter-relationship between skin vulnerability and urinary incontinence and related nursing intervention. *International Journal of Nursing Studies, 2*, 823–835.

Ertl, J. P. (2012). *Amputations of the lower extremity treatment & management.* Retrieved from http://emedicine.medscape.com/article/1232102-treatment#a1135

Esche, C. A. (2005). Resiliency: A factor to consider when facilitating the transition from the hospital to home in older adults. *Geriatric Nursing, 26*(4), 218–222.

Eslinger, P. (2002). Empathy and social-emotional factors in recovery from stroke. *Current Opinion in Neurology, 15*(1), 91–97.

European Pressure Ulcer Advisory Panel and National Pressure Ulcer Advisory Panel. (2009). *Prevention and treatment of pressure ulcers: Quick reference guide.* Washington, DC: National Pressure Ulcer Advisory Panel.

Evans, B. (2005). Best practice protocols: VAP prevention. *Nursing Management, 36*(12), 10–15.

Ewing, J. A. (1984). Detecting alcoholism: The CAGE questionnaire. *Journal of American Medical Association, 252*, 1905–1907.

Ezzone, S., Baker, C., Rosselet, R., & Terepka, E. (1998). Music as an adjunct to antiemetic therapy. *Oncology Nursing Forum, 25*(9), 1551–1556.

Farrell, S., Harmon, R., & Hastings, S. (1998). Nursing management of acute psychotic episodes. *Nursing Clinics of North America, 33*(1), 187–200.

Fazia, A., Lin, J., & Staros, E. (2012). *Urine sodium.* Emedicine. Retrieved from http://emedicine.medscape.com/article/2088449-overview#showall

Fellowes, D., Barnes, K., & Wilkinson, S. (2004). Aromatherapy and massage for symptom relief in patients with cancer. *Cochrane Database of Systematic Reviews 2*, CD002287

Ferrell, B. R. (1995). The impact of pain on quality of life. *Nursing Clinics of North America, 30*, 609–624.

Fetterman, L. G., & Lemburg, L. (2004). A silent killer—Often preventable. *American Journal of Critical Care, 13*(5), 431–436.

Field, J. B. (1989). *Hypoglycemia: Definition, clinical presentations, classification, and laboratory tests.* Retrieved from http://www.ncbi.nlm.nih.gov/pubmed/2645129

Fields, L. (2008). Oral care intervention to reduce incidence of ventilator-associated pneumonia in the neurologic intensive care unit. *American Association of Neuroscience Nurses, 40*(5), 291–298.

File, T. M., Jr. (2012). *Treatment of community-acquired pneumonia in adults who require hospitalization.* Retrieved from http://www.uptodate.com/contents/treatment-of-community-acquired-pneumonia-in-adults-who-require-hospitalization

Fineman, L. D., LaBrecque, M. A., Shih, M., & Curley, M. A. Q. (2006). Prone positioning can be safely performed in critically ill infants and children. *Pediatric Critical Care Medicine, 7*(5), 413–422.

Finkelman, A. W. (2000). Self-management for psychiatric patient at home. *Home Care Provider, 5*(6), 95–101.

Fitch, M. I. (2006). Programmatic approaches to psychological support. In R. M. Carroll Johnson, L. M. Gorman, & N. J. Bush (Eds.), *Psychosocial nursing care along the cancer continuum* (2nd ed., pp. 419–438). Pittsburgh, PA: Oncology Nursing Society.

Fitzmaurice, D., Blann, A., & Lip, G. (2002). Bleeding risks of antithrombotic therapy. *BMJ, 12*(325)(7368), 828–831. Retrieved from http://www.ncbi.nlm.nih.gov/pmc/articles/PMC1124331/

Fletcher, L. (2006). Management of patients with intermittent claudication. *Nursing Standard, 20*(31), 59–65.

Foltz, A. (2000). Nutritional disturbances. In S. Groenwald, M. Frogge, M. Goodman, & C. Yarbro (Eds.), *Cancer nursing: Principles and practice* (5th ed.). Boston, MA: Jones & Bartlett.

Forsythe, B., & Faulkner, K. (2004). Overview of the tolerability of gefitinib (IRESSA) monotherapy: Clinical experience in non-small-cell-lung cancer [Electronic version]. *Drug Safety, 27*(14), 1081–1092. Retrieved from http://ebsco.waldenu.edu/ehost/pdf?vid=144&hid=102&sid=781c7c0c-696c-44ec- 9c5d-f6382763aca4%40sessionmgr106

Fouque, D., & Juillard, L. (2011). Protein intake. In J. T. Daugirdas (Ed.), *Handbook of chronic kidney disease management.* Philadelphia, PA: Lippincott Williams & Wilkins.

Franz, M. G., Steed, D. L., & Robson, M. C. (2007). Optimizing healing of the acute wound by minimizing complications. *Current Problems in Surgery, 44*, 691–763.

French, K., Beynon, C., & Delaforce, J. (2007). Alcohol is the true "rape drug." *Nursing Standard, 21*(29), 26–27.

Fried, L. P., Ferrucci, L., Darer, J., Williamson, J. D., & Anderson, G. (2004). Untangling the concepts of disability, frailty, and comorbidity: Implications for improved targeting and care. *Journals of Gerontology—Series A Biological Sciences and Medical Sciences, 59*(3), 255–263.

Fried, L. P., Tangen, C. M., Walston, J., Newman, A. B., Hirsch, C., Gottdiener, J., . . . Cardiovascular Health Study Collaborative Research Group. (2001). Frailty in older adults: Evidence for a phenotype. *Journals of Gerontology—Series A Biological Sciences and Medical Sciences, 56*(3), M146–M156.

Frossard, J. L., Steer, M. L., & Pastor, C. M. (2008). *Acute pancreatitis. Lancet, 371*(9607), 143–152.

Funnell, M. M., Kruger, D. F., & Spencer, M. (2004). Self-management support for insulin therapy in type 2 diabetes. *Diabetes Educator, 30*(2), 274–280.

Furie, K., Kasner, S., Adams, R., Albers, G., Bush, R., Fagan, S.,…Wentworth, D. (2011). *Guidelines for the prevention of stroke in patients with stroke or transient ischemic attack.* A Guideline for Healthcare Professionals From the American Heart Association/American Stroke Association. Retrieved from http://stroke.ahajournals.org/content/early/2010/10/21/STR.0b013e3181f7d043.full.pdf+html

Gallagher, P., Horgan, O., Franchignoni, F., Giordano, A., & MacLachlan, M. (2007). Body image in people with lower-limb amputation: A Rasch analysis of the amputee body image scale. *American Journal of Physical Medicine and Rehabilitation, 86*(3), 205–215.

Garcia-Tsao, G. (2011). Cirrhosis and its sequelae. In L. Goldman & A. I. Schafer (Eds.), *Cecil medicine* (24th ed., Chapter 156). Philadelphia, PA: Saunders Elsevier.

Garcia-Tsao, G., Sanyal, A. J., Grace, N. D., & Carey, W. D. (2007). Practice Guidelines Committee of American Association for Study of Liver Diseases; Practice Parameters Committee of American College of Gastroenterology. Prevention and management of gastroesophageal varices and variceal hemorrhage in cirrhosis. *American Journal of Gastroenterology, 102*, 2086–2102.

Gary, R., & Fleury, J. (2002). Nutritional status: Key to preventing functional decline in hospitalized older adults. *Topics in Geriatric Rehabilitation, 17*(3), 40–71.

Geary, C. M. B. (1987). Nursing grand rounds: The patient with viral cardiomyopathy. *Journal of Cardiovascular Nursing, 2*(1), 48–52.

Geerlings, S. E., & Hoepelman, A. I. (1999). Immune dysfunction in patients with diabetes mellitus (DM). *FEMS Immunology and Medical Microbiology, 26*(3–4), 259–265.

Ghotkar, S. V., Grayson, A. D., Fabri, B. M., Dihmis, W. C., & Pullan, D. M. (2006). Preoperative calculation of risk for prolonged intensive care unit stay following coronary artery bypass grafting. *Journal of Cardiothoracic Surgery, 1*(14), 8090–8091.

Giardina, E. (n.d.). Cardiovascular effects of nicotine. Retrieved from http://cmbi.bjmu.edu.cn/uptodate/coronary%20heart%20disease/Miscellaneous/Cardiovascular%20effects%20of%20nicotine.htm

Gil, K., Carson, J., Sedway, J., Porter, L., Schaeffer, J., & Orringer, E. (2000). Follow-up of coping skills training in adults with sickle cell disease. *Health Psychology, 19*(1), 85–90.

Gillenwater, J. Y., Grayhack, J. T., Howards, S. S., & Duckett, J. W. (1996). *Adult and pediatric urology* (3rd ed.). St. Louis, MO: Mosby-Year Book.

Ginzler, E., & Tayar, J. (2004). *Systemic lupus erythematosus.* Retrieved from http://rheumatolgy.org/public/factsheets/sle_new.asp

Giuliano, A. E., & Hurvitz, S. A. (2012). Breast disorders. In S. McPhee & M. Papadakis (Eds.), *2012 Current medical diagnosis & treatment* (pp. 699–726). New York, NY: McGraw-Hill Lange.

Glantz, M., Chamberlain, M., Liu, Q., Hsieh, C., Edwards, K., VanHorn, A., & Recht, L. (2009). Gender disparity in the rate of partner abandonment in patients with serious medical illness. *Cancer, 115*(22), 5237–5242.

Gooszen, A. W., Geelkerken, R. H., Hermans, J., Lagaay, M. B., & Gooszen, H. G. (2000). Quality of life with a temporary stoma: Ileostomy vs. colostomy. *Diseases of Colon and Rectum, 43*(5), 650–655.

Glaser, V. (2000). Topics in geriatrics: Effective approaches to depression in older patients. *Patient Care, 17,* 65–80.

Gobel, B. H. (2005). Bleeding disorder. In S. Groenwald, M. Frogge, M. Goodman, & C. Yarbro (Eds.), *Cancer nursing: Principles and practice* (6th ed.). Boston, MA: Jones & Bartlett.

Gonzalez, E. L., Patrignani, P., Tacconelli, S., & Rodriquez, L. A. (2010). Variabililily among nonsteriodial Antiinflammatory drugs in risk for upper GI bleedinng. *Arthritis & Rheumatism, 62*(6), 1592–1601.

Goodman, M., & Hayden, B. K. (2000). Chemotherapy: Principles of administration. In C. H. Yarbo, M. H. Frogge, & M. Goodman (Eds.), *Comprehensive cancer nursing review* (6th ed.). Boston, MA: Jones & Bartlett.

Gor, H. (2012). *Hysterectomy.* Retrieved from http://emedicine.medscape.com/article/267273-overview

Gordon, A. J. (2006). Identification and treatment of alcohol-use disorders in the perioperative period. *Post Graduate Medicine, 199*(2), 46–55.

Gorski, L. A. (2002, October). Effective teaching of home IV therapy [Electronic version]. *Home Healthcare Nurse, 20*(10), 666–674. Retrieved from http://gateway.tx.ovid.com.library.gcu.edu:2048/gw2/ovidweb.cgi

Goshorn, J. (2000). Management of patients with urinary and renal dysfunction. In S. Smeltzer & B. Bare (Eds.), *Brunner & Suddarth's textbook of medical-surgical nursing* (9th ed.). Philadelphia, PA: Lippincott Williams & Wilkins.

Goss, L., Coty, M. B., & Myers, J. A. (2011). A review of documented oral care practices in an intensive care unit. *Clinical Nursing Research, 20,* 181–196.

Graf, J., & Janssens, U. (2007). Recognizing shock: Who cares, and when? *Critical Care Medicine, 35*(11), 2651–2652.

Grainger, R. (1990). Anxiety interrupters. *American Journal of Nursing, 90*(2), 14–15.

Graul, T. (2002). Total joint replacement: Baseline benchmark data for interdisciplinary outcomes management. *Orthopaedic Nursing, 21*(3), 57–67.

Gray-Miceli, D., Johnson, J. C., & Strumpf, N. E. (2005). A step-wise approach to a comprehensive post-fall assessment. *Annals of Long-Term Care: Clinical Care and Aging, 13*(12), 16–24.

Greelish, J., Mohler, E., & Fairman, R. (2006a). *Carotid endarectomy in asymptomatic patients.* Retrieved from UpToDate.com

Greelish, J., Mohler, E., & Fairman, R. (2006b). *Carotid endarectomy: Preoperative evaluation; surgical technique; and complications.* Retrieved from UpToDate.com

Greenberger, P. A. (2002). Anaphylaxis. In *Manual of Allergy & Immunology (10).* Retrieved from Ovid database.

Greenberger, P. A. (2007). Idiopathic anaphylaxis. *Immunology Allergy Clinician North America, 27,* 273.

Greene, J. H. (2011). Restricting dietary sodium and potassium: A dietitian's perspective. In J. T. Daugirdas (Ed.), *Handbook of chronic kidney disease management.* Philadelphia, PA: Lippincott Williams & Wilkins.

Griebling, T. L. (2009). Urinary incontinence in the elderly. *Clinics in Geriatric Medicine, 25*(3), 445–457.

Griffin-Broan, J. (2000). Diagnostic evaluation, classification, and staging. In C. Yarbo, M. H. Frogge, M. Goodman, & S. Groenwald (Eds.), *Cancer nursing: Principles and practice* (5th ed.). Boston, MA: Jones & Bartlett.

Grisham, K., & Estes, N. (1982). Dynamics of alcoholic families. In N. Estes & M. E. Heinemann (Eds.), *Alcoholism: Development, consequences and interventions.* St. Louis, MO: Mosby-Year Book.

Guideline for the prevention and management of pressure ulcers. (2010, June). Mt. Laurel, NJ: Wound Ostomy and Continence Nurses Society.

Guillain-Barre syndrome fact sheet. (n.d.). Retrieved from http://www.ninds.nih.gov/disorders/gbs/detail_gbs.htm

Guo, S., & DiPietro, L. A. (2010). Factors affecting wound healing. *Journal of Dental Research, 89*(3), 219–229.

Gupta, A., & Reilly, C. (2007). Fat embolism. *Continuing Education in Anaesthesia, Critical Care & Pain, 7*(5), 148–151. Retrieved from http://ceaccp.oxfordjournals.org/content/7/5/148.full

Gutekunst, L. (2011). Restricting protein and phosphorus: A dietitian's perspective. In J. T. Daugirdas (Ed.), *Handbook of chronic kidney disease management.* Philadelphia, PA: Lippincott Williams & Wilkins.

Hadley, S. K., & Gaarder, S. M. (2005). Treatment of irritable bowel syndrome. *American Family Physician, 72*(12), 2501–2506.

Hahn, B. H., McMahon, M. A., Wilkinson, A., Wallace, W. D., Daikh, D., Fitzgerald, J. D., . . . American College of Rheumatology. (2012). American College of Rheumatology guidelines for screening, treatment, and management of lupus nephritis. *Arthritis Care & Research, 64*(6), 797–808.

Haire, W. D. (2007). *Catheter-induced upper extremity venous thrombosis.* Retrieved from www.UpToDate.com

Hall, B. (1990). The struggle of the diagnosed terminally ill person to maintain hope. *Nursing Science Quarterly, 3*, 177–184.

Hall, G. R. (1991). Altered thought processes: Dementia. In M. Maas, K. Buckwalter, & M. Hardy (Eds.), *Nursing diagnoses and interventions for the elderly*. Menlo Park, CA: Addison-Wesley.

Hall, G. R. (1994). Caring for people with Alzheimer's disease using the conceptual model of progressively lowered stress threshold in the clinical setting. *Nursing Clinics of North America, 29*, 129–141.

Hall, G. R., & Buckwalter, K. C. (1987). Progressively lowered stress threshold: A conceptual model for care of adults with Alzheimer's disease. *Archives of Psychiatric Nursing, 1*, 399–406.

Halloran, R. (2009). Caring for the patient with inflammatory response, shock, and severe sepsis. In K. Osborn (Ed.), *Medical surgical nursing: Preparation for practice* (Volume 1, Chapter 61). Upper Saddle River, NJ: Prentice Hall.

Halm, M. A., & Krisko-Hagel, K. (2008). Instilling normal saline with suctioning: Beneficial technique or potentially harmful sacred cow? *American Journal of Critical Care, 17*(5), 469–472.

Halter, M. J., & Carson, V. B. (2010). Sexual assault. In E. Varcarolis (Ed.), *Foundations of psychiatric mental health nursing* (6th ed.). Philadelphia, PA: Saunders.

Halyard, M., & Ferrans, C. (2008). Quality of life assessment for routine clinical practice. *Journal of Supportive Oncology, 6*(5), 221–229, 233.

Hamdy, O. (2012). *Hypoglycemia*. Retrieved from http://emedicine.medscape.com/

Hamric, A. B. (2000.) Moral distress in everyday ethics. *Nursing Outlook, 49*(2), 199–201.

Headley, C. M., & Wall, B. M. (2007). Flash pulmonary edema in patients with chronic kidney disease and end stage renal disease. *Nephrology Nursing Journal, 34*(1), 15–26, 37; quiz 27–28.

Hamilton, H. (2006). Complications associated with venous access devices: Part one. *Nursing Standard, 20*(26), 43–50. Retrieved from http://ebscohost.com/ehost/pdf?vid=140&hid=106&sid=c7e5d2b4-a693-4480-a27f-fdf75c59b820%40sessionmgr106

Hampton, S. (2005). Importance of the appropriate selection and use of continence pads. *British Journal of Nursing, 14*(5), 265–269.

Hanna, D. (2004). Moral distress: The state of the science. *Research and Theory for Nursing Practice: An International Journal, 18*(1), 73–79.

Hansen, L. B., & Vondracek, S. F. (2004). Prevention and treatment of nonpostmenapausal osteoporosis. *American Journal of Health-System Pharmacy, 61*(24), 2637–2654.

Hansen, L. B., & Vondracek, S. F. (2006). Prevention and treatment of nonpostmenopausal osteoporosis. *American Journal of Health-System Pharmacy, 61*(24), 2637–2654.

Happ, M. B., Swigert, V. A., Tate, J. A., Arnold, R. M., Serelka, S. M., & Hoffman, L. A. (2007). Family presence and surveillance during weaning from prolonged mechanical ventilation. *Heart & Lung, 36*(1), 47–57.

Harari, D., Coshall, C., Rudd, A., & Wolfe, C. (2003). New-onset fecal incontinence after stroke. *Prevalence, Natural History, Risk Factors, and Impact Stroke. 34*, 144–150.

Hardt, J., Jacobsen, C., Goldberg, J., Nickel, R., & Buchwald, D. (2008). Prevalence of chronic pain in a representative sample in the United States. *Pain Medicine Pain Medicine, 9*(7), 803–812.

Harker, J. (2006). *Wound healing complications associated with lower limb amputation*. World Wide Wounds. Retrieved from http://www.worldwidewounds.com/2006/september/Harker/Wound-Healing-Complications-Limb-Amputation.html

Harman, E., & Dutka, P. (2007). Hemolysis: A hidden danger. *Nephrology Nursing Journal, 34*(2), 219–224.

Harmanli, O. H., Khilnani, R., Dandolu, V., & Chatwani, A. J. (2004). Narrow pubic arch and increased risk of failure for vaginal hysterectomy. *Obstetrics & Gynecology, 104*(4), 697–700.

Harrington, K. D. (1985). Metastatic disease of the spine. *Clinical Orthopaedics, 192*, 222–228.

Hartley, J. (2007). Compartment syndrome. Retrieved from http://www.ceufast.com/courses/viewcourse.asp?id=176

Harvey, S., & Whelan, C. A. (2008). Pneumonia. In T. M. Buttaro, J. Trybulski, P. P. Bailey, & J. Sandberg-Cook (Eds.), *Primary care: A collaborative practice* (3rd ed., pp. 466–475). St. Louis, MO: Mosby.

Haugen, V., Bliss D. Z., & Savik, K. (2006). Perioperative factor that affect long-term adjustment to an incontinent ostomy. *Journal of Wound, Ostomy and Continence Nursing, 33*(5), 525–535.

Haughney, A. (2004). Nausea and vomiting in end-stage cancer: These symptoms can be treated most effectively if the underlying cause is known. *American Journal of Nursing, 104*(11), 40–48.

Heard, L., & Buhrer, R. (2005). How do we prevent UTI in people who perform intermittent catheterization? *Rehabilitation Nursing, 30*, 44–45.

Heard, L., & Buhrer, R. (2005). How do we prevent UTI in people who perform intermittent catheterization? *Rehabilitation Nursing, 30*(2), 44–61.

Heeney, M., & Mahoney, D. H. (2011). *The acute chest syndrome in children and adolescents with sickle cell disease*. Retrieved from UpToDate.com

Heidelbaugh, J. J., & Sherbondy, M. (2006). Cirrhosis and chronic liver failure: Part II. Complications and treatment. *American Family Physician, 74*(5), 767–776. Retrieved from http://www.aafp.org/afp/2006/0901/p767.html

Heidenreich, P. A., Trogdon, J. G., Khavjou, O. A., Butler, J., Dracup, K., Ezekowitz, M. D., . . . Council on Cardiovascular Surgery and Anesthesia, and Interdisciplinary Council on Quality of Care and Outcomes Research. (2011). Forecasting the future of cardiovascular disease in the United States: A policy statement from the American Heart Association. *Circulation, 123*(8), 933–944.

Heinrich, L. (1987). Care of the female rape victim. *Nurse Practitioner, 12*(11), 9–27.

Heitman, J. (2012). Acute ischemic stroke management. RN.com. Retrieved from http://www.rn.com/getpdf.php/1739. pdf?Main_Session=3025b55ccecb8a9bf3bfa10ece7f06ce

Held-Warmkessel, J. (2005). Prostate cancer. In C. Yarbo, M. Frogge, & M. Goodman (Eds.), *Cancer nursing: Principles and practice* (5th ed.). Boston, MA: Jones & Bartlett.

Heller, L., Levin, S. L., & Butler, C. E. (2006). Management of abdominal wound dehiscence using vacuum assisted closure in patients with compromised healing. *The American Journal of Surgery, 191*(2), 165.

Hemphill, R. (2012). *Hyperosmolar hyperglycemic state Medscape.* Retrieved from http://emedicine.medscape.com/article/1914705-overview

Hernán, M. A., Jick, S. S., Logroscino, G., Olek, M. J., Ascherio, A., & Jick, H. (2005). Cigarette smoking and the progression of multiple sclerosis. *Brain, 128*(Pt. 6), 1461–1465.

Hernigou, P., Bachir, D., & Galacteros, F. (2003). The national history of symptomatic osteonecrosis in adults with sickle cell disease. *Journal of Bone and Joint Surgery, 85*(3), 500–504.

Hess, C. (2011). Checklist for factors affecting wound healing. *Advances in Skin & Wound Care, 24*(4), 192.

Hickey, J. V. (2009). *The clinical practice of neurological and neurosurgical nursing* (6th ed.). Philadelphia, PA: Lippincott Williams & Wilkins.

Hickey, J. V. (2009). *The clinical practice of neurosurgical nursing* (6th ed.). Philadelphia, PA: Lippincott Williams & Wilkins.

Hilderley, L. (2000). Radiotherapy. In S. Groenwald, M. Frogge, M. Goodman, & C. Yarbro (Eds.), *Cancer nursing: Principles and practice* (5th ed.). Boston, MA: Jones & Bartlett.

Hillis, L. D., Smith, P. K., Anderson, J. L., Bittl, J. A., Bridges, C. R., Byrne, J. G., . . . American Heart Association Task Force on Practice Guidelines. (2011). 2011 ACCF/AHA Guideline for Coronary Artery Bypass Graft Surgery. A Report of the American College of Cardiology Foundation/American Heart Association Task Force on Practice Guidelines. *Circulation, 124*, e652–e735. Retrieved from http://circ.ahajournals.org/content/124/23/e652

Himiak, L. (2007). *The amputee community continues to face undue hardships and discrimination.* Retrieved from http://nursing.advanceweb.com/Editorial/Content/Editorial.aspx?CC=100852&CP=2

Hirsch, A. T., Haskal, Z. J., Hertzer, N. R., Bakal, C. W., Creager, M. A., Halperin, J. L., . . . Vascular Disease Foundation. (2006). ACC/AHA guidelines for the management of patients with peripheral arterial disease (lower extremity, renal mesenteric, and abdominal aortic). *Journal of Vascular Interventional Radiology,* (17), 1383–1398.

Hlebovy, D. (2008). Hemodialyis: Fluid removal: Obtaining estimated dry weight during hemodilaysis. In C. S. Counts (Ed.), *Core curriculum for nephrology nursing* (5th ed.). Pitman, NJ: American Nephrology Nurses' Association.

Hlebovy, D., & King, B. (2008). Complications of hemodialysis. In C. S. Counts (Ed.), *Core curriculum for nephrology nursing* (5th ed.). Pitman, NJ: American Nephrology Nurses' Association.

Hockenberry, M. J., & Wilson, D. (2009). *Wong's essentials of pediatric nursing.* St. Louis, MO: Elsevier.

Hockenberry, M. J., Wilson, D., & Winkelstein, M. L. (2007). *Wong's nursing care of infants and children* (8th ed.). St. Louis, MO: Elsevier.

Hoffman, R., & Weinhouse, G. (2012). *Management of moderate and severe alcohol withdrawal syndromes.* Retrieved from http://www.uptodate.com/contents/management-of-moderate-and-severe-alcohol-withdrawal-syndromes

Holditch-Davis, D., & Blackburn, S. (2007). Neurobehavioral development. In C. Kenner & J W. Lott (Eds.), *Comprehensive neonatal care: an interdisciplinary approach* (4th ed., pp. 448–479). St. Louis, MO: Saunders Elsevier.

Holland, J. C., & Reznik, I. (2005). Pathways for psychosocial care of cancer survivors. *Cancer, 104*(Suppl. 11), 2524–2637. doi:10.1002/cncr.21252

Holman, J. S., & Shwed, J. A. (1992). Influence of sucralfate on the detection of occult blood in simulated gastric fluid by two screening tests. *Clinical Pharmacology, 11*(7), 625–627.

Holt, P. R. (2001). Diarrhea and malabsorption in the elderly. *Gastroenterology Clinics of North America, 30*, 427–444.

Hooyman, N. R. & Kramer, B. J. (2006). *Living through loss: Interventions across the life span.* New York, NY: Columbia University Press.

Horwitz, M. (2012). *Hypercalcemia of malignancy.* Retrieved from http://www.uptodate.com/contents/hypercalcemia-of-malignancy

Hoskins, C. N., & Budin, W. C. (2000). Measurement of psychosocial adjustment to breast cancer: A unidimensional or multidimensional construct? *Psychological Reports, 87*(2), 649–663.

Hoskins, C. N., & Haber, J. (2000). Adjusting to breast cancer. *American Journal of Nursing, 100*(4), 26–33.

Hospice and Palliative Nurses Association. (2013). *Final days* (patient/family teaching sheet). Retrieved from http://www.hpna.org/DisplayPage.aspx?Title=Patient/Family%20Teaching%20sheets

Howard, J. F. (2006). *Clinical overview of MG. Myasthenia gravis: A summary.* Retrieved from http://www.myasthenia.org/HealthProfessionals/ClinicalOverviewofMG.aspx

Hudman, L., & Bodenham, A. (2013). Practical aspects of long-term venous access. *Continuing Education in Anaesthesia, Critical Care & Pain, 13*(1), 6–11. Retrieved from http://www.medscape.com/viewarticle/782389_4

Huffman, G. B. (2002). Evaluating and treating unintentional weight loss in the elderly [Electronic Version]. *American Family Physician, 65*(4). Retrieved from http://web.ebscohost.com/ehost/detail?vid=4%hid=106&sid=c7e5d2b4-****3-4480-a27f-fdf75c59b820%40sessionmgr106.

Hull, R. D., Pineo, G. F., Stein, P. D., Mah, A. F., MacIsaac, S. M., Dahl, O. E., . . . Raskob, G. E. (2001). Timing of initial administration of low-molecular-weight heparin prophylaxis against deep vein thrombosis in patients following elective hip arthroplasty: A systematic review. *Archives of Internal Medicine, 161*(16), 1952–1960.

Hunter, K. F., Moore, K. N., & Glazner, C. M. A. (2007). Conservative management for postprostectomy urinary incontinence [Systematic Review]. *Cochrane Database of Systematic Reviews, 3.*

Hunter, M., & King, D. (2001). COPD: Management of acute exacerbations and chronic stable disease. *American Family Physician, 64*(4), 603–612.

Hurkmans, E., van der Giesen, F. J., Vliet Vlieland, T. P. M., Schoones, J., & Van den Ende, E. C. H. M. (2009). Dynamic exercise programs (aerobic capacity and/or muscle strength training) in patients with rheumatoid arthritis. *Cochrane Database of Systematic Review.* Retrieved from http://summaries.cochrane.org/CD006853/dynamic-exercise-programs-aerobic-capacity-andor-muscle-strength-training-in-patients-with-rheumatoid-arthritis

Huskamp, H., Keating, N., Malin, J., Zaslavsky, A., Weeks, Earle, C. C.,...Ayanian, J. Z. (2009). Discussions with physicians about hospice among patients with metastatic lung cancer. *Archives of Internal Medicine, 169*(10), 954–962.

Hyland, J. (2002). The basics of ostomies. *Gastroenterology Nursing, 25*(6), 241–244.

Iezzoni, L. F., O'Day, B., Keleen, M. A., & Harker, H. (2004). Improving patient care: Communicating about health care: Observations from persons who are deaf or hard of hearing. *Annals of Internal Medicine, 140*(5), 356–362.

Institute for Healthcare Improvement. (2008). Implement the ventilator bundle: Elevation of the head of the bed. Retrieved from www.ihi.org/IHI/Topics/CriticalCare/IntensiveCare/Changes/IndividualChanges/Elevationoftheheadofthebed.htm

Institute of Medicine. (2007). *Cancer care for the whole patient: Meeting psychosocial health needs.* Washington, DC: National Academies Press.

Institute of Medicine. (2009a). Sleep disorders and sleep deprivation: An unmet public health problem. *Gerontology, 55*(2), 162–168.

Institute of Medicine. (2009b). *Weight gain during pregnancy: Reexamining the guideline.* Retrieved from http://www.iom.edu

International Association of the Study of Pain. (2011). Part III: Pain terms, a current list with definitions and notes on Usage. In *Classification of chronic pain* (2nd ed.). Washington, DC: International Association of the Study of Pain.

International League Against Epilepsy. (2007). *Classifications of seizures.* Retrieved from http://www.ilae-epilepsy.org

Inzucchi, S. (2012). *Diabetes facts and guidelines.* Yale Diabetes Center.

Ioannidis, O., Lavrentieva, A., & Botsios, D. (2008). Nutrition support in acute pancreatitis. *Journal of Periodontology, 9*(4), 375–390.

Inzucchi, S., Bergenstal, R., Buse, J., Diamant, M., Ferrannini, E., Nauck, M., . . . Mathews, D. (2012). Position statement of the American Diabetes Association (ADA) and the European Association for the Study of Diabetes (EASD). Retrieved from http://care.diabetesjournals.org/content/early/2012/04/17/dc12-041.full.pdf+html

Jablonski, R. (2001). Discovering asthma in the older adult. *Nurse Practitioner, 25*(1), 14, 24–25, 29–32.

Jain, S., Mittal, M., Kansal, A., Singh, Y., Kolar, P. R., & Saigal, R. (2008). Fat embolism syndrome. *JAPI, 56*, 245–249. Retrieved from http://www.japi.org/april2008/R-245.pdf and http://www.japi.org/april2008/R-245.pdf

James, M. L. (2007). Prostate cancer (early). In G. F. G. (Ed.), *Clinical evidence.* London, UK: BMJ Publishing Group.

Jauch, E. C., Cucchiara, B., Adeoye, O., Meurer, W., Brice, J., Chan, Y., & Hazinski, M. (2010). American Heart Association guidelines for cardiopulmonary resuscitation and emergency cardiovascular care. *Circulation, 122*(Suppl. 3), S818–S828.

Jauch, E. C., Saver, J. L., Adams, H. P., Jr., Bruno, A., Connors, J. J., Demaerschalk, B. M., . . . Yonas, H. (2013). AHA/ASA Guideline: Guidelines for the early management of patients with acute ischemic stroke: A guideline for healthcare professionals from the American Heart Association *Stroke, 44*, 870–947.

Jenkins, T. (2002). Sickle cell anemia in pediatric intensive care unit. *AACN Clinical Issues, 13*(2), 154–168.

Jennings-Ingle, S. (2007). The sobering facts of alcohol withdrawal. *Nursing Made Incredibly Easy, 5*(1), 50–60.

Jepson, R. G., & Craig, J. C. (2008). Cranberries for preventing urinary tract infections. *Cochrane Database of Systematic Review, 2*, CD00132.

Johns Hopkins Breast Cancer Center. (2007). *Johns Hopkins decision of plastic and reconstructive surgery: Breast reconstruction.* Retrieved from http://www.hopkinsbreastcenter.org/services/patientcare/plasticsurgery.shtml

Johnson, J. E., Rice, V., Fuller, S., & Endress, P. (1978). Sensory information instruction in coping strategy and recovery from surgery. *Research in Nursing and Health, 1*(1), 4–17.

Joint Commission. (2006). Sentinel event alert. *Tubing Misconnections – A Persistent and Potentially Deadly Occurrence, Issue 36.* Retrieved from http://www.jointcommission.org/SentinelEvents/SentinelEventAlert/sea_36.htm

Joint Commission. (2010). *Achieving effective communication, cultural competence, and patient-centered care: A roadmap for hospitals.* Oakland Terrace, IL: Author.

Joyce, N. (2002). *Eye care for intensive care patients.* A systematic review (No. 21). Adelaide, Australia: The Joanna Briggs Institute for Evidence-Based Nursing and Midwifery. Retrieved from www.graphics.ovid.com/db/cinahl/pdf20020444

Junkin, J., & Beitz, J. M. (2005). Sexuality and the person with a stoma: Implications for comprehensive WOC nursing practice. *Journal of Wound, Ostomy and Continence Nursing, 32*(2), 121–128.

Kahn, S. R. (2013). Elastic compression stockings failed to prevent post-thrombotic syndrome. *HemOnc Today*, *14*(3), 31.

Kahn, S. R. Lim, W., Dunn, A. S., Cushman, M., Dentali, F., Akl, E. A., . . . American College of Chest Physicians. (2012). Prevention of VTE in nonsurgical patients. American College of Chest Physicians Evidence-Based Clinical Practice Guidelines. CHEST. accessed5/3/2013 at 2):e195S–e226S.

Kalichman, S. C., Cain, D., Fuhel, A., Eaton, L., Di Fonzo, K., & Ertl, T. (2005). Assessing medication adherence self-efficacy among low-literacy patients: Development of a pictographic visual analogue scale. *Health Education Research*, *20*(1), 24–35.

Kannel, W. B., & Belanger, A. J. (1991). Epidemiology of heart failure. *American Heart Journal*, *121*, 951–957.

Kantaff, P., Carroll, P., D'Amico, A., Isaacs, J., Ross, R., & Schertt, C. (2001). *Prostate cancer: Principles and practice*. Philadelphia, PA: Lippincott Williams & Wilkins.

Kaplan, J. E., Masur, H., & Holmes, K. K. (2002). USPHS Infectious Disease Society of America: Guidelines for preventing opportunistic infections in HIV infected groups. *MMWR*, *51*(RR8), 1–52.

Kappas-Larson, P., & Lathrop, L. (1993). Early detection and intervention for hazardous ethanol use. *Nurse Practitioner*, *18*(7), 50–55.

Karalis, M. (2008), Nutrition intervention. In C. S. Counts (Ed.), *Core curriculum for nephrology nursing* (5th ed.). Pitman, NJ: American Nephrology Nurses' Association.

Katz, A. (2005). Sexually speaking: Sexuality and hysterectomy: Finding the right words: Responding to patients' concerns about the potential effects of surgery. *American Journal of Nursing*, *105*(12), 65–68.

Katz, A. (2006). What have my kidneys got to do with my sex life? The impact of late stage chronic kidney disease on sexual function. *American Journal of Nursing*, *106*(9), 81–83.

Katz, J. (1996). The role of the sympathetic nervous system in phantom limb pain. *Physical Medicine and Rehabilitation: State of the Art Reviews*, *10*(1), 153–175.

Katz, P. (2003). Peptic ulcer disease. In L. R. Baker, J. Burton, & P. Zieve. *Principles of ambulatory medicine* (6th ed.). Philadelphia, PA: Lippincott Williams & Wilkins.

Kawada, E., Moridaira, K., Itoh, K., Hoshino, A., Tamura, J., & Morita, T. (2006). Long-term bedridden elderly patients [Electronic version]. *Annals of Nutrition & Metabolism*, *50*(5), 420–424. Retrieved from http://ebsco.waldenu.edu/ehost/pdf?vid=11&hid=102&sid=b2fae363-688a-4e54-96d6-e87f0fde711c%40ses sionmgr103

Kee, J. L. (2004). *Handbook of laboratory & diagnostic tests with nursing implications* (5th ed.). Upper Saddle River, NJ: Pearson Education, Prentice Hall.

Keenan G. (1997). Management of complications of glucocorticoid therapy. *Clinics In Chest Medicine*, *18*, 507–520.

Kelly, K. J., Kurup, V. P., Reijula, K. E., & Fink, J. N. (1994). The diagnosis of natural rubber latex allergy. *Journal of Allergy and Clinical Immunology*, *93*, 813–816.

Kemp, C. (2006). Spiritual care interventions. In B. Ferrell & N. Coyle (Eds.), *Textbook of palliative nursing* (2nd ed., pp. 440–455). New York, NY: Oxford University Press.

Khardori, R. (Ed.). (n.d.). *Infection in patients with diabetes mellitus*. Retrieved from http://emedicine.medscape.com/article/2122072-overview

Khraim, F. M. (2007). The wider scope of video-assisted thoracoscopic surgery. *AORN Journal*, *85*(6), 1199–1208.

King, B. (2008). Principles of dialysis. In C. S. Counts (Ed.), *Core curriculum for nephrology nursing* (5th ed.). Pitman, NJ: American Nephrology Nurses' Association.

Kirkeby-Garstad, I., Wisloff, U., Skogvoll, E., Stolen, T., Tjonna, A. E., Stenseth, R., & Sellevold, O. F. (2006). The marked reduction in mixed venous oxygen saturation during early mobilization after cardiac surgery: The effect of posture or exercise? *Anesthesia & Analgesia*, *102*(6), 1609–1616.

Kitabchi, A. E., Haerian, H., & Rose, B. D. (2008). *Treatment of diabetic ketoacidosis and hyperosmolar hyperglycemic state*. Retrieved from www.UpToDate.com

Knodrup, J., Allison, S. P., Elia, M., Vellas, B., & Plauth, M. (2003). ESPEN guidelines for nutrition screening 2002. *Clinical Nutrition*, *22*(4), 415–442.

Koch, A. (2003). Angiogenesis as a target in rheumatoid arthritis. *Annals of Rheumatic Diseases*, *62*(Suppl. 2), ii60–ii67.

Kohtz, C., & Thompson, M. (2007). Preventing contrast medium-induced nephrology. *The American Journal of Nursing*, *107*(9).

Kok, N., Alwayn, I., Tran, K., Hop, W., Weimar, W., & Ijzermans, J. (2006). Psychosocial and physical impairment after mini-incision open and laparoscopic donor nephrectomy: A positive study [Electronic version]. *Transplantation*, *82*(10), 1291–1297. Retrieved from http://gateway.uk.ovid.com/gw1/ovidweb.cgi

Koul, R., Dufan, T., Russell, C., Guenther, W., Nugent, Z., Sun, X., & Cookie, A. L. (2007). Efficacy of complete decongestive therapy and manual lymphatic drainage on treatment-related lymphedema in breast cancer. *International Journal of Radiation Oncology, Biology, Physics*, *67*, 841–846.

Krebs, L. U. (2000). Sexual and reproductive dysfunction. In S. L. Groenwald, M. H. Frogge, M. Goodman, & C. Yarbro (Eds.), *Cancer nursing: Principles and practice* (5th ed.). Boston, MA: Jones & Bartlett.

Kuntzsch, T., & Voge, C. (2009). Hypersensitivity reactions to chemotherapy in acute care oncology. In C. Chernecky, & K. Murphy-Ende (Ed.), *Nursing* (2nd ed.). St. Louis, MO: Saunders

Ladd, A., Jones, H. H., & Otanez, O. (2003). *Osteomyelitis*. Retrieved from http:// osteomyelitis.stanford.edu

Lankshear, A., Harden, J., & Simms, J. (2010). Safe practice for patients receiving anticoagulant therapy. *Nursing Standard, 24*(20), 47–55.

Lanza, F. L., Chan, F. M., & Quigley, E. M. (2009). Practice Parameters Committee of the American College of Gastroenterology. Prevention of NSAID-Related Ulcer Complications. *American Journal of Gastroenterology, 104*(3), 728–738.

LaReau, R., Bensen, L.,Watcharotone, K., & Manguba, G. (2008). Examining the feasibility of implementing specific nursing interventions to promote sleep in hospitalized elderly patients. *Geriatric Nursing, 29*(3), 197–206.

Larsson, G. U., Johannesson, A., & Oberg, T. (2004). From major amputation to prosthetic outcome: A prospective study of 190 patients in a defined population. *Prosthetics and Orthotics International, 28*(1), 9–21.

LaSala, C. A., & Bjarnason, D. (2010). Creating workplace environments that support moral courage. *Online Journal of Issues in Nursing, 15*(3), 1–11. Retrieved from http://www.nursingworld.org/OJIN

Lazarus, R. (1985). The costs and benefits of denial. In A. Monat & R. Lazarus (Eds.), *Stress and coping: An anthology* (2nd ed.). New York, NY: Columbia University Press.

Ledford, D. K. (1998). Immunologic aspects of vasculitis and cardiovascular disease. *International Journal of Cardiology, 66*(1), 101–105.

Ledray, L. E. (2001). Evidence collection and care of the sexually assault survivor: SANE-SART response. Retrieved from www.vaw.umn.edu/documents/commissioned/2forensicvidence.htlm

Lee, I. M., Haskell, W. L., Pate, R. R., Powell, K. E., Blair, S. N., Franklin, B. A.,…Bauman, A. (2007). Physical activity and public health: Updated recommendation for adults from the American College of Sports Medicine and the American Heart Association. *Medicine and Science in Sports and Exercise, 39*(8), 1423–1434.

Lee, R. K. (2012). Compartment syndrome: A comprehensive overview. *Critical Care Nurse, 32*(1), 19–31.

Leenerts, M. H., Teel, C. S., & Pendelton, M. K. (2002). Building a model of self-care for health promotion in aging [Electronic version]. *Journal of Nursing Scholarship, 34*(4), 355–361. Retrieved from http://web.ebscohost.com/ehost/detail?vid=21&hid=106&sid=c7e5d2b4-****3-4480-a27f-fdf75c59b820%40session mgr106

Lehne, R. A. (2004). *Pharmacology for nursing care* (5th ed.). St. Louis, MO: W. B. Saunders.

Lehrner, J., Marwinski, G., Lehr, S., Johren, P., & Deecke, L. (2005). Ambient odors of orange and lavender reduce anxiety and improve mood in a dental office. *Physiology and Behaviour, 86*(1–2), 92–95.

Lemming, M. R., & Dickinson, G. E. (2010). *Understanding dying, death, and bereavement* (7th ed.). Belmont, CA: Wadsworth.

LeMone, P., Burke, K., & Bauldoff, G. (2011). *Medical-surgical nursing: Critical thinking in patient care* (5th ed.). Upper Saddle River, NJ: Pearson.

Leng, G., Fowler, B., & Ernst, E. (2000). Exercise for intermittent claudication. *Cochrane Database of Systematic Reviews.* Art. No: CD000990. doi:10.002/14651858.CD000990(2)

Leonard, M., Graham, S., & Bonacum, D. (2004). The human factor: The critical importance of effective teamwork and communication in providing safe care. *Quality and Safety in Health Care, 13*(Suppl. 1), i85–i90.

Leukemia & Lymphoma Society. (2007a). *Hairy cell leukemia.* Retrieved from http://www.leukemia-lymphoma.org/all_page?itemid=8507

Leukemia & Lymphoma Society. (2007b). *Leukemia.* Retrieved from http://www.leukemia-lymphoma.org/all_page?itemid=7026

Levin, R. F., Krainovitch, B. C., Bahrenburg, E., & Mitchell, C. A. (1989). Diagnostic content validity of nursing diagnoses. *Image: The Journal of Nursing Scholarship, 21*(1), 40–44.

Lew, D. P., & Waldvogel, F. A. (2004). Osteomyelitis. *Lancet, 364*(9431), 369–379.

Lewis, S. L., Dirksen, S. R., Heitkemper, M. M., Bucher, L., & Camera, I. M. (2011). *Medical-surgical nursing: Assessment and management of clinical problems* (8th ed.). St. Louis, MO: Elsevier.

Lewis, S. M., Heitkemper, M. M., Dirksen, S. R., O'Brien, P. G., Giddens, J. F., & Bucher, L. (2004). *Medical-surgical nursing: Assessment and management of clinical problems* (6th ed.). St. Louis, MO: Mosby.

Licker, M., de Perrot, M., Spiliopoulos, A., Robert, J., Diaper, J., Chevalley, C., & Tschopp, J. M. (2003). Risk factors for acute lung injury after thoracic surgery for lung cancer. *Anesthesia & Analgesia, 97*(6), 1558–1565.

Lieberman, P., Kemp, S. F., Oppenheimer, J., Lang, D. M., Bernstein, I. L., & Nicklas, R. A. (2005). The diagnosis and management of anaphylaxis: An updated practice parameter. *Journal of Allergy and Clinical Immunology, 115*(3), 483–523.

Liebeskind, D. A. (2013). *Hemorrhagic stroke.* Retrieved from http://emedicine.medscape.com/article/1916662-overview

Lim, W. S., van der Eerden, M. M., Laing, R., Boersma, W. G., Karalus, N., Town, G. I., . . . Macfarlane, J. T. (2003). Defining community acquired pneumonia severity on presentation to hospital: An international derivation and validation study. *Thorax, 58*(5), 377–382.

Lindqvist, O., Widmark, A., & Rasmussen, B. H. (2006). Reclaiming wellness—Living with bodily problems, as narrated by men with advanced prostate cancer. *Cancer Nursing: An International Journal for Cancer Care, 24*(9), 327–337.

Lloyd-Jones, D., Adams, R. J., Brown T. M., Carnethon, M., Dai, S., De Simone, G., . . . American Heart Association Statistics Committee and Stroke Statistics Subcommittee. (2010). Heart disease and stroke statistics—2010 update: A report from the American Heart Association. *Circulation, 126,* e46–e215.

Longino, C. F., & Kart, C. S. (1982). Explicating activity theory: A formal replication. *Journal of Gerontology, 37,* 713–722.

Lopez-Bushnell, K., Gary, G., Mitchell, P., & Reil, E. (2004). Joint replacement and case management in indigent hospitalized patients. *Orthopaedic Nursing, 23*(2), 113–117.

Lord, R., & Dayhew, J. (2001). Visual risks factors for falls in older people. *American Journal of Geriatric Society, 49,* 58–64.

Lowitz, M., & Casciato, D. (2009). *Manual of clinical oncology* (5th ed.). Philadelphia, PA: Lippincott Williams & Wilkins

Lupus Foundation of America. (2013). *What is lupus?* Retrieved from http://www.lupus.org/webmodules/webarticlesnet/templates/new_learnunderstanding.aspx?articleid=2232&zoneid=523

Lusardi, P., Jodka, P., Stambovsky, M., Stadnicki, B., Babb, B., Plouffe, D., . . . Montonye, M. (2011). The going home initiative: Getting critical care patients home with hospice. *Critical Care Nurse, 31*(5), 46–57.

Lussier-Cushing, M., Repper-Del, J., Mitchell, M. T., Lakatos, B. E., Mahoud, F., & Lipkis-Oralando, R. (2007). Is your medical/surgical patient withdrawing from alcohol? *Nursing, 37*(10), 50–55.

Lutz, C., & Przytulski, K. (2011). Nutrition and diet therapy (5th ed.). Philadelphia, PA: F. A. Davis.

Lynch, C. S., & Phillips, M. W. (1989). Nursing diagnosis: Ineffective denial. In R. M. Carroll-Johnson (Ed.), *Classification of nursing diagnosis: Proceedings of the eighth conference.* Philadelphia, PA: J. B. Lippincott.

Lynn-McHale Wiegand, D. J. (2010). *AACN procedure manual for critical care.* St. Louis, MO: Elsevier.

Maakaron, J. (2013). *Sickle cell anemia Medscape.* Retrieved from http://emedicine.medscape.com/article/205926-overview

Macdougall, I. C. (2011). Anemia. In J. T. Daugirdas (Ed.), *Handbook of chronic kidney disease management.* Philadelphia, PA: Lippincott Williams & Wilkins.

MacFie, J. (2004). Current status of bacterial translocation as a cause of surgical sepsis. *British Medical Bulletin, 71*(1), 1–11.

MacGregor, M. S., & Methven, S. (2011). Assessing kidney function. In J. T. Daugirdas (Ed.), *Handbook of chronic kidney disease management* (pp. 1–18). Philadelphia, PA: Lippincott Williams & Wilkins.

MacGregor, M. S., & Methven, S. (2011). Assessing kidney function. In J. T. Daugirdas (Ed.), *Handbook of chronic kidney disease management* (pp. 1–18). Philadelphia, PA: Lippincott Williams & Wilkins.

Mack, J. W., & Smith, T. J. (2012). Reasons why physicians do not have discussions about poor prognosis, why it matters, and what can be improved. *Journal of Clinical Oncology, 30*(22), 2715–2717.

Mackowaik, P. (2007). *Diagnosis of osteomyelitis in adults.* Retrieved from UpToDate.com

Maclean, C., Louie, R., Leake, B., McCaffery, D., Paulus, H., Brook, R., & Shekelle, P. G. (2000). Quality of care for patients with rheumatoid arthritis. *Journal of the American Medical Association, 284*(8), 984–992.

Maher, A. B., Salmond, S. W., & Pellino, T. (1998). *Orthopedic nursing* (2nd ed.). Philadelphia, PA: W. B. Saunders.

Maher, K. (2005). Radiation therapy: Toxicities and management. In C. H. Yarbro, M. H. Frogge, & M. Goodman (Eds.), *Cancer nursing: Principle and practice* (6th ed.). Boston, MA: Jones & Bartlett.

Mairis, E. (1994). Concept clarification of professional practice—Dignity. *Journal of Advanced Nursing, 19*(5), 947–953.

Maklebust, J. (1990). Assisting with adjustment following ostomy surgery. *Hospital Home Health, 7*(7), 91–94.

Maklebust, J., & Sieggreen, M. (2001). *Pressure ulcers: Guidelines for prevention and nursing management* (3rd ed.). West Dundee, IL: SN Publications.

Maliski, S., Heilemann, M. S., & McCorkle, R. (2001). Mastery of postprostatectomy incontinence and impotence: His work, her work, our work. *Oncology Nursing Forum, 28*(6), 985–992.

Mallinson, R. K. (1999). The lived experience of AIDS-related multiple losses by HIV-negative gay men. *Journal of Association of Nurses in AIDS Care, 10*(5), 22–31.

Maloni, H. (2012). Pain in multiple sclerosis clinical bulletin information for health professionals. Retrieved from http://www.nationalmssociety.org/ms-clinical-care-network/clinical-resources-and-tools/pub

Maltoni, M., Scarpi, E., Rosati, M., Derni, S., & Fabbri, L. (2012). Palliative sedation in end-of-life care and survival: A systematic review. *Journal of Clinical Oncology, 30*(12), 1378–1383.

Manack, A., Motsko, S. P., Haag-molkenteller, C., Dmochowski, R. R., Goehring, E. L. Jr., Nguyen-Khoa, B. A., & Jones, J. K. (2011). Epidemiology and healthcare utilization of neurogenic bladder patients in a U.S. claims database. *Neurourology and Urodynamics, 30*(3), 395–401. doi:10.1002/nau.21003

Marchiondo, K., & Thompson, A. (1996). Pain management in sickle cell disease. *MEDSURG Nursing, 5*(1), 29–33.

Margaretten, M., Kohlwes, J., Moore, D., & Bent, S. (2007). Synovial lactic acid and septic arthritis. *Journal of the American Medical Association, 298*(1), 40.

Marinell, M. A. (2008). Refeeding syndrome in cancer patients. *International Journal of Clinical Practice, 62*(3), 460–465.

Marshall, K. (2011). Acute coronary syndrome: Diagnosis, risk assessment and management. *Nursing Standard, 25*(23), 47–57.

Martin, C. G., & Turkelson, S. L. (2006). Nursing care of the patient undergoing coronary artery bypass grafting. *Journal of Cardiovascular Nursing, 21*(2), 109–117.

Massey, R., & Jedlicka, D. (2002). The Massey bedside swallowing screen. *Journal of Neuroscience Nursing, 34,* 252–253, 257–260.

Massó González, E. L., Patrignani, P., Tacconelli, S., & García Rodríguez, L. A. (2010). Variability among nonsteroidal antiinflammatory drugs in risk of upper gastrointestinal bleeding. *Arthritis & Rheumatism, 62*(6), 1592–1601. doi:10.1002/art.27412

Mathew, J. P., Fontes, M. L., Tudor, I. C., Ramsay, J., Duke, P., Mazer, C. D., . . . Mangano, D. T. (2004). Multicenter Study of Perioperative Ischemia Research Group. *JAMA, 291*(14), 1720–1729.

Matsuda, P. N., Shumway-Cook, A., Ciol, M. A., Bombardier, C. H., & Kartin, D. A. (2012). Understanding falls in multiple sclerosis: Association of mobility status, concerns about falling, and accumulated impairments. *Physical Therapy, 92*(3), 407–415.

Mattar, K., & Finelli, A. (2007). Expanding the indications of laparoscopic radical nephrectomy [Electronic version]. *Current Opinion in Urology, 17*(2), 88–92. Retrieved from http://www.kidney.org

Matzo, M., & Sherman, D. (Eds.), *Palliative care nursing: Quality care to the end of life* (3rd ed.). New York, NY: Springer.

Mauer, K. A., Abrahams, E. B., Arslanian, C., Schoenly, L., & Taggart, H. M. (2002). National practice patterns for the care of the patient with total joint replacement. *Orthopedic Nursing, 21*(3), 37–47.

Mauk, K. L., & Schmidt, N. A. (2004). *Spiritual care in nursing practice.* Philadelphia, PA: Lippincott Williams & Wilkins.

Mayor, S. (2007). Breathing and relaxation technique cut asthma symptoms by one third. *British Medical Journal, 335*(7611), 119.

McCafferty, M. (2003). *Pain: Clinical manual for nursing practice.* St. Louis, MO: Mosby.

McCafferty, M., & Pasero, C. (2011). *Pain assessment and pharmacological management.* New York, NY: Mosby.

McClave, S. A., DeMeo, M. T., DeLegge, M. H., DiSario, J. A., Heyland, D. K., Maloney, J. P., . . . Zaloga, G. P. (2002). North American Summit on Aspiration in the Critically Ill Patient: Consensus statement. *Journal of Parenteral and Enteral Nutrition, 26*(6 Suppl.), S80–S85.

McCullough, J., & Ownby, D. (1993). A comparison of three in vitro tests for latex specific IgE [Abstract]. *J Allergy Clin Immunol* 91(1993): 242.

McDermott, M. M., Mehta, S., & Greenland, P. (1999). Exertional leg symptoms other than intermittent claudication are common in peripheral arterial disease. *Archives of Internal Medicine, 159*(4), 387–392.

McDermott, M. M., Tiukinhoy, S., Greenland, P., Liu, K., Pearce, W. H., Guralnik, J. M., . . . Ferrucci, L. (2004). A pilot exercise intervention to improve lower extremity functioning in peripheral arterial disease unaccompanied by intermittent claudication. *Journal of Cardiopulmonary Rehabilitation, 24*(3), 187–196.

McGrory, B., Callaghan, J., Kraay, M., Jacobs, J., Robb, W., Brand, R. A., & Wasielewski, R. (2005). Editorial: Minimally invasive and small-incision joint replacement surgery—What surgeons should you consider. *Clinical Orthopaedics and Related Research, 440,* 251–254.

McGuire, D., Sheidler, V., & Polomano, R. C. (2000). Pain. In S. Groenwald, M. Frogge, M. Goodman, & C. Yarbo (Eds.), *Cancer nursing: Principles and practice* (5th ed.). Boston, MA: Jones and Bartlett.

McKinley, M. (2005). Alcohol withdrawal syndrome: Overlooked and mismanaged? *Critical Care Nurse, 25*(3), 40–49.

McMenamin, E. (2011). Pain management principles. *Current Problems in Cancer, 35*(6), 317–323.

McQuellon, R. P., Wells, M., Hoffman, S., Craven, B., Russell, G., Cruz, J., . . . Savage, P. (1998). Reducing distress in cancer patients with an orientation program. *Psycho-Oncology, 7*(3), 207–217.

Menon, M., Shrivastava, A., Kaul, S., Badani, K. K., Bhandani, M., & Peabody, J. O. (2007). Vattikuti Institute prostatectomy: Contemporary technique and analysis of results. *European Urology, 51*(3), 648–657.

Mercadante, S., Intravaia, G., Villari, P., Ferrera, P., David, F., & Casuccio, A. (2009). Controlled sedation for refractory symptoms in dying patients. *Journal of Pain Symptom Management, 37*(5), 771–779.

Mercandetti, M. (2013). *Wound healing and repair.* Retrieved from http://emedicine.medscape.com/article/1298129-overview#aw2aab6b5

Merck Manual Online Library. (2005). *Osteomyelitis.* Retrieved from http://www.merck.com/mmpe/sec04/ch039/ch039d.html

Metheny, N. A., Mueller, C., Robbins, S., Wessel, J., & the A.S.P.E.N. Board of Directors. (2009). A.S.P.E.N. Enteral Nutrition Practice Recommendations. *Journal of Parenteral Enteral Nutrition, 33*(2), 122–167.

Meurman, J., Odont, D., Sorvari, R., Pelttari, A., Rytömaa, I., Odont, R., . . . Kroon, L. (1996). Hospital mouth-cleaning aids may cause dental erosion. *Special Care in Dentistry, 16*(6), 247–250.

Miller, C. A. (2009). *Nursing care of older adults* (5th ed.). Philadelphia, PA: Lippincott Williams & Wilkins.

Miller, C. A. (2013). *Nursing care of older adults* (6th ed.). Philadelphia, PA: Lippincott Williams & Wilkins.

Miller, E., Murray, L., Richards, L., Zorowitz, R., Bakas, T., Clark, P., & Billinger, S. (2010). Comprehensive overview of nursing and interdisciplinary rehabilitation care of the stroke patient: A scientific statement from the American Heart Association. *Stroke, 41,* 2402–2448.

Miller, J., & Mink, J. (2009). Acute ischemic stroke: Not a moment to lose. *Nursing2009, 39*(5), 37–42.

Miller, M., & Kearney, N. (2004). Chemotherapy-related nausea and vomiting—past reflections, present practice and future management. *European Journal of Cancer Care (England), 13*(1), 71–81.

Miller, N. C., & Askew, A. E. (2007). Tibia fractures: An overview of evaluation and treatment. *Orthopaedic Nursing, 26*(4), 216–223.

Miller, N., Allcock, L., Hildreth, A. J., Jones, D., Noble, E., & Burn, D. J. (2009). Swallowing problems in Parkinson disease: Frequency and clinical correlates. *Journal of Neurological Neurosurgical Psychiatry, 80*(9), 1047–1049.

Mink, J., & Miller, J. (2011). Opening the window of opportunity. *Nursing2011, 41*(1), 24–33.

Minkes, R. (2013). *Stomas of the small and large intestine treatment & management.* Retrieved from http://emedicine.medscape.com/article/939455-treatment#a17

Mitchell, A. J. (2007). Pooled results from 38 analyses of the accuracy of distress thermometer and other ultra-short methods of detecting cancer-related mood disorder. *Journal of Clinical Oncology, 25*, 4670–4681.

Mitchell, M., Mohler, E., & Carpenter, J. (2007). *Acute arterial occlusion of the lower extremity*. Retrieved from UpTo-Date.com

Miura, H. (2012). An exercise program for improving and/or maintaining arterial function in middle-aged to older individuals. *Advanced Exercise Sports Physiology, 18*(3), 47–51.

Mokdad, A., Balluz, L. S., & Okoro, C. A. (2008). Association between selected unhealthy lifestyle factors, body mass index, and chronic health conditions among individuals 50 years of age or older, by race/ethnicity. *Ethnicity and Disease, 18*(4), 450–457.

Montgomery, G. H., & Bowbjerg, D. H. (2004). Presurgery distress and specific response expectations predict postsurgery outcomes in surgery patients confronting breast cancer. *Health Psychology, 270*, 825–827.

More, K. N., Truong, V., Estey, E., & Voaklander, D. C. (2007). Urinary incontinence after prostatectomy: Can men at risk be indentified preoperatively? *Journal of Wound, Ostomy and Continence, 34*(3), 270–279; quiz 280–281.

Morse, J. (2007). Enhancing the safety of hospitalization by reducing patient falls. *American Journal of Infection Control, 30*, 376–380.

Morton, K., & Gambier, E. (2000). Guidelines for prescribing nutritional supplements in primary care. Retrieved from http://www.bolton.nhs.uk/Library/Leaflets/patient/nutrition/guidelines.pdf

Mueller, A. C., & Bell, A. E. (2008). Electrolye update: Potassium, chloride, and magnesium. *Nursing Critical Care, 3*(1), 5–7.

Mukherjee, D. (2003). Perioperative cardiac assessment for noncardiac surgery: Eight steps to the best possible outcome. *Circulation, 107*, 2771–2774. doi: 10.1161/Circulation. 107: 2771-2774 /.

Mulhauser, G. (2007). *Welcome to the CAGE questionnaire, a screening test for alcohol dependence*. Retrieved from http://counsellingresource.com/quizzes/alcohol-cage/index.html

Munoz, A., & Katerndahl, D. (2000). Diagnosis and management of acute pancreatitis. *American Family Physician, 62*(1), 164–174.

Murphy, S. A. (1993). Coping strategies of abstainer from alcohol up to three years post-treatment. *Image: Journal of Nursing Scholarship, 25*(2), 87.

Murray, J. (2001). Loss as a universal concept: A review of the literature to identify common aspects of loss in diverse situations. *Journal of Loss and Trauma: International Perspectives on Stress & Coping, 6*(3).

Murray, R. B., Zentner, J. P., & Yakimo, R. (2009). *Health promotion strategies through the life span* (8th ed.). Upper Saddle River, NJ: Pearson Prentice Hall.

Murray, S. A., Boyd, K., & Sheikh, A. (2005). Palliative care in chronic illness. *British Medical Journal, 330*(7492), 611–612.

Mutlu, G., & Mutlu, E., & Factor, P. (2001). GI complications in patients receiving mechanical ventilation. *CHEST, 119*(4). Retrieved from http://journal.publications.chestnet.org/data/Journals/CHEST/21961/1222.pdf

Myasthenia Gravis Foundation of America. (2010). *Myasthnai gravis: A manual for health care providers*. New York, NY: MGFA.

Myasthenia Gravis Foundation of America. (2010). *Ocular myasthenia gravis* [Brochure]. New York, NY: Author.

Nation Stroke Association. (2013). Recovery & rehabilitation. Retrieved from http://www.stroke.org/site/PageServer?pagename=rehabt

National Cancer Institute. (2003b). *Types of leukemia*. Retrieved from http://www.cancer.gov/cancertopics/wyntk/leukemia/page5

National Cancer Institute. (2007). *Lymphedema management*. Retrieved from http://www.cancer.gov/cancertopics/pdq/supportivecare/lymphedema/HealthProfessional/page2

National Cancer Institute. (2008). *Support and resources*. Retrieved from http://www.cancer.gov/cancertopics/support

National Cancer Institute. (2010). *Palliative care in cancer*. Retrieved from http://www.cancer.gov/cancertopics/factsheet/Support/palliative-care

National Cancer Institute. (2013). *Adjustment to cancer: Anxiety and distress (PDQ®)* [Comprehensive cancer information]. Bethesda, MD: Author. Retrieved from http://www.cancer.gov/cancertopics/pdq/supportivecare/adjustment/HealthProfessional/page3#Reference3.3

National Cholesterol Education Program. (2004). *Third Report of the National Cholesterol Education Program (NCEP)*. Expert Panel on Detection, Evaluation and Treatment of High Blood Cholesterol in Adults (Adult Treatment Panel III). Retrieved from National http://www.scymed.com/en/smnxdj/edzr/edzr9610.htm

National Comprehensive Cancer Network. (2008). Oral mucositis is often underrecognized and undertreated. Retrieved from http://bestpractice.bmj.com/best-practice/monograph/1135/treatment/guidelines.html

National Digestive Diseases Information Clearinghouse. (n.d.). *Viral gastroenteritis*. Retrieved from http://digestive.niddk.nih.gov/ddiseases/pubs/viralgastroenteritis/

National Guideline Clearinghouse. (2009). Guideline for prevention of catheter-associated urinary tract infections. Retrieved from guideline.gov/content.aspx?id=15519

National Institute of Arthritis and Musculoskeletal and Skin Diseases. (2003). *Lupus*. Retrieved from http://www.niams.nih.gov/Health_Info/Lupus/default.asp

National Institute of Arthritis and Musculoskeletal and Skin Diseases. (2008). *Health information page*. Retrieved from http://www.naims.nih.gov/Health_Info/Fibromyalgia/fibrmyalgia_ff.asp

National Institute of Health. (2012). *Urostomy and continent urinary diversion.* Retrieved from http://kidney.niddk.nih.gov/kudiseases/pubs/urostomy/

National Institute of Health. (2013). *Parkinson's disease.* Retrieved from http://www.nlm.nih.gov/medlineplus/parkinsonsdisease.html

National Institute of Neurological Disorders and Stroke. (2007). *Multiple sclerosis.* Retrieved from http://www.commondataelements.ninds.nih.gov/ms.aspx#tab=Data_Standards

National Institute of Neurological Disorders and Stroke. (2011, August 19). *Guillain-Barre syndrome fact sheet.* Retrieved from http://www.ninds.nih.gov/disorders/gbs/detail_gbs.htm

National Institutes of Health. (2007). *Asthma action plan.* Retrieved from http://www.nhlbi.nih.gov/health/public/lung/asthma/asthma_actplan.pdf

National Kidney Foundation. (2007). *Facts about chronic kidney disease.* Retrieved from www.kidney.org

National Library of Medicine. (2006). *Leukemia.* Retrieved from http://www.nlm.nih.gov/medlineplus/tutorials/leukemia/htm/index.htm

National Pressure Ulcer Advisory Panel, European Pressure Ulcer Advisory Panel. (2007). Pressure ulcer stages/categories. Retrieved from http://www.npuap.org/resources/educational-and-clinical-resources/npuap-pressure-ulcer-stagescategories/

National Pressure Ulcer Advisory Panel, European Pressure Ulcer Advisory Panel. (2009). Pressure ulcer prevention recommendations (pp. 21–50). In *Prevention and treatment of pressure ulcers: Clinical practice guideline.* Washington, DC: National Pressure Ulcer Advisory Panel.

National Pressure Ulcer Advisory Panel. (2007). *Pressure ulcer category/staging illustrations.* Retrieved from http://www.npuap.org/resources/educational-and-clinical-resources/pressure-ulcer-categorystaging-illustrations/

National Spinal Cord Injury Association. (2007). Retrieved from http://www.spinalcord.org

National Stroke Association. (2013). *Stroke 101 and prevention.* Retrieved from http://www.stroke.org/site/PageServer?pagename=factsheets

NCCN Clinical Practice Guidelines in Oncology. (2013). *NCCN – Evidence-based cancer guidelines, oncology drug compendium, oncology continuing medical education: Distress management.* Retrieved from http://www.nccn.org

Nead, K. G., Halterman, J. S., Kaczorowski, J. M., Auinger, P., & Weitzman, M. (2004). Overweight children and adolescents: A risk group for iron deficiency. *Pediatrics, 114,* 104–108.

Nelson, K. A., Walsh, D., Behrens, C., Zhukovsky, D. S., Lipnickey, V., & Brady, D. (2000). The dying cancer patient. *Seminars in Oncology, 27*(1), 84–89.

NeSmith, E., Weinrich, S., Andrews, J., Medeiros, S., Hawkins, M., & Weinrich, M. (2009). Systemic inflammatory response syndrome score and race as predictors of length of stay in the intensive care unit. *American Journal of Critical Care, 18*(4), 339–345.

Ness, J., Aronow, W. S., Newkirk, E., & McDanel, D. (2005). Prevalence of symptomatic peripheral arterial disease, modifiable risk factors, and appropriate use of drugs in the treatment of peripheral arterial disease in older persons seen in a university general medicine clinic. *Journals of Gerontology Series A: Biological Sciences and Medical Sciences, 60*(2), 255–257.

Nettina, S. M. (2006). *Lippincott manual of nursing practice* (8th ed.). Ambler, PA: Lippincott Williams & Wilkins.

Neubauer, A. C., & Fink, A. (2009). Intelligence and neural efficiency. *Neuroscience and Biobehavioral Reviews, 33,* 1004–1023.

Newcombe, P. (2002). Pathophysiology of sickle cell disease crisis. *Emergency Nurse, 9*(9), 9–22.

Newman, D. K. (2005, June). Urinary incontinence and indwelling catheters: CMS guidance for long-term care. *ECPN,* 50–56. Retrieved from http://www.health.state.mn.us/divs/fpc/profinfo/urinconcath/p50_54_ecpn06_newmance.pdf

Newman, D. K., & Willson, M. M. (2011). Review of intermittent catheterization and current best practices. *Urologic Nursing, 31*(1), 12–28, 48; quiz 29.

Newman, D., & Willson, M. (2011). Review of intermittent catheterization and current best practices. *Urologic Nursing, 31*(1), 1–19.

Newswanger, D. L., & Warren, C. R. (2004). Guillain-Barre syndrome. *American Family Physician, 69*(10), 2405–2410.

Ng, B. L., & Anpalahan, M. (2011). Management of chronic kidney disease in the elderly. *Internal Medicine Journal, 41*(11), 761–768.

Nguyen, T., Gwynn, R., Kellerman, S., Begier, E., Garg, R., Konty, K., . . . Thorpe, L. (2008). Population prevalence of reported and unreported HIV and related behaviors among the household adult population in New York City, 2004. *AIDS: Official Journal of the International AIDS Society, 22*(2), 281–287.

Nichols, R. I. (1991). Surgical wound infections. *American Journal of Medicine, 91*(Suppl. 3B), 54–64.

Nickloes, T. A. (2012). *Superior vena cava syndrome treatment & management.* Retrieved from http://emedicine.medscape.com/article/460865-treatment

Nighorn, S. (1988). Narcissistic deficits in drug abusers: A self-psychological approach. *Journal of Psychosocial Nursing & Mental Health Services, 26*(9), 22–26.

Norton, B., Homer-Ward, M., Donnelly, M. T., Long, R. G., & Holmes, G. K. (1996). A randomized prospective comparison of percutaneous endoscopic gastrostomy and nasogastric tube feeding after acute dysphagic stroke. *BMJ, 3*(12), 13–16.

Nostrant , T. T. (2012). *Clinical features, diagnosis, and treatment of radiation proctitis.* In L. Friedman & C. Willett (Eds.), *UpToDate.* Retrieved from http://www.uptodateonline.com

Nucifora, G., Hysko, F., Vit, A., & Vasciaveo, A. (2007). Pulmonary fat embolism: Common and unusual computed tomography findings. *Journal of Computer Assisted Tomography, 31*(5), 806–807.

O'Brien, M. E. (2010). *Spirituality in nursing: Standing on holy ground* (4th ed.). Boston, MA: Jones and Bartlett.

O'Donnell, P. (2012). *Impending fracture & prophylactic fixation.* Retrieved from http://www.orthobullets.com/pathology/8002/impending-fracture-and-prophylactic-fixation

O'Mallon, M. (2009). Vulnerable populations: Exploring a family perspective of grief. *Journal of Hospice & Palliative Nursing, 11*(2), 91–98.

Oka, R. K. (2006). Peripheral arterial disease in older adults: Management of cardiovascular disease risk factors. *Journal of Cardiovascular Nursing, 21*(5) supplement, S15–S20.

Olek, M. J. (2007a). *Comorbid problems associated with multiple sclerosis in adults.* Retrieved from UpToDate.com

Olek, M. J. (2007b). *Diagnosis of multiple sclerosis in adults.* Retrieved from UpToDate.com

Olek, M. J. (2007c). *Epidemiology, risk factors, and clinical features of multiple sclerosis in adults.* Retrieved from UpToDate.com

Olek, M. J. (2007d). *Treatment of progressive multiple sclerosis in adults.* Retrieved from UpToDate.com

Oliveira-Filho, J., & Koroshetz, W. J. (2007). *Initial assessment and management of acute stroke.* Retrieved from UpToDate.com

Oliver, M. J. (2007). *Chronic hemodialysis vascular access: Types and placement.* Retrieved from www.UpToDate.com

Oncology Nursing Society. (2007). *Mucositis: What interventions are effective for managing oral mucositis in people receiving treatment for cancer* [ONS PEP Cards]. Pittsburgh, PA: Author.

Onizuka, Y., Mizuta, Y., Isomoto, H., Takeshima, F., Murase, K., Miyazaki, M., ... Kohno, S. (2001). Sludge and stone formation in the gallbladder in bedridden elderly patients with cerebrovascular disease: Influence of feeding method [Electronic version]. *Journal of Gastroenterology, 36*(5), 330–337. Retrieved from http://web.ebscohost.com/ehost/pdf?vid=132&hid=106&sid=c7e5d2b4-a****3-4480-a27f-fdf75c59b820%40session mgr106

Osborn, K. S., Wraa, C. E., & Watson, A. (2010). *Medical-surgical nursing: Preparation for practice.* Upper Saddle River, NJ: Pearson.

Osinbowale, O. O., & Milani, R. V. (2011). Benefits of exercise therapy in peripheral arterial disease. *Progress in Cardiovascular Diseases, 53*(6), 447–453.

Oxman, A. D., Lavis, J. N., Lewin, S., & Fretheim, A. (2009). SUPPORT Tools for evidence-informed health Policymaking (STP) 10: Taking equity into consideration when assessing the findings of a systematic review. *Health Research Policy and Systems, 7*(S1), S10.

Pace, R. C. (2007). Fluid management in patients on hemodialysis. *Nephrology Nursing Journal, 34*(5), 557–559.

Pajeau, A. (2002). Identifying patients at high risk of ischemic stroke. *Patient Care, 36*(5), 36–51.

Paparella, P., Sizzi, O., De Benedittis, F., Rossetti, A., & Paparella, R. (2004). Vaginal hysterectomy in generally considered contraindications to vaginal surgery. *Archives of Gynecological Obstetrics, 270*(2), 104–109.

Parekattil, S. J., Gill, I. S., Castle, E. P., Burgess, S. V., Walls, M. M., Thomas, R.,...Andrews, P. E. (2005). Multi-institutional validation study of neural networks to predict duration of stay after laparoscopic radical/simple or partial nephrectomy. *Journal of Urology, 174*(4 Pt. 1), 1380–1384.

Parikh, S., Koch, M., & Narayan, R. (2007). Traumatic brain injury. *International Anesthesiology Clinics, 45*(3), 119–135.

Park, J. J., Del Pino, A., Orsay, C. P., Nelson, R. L., Pearl, R. K., Cintron, J. R., & Abcarian, H. (1999). Stoma complications: The Cook County Hospital experience. *Diseases of the Colon and Rectum, 42*, 1575–1580.

Park, R. H. R., Allison, M. C., Lang, J., Spence, E., Morris, A. J., Danesh, B. J., . . . Mills, P. R. (1992). Randomised comparison of percutaneous endoscopic gastrostomy and nasogastric tube feeding in patients with persisting neurological dysphagia. *BMJ, 304*, 1406–1409. doi:10.2337/dc09-1748

Parker-Frizzell, J. (2005). Acute stroke. *AACN Clinical Issues, 16*(4), 421–440.

Parkinson's Disease Foundation. (2007). *Parkinson's disease: An overview. What is Parkinson's disease?* Retrieved from http://www.pdf.org/AboutPD

Pasacreta, J. V., & Massie, M. J. (1990). Nurses' reports of psychiatric complications in patients with cancer. *Oncology Nursing Forum, 17*(3), 347–353.

Pasacreta, J. V., Kenefick, A. L., & McCorkle, R. (2008). Managing distress in oncology patients. *Cancer Nursing, 31*(6), 485–490.

Pasero, C., & McCaffery, M. (2004). Comfort–function goals: A way to establish accountability for pain relief. *American Journal of Nursing, 104*(9), 77–81.

Pasero, C., & McCaffery, M. (2011). *Pain assessment and pharmaceutical management.* New York, NY: Mosby.

Pasero, C., Paice, J., & McCaffery, M. (2004). Basic mechanisms underlying the causes and effects of pain. In M. McCaffery & C. Pasero (Eds.), *Clinical pain manual* (pp. 15–34). New York, NY: Mosby.

Pasquel, F., Spiegelman, R., Smiley, D., Umpierrez, D., Johnson, R., . . . Umpierrez, G. (2010). Hyperglycemia during total parenteral nutrition. *Diabetes Care, 33*(4), 739–741.

Patel, A., Lall, C. G., Jennings, S. G., & Sandrasegaran, K. (2007). Abdominal compartment syndrome. *American Journal of Roentgenology, 189*, 1037–1043.

Pearce, H. (2011). *Abdominal aortic aneurysms*. Retrieved from http://emedicine.medscape.com/article/1979501-overview#aw2aab6b2b7aa

Pearce, J. M. (2007). Documenting peritoneal dialysis. *Nursing 2007, 37*(10), 28.

Pearson, L., & Hutton, J. (2002). A controlled trial to compare the ability of foam swabs and toothbrushes to remove dental plaque. *Journal of Advanced Nursing, 39*(5), 480–489.

Pellino, T., Polacek, L. P., Preston, A., Bell, N., & Evans, R. (1998). Complications of orthopedic disorders and orthopedic surgery. In A. Maher, S. Salomond, & T. Pellino (Eds.), *Orthopaedic nursing* (2nd ed.). Philadelphia, PA: W. B. Saunders.

Pennsylvania Patient Safety Advisory. (2012). Analysis of the multiple risks involving the use of IV Fentanyl. *Pennsylvania Patient Safety Advisory, 9*(4), 122–129.

Pepys, M. B., & Hirschfield, G. M. (2003, June). C-reactive protein: A critical update. *Journal of Clinical Investigation, 111*(12), 1805–1812.

Pereira, J. de M. V., Cavalcanti, A. C. D., Santana, R. F., Cassiano, K. M., Queluci, G. de C., & Guimarães, T. C. F. (2011). Nursing diagnoses for inpatients with cardiovascular diseases. *Escola Anna Nery [online], 15*(4)737–745.

Peripheral artery disease. This increasingly common disorder often goes undetected in women until serious problems arise. *Harvard Women's Health Watch, 19*(8), 4–6.

Perry, D., Borchert, K., Burke, S., Chick, K., Johnson, K., Kraft, W., . . . Thompson, S. (2012). Institute for Clinical Systems Improvement. Pressure Ulcer Prevention and Treatment Protocol. Retrieved from https://www.icsi.org/_asset/6t7kxy/

Persson, E., & Hellström, A. L. (2002). Experiences of Swedish men and women 6 to 12 weeks after ostomy surgery. *Journal of Wound Ostomy and Continence Nursing 29*(2), 103–108.

Persson, E., & Larsson, B. (2005). Quality of care after ostomy surgery: A perspective study of patients. *Ostomy Wound Management, 51*(8), 40–48.

Petterson, R., Haig, Y., Nakstad, P. H., & Wyller, T. B. (2008). Subtypes of urinary incontinence after stroke: Relation to size and location of cerebrovascular damage. *Age and Ageing, 37*(3), 324–327.

Pezzilli, R., Corinaldesi, R., & Morselli-Labate, A. (2010). Pancreatic cancer and cancer screening programs: From nihilism to hope. *Journal of the Pancreas, 11*, 654–645.

Philbin, T. M., DeLuccia, D. M., Nitsch, R. F., & Maurus, P. B. (2007). Syme amputation and prosthetic fitting challenges. *Techniques in Foot and Ankle Surgery, 6*, 147–155.

Piasecki, P. A. (2000). Bone and soft tissue sarcoma. In S. Groenwald, M. Frogge, M. Goodman, & C. Yarbro (Eds.), *Cancer nursing: Principles and practice* (5th ed.). Boston, MA: Jones and Bartlett.

Picard, K., Donoghue, S., Young-Kershaw, D., & Russell, K. (2006). Development and implementation of a multidisciplinary sepsis protocol. *Critical care nurse, 26*(3), 42–54.

Pieper, B., & Mikols, C. (1996). Predischarge and postdischarge concerns of persons with an ostomy. *Journal of WOCN, 23*(2), 105–109.

Piette, J. D. (2005). *Using telephone support to manage chronic disease*. Retrieved from http://www.chef.org/topics/chronicdisease/index.cfm

Pike, N. A., & Gundry, S. R. (2003). Robotically assisted cardiac: Minimally invasive technology to totally endoscopic heart surgery. *Journal of Cardiovascular Nursing, 18*(5), 238–388.

Pillitteri, A. (2010). *Maternal and child health nursing* (6th ed.). Philadelphia, PA: Lippincott Williams & Wilkins.

Podsiadlo, D., & Richardson, S. (1991). The timed "Up and Go" test: A test of basic functional mobility for frail elderly persons. *Journal of American Geriatric Society, 39*, 142–148. Retrieved from www.fallrventiontaskforce.orgpdf.Timed UpandGoTest.pdf

Pollack, A. (2010). *Radiation therapy for prostate cancer*. Retrieved from http://www.whcenter.org/documents/CME/prostatecancer/RadiationTherapyIMRT_IGRTAlanPollack.pdf

Ponferrada, L. P., & Prowant, B. F. (2008). Peritoneal dialysis: Peritoneal dialysis therapy. In C. S. Counts (Ed.), *Core curriculum for nephrology nursing* (5th ed.). Pitman, NJ: American Nephrology Nurses' Association.

Pontieri-Lewis, V. (2006). Basics of ostomy care. *Medical and Surgical Nursing, 15*(4), 199–202.

Porth, C. M. (Ed.). (2009). *Pathophysiology: Concepts of altered health states* (8th ed.). Philadelphia, PA: Lippincott Williams & Wilkins.

Porth, C. M. (Ed.). (2011). *Essentials of Pathophysiology: Concepts of altered health states* (3rd ed.). Philadelphia, PA: Lippincott Williams & Wilkins.

Powell-Cope, G., & Brown, M. A. (1992). Going public as an AIDS family caregiver. *Social Science & Medicine, 34*(5), 571–580.

Price, C. S., Williams, A., Philips, G., Dayton, M., Smith, W., & Morgan, S. (2008). *Staphylococcus aureus* nasal colonization in preoperative orthopaedic outpatients. *Clinical Orthopedic Related Research, 466*(11), 2842–2847.

Prommer, E. (2009). Talking with cancer patients and their families. In D. A. Casciato, & M. C. Territo (Eds.), *Manual of clinical oncology* (6th ed.). Philadelphia, PA: Lippincott Williams & Wilkins.

Prowant, B. F. (2008). Peritoneal dialysis: Peritoneal dialysis access. In C. S. Counts (Ed.), *Core curriculum for nephrology nursing* (5th ed.). Pitman, NJ: American Nephrology Nurses' Association.

Puchalski, C. M., & Ferrell, B. (2010). *Making health care whole: Integrating spirituality into patient care*. West Conshohocken, PA: Templeton Press.

Puchalski, C. M., & McSkimming, S. (2006). Creating healing environments. *Health Progress, 87*(3), 30–35.

Pugh, S., Mathiesen, C., Meighan, M., Summers, D., & Zrelak, P. (2009). *Guide to the care of the hospitalized patient with ischemic stroke* (AANN Clinical Practice Guideline Series, 2nd ed.). Retrieved from www.aann.org/pdf/cpg/aannischemicstroke.pdf

Pullen, R. (2007). Replacing a urostomy drainage pouch. *Nursing, 37*(6), 14.

Purkayastha, S., Zhang, G., & Cai, D. (2011). Uncoupling the mechanisms of obesity and hypertension by targeting hypothalamic IKK-β and NF-B. *National Medicine, 17*(7), 883–887. doi: 10.1038/nm.2372

Rackley, R. (2011, November). *Neurogenic bladder*. Retrieved from http://emedicine.medscape.com/article/453539-overview#a30

Raghavan, V. A., & Hamdy, O. (2012). *Diabetic ketoacidosis treatment & management.* Retrieved from http://emedicine.medscape.com/article/118361-treatment

Rando, T. A. (1984). *Grief, dying, and death: Clinical interventions for caregivers.* Champaign, IL: Research Press.

Rangel-Castillo, L., Gopinath, S., & Robertson, C. S. (2008). Management of intracranial hypertension. *Neurologic Clinics, 26,* 521–541.

Rangel-Castillo, L., Gopinath, S., & Robertson, C. S. (2008). Management of Intracranial Hypertension. *Neurologic Clinics, 26*(2), 521–541. Retrieved from http://www.ncbi.nlm.nih.gov/pmc/articles/PMC2452989/

Ray, R. I. (2000). Complications of lower extremity amputations. *Topics in Emergency Medicine, 22*(3), 35–42.

Registered Nurses' Association of Ontario. (2005, March). *Risk assessment and prevention of pressure ulcers.* Toronto, Ontario, Canada: Author.

Registered Nurses' Association of Ontario. (2009). *Ostomy care and management.* Toronto, Ontario, Canada: Author.

Richardson, C., Glenn, S., Nurmikko, T., & Horgan, M. (2006). Incidence of phantom phenomena including phantom limb pain 6 months after major lower limb amputation in patients with peripheral vascular disease. *Journal: Clinical Journal of Pain 22*(4), 353–358.

Richbourg, L., Thorpe, J. M., & Rapp, C. G. (2007). Difficulties experienced by the ostomate after hospital discharge. *Journal of Wound, Ostomy and Continence Nursing, 34*(1), 70–79.

Riefkohl, E. Z., Heather, L., Bieber, H. L., Burlingame, M. B., & Lowenthal, D. T. (2003). Medications and falls in the elderly: A review of the evidence and practical considerations. *Pharmacy & Therapeutics, 28*(11), 724–733.

Rigdon, J. L. (2006). Robotic-assisted laparoscopic radical prostatectomy. *AORN, 84*(5), 759–762, 764, 766–770.

Rindfleisch, J., & Muller, D. (2005). Diagnosis and management of rheumatoid arthritis. *American Family Physician, 72*(6), 1037–1047.

Roberts, I. (2012). Diagnosis and management of chronic radiation enteritis. Retrieved from http://www.aboutcancer.com/radiation_enteritis_utd_807.htm

Robinson, A. (2008). Review article: Improving adherence to medication in patients with inflammatory bowel disease. *Alimentary Pharmacology & Therapeutics, 27,* 9–14.

Rockman, C. B., Cappadona, C., Riles, T. S., Lamparello, P. J., Giangola, G., Adelman, M. A., & Landis, R. (1997). Causes of the increased stroke rate after carotid endarterectomy in patients with previous strokes. *Annals of Vascular Surgery, 11*(1), 28–34.

Roe, B., Flanagan, L. B., Barrett, J., Chung, A., Shaw, C., & Williams, K. (2011). Systematic review of the management of incontinence and promotion of continence in older people in care homes: Descriptive studies with urinary incontinence as primary focus. *Journal of Advanced Nursing, 67*(2), 228–250.

Roger, V. L., Go, A. S., Lloyd-Jones, D. M., Benjamin, E. J., Berry, J. D., Borden, W. B., . . . American Heart Association Statistics Committee and Stroke Statistics Subcommittee. (2012). Heart disease and stroke statistics—2012 update: A report from the American Heart Association. *Circulation, 125*(1), e2–220.

Rogers, B. (2005). Looking at lymphoma and leukemia. *Nursing 2005, 35*(7), 56–64.

Rolim de Moura, C., Paranhos, A., Jr., & Wormald, R. (2007). Laser trabeculoplasty for open angle glaucoma [Systematic Review]. *Cochrane Database of Systematic Reviews,* (4). doi:10.1002/14651858.CD003919.pub2

Rollnick, S., Mason, P., & Butler, C. (2000). *Health behavior change: A guide for practitioners.* Edinburgh, UK: Churchill Livingstone.

Roman, M., Weinstein, A., & Macaluso, S. (2003). Primary spontaneous pneumothorax. *Medical and Surgical Nursing, 12*(3), 161–169.

Rosamond, W., Flegal, K., Friday, G., Furie, K., Go, A., Grenlund, K., . . . American Heart Association Statistics Committee and Stroke Statistics Subcommittee. (2007). Heart disease and stroke statistics—2007 update: A report from the American Heart Association Statistics Committee and Stroke Statistics Subcommittee. *Circulation, 115*(5), e69–171.

Rowley, H. A. (2005). Extending the time window for thrombolysis: Evidence from acute stroke trials. *Neuroimaging Clinics of North America, 15*(3), 575–587, x.

Rowley, H. A. (2009). *Comprehensive stroke imaging: The time is now.* Retrieved from http://my.americanheart.org/professional/General/Comprehensive-Stroke-Imaging-The-Time-is-Now_UCM_432617_Article.jsp

Roy, P. (2011). *Hepatitis D.* Retrieved from http://emedicine.medscape.com/article/178038-overview

Runyon, B. A. (2009). Management of adult patients with ascites due to cirrhosis: An update. Retrieved from http://www.aasld.org/practiceguidelines/Documents/Bookmarked%20Practice%20Guidelines/Ascites%20Update6-2009.pdf

Runyon, B. A., & AASLD Practice Guidelines Committee. (2009). Management of adult patients with ascites due to cirrhosis: An update. Hepatology, 49(6), 2087–2107. doi:10.1002/hep.22853

Russo, C. A., & Elixhauser, A. (2006). Hospitalizations related to pressure sores, 2003 (HCUP Statistical Brief #3). Retrieved from www.hcup-us.ahrq.gov/reports/statsbrief/sb3.jsp

Russo, C. A., Steiner, C., & Spector, W. (2006). Hospitalizations related to pressure ulcers among adults 18 years and older. Retrieved from http://www.hcup-us.ahrq.gov/reports/statbriefs/sb64.pdf

Saberi A., & Pouresmail, Z. (2007). The effect of acupressure on phantom pain in client with extremities amputation. European Journal of Pain, 11(S1), 127–128.

Sabia, S., Elbaz, A., Dugravot, A., Head, J., Shipley, M., Hagger-Johnson, G. . . . Singh-Manoux, A. (2010). Impact of smoking on cognitive decline in early old age. The Whitehall II Cohort Study. Archives of General Psychiatry, 69(6), 627–635.

Sacco, R. L., Adams, R., Albers, G., Alberts, M. J., Benavente, O., Furie, K., ... Tomsick, T. (2006). Guidelines for prevention of strokes in patients with ischemic stroke or transient ischemic attach: A statement for healthcare professionals from the American Heart Association/American Stroke Association Council on Stroke: Co-sponsored by the Council on Cardiovascular Radiology and Intervention: The American Academy of Neurology affirms the value of this guideline. Stroke, 37, 577–617.

Sacco, R. L., Adams, R., Albers, G., Alberts, M., Benavente, O., Furie, K.,...Tomsick, T. (2006). Guidelines for prevention of stroke in patients with ischemic stroke or ransient ischemic attack. Stroke, 37(2), 577–617.

Sahjian, M., & Frakes, M. (2007). Crush injuries: Pathophysiology and current treatment. Nurse Practitioner: The American Journal of Primary Health Care, 32(9), 13–18.

Salai, P. B. (2008). Patient management: The dialysis procedure. In C. S. Counts (Ed.), Core curriculum for nephrology nursing (5th ed.). Pitman, NJ: American Nephrology Nurses' Association.

Salcido, R. (2012). Pressure ulcers and wound care. Retrieved from http://emedicine.medscape.com/article/319284-overview

Salmond, S. (Ed.). (1996). Core curriculum for orthopedic nursing (3rd ed.). Pitman, NJ: National Association of Orthopedic Nurses.

Sampson, H. W. (2002). Alcohol and other factors affecting osteoporosis risk in women [Electronic version]. Alcohol Research and Health, 26(4), 292–298. Retrieved from http://ebsco.waldenu.edu/ehost/pdf?vid=6&hid=102&sid=55fdd3ae-a6d5-4629-8fa9-fd330627fcf%40sessionmgr103

Sanofi-Aventis US. (2011). Lovenox (enoxaparin sodium) injection prescribing information. Bridgewater, NJ: Author.

Santoni-Reddy, L. (2006). Heads up on cerebral bleeds. ED Insider, (Spring), 4–9.

Satalowich, R. J., & Prowant, B. F. (2008). Peritoneal dialysis: Peritoneal dialysis complications. In C. S. Counts (Ed.), Core curriculum for nephrology nursing (5th ed.). Pitman, NJ: American Nephrology Nurses' Association.

Satin, J. R., Linden, W., & Phillips, M. J. (2009). Depression as a predictor of disease progression and mortality in cancer patients. Cancer, 115(22), 5349–5361. doi:10.1002/cncr.24561

Sax, P., Cohen, C., & Kuritzkes, D. (2012). HIV essentials. Boston: Jones & Bartlett.

Scardillo, J., & Aronovitch, S. A. (1999). Successfully managing incontinence-related irritant dermatitis across the lifespan. Ostomy Wound Management, 45(4), 36–44.

Schira, M. (2008a). The kidney: Anatomy and physiology. In C. S. Counts (Ed.), Core curriculum for nephrology nursing (5th ed., pp. 4–32). Pitman, NJ: American Nephrology Nurses' Association.

Schira, M. (2008b). The kidney: Pathophysiology. In C. S. Counts (Ed.), Core curriculum for nephrology nursing (5th ed., pp. 33–62). Pitman, NJ: American Nephrology Nurses' Association.

Schmidt, A., & Mandel, J. (2012). Management of severe sepsis and septic shock in adults. Retrieved from http://www.uptodate.com/contents/management-of-severe-sepsis-and-septic-shock-in-adults

Schmidt, L. M. (2004). Herbal remedies: The other drugs your patients take [Electronic version]. Home Healthcare Nurse, 22(3), 169–175. Retrieved from http://gateway.tx.ovid.com.library.geu.edu:2048/gw2/ovidweb.cgi

Schmulson, M. J. (2001). Brain-gut interaction in irritable bowel syndrome: New findings of a multicomponent disease model. IMAJ. Retrieved from http://www.ima.org.il/imaj/ar01feb-5.pdf

Schmulson, M. J., Ortiz-Garrido, O. M., Hinojosa, C., & Arcila, D. (2006). A single session of reassurance can acutely improve the self-perception of impairment in patients with IBS. Journal of Psychosomatic Research, 61, 461–467.

Schonder, K., & Cincotta, E. (2008). Pharmacologic aspects of chronic kidney disease. In C. Counts (Ed.), Core curriculum for nephrology nursing (5th ed.). American Nephrology Nurses' Association.

Schulman, M., Lowe, L. H., Johnson, J., Neblett, W. W., Polk, D. B., Perez, R. Jr.,...Cywes, R. (2001). In vivo visualization of pyloric mucosal hypertrophy in infants with hypertrophic pyloric stenosis: Is there an etiologic role? American Journal of Roentgenology, 177(4), 843–848.

Schummer, W., Schummer, C., & Schelenz, C. (2003). Case report: The malfunctioning implanted venous access device [Electronic version]. British Journal of Nursing, 12(4), 210–214. Retrieved from http://web.ebscohost.com/ehost/pdf?vid=139&hid=106&sid=c7e5d2b4-a693-4480-a27f-fdf75c59b820%40session mgr106

Schwamm, L. H., Pancioli, A., Acker, J. E., Goldstein, L. B., Zorowitz, R. D., Shephard, T. J., . . . American Stroke Association's Task Force on the Development of Stroke Systems. (2005). Recommendations for the establishment of stroke systems of care: Recommendations from the American Stroke Association's Task Force on the development of stroke systems. Stroke, 36, 690–703.

Seamon, M. J., Wobb, J., Gaughan, J. P., Kulp, H., Kamel, I., & Dempsey, D. T. (2012). The effects of intraoperative hypothermia on surgical site infection: An analysis of 524 trauma laparotomies. *Annals of Surgery, 255*(4), 789–795.

Selius, B. A., & Subedi, R. (2008). Urinary retention in adults: Diagnosis and initial management. *American Family Physician, 77*(5), 643–650. Retrieved from http://www.aafp.org/afp/2008/0301/p643.html

Selius, B., & Subedi, R. (2008). Urinary retention in adults: Diagnosis and initial management. *American Family Physician, 77*(5), 643–650. Retrieved from http://www.aafp.org/afp/2008/0301/p643.html

Sesler, J. M. (2007). Stress-related mucosal disease in the intensive care unit: An update on prophylaxis. *AACN Advanced Critical Care, 18*(2), 119–128.

Sessler, D. (2006). Non-pharmacologic prevention of surgical wound infection. *Anesthesiology Clinics, 24*(2), 279–297.

Shafir, A., & Rosenthal, J. (2012). Shared decision making: Advancing patient-centered care through state and federal implementation. Informed Medical Decisions Foundation. Retrieved from http://www.nashp.org/sites/default/files/shared.decision.making.report.pdf

Shaikh, N. (2009). Emergency management of fat embolism syndrome. *Journal of Emergency Trauma and Shock, 2*, 29–33.

Shatzer, M. B., George, E. L., & Wei, L. (2007). To pump or not to pump? *Critical Care Nursing Quarterly, 30*(1), 67–73.

Sheppard, C. M., & Brenner, P. S. (2000). The effects of bathing and skin care practices on skin quality and satisfaction with an innovative product. *Journal of Gerontological Nursing, 26*(10), 36–45.

Shaughnessy, K. (2007). Massive pulmonary embolism. *Critical Care Nurse, 27*(1), 39–51.

Sheahan, S. L. (2002). How to help older adults quit smoking [Electronic version]. *Nurse Practitioner, 27*(12), 27–34. Retrieved from http://web.ebscohost.com/ehost/results?vid=14&hid=106&sid=c7e5 d2b4-a****3-4480-a27f-fdf75c59b820%40sessionmgr106

Shelton, B. K. (2005). Infection. In C. H. Yarbo, M. H. Frogge, & M. Goodman (Eds.), *Cancer nursing: Principles and practice* (6th ed.). Boston, MA: Jones & Bartlett.

Sheth, K. (2007). *Increased intracranial pressure.* Retrieved from http://www.nlm.nih.gov/medlineplus/ency/article/000793.htm

Shigehiko, U., Kellum, J., Bellomo, R., Doig, G., Morimatsu, H., Morgera, S., . . . Ronco, C. (2005). Acute renal failure in critically ill patients. *Journal of the American Medical Association, 294*(7), 813–818.

Shipes, E. (1987). Psychosocial issues: The person with an ostomy. *Nursing Clinics of North America, 22*(2), 291–302.

Shirato, S. (2005). How CAM helps systemic lupus erythematosus. *Holistic Nursing Practice, 19*(1), 36–39.

Siedliecki, S. L., & Good, M. (2006). Effect of music on power, pain, depression and disability. *Journal of Advanced Nursing, 54*(5), 553–562.

Siegel, J. D., Rhinehart, E., Jackson, M., Chiarello, L., & the Healthcare Infection Control Practices Advisory Committee. (2007, June). 2007 guideline for isolation precautions: Preventing transmission of infectious agents in healthcare settings. Retrieved from www.cdc.gov/ncidod/dhqp/pdf/isolation2007.pdf

Siegel, J., Rhinehart, E., Jackson, M., & Chiarello, L. (2007). Guideline for isolation precautions: Preventing transmission of infectious agents in healthcare settings. Retrieved from www.Premerinc.com/safety/topics/guidelines/downloads/cdc.isolation-2007.pdf

Sieggreen, M. (2006). A contemporary approach to peripheral arterial disease. *Nurse Practitioner, 31*(7), 14–25.

Sieggreen, M. (2007). Recognize acute arterial occlusion. *Nursing2007 Critical Care, 2*(5), 50–59.

Simmons, S. F., & Levy-Storms, L. (2005). The effect of dining location on nutritional care quality in nursing homes. *Journal of Nutrition Health and Aging, 9*(6), 434–439.

Sims, J. M. (2006). An overview of asthma [Electronic version]. *Dimensions of Critical Care Nursing, 25*(6), 264–268. Retrieved from http://gateway.tx.ovid.com.library.gcu.edu:2048/gw2/ovidweb.cgi

Singer, P., & Martin, D. (1999). Quality of life care patient's perspectives. *The Journal of the American Medical Association, 281*(2), 166–168.

Sjogren's Syndrome Foundation. (2008). Home page. Sjogren's Syndrome Foundation. Retrieved from http://www.sjogrens.org

Skillman, J. J., Bushnell, L. S., Goldman, H., & Silen, W. (1969). Respiratory failure, hypotension, sepsis, and jaundice: A clinical syndrome associated with lethal hemorrhage from acute stress ulceration of the stomach. *American Journal of Surgery, 117*(4), 523–530.

Slater, J. E. (1989). Rubber anaphylaxis. *New England Journal of Medicine, 320*, 1126–1130.

Smeltzer, S., & Bares, B. (2008). *Textbook of medical-surgical nursing* (10th ed.). Philadelphia, PA: Lippincott Williams & Wilkins.

Söderberg, A., Gilje, F., & Norberg, A. (1998). Dignity in situations of ethical difficulty in ICU. *Intensive Critical Care Nursing Journal Palliative Care, 14*(1), 36–42.

Smith-DiJulio, K. (2001). Rape. In E. Varcarolis (Ed.), *Foundations of psychiatric mental health nursing* (4th ed.). Philadelphia, PA: W. B. Saunders.

Smith, M. (2007). Intensive care management of patients with subarachnoid hemorrhage. *Current Opinion in Anesthesiology, 20*(5), 400–407.

Smith, M., Robinson, L., & Segal, R. M. A. (2012). Memory loss and aging: Causes, treatment, and help for memory problems. Retrieved from http://www.helpguide.org/life/prevent_memory_loss.htm#reversible

Snyder, M. (1983). Relation of nursing activities to increases in intracranial pressure. *Journal of Advanced Nursing, 8(4)*, 273–279. Retrieved from http://onlinelibrary.wiley.com/doi/10.1111/j.1365-2648.1983.tb00326.x/abstract

Society for Vascular Surgery. (2007). *Amputation.* Retrieved from http://vascularweb.org/_CONTRIBUTION_PAGES/Patient_Information/NorthPoint/Amputation.html

Society for Vascular Surgery. (2007). *Amputation.* Retrieved from http://vascularweb.org/vascularhealth/Pages/amputation.aspx

Soholt, D. (1990). *A life experience: Making a health care treatment decision* (Unpublished master's thesis). South Dakota State University, Brookings, SD.

Solomon, J., Yee, N., & Soulen, M. (2000). Aortic stent grafts: An overview of devices, indications and results. *Applied Radiology Supplement, 7,* 43–51.

Sørensen, L. T. (2012). Wound healing and infection in surgery: the pathophysiological impact of smoking, smoking cessation, and nicotine replacement therapy: a systematic review. *Annals of Surgery, 255*(6), 1069–1079.

Sotir, M. J., Lewis, C., Bisher, E. W., Ray, S. M., Soucie, M., & Blumberg, H. M. (1999). Epidemiology of device-associated infections related to a long-term implantable vascular access device. *Infection Control and Hospital Epidemiology, 20*(3), 187–191.

South Carolina Department of Disabilities and Special Needs. (2006). *Nursing management of seizures.* Retrieved from http://ddsn.sc.gov/providers/manualsandguidelines/Documents/HealthCareGuidelines/NursingMgmtSeizures.pdf

Speaar, M. (2008). Wound care management: Risk factors for surgical site infections. *Plastic Surgical Nursing, 28*(4), 201–204.

Spies, L. (2009). Diarrhea A to Z: America to Zimbabwe. *Journal of the American Academy of Nurse Practitioners, 21*(6), 307–313.

Spiller, R. (2008). Review article: Probiotics and prebiotics in irritable bowel syndrome. *Alimentary Pharmacology & Therapeutics, 28,* 385–396.

Spiller, R., & Garsed, K. (2009). Postinfectious irritable bowel syndrome. *Gastroenterology, 136*(6), 1979–1988.

Stacy, M. (2009). Medical treatment of Parkinson disease. *Neurologic Clinics, 27*(3), 605–631.

Stajduhar, K. I., Martin, W. L., & Barwich, D. (2008). Factors influencing family caregivers ability to cope with providing end-of-life cancer at home. *Cancer Nursing: An International Journal for Cancer Care, 31*(1), 77–85.

Stanbridge, R., Hon, J. K. F., Bateman, E., & Roberts, S. (2007). Minimally invasive anterior thoracotomy for routine lung cancer resection. *Innovations, 2*(2), 76–83.

Stanley, M. M., Ochi, S., Lee, K. K., Nemchausky, B. A., Greenlee, H. B., Allen, J. I., . . . Camara, D. S. (1989). Peritoneovenous shunting as compared with medical treatment in patients with alcoholic cirrhosis and massive ascites. *New England Journal of Medicine, 321,*1632–1638.

Starling, B. P., & Martin, A. C. (1990). Adult survivors of parental alcoholism: Implications for primary care. *Nursing Practice, 15*(7), 16–24.

Starnes, D. N., & Sims, T. W. (2006). Care of the patient undergoing robotic-assisted prostatectomy. *Urology Nursing, 26*(2), 129–136.

Starr, S. P., & Raines, D. (2011). Cirrhosis: Diagnosis, management, and prevention. *American Family Physician, 84*(12), 1353–1359.

Steeves, R. H. (1992). Patients who have undergone bone marrow transplantation: Their quest for meaning. *Oncology Nursing Forum, 19*(6), 899–905.

Stein, J. (2008). Stroke. In W. R. Frontera, J. K. Silver, & T. D. Rizzo, Jr. (Eds.), *Essentials of physical medicine and rehabilitation* (2nd ed., Chapter 149). Philadelphia, PA: Saunders.

Stone, M. S., Bronkesh, S. J., Gerbarg, Z. B., & Wood, S. D. (1998). Improving patient compliance. Strategic Medicine. Retrieved from http://www.patientcompliancemedia.com/Improving_Patient_Compliance_article.pdf

Story, K. T. (2006). Malignant pleural effusion. In M. Kaplin (Ed.), *Understanding and managing oncologic emergencies: A resource for nurses* (pp. 123–155). Pittsburgh, PA: Oncology Nursing Society.

Strobik, Y. (2007). Protocols, practice and patients: The case of alcohol withdrawal. *Critical Care Medicine, 35*(3), 955.

Strobl, R. A. (2009). Radiation therapy. In S. Newton, M. Hickey, & J. Marrs (Eds.), Mosby's oncology nursing advisor: A comprehensive guide to clinical practice (p. 141). St. Louis, MO: Mosby Elsevier.

Stroke Association. (2012). Communication problems after a stroke. Retrieved from http://www.stroke.org.uk/sites/default/files/Communication%20problems%20after%20stroke.pdf

Stuart, G. W., & Sundeen, S. (2002). *Principles and practice of psychiatric nursing* (6th ed.). St. Louis, MO: Mosby-Year Book.

Su, Y-H., & Ryan-Wenger, N. A. (2007). Children's adjustment to parental cancer: A theoretical model development. *Cancer Nursing, 30*(5), 362–381.

Sublett, C. M. (2007). Critique of "Effects of advanced practice nursing on patient and spouse depressive symptoms, sexual function, and marital interaction after radical prostatectomy." *Urology Nursing, 27*(1), 78–80.

Sullivan, M. J., & Hawthorne, M. H. (1996). Nonpharmacologic interventions in the treatment of heart failure. *Journal of Cardiovascular Nursing, 10*(2), 47–57.

Sullivan, M. J., Reesor, K., Mikail, S., & Fisher, R. (1992). The treatment of depression in chronic low back pain: Review and recommendations. *Pain, 50*(1), 5–13. Retrieved from http://www.ncbi.nlm.nih.gov/pubmed/1387469

Summers, D., Leonard, A., Wentworth, D., Saver, J., Simpson, J., Spilker, J. A., . . . American Heart Association Council on Cardiovascular Nursing and the Stroke Council. (2009). Comprehensive overview of nursing and interdisciplinary care of the acute ischemic stroke patient: Scientific statement from the American Heart Association. *Stroke, 40*, 2911–2944.

Support Study. (1995). The SUPPORT prognostic model. Objective estimates of survival for seriously ill hospitalized adults. Study to understand prognoses and preferences for outcomes and risks of treatments. *Annals of Internal Medicine, 122*(3), 191–203.

Susan B. Komen for the Cure. (2007c). *Lymphedema.* Retrieved from http://cms.komen.org/komen/aboutbreastcancer/aftertreatment/3-6-3?ssSourceNodeld=301&ssSourceSiteld=Komen

Susan B. Komen for the Cure (2007d). *Sex and sexuality.* Retrieved from http://cms.komen.org/komen/aboutbreastcancer/aftertreatment/3-3-4?ssSourceNodeld=301&ssSourceSiteld=Komen

Sussman, G., & Gold, M. (1996). *Guidelines for the management of latex allergies and safe latex use in health care facilities.* Arlington Heights, IL: American College of Allergy, Asthma & Immunology. Retrieved from http://www.acaai.org/allergist/allergies/Types/latexallergy/Pages/latex-allergies-safe-use.aspx#anchor408950

Swadener-Culpepper, L. (2010). Continuous lateral rotation therapy. *Critical Care Nurse, 30*(2), S5–S7. Retreived from Medline Database.

Swanson, J., & Koch, L. (2010). The role of the oncology nurse navigator in distress management of adult in patients with cancer: A retrospective study. *Oncology Nursing Forum, 37*(1), 69–76.

Swanson, K. M. (1991). Empirical development of a middle range theory of caring. *Nursing Research, 40*, 161–166.

Swanson, M. C. (2004). Encouraging adherence to treatment regimen in a CCPD patient. *Nephrology Nursing Journal, 31*(1), 80.

Symes, L. (2000). Arriving at readiness to recover emotionally after sexual assault. *Archives of Psychiatric Nursing, 14*(1), 30–38.

Tang, N. K. Y., Wright, K., & Salkovskis, P. M. (2007). Prevalence and correlates of clinical insomnia co-occurring with chronic pain. *Journal of Sleep Research, 16*(1), 85–95.

Tapasi, S., & Harmeet, S. (2007). Noninfectious complications of peritoneal dialysis. *Southern Medical Journal, 100*(1), 54–58.

Task Force for Diagnosis and Treatment of Non-ST-Segment Elevation Acute Coronary Syndromes of European Society of Cardiology, Bassand, J-P., Hamm, C. W., Ardissino, D., Boersma, E., Budaj, A., . . . Wijns, W. (2007). Guidelines for the diagnosis and treatment of non-ST-segment elevation acute coronary syndromes. *European Heart Journal, 28*(13), 1598–1660.

Tattersall, J. E., & Daugirdas, J. T. (2011). Preparing for dialysis. In J. T. Daugirdas (Ed.), *Handbook of chronic kidney disease management.* Philadelphia, PA: Lippincott Williams & Wilkins.

Taylor, J. (1993). *Discretion versus policy rules in practice.* Retrieved from http://www.stanford.edu/~johntayl/Papers/Discretion.PDF

Tewari, A., Peabody, J., Sarle, R., Balakrishnan, G., Hemal, A., Shrivastava, A., & Menon, M. (2002). Technique of Da Vinci robot-assisted anatomic radical prostatectomy. *Urology, 60*(4), 569–572.

Thakar, R., Ayers, S., Clarkson, P., Stanton, S., & Manyonda, I. (2002). Outcomes after total versus subtotal abdominal hysterectomy. *New England Journal of Medicine, 347*, 1318–1325.

The American Society of Colon & Rectal Surgeons and the Wound Ostomy Continence Nurse Society. (2007). *Joint position statement on the value of preoperative stoma marking for patients undergoing fecal ostomy surgery.* Retrieved from http://www.ostomy.org/ostomy_info/wocn/wocn_preoperative_stoma_marking.pdf

The World Society of the Abdominal Compartment Syndrome. (2013). Intra-abdominal hypertension and the abdominal compartment syndrome: Updated consensus definitions and clinical practice guidelines from the World Society of the Abdominal Compartment Syndrome. *Intensive Care Medicine, 39*(7), 1190–1206.

Thompson, C., & Fuhrman, M. P. (2005). Nutrients and wound healing: Still searching for the magic bullet. *Nutrition in Clinical Practice, 20*, 331–347.

Thompson, P., Langemo, D., Anderson, J., Hanson, D., & Hunter, S. (2005). Skin care protocols for pressure ulcers and incontinence in long-term care: A quasi-experimental study. *Advances in Skin & Wound Care, 18*(8), 422–429.

Tilden, V. P., & Weinert, C. (1987). Social support and the chronically ill individual. *Nursing Clinics of North America, 22*, 613–620.

Timoney, J. P., Eagan, M. M., & Sklarin, N. T. (2003). Establishing clinical guidelines for the management of acute hypersensitivity reactions secondary to the administration of chemotherapy/biologic therapy. *Journal of Nursing Care Quality, 18*(1), 80–86.

Tisminetzky, M., Bray, B. C., Miozzo, R., Aupont, O., & McLaughlin, T. (2012). Classes of depression, anxiety, and functioning in acute coronary syndrome patients. *American Journal of Health Behavior, 36*(1), 20–30.

Titler, M., Dochterman, J., Xie, X., Kanak, M., Fei, Q., Picone, D., & Shever, L. (2006). Nursing interventions and other factors associated with discharge disposition in elderly patients after hip surgery. *Nursing Research, 55*(4), 231–242.

Torpy, J., Glass, T. J., & Glass, R. M. (2005). Myasthenia Gravis. *Journal of the American Medical Association, 293*(15), 1940.

Townsend, C. M., Beauchamp, R. D., Evers, B. M., & Mattox, K. L. (Eds.). (2012). *Sabiston textbook of surgery* (19th ed.). St. Louis, MO: W. B. Saunders.

Truscott, W. "The industry perspective on latex." *Immunology and Allergy Clinics of North America* 15(1995): 89–115.

Turban, S., & Miller, E. R., III. (2011). Sodium and potassium intake. In J. T. Daugirdas (Ed.), *Handbook of chronic kidney disease management*. Philadelphia, PA: Lippincott Williams & Wilkins.

Turner, J. R. (2010). The gastrointestinal tract. In V. Kumar, A. K. Abbas, N. Faisto, et al. (Eds.), *Robbins and Cotran pathologic basis of disease* (8th ed., pp. 763–831). Philadelphia, PA: Saunders Elsevier.

Tusaie, K., & Dyer, J. (2004). Resilience: A historical review of construct. *Holistic Nursing Practice, 18*(1), 3–8.

U. S. Department of Health and Human Services. (1992). *Management and therapy of sickle cell disease* (NIH Publication No. 92-2117). Washington, DC: Author.

U.S. National Library of Medicine. (2006). *Osteomyelitis.* Retrieved from http://www.nlm.nih.gov/medlineplus/ency/article/000437.htm

Underwood, C. (2004). How can we best deliver an inclusive health service? *Primary Health Care, 14*(9), 20–21.

United Ostomy Association. (2006). *Urostomy: A guide.* Retrieved from http://cancer.org/docroot/CRI/content/CRI_2_6x_Urostomy.asp

University of Michigan Health System. (2007). Instructions for care following conventional prostatectomy/Robotic prostatectomy. Retrieved from http://www.med.umich.edu/1libr/urology/postcare/rprostatectomy.htm

Urbano, F. (2001). Homans' sign in the diagnosis of deep venous thrombosis. *Hospital Physician, 3*, 22–24. Retrieved from www.turner-white.com

Urinary retention. (2012, June) Retrieved from http://kidney.niddk.nih.gov/kudiseases/pubs/UrinaryRetention/

Vacco v. Quill–521 U.S. 793. (1997). *Assisted suicide.* Retrieved from http://supreme.justia.com/cases/federal/us/521/793/

Valente, S. (2004). End-of-life challenges: Honoring autonomy. *Cancer Nursing: An International Journal for Cancer Care, 27*(4), 314–319.

van Kimmenade, R. R. J., & Januzzi, J. L., Jr. (2011). Heart failure. In J. T. Daugirdas (Ed.), *Handbook of chronic kidney disease management*. Philadelphia, PA: Lippincott Williams & Wilkins.

van Ramshorst, G. H., Nieuwenhuizen, J., Hop, W. C. J., Arends, P., Broom, J., Jeekel, J., & Lange, J. H. (2010). Abdominal wound dehiscence in adults: Development and validation of a risk model. World Journal of Surgery, *34*(1), 20–27. doi:10.1007/s00268-009-0277-y

Vanezis, M., & McGee, A. (1999). Mediating factors in the grieving process of the suddenly bereaved. *British Journal of Nursing, 8*(14), 932–937.

Varcarolis, E. M. (2011). *Manual of psychiatric nursing care planning* (4th ed.). St. Louis, MO: Saunders.

Vasavada, S. (2013). *Urinary incontinence.* Retrieved from http://emedicine.medscape.com/article/452289-overview#a0156

Vassar, T., Batenjany, M., Kooman, W., & Ricci, M. (2008). Nursing issues. In J. F. Howard (Ed.), *Myasthenia gravis: A manual for health care providers* (pp. 32–53). St. Paul, MN: Myasthenia Gravis Foundation of America.

Vasterling, J., Jenkins, R. A., Tope, D. M., & Burish, T. G. (1993). Cognitive distraction and relaxation training for the control of side effects due to cancer chemotherapy. *Journal of Behavioral Medicine, 1*, 65–80.

Vasudevan, J. M., Baheti, N. D., Naber, R. I., & Fredericson, M. (2012). Physiotherapy, pain management, and surgical interventions for low back pain: Initial review. *Current Sports Medicine Reports, 11*(1), 35–42.

Vere-Jones, E. (2007). Nursing the survivors of sexual assault. *Nursing Times, 103*(35), 18–19.

Vermeer, S., Hollander, M., van Dijk, E., Hofman, A., Koudstaal, P., & Breteler, M. (2001). Silent brain infarcts and white matter lesions increase stroke risk in the general population. *The Rotterdam Scan Study Stroke, 34*, 1126–1129.

Vernava, A. M., III, Moore, B. A., Longo, W. E., & Johnson, F. E. (1997). Lower gastrointestinal bleeding. *Diseases of the Colon & Rectum, 40*(7), 846–858.

Vinik, A. I., Maser, R. E., Mitchell, B. D., & Freeman, R.(2003). Diabetic autonomic neuropathy. *Diabetes Care, 26*(5), 1553–1579.

Volker, D. (2000). Palliative sedation and terminal weaning are ethical and realistic interventions in a percentage of dying patients whose symptoms remain unbearable despite aggressive palliative. *Clinical Journal of Oncology Nursing, 7*, 653–667, 8.

Wagner, K. D., Johnson, K., & Kidd, P. S. (2006). *High acuity nursing* (4th ed.). Upper Saddle River, NJ: Prentice Hall.

Walker, C., Hogstel, M. O., & Curry, L. (2007). Hospital discharge of older adults: How nurses can ease the transition. *American Journal of Nursing, 107*(6), 60–70.

Walker, T. G., Kalva, S. P., Yeddula, K., Wicky, S., Kundu, S., Drescher, P., . . . Canadian Interventional Radiology Association. (2010). Clinical practice guidelines for endovascular abdominal aortic aneurysm repair. Written by the Standards of Practice Committee for the Society of Interventional Radiology and Endorsed by the Cardiovascular and Interventional Radiological Society of Europe and the Canadian Interventional Radiology Association. *Journal of Vascular International Radiology, 21*, 1632–1655.

Walker, T., Kalva, S.,Yeddula, K., Wicky, S., Kundu, S., Drescher, P.,...Cardella, J. (2010). Clinical practice guidelines for endovascular abdominal aortic aneurysm repair: Written by the Standards of Practice Committee for the Society of Interventional Radiology and Endorsed by the Cardiovascular and Interventional Radiological Society of Europe and the Canadian Interventional Radiology Association. *Journal of Vascular and Interventional Radiology, 21*, 1632–1655.

Walsh, P. C., Marschke, P., Ricker, D., & Burnett, A. L. (2000). Patient-reported urinary continence and sexual function after anatomic radical prostatectomy. *Urology, 55*(1), 58–61.

Warrington, T., & Bostwick, M. (2006). Psychiatric adverse effects of corticosteroids. *Mayo Clinic Proceedings*, *81*(10), 1361–1367.

Washington V. Glucksberg. (1997). *Legatal Information Institute*. Retrieved from http://www.law.cornell.edu/supct/html/historics/USSC_CR_0521_0702_ZO.html

Wasserman, A. M. (2011). Diagnosis and management of rheumatoid arthritis. *American Family Physician*, *84*(11), 1245–1252.

Waterbury, L. (2007). Anemia. In N. H. Fiebach, D. E. Kern, P. A. Thomas, & R. C. Ziegelstein (Eds.), *Principles of ambulatory medicine* (7th ed.). Baltimore, MD: Williams & Wilkins.

Weaver, T., & Narsavage, G. (1992). Physiological and psychological variables related to functional status in chronic obstructive pulmonary disease. *Nursing Research*, *41*(5), 286–291.

Weeks, J. C., Catalano, P. J., Cronin, A., Finkelman, M. D., Mack, J. W., Keating, N. L., & Schrag, D. (2012). Patients' expectations about effects of chemotherapy for advanced cancer. *New England Journal of Medicine*, *367*, 1616–1625.

Weisberg, J. N., & Boatwright, B. A. (2007). Mood, anxiety and personality traits and states in chronic pain. *Pain*, *133*(1–3), 1–2.

Weissman, D. (2009). What is palliative care? Retrieved from http://www.getpalliativecare.org

Welch, P., Porter, J., & Endres, J. (2003). Efficacy of a medication pass supplement program in the long term-care compared to a traditional system. *Journal of Nutrition in Elderly*, *22*(3), 19–29.

Whelton, S. P., Chin, A., Xin, X., & He, J. (2002). Effect of aerobic exercise on blood pressure: A meta-analysis of randomized, controlled trials. *Annals of Intern Medicine*, *136*, 493–503.

Wilkins, K. L., McGrath, P. J., Finley, G. A., & Katz, J. (2004). Prospective diary study of nonpainful and painful phantom sensations in a preselected sample of child and adolescent amputees reporting phantom limbs. *The Clinical Journal of Pain*, *20*(5), 293–301.

Wilkinson, J., & Van Leuven, K. (2007). *Fundamentals of nursing: Theory, concepts & applications*. Philadelphia, PA: F. A. Davis.

Willett, C. (Ed.). (n.d.). *UpToDate*. Retrieved from http://www.uptodateonline.com.

Williams, H. F., Bogle, J. L., & Davey-Tresemer, J. (2008). Acute kidney injury and acute renal failure. In C. S. Counts (Ed.), *Core curriculum for nephrology nursing* (5th ed., pp. 144–175). Pitman, NJ: American Nephrology Nurses' Association.

Williams, J. Z., & Barbul, A. (2003). Nutrition and wound healing. *Surgical Clinics of North America*, *83*, 571–596.

Williams, L. S., Brizendine, E. J., Plue, L., Bakas, T., Tu, W., Hendrie, H., & Kroenke, K. (2005). Performance of the PHQ-9 as a screening tool for depression after stroke. *Stroke*, *36*, 635–638.

Williamson, D. F., Serdula, M. K., & Anda, R. F., Levy, A., & Byers, T. (1992). Weight loss attempts in adults: Goals, duration, and rate of weight loss. *American Journal of Public Health*, *82*(9), 1251–1257.

Wilson, J. A., & Clark, J. J. (2004). Obesity: Impediment to postsurgical wound healing. *Adv Skin Wound Care*, *17*, 426–435.

Wilson, K. G., Eriksson, M. Y., D'Eon, J. L., Mikail, S. F., & Emery, P. C. (2002). Major depression and insomnia in chronic pain. *Clinical Journal of Pain*, *18*(2), 77–83.

Wilson, L. D., Detterbeck, F. C., & Yahalom, J. (2007). Clinical practice: Superior vena cava syndrome with malignant causes. *New England Journal of Medicine*, *356*(18), 1862–1869.

Wilson, P., Berghmans, B., Hagen, S., Hay-Smith, J., Moore, K., Nygaard, I.,…Wyman, J. (2005). Adult conservative management in incontinence. *Incontinence Volume 2: Management*. Paris: International Continence Society Health Publication Ltd.

Wiseman, K. C., Arduino, M. J., Arnold, E., Axley, B., Butera, E., Curry, G., & Peacock, E. J. (2008). Infection control. In C. S. Counts (Ed.), *Core curriculum for nephrology nursing* (5th ed.). Pitman, NJ: American Nephrology Nurses' Association.

Witting, M. D., Magder, L., Heins, A. E., Mattu, A., Granja, C. A., & Baumgarten, M. (2006). Usefulness and validity of diagnostic nasogastric aspiration in patients without hematemesis. *Annals of Emergency Medicine*, *43*(4), 280–285. Retrieved from http://www.ncbi.nlm.nih.gov/pubmed/16635697

Wityk, R. J. (2007). The management of blood pressure after stroke. *Neurologist*, *13*, 171–181.

Women's Health. (2005). Women's support center for rape victims. Retrieved from www.womenshealth.gov

Woodbury, M. G., Hayes, K. C., & Askes, H. K. (2008). Intermittent catheterization practices following spinal cord injury: A national survey. *Canadian Journal Urology*, *15*(3), 4065–4071.

Worden, W. (2002). *Grief counseling and grief therapy* (3rd ed.). New York, NY: Springer.

World Health Organization. (2011). Indoor air pollution and health (Fact sheet #292). Retrieved from http://www.who.int/mediacentre/factsheets/fs292/en/

World Health Organization. (2011). *World Health Statistics 2011*. Retrieved from *ww.who.int/whosis/whostat/2011*

Wound Ostomy Continence Nursing. (2003). *Guideline for prevention and management of pressure ulcers*. Glenview, IL: Author.

Wound, Ostomy and Continence Nurses' Society. (2011). *Management of the patient with a fecal ostomy: Best practice for clinicians*. Mount Laurel, NJ: Author.

Wound, Ostomy, and Continence Nurses Society. (2010). Guideline for prevention and management of pressure ulcers. Mount Laurel (NJ): Wound, Ostomy, and Continence Nurses Society (WOCN); 1.96 p. (WOCN clinical practice guideline; no. 2)

Wright, L. M. (2004). *Spirituality, suffering, and illness: Ideas for healing*. Philadelphia, PA: F. A. Davis.

Wright, M., Wood, J., Lynch, T., & Clark, D. (2008b). Mapping levels of palliative care development: A global view. *Journal of Pain and Symptom Management, 35*(5), 469–485.

Wright, P. M., & Hogan, N. S. (2008). Grief theories and models: Applications to hospice nursing practice. *Journal of Hospice & Palliative Nursing, 10*(6), 350–355.

Wu, L., Li, W., Hu, Z., Rao, N. Y., Song, C. G., Zhang, B.,…Shao, Z. M. (2008). The prevalence of *BRCA1* and *BRCA2* germline mutations in high-risk breast cancer patients of Chinese Han nationality: Two recurrent mutations were identified. *Breast Cancer Research and Treatment, 110*(1), 99–109.

Yakimo, R., (2006). Perspectives on psychiatric consultation liaison nursing. *Perspectives in Psychiatric Care, 42*(1), 59–62.

Yaklin, K. M. (2011). Acute kidney injury: An overview of pathophysiology and treatments. *Nephrology Nursing Journal, 38*(1), 13–18.

Yanoff, J., & Duker, M. (2009). *Ophthalmology* (3rd ed.). New York, NY: Mosby.

Yarbro, C., Wujeck, D., & Gobel, B. (2011). *Cancer nursing: Principles and practice* (7th ed.). Boston, MA: Jones & Bartlett.

Yates, P. C. (1993). Toward a reconceptualization of hope for patients with a diagnosis of cancer. *Journal of Advanced Nursing, 18*(4), 701–708.

Yazicioglu, K., Taskaynatan, M. A., Guzelkucuk, U., & Tugcu, I. (2007). Effect of playing football (soccer) on balance, strength, and quality of life in unilateral below-knee amputees. *American Journal of Physical Medicine and Rehabilitation, 86*(10), 800–805.

Yetzer, E. A. (1996). Helping the patient through the experience of an amputation. *Orthopaedic Nursing, 15*(6), 45–49.

Young, M. G. (2001). Providing care for the caregiver. *Patient Care for the Nurse Practitioner, 2*, 36–47.

Zagaria, M. E. (2011). Acute pancreatitis: Risks, causes, and mortality in older adults. *US Pharmacist, 36*(12), 24–27.

Zalon, M. (2004). Correlates of recovery among older adults after major abdominal surgery. *Nursing Research, 53*(2), 99-106.

Zeller, J., Lynm, C., & Glass, R. M. (2007). Septic arthritis. *Journal of the American Medical Association, 297*(13), 1510.

Zidan, J., Hussein, O., Abzah, A., Tamam, S., & Farraj, Z. (2008). Oral premedication for the prevention of hypersensitivity reactions to paclitaxel. *Medical Oncology, 25*, 274–278.

Zisman, A. L., Worcester, E. M., & Coe, F. L. (2011). Evaluation and management of stone disease. In J. T. Daugirdas (Ed.), *Handbook of chronic kidney disease management* (pp. 482–492). Philadelphia, PA: Lippincott Williams & Wilkins.

Appendix A

Nursing Diagnoses Grouped by Functional Health Pattern*

1. Health Perception—Health Management

Contamination, Individual
    Contamination, Risk for Individual
Contamination: Community
    Contamination: Community, Risk for
Contamination: Family
    Contamination: Family, Risk for
Energy Field, Disturbed
Growth and Development, Delayed
    Development, Risk for Delayed
    Failure to Thrive, Adult
    Growth, Risk for Disproportionate
Health, Deficient Community
Health Behavior, Risk-Prone
Health Maintenance, Ineffective
Immunization Status, Readiness for
    Enhanced
Injury, Risk for
    Aspiration, Risk for
    Falls, Risk for
    Perioperative Positioning Injury,
        Risk for
    Poisoning, Risk for
    Suffocation, Risk for
    Thermal Injury, Risk for
    Trauma, Risk for
Noncompliance
Self-Health Management, Ineffective
†Self-Health Management, Ineffective
    Community
†Self-Health Management, Ineffective
    Family
Self-Health Management, Readiness for
    Enhanced
Surgical Recovery, Delayed

2. Nutritional—Metabolic

Adverse Reaction to Iodinated Contrast
    Media, Risk for
Allergy Response, Risk for
Blood Glucose Level, Risk for
    Unstable
Body Temperature, Risk for
    Imbalanced
    Hyperthermia
    Hypothermia
    Thermoregulation, Ineffective
Breastfeeding, Ineffective
Breastfeeding, Interrupted
Breastfeeding, Readiness for Enhanced
Breast Milk, Insufficient
Electrolyte Imbalances, Risk for
Fluid Balance, Readiness for Enhanced
Fluid Volume, Deficient
Fluid Volume, Excess
Fluid Volume, Risk for Imbalance
Infection, Risk for
†Infection Transmission, Risk for
Intracranial Adaptive Capacity,
    Decreased
Jaundice, Neonatal
    Jaundice, Risk for Neonatal
Latex Allergy Response
    Latex Allergy Response, Risk for
Liver Function, Risk for Impaired
Nutrition, Imbalanced: Less Than Body
    Requirements
    Dentition, Impaired
    Infant Feeding Pattern, Ineffective
    Swallowing, Impaired
Nutrition, Imbalanced: More Than
    Body Requirements
Nutrition, Imbalanced: More Than
    Body Requirements, Risk for
Nutrition, Readiness for Enhanced
Protection, Ineffective
    Dry Eye, Risk for
    Oral Mucous Membrane, Impaired
    Skin Integrity, Impaired
    Skin Integrity, Risk for Impaired
    Tissue Integrity, Impaired

3. Elimination

Bowel Incontinence
Constipation
    Constipation, Perceived
Diarrhea
Gastrointestinal Motility, Dysfunctional
    Gastrointestinal Motility, Risk for
        Dysfunctional
Urinary Elimination, Impaired
    †Continuous Urinary Incontinence
    Functional Urinary Incontinence
    Maturational Enuresis
    Overflow Urinary Incontinence
    Reflex Urinary Incontinence
    Stress Urinary Incontinence
    Urge Urinary Incontinence
Urinary Elimination, Readiness for
    Enhanced

4. Activity—Exercise

Activity Intolerance
Activity Planning, Ineffective
    Activity Planning, Risk for Ineffective
Bleeding, Risk for
Cardiac Output, Decreased

---

*The Functional Health Patterns were identified in Gordon, M. (1994). *Nursing diagnosis: Process and application.* New York: McGraw-Hill, with minor changes by the author.
†These diagnoses are not currently in the NANDA-I taxonomy but have been included for clarity and usefulness.

Nursing Admission Data Base

Nursing Admission Data Base

Date _____ Arrival Time _____ Contact Person _____ Phone _____

ADMITTED FROM: ____ Home alone ____ Home with relative ____ Long-term care
____ Homeless ____ Home with ____ (Specify) facility
____ ER ____ Other _____

MODE OF ARRIVAL: ____ Ambulatory _____ Wheelchair _____ Ambulance _____ Stretcher

REASON FOR HOSPITALIZATION: _____

_____

Analysis: Does the individual understand why he is in the hospital?

LAST HOSPITAL ADMISSION: Date _____ Reason _____

_____

Analysis: Was this hospitalization related to the last admission?

PAST MEDICAL HISTORY: _____

_____

MEDICATION

(Prescription/Over-the-Counter)	DOSAGE	LAST DOSE	FREQUENCY

Analysis: Ask if taking the med and if missing doses? Why?

Health Maintenance–Perception Pattern

USE OF:

Tobacco: ____ None ____ Quit (date) ____ Smokeless ____ Pipe ____ Cigar ____ <1 pk/day
____ 1–2 pks/day _____ >2 pks/day pks/year History _____

Want to quit? Have you tried to quit? When? How long?

Alcohol: ____ Date of last drink ____ Amount/Type
____ No. of days in a month when alcohol is consumed

Should you cut down?

Drug Use: _____ No _____ Yes Type _____ Use _____

Would you like help?

Allergies (drugs, food, tape, dyes): _____ Reaction _____

_____

Side One

Activity–Exercise Pattern

SELF-CARE ABILITY:

0 = Independent   1 = Assistive device   2 = Assistance from others
3 = Assistance from person and equipment   4 = Dependent/Unable

	0	1	2	3	4
Eating/Drinking					
Bathing					
Dressing/Grooming					
Toileting					
Bed Mobility					
Transferring					
Ambulating					
Stair Climbing					
Shopping					
Cooking					
Home Maintenance					

ASSISTIVE DEVICES: ____ None ____ Crutches ____ Bedside commode ____ Walker
____ Cane ____ Splint/Brace ____ Wheelchair ____ Other

CODE: (1) Not applicable (2) Unable to acquire (3) Not a priority at this time
(4) Other (specify in notes)

Is this person at risk for a complex transition?

Nutrition–Metabolic Pattern

Special Diet/Supplements _____

Previous Dietary Instruction: ____ Yes ____ No

Appetite: ____ Normal ____ Increased ____ Decreased ____ Decreased taste sensation
____ Nausea ____ Vomiting

Weight Fluctuations Last 6 Months: ____ None _____ lbs. Gained/Lost

Swallowing difficulty: ____ None ____ Solids ____ Liquids

Dentures: ____ Upper (___ Partial ___ Full) ____ Lower (___ Partial ___ Full)
With Person ____ Yes ____ No

History of Skin/Healing Problems: ____ None ____ Abnormal Healing ____ Rash
____ Dryness ____ Excess Perspiration

Elimination Pattern

Bowel Habits: ____ # BMs q __/day ____ Date of last BM ____ Within normal limits
____ Constipation ____ Diarrhea ____ Incontinence
____ Ostomy: Type: ____ Appliance ____ Self-care ____ Yes ____ No

Bladder Habits: ____ WNL ____ Frequency ____ Dysuria ____ Nocturia ____ Urgency
____ Hematuria ____ Retention

Incontinence: ____ No ____ Yes ____ Total ____ Daytime ____ Nighttime
____ Occasional ____ Difficulty delaying voiding
____ Difficulty reaching toilet ____ Difficulty perceiving cues

Assistive Devices: ____ Intermittent catheterization
____ Indwelling catheter ____ External catheter
____ Incontinent briefs

Side Two

Sleep–Rest Pattern

Habits: _____ hrs/night _____ AM nap _____ PM nap
           Feel rested after sleep _____ Yes _____ No
Problems: _____ None _____ Early waking _____ Difficulty falling asleep _____ Nightmares

Cognitive–Perceptual Pattern

Mental Status: _____ Alert _____ Receptive aphasia _____ Poor historian
                    _____ Oriented _____ Confused _____ Combative _____ Unresponsive
Speech: _____ Normal _____ Slurred _____ Garbled _____ Expressive aphasia
           Spoken language _____ Interpreter _____
Language Spoken: _____ English _____ Spanish _____ Other _____
Ability to Read English: _____ Yes _____ No _____
Ability to Communicate: _____ Yes _____ No _____ Verbally _____ Written _____ Interpreter _____
Ability to Comprehend: _____ Yes _____ No Memory intact _____ Yes _____ No _____
Level of Anxiety: _____ Appropriate _____ Mild _____ Moderate _____ Severe _____ Panic
Interactive Skills: _____ Appropriate _____ Other _____
Hearing: _____ WNL _____ Impaired (_____ Right _____ Left) _____ Deaf (_____ Right _____ Left)
           _____ Hearing Aid
Is this individual capable to learning and performing self-care?
Vision: _____ WNL _____ Eyeglasses _____ Contact lens
           _____ Impaired _____ Right _____ Left
           _____ Blind _____ Right _____ Left
           _____ Prosthesis _____ Right _____ Left
Vertigo: _____ Yes _____ No
Discomfort/Pain: _____ None _____ Acute _____ Chronic _____ Description _____
_____

Pain Management: Meds, other the rapies _____

Coping–Stress Tolerance/Self-Perception/Self-Concept Pattern

Major concerns regarding hospitalization or illness (financial, self-care): _____
Does the person need a referral to social services? _____
Major loss/change in past year: _____ No _____ Yes   Specify _____
Do you feel safe? _____ Yes _____ No Why? _____
CODE: (1) Not applicable (2) Unable to acquire (3) Not a priority at this time
           (4) Other (specify in notes)

Sexuality–Reproductive Pattern

LMP: _____ Gravida _____ Para _____ Birth Control _____
Menstrual/Hormonal Problems: _____ Yes _____ No _____
Last Pap Smear: _____ Dx of Abnormal PAP _____
Last Mammogram:
Sexual Concerns: _____
_____

Role–Relationship Pattern

Single____ Married ____ Widowed _____ Divorced _____ Separated _____ Lives with _____
Occupation:_____
Employment Status: ____ Employed ____ Short-term disability ____ Long-term disability
                    ____ Unemployed
Support System: ____ Spouse ____ Neighbors/Friends ____ None
                ____ Support in same residence ____ Support in separate residence____ Other
Will the person need assistance at home? How much? 24/7
Family concerns regarding hospitalization:

Value–Belief Pattern

Religion: _____
Religious Restrictions: _____ No _____ Yes (Specify)_____
Request Chaplain Visitation at This Time: _____ Yes _____ No

PHYSICAL ASSESSMENT (Objective)

1. CLINICAL DATA
Age _____ Height _____ Weight ____ BMI Temperature_____
Pulse: ____ Strong ____ Weak ____ Regular ____ Irregular____
Blood Pressure: Right Arm ____ Left Arm ____ Sitting ____ Lying ____

2. RESPIRATORY/CIRCULATORY
Rate_____
Quality: ____ WNL ____ Shallow ____ Rapid ____ Labored ____ Other_____
Cough: ____ No ____ Yes/Describe_____
Auscultation:
    Upper rt lobes ____ WNL ____ Decreased ____ Absent ____ Abnormal sounds ____
    Upper lt lobes ____ WNL ____ Decreased ____ Absent ____ Abnormal sounds ____
    Lower rt lobes ____ WNL ____ Decreased ____ Absent ____ Abnormal sounds ____
    Lower lt lobes ____ WNL ____ Decreased ____ Absent ____ Abnormal sounds ____
Right Pedal Pulse: ____ Strong ____ Weak ____ Absent
Left Pedal Pulse: ____ Strong ____ Weak ____ Absent

3. METABOLIC–INTEGUMENTARY
SKIN:
    Color: ____ WNL ____ Pale ____ Cyanotic ____ Ashen ____ Jaundice ____ Other ____
    Temperature: ____ WNL ____ Warm ____ Cool
    Edema: ____ No ____ Yes/Description/location_____
    Lesions: ____ None ____ Yes/Description/location_____
    Bruises: ____ None ____ Yes/Description/location_____
    Reddened: ____ No ____ Yes/Description/location_____
    Pruritus: ____ No ____ Yes/Description/location_____
    Is the person at risk for Pressure Ulcer?
MOUTH:
    Gums: ____ WNL ____ White plaque ____ Lesions ____ Other_____
    Teeth: ____ WNL ____ Other_____
ABDOMEN:
    Bowel Sounds: ____ Present ____ Absent

4. NEURO/SENSORY

Pupils: _____ Equal _____ Unequal describe

Reactive to light:

    Left: _____ Yes _____ No/Specify _____

    Right: _____ Yes _____ No/Specify _____

Eyes: _____ Clear _____ Draining _____ Reddened _____ Other_____

5. MUSCULAR–SKELETAL

Range of Motion: _____ Full _____ Other Balance and Gait: _____ Steady _____ Unsteady

Hand Grasps: _____ Equal _____ Strong _____ Weakness/Paralysis (_____ Right _____ Left)

Leg Strength: _____ Equal _____ Strong _____ Weakness/Paralysis (_____ Right _____ Left)

Is this person at risk for fall?

6. OTHER SIGNIFICANT OBSERVATIONS

TRANSITION PLANNING

Intended Destination Post transition: _____ Home _____ Undetermined _____ Other _____

Previous Utilization of Community Resources:

    _____ Home care/Hospice _____ Adult day care _____ Church groups _____ Other _____

    _____ Meals on Wheels _____ Homemaker/Home health aide _____ Community support group

Postdischarge Transportation:

    _____ Car _____ Ambulance _____ Bus/Taxi

    _____ Unable to determine at this time

Anticipated Financial Assistance Postdischarge?:_____ No _____ Yes_____

Anticipated Problems with Self-care Postdischarge?: _____ No _____ Yes_____

Assistive Devices Needed Postdischarge?: _____ No _____ Yes_____

Referrals: (record date)

    Discharge Coordinator_____Home Health_____

    Social Service_____

SIGNATURE/TITLE _____ Date_____

Side Five

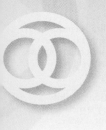

Nursing Diagnoses Index

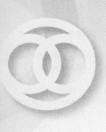

Collaborative Problems Index

General Index

Note: Page numbers followed by *f*, *t*, and *b* indicate figures, tables and boxes, respectively.

High Risk for Falls

Fall Risk Assessment

Assess for the following risk factors. Record the number of checks in the Fall assessment scores in the ( ) as High Risk for Falls (score) or add the risk factors for example as High Risk for Falls related to instability, postural hypotension and IV equipment.

Assess all individuals for risk factors for falls, using the assessment tool in the institution. The following represents one assessment tool:

Variables Score
History of falling
No (score as 0).
Yes (score as 25).
Secondary diagnosis
No (score as 0).
Yes (score as 15).
Ambulatory aid
Bed rest/nurse assist (score as 0).
Crutches/cane/walker (score as 15).
Furniture (score as 30).
IV or IV access
No (score as 0).
Yes (score as 20).
Gait
Normal/bed rest/immobile (score as 0).
Weak (score as 10).
Impaired (score as 20).
Mental status
Knows own limits (score as 0).
Overestimates or forgets limits (score as 15).
Total Score _____

Risk Level MFS Score Action
No risk
0–24 Good basic nursing care
Low to moderate risk
25–45 Implement standard fall prevention interventions
High risk
46 + Implement high-risk fall prevention interventions

Morse Fall Scale (Morse, 2009). Used with permission

Timed Up and Go (TUG): (Podsiadlo & Richardson, 1991)

For individuals who are independent and ambulatory but frail, fatigued and/or with possible compromised ambulation, assess the person's ability to Timed Up and Go (TUG):

- Have the person wear their usual footwear and use any assistive device they normally use.
- Have the person sit in the chair with their back to the chair and their arms resting on the arm rests.
- Ask the person to stand up from a standard chair and walk a distance of 10 ft (3m).
- Have the person turn around, walk back to the chair, and sit down again.
- Timing begins when the person starts to rise from the chair and ends when he or she returns to the chair and sits down.

The person should be given one practice trial and then three actual trials if needed. The times from the three actual trials are averaged.

Predictive Results
Seconds Rating
<10 Freely mobile
10–19 Mostly independent
20–29 Variable mobility
>29 Impaired mobility

Risk Factors for Surgical Site Infection

The Risk of Surgical Site Infection is influenced by the amount and virulence of the microorganism and the ability of the individual to resist it (Pear, 2007).

Assess for the following risk factors. Record the number of Risk Factors in the ( ) as High Risk for Surgical Site Infection (1–10) or add the risk factors for example as as High Risk for Surgical Site Infection related to obesity, diabetes mellitus, and tobacco use.

Infection colonization of microorganisms (1)
Pre-Existing Remote Body Site Infection (1)
Pre-operative contaminated or dirty wound (e.g., post trauma) (1)
Glucocorticoid Steroids (2)
Tobacco Use (3)
Malnutrition (4)
Obesity (5)
Perioperative Hyperglycemia (6)
Diabetes Mellitus (7)
Altered immune response (8)
Chronic alcohol use/acute alcohol intoxication (9)

1. Preoperative nares colonization with *Staphylococcus aureus* noted in 30% of most healthy populations, and especially methicillin-resistant *staph aureus* (MRSA), predisposes individuals to have higher risk of SSI (Price et al., 2008).
2. Systemic glucocorticoids (GC), which are frequently used as anti-inflammatory agents, are well-known to inhibit wound repair *via* global anti-inflammatory effects and suppression of cellular wound responses, including fibroblast proliferation and collagen synthesis. Systemic steroids cause wounds to heal with incomplete granulation tissue and reduced wound contraction (Franz *et al.*, 2007).
3. "Smoking has a transient effect on the tissue microenvironment and a prolonged effect on inflammatory and reparative cell functions leading to delayed healing and complications" (Sørensen, 2012). Quit smoking four weeks before surgery "restores tissue oxygenation and metabolism rapidly" (Ibid).
4. Malnourished individuals have been found to have less competent immune response to infection and decreased nutritional stores which will impair wound healing (Speaar, 2008).
5. An obese individuals may experience a compromise in wound healing due to poor blood supply to adipose tissue. In addition, antibiotics are a not absorbed well by adipose tissue. Despite excessive food intake, many obese individuals have protein malnutrition, which further impedes the healing (Cheadle, 2006).
6. There are two primary mechanisms that place individuals experiencing acute perioperative hyperglycemia at increased risk for SSI. The first mechanism is the decreased vascular circulation that occurs reducing tissue perfusion and impairing cellular-level functions. A clinical study by Akbari et al. noted that when healthy, non-diabetic subjects ingested a glucose load, the endothelial-dependent vasodilatation in both the micro and macro circulations were impaired similar to that seen in diabetic patients (1998). The second affected mechanism is the reduced activity of the cellular immunity functions of chemotaxis, phagocytosis, and killing of polymorphonuclear cells as well as monocytes/macrophages that have been shown to occur in the acute hyperglycemic state (Akbari et al., 1998).
7. Postsurgical adverse outcomes related to DM are believed to be related to the pre-existing complications of chronic hyperglycemia, which include vascular atherosclerotic disease and peripheral as well as autonomic neuropathies (Geerlings et al., 1999).
8. Suppression of the immune system by disease, medication, or age can delay wound healing (Cheadle, 2006).
9. Chronic alcohol exposure causes impaired wound healing and enhanced host susceptibility to infections. Wounds from trauma in the presence of acute alcohol exposure have a higher rate of post-injury infection due to decreased neutrophil recruitment and phagocytic function (Guo & DiPietro, 2010).